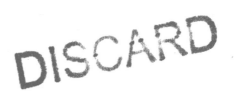

GLENN'S UROLOGIC SURGERY

Sixth Edition

GLENN'S UROLOGIC SURGERY

Sixth Edition

Editor-in-Chief

Sam D. Graham, Jr., M.D.

Virginia Urology Center
Richmond, Virginia

LIPPINCOTT WILLIAMS & WILKINS
A **Wolters Kluwer** Company

Philadelphia • Baltimore • New York • London
Buenos Aires • Hong Kong • Sydney • Tokyo

Acquisitions Editor: Craig Percy
Developmental Editor: Joanne Bersin
Production Manager: Toni Ann Scaramuzzo
Supervising Editors: Steve Martin, Michael Mallard
Production Editor: Kathy Cleghorn, Chernow Editorial Services, Inc.
Manufacturing Manager: Benjamin Rivera
Cover Designer:
Compositor: Lippincott Williams & Wilkins Desktop Division
Prepress: Maryland Composition
Printer: Edwards Brothers

© 2004 by LIPPINCOTT WILLIAMS & WILKINS
530 Walnut Street
Philadelphia, PA 19106 USA
LWW.com

ISBN: 0-7817-4082-7

Care has been taken to confirm the accuracy of the information presented and to describe generally accepted practices. However, the authors, editors, and publisher are not responsible for errors or omissions or for any consequences from application of the information in this book and make no warranty, expressed or implied, with respect to the currency, completeness, or accuracy of the contents of the publication. Application of this information in a particular situation remains the professional responsibility of the practitioner.

The authors, editors, and publisher have exerted every effort to ensure that drug selection and dosage set forth in this text are in accordance with current recommendations and practice at the time of publication. However, in view of ongoing research, changes in government regulations, and the constant flow of information relating to drug therapy and drug reactions, the reader is urged to check the package insert for each drug for any change in indications and dosage and for added warnings and precautions. This is particularly important when the recommended agent is a new or infrequently employed drug.

Some drugs and medical devices presented in this publication have Food and Drug Administration (FDA) clearance for limited use in restricted research settings. It is the responsibility of the health care provider to ascertain the FDA status of each drug or device planned for use in their clinical practice.

10 9 8 7 6 5 4 3 2 1

Contents

Section III. Bladder
edited by James E. Montie

ANATOMY

Section IV. Prostate
edited by Randall G. Rowland

ANATOMY

Section VI. Vas Deferens and Seminal Vesicle
edited by Larry Lipshultz

Section VII. Testis
edited by David A. Swanson

ANATOMY

Section VIII. Penis/Scrotum
edited by Gerald H. Jordan

ANATOMY

Section IX. Urinary Diversion
edited by Urs E. Studer

Section XI. Laparoscopic Surgery
edited by Leonard G. Gomella

Section XII. Frontiers in Urology
edited by Louis Kavoussi

Editors

Editor-in-Chief
Sam D. Graham, Jr., M.D.
Virginia Urology Center
9105 Stony Point Drive
Richmond, Virginia, 23235

Consultant Editor
Thomas E. Keane, M.D.
Department of Urology
Medical University of South Carolina
96 Jonathan Lucas Street
P.O. Box 250620
Charleston, South Carolina 29425

Consultant Editor
James F. Glenn, M.D.
Professor of Surgery
Department of Surgery
Division of Urology
University of Kentucky Medical Center
800 Rose Street
Lexington, Kentucky 40536

Associate Editors
Charles B. Brendler, M.D.
Professor and Chief
Section of Urology MC6038
University of Chicago Hospitals
5841 South Maryland Avenue
Chicago, Illinois 60637
Section: Ureter and Pelvis

Leonard G. Gomella, M.D.
The Bernard W. Goodwin
Professor of Prostate Cancer
Chairman, Department of Urology
Thomas Jefferson University
1025 Walnut Street
Philadelphia, Pennsylvania 19107
Section: Laparoscopic Surgery

E. Ann Gormley, M.D.
Section of Urology
Dartmouth-Hitchcock Medical Center
1 Medical Center Drive
Lebanon, New Hampshire 03766
Section: Urethra

Gerald H. Jordan, M.D.
Professor of Urology
Eastern Virginia Medical School
Director of Adult Reconstructive Surgery
The Devine Center for Genitourinary
 Reconstruction
Sentara Norfolk General Hospital
Devine-Fiveash Urology, Ltd.
P.O. Box 1980
Norfolk, Virginia 23501
Section: Penis/Scrotum

Louis R. Kavoussi, M.D.
Vice Chairman of Urology
The James Buchanan Brady Urological
 Institute
Chief of Urology
Department of Urology
Johns Hopkins Hospital
600 N. Wolfe Street
Jefferson Street Building
Baltimore, M.D. 21287
Section: Frontiers in Urology

Larry Lipshultz, M.D.
Professor, Division of Male Reproductive
 Medicine and Surgery
Scott Department of Urology
Baylor College of Medicine
6560 Fannin #2100
Houston, Texas 77030
Section: Vas Deferens and Seminal Vesicle

James E. Montie, M.D.
George F. and Nancy P. Valassis Professor of
*   Urologic Oncology*
Chairman
Department of Urology
University of Michigan Health System
1500 East Medical Center Drive
Ann Arbor, Michigan 48109
Section: Bladder

Jerome P. Richie, M.D.
Chief, Division of Urology
Brigham and Women's Hospital
Harvard Medical School
45 Francis Street, ASB II-3
Boston, Massachusetts 02115
Section: Adrenal and Renal

Randall G. Rowland, M.D.
Professor and Chief of Surgery (Urology)
Program Director (Urology)
University of Kentucky College of Medicine
UK Chandler Medical Center MS-283
800 Rose Street
Lexington, Kentucky 40536
Section: Prostate

H. Gil Rushton, M.D.
Department of Urology
George Washington University
Chairman, Urology
Children's National Medical Center
2300 Eye Street, N.W.
Washington, DC 20037
Section: Pediatric Urology

Urs E. Studer, M.D.
Professor and Chairman
Department of Urology
University of Berne
3010 Bern, Switzerland
Section: Urinary Diversion

David A. Swanson, M.D
Professor and Chairman
Department of Urology
M.D. Anderson Cancer Center
The University of Texas
1515 Holcombe Blvd.
Houston, Texas 77030
Section: Testis

Contributors

Hassan Abol-Enein, M.D., Ph.D.
Associate Professor of Urology
Urology & Nephrology Center
Mansoura University
Mansoura, Egypt
Chapter 86

A. Rolf Ackermann, M.D.
Heinrich-Heine-Universität Düsseldorf
Universitätsstr. 1
Gebäude 25.41
D 40225 Düsseldorf
Germany
Chapter 17

Mark C. Adams, M.D.
Vanderbilt Children's Hospital
Pediatric Urology
435 Medical Arts Building
Nashville, Tennessee 37212
Chapter 101

David M. Albala, M.D.
Professor, Department of Urology
Duke University Medical Center
Durham, North Carolina 27710
Chapter 113

Michael Aleman, M.D.
Cleveland Clinic Foundation
9500 Euclid Avenue
Cleveland, Ohio 44195
Chapters 78

Bradley W. Anderson, M.D.
Division of Urology
St. Vincent Healthcare
2900 12th Avenue North, Suite 503E
Billings, Montana 59101
Chapter 115

Kenneth W. Angermeier, M.D.
The Urological Institute
Cleveland Clinic Foundation
9500 Euclid Avenue
Cleveland, Ohio 44195
Chapter 26

Elizabeth J. Anoia, M.D.
University Hospitals of Cleveland
11100 Euclid Avenue
Cleveland, Ohio 44106-5046
Chapter 8

Rodney A. Appell, M.D.
Scott Department of Urology
Baylor College of Medicine
6560 Fannin, Sute Z100
Houston, Texas 77030
Chapter 38

J. Christopher Austin
Department of Urology
Children's Hospital of Iowa
Iowa City, Iowa 52242
Chapter 95

Gopal Badlani, M.D., F.A.C.S.
Associate Chairman, Professor of Urology
Department of Urology
Long Island Jewish Medical Center
New Hyde Park, New York 11040
Chapter 39

Robert R. Bahnson, M.D.
Chapter 27

Linda A. Baker, M.D.
Assistant Professor of Urology
University of Texas Southwestern at Dallas
Children's Medical Center of Dallas
Bank One Building, Suite 1401
6300 Harry Hines Blvd.
Dallas, Texas 75235
Chapter 132

David M. Barrett, M.D.
Department of Urology
Lahey Clinic
41 Mall Road
Burlington, MA 01805-3947
Chapter 50

Pierfrancesco Bassi, M.D.
Chapter 83

Stephen M. Baughman
Chapter 135

Ricardo Beduschi, M.D.
Chapter 1

Arnold M. Belker, M.D.
250 East Liberty Street, Suite 602
Louisville, Kentucky 40202
Chapter 56

Barry Belman, M.D.
Chair
Department of Urology
Children's National Medical Center
111 Michigan Avenue, NW
Washington, DC 20010
Chapter 103

Richard E. Berger, M.D.
Professor of Urology
University of Washington
Box 356510
Seattle, Washington 98195-6510
Chapter 55

Vincent G. Bird, M.D.
Endourology/Laparoscopy Fellow
University of Iowa Hospitals and Clinics
Department of Urology
#3236 RCP
200 Hawkins Drive
Iowa City, Iowa 52242-1089
Chapter 130

Jay T. Bishoff, M.D.
LT COL, USAF, MC
Director, Endourology Section
Department of Urology
Wilford Hall Medical Center
2200 Berquist Drive, Suite 1
Lackland AFB, Texas 78236-5300
Chapter 135

Jerry G. Blaivas, M.D., Director
Clinical Professor of Urology
Joan and Sanford Weill College of Medicine
Cornell University
Director of Urogynecology, Lenox Hill Hospital
New York, NY
The Urocenter
400 E. 56th Street
New York, New York 10022
Chapter 47

Derek J. Bochinski, M.D.
Department of Urology, UCSF
1412- 29th Avenue
San Francisco, California 94143
Chapter 69

James A. Brown, M.D.
Assistant Professor
Head of the Sub-Section of Urologic Oncology
Section of Surgery/Urology
Medical College of Georgia
1120 15th Street, BA-8415
Augusta, Georgia 30912-4050
Chapter 117

Scott V. Burgess, M.D.
Urology Resident
William Beaumont Hospital
3535 W. 13 Mile Road, Suite 438
Royal Oak, Michigan 48073
Chapter 94

Jeffrey A. Cadeddu, M.D.
Department of Urology
University of Texas Southwestern Medical
  Center
5323 Harry Hines Blvd.
Dallas, Texas 75390-9110
Chapter 133

Mark P. Cain, M.D.
Associate Professor, Department of Urology
Indiana University School of Medicine
JW Riley Hospital for Children
702 Barnhill Drive #1739
Indianapolis, Indiana 46202
Chapter 112

Anthony A. Caldamone, M.D.
Department of Urology
Brown University School of Medicine
2 Dudley Street, Suite 174
Providence, Rhode Island 02905
Chapter 100

Douglas A. Canning, M.D.
Chief
Division of Urology
The Children's Hospital of Philadelphia
34th Street and Civic Center Boulevard
Philadelphia, Pennsylvania 19104
Chapter 95

Jeffrey M. Carey, M.D.
Fellow, Urodynamics/Pelvic Reconstruction
Tower Urology Institute for Continence
Cedars-Sinai Medical Center
Tower Urology Institute for Continence
8631 West Third Street, Suite 900 East
Los Angeles, California 90048-2926
Chapter 45

Culley C. Carson, M.D.
*University of North Carolina School of
   Medicine*
Division of Urology
University of North Carolina at Chapel Hill
2140 Bioinformatics Building
Chapel Hill, North Carolina 27599
Chapter 70

Anthony J. Casale, M.D.
Professor of Urology
Indiana University School of Medicine
Riley Hospital for Children
702 Barnhill Drive, #4230
Indianapolis, Indiana 46202
Chapter 109

Pasquale Casale, M.D.
Chief Resident
Department of Urology
Thomas Jefferson University
1025 Walnut Street
Philadelphia, Pennsylvania 19107
Chapter 114

John R. Case, M.D.
Resident, Department of Urology
Northwestern University
Tarry #11-715,
303 E. Chicago Avenue.
Chicago, IL 60611-3008
Chapter 9

William A. Cavanagh, M.D.
Northwest Biotherapeutics
21720 23rd Drive, SE
Suite 100
Bothell, Washington 98021
Chapter 34

R. Duane Cespedes, M.D.
Assistant Professor of Urology
University of Texas-San Antonio
Director, Female Urology and Urodynamics
Wilford Hall Medical Center
Lackland AFB, Texas
8843 Goodwick Heights
San Antonio, Texas 78254
Chapters 23 and 37

Toby C. Chai, M.D. F.A.C.S.
Associate Professor of Urology
University of Maryland School of Medicine
*Director, University of Maryland Continence
   Center*
22 S. Greene Street, S8D18
Baltimore, Maryland 21201
Chapter 35

David Y. Chan, M.D.
Assistant Professor of Urology
James Buchanan Brady Urological Institute
The Johns Hopkins Hospital
600 North Wolfe Street
Jefferson Street Bldg
Suite 171
Baltimore, Maryland 21209
Chapter 138

Sam S. Chang, M.D.
Assistant Professor
Department of Urologic Surgery
Vanderbilt University, MCN A1302
2201 West End Avenue
Nashville, Tennessee 37235
Chapters 4 and 22

Ralph V. Clayman, M.D.
Chairman and Professor
Department of Urology
UCI Medical Center
101 The City Drive South
Orange, California 92868
Chapter 116

William T. Connor, M.D.
Associate Professor of Surgery
Division of Urology
University of Kentucky Medical Center
800 Rose Street, MS-283
Lexington, Kentucky 40536-0298
Chapter 30

Michael S. Cookson, M.D.
Associate Professor
Department of Urologic Surgery
Vanderbilt University Medical Center
2201 West End Avenue, MCN A-1302
Nashville, Tennessee 37232
Chapters 4 and 22

Christopher S. Cooper, M.D.
Assistant Professor of Urology
The University of Iowa
Director, Pediatric Urology
Children's Hospital of Iowa
University of Iowa Hospitals and Clinics
200 Hawkins Drive, 3RCP
Iowa City, Iowa 52242-1089
Chapter 107

Monisha S. Crisell, M.D.
Chief Resident, Urology
Georgetown University Hospital
7th floor PHC
3800 Reservoir Road
Washington, DC 20007
Chapter 93

Hansjörg Danuser, M.D.
Chapter 81

Ross M. Decter, M.D.
Professor of Surgery, Chief Division of Urology
Penn State Milton S. Hershey Medical Center
500 University Drive, MC H055
Hershey, Pennsylvania 17033-0850
Chapter 92

Serdar Deger, M.D.
Department of Urology
Campus Charité Mitte
Schumannstrasse 20/21
10117 Berlin
Germany
Chapter 125

G. D'elia, M.D.
Chapter 88

Ralph W. deVere-White, M.D.
Department of Urology
UC Davis Medical Center
4860 Y Street, Suite 3500
Sacramento, California 95817
Chapter 31

David A. Diamond, M.D.
Associate Professor of Surgery
Department of Urology
Children's Hospital of Boston
Harvard Medical School
300 Longwood Avenue
Boston, Massachusetts 02115
Chapter 99

Stuart Diamond, M.D.
Assistant Professor
Department of Urology
Thomas Jefferson University
1025 Walnut Street
Philadelphia, Pennsylvania 19107
Chapter 118

Ananias C. Diokno, M.D.
Chief, Department of Urology
William Beaumont Hospital
3535 W. 13 Mile Road, Suite 438
Royal Oak, Michigan 48073
Chapter 28

Roger R. Dmochowski, M.D., F.A.C.S.
Department of Urologic Surgery
Room A1302, Medical Center North
Vanderbilt University Medical Center
2201 West End Avenue
Nashville, Tennessee 37232
Chapter 41

Steven G. Docimo, M.D.
Director, Pediatric Urology
Professor, Department of Urology
University of Pittsburgh
Children's Hospital of Pittsburgh
4A-424 De Soto Wing
3705 Fifth Avenue
Pittsburgh, Pennsylvania 15213
Chapter 107

Sherri M. Donat, M.D.
Assistant Attending Surgeon
Memorial Sloan Kettering Cancer
*   Center/Urology*
1275 York Avenue
New York, New York 10021
Chapter 60

James F. Donovan, M.D.
Professor of Surgery
Chief, Division of Urology
Department of Surgery
University of Cincinnati
231 Albert Sabin Way, ML 0589
P.O. Box 670589
Cincinnati, OH 45267-0589

Karyn S. Eilber, M.D.
Assistant Attending Surgeon
Department of Urology
Memorial Sloan-Kettering Cancer Center
1275 York Avenue, Box 27
New York, New York 10021
Chapters 43 and 44

Paul G. Espy, M.D.
Chapter 64

Michael D. Fabrizio, M.D.
Assistant Professor in Urology
Eastern Virginia Medical School
Devine-Tidewater Urology
P.O. Box 1980
Norfolk, Virginia 23501
Chapter 125

Michael P. Federle, M.D.
Chapter 27

Margit Fisch, M.D.
Professor of Urology
Director, Department of Urology and Pediatric
*   Urology*
Allgemeines Krankenhaus Harburg
Eissendorfer Pherdeweg 52
21075 Hamburg, Germany
Chapters 79 and 88

John M. Fitzpatrick, M.D.
Chapter 15

Adam J. Flisser, M.D.
Clinical Instructor in Obstetrics and
   Gynecology
Joan and Sanford Weill College of Medicine
Cornell University, New York, NY
The Urocenter
400 E. 56th Street
New York, New York 10022
Chapter 47

Brian J. Flynn, M.D.
Department of Surgery, Division of Urology
University of Colorado Health Sciences Center
4200 East 9th Avenue, Box C319
Denver, Colorado 80262
Chapter 48

Randy A. Fralick, M.D.
Scott Department of Urology
Baylor College of Medicine
6560 Fannin, Suite 2100
Houston, Texas 77030
Chapter 38

Robert W. Frederick, M.D.
University of Texas Southwestern Medical
   Center
5323 Harry Hines Blvd.
Dallas, Texas 75390-9110
Chapter 46

Dominic Frimberger, M.D.
Department of Urology
Johns Hopkins Hospital
149 Marburg
600 N. Wolfe Street
Baltimore, Maryland 21287
Chapter 105

John P. Gearhart, M.D.
Department of Urology
Johns Hopkins Hospital
149 Marburg
600 N. Wolfe Street
Baltimore, Maryland 21287
Chapter 105

Glenn S. Gerber, M.D.
Associate Professor, Surgery
Section of Urology MC6038
University of Chicago
5841 S. Maryland Avenue
Chicago, Illinois 60637
Chapter 18

Elmar W. Gerharz, M.D.
Associate Professor of Urology
Department of Urology
Julius Maximilians-University
Medical School
Josef Schneider Strasse 2
97080 Wurzburg
Germany
Chapter 87

Matthew T. Gettman, M.D.
Department of Urology
Mayo East 17
200 1st Street SW
Rochester, Minnesota 55905-0001
Chapter 133

Mohamed A. Ghoneim, M.D.
Professor of Urology
Director, Urology-Nephrology Center
Mansoura, Egypt
Chapters 20 and 86

Inderbir S. Gill, M.D., MCh
Section of Laparoscopic and Minimally
   Invasive Surgery
Urologic Institute, A-100
The Cleveland Clinic Foundation
9500 Euclid Avenue
Cleveland, Ohio 44195
Chapter 124

Kenneth I. Glassberg, M.D.
Professor of Urology
Director, Division of Pediatric Urology
State University of New York – Downstate
   Medical School
470 Clarkson Avenue, Box 79
Brooklyn, New York 11203
Chapter 102

Deborah Glassman, M.D.
Thomas Jefferson University
Department of Urology
1025 Walnut Street, Suite 1112
Philadelphia, Pennsylvania 19107-5083
Chapter 120

Irwin Goldstein, M.D.
Professor, Department of Urology
Boston University
770 Harrison Avenue, Suite 606
Boston, Massachusetts 02118
Chapter 72

Marc Goldstein, M.D.
Cornell Institute for Reproductive Medicine and
*   Department of Urology*
New York Weill Cornell Medical Center
525 East 68th Street, Box 580
New York, New York 10021
Chapter 75

Leonard G. Gomella, M.D.
The Bernard W. Goodwin
Professor of Prostate Cancer
Chairman, Department of Urology
Thomas Jefferson University
1025 Walnut Street
Philadelphia, Pennsylvania 19107
Chapters 113, 114, and 117

Alexander Gomelsky, M.D.
Department of Urologic Surgery
Vanderbilt University Medical Center
A-1302, Medical Center North
Nashville, Tennessee 37232
Chapter 41

María Fernanda Lorenzo Gómez, M.D.,
**   Ph.D.**
Fellow, Pediatric Urology
Division of Pediatric Urology
University of Miami
1400 NW 10th Avenue (M-814)
Miami, Florida 33136
Chapter 131

Ricardo González, M.D. F.A.A.P
Chief, Division of Pediatric Urology
Jackson Memorial Hospital
Professor of Urology and Pediatrics
Department of Urology
University of Miami School of Medicine
1400 NW 10th Avenue (M-814)
Miami, Florida 33136
or
Attending Urologist/Director Fellowship
*   Program*
Division of Urology
Al duPont Hospital for Children
1600 Rockland Road
Wilmington, Delaware 19899
Chapter 131

Richard W. Grady, M.D.
Assistant Professor of Urology
The University of Washington Medical Center
Children's Hospital and Regional Medical
*   Center*
Box 356510
Seattle, Washington 98195-6510
Chapter 104

Sam D. Graham, Jr., M.D.
Virginia Urology Center
9105 Stony Point Drive
Richmond, Virginia 23235
Chapter 33

Marc-Oliver Grimm, M.D.
Department of Urology
Heinrich Heine University
Moorenstrasse
540225 Dusseldorf
Germany
Chapter 17

Richard E. Hautmann, M.D.
Professor/Chairman
Department of Urology
University of Ulm
Chief, Department of Urology
Urologische Universitatsklinik Ulm
Prittwitzstrasse 43
89075 Ulm
Germany
Chapter 82

John A. Heaney, M.D.
Professor of Surgery, Urology
Chief, Section of Urology
Dartmouth-Hitchcock Medical Center
1 Medical Center Drive
Lebanon, New Hampshire 03756
Chapters 51 and 52

Axel Heidenreich, M.D.
Associate Professor of Urology
Department of Urology and Pediatric Urology
Philipps-University
Baldingerstrasse
35043 Marburg
Germany
Chapter 62

C.D. Anthony Herndon, M.D.
Indiana University School of Medicine
702 Barnhill Drive, #4230
Indianapolis, Indiana 46202
Chapter 109

Markus Hohenfellner, M.D.
Professor of Urology
Department of Urology
Mainz Medical School
Langenbeckstrasse 1
55131 Mainz
Germany
Chapter 85

Rudolf Hohenfellner, M.D.
Professor of Urology
Department of Urology
Johannes Gutenberg University
55131 Mainz Germany
Langenbeckstrasse 1
55131 Mainz
Germany
Chapters 79 and 88

Carin V. Hopps, M.D.
Department of Urology
Medical College of Ohio
3000 Arlington Avenue
Toledo, Ohio 43614
Chapters 58 and 75

Stephen C. Jacobs, M.D.
University of Maryland Hospital
Division of Urology
22 S. Greene Street, Room S8D18
Baltimore, Maryland 21230
Chapter 120

Thomas W. Jarrett, M.D.
Associate Professor of Urology
James Buchanan Brady Urological Institute
Johns Hopkins University
Suite 165 Jefferson Street Building
600 North Wolfe Street
Baltimore, Maryland 21287-8915
Chapter 123

Michael A.S. Jewett, M.D.
Department of Surgery
University of Toronto
610 University Avenue, 3-130
Toronto, Ontario M5G 2M9
Canada
Chapter 63

Gerald H. Jordan, M.D.
Professor of Urology
Eastern Virginia Medical School
Director of Adult Reconstructive Surgery
The Devine Center for Genitourinary
  Reconstruction
Sentara Norfolk General Hospital
Devine-Fiveash Urology, Ltd.
P.O. Box 1980
Norfolk, Virginia 23501
Chapter 65, 68, 74, and 132

David B. Joseph, M.D.
Professor of Surgery
Chief, Pediatric Urology
The University of Alabama at Birmingham
318 Ambulatory Care Center
1600 7th Avenue South
Birmingham, Alabama 35233-1711
Chapter 96

Jihad H. Kaouk, M.D.
Fellow
Section of Laparoscopic and Minimally
  Invasive Surgery
Urologic Institute
Cleveland Clinic Foundation
9500 Euclid Avenue
Cleveland, Ohio 44195
Chapter 124

George W. Kaplan
7930 Frost Street
Suite 407
San Diego, California 92123
Chapter 110

Evan J. Kass, M.D., F.A.A.P., F.A.C.S.
Clinical Professor
Department of Urology
Wayne St. University
Chief of Pediatric Urology
Department of Urology
William Beaumont Hospital
3535 W. 13 Mile Drive, Suite 438
Royal Oak, Michigan 48073
Chapter 94

Francis X. Keeley Jr., M.D.
Consultant Urological Surgeon
Bristol Urological Institute
Southmead Hospital
Bristol BS10 5NB
UK
Chapter 122

Stephen R. Keoghane, M.B.B.S, M.S.,
  F.R.C.S.
The Old Bakery Chedworth
Glos GL54 4AA
UK
Chapter 122

Richard T. Kershen, M.D.
Instructor, Scott Department of Urology
Baylor College of Medicine
6560 Fannin, Suite 2100
Houston, Texas 77030
Chapter 38

Fernando J. Kim, M.D.
Chief of Urology
Denver Health Medical Center
Assistant Professor of Surgery/Urology
Urology, MC 206
University of Colorado Health Sciences Center
777 Bannock Street
Denver, CO 8020
Chapter 123

Eric A. Klein, M.D.
Head, Section of Urologic Oncology
The Cleveland Clinic Foundation
9500 Euclid Avenue, A100
Cleveland, Ohio 44195
Chapters 26 and 78

Frederick A. Klein, M.D.
Professor, Department of Surgery
Chief, Division of Urology
University of Tennessee Medical Center
1928 Alcoa Highway, MOB-B Suite 127
Knoxville, Tennessee 37920
Chapter 2

Chester J. Koh, M.D.
Department of Urology
Harvard Medical School and Children's
    Hospital
Hunnewell 3
300 Longwood Avenue
Boston, Massachusetts 02115
Chapter 99

Badrinath R. Konety, M.D.
Chapter 27

Harry P. Koo, M.D.
Chapter 64

Karl J. Kreder, M.D.
Department of Urology
University of Iowa Health Care
3235 RCP
200 Hawkins Drive
Iowa City, Iowa 52242-1089
Chapter 129

Sanjaya Kumar, M.D.
Brigham and Women's Hospital
Harvard Medical School
45 Francis Street ASB2-3
Boston, Massachusetts 02115
Chapter 6

Peter O. Kwong, M.D.
Urology of Virginia
Devine-Tidewater Urology
6333 Center Drive
Building 16
Norfolk, Virginia 23502
Chapter 25

Jaime Landman, M.D.
Assistant Professor of Urology
Washington University School of Medicine
4960 Children's Place
Campus Box 8242
St. Louis, Missouri 63110
Chapters 116 and 137

Jerilyn M. Latini, M.D.
Clinical Fellow, Department of Urology
University of Iowa Hospitals and Clinics
200 Hawkins Drive, 3RCP
Iowa City, Iowa 52242-1089
Chapter 129

Gary E. Leach, M.D.
863 W. Third Street
Suite 900 East
Los Angeles, California 90048
Chapter 45

Benjamin R. Lee, M.D.
Assistant Professor of Urology
Department of Urology
Long Island Jewish Medical Center
270-05 76th Avenue
New Hyde Park, New York 11040
Chapter 139

Cheryl T. Lee, M.D.
Assistant Professor, Urology
University of Michigan & Hospital
1500 E. Medical Center Drive, Box 0330
Ann Arbor, Michigan 48109-0330
Chapter 21

David I. Lee, M.D.
Endocrinology Fellow
Department of Urology
University of California, Irvine Medical Center
101 The City Drive
Bldg. 55, Room 304, Rt. 81
Orange, California 92868
Chapter 116

Richard S. Lee, M.D.
Urology Resident
University of Washington
Box 356510
Seattle, Washington 98195-6510
Chapter 55

Thomas S. Lendvay, M.D.
Senior Resident
Department of Urology
Emory University/Hospital
2425 Hosea L. Williams Drive
Atlanta, Georgia 30317
Chapter 19

Ronald W. Lewis, M.D.
Chief, Section of Urology
Medical College of Georgia
1120 15th Street, Room BA 8412
Augusta, Georgia 30912
Chapter 71

John A. Libertino, M.D.
Lahey Hitchcock Medical Center
41 Mall Road
Burlington, Massachusetts 01805
Chapter 7

Mark R. Licht, M.D.
Boca Urology, PA
851 Meadows Road, Suite 212
Boca Raton, Florida 33486
Chapter 71

Larry I. Lipshultz, M.D.
Professor, Division of Male Reproductive
  Medicine and Surgery
Scott Department of Urology
Baylor College of Medicine
6560 Fannin #2100
Houston, Texas 77030
Chapters 59

Stefan A. Loening, M.D., F.R.C.S
Professor, Director of the Department
Department of Urology
Charite Hospital
Medical School of the Humboldt-University of
  Berlin
Germany
Chapter 128

Bruce A. Lucas, M.D.
Department of Surgery
Division of Urology
Kentucky University Medical Center
800 Rose Street
Lexington, Kentucky 40536-0001
Chapter 11

Tom F. Lue, M.D.
Department of Urology U-575
University of California
Box 0738
San Francisco, California 94143
Chapter 69

Michael J. Manyak, M.D.
Department of Urology George Washington
  University
2150 Pennsylvania Avenue NW, Suite 9-41
Washington, DC 20037
Chapter 140

Michael Marberger, M.D.
Professor and Chairman, Department of
  Urology
Klinik fur Urologie der Universitat Wien
Allgemeines Krankenhaus
Wahringer Gurtel 18-20
A-1090 Wien
Austria
Chapter 16

Fray F. Marshall, M.D.
Professor and Chairman, Department of
  Urology
Emory University School of Medicine
Building A, Room 3225
1365 Clifton Road, NE
Atlanta, Georgia 30322
Chapter 5

Irene M. McAleer
7930 Frost Street
Suite 407
San Diego, California 92123
Chapter 110

Jack W. McAninch, M.D.
Professor
Department of Urology
San Francisco General Hospital
1001 Potero Avenue
San Francisco, California 94110
Chapters 10, 49, and 73

Kurt A. McCammon, M.D.
Devine-Tidewater Urology
400 W. Brambleton Avenue, Suite 100
Norfolk, Virginia 23510-1196
Chapter 77

W. Scott McDougal, M.D.
Chief of Urology
Massachusetts General Hospital
55 Fruit Street, GRB-1102
Boston, Massachusetts 02114-2696
Chapter 67

Edward J. McGuire, M.D.
Professor of Urology
The University of Michigan Health Systems
Department of Urology-Room #2918B Taubman
  Center
1500 East Medical Center Drive
Ann Arbor, Michigan 48109-0330
Chapters 23 and 37

Hunter A. McKay, M.D., F.A.C.S.
Associated Urologists
4011 Talbot Road, South #440
Renton, Washington 98055
Chapter 40

Mani Menon, M.D.
Director Henry Ford Vattikuti Urology Institute
Henry Ford Health System
Department of Urology
2799 W. Grand Blvd.
Detroit, Michigan 48202-2608
Chapters 13 and 126

Shafquat Meraj, M.D.
Chief Resident
Department of Urology
Beth Israel Medical Center
10 Union Square East, Suite 3A
New York, New York 10003
Chapter 57

Michael J. Metro, M.D.
Department of Urology
University of California School of Medicine
San Francisco, California 94110
Chapter 49

Aaron J. Milbank, M.D.
The Urological Institute
Cleveland Clinic Foundation
9500 Euclid Avenue
Cleveland, Ohio 44195
Chapter 26

Rosalia Misseri, M.D.
Pediatric Urology Fellow
Department of Urology
James Whitcomb Riley Hospital for Children
Indiana University School of Medicine
702 Barnhill Drive, Box 1739
Indianapolis, Indiana 46202
Chapter 102

Michael E. Mitchell, M.D.
Professor of Urology
Children's Hospital and Regional Medical
  Center
The University of Washington Medical Center
Box 356510
Seattle, Washington 98195-6510
Chapter 104

James E. Montie, M.D.
George F. and Nancy P. Valassis Professor of
  Urologic Oncology
Chairman
Department of Urology
University of Michigan Health System
1500 East Medical Center Drive
Ann Arbor, Michigan 48109
Chapter 21

Allen F. Morey
Chapters 10 and 73

John Mulhall, M.D.
Associate Professor, Urology
Cornell University
New York Hospital
525 E. 68th Street
New York, New York 10021
Chapter 72

Ricardo Munarriz, M.D.
Assistant Professor, Urology
Boston University and Medical Center
720 Harrison Avenue, Suite 606
Boston, Massachusetts 02118
Chapter 72

Larry C. Munch, M.D., F.A.C.S.
Methodist Urology, LLC
1801 N. Senate Blvd., Suite 220
Indianapolis, Indiana 46240
Chapter 127

Harris M. Nagler, M.D., F.A.C.S.
Professor of Urology
Albert Einstein College of Medicine
Chair, Department of Urology
Beth Israel Medical Center
10 Union Square East, Suite 3A
New York, New York 10003
Chapter 57

Stephen Y. Nakada, M.D.
The David T. Uehling Professor of Urology
Chairman of Urology
Department of Surgery, Division of Urology
University of Wisconsin Medical School
G5/339 Clinical Science Center
600 Highland Avenue
Madison, Wisconsin 53792
Chapter 119

John A. Nesbitt, M.D.
Assistant Professor of Surgery
Department of Surgery
Division of Urologic Surgery
550 South Jackson Street
2ⁿᵈ floor ACB
Louisville, Kentucky 40202
Chapter 76

Victor W. Nitti, M.D.
Associate Professor and Vice Chairman
Department of Urology
New York University School of Medicine
150 East 32 Street, Second Floor
New York, New York 10016
Chapter 42

Andrew C. Novick, M.D.
Chairman
The Cleveland Clinic Foundation Urological
   Institute
9500 Euclid Avenue
Cleveland, Ohio 44195
Chapter 3

Unyime O. Nseyo, M.D.
Professor and Chairman
Division of Urology, Department of Surgery
Virginia Commonwealth University-Medical
   College of VA
Chairman
Department of Surgery
Division of Urology
VCU Health Systems
West Hospital, 7ᵗʰ floor
1200 East Broad Street
PO Box 980118
Richmond, Virginia 23298
Chapter 1

David M. Nudell, M.D.
Staff Physician
Department of Surgery
Good Samaritan Hospital
Urology Associates of Silicon Valley
555 Knowles #211
Los Gatos, California 95032
Chapter 59

Francesco Pagano, M.D.
Professor/Chairman
Department of Urology
Instituto di Urologia
Universita di Padova
Monoblocco Ospedaliero
2, Via Giustiniani
35001 Padova
Italy
Chapter 83

Michael L. Paik, M.D.
Department of Urology
University Hospitals of Cleveland
11100 Euclid Avenue
Cleveland, Ohio 44106-5046
Chapter 8

Rishikesh R. Pandya, M.D.
Chapter 63

Eugene L. Park, M.D.
Urology Resident
University of Arizona/Arizona Health Sciences
   Center
P.O. Box 245077
1501 N. Campbell Avenue
Tucson, Arizona 85724-5077
Chapter 136

Kent Perry, M.D.
Department of Urology
University of California, Los Angeles
924 Westwood Boulevard, Suite 520
Los Angeles, California 90024
Chapter 134

Kenneth M. Peters, M.D.
Director of Clinical Research
Department of Urology
William Beaumont Hospital
3535 W. 13 Mile Road, Suite 438
Royal Oak, Michigan 48073
Chapter 28

John A. Petros, M.D.
The Emory Clinic B
1365 Clifton Road, NE
Atlanta, Georgia 30322
Chapter 19

Michael W. Phelan, M.D.
Department of Urology
University of California, Los Angeles
924 Westwood Boulevard, Suite 520
Los Angeles, California 90024
Chapter 134

Paul K. Pietrow, M.D.
Assistant Professor
Department of Urology
Kansas University Medical Center
3901 Rainbow Boulevard
Kansas City, Kansas 66160-7300
Chapter 113

Hans G. Pohl, M.D.
Department of Urology and Pediatrics
Children's National Medical Center
George Washington University
2300 Eye Street, N.W.
Washington, DC 20037
Chapter 111

Thomas J. Polascik, M.D.
3914 Chippenham Road
Durham, North Carolina 27707-5093
Chapter 5

John C. Pope, IV, M.D.
Assistant Professor
Departments of Urologic Surgery and
  Pediatrics
Vanderbilt University Medical Center and
  Children's Hospital
A-1302 Medical Center North
Nashville, Tennessee 37232-3765
Chapter 101

Jon L. Pryor, M.D.
Department of Urologic Surgery
Reproductive Health Association
University of Minnesota
420 Delaware Street, SE
PO Box 394 FUMC, MMC 394
Minneapolis, Minnesota 55455
Chapter 54

Antonio Puras Baez, M.D.
University of Puerto Rico School of Medicine
1431 Ponce de Leon Avenue, Suite 601
Santurce, Puerto Rico 00907
Chapter 66

Haakon Ragde, M.D.
Grado Ragde Clinics
10330 Meridian Avenue, No.
Suite 300
Seattle, Washington 98133
Chapter 34

Sanjay Ramakumar, M.D.
Assistant Professor of Surgery/Urology
University of Arizona/Arizona Health Sciences
  Center
PO Box 245077
1501 N. Campbell Avenue
Tucson, Arizona 85724-5077
Chapter 136

Shlomo Raz, M.D.
Professor of Urology
Director, Pelvic Medicine, Reconstructive
  Surgery and Urodynamics
University of California, Los Angeles
924 Westwood Blvd., Suite 520
Los Angeles, CA 90024
Chapters 43 and 44

Pramod P. Reddy, M.D.
Division of Pediatric Urology
Cincinnati Children's Hospital
3333 Burnet Avenue
Cincinnati, Ohio 45229
Chapter 90

Martin I. Resnick, M.D.
Chapter 8

Hubertus Riedmiller, M.D.
Professor and Chairman
Department of Urology
Julius Maximilians University
Chief, Department of Urology
Luitpold Hospital
Josef Schneider Strasse 2
97080 Wurzburg
Germany
Chapter 87

Richard C. Rink, M.D.
Indiana University School of Medicine
Indianapolis, Indiana
Chapter 108

Michael L. Ritchey, M.D.
Professor of Surgery and Pediatrics
Director, Division of Urology
University of Texas-Houston Medical School
6431 Fannin 601B
Houston, Texas 77030
Chapter 91

Omid Rofeim, M.D.
Resident
Department of Urology
Long Island Jewish Medical Center
New Hyde Park, New York 11040
Chapter 34

Nirit Rosenblum, M.D.
Assistant Professor
Department of Urology
New York University School of Medicine
Associate Director of Urology
Bellevue Hospital
150 E. 32 Street, 2nd floor
New York, New York 10016
Chapters 43 and 44

Daniel I. Rosenstein, M.D.
Department of Urology
Santa Clara Valley Medical Center
751 S. Bascom Avenue
San Jose, California 95128
Chapters 10, 73, and 74

David R. Roth, M.D.
Associate Professor
Department of Pediatric Urology
6621 Fannin, CCC 660
Houston, Texas 77030
Chapter 106

Stephan Roth, M.D.
Department of Adult and Pediatric Urology
University of Witten/Herdecke
Klinikum Wuppertal GmbH
Heusnerstrasse 40
42283 Wuppertal
Germany
Chapter 89

Keith F. Rourke, M.D.
Eastern Virginia Graduate School of Medicine
400 West Brambleton Avenue, Suite 100
Norfolk, Virginia 23510
Chapter 68

Randall G. Rowland, M.D., Ph.D.
Professor and James F. Glenn Chair of Urology
University of Kentucky Medical Center
800 Rose Street, MS-283
Lexington, Kentucky 40536-0298
Chapter 30

H. Gil Rushton, M.D.
Department of Urology
George Washington University
Chairman, Urology
Children's National Medical Center
2300 Eye Street, N.W.
Washington, DC 20037
Chapter 93

Harriette M. Scarpero, M.D.
Assistant Professor, Department of Urology
Vanderbilt University School of Medicine
A-1302 Medical Center North
Nashville, TN 37232-2765
Chapter 42

Anthony J. Schaeffer, M.D.
Chief, Department of Urology
Northwestern Memorial Hospital
Professor and Chair
Department of Urology
Feinberg School of Medicine
Northwestern University
Tarry 11-715
303 E. Chicago Avenue
Chicago, Illnois 60611
Chapter 9

Peter N. Schlegel, M.D.
Department of Urology and Cornell
Institute for Reproductive Medicine
New York Weill Cornell Medical Center
525 East 68th Street, Starr 900
New York, New York 10021
Chapter 58

Peter G. Schulam, M.D.
Department of Urology
University of California, Los Angeles
924 Westwood Blvd., Suite 520
Los Angeles, California 90024
Chapter 134

Brian D. Seifman, M.D.
Department of Urology
University of Michigan Health System
1500 E. Medical Center Drive
Ann Arbor, MI 48109-0330
Chapter 24

Darshan K. Shah, M.D., M.Ch.
Post Doctorate Fellow
Department of Urology
Long Island Jewish Medical Center
New Hyde Park, New York 11040
Chapter 39

Curtis A. Sheldon, M.D.
Cincinnati Children's Hospital
3333 Burnet Avenue
Cincinnati, Ohio 45229
Chapter 90

Donald G. Skinner, M.D.
Professor and Chairman
Department of Urology
University of Southern California
Norris Comprehesive Cancer Center
1441 Eastlake Avenue, Suite 7416
Los Angeles, California 90089
Chapter 84

John J. Smith III, M.D.
Department of Urology
Lahey Clinic
41 Mall Road
Burlington, Massachusetts 01805-3947
Chapter 50

Joseph A. Smith, Jr., M.D.
Department of Urologic Surgery
Vanderbilt University Medical Center
A1302 Medical Center North
Nasvhille, Tennessee
Chapter 32

Howard M. Snyder, III, M.D.
Professor of Urology
Department of Surgery
University of Pennsylvania
Associate Director, Pediatric Urology
Children's Hospital of Philadelphia
3rd floor Wood Building
Philadelphia, Pennsylvania 19104-4399
Chapter 97

Stephen B. Solomon, M.D.
Assistant Professor of Radiology
The Johns Hopkins University School of
  Medicine
Baltimore, Maryland 21287
Chapter 138

John P. Stein, M.D.
Associate Professor
Department of Urology
University of Southern California
Norris Comprehensive Cancer Center
1441 Eastlake Avenue, MS #74
Suite #7416
Los Angeles, California 90089
Chapter 84

Gary D. Steinberg, M.D.
Associate Professor
Section of Urology
University of Chicago
Director of Urology
Weiss Memorial Hospital
4646 N. Marine Drive
Chicago, Illinois 60640
Chapter 14

Lynn Stothers, M.D., F.R.C.S.C
Assistant Professor, Division of Urology
Associate Member Department of Health Care
  and Epidemiology
University of British Columbia
1081 Burrard Street
Vancouver, B.C. V6Z1Y6
Canada
Chapter 36

Stephen E. Strup, M.D.
Associate Professor
Department of Urology
Thomas Jefferson University
1025 Walnut Street
Philadelphia, Pennsylvania 19107
Chapter 118

Urs E. Studer, M.D.
Professor and Chairman
Department of Urology
University of Berne
3010 Bern, Switzerland
Chapter 80 and 81

Ray E. Stutzman, M.D.
Department of Urology
The Johns Hopkins University
601 North Caroline Street
Baltimore, Maryland 21287
Chapter 29

David A. Swanson, M.D.
Professor and Chairman
Department of Urology
M.D. Anderson Cancer Center
The University of Texas
1515 Holcombe Blvd.
Houston, Texas 77030-4009
Chapter 61

Shahin Tabatabaei, M.D.
Senior Urology Resident
Massachusetts General Hospital
55 Fruit Street, GRB-1102
Boston, Massachusetts 02114-2696
Chapter 67

Leslie D. Tackett, M.D.
Department of Urology
University Urologic Associates
2 Dudley Street, Suite 174
Providence, Rhode Island 02905
Chapter 100

Rodney J. Taylor, M.D.
Professor of Surgery
University of Louisville
Chief, Urologic Surgery
University of Louisville Medical Center
550 South Jackson Street, ACB
Louisville, Kentucky 40292
Chapter 12

Ashutosh Tewari, M.D.
Director
Robotic Prostatectomy and Urologic
*   Outcomes*
Brady Urologic Health Center
Weill Medical College of Cornell University
New York Presbyterian Hospital
New York, NY 10021

Joachim W. Thüroff, M.D.
Professor of Urology
Director, Department of Urology
Mainz Medical School
Langenbeckstrasse 1
55131 Mainz
Germany
Chapter 85 and 88

Ingolf A. Türk, M.D., Ph.D.
Professor, Director of Minimally Invasive
*   Urologic Surgery*
Department of Urology
Lahey Clinic
41 Mall Road
Burlington, Massachusetts 01805
Chapter 125 and 128

Paul J. Turek, M.D.
Associate Professor
Director, Male Reproductive Laboratory
Department of Urology
University of California San Francisco
2330 Post Street, 6ᵗʰ floor
San Francisco, California 94115-1695
Chapter 53

Burkhard Ubrig, M.D.
Klinik fuer Urologie und Kinderurologie
Witten/Herdecke University
Klinikum Wuppertal GmbH
Heusnerstr. 40
42283 Wuppertal
Germany
Chapter 89

C. Varol, M.D.
Chapter 80

Ramakrishna Venkatesh, M.D., F.R.C.S
Fellow in Minimally Invasive Urology
Division of Urology
Barnes-Jewish Hospital
Washington University School of Medicine
4960 Children's Place
Campus Box 8242
St. Louis, Missouri 63110
Chapter 137

Michael Waldner, M.D.
Department of Adult and Pediatric Urology
University of Witten/Herdecke
Klinikum Wuppertal GmbH
Heusnerstr. 40
42283 Wuppertal
Germany
Chapter 89

Brad W. Warner, M.D.
Chapter 90

John W. Warner, M.D.
Chapter 140

W. Bedford Waters, M.D.
Professor, Department of Surgery
Associate Chief, Division of Urology
University of Tennessee Medical Center
1928 Alcoa Highway, MOB-B Ste 127
Knoxville, Tennessee 37920
Chapter 2

George D. Webster, M.D.
Professor of Urology
Department of Surgery, Division of Urology
Duke University Medical Center
Durham, North Carolina 27710
Chapter 48

O. Lenaine Westney, M.D.
Assistant Professor
Department of Surgery
Division of Urology
UT-Houston Medical School
Medical Director
Memorial Hermann Urology and Continence
*   Center*
6431 Fannin, Suite 6018
Houston, Texas 77030
Chapter 25

Michael Wilkin, M.D.
Resident in Urology
University of Wisconsin Medical School
600 Highland Avenue
Madison, Wisconsin 53792
Chapter 119

Howard N. Winfield, M.D.
Professor of Urology
#3236 RCP
University of Iowa Hospitals and Clinics
200 Hawkins Drive
Iowa City, Iowa 52242-1089
Chapter 130

J. Stuart Wolf, Jr., M.D.
Department of Urology
University of Michigan
1500 E. Medical Center Drive
Ann Arbor, Michigan 48109-0330
Chapters 24 and 121

Hsi-Yang Wu, M.D.
Fellow, Division of Urology
Children's Hospital of Philadelphia
University of Pennsylvania
34th Street and Civic Center Boulevard
Philadelphia, Pennsylvania 19104
Chapter 97

Paulos Yohannes, M.D.
Assistant Professor of Surgery (Urology)
Department of Surgery
Division of Urology
Creighton University
601 North 30th Street, Suite 3703
Omaha, Nebraska 68131
Chapter 139

Robin L. Zagone, M.D.
Resident in Urology
University of Texas-Houston Medical
*   School*
6431 Fannin, Suite 6018
Houston, Texas 77030
Chapter 91

Mark R. Zaontz, M.D.
Associate Professor of Surgery and
*   Pediatrics*
Temple University Medical School
Director, Pediatric Surgical Subspecialties
Virtua Health System
120 Carnie Blvd., Suite 2
Voorhees, New Jersey 08043
Chapter 98

Philippe E. Zimmern, M.D.
Department of Urology
University of Texas Southwestern Medical
*   Center*
4323 Harry Hines Boulevard
Dallas, TX 75390-9110
Chapter 46

Adrenal and Renal

SECTION EDITOR: Jerome P. Richie

Adrenal

Ricardo Beduschi and
Unyime O. Nseyo

The adrenal glands are paired and located high in the retroperitoneum, on anterior craniomedial aspect of the kidney (Figures SI-1, S1-2, and S1–3). Their characteristic yellow color distinguishes them from the surrounding fat or pancreas. They weigh approximately 5 g, but weight and size may change significantly after prolonged illness or as the result of prolonged adrenocorticotropic hormone (ACTH) stimulation. The atrophic gland is thin and pale and its easily recognizable hyperplasia makes it readily visible. The left adrenal gland has a semicircular, or crescent shape. The right gland has an inverted pyramidal, or V-shape. The adrenal gland consists of the cortex and medulla and arose from the mesoderm (cortex) and ectodermal (medulla) elements in the medial aspect of the ceolomic cavity.

Embryology

Embryologically, the ectodermal medullary elements migrate from the same primordial neural crest that gives rise to the sympathetic chain. The mesodermal cortical tissues arise from the dorsal cells of the blastema cord at the medial aspect of the mesonephric bodies. However, the ventral cells of these bodies are the origin of the interstitial cells of the testis or the theca cells of the ovary. The 8-week embryo has massive adrenals, approximately the size of the kidney, and they remain enlarged and very vascular until birth. Rapid regression occurs in the adrenal size during the first month. The large adrenal size with hypervascularity may predispose to adrenal hemorrhage in the newborn as well as misdiagnosis for Wilm's tumor or neuroblastoma. The medullary tissue within the gland imparts a unique tripartite structure of the head (most medial), body and tail (most lateral). Each adrenal gland resides within the Gerota's fascia with the kidney. However, in the case of renal ectopy the adrenal remains in its natural position.

Ectopic adrenal tissues may develop in certain locations of the body. Although rare, they may undergo neoplastic changes or hyperplasia. Ectopic adrenal tissues in most cases consist of cortex only, rarely do they contain cortex and medulla. Embryological relationship in the urogenital ridge predisposes to adrenal ectopy in the retroperironeum, the testis, spermatic cord, and in the region of the celiac ganglion.

Vascular Anatomy

The arterial supply remains variable; the main sources include primarily the branches from the aorta, inferior phrenic artery, and renal artery. The multiple small caliber arterial branches must be appreciated for hemostasis during surgery. The venous drainage, although less variable, usually represents a bigger challenge, especially during operations of large adrenal masses. The right adrenal vein is short and empties directly into the inferior vena cava (IVC) in its most posterolateral aspect. Large adrenal tumors may obscure its visualization, making identification of this vein very challenging. Bleeding from this site can be profuse and even life threatening if not identified and controlled immediately. The left adrenal vein is much smaller than the right adrenal vein. It usually exits anteroinferiorly, draining into the ipsilateral renal vein.

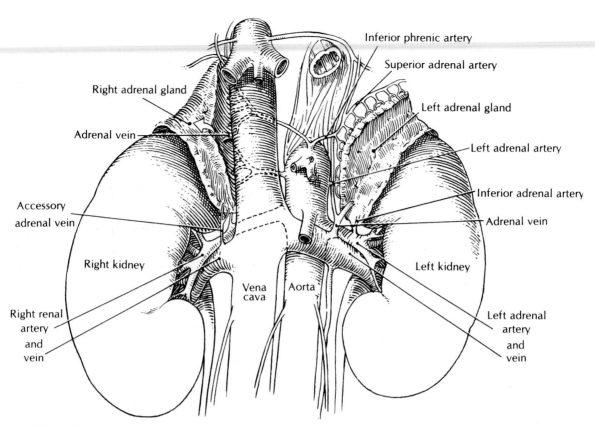

FIG. SI–1. The anatomic relationship of the adrenal glands to the aorta and inferior vena cava. Multiple arterial vessels entering the glands indicate the rich arterial supply, while a single central adrenal vein illustrates the limited and relatively constant venous damage.

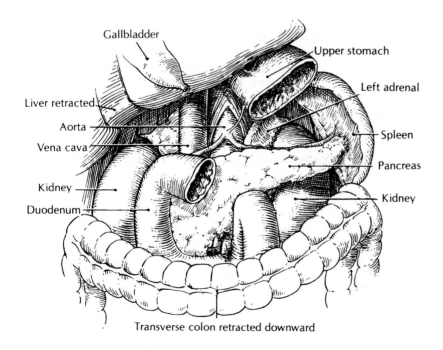

FIG. SI–2. An anterior view of the abdomen illustrating the anatomic relationship of the adrenal glands to surrounding gastrointestinal tract and organs.

Contiguous Structures

Thorough knowledge of the anatomic relationships holds the key to preventing injury to the contiguous structures during surgical dissection (Figure SI-2). The right adrenal gland lies superior to the upper pole of the right kidney, posterolateraly to the IVC. Dissection of the right adrenal gland is limited medially by the duodenum and superiorly by the right hepatic lobe. Access to the right adrenal gland is more easily obtained by entering the retroperitoneum behind the liver. The right hepatic lobe can be mobilized from the colon and diaphragm by transecting the triangular, coronary, and hepatocolic ligaments, allowing visualization of the right adrenal gland just superior to the upper pole of the right kidney. Mobilization of the duodenum is also required for easier identification of the right adrenal vein. This step is of special interest for large pheochromocytomas, in which early access to the adrenal vein is essential. Using the Kocher maneuver, the duodenum can be retracted medially allowing easier access to the IVC and a complete dissection of the right adrenal vein. Once the right adrenal vein is controlled, an avascular plane can be developed towards the lateral aspect of the gland allowing quick and bloodless removal of the gland. Attention should be paid to the main arterial trunks as well as the multiple small calibered arteries which can be easily controlled with electrocautery, and/or surgical clips.

The left adrenal gland is usually more medial than the right gland, and it lies on the upper pole of the left kidney, just lateral to the aorta. The left adrenal gland lies in close contact with the spleen and stomach, and is crossed on its anterior inferior surface by the body of the pancreas, and the splenic artery and vein. A special technical effort must be made to prevent inadvertent injury to the tail of the pancreas and/or capsule of the spleen. Releasing the splenocolic ligament allows free mobilization of the spleen, and gentle blunt dissection allows medial mobilization of the left abdominal viscera and adequate exposure of the left adrenal gland. The left adrenal vein is usually isolated in the anteroinferior aspect of the gland and control of this vein is usually less of a problem, with minimal blood loss (Figure SI-3). The lowest extent of this gland is close to the renal vessel, which remains at risk of injury during adrenalectomy.

Kidney

Sam D. Graham, Jr.

The abdominal wall is comprised of three layers of muscle and fascia that are derived from the same embryonic muscle sheets as the intercostal muscles. Each muscle is covered by its own layer of deep fascia and is innervated by the intercostal nerves. The external oblique fibers are oriented anteriorly and inferiorly, attaching posteriorly to the iliac crest, while the anterior fibers attach to the linea alba in the midline (Figure SI-4a). The internal oblique fibers are oriented anteriorly and superiorly (Figure SI-4b). Posteriorly, the fibers of the internal oblique attach to the lower four ribs, while anteriorly they attach to the linea alba. In the upper abdomen, the internal oblque fascia splits to enclose the rectus muscle, while inferiorly, the fascia only covers the rectus muscle anteriorly. The ilioinguinal and iliohypogastric nerves are found in the interior oblique fascia anterior to the internal oblique muscle. The transversus abdominus are horizontally oriented fibers that attach to the linea alba (Figure SI-4c). The ribs are supported by the intercostals muscles and fascia as well as the costovetebral (costotransverse) ligament, which must be divided if the rib is to be retracted inferiorly (Figure SI-5) .

The kidneys are located on either side of the vertebral column in the lumbar fossa of the retroperitoneum and vary in length in adults from 11 cm to 14 cm or approximately 3 to 4.5 times the height of the second lumbar vertebrae (Figure SI-1). The parenchyma of the kidney is covered by a thin transparent capsule which in turn is covered by a layer of perinephric fat enclosed in a distinct layer of fascia. (Gerota's fascia) (Figure SI-6). The capsule is attached to Gerota's fascia by fibrous trabeculae (1). Gerota's fascia is completely fused superiorly and laterally, but open inferiorly and to some extent medially where it is adherent to the adventitia of the renal vessels, aorta, and inferior vena cava. Gerota's fascia extends above the kidney to form a special compartment for the adrenal gland (2). Posteriorly, Gerota's fascia is connected to the sheaths of the psoas and quadratus lumborum muscles by connective tissue septae. Anteriorly, Gerota's fascia is closely applied to the peritoneum. On the left, the hilum of the spleen is attached to the ventral aspect of the kidney by a double layer of peritoneum known as the splenorenal ligament (2).

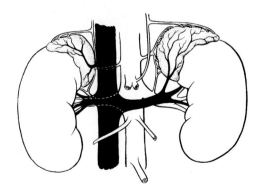

FIG. SI–3.

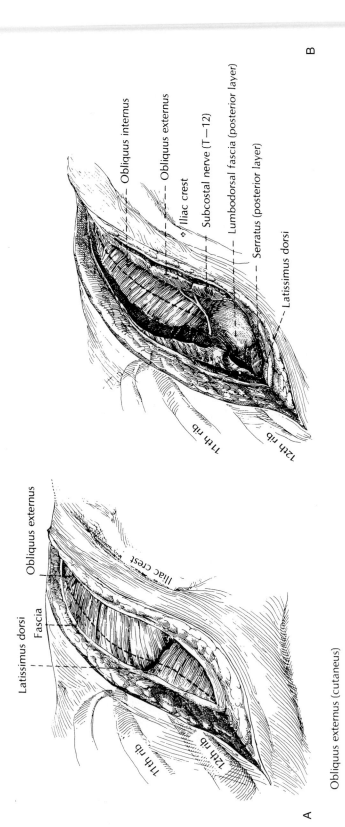

Obliquus externus

Latissimus dorsi
Fascia

Iliac crest

11th rib
12th rib

A

Obliquus internus

Obliquus externus

Iliac crest

Subcostal nerve (T−12)

Lumbodorsal fascia (posterior layer)

Serratus (posterior layer)

Latissimus dorsi

11th rib
12th rib

B

Transversus and its aponeurosis

Obliquus externus (cutaneus)

Obliquus interior (cutaneus)

Paranephric fat

Penrose drain

Latissimus dorsi
and serratus posterior inferior

Erector spinae and quadratus lumborum

11th rib
12th rib

C

FIG. SI–4. (A) Flank incision showing the orientation of the external oblique. This incision is subcostal and also shows the relationships of the latissimus dorsi posteriorly. **(B)** Exposure of the internal oblique showing the relationship to the intercostal nerve. **(C)** Exposure of the transversus abdominus and its aponeurosis.

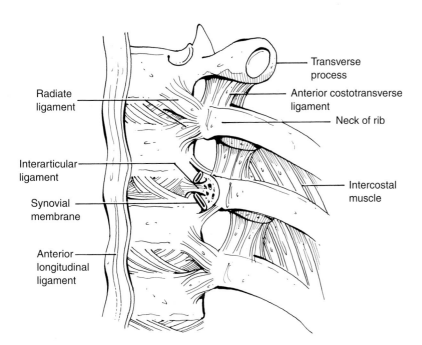

FIG. SI–5. Costovetebral (costotransverse) ligaments extend from the transverse process of the vertebra immediately above the rib to the neck of the rib. In order to gain exposure during a thoracolumbar or supracostal approach, this must be divided to allow the rib to rotate inferiorly.

Vascular Anatomy

The main renal arteries are branches of the aorta emanating from the lateral portion of the aorta at approximately L-2. In general, the renal arteries divide into segmental branches at the junction of the middle and final third of their course. A single left artery most commonly lies dorsal to the renal vein, and a long right renal artery lies dorsal to the vena cava and the renal vein. Up to 35% of kidneys have an accessory renal artery with 1.5% more than one accessory artery (2). As the renal artery approaches the hilum it has two branches, the inferior suprarenal (adrenal) and the ureteric arteries. (Figure SI-6) At the hilus, the main renal artery divides into an anterior and posterior branch which further divide into segmental arteries. The kidney can be divided into 4 segments based upon the arterial supply. (Figure SI-7). Both the apical and basilar segmental arteries supply each respective pole of the kidney anteriorly and posteriorly. The largest segment is the anterior segment

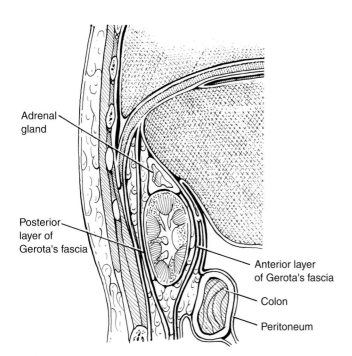

FIG. SI–6. Retroperitoneal anatomy showing Gerota's fascia in sagittal section.

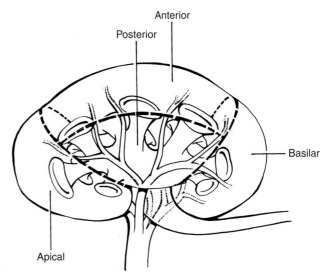

FIG. SI–7. Segmental anatomy of the kidney. The relatively avascular plane between the anterior and posterior segments is the line of Brödel. In general, calyces tend to extend from the renal pelvis to the central mass of the segment they supply.

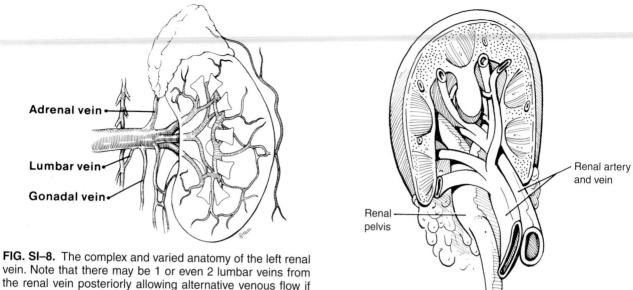

FIG. SI–8. The complex and varied anatomy of the left renal vein. Note that there may be 1 or even 2 lumbar veins from the renal vein posteriorly allowing alternative venous flow if the vena cava is occluded.

Adrenal vein

Lumbar vein

Gonadal vein

Renal artery and vein

Renal pelvis

FIG. SI–9. Transverse section of kidney showing relative anatomy of vascular structures in the renal hilum.

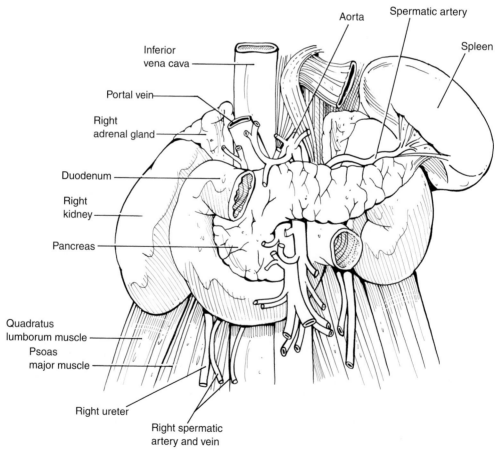

Aorta

Spermatic artery

Spleen

Inferior vena cava

Portal vein

Right adrenal gland

Duodenum

Right kidney

Pancreas

Quadratus lumborum muscle

Psoas major muscle

Right ureter

Right spermatic artery and vein

FIG. SI–10. The kidney in relation to contiguous structures.

which is supplied by two segmental arteries and extends posteriorly to the avascular plane at Brödel's line where it meets the posterior segment (3).

The renal veins directly join the vena cava. The right renal vein is usually less than one-half the length of the left renal vein and has no significant branches. The left renal vein, however, is usually joined by the adrenal and inferior phrenic vein superiorly, the gonadal vein inferiorly, and frequently by lumbar vein(s) posteriorly. (Figure SI-8). These collaterals are of great importance in patients in whom the vena caval ligation or resection is contemplated.

The renal vein is usually the most anterior structure in the renal hilum. Posterior to the vein is the renal artery, and the most posterior structure in the hilum is the renal pelvis. The hilum is filled with fibrofatty tissue that can usually be easily dissected from these structures to allow access into the renal sinus. (Figure SI-9).

Lymphatic Anatomy

Parenchymal and capsular lymphatics coalesce and drain into the right lumbar or para-aortic chains respectively. These lymphatics become part of the cisterna chylae superior to the renal artery.

Contiguous Structures (Figure SI-10)

Posterior to the kidney lies the psoas major and quadratus lumborum muscles. Posteriorly and superiorly, the upper pole of each kidney is in contact with the diaphragm. The pleura is also adjacent to the upper poles of both kidneys, usually extending down below the level of the 12th rib posteriorly and to the 11th rib anteriorly (1).

Embryologically, when the gut rotates, this leaves the posterior parietal peritoneum covering the upper three quarters of the right kidney and is directly related to the hepatorenal pouch of Morrison. The duodenum is fixed to the original peritoneal covering of the lower pole of the right kidney by fusion of the embryonic dorsal mesentery to the posterior parietal peritoneum (2). On the left, the rotation of the foregut causes a fusion of the embryonic mesogastrium with the original peritoneal covering of the upper anterior kidney and thereby causing the relationship of the left kidney to the omental bursa (2). The midportion of the left kidney loses its contact with the peritoneum due to growth of the tail of the pancreas.

Superiorly, the anterior medial surface of the right kidney is in contact with the right adrenal gland. The liver overlies the anterior two-thirds of the right kidney, and the hepatic flexure of the colon overlies the lower one-third of the right kidney. The second portion of the duodenum overlies the renal hilum. In more than 90% of patients, the right kidney is lower than the left (2).

The medial surface of the left kidney is also in contact with the left adrenal gland. Other structures anterior and in close approximation to the left kidney are the spleen, tail of the pancreas, stomach, and the splenic flexure of the colon.

REFERENCES

1. Bergman EV, Bruns P, von Mikulicz J. A System of Practical Surgery, Vol. 5. Trans. by Bull WT, Foote EM. New York: Lea Brothers, New York 1904.
2. Healey JE Jr, Seybold WD. A Synopsis of Clinical Anatomy. Philadelphia: WB Saunders, 1969.
3. Stewart BH. Operative Urology: The Kidneys, Adrenal Glands, and Retroperitoneum. Baltimore: Williams and Wilkins, 1975.

CHAPTER 1

Adrenal Surgery

Ricardo Beduschi and Unyime O. Nseyo

Adrenalectomy is indicated for adrenal tumors that may or may not be functional. The traditional approach has been an open procedure, although laparoscopic adrenalectomy has gained increased popularity due to the purported benefits of its minimal invasiveness. Parameters such as size of the tumor, bilaterality of the adrenal disorder, tumor pathology, and patient's body habitus can influence the choice of surgical approach.

DIAGNOSIS

Pheochromocytoma

Pheochromocytomas are diagnosed utilizing static and functional biochemical tests. Urine-based biochemical tests include vanillylmandelic acid (VMA), total metaphrines (normetaphrine and metaphrine), and free catecholamines. When all three tests are employed concurrently, pheochromocytomas may be diagnosed in 95% of patients. Radioenzymatic assay for catecholamines have replaced the urinary tests, allowing direct measurement of plasma serum norepinephrine (NE) and other important metabolites of catecholamines in serum. The clonidine suppression test is also utilized in the diagnosis of pheochromocytoma. While clonidine will suppress the elevated peripheral catecholamines found in essential hypertension, patients with a pheochromocytoma will not demonstrate suppression.

In addition to diagnosis, pheochromocytomas must be localized preoperatively (Fig. 1–1). While computed tomography (CT) scans can delineate most adrenal pheochromocytomas, magnetic resonance imaging (MRI) has a significant benefit because pheochromocytomas show a high signal intensity on T2-weighted images that differentiates them from benign adrenal adenomas (6) (Fig. 1–2). Another option for localization studies is isotopic scanning with iodine-131-meta-iodo-benzyl guanidine (I^{131}-MIBG) (3,6) (Fig. 1–3).

Hyperaldosteronism

Primary hyperaldosteronism (Conn's syndrome) results in increased secretion of aldosterone by the cells of the zona glomerulosa of the adrenal cortex. This condition primarily is the result of functional adrenal adenoma and leads to suppressed plasma renin activity, hypokalemia, and metabolic alkalosis. Bilateral micronodular hyperplasia of zona glomerulosa cells exhibits hypersecretion in 20% of patients with clinical aldosteronism. The most common sign is hypertension and the most common symptom is relative muscle weakness.

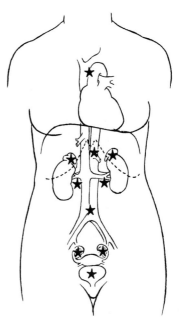

FIG. 1–1. Pheochromocytoma (paraganglioma) may occur wherever neural crest (chromaffin) tissue is found. The most common sites are indicated.

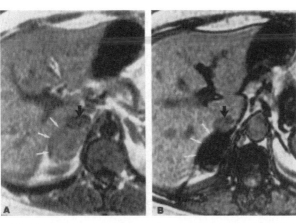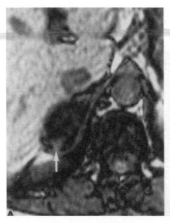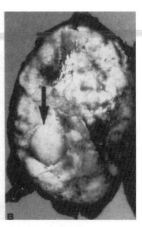

FIG. 1–2. A: Magnetic resonance imaging (MRI) appearance of an adrenal adenoma illustrating its isointense appearance on T1-weighted image. **B:** Its hypointense appearance following the dramatic subtraction of its microlipid signal. White arrows point to the adrenal mass and the black arrow to the inferior vena cava. (Courtesy of Roger Y. Shifrin, MD.) **C:** MRI appearance of a small isointense malignant lesion (marked by white arrow) in a hypointense right adrenal adenoma. This image illustrates the value of MRI in accurately detecting a small metastatic deposit in an adenomatous gland. **D:** Cross-section gross appearance of the adrenal gland following surgical excision illustrating the lesion (black arrow). The lesion was a deposit from primary bronchogenic adenocarcinoma. (Courtesy of Roger Y. Shifrin, MD.)

Finding elevated urinary and plasma aldosterone associated with hypokalemia remains the key to the diagnosis of primary aldosteronism. Additional tests include renal vein renin, saline infusion failing to suppress plasma aldosterone, and furosemide stimulation or captopril infusion test failing to stimulate plasma renin. Localization of the tumor is usually by CT scanning using thin section (l.5 to 3 mm),

which shows an accuracy of 75% to 90% (13). MRI with or without gadolinium yields similar results as CT.

Cushing's syndrome

Cushing's syndrome is due to excess circulating glucocorticosteroids. Cushing's disease refers to the form of Cushing's syndrome caused by basophilic pituitary adenoma, which accounts for about 75% to 80% of the cases of Cushing's syndrome. Exogenous steroids, glucocorticoid-producing adrenal tumors, and ectopic adrenocorticotropic hormone (ACTH) production account for the other causes of Cushing's syndrome. The classic clinical presentation includes such prominent findings as truncal obesity with peripheral extremity muscle wasting, plethora, hypertension, and increased bruising and characteristic purple striae. Hirsutism and amenorrhea may present in females.

Cushing's syndrome caused by benign adrenal adenomas is associated with elevated plasma cortisol values with loss of diurnal variations and ACTH suppression. Excess cortisol production in adrenal tumors is not suppressed by dexamethasone. CT scanning helps in localizing small adrenal adenomas. Alternative imaging studies include arteriography or radioisotopic C-19 I^{131} scans.

Adrenocortical Carcinoma

Primary adrenocortical carcinoma is an uncommon tumor that is metabolically active in 50% of patients. Cushing's syndrome, virilization, and feminization occur in 20%, 9%, and 3% of these patients, respectively. About one-third are localized to the adrenal gland at diagnosis. Staging includes three levels (Table 1–2).

FIG. 1–3. Iodine-131- meta-iodobenzyl guanidine scan of a pheochromocytoma.

TABLE 1–1. *Diagnostic tests for surgical adrenal disorders*

Tests	Aldosteronism	Cushing's syndrome	Virilization	Pheochromocytoma	Neuroblastoma	1°/2° Carcinoma	Incidental adenoma
Plasma renin activity (PRA)	+						–
Lasix stimulation (PRA, Aldo)	–						–
Serum electrolytes (K+,CO2)	+						–
Plasma aldosterone (PA)	+						–
Urine aldosterone (UA)	+						–
Differential adrenal venous samples (diff. adr. VV)	+	±					+
Isotopic scan (19-iodo cholesterol)	+	+					+
Isotopic scan (M-BIG)				+			
Computed tomography (CT scan)	+	+	+	+	+	+	+
Magnetic resonance imaging (MRI)		+		+			
Plasma 17-ketosteroids (17-Ketos)			+				
Serum testosterone (T)			+				
Clonidine suppression test				+			–
Catecholamines (VMA, HVA)				+			–
Serum Norepinephrine (NE)				+	+		–
Serum epinephrine (E)				+	+		–
Urine Norepinephrine (U/NE)				+	+		–
Urine epinephrine (U/E)				+	+		–
Selective venous IVC/SVS samples							–
Serum ACTH		+					–
Dexamethasone suppression		+					–

Modified from Donohue JP, Surgery of the adrenal. In: Crawford ED, Das S, eds. *Current genitourinary cancer surgery,* 2nd ed. Baltimore: Williams & Wilkins 1997:11–23.

INDICATIONS FOR SURGERY

Surgical excision remains the treatment of choice for most solitary adrenal masses as well as adrenal and extraadrenal pheochromocytoma. Because adrenal tumors are frequently endocrinologically active, the surgeon must be prepared to deal with the medical consequences of the removal of the tumor, including adrenal insufficiency and changes in blood pressure.

Preoperative medical management of patients with pheochromocytoma is imperative to minimize cardiovascular morbidity. Preoperative alpha blockade with either oral phenoxybenzamine or prazosin (short-acting alpha blocker) is indicated for 2 to 3 weeks to control the blood pressure as well as facilitate intravascular volume expansion at the time of surgery. Calcium channel blockers are also used to aid in normalization of blood pressure as well as minimization of the profound hypotension that may follow acute catecholamine withdrawal after removal of the tumor. The alternative protocol includes transfusion, aggressive hydration with colloid, and normal saline right before the surgery. The newest paradigm is that blockade is not essential in pheochromocytoma patients; calcium channel blockers are effective and safer as primary antihypertensive agents.

ALTERNATIVE THERAPY

Medical management of hyperaldosteronism with spironolactone (200 mg per day) remains appropriate treatment for those patients with bilateral adrenal hyperplasia in the absence of any adenoma. Bilateral adrenalectomy plays no role in the management of these patients because of the untoward consequence of adrenal insufficiency.

Incidental adrenal tumors are found serendipitously in 0.3% to 5% of patients undergoing abdominal CT scanning for nonurologic indications. Approximately 70% to 94% of these tumors are benign and biochemically inactive. Adrenalectomy is indicated for endocrinologic tumors, tumors 3 cm or greater, tumors with specific characteristics on CT or MRI, and masses that show temporal changes in size. Observation with periodic (every 6 to 12 months) radiological imaging is recommended for those patients who are excluded by the above criteria (Fig. 1–4).

SURGICAL TECHNIQUE

The surgical approach to adrenalectomy depends upon the type of adrenal disorder and its functional status (Table 1–1). The choice of optimal technique must be individualized according to the adrenal disease, surgical history, patient's body habitus, and surgeon's preference.

Anterior Approach

The anterior transabdominal involves bilateral subcostal (modified Chevron) or a midline incision. This approach is indicated for large pheochromocytomas, suspected or proven large adrenal cortical adenomas, adrenal cortical carcinomas, and adrenal malignancy with inferior vena cava involvement. The transabdominal approach allows for exploration for intraabdominal metastatic deposits and provides an excellent access to both adrenals, the vascular pedicles, and the retroperitoneum. This is an indirect approach to the adrenals, and exposure may be more difficult in an obese patient.

In the Chevron incision, the patient is placed in the supine position with a rolled towel beneath the lumbar back with the trunk slightly hyperextended (Fig. 1–5). A unilateral subcostal (hemi-Chevron) or bilateral subcostal (Chevron) incision allows access to the peritoneal cavity and inspection is performed to rule out metastasis and/or extraadrenal disease.

Exposure of the right adrenal gland begins with incising the posterior peritoneum lateral to the ascending colon and taking down the hepatocolic ligament (Fig. 1–6). The colon is displaced medially and the liver is reflected superiorly. With the Kocher maneuver the duodenum and the head of the pancreas are dissected and retracted medially to expose the right kidney. With a sponge stick a gentle caudal retraction of the kidney brings the anterior surface of the right adrenal gland into view.

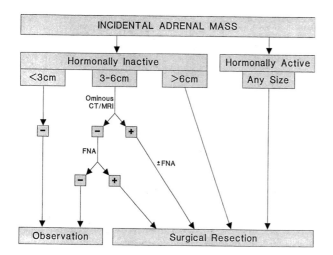

FIG. 1–4. Algorithm for management strategy of incidentally discovered adrenal masses.

TABLE 1–2. *Staging of adrenal cortical carcinoma*

Stage I:	Tumor confined to the adrenal gland
Stage II:	Direct tumor spread into adjacent and cartigous structures
Stage III:	Tumor has distant metastasis

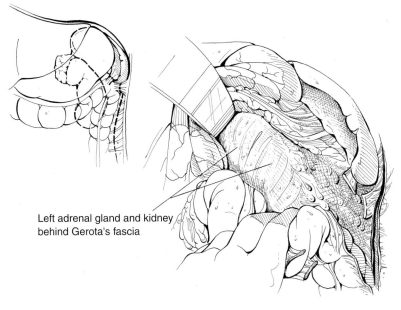

Left adrenal gland and kidney
behind Gerota's fascia

FIG. 1–5. Lateral approach to the left adrenal and the lines of paracolic incision, including lienocolic and lienophrenic attachments (inset). This approach permits retraction of the colon medically and retraction of the pancreas medially and cephalad to expose the underlying adrenal.

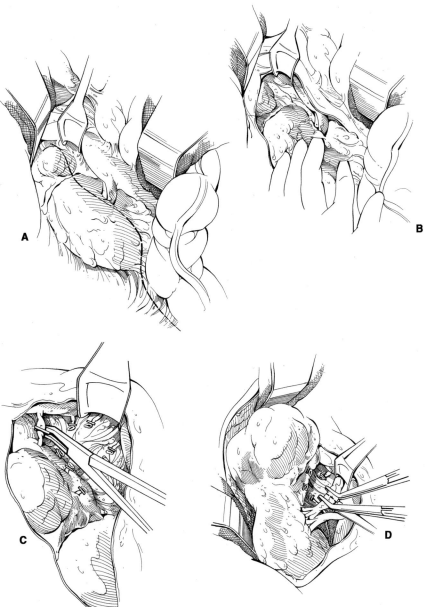

FIG. 1–6. Anterior approach to the right adrenal gland. **A:** The posterior peritoneum lateral to the right colon is incised and the mobilization is carried along the vena cava to the level of the hepatic veins. **B:** With the duodenum and colon reflected medially, the liver and gallbladder are retracted upward. Gentle downward retraction on the kidney brings the anterior surface of the right adrenal gland into view. Small veins draining the caudate lobe of the liver to the vena cava may be injured with excessive retraction, and a self-retaining ring retractor is ideal at this stage. **C:** The adrenal vein should be ligated early in the procedure. In many cases, the vein may lie high and enter the cava posterolaterally. Extensive dissection of the arterial supply medially and laterally may be necessary to adequately expose the vein. Exposure is facilitated by medial and downward traction on the cava. The remaining lateral and inferior attachments are readily divided to complete the procedure. **D:** In rare cases where the kidney is invaded, nephrectomy and adrenalectomy are the treatments of choice.

The attachment of the adrenal gland to the undersurface of the liver is mobilized sharply. Deep Harrington retractors are useful in retracting the liver during the direct dissection along the inferior vena cava (IVC). The IVC must be mobilized by sharp dissection from caudad to cephalad and carried to the level of the right adrenal vein. The renal venous structures are also mobilized by sharp dissection to facilitate superior exposure of the gland. Vein retractors are employed to retract the IVC medially to facilitate surgical exposure of the common right adrenal vein. The right adrenal vein is secured with a suture ligature and transected. Gerota's fascia is incised sharply to expose the adrenal gland and mobilized from the kidney along the avascular plane between the two structures. The adherent inferior and lateral attachments are divided using clips and silk ligatures. The several small arterial structures and fatty attachments are controlled and divided in the superior and medial portions to complete the right adrenalectomy.

Access to the left adrenal gland is obtained through incision of the posterior parietal peritoneum along the white line of Toldt and lateral to the descending colon (Fig. 1–7). The splenocolic and lienorenal ligaments are divided to allow medial retraction of the colon and superior retraction of the spleen. This also exposes the tail of the pancreas and fourth portion of the duodenum, which are reflected medially to access the inferior surface of the left adrenal gland. Gerota's fascia is incised and the adrenal gland is reflected from the kidney. The left adrenal vein is encountered at its tributary off the left renal vein; it is ligated and divided. The inferior attachments are mobilized, ligated, and divided. The blunt and sharp dissection of the gland is continued laterally and posteriorly and the gland rotated laterally to mobilize its vascular medial surface. The downward retraction of the adrenal gland exposes the vascular superior surface. The small arteries on these surfaces are clipped and/or ligated with silk. The remaining attachments are mobilized by

sharp and blunt discretion to remove the adrenal gland. Homeostasis is controlled with electrocautery, clip, or suture ligatures. In thin patients with small tumors the adrenal can be exposed through an incision of the mesentry of the transverse colon to the left of the middle colic artery.

When the adrenal cancer invades the kidney, an *en-bloc* removal of the adrenal gland and the kidney is indicated. The technique is described in Chapter 20.

Flank Approach

The flank approach provides an alternative extraperitoneal technique for excision of small benign and unilateral tumors. The extraperitoneal incision is preferred for performing adrenalectomy in obese patients.

Adequate exposure of the adrenal gland through the flank requires resection of either the eleventh or twelfth rib or a tenth or eleventh intercostal incision. The classic subcostal flank incision is too low for adrenalectomy. The patient is placed in the lateral position on the operating table with an axillary roll. The kidney rest is elevated; the table is flexed slightly, and the patient is secured in place with tapes across the shoulder and the hip. The skin incision is made over or along the chosen rib(s) toward the umbilicus and deepened through the latissimus dorsi, external and internal oblique, and transversus abdominis muscles (Fig. 1–8). The retroperitoneum is entered through the intercostals muscles, which are divided cautiously to avoid entry into the pleura or peritoneum. The attachments of the diaphragm are mobilized early to avoid injury to the pleura.

In gaining access to the right adrenal the duodenum and the colon are retracted medially and the kidney is retracted caudad to bring the adrenal gland down. The adrenal gland is mobilized from the surrounding organs with sharp and blunt dissection. The apical attachment is mobilized, ligated, and divided. The vena cava is dis-

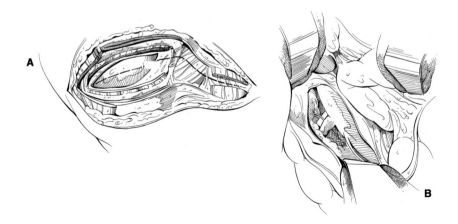

FIG. 1–7. Anterior approach for left adrenalectomy. **A:** The adrenal vein is divided and can be used for traction, although excessive traction may provoke a sharp elevation in the blood pressure even in the adequately blocked patients. **B:** The kidney can be used to provide excellent traction of the adrenal, allowing the lateral attachments to be divided.

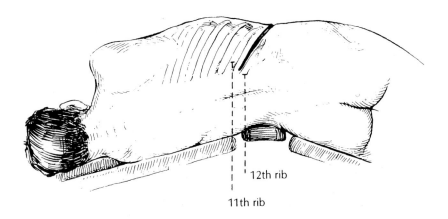

12th rib

11th rib

FIG. 1–8. Supracostal incision with a modification of the interspace approach in which the incision is made along the superior margin of the rib. The rib should be freed to allow it to be hinged downward.

sected to expose the right adrenal vein and up to its drainage into the IVC. The adrenal vein is secured with silk sutures and divided. The gland is retracted laterally to expose the medial surface and the tiny arteries as they course beneath the vena cava. These vessels are divided between surgical clips.

In accessing the left adrenal gland, the peritoneum and the descending colon are mobilized and pushed medially to expose the left kidney and the left adrenal gland. Gerota's fascia is entered sharply and the kidney is retracted caudally to lower the adrenal gland into the operative field. The left adrenal vein is localized, secured, and ligated as it enters the left renal vein. The surgical excision of the gland is completed with blunt and sharp dissection and securing the multiple small arteries with surgiclips and ligatures in the medial and superior vascular surfaces.

Iatrogenic injury of the pleura is a possibility in the flank approach and is repaired by placing a red Robinson catheter in the pleural cavity, which allows continuous aspiration of air from the chest cavity while the laceration is repaired with a running absorbable suture. Once the repair is complete the anesthetist is asked to hyperinflate the lungs manually and hold while the catheter is removed quickly and the suture is tied to prevent air reentry and pneumothorax. A chest x-ray in the recovery room may show a small inconsequential apical pneumothorax that often resolves within 48 hours.

Thoracoabdominal Approach

The thoracoabdominal approach is an appropriate alternative approach to the adrenal gland in patients with large tumors. This is an excellent exposure for inspection of the abdominal cavity and retroperitoneum; however, access to the contralateral adrenal gland is limited.

The patient is placed in a semioblique position (30- to 45-degree angle) with a roll of towel placed longitu-

dinally between the patient's flank and hemithorax. The incision is originated in the eighth or ninth intercostal space near the angle of the rib and continued across the costal margin and the umbilicus (Fig. 1–9). The incision is extended deep through the latissimus dorsi, external and internal oblique, and transversus abdominis and abdominus rectus muscles. The intercostal muscles and costal cartilages are divided to expose the diaphragm and the pleura. Care is taken to avoid injury to the phrenic nerve while dividing the diaphragm circumferentially. The peritoneal and chest cavities are entered and a large retractor is used to expose the operative field.

After the tumor has been excised, a chest tube is often placed under direct vision and the diaphragm closed with either interrupted or running sutures. The incision is closed in layers. Drainage of the abdominal cavity is indicated following injury or resection of the liver or pancreas and/or excision of a very large tumor.

Posterior Approach

The major advantage of the posterior approach is the relative ease of exposing the adrenal glands with direct access to the adrenal vein in particular on the right (Figs. 1–10 to 1–14). The other advantages include simultaneous exposure of both glands, extraperitoneal dissection through a limited incision, and minimal incisional pain. This incision is suitable for the obese patient. The primary indication for this posterior approach is in patients with bilateral hyperplasia secondary to Cushing's disease and small benign adrenal lesions that are not yet the primary targets of laparoscopic adrenalectomy. The major disadvantages of this approach include limited operative field, which is unsuitable for removal of large tumors, and lack of access to explore the abdominal cavity, in particular in patients with adrenal carcinomas or pheochromocytomas.

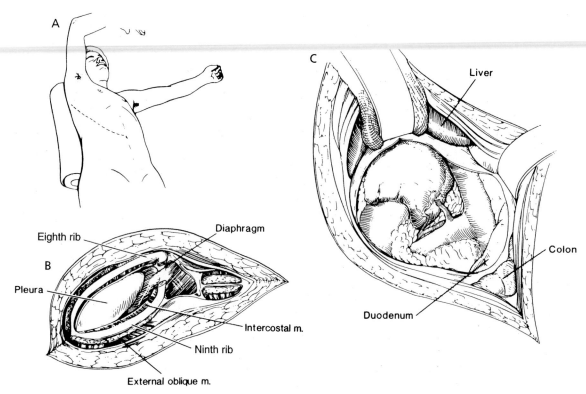

FIG. 1–9. Thoracoabdominal approach. The incision is originated in the eighth or ninth intercostal space near the angle of the rib and continued across the costal margin and the umbilicus.

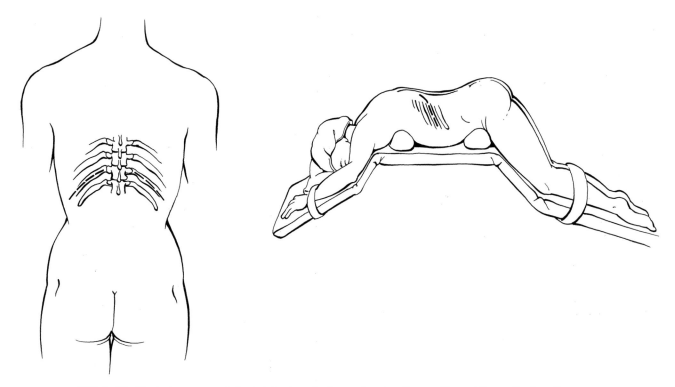

FIG. 1–10. Posterior approach for total adrenalectomy showing the position of the patient on the operating table and bilateral incision over the eleventh rib. The medial end of the incision should be extended superiorly along the paravertebral musculature.

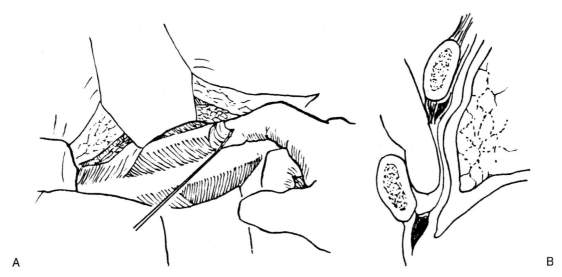

A   B

FIG. 1–11. A: Mobilization of the rib in the supracostal approach. The intercostal muscle is divided, with a finger behind to protect the deep structures. **B:** Extrapleural fascia dissects away from the posterior surface of the rib with exposure of the insertion of the diaphragm and the pleura.

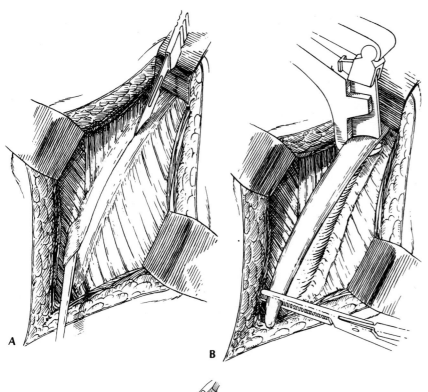

FIG. 1–12. Rib resection in any of the surgical approaches to the adrenal involves **(A)** incision and elevation of the periosteum with **(B)** mobilization and resection of the rib as medially as is convenient.

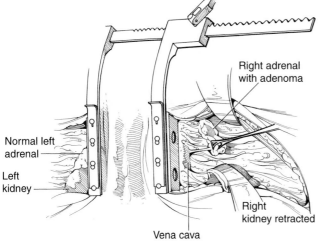

FIG. 1–13. Simultaneous bilateral exposure of the adrenals is facilitated by use of a self-retaining retractor.

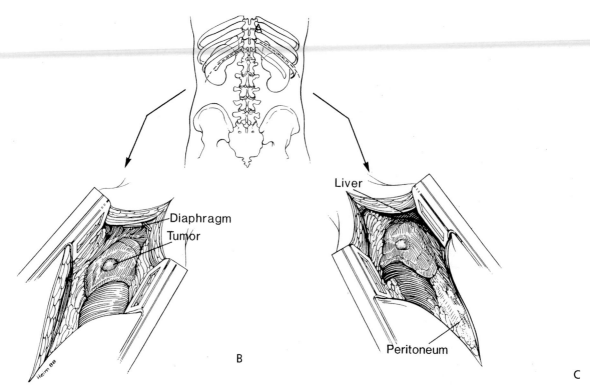

FIG. 1–14. Sketch illustrating **(A)** the posterior approach for adrenal surgery, **(C)** through the eleventh rib on the right side, and **(B)** through the twelfth rib on the right side. (From Novick AC. Surgery for primary hyperaldosteronism. *Urol Clin North Am* 1989;16:535, with permission.)

OUTCOMES

Complications

The incidence rate of general complications such as pneumonia, wound dehiscence, fascial dehiscence, and pulmonary embolism is no higher than that seen in other major surgeries. The most significant intraoperative complications during open surgery of adrenal glands include hemorrhage, laceration of the IVC or left renal vein, ligation of the renal artery, inadvertent injury to the pleura with pneumothorax, and injury to adjacent organs such as the tail of the pancreas, spleen, liver, colon, duodenum, and kidney. The complication rates are extremely variable and likely to be directly proportional to the pathology and the surgeon's experience with the procedure. These complications are in general preventable with careful anatomic dissection and mobilization of adjacent/contiguous structures in open surgical excision of the adrenal tumor. Avulsion of the adrenal vessels can cause significant bleeding and can be controlled by packing and suture ligation. The rate of blood transfusion is low, with less than 1% of patients requiring blood replacement after surgery. The reported perioperative mortality after adrenalectomy is also very low (less than 0.25%).

Cardiovascular crises can occur during resection of pheochromocytomas and paragangliomas. Early control of the adrenal vein prior to manipulation of the gland minimizes the occurrences of these potentially lethal adverse events. Severe persistent hypertension following ligation and division of the adrenal vein for pheochromocytoma indicates that an extraadrenal tumor might have been overlooked.

Adrenal insufficiency after unilateral adrenalectomy is not uncommon and corticosteroid replacement should be immediately instituted at the first sign of steroid deficiency. Steroid supplementation should be considered for all patients with functional adrenocortical tumors because preoperative atrophy of the contralateral gland is expected.

Patients with Cushing's syndrome are more prone to complications related to chronic hyperadrenocortisol secretion leading to poor wound healing, impaired resistance to infection, and thromboembolic events. Glucocorticoid replacement begins immediately and is continued postadrenalectomy to allow the slow recovery of the contralateral adrenal gland. A rare but serious condition following bilateral adrenalectomy for Cushing's disease is hyperpituitarism (Nelson's syndrome), occurring in 5% to 10% of patients. Immediate diagnosis is mandatory because the condition may require treatment with resection of the pituitary gland.

Results

In general, patients who undergo adrenalectomy have a favorable outcome. Patients with low-stage adrenocortical carcinomas have 50% or greater chances of complete tumor resection. The 5-year survival remains 50%, 15%, and 5% for stages I, II, and III, respectively.

REFERENCES

1. Atuk NO. Pheochromocytomas diagnosis, localization, and treatment. *Hosp Pract* 1983;18(4):187–202.
2. Bloom LS, Libertino JA. Surgical management of Cushing's syndrome. *Urol Clin North Am* 1989;16:547–565.
3. Brennam M. Cancer of the endocrine system. In: Devita V, Hellman S, Rosenberg S, eds. *Cancer, principles and practice of oncology*, 2nd ed. Philadelphia: JB Lippincott, 1985:198.
4. Donohue JP. Primary aldosteronism. In: Kauffman, JJ, ed. *Current urology practice*, 2nd ed. Philadelphia: WB Saunders, 1986:3.
5. Donohue JP. Surgery of the adrenal. In: Crawford ED, Das S, eds. *Current genitourinary cancer surgery*, 2nd ed. Baltimore: Williams & Wilkins 1997:11–23.
6. Glazer GM, Francis IR, Quint LE. Imaging of the adrenal glands. *Invest Radiol* 1988;23:3–11.
7. Glenn JF. Adrenal surgery. In: Glenn JR, ed. *Urologic surgery*, 4th ed. Philadelphia: JB Lippincott Co, 1993:1–21.
8. Gonzales-Serva L, Glenn JF. Adrenal surgical techniques. *Urol Clin North Am* 1977;4:327–336.
9. Hume DM. Pheochromocytoma and hypertension analysis of 207 cases. *Int Abstr Surg* 1960;99:458–470.
10. Novick AC, Howards SS. The adrenals. In: Gillenwater JY et al., eds. *Adult and pediatric urology*, 4th ed. Philadelphia: JB Lippincott Co, 2002:531–562.
11. Roake JA. The adrenal gland. In: Morris PJ, Wood WC, eds. *Oxford textbook of surgery*, 2nd ed. New York: Oxford University Press, 2000: 1143–1165.
12. Stackpole RH, Melicow MM, Uson AC. Pheochromocytoma in children. *J Pediatr* 1963;66:515–527.
13. Young WF Jr., Hogan MJ, Klee GG, et al. Primary aldosteronism diagnosis and treatment. *Mayo Clin Proc* 1990,65:96–110.

CHAPTER 2

Simple Nephrectomy

Frederick A. Klein and W. Bedford Waters

Simple nephrectomy is defined as the technique of removing the kidney from within Gerota's fascia. It is usually performed for nonneoplastic disease. However, it is often performed as an end operation after other surgeries have failed. Therefore, a simple nephrectomy may often be technically challenging.

The first planned nephrectomy was credited to Gustave Simon in 1869 for treatment of a ureterovaginal fistula. Since then, there has been considerable controversy over the merits of transperitoneal vs retroperitoneal exposure of the kidney. Because of possible complications of peritonitis and intestinal obstruction, the retroperitoneal approach was the exposure of choice in the first half of the twentieth century. With the advent of antibiotics and modern vascular techniques, the anterior approach was repopularized in the early 1960s (3).

INDICATIONS FOR SURGERY

Simple nephrectomy is indicated for the patient with a nonneoplastic irreversibly damaged kidney. Common specific disease states would include obstruction, calculus disease, symptomatic chronic infection, severe trauma, nephrosclerosis associated with pyelonephritis, reflux, or congenital dysplasia, nonreconstructible renal artery stenosis, or renovascular hypertension.

SURGICAL ANATOMY

The kidneys are located on either side of the vertebral column in the lumbar fossa of the retroperitoneum. Each kidney is surrounded by a layer of perinephric fat and a distinct layer termed Gerota's fascia. Posteriorly lies the psoas major and quadratus lumborum muscles. Posteriorly and superiorly, the upper pole of each kidney is in contact with the diaphragm.

The anterior medial surface of the right kidney is in contact with the right adrenal gland. The liver overlies the anterior two-thirds of the right kidney, and the hepatic flexure of the colon overlies the lower one-third of the right kidney. The second portion of the duodenum overlies the renal hilum. In over 90% of patients, the right kidney is lower than the left (2).

The medial surface of the left kidney is also in contact with the left adrenal gland. Other structures anterior and in close approximation to the left kidney are the spleen, tail of the pancreas, stomach, and the splenic flexure of the colon. The main renal arteries are branches of the aorta. The renal veins join the vena cava. In general, the renal arteries divide into segmental branches at the junction of the middle and final third of their course. A single left artery most commonly lies dorsal to the renal vein, and a long right renal artery lies dorsal to the vena cava and the renal vein. Approximately 25% of kidneys have an accessory renal artery with 1.5% more than one accessory artery (1).

The right renal vein is usually less than one-half the size of the left. Most commonly, the right renal vein receives no tributaries. The left renal vein, however, is usually joined by the adrenal and inferior phrenic vein superiorly, the gonadal vein inferiorly, and frequently by lumbar veins posteriorly.

PERIOPERATIVE EVALUATION

Nephrectomy as well as other operations on the kidney should be considered as major surgery. Therefore, the patient deserves a through preoperative evaluation to be sure there are no significant ancillary problems that will affect a successful outcome. Important historical data should be obtained with regard to cardiac, vascular, pulmonary, and gastrointestinal (GI) status as well as any bleeding abnormalities. In addition to routine physical examination, particular attention should be paid to the patient's body habitus and sites of previous abdominal and/or flank surgery to choose the best incision for surgical exposure.

Routine preoperative studies in adults who will be undergoing nephrectomy would include a complete blood count, complete metabolic profile, electrocardiogram, urinalysis with possible culture and sensitivity, and recent chest x-ray. Coagulation studies may commonly be ordered.

It is, of course, essential to be sure the functional status of the remaining kidney be assessed. This is routinely accomplished by obtaining a serum creatinine measure and looking at the excretory function of the life-sustaining kidney on the intravenous (IV) pyelogram or computerized axial tomography scan performed at the initial diagnosis of the renal abnormality requiring nephrectomy. If there is any question of renal compromise, differential creatinine clearance or a radionuclide renal scan to determine differential function is essential.

Finally, preoperative referral to the anesthesia preoperative clinic should be encouraged with a discussion regarding pain management and a possible epidural for pain control. Likewise, the use of compression hose during surgery and postoperatively until the patient is mobile should be mandatory. If there is any anticipation of possible blood loss, type and hold or type and screen should also be performed.

SURGICAL TECHNIQUE

There are numerous approaches to exposing the kidney for nephrectomy, including flank (subcostal, eleventh rib, twelfth rib, thoracoabdominal tenth rib), transabdominal (subcostal, midline, rooftop), and posterior (lumbotomy). Laparoscopic nephrectomy is now also a common approach and may be performed transperitoneal or retroperitoneal. Which surgical approach is used depends on the reason for the nephrectomy, the patient's body habitus, previous surgery, and, perhaps more importantly, the surgeon's preference, ability, and experience. It is uniformly recommended that the flank approach be used for infectious processes so that the peritoneal contents are not contaminated and the abdominal approach be used for trauma to have better access to the renal vasculature and for the necessity of thorough abdominal exploration.

Flank Approach

The flank approach provides good access to the renal parenchyma and collecting system and is extraperitoneal so there is minimal disturbance to other viscera and no peritoneal contamination if the reason for nephrectomy is infection or abscess. This incision may be more attractive in obese patients as the panniculus falls forward. Disadvantages of this approach are less exposure to the renal pedicle and the patient positioning can be compromised by spinal deformities or cardiopulmonary problems.

Procedure

The patient is placed on the operating table so that the kidney rest is just above the anterior superior iliac spine. After placement of the Foley catheter and nasogastric tube if desired, the patient is placed in a lateral decubitus position with the back placed close to the edge of the operating table. The bottom leg is flexed 90 degrees and the top leg straightened to maintain stability. Pillows are placed between the legs for padding as well as a jellyroll or roll of towels under the axilla to prevent compression of the axillary vessels and nerves. The kidney rest is elevated, the table flexed, and the patient secured in place with wide adhesive tape passed over the greater trochanter. Some surgeons prefer to use a beanbag, which can be inflated to help hold the patient in the proper position after the table is flexed. The extended lower arm is secured to an arm board and the upper arm supported either on a padded Mayo stand, by a sling, or on several pillows.

The incision may be made subcostal approximately 2 cm inferior to the twelfth rib or directly over the tenth, eleventh, or twelfth rib beginning at the lateral border of the sacrospinalis muscle. The level of the incision obviously depends on the patient body habitus and size and the position of the kidney. The incision is gently curved toward the umbilicus to the lateral edge of the rectus muscle. The latissimus dorsi and external oblique are divided with cautery exposing the serratus posterior inferior and internal oblique, which are then divided. The subcostal nerve or intercostal nerve is usually seen exiting superficial to the transversalis muscle. An incision is made in the lumbodorsal fascia providing access to the retroperitoneum. The peritoneum is then dissected medially off of the transversalis fascia bluntly. The transverses can then usually be divided bluntly between muscle fibers. Gerota's fascia can be identified underneath the perinephric fat and then excised (Fig. 2–1). For additional exposure, a Finochietto type retractor can be used. The kidney is then dissected free from surrounding perinephric fat using blunt, sharp dissection or cautery. The ureter is identified at the lower end of Gerota's fascia on the posterior surface of the peritoneum and can be traced to the pelvis to identify and dissect free the renal pedical vessels. It is preferable to ligate the renal arterial and venous vessels separately. However, for the sake of convenience or in difficult cases, an endovascular stapler can certainly be used to take the vessels *en bloc*. Likewise, complete hilar ligature with absorbable suture can be used to take all of the vessels at one time. The use of nonabsorbable sutures, such as silk, for a complete hilar ligation is not recommended secondary to the possible development of an arteriovenous fistula.

The technique of rib resection is similar regardless of what level is selected. The incision is made directly over the selected rib from the costovertebral angle over the tip

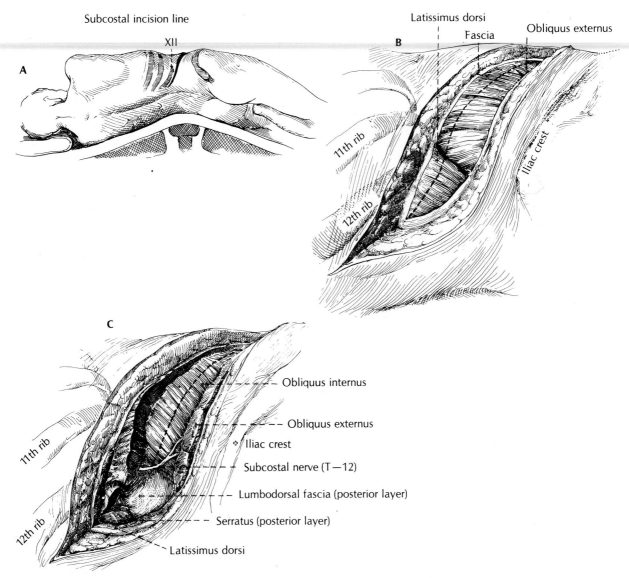

Subcostal incision line

XII

A

B

Latissimus dorsi

Fascia

Obliquus externus

11th rib

12th rib

Iliac crest

C

11th rib

12th rib

— Obliquus internus

— Obliquus externus

— Iliac crest

— Subcostal nerve (T—12)

— Lumbodorsal fascia (posterior layer)

— Serratus (posterior layer)

— Latissimus dorsi

FIG. 2–1. A: The subcostal incision begins below the tip of the twelfth rib and extends toward the umbilicus, ending at the rectus and running parallel to the rib. **B:** The external oblique edges of the latissimus dorsi muscles are divided in the direction of the incision. The twelfth nerve usually is seen beneath this layer as it penetrates the lumbodorsal fascia. The nerve can be freed from its subcostal tunnel medially by sharp dissection until it is slack enough to be drawn out of the way (see **D**). **C:** The internal oblique muscle is incised and can be seen to originate from the posterior layer of the lumbodorsal fascia.

of the rib medially to the edge of the rectus muscle (Fig. 2–2). Once the rib is exposed, the periosteum is incised with a knife or cautery. The periosteum is dissected off the rib with a periosteal elevator (Alexander) and a Doyan periosteal elevator may be guided beneath the rib to complete the dissection posteriorly. Once free, the rib is resected with a rib cutter and the sharp edges smoothed with a bone ronguer or the Alexander (Fig. 2–3). At this point, the posterior peritoneum is incised and the fascial attachments of the pleura divided so the pleura can be reflected superiorly (Fig. 2–4). The remainder of the pro-

cedure is as described above (Fig. 2–5). If the pleura is inadvertently entered, it needs to be repaired and water tight. This may be accomplished by placing a 14 Fr red rubber catheter into the chest cavity placing a running suture of 2-0 or 3-0 Dexon around the tube, having anesthesia inflate the lungs and hold in inspiration. The red rubber catheter on suction is then removed and the suture tied. Testing for an air leak can simply be done by filling the wound cavity with water and looking for bubbles. Rarely, if the pleural injury is significant, a chest tube might need to be placed for several days postoperatively.

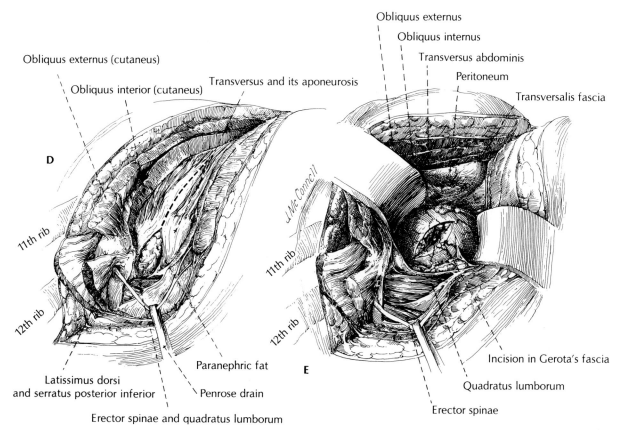

FIG. 2–1. *Continued.*

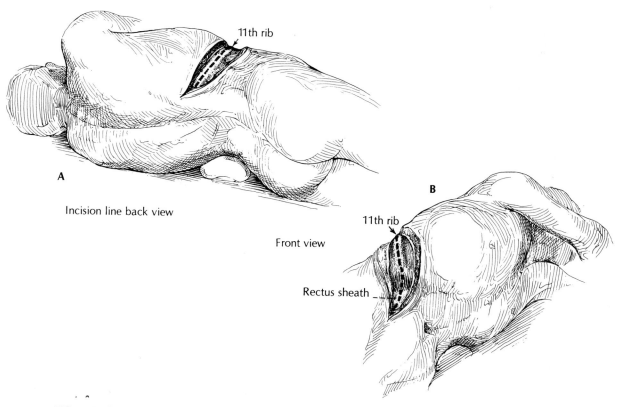

FIG. 2–2. Technique of eleventh-rib resection. **A and B:** The incision is made over the eleventh rib.

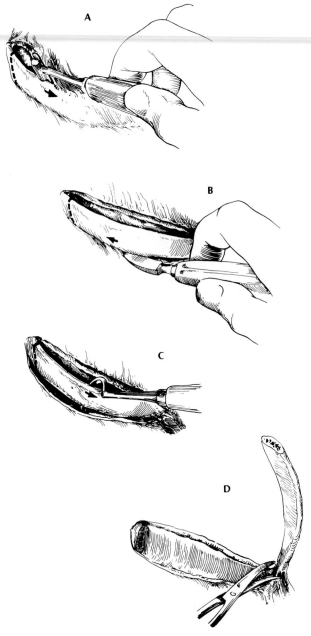

FIG. 2–3. Rib resection technique. **A:** After exposure of the rib, the intercostal muscles are stripped from the upper and lower rib surfaces with an Alexander–Farabeuf costal periosteotome. **B:** The rib is freed from the periosteum by subperiosteal resection or from the pleura with a periosteum elevator. **C:** A Doyan costal elevator is slipped beneath the rib to free it. The proximal and distal portions of the rib are immobilized with Kocher clamps, and the rib is divided proximal to its angle with a right-angled rib cutter. **D:** The costal cartilage is cut free with scissors. The cut surface of the rib is inspected for spicules, which are removed with a rongeur.

Subcostal Abdominal Incision

Anterior subcostal incisions can have several advantages over other approaches as outlined below:

1. The position has less effect on ventilatory function in patients in the lateral decubitus position.

2. There is significantly less risk of inadvertent pleurotomy.
3. It provides easier and more direct access to the renal pedicle.
4. It allows exploration of the other kidney as well as easy abdominal exploration and performance of other possible intraabdominal procedures that may be necessary.
5. Postoperative pain and ileus are less.
6. It can be easily extended to the other side for additional exposure if necessary.

Technique

The patient is placed supine over the kidney rest at the level of the twelfth rib. A jellyroll or rolled sheet is placed longitudinally under the flank, the kidney rest elevated, and the table flexed for maximum exposure.

The incision is made two finger breadths below the costal margin and extends medially from the xiphoid laterally (Fig. 2–6). Length would depend on the body habitus of the patient, size of the kidney, and size of the surgeon's hand. The peritoneal cavity is entered after dividing the rectus fascia and muscle, external oblique, internal oblique, transversalis, and lumbodorsal fascia. Most commonly, a self-retaining retractor such as a Buckwalter may then be used to provide excellent exposure.

There are two possible approaches to the renal vessels: Either the posterior parietal peritoneum is incised or the right or left colon can be incised along the white line of Toldt and reflected medially. In renal trauma, it is preferable to obtain control of the vessels before opening Gerota's fascia as the hemorrhagic tamponade effect is lost.

The approach to the left renal hilum through the posterior parietal peritoneum is by vertical incision over the aorta just below the duodenojejunal flexure, avoiding the inferior mesenteric vein. The renal vein can be seen in front of the aorta and should be dissected free and elevated with a vein retractor to find the artery, which usually lies below and slightly superior to the renal vein. The right renal vessels are approached by making an incision over the inferior cava so the vein may be retracted medially or laterally to expose the artery. Usually, control of the artery is obtained on the medial side of the vena cava because the vein is short.

In a standard simple nephrectomy during reflection of the colon, dissection should be carried around the splenic and/or hepatic flexure to ensure adequate mobilization. Usually, the colon and mesenteric vessels may be easily separated from Gerota's fascia along a natural cleavage plane (Figs. 2–7 and 2–8). There are numerous approaches to freeing up the kidney for nephrectomy depending on surgeon preference, reason for nephrectomy, and history of previous surgery. By initially staying

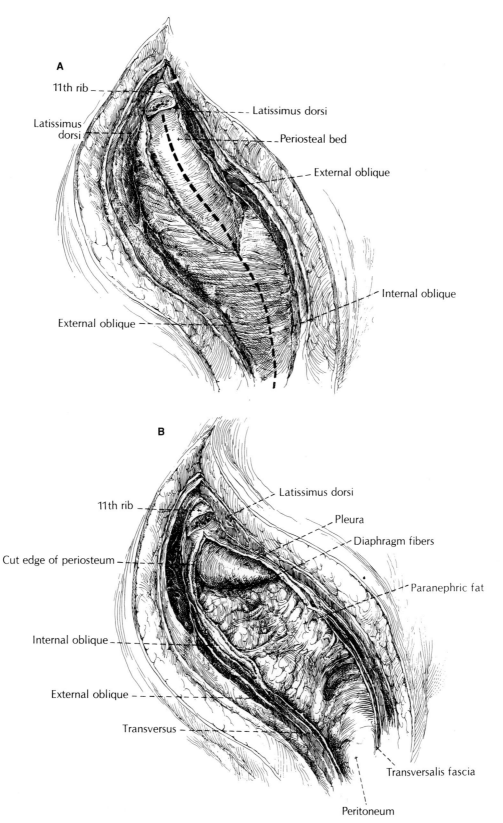

A

11th rib

Latissimus dorsi

External oblique

Latissimus dorsi

Periosteal bed

External oblique

Internal oblique

B

11th rib

Cut edge of periosteum

Internal oblique

External oblique

Transversus

Latissimus dorsi

Pleura

Diaphragm fibers

Paranephric fat

Transversalis fascia

Peritoneum

FIG. 2–4. A: After division of the latissimus and external oblique muscles, subperiosteal resection of the rib is performed. **B:** The incision is carried through the periosteum posteriorly and the internal oblique and transversus muscles medially, exposing the paranephric space. A tongue of pleura lies in the upper portion of the wound. Diaphragmatic slips that come into view are divided, and the pleura can be retracted upward.

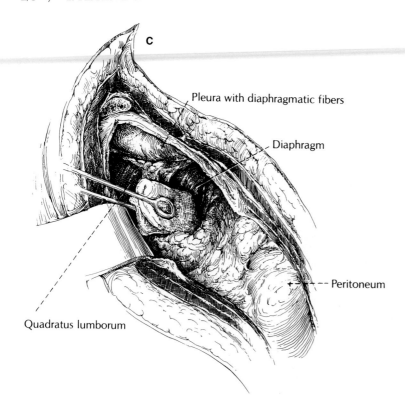

C

Pleura with diaphragmatic fibers

Diaphragm

Peritoneum

Quadratus lumborum

FIG. 2–4. *Continued.* **C:** The paranephric fat is dissected bluntly.

outside Gerota's fascia, it is easy to separate the fascia from the psoas muscle by blunt dissection and use of cautery. The ureter is identified easily at the lower end of Gerota's fascia on the posterior side of the peritoneum. The ureter may be divided at this point after tying each end, or clipping and then dividing, or may be isolated and a vessel loop or Penrose drain placed around it for traction.

After Gerota's fascia is incised, the kidney is dissected free from surrounding perinephric fat and the renal hilum identified. Care should be taken to identify aberrant vessels, especially to the lower pole. The renal artery should be dissected free and ligated first to prevent renal congestion. Typically, two size 0 silk ties are placed, one proximally and one distally before division. To minimize any risk of the tie coming off the proximal end, some surgeons place a suture ligature; others prefer to place a proximal right angle clamp and place the second tie after dividing the vessel. The renal veins may be handled in a similar fashion, paying particular attention to the gonadal vein, adrenal vein, and lumbar branches in particular on the left. Finally, the adrenal gland can be dissected off the upper pole using scissors or cautery to handle small vessels or clips to control larger vessels.

Although in general it is not recommended, in cases where it is difficult to separate the artery and vein a common suture—preferably absorbable—may be placed around the entire hilum or, if preferred, the renal vessels may be stapled individually or together using a vascular stapler commonly used in laparoscopic nephrectomy.

Vertical Abdominal Incision

A vertical abdominal incision is rarely used for elective simple nephrectomy but it still must be in the surgeon's armamentarium. This incision is most commonly used for abdominal exploration for trauma or for other procedures where nephrectomy is secondary. After the abdomen is entered, the approach to the kidney is the same as described above with the colon reflected medially to expose Gerota's fascia.

A paramedian incision likewise is rarely used but may be helpful if one tries to remain extraperitoneal or if a two-layer closure of the abdomen is preferred. It is typically made two finger breadths lateral to the midline. The rectus muscle fibers are dissected off of the linea alba and retracted laterally. Gerota's fascia is incised and the kidney dissected free from the surrounding fat. If the peritoneum is opened, the colon must be reflected medially.

Subcapsular Approach

For patients undergoing simple nephrectomy where dissection is extremely difficult secondary to scarring from previous surgery, infections, or stone disease with chronic inflammation, dissection can be carried down to

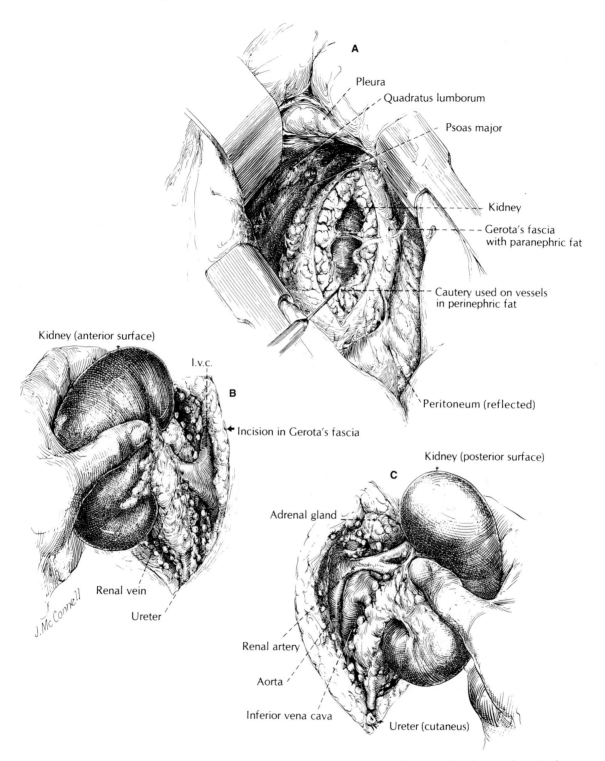

FIG. 2–5. A: Gerota's fascia is incised and entered. In nephrectomy for renal donation, a sharp technique is used to dissect the paranephric fat. **B:** The renal vein is exposed to its entrance into the vena cava anteriorly. The tissue between the ureter laterally and the vena cava medially is dissected free, with care taken to preserve the periureteral blood supply. The hilar region of the kidney is avoided in dissection. **C:** The kidney is rotated anteromedially, and the renal artery is isolated as far as possible. The ureter is divided as far inferiorly as possible.

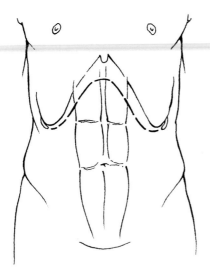

FIG. 2–6. Simple nephrectomy is performed through an anterior subcostal incision, which can be easily extended to the other side for additional exposure if necessary.

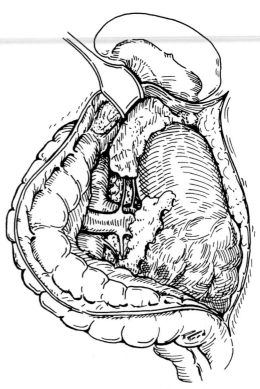

FIG. 2–8. The colon is mobilized medially after the splenic flexure has been taken down. Special care should be taken to keep the proper plane between the mesocolon and the anterior aspect of Gerota's fascia. Mesenteric injuries can occur during this phase of the procedure. If the major vessel of the mesentery is injured and ligation is necessary, careful inspection of the colon in regard to viability must be made. (From Natioh J, Smith RB. Complications of renal surgery. In: Taneja SS, Smith RB, Ehrlich RM, eds. *Complications of urologic surgery*, 3rd ed. Philadelphia: WB Saunders; 2001:307, with permission.)

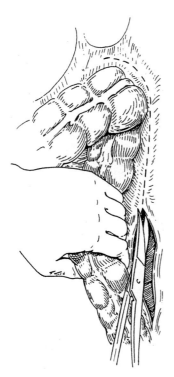

FIG. 2–7. The left kidney is approached by mobilizing the descending colon medially and taking down the splenic flexure. The renocolic ligament is divided. All attachments between the colon and spleen must be completely divided to prevent inadvertent splenic injury from traction on the spleen. The spleen should be carefully inspected at the end to ensure that inadvertent injury has not occurred. (From Natioh J, Smith RB. Complications of renal surgery. In: Taneja SS, Smith RB, Ehrlich RM, eds. *Complications of urologic surgery*, 3rd ed. Philadelphia: WB Saunders; 2001:307, with permission.)

the capsule, which can be incised. A plane is developed between the renal parenchyma and the capsule over the entire surface of the kidney down to the hilum. The vascular branches are ligated and transected as far laterally as possible to allow proximal control of each branch.

Wound Closure

Techniques of wound closure vary considerably depending on the incision, pathology, patient condition, and surgeon preference. In principal, whatever muscle layers are incised on entering should be closed individually on exit. In general, for midline incisions a running double-looped polydioxanone suture (PDS) is preferred. For subcostal anterior incisions, a double-looped PDS is used on the posterior rectus and internal oblique and transversalis muscles together with interrupted PDS on the anterior rectus and external oblique fascia. For flank incisions, we prefer a running PDS to close the posterior layers and interrupted PDS to close the external oblique.

POSTOPERATIVE CARE

Postoperative care for simple nephrectomy should be on a pathway system where overall management is standardized. The principles of postoperative care should be focused on preventing complications and ensuring adequate pain control. The major factor that prolongs hospitalization is return of bowel function, the delay of which can be associated with pain management, so standards seem appropriate. Although we favor epidural morphine for 36 hours, IV narcotics are acceptable. The routine use of Toradol is controversial secondary to possible nephrotoxicity.

Standard management includes postoperative compression hose for prevention of emboli and deep vein thrombosis, perioperative antibiotics for clean cases and prolonged antibiotics for infected cases, aggressive pulmonary toilet, and daily bowel stimulation with suppositories. Significant oral intake is withheld until passage of flatus is noted. The average postoperative stay for anterior approaches is 48 to 96 hours and for flank approaches 96 to 120 hours (4 to 5 days).

COMPLICATIONS

The operative mortality of nephrectomy for benign disease is less than 1% (5). Complications can be divided into operative and postoperative. The most common operative problems include hemorrhage and shock, pneumothorax with rib incisions, and various visceral injuries to surrounding organs such as the liver, spleen, adrenal gland, pancreas, duodenum, and colon. Careful technique and adequate exposure should prevent undue harm. However, if an injury occurs it is mandatory that it be recognized and usually can be repaired without significant morbidity.

Postoperative complications include would dehiscence; infection; hernia; GI problems such as ileus or fistula; pulmonary problems such as pneumothorax, pneumonia, and atelectasis; renal function impairment; and cardiovascular complications including myocardial infarct, phlebitis, pulmonary embolism, cerebrovascular accident, septicemia, and blood loss. Significant sequelae of the above problems are rare. Recognition and management of the above is beyond the scope of this text.

Patients should be counseled on possible postoperative protrusion of abdominal or flank muscles secondary to injury to the subcostal nerve. The nerve lies below the internal oblique muscle and above the transverse abdominus muscle. Careful identification, proximal and distal dissection, and gentle retraction of the nerve can minimize this problem. These bulges are rarely incisional hernias, where a fascial defect is usually palpable (4).

In general, a simple nephrectomy can be performed safely with minimal morbidity as long as attention to detail and meticulous techniques are employed.

REFERENCES

1. Davies ER, Sutton D. Hypertension and multiple renal arteries. *Lancet* 1965;1:341–344.
2. Moell H. Kidney size and its deviation from normal in acute failure. *Acta Radiol* 1961;206[Suppl]:1–74.
3. Novick AC, Campbell SC. Renal tumors. In: Walsh PC, Retik AB, Vaughan ED Jr, Wein AJ, eds. *Campbell's urology*, 8th ed. Philadelphia: WB Saunders, 2002:2672–2673.
4. Sanders WH, Anderson C. Simple nephrectomy. In: Graham SD Jr, ed. *Glenn's urologic surgery*, 5th ed. Philadelphia: Lippincott Williams & Wilkins, 1998:49.
5. Scott RF Jr, Selzman HM. Complications of nephrectomy: review of 450 patients and a description of the modification of the transperitoneal approach. *J Urol* 1966;95:307–312.

CHAPTER 3

Partial Nephrectomy

Andrew C. Novick

Recent interest in partial nephrectomy or nephron-sparing surgery for renal cell carcinoma (RCC) has been stimulated by advances in renal imaging, improved surgical techniques, the increasing number of incidentally discovered low-stage RCCs, and good long-term survival in patients undergoing this form of treatment. Partial nephrectomy entails complete local resection of a renal tumor while leaving the largest possible amount of normal functioning parenchyma in the involved kidney.

DIAGNOSIS

The evaluation of patients with RCC prior to partial nephrectomy must include a detailed history and physical examination, a laboratory evaluation including serum creatinine, liver function tests, and urinalysis or urine dipstick check to screen for preoperative proteinuria. Radiographic testing is used to rule out locally extensive or metastatic disease, including chest x-ray and abdominal computed tomography (CT), as well as possible bone scan and chest or head CT depending on the clinical circumstances.

Partial nephrectomy requires a more detailed understanding of renal anatomy than radical nephrectomy. Therefore, more extensive and invasive preoperative imaging studies are often obtained before partial nephrectomy, including arteriography and on occasion venography. Arteriography is most useful for nonperipheral tumors encompassing two or more renal arterial segments. Selective renal venography is performed in patients with large or centrally located tumors to evaluate for intrarenal venous thrombosis and assess the adequacy of venous drainage of the planned renal remnant. Advances in helical CT and computer technology now allow the production of high-quality, 3D images of the renal vasculature and soft-tissue anatomy in any plane. New volume-rendering software allows real-time interactive stereoscopic viewing of these images and provides a topographical road map of the renal surface and multiplanar views of the intrarenal anatomy. This permits the complex renal anatomy to be evaluated by using a single unified study in a format that is familiar to the surgeon and consistent with intraoperative findings, thereby obviating mental reconstruction of several 2D imaging studies.

INDICATIONS FOR SURGERY

Accepted indications for partial nephrectomy include situations in which radical nephrectomy would render the patient anephric, with subsequent immediate need for dialysis. This encompasses patients with bilateral RCC or RCC involving a solitary functioning kidney. The latter circumstance may result from unilateral renal agenesis, prior removal of the contralateral kidney, or irreversible impairment of contralateral renal function. Partial nephrectomy is also indicated for patients with unilateral RCC and a functioning opposite kidney when the opposite kidney is affected by a condition that might threaten its future function, such as calculus disease, chronic pyelonephritis, renal artery stenosis, ureteral reflux, or systemic diseases (e.g., diabetes and nephrosclerosis) (10).

Recent studies have clarified the role of partial nephrectomy in patients with localized unilateral RCC and a normal contralateral kidney. The data indicate that radical nephrectomy and partial nephrectomy provide equally effective curative treatment for patients who present with a single, small (less than 4 cm), and clearly localized RCC. The results of partial nephrectomy are less satisfactory in patients with larger (greater than 4 cm) or multiple localized RCCs, and radical nephrectomy remains the treatment of choice in such cases when the opposite kidney is normal. The long-term renal functional advantage of partial nephrectomy with a normal opposite kidney requires further study.

ALTERNATIVE THERAPY

Alternatives to open partial nephrectomy include radical nephrectomy and laparoscopic nephrectomy or partial nephrectomy.

SURGICAL TECHNIQUE

Anatomic Considerations

Figure 3–1 illustrates the normal renal arterial supply. The kidney has four constant vascular segments, which are termed apical, interior, posterior, and basilar. Each of these segments is supplied by one or more major arterial branches. Although the origin of the branches supplying these segments may vary, the anatomic position of the segments is constant. All segmental arteries are end arteries with no collateral circulation; therefore, all branches supplying tumor-free parenchyma must be preserved to avoid devitalization of functioning renal tissue.

The normal renal venous anatomy is depicted in Figure 3–2 (for the left kidney). The renal venous drainage system differs significantly from the arterial blood supply in that the intrarenal venous branches intercommunicate freely between the various renal segments. Ligation of a branch of the renal vein, therefore, will not result in segmental infarction of the kidney because collateral venous blood supply will provide adequate drainage. This is important clinically because it enables one to obtain surgical access safely to tumors in the renal hilus by ligating and dividing small adjacent or overlying venous branches. This allows major venous branches to be completely mobilized and freely retracted in either direction to expose the tumor with no vascular compromise of uninvolved parenchyma (Fig. 3–3).

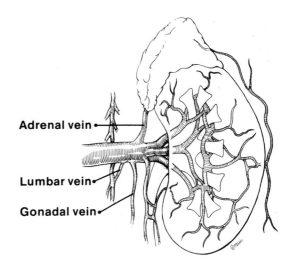

FIG. 3–2. Renal venous anatomy depicted here for the left kidney.

Timing of Surgery in Bilateral Tumors

In patients with bilateral synchronous RCC, the kidney most amenable to a partial nephrectomy is usually approached first by the author. Then, approximately 1 month after a technically successful result has been documented, radical nephrectomy or a second partial nephrectomy is performed on the opposite kidney. Staging surgery in this fashion obviates the need for temporary dialysis if ischemic renal failure occurs following nephron-sparing excision of RCC.

General Operative Considerations

It is usually possible to perform partial nephrectomy for malignancy *in situ* by using an operative approach that optimizes exposure of the kidney and combining meticulous surgical technique with an understanding of the renal vascular anatomy in relation to the tumor (11). We employ an extraperitoneal flank incision through the bed of the eleventh or twelfth rib for almost all of these

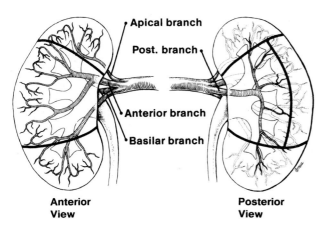

FIG. 3–1. Normal arterial supply for the right kidney with anterior and posterior views.

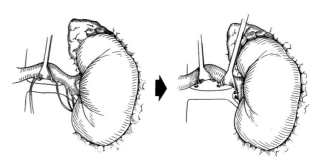

FIG. 3–3. Mobilization of the left renal vein to obtain better exposure of the renal hilus by ligating and dividing small renal venous branches.

operations; we on occasion use a thoracoabdominal incision for very large tumors involving the upper portion of the kidney. These incisions allow the surgeon to operate on the mobilized kidney almost at skin level and provide excellent exposure of the peripheral renal vessels. With an anterior subcostal transperitoneal incision, the kidney is invariably located in the depth of the wound and the surgical exposure is simply not as good. In partial nephrectomy for benign disease the preferred surgical approach is usually through an extraperitoneal flank incision, except for cases of renal trauma, which are best approached anteriorly.

When performing *in situ* partial nephrectomy for malignancy, the kidney is mobilized within Gerota's fascia while leaving intact the perirenal fat around the tumor. For small peripheral renal tumors, it may not be necessary to control the renal artery. In most cases, however, partial nephrectomy is most effectively performed after temporary renal arterial occlusion. This measure not only limits intraoperative bleeding but, by reducing renal tissue turgor, also improves access to intrarenal structures. In most cases, we believe that is important to leave the renal vein patent throughout the operation. This measure decreases intraoperative renal ischemia and, by allowing venous backbleeding, facilitates hemostasis by enabling identification of small transected renal veins. In patients with centrally located tumors, it is helpful to occlude the renal vein temporarily to minimize intraoperative bleeding from transected major venous branches.

When the renal circulation is temporarily interrupted, *in situ* renal hypothermia can be used to protect against postischemic renal injury. This approach is only necessary if the warm renal ischemia time is likely to exceed 30 minutes. We have found that with careful preliminary dissection of the tumor and related segmental vascular branches the time for actual tumor resection and renal reconstruction is often less than 30 minutes, even for central tumors. Surface cooling of the kidney with ice slush allows up to 3 hours of safe ischemia without permanent renal injury. An important caveat with this method is to keep the entire kidney covered with ice slush for 10 to 15 minutes immediately after occluding the renal artery and before commencing the nephron-sparing operation. This amount of time is needed to obtain core renal cooling to a temperature (approximately 20°C) that optimizes *in situ* renal preservation. During the excision of the tumor, large portions of the kidney invariably are no longer covered with ice slush and, in the absence of adequate prior renal cooling, rapid rewarming and ischemic renal injury can occur. Cooling by perfusion of the kidney with a cold solution instilled via the renal artery is not recommended because of the theoretic risk of tumor dissemination. Mannitol is given intravenously 5 to 10 minutes before temporary renal artery occlusion. Systemic or regional anticoagulation to prevent intrarenal vascular thrombosis is not necessary.

Several surgical techniques are available for performing partial nephrectomy in patients with malignancy. These include polar (apical and basilar) segmental nephrectomy, wedge resection, and transverse resection. All of these techniques require adherence to basic principles of early vascular control, avoidance of ischemic renal damage, complete tumor excision with free margins, precise closure of the collecting system, careful hemostasis, and closure or coverage of the renal defect with adjacent fat, fascia, peritoneum, or hemostatic collagen. Whichever technique is used, the tumor is removed with a small surrounding margin of grossly normal renal parenchyma. Intraoperative ultrasonography is helpful in achieving accurate tumor localization, in particular for intrarenal lesions that are not visible or palpable from the external surface of the kidney. A recent ultrasonography is of limited value for detecting occult multicentric tumors in the kidneys (2).

Whichever nephron-sparing technique is used, the parenchyma around the tumor is divided with a combination of sharp and blunt dissection. In many cases, the tumor extends deep into the kidney and the collecting system is entered. Often, renal arterial and venous branches supplying the tumor can be identified as the parenchyma is being incised; these should be directly suture-ligated at that time while they are most visible. If the portion of kidney or tumor supplied by a segmental artery is not readily apparent, then temporary occlusion of the branch with a minivascular clamp can resolve the question by enabling direct visualization of the ischemic-supplied renal tissue. Similarly, in many cases direct entry into the collecting system may be avoided by isolating and ligating major infundibula draining the tumor-bearing renal segment as the incision into the parenchyma is developed. Although a surrounding margin of normal parenchyma should be removed with the tumor, a 5- to 10-mm margin of normal renal tissue is often not available for hilar tumors, which may in part impinge directly on the central collecting system. It is sufficient to remove these tumors with all adjacent renal sinus fat and with a 3- to 4-mm margin of surrounding normal parenchyma where this is available.

After excision of the tumor, the remaining transected blood vessels on the renal surface are secured with figure-of-eight 4-0 chromic sutures. At this point, with the renal artery still clamped but with the renal vein open, the anesthesiologist hyperinflates the lungs and thereby raises the central and renal venous pressure. This forces blood out through residual unsecured transected veins on the renal surface and thereby facilitates their detection. Once identified, these veins are secured with interrupted figure-of-eight 4-0 chromic sutures. The argon beam coagulator is a useful adjunct for achieving hemostasis on the transected peripheral renal surface.

In most cases, after securing the renal vasculature and collecting system, the kidney is closed upon itself by approximating the transected cortical margins with simple interrupted 3-0 chromic sutures after placing a small piece of Oxycel at the base of the defect. This is an important additional hemostatic measure. When this is done, the suture line must be free of tension and the blood vessels supplying the kidney must be free of significant angulation or kinking. After closure of the renal defect, the renal artery is unclamped and circulation to the kidney is restored. When the remnant kidney resides within a large retroperitoneal fossa, the kidney is fixed to the posterior musculature with interrupted 3-0 chromic sutures to prevent postoperative movement or rotation of the kidney, which may compromise the blood supply. A retroperitoneal drain is always left in place for at least 7 days, and an intraoperative ureteral stent is placed only when major reconstruction of the intrarenal collecting system has been performed.

In patients with RCC, partial nephrectomy is contraindicated in the presence of lymph node metastasis because the prognosis is poor. Enlarged or suspicious-looking lymph nodes should be biopsied before initiating the renal resection. When partial nephrectomy is performed, after excision of all gross tumor, the absence of malignancy in the remaining portion of the kidney should be verified intraoperatively by frozen section examinations of biopsy specimens obtained at random from the renal margin of excision. It is unusual for such biopsies to show residual tumor, but if so then additional renal tissue must be excised.

Segmental Polar Nephrectomy

In a patient with malignancy confined to the upper or lower pole of the kidney, partial nephrectomy can be performed by isolating and ligating the segmental apical or basilar arterial branch while allowing unimpaired perfusion to the remainder of the kidney from the main renal artery. This procedure is illustrated in Figure 3–4 for a tumor confined to the apical vascular segment. The apical artery is dissected away from the adjacent structures, ligated, and divided. An ischemic line of demarcation will then in general appear on the surface of the kidney and outline the segment to be excised. If this area is not obvious, a few milliliters of methylene blue can be directly injected distally into the ligated apical artery to better outline the limits of the involved renal segment. An incision is then made in the renal cortex at the line of demarcation, which should be several millimeters away from the visible edge of the cancer. The parenchyma is divided by sharp and blunt dissection and the polar segment is removed. In cases of malignancy, it is not possible to preserve a strip of capsule beyond the parenchymal line of resection for use in closing the renal defect.

Often, a portion of the collecting system will have been removed with the cancer during a segmental polar nephrectomy. The collecting system is carefully closed

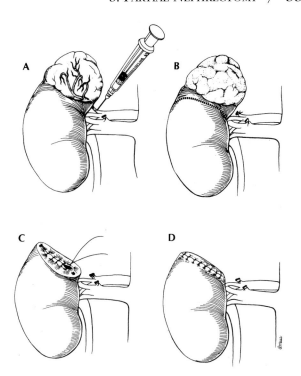

FIG. 3–4. Technique of segmental polar nephrectomy for a tumor confined to the apical vascular renal segment.

with interrupted or continuous 4-0 chromic sutures to ensure a watertight repair. Small transected blood vessels on the renal surface are identified and ligated with shallow figure-of-eight 4-0 chromic sutures. The edges of the kidney are reapproximated as an additional hemostatic measure, using simple interrupted 3-0 chromic sutures inserted through the capsule and a small amount of parenchyma. Before these sutures are tied, perirenal fat or Oxycel can be inserted into the defect for inclusion in the renal closure. If the collecting system has been entered, a Penrose drain is left in the perinephric space.

When performing an apical or basilar partial nephrectomy for benign disease, the segmental apical or basilar arterial branch is secured and the parenchyma is divided at the ischemic line of demarcation, without the need for temporary renal arterial occlusion. More complex transverse or wedge renal resections are best performed with temporary renal arterial occlusion and ice slush surface hypothermia. The technical aspects of partial nephrectomy for benign disease are otherwise the same as those described for malignancy with adherence to the same basic principles of appropriate vascular control, avoidance of ischemic renal damage, precise closure of the collecting system, careful hemostasis, and closure or coverage of the renal defect. In benign conditions necessitating partial nephrectomy, however, the renal capsule is excised and reflected off the diseased parenchyma for subsequent use in covering the renal defect.

Wedge Resection

Wedge resection is an appropriate technique for removing peripheral tumors on the surface of the kidney, in particular ones that are larger or not confined to either renal pole. Because these lesions often encompass more than one renal segment, and because this technique is in general associated with heavier bleeding, it is best to perform wedge resection with temporary renal arterial occlusion and surface hypothermia.

In performing a wedge resection, the tumor is removed with a surrounding margin of grossly normal renal parenchyma (Fig. 3–5). The parenchyma is divided by a combination of sharp and blunt dissection. Invariably, the tumor extends deeply into the kidney and the collecting system is entered. Often, prominent intrarenal vessels are identified as the parenchyma is being incised. These may be directly suture-ligated at that time, while they are most visible. After excision of the tumor, the collecting system is closed with interrupted or continuous 4-0 chromic sutures. Remaining transected blood vessels on the renal surface are secured with figure-of-eight 4-0 chromic sutures. Bleeding at this point is usually minimal and the operative field can be kept satisfactorily clear by gentle suction during placement of hemostatic sutures.

The renal defect can be closed in one of two ways. The kidney may be closed upon itself by approximating the transected cortical margins with simple interrupted 3-0 chromic sutures, after placing a small piece of Oxycel at the base of the defect. If this is done, there must be no tension on the suture line and no significant angulation or kinking of blood vessels supplying the kidney. Alternatively, a portion of perirenal fat may simply be inserted into the base of the renal defect as a hemostatic measure and sutured to the parenchymal margins with interrupted

4-0 chromic sutures. After closure or coverage of the renal defect, the renal artery is unclamped and circulation to the kidney is restored. A Penrose drain is left in the perinephric space.

Transverse Resection

A transverse resection is done to remove large tumors that extensively involve the upper or lower portion of the kidney. This technique is performed using surface hypothermia after temporary occlusion of the renal artery (Fig. 3–6). Major branches of the renal artery and vein supplying the tumor-bearing portion of the kidney are identified in the renal hilus, ligated, and divided. If possible, this should be done before temporarily occluding the renal artery to minimize the overall period of renal ischemia.

When performing a transverse resection of the upper part of the kidney, one must be careful to avoid injury to the posterior segmental renal arterial branch, which may also on occasion supply the basilar renal segment. Preoperative selective renal arteriography with oblique views is integral for identifying and preserving the posterior segmental artery at surgery, which thereby avoids devascularizing a major portion of the healthy remnant kidney.

After occluding the renal artery, the parenchyma is divided by blunt and sharp dissection, leaving a margin of grossly normal tissue around the tumor. Transected blood vessels on the renal surface are secured as previously described and the hilus is inspected carefully for remaining unligated segmental vessels. An internal ureteral stent may be inserted if extensive reconstruction of the collecting system is necessary. If possible, the renal defect is sutured together with one of the techniques previously

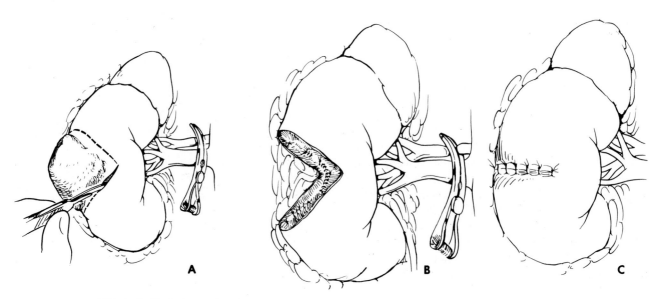

FIG. 3–5. Technique of wedge resection for a tumor on the midlateral aspect of the kidney.

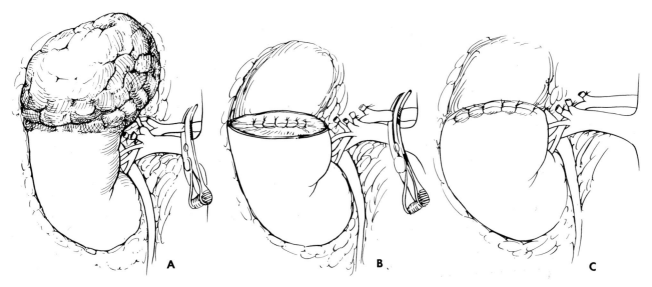

FIG. 3–6. Technique of transverse resection for a tumor involving the upper half of the kidney.

described. If this suture cannot be placed without tension or without distorting the renal vessels, a piece of peritoneum or perirenal fat is sutured in place to cover the defect. Circulation to the kidney is restored and a Penrose drain is left in the perirenal space.

Simple Enucleation

Some RCCs are surrounded by a distinct pseudocapsule of fibrous tissue. The technique of simple enucleation implies circumferential incision of the renal parenchyma around the tumor simply and rapidly at any location, often with no vascular occlusion and with maximal preservation of normal parenchyma.

Initial reports indicated satisfactory short-term clinical results after enucleation with good patient survival and a low rate of local tumor recurrence. However, most recent studies have suggested a higher risk of leaving residual malignancy in the kidney when enucleation is performed. These latter reports include several carefully done histopathologic studies that have demonstrated frequent microscopic tumor penetration of the pseudocapsule that surrounds the neoplasm. These data indicate that it is not always possible to be assured of complete tumor encapsulation prior to surgery. Local recurrence of tumor in the treated kidney is a grave complication of partial nephrectomy for RCC, and every attempt should be made to prevent it. Therefore, it is the author's view that a surrounding margin of normal parenchyma should be removed with the tumor whenever possible. This provides an added margin of safety against the development of local tumor recurrence and, in most cases, does not appreciably increase the technical difficulty of the operation. The technique of enucleation is currently employed only in occasional patients with von Hippel–Lindau disease who have multiple low-stage encapsulated tumors involving both kidneys.

Partial Nephrectomy in Duplex Collecting Systems

On occasion, heminephrectomy in a kidney with a duplicated collecting system is indicated due to hydronephrosis and parenchymal atrophy of one of the two segments. In these cases, the demarcation of the tissue to be removed is usually very evident. The atrophic parenchyma lining the dilated system can be further delineated by blue pyelotubular backflow if the ureter is ligated and the affected collecting system is distended by blue dye under pressure. In such cases, often there is also a dual arterial supply with distinct segmental branches to the upper and lower halves of the kidney. Segmental arterial and venous branches to the diseased portion of the kidney are ligated and divided. After preserving a strip of renal capsule, the parenchyma is divided at the observed line of demarcation. There is usually minimal bleeding from the renal surface, and temporary occlusion of the arterial supply to the nondiseased segment is often unnecessary. There should be no entry into the collecting system over the transected renal surface, which is then closed or covered as described above.

Surgical Complications

Complications of partial nephrectomy include hemorrhage, urinary fistula formation, ureteral obstruction, renal insufficiency, and infection. Significant intraoperative bleeding can occur in patients who are undergoing partial nephrectomy. The need for early control and ready access to the renal artery is emphasized. Postoperative hemorrhage may be self-limiting, if confined to the retroperitoneum, or associated with gross hematuria. The initial management of postoperative hemorrhage is expectant with bedrest, serial hemoglobin and hematocrit determinations, frequent monitoring of vital signs, and blood transfusions as needed. Angiography may be helpful in some patients to localize actively bleeding segmental renal arteries, which may be controlled via angioinfarction. Severe intractable hemorrhage may necessitate reexploration with early control of the renal vessels and ligation of the active bleeding points.

Postoperative urinary flank drainage after a partial nephrectomy on occasion occurs and usually resolves as the collecting system closes with healing. Persistent drainage suggests the development of a urinary cutaneous fistula. This diagnosis can be confirmed by determination of the creatinine level of the drainage fluid and intravenous (IV) injection of indigo carmine with subsequent appearance of the dye in the drainage fluid. The majority of urinary fistulas resolve spontaneously if there is no obstruction of urinary drainage from the involved renal unit. If the perirenal space is not adequately drained, a urinoma or abscess may develop. An IV pyelogram or retrograde pyelogram should be obtained to rule out obstruction of the involved urinary collecting system. In the event of hydronephrosis or persistent urinary leakage, an internal ureteral stent is placed. If this is not possible, a percutaneous nephrostomy may be inserted. The majority of urinary fistulas resolve spontaneously with proper conservative management, although this may take several weeks in some cases. A second operation to close the urinary fistula is rarely necessary.

Ureteral obstruction can occur after partial nephrectomy because of postoperative bleeding into the collecting system with resulting clot obstruction of the ureter and pelvis. This obstruction can lead to temporary extravasation of urine from the renal suture line. In most cases, expectant management is appropriate and the obstruction resolves spontaneously with lysis of the clots. When urinary leakage is excessive, or in the presence of intercurrent urinary infection, placement of an internal ureteral stent can help maintain antegrade ureteral drainage.

Varying degrees of renal insufficiency often occur postoperatively when partial nephrectomy is performed in a patient with a solitary kidney. This insufficiency is a consequence of both intraoperative renal ischemia and removal of some normal parenchyma along with the diseased portion of the kidney. Such renal insufficiency is usually mild and resolves spontaneously with proper fluid and electrolyte management. Also, in most cases the remaining parenchyma undergoes compensatory hypertrophy that serves to further improve renal function. Severe renal insufficiency may require temporary or permanent hemodialysis, and the patient should be aware of this possibility preoperatively.

Postoperative infections are usually self-limiting if the operative site is well drained and in the absence of existing untreated urinary infection at the time of surgery. Unusual complications of partial nephrectomy include transient postoperative hypertension and aneurysm or arteriovenous fistula in the remaining portion of the parenchyma.

A recent study detailed the incidence and clinical outcome of technical or renal-related complications occurring after 259 partial nephrectomies for renal tumors at the Cleveland Clinic (3). In the overall series, local or renal-related complications occurred after 78 operations (30.1%). The incidence of complications was significantly less for operations performed after 1988 and significantly less for incidentally detected versus suspected tumors. The most common complications were urinary fistula formation and acute renal failure. A urinary fistula occurred after 45 of 259 operations (17%). Significant predisposing factors for a urinary fistula included central tumor location, tumor size greater than 4 cm, the need for major reconstruction of the collecting system, and *ex vivo* surgery. Only one urinary fistula required open operative repair while the remainder resolved either spontaneously (n=30) or with endoscopic management (n=14).

Acute renal failure occurred after 30 of 115 operations (26%) performed on a solitary kidney. Significant predisposing factors for acute renal failure were tumor size greater than 7 cm, greater than 50% parenchymal excision, greater than 60 minutes ischemia time, and *ex vivo* surgery. Acute renal failure resolved completely in 25 patients, 9 of whom (8%) required temporary dialysis; 5 patients (4%) required permanent dialysis.

Overall, only eight complications (3.1%) required repeat open surgery for treatment while all other complications resolved with noninterventive or endourologic management. Surgical complications contributed to an adverse clinical outcome in only seven patients (2.9%). These data indicate that partial nephrectomy can be performed safely with preservation of renal function in most patients with renal tumors.

OUTCOMES

Results

The technical success rate with partial nephrectomy is excellent, and long-term patient survival rates free of cancer are comparable with those obtained after radical nephrectomy, in particular for low-stage RCC (Table 3–1) (1,7,9,15). The major disadvantage of partial nephrectomy for RCC is the risk of postoperative local tumor recurrence in the operated kidney, which has occurred in 4% to 6% of patients. These local recurrences are most likely a manifestation of undetected microscopic multifocal RCC in the remnant kidney. The risk of local tumor recurrence after radical nephrectomy has not been studied, but it is presumably very low.

We recently reviewed the results of partial nephrectomy for treatment of localized sporadic RCC in 485

TABLE 3–1. *Results of partial nephrectomy for renal cell carcinoma*

Series	No. of patients	Local tumor recurrence (%)	5-yr cancer specific survival (%)
Steinbach et al. (15)	121	4.1	90
Lerner et al. (9)	185	5.9	89
Belldegrun et al. (1)	146	2.7	93
Campbell et al. (9)	485	3.2	92

patients managed at the Cleveland Clinic before December 1996 (7). A technically successful operation with the preservation of function in the treated kidney was achieved in 476 patients (98%). The overall and cancer-specific 5-year patient survival rate in the series was 81% and 93%, respectively. Recurrent RCC developed postoperatively in 44 of 485 patients (9%). Sixteen patients (3.2%) developed local recurrence in the remnant kidney, whereas 28 patients (5.8%) developed metastatic disease.

More recently, we received the long-term (10-year) results of partial nephrectomy in 107 patients with localized sporadic RCC treated before 1988 (6). All patients were followed up for a minimum of 10 years or until death. Cancer-specific survival was 88.2% at 5 years and 73% at 10 years. Long-term preservation of renal function was achieved in 100 patients (93%). These results attest that partial nephrectomy is an effective therapy for localized RCC that can provide both long-term tumor control and the preservation of renal function.

POSTOPERATIVE FOLLOW-UP

Patients who undergo partial nephrectomy for RCC are advised to return for initial follow-up 4 to 6 weeks postoperatively. At that time, a serum creatinine measurement and IV pyelogram are obtained to document renal function and anatomy. In patients with impaired overall renal function, a renal ultrasound or magnetic resonance imaging study is obtained instead of an IV pyelogram.

We recently completed a detailed analysis of tumor recurrence patterns after partial nephrectomy for sporadic localized RCC in 327 patients at the Cleveland Clinic (8). The purpose of this study was to develop appropriate guidelines for long-term surveillance after partial nephrectomy for RCC. Recurrent RCC occurred postoperatively in 38 patients (11.6%), including 13 (4.0%) who developed local tumor recurrence and 25 (7.6%) who developed metastatic disease. The respective incidences of postoperative local tumor recurrence and metastatic disease according to initial pathologic tumor stage was as follows: 0% and 4.4% for T1 RCC, 2.0% and 5.3% for T2 RCC, 8.2% and 11.5% for T3a RCC, and 10.6% and 14.9% for T3b RCC. The peak postoperative intervals for

developing local tumor recurrence were 6 to 24 months (in T3 RCC patients) and more than 48 months (in T2 RCC patients).

Such data indicate that surveillance for recurrent malignancy after partial nephrectomy for RCC can be tailored according to the initial pathologic tumor stage. The recommended surveillance scheme is shown in Table 3–2. All patients should be evaluated with a medical history, physical examination, and selected blood studies on a yearly basis. The latter should include serum calcium, alkaline phosphatase, liver function tests, blood urea nitrogen, serum creatinine, and electrolytes. A 24-hour urinary protein measurement should be obtained for patients with a solitary remnant kidney to screen for hyperfiltration nephropathy (12). Patients who have proteinuria may be treated with a low-protein diet and a converting enzyme inhibitor agent, which appear to be beneficial in preventing glomerulopathy caused by reduced renal mass (13).

The need for postoperative radiographic surveillance studies varies according to the initial pathologic tumor (pT) stage. Patients who undergo partial nephrectomy for pT1 RCC do not require radiographic imaging postoperatively because of the very low risk of recurrent malignancy. A yearly chest radiograph is recommended after partial nephrectomy for pT2 or pT3 RCC because the lung is the most common site of postoperative metastasis in both groups. Abdominal or retroperitoneal tumor recurrence is uncommon in pT2 patients, in particular early after nephron-sparing surgery, and these patients require only occasional follow-up abdominal CT scanning. We recommend that this be done every 2 years in this category. Patients with pT3 RCC have a higher risk of developing local tumor recurrence, in particular during the first 2 years after partial nephrectomy, and they may benefit from more frequent follow-up abdominal CT scanning. We recommend that this be done every 6 months for 2 years and every 2 years thereafter.

TABLE 3–2. *Recommended postoperative surveillance after nephron-sparing surgery for sporadic localized renal cell carcinoma*

	Pathologic history		
Tumor stage	Exam, blood tests[a]	Chest x-ray	Abdominal computed tomography scan
T1	Yearly	B	B
T2	Yearly	Yearly	Every 2 yr
T3	Yearly	Yearly	Every 6 mo for 2 yr, Then every 2 yr

[a]Medical history, physical examination, and measurement of serum calcium, alkaline phosphatase, liver function, and renal function.

PARTIAL NEPHRECTOMY FOR RENAL ANGIOMYOLIPOMA

Renal angiomyolipomas (AMLs) are benign hematomas whose course may be complicated by pain, hematuria, hemorrhage, rupture, and even death (16). They may develop spontaneously or be part of the tuberous sclerosis complex, where they are often multiple and bilateral. These tumors have a propensity to grow, and treatment has been recommended for asymptomatic AMLs larger than 4 cm and symptomatic AMLs of any size (14). Partial nephrectomy and selective angioembolization are two renal-preserving treatment modalities available for patients with these benign neoplasms. Currently, there are few data reporting the efficacy and ability to preserve renal function by using selective embolization, and it is therefore best suited when a distinct and accessible renal arterial branch supplies the tumor exclusively and not the adjacent normal parenchyma. Partial nephrectomy is considered the preferred treatment in cases of bilateral tumors or tumors in a solitary kidney. Angiomyolipomas are well suited to a nephron-sparing approach for several reasons. Because these lesions are benign, the risk of residual microfocal disease is of less long-term significance. Further, most angiomyolipomas are exophytic and maintain a distinct pseudocapsule that is readily identified and can be dissected to a narrow base. The amount of renal parenchyma that can be spared with an open procedure is usually much greater than one would predict radiographically. There are few published studies evaluating the efficacy of partial nephrectomy for patients with AMLs. Fazeli-Matin and Novick reported the largest series of 27 patients undergoing partial nephrectomy for renal AMLs ranging in size up to 26 cm (5). All kidneys maintained good function postoperatively, no patient required dialysis, and there were no recurrent AMLs or related symptoms identified at a mean follow-up time of 39 months. When surgical treatment for renal AMLs is indicated, partial nephrectomy can be performed with a high rate of success, even in patients with larger tumors involving a solitary kidney.

REFERENCES

1. Belldegrun A, Tsui KH, deKernion JB, et al. Efficacy of nephron-sparing surgery for renal cell carcinoma: Analysis based on the new 1997 tumor–node–metastasis staging system. *J Clin Oncol* 1999;17: 2868–2875.
2. Campbell SC, Fichtner J, Novick AC, et al. Intraoperative evaluation of renal cell carcinoma: A prospective study of the role of ultrasonography and histopathological frozen sections. *J Urol* 1996;155:1191–1195.
3. Campbell SC, Novick AC, Streem SB, et al. Complications of nephron-sparing surgery for renal tumors. *J Urol* 1994;151:1177–1180.
4. Coll DM, Uzzo RG, Herts BR, et al. 3-dimensional volume-rendered computerized tomography for preoperative evaluation and intraoperative treatment of patients undergoing nephron-sparing surgery. *J Urol* 1999;161:1097–1102.
5. Fazeli-Matin S, Novick AC. Nephron-sparing surgery for renal angiomyolipoma. *Urology* 1998;52:577–583.
6. Fergany AF, Hafez KS, Novick AC. Long-term results of nephron-sparing surgery for localized renal cell carcinoma: 10-year follow-up. *J Urol* 2000;163:442–445.
7. Hafez KS, Fergany AF, Novick AC. Nephron-sparing surgery for localized renal cell carcinoma: Impact of tumor size on patient survival, tumor recurrence and TNM staging. *J Urol* 1999;162:1930–1933.
8. Hafez KS, Novick AC, Campbell SC. Patterns of tumor recurrence and guidelines for follow-up after nephron-sparing surgery for sporadic renal cell carcinoma. *J Urol* 1997;157:2067–2070.
9. Lerner SE, Hawkins CA, Blute ML, et al. Disease outcome in patients with low-stage renal cell carcinoma treated with nephron-sparing or radical surgery. *J Urol* 1996;155:1868–1873.
10. Licht MR, Novick AC. Nephron-sparing surgery for renal cell carcinoma. *J Urol* 1993;149:1–7.
11. Novick AC. Anatomic approaches in nephron-sparing surgery for renal cell carcinoma. *Atlas Urol Clin North Am* 1998;6:39.
12. Novick AC, Gephardt G, Guz B, et al. Long-term follow-up after partial removal of a solitary kidney. *N Engl J Med* 1991;325:1058–1062.
13. Novick AC, Schreiber JM Jr. Effect of angiotensin-converting enzyme inhibition on nephropathy in patients with a remnant kidney. *Urology* 1995;46:785–789.
14. Oesterling JE. The management of renal angiomyolipoma. *J Urol* 1986;135:1121–1124.
15. Steinbach F, Stockle M, Muller SC, et al. Conservative surgery of renal cell tumors in 140 patients: 21 years of experience. *J Urol* 1992;148: 24–29.
16. Steiner MS, Goldman SM, Fishman EK, et al. The natural history of renal angiomyolipoma. *J Urol* 1993;150:1782–1786.

CHAPTER 4

Radical Nephrectomy

Michael S. Cookson and Sam S. Chang

Renal cell carcinoma (RCC) is the most common malignancy of the kidney and accounts for about 3% of all adult neoplasms. The estimated number of new cases of RCC in the United States in 2002 was 31,800 with a projected 11,600 deaths, and this incidence is expected to increase as a result of the expanded use of radiographic imaging (6). RCC is refractory to radiation and chemotherapy, and therefore surgery has evolved as the primary treatment in patients with clinically localized and locally advanced disease.

Radical nephrectomy is classically defined as resection of Gerota's fascia and its entire contents including the kidney, perinephric fat, lymphatics, and ipsilateral adrenal gland (2). However, the routine removal of the ipsilateral adrenal gland at the time of radical nephrectomy has been questioned, in particular in smaller tumors and those tumors not involving the upper pole. In theory, complete surgical excision of all tumor with negative surgical margins offers the best opportunity for cure in patients with RCC. This argument would favor radical nephrectomy over simple nephrectomy, given the frequent propensity of the tumor to extend microscopically outside the renal capsule and into perinephric fat. Thus, although no randomized trial has demonstrated the superiority of radical nephrectomy over simple nephrectomy, multiple series have documented improved survival in patients with RCC treated with radical nephrectomy over the past 30 years (4,5).

DIAGNOSIS

Between 85% and 90% of all solid renal masses are RCCs. Accordingly, the diagnosis of RCC should be considered in all patients with a suspected solid renal mass. A renal mass detected on either intravenous (IV) pyelography or ultrasound is usually confirmed by computed tomography (CT) scan. Typically, RCCs are characterized on CT scan by a solid parenchymal mass with a hetero-

geneous density and enhancement with IV contrast injection (between 15 and 40 Hounsfield units). However, despite modern imaging, some benign tumors and complex cysts may be indistinguishable from cancer and confirmed only after surgical excision. In addition, metastatic deposits from a variety of malignancies including breast, lung, and gastrointestinal cancers may involve the kidney and should be considered in patients with a known or suspected other malignancy. The role of percutaneous biopsy or needle aspiration in differentiating an indeterminate renal mass remains controversial, and the absence of malignant cells on biopsy does not rule out the possibility of a neoplasm. In addition, there is the potential for seeding the biopsy tract with cancer. For these reasons, percutaneous renal biopsy for the purpose of diagnosis should be used only in selected cases.

Preoperative evaluation usually includes a complete metabolic panel, which includes serum creatinine and liver function studies. Clinical staging in patients suspected of RCC usually includes a contrast-enhanced CT scan of the abdomen including three dimensional reconstructions; however, magnetic resonance imaging (MRI) is used on occasion and is in particular useful in patients with a history of an IV iodinated contrast allergy, renal insufficiency, or a suspected vena caval thrombus. From these imaging modalities, a number of factors can be determined. This includes the size and potential resectability of the primary, the presence or absence of lymphadenopathy and/or metastasis, involvement of adjacent structures, and the status of the contralateral kidney, including its function. A chest x-ray is obtained to rule out lung metastasis. Bone scans are performed in any patients with symptoms referable to the bone, as well as an elevation in serum alkaline phosphatase or hypercalcemia. In cases of suspected vena caval involvement, Doppler ultrasound is a useful screening tool. However, if results are equivocal or if a vena caval thrombus is confirmed a vascular phase MRI is usually able to determine the level of extension of the tumor thrombus, which then allows the surgeon to properly plan an operative strategy.

INDICATIONS FOR SURGERY

The indication for radical nephrectomy is a clinically localized solid renal mass in a patient with a normal contralateral kidney. Patients with solitary kidneys, renal insufficiency, or bilateral renal masses should be considered candidates for nephron-sparing surgery. A thorough preoperative history and physical examination should be performed before the procedure. If significant comorbidities are suspected, preoperative consultation with the appropriate physician is recommended. In an elective radical nephrectomy, the patient should be expected to physically withstand the operation, have a reasonable overall performance status, and have a 5-year life expectancy.

Radical nephrectomy in combination with immunotherapy has been demonstrated to improve survival among patients with metastatic RCC over immunotherapy alone (3). Accordingly, radical nephrectomy is being offered to an increasing number of patients with a resectable primary tumor in the setting of metastatic disease as an initial treatment strategy prior to immunotherapy. Radical nephrectomy may also be performed for palliation, such as those patients with intractable pain or life-threatening hemorrhage who fail conservative treatment despite the presence of metastases. The role of radical nephrectomy among patients with a solitary metastatic site is controversial; however, 5-year survival rates of 30% have been reported in selected patients, with best results reported in patients with solitary pulmonary metastases (2).

Although local extension of primary RCC into the perinephric fat, vena cava, or ipsilateral adrenal gland may portend a worse prognosis, in the absence of metastatic disease these factors alone should not dissuade the surgeon from attempting a radical nephrectomy. In addition, radical nephrectomy has been successfully performed in the setting of direct extension of the tumor into adjacent organs such as the liver, colon, spleen, pancreas, or psoas muscle. However, surgical removal in this setting is technically difficult and associated with a higher morbidity and a potentially poor prognosis. Therefore, it should be attempted only after careful preparation and in cooperation with appropriate surgical consultants. The role of regional lymphadenectomy at the time of radical nephrectomy remains controversial, and at present most patients undergo only a limited unilateral lymphadenectomy for the purpose of staging (2).

ALTERNATIVE THERAPY

Surgery remains the only effective and potentially curative form of therapy for primary RCC. Along this line, the main challenge to radical nephrectomy in the near future appears to be from more conservative surgical approaches, including nephron-sparing surgery and minimally invasive approaches. Elective partial nephrectomy, enucleation, and wedge resection have been proven to be near equivalent in terms of cancer control and may afford potential advantages in terms of preserved renal function and quality of life in properly selected patients (10). Radical nephrectomy is also being performed through laparoscopic approaches including hand-assisted techniques, which again have shown equivalent cancer control and significant advantages in terms of reduced pain, shorter convalescence, and improvements in quality of life (8). Despite these competing approaches, open radical nephrectomy will continue to play an important role in the management of RCC and it is essential that any surgeon who employs minimally invasive techniques be well versed in its performance.

SURGICAL TECHNIQUE

There are a variety of factors that influence the choice of incision during radical nephrectomy. These include location of the affected kidney, tumor size and characteristics, body habitus, and physician preference. There are advantages and disadvantages to each incision, and it is important to be familiar with several approaches to the kidney as no one incision is appropriate in all settings. The most commonly used incisions for radical nephrectomy are the flank, thoracoabdominal, and transabdominal (subcostal or chevron) (Fig. 4–1).

Flank Incision

The flank approach is an excellent choice for a variety of reasons. First, it allows direct access to the retroperitoneum and kidney, and the entire procedure can often be performed in an extrapleural and extraperitoneal fashion. In addition, the incision is anatomic in that it follows the track of the intercostal nerves with minimal risk of denervation. However, in large tumors, tumors involving the upper pole, or situations where vena cava access is critical, a flank approach may be suboptimal. Although a flank approach may be performed through a subcostal incision, an eleventh or twelfth rib incision is superior for exposure of the upper pole and ipsilateral adrenal gland during radical nephrectomy.

The patient is positioned in the lateral decubitus position with the upper chest at about a 45-degree angle. An axillary roll is placed under the patient to cushion against pressure on the brachial plexus, and the elbows are padded to prevent ulnar nerve injury. The upper arm is draped across the body and placed on a Mayo stand or padded support. The lower leg is flexed at 90 degrees, and the upper leg is extended over one or two pillows. The kidney rest is raised and the table is flexed to elevate the flank and adjusted to make the flank horizontal to the floor. The beanbag or inflatable mattress may be helpful,

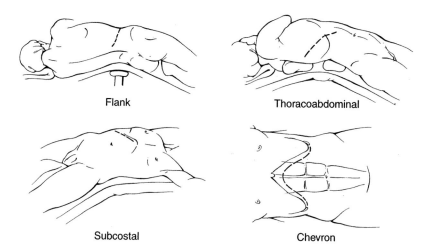

FIG. 4–1. Types of incisions during radical nephrectomy.

Flank

Thoracoabdominal

Subcostal

Chevron

and if utilized can be activated to further support the patient. The patient is then secured with wide adhesive tape and safety straps.

An eleventh or twelfth rib incision is made based on several factors including the kidney position, the cephalad extent of the tumor, and the patient's body habitus. A general rule is to incise over the rib that, when extended medially, will position the incision over the renal hilum. The incision is then made off of the tip or over the rib from the posterior axillary line to the tip and extended medially as far as necessary, which usually stops short of the lateral border of the rectus abdominis (Fig. 4–2). The latissimus dorsi is divided, and the upper portion of the incision is carried down to the rib or near its tip. At this point, a partial rib resection may be accomplished as shown in Fig. 4–3. An Alexander periosteal elevator is used to deflect the periosteum from the bone to avoid injury to the intercostal bundle located under the inferior portion of the rib. A Doyen elevator is then used to strip the periosteum from the entire undersurface of the rib to be resected. Next, a rib cutter is used to divide the proximal segment of the rib. Alternatively, the incision may be created between the ribs in the intercostal space and additional exposure may be obtained by incising the costovertebral ligament.

The posterior layer of the periosteum is then incised carefully, and the pleura is protected superiorly. Anteriorly, the external and internal oblique muscles are divided and the transversus abdominis muscle is split in the direction of its fibers, taking care not to enter the peritoneum. The peritoneum is swept medially, and the intermediate stratum of the retroperitoneal connective tissue is incised sharply to expose the paranephric space. Approaching this in a posterior fashion with early identification of the psoas muscle helps keep proper orientation. A self-retaining retractor such as a Balfour, Buckwalter or Finochetto helps maintain exposure. A radical nephrectomy is then performed.

The wound is closed after checking to ensure that no injury to the pleura has occurred (see complications). The table flex is released and the kidney rest is lowered. The posterior layer consisting of the fascia of the transversus abdominis and the internal oblique is closed in a running fashion with no. 1 PDS (polydioxanone suture) or Prolene. The anterior layer of external oblique fascia is closed with a running no. 1 PDS or Prolene. Alternatively, interrupted figure-of-eight sutures of no. 1 Vicryl can be used for both layers. The skin is closed in accordance with surgeon preference.

Thoracoabdominal Incision

The thoracoabdominal approach allows for excellent exposure of large tumors as well as upper-pole tumors, in particular on the left. In addition, it affords easy access to the adrenal gland and thoracic cavity. The patient is positioned with the hips flat and with the break of the table located just above the iliac crest. The pelvis can be torqued up to about 30 degrees if necessary. The patient's ipsilateral shoulder is rotated 45 degrees, and the ipsilateral arm is extended over the table and properly supported on a Mayo stand or padded armrest (Fig. 4–4). It is important to properly pad all pressure points including between the legs and the contralateral shoulder. The kidney rest may be elevated to accentuate the proper extension, and the break in the table is made to optimize the incision. After positioning, the patient is secured with wide adhesive tape and safety straps.

The thoracoabdominal incision is made over the bed of the eighth, ninth, or tenth rib, depending on the surgeon's preference based on patient and tumor characteristics. The incision may be made between the ribs or a portion of the rib may be removed. The incision is made over the rib beginning at the posterior axillary line. The incision is carried medially across the costal cartilage margin to the midline and then carried down the midline to the umbilicus. Alternatively, the medial portion of the incision may be carried across the midline or combined with a low midline to form a T shape. The latissimus dorsi is divided,

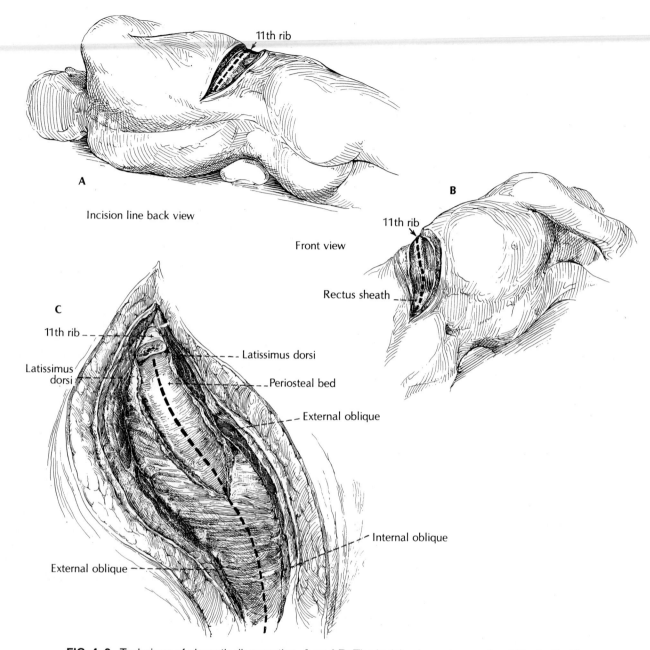

Incision line back view

Front view

11th rib

Rectus sheath

11th rib

Latissimus dorsi

Latissimus dorsi

Periosteal bed

External oblique

Internal oblique

External oblique

FIG. 4–2. Technique of eleventh-rib resection. **A and B:** The incision is made over the 11th rib. **C:** After division of the latissimus dorsi and external oblique muscles, subperiosteal resection of the rib is performed.

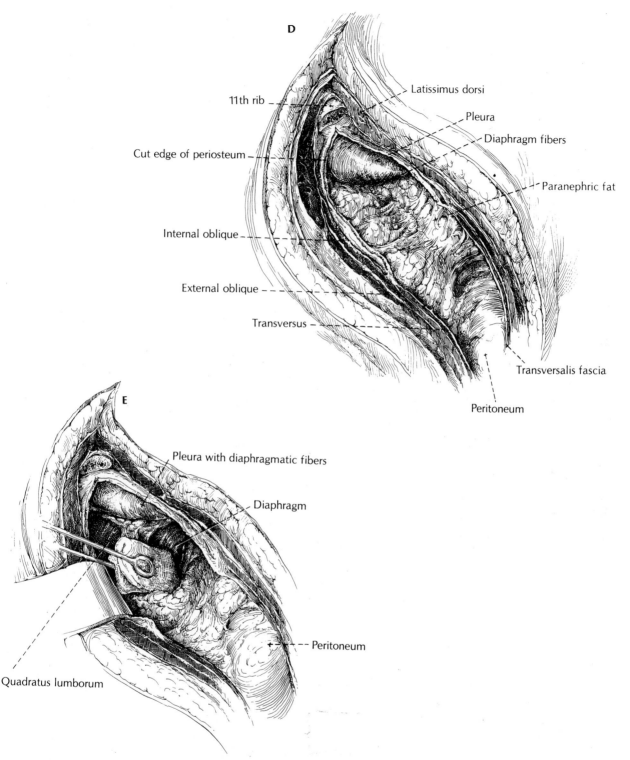

FIG. 4–2. *Continued.* **D:** The incision is carried through the periosteum posteriorly and the internal oblique and transversus muscles medially, exposing the paranephric space. A tongue of pleura lies in the upper portion of the wound. Diaphragmatic slips that come into view are divided, and the pleura can be retracted upward. **E:** The paranephric fat is dissected bluntly.

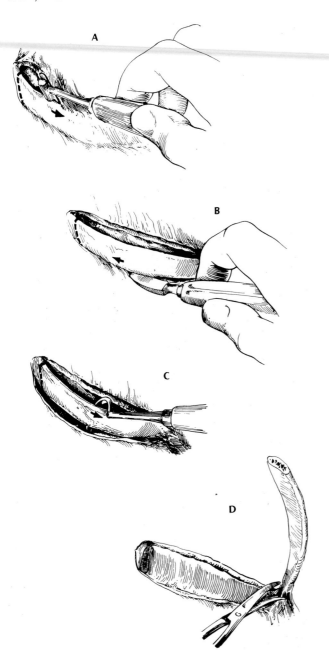

FIG. 4–3. Rib resection technique. **A:** After exposure of the rib, the intercostal muscles are stripped from the upper and lower rib surfaces with an Alexander–Farabeuf costal periosteotome. **B:** The rib is freed from the periosteum by subperiosteal resection or from the pleura with a periosteum elevator. **C:** A Doyen costal elevator is slipped beneath the rib to free it. The proximal and distal portions of the rib are immobilized with Kocher clamps, and the rib is divided proximal to its angle with a right-angled rib cutter. **D:** The costal cartilage is cut free with scissors. The cut surface of the rib is inspected for spicules, which are removed with a rongeur, and covered with bone wax.

FIG. 4–4. Thoracoabdominal incision. **A:** The patient is placed in a semirecumbent position using sandbags. If the chest is entered through the ninth intercostal space, the incision extends from the midaxillary line across the costal margin at the intercostal space to the midline or across it just above the umbilicus. **B:** The anterior rectus sheath and the external oblique and latissimus dorsi muscles are divided. **C:** The intercostal muscles parallel the direction of the three abdominal layers and are divided. The costal cartilage and the internal oblique and rectus muscles are incised. If more exposure is desired, the linea alba and opposite rectus can be divided. **D:** The pleural reflection *(shaded areas)* lies progressively closer to the costal margin in the more cephalic intercostal spaces. **E:** The pleura, reflecting as the costophrenic sinus near the costal margin, is exposed beneath the intercostal muscles. The diaphragm can be seen inferior and dorsal to the pleura. The pleura is opened with care to avoid injuring the lung, which comes into view with inspiration. After the lung is packed away gently, the diaphragmatic surface of the pleura is seen. The diaphragm is incised on its thoracic surface, avoiding the phrenic nerve.

(continued on page 46)

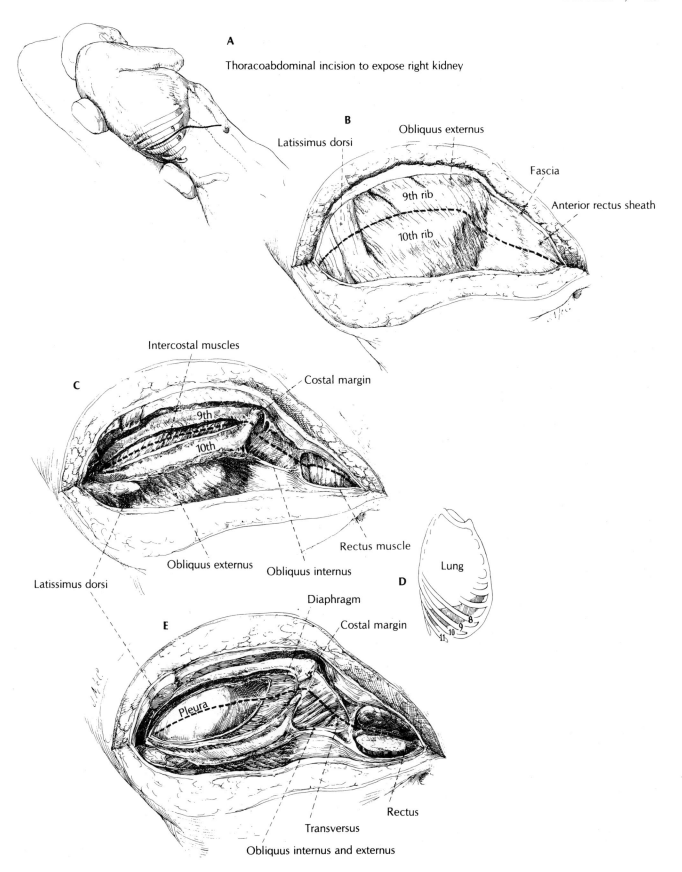

A

Thoracoabdominal incision to expose right kidney

B

Latissimus dorsi

Obliquus externus

Fascia

Anterior rectus sheath

9th rib

10th rib

Intercostal muscles

Costal margin

C

9th

10th

Rectus muscle

Latissimus dorsi

Obliquus externus

Obliquus internus

Diaphragm

D

Lung

Costal margin

8

9

10

11

E

Pleura

Rectus

Transversus

Obliquus internus and externus

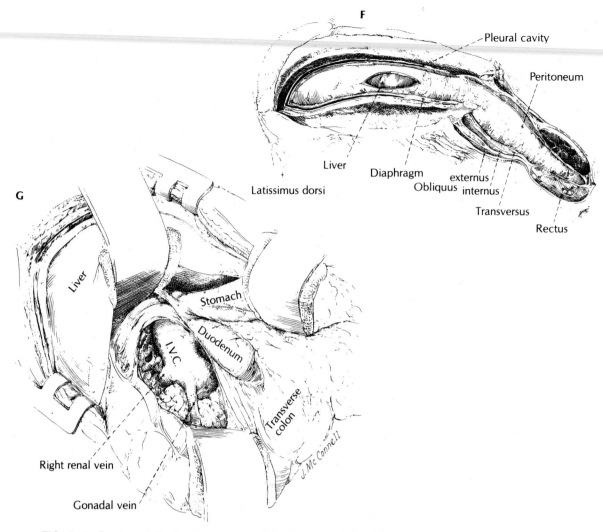

FIG. 4–4. *Continued.* **F:** The transversus abdominis muscle is divided, exposing the peritoneum with the liver lying beneath it. **G:** The peritoneum is incised, and a rib-spreading retractor (Finochetto) is inserted, enabling upward displacement of the liver (or the spleen on the left) into the thoracic cavity and giving wider access to the posterior peritoneum than in an anterior abdominal incision.

and the upper portion of the incision is carried down to the rib. At this point, a rib resection can be performed as previously described (Fig. 4–3).

The peritoneum may be entered by incising the external and internal obliques, the transversus abdominis, and the ipsilateral rectus abdominus. Next, the costochondral cartilage at the inferior portion of the upper thoracic incision is divided, and the chest is entered along the entire length of the periosteal bed. The pleural space is entered, and care should be taken not to injure the lung. The lung is protected, and the diaphragm is divided in the direction of the muscle fibers, which helps avoid injury to the phrenic nerve. A self-retaining retractor such as a Balfour, Buckwalter, or Finochetto is properly padded and placed to maintain exposure. A radical nephrectomy is then performed.

After completion of the radical nephrectomy, the table flex is removed and the diaphragm is closed with interrupted 2-0 silk sutures with knots placed on the inferior side. After a 24 to 32 Fr chest tube has been inserted through a separate incision and properly positioned, the ribs are reapproximated with 2-0 chromic pericostal sutures. The thoracic portion of the incision is closed with interrupted figure-of-eight 1-0 Vicryl sutures through all layers of the chest wall. The medial portion of the intercostal muscle closure should include at least a small portion of the diaphragm. An intercostal nerve block is administered before closure and may be accomplished by injecting approximately 10 mL of 1.0% lidocaine or 0.5% bupivacaine hydrochloride into the intercostal space of the incision and two interspaces above and below. The costal cartilage can be reapproximated with 0 chromic sutures. The peritoneum is closed with a running 2-0 chromic, although this is optional. The posterior rectus fascia, the fascia of the transversus abdominis, and the internal oblique muscles are closed with a running or interrupted no. 1 PDS suture. The anterior rectus and the external oblique fascia are closed with either a running or interrupted no. 1 PDS or Prolene suture. Skin closure is determined by surgeon preference. The chest tube is secured in place with a 0 silk and taped securely in place.

Transabdominal (Chevron or Anterior Subcostal)

Anterior incisions offer several advantages, including excellent exposure of the renal pedicle and access to the entire intraperitoneal contents and contralateral retroperitoneum. With the patient in the supine position, the operative side is elevated slightly with a flank roll and the patient hyperextended to accentuate the line of incision. An incision is made from near the tip of the eleventh or twelfth rib on the ipsilateral side two finger breadths below the costal margin and extended medially to the xiphoid process. The incision is then gently curved across the midline and as far laterally as necessary for exposure up to near the tip of the contralateral eleventh rib.

On occasion, only a portion of the contralateral side will be incised just across the rectus abdominis. The incision is carried down to the anterior rectus fascia, which is then divided (Fig. 4–5). Next, the external and internal oblique fascia and muscles are divided and the fibers of the transversus abdominis split. The rectus muscle and posterior rectus sheath are divided with electrocautery by placing a straight clamp underneath and gently elevating it. The superior epigastric artery is ligated with 2-0 silk and divided when encountered. The peritoneal cavity is then entered, and the falciform ligament is ligated between two Kelly clamps, divided, and tied with 0 silk suture. To facilitate exposure, use of a self-retaining retractor such as a Buckwalter (oval or segmented) or an Omni-Tract is helpful. A radical nephrectomy is then performed.

Closure of the wound is performed after the table is returned to the horizontal position. The wound is then closed in two layers. The posterior layer consisting of the fascia of the transversus abdominis and the internal oblique laterally along with the posterior rectus fascia medially is closed with two running no. 1 PDS sutures, each starting at the lateral aspect and running medially to the midline. The anterior layer of external oblique and anterior rectus fascia is closed in a similar fashion with no. 1 PDS. Alternatively, the layers can be closed with interrupted no. 1 Vicryl. On occasion, it is helpful to place a U stitch of no. 1 Prolene at the apex of the chevron incision before closure, which includes the rectus fascia on either side of the midline, securing this suture after the anterior fascia has been approximated. The skin is then closed according to the surgeon's preference.

Radical Nephrectomy

Irrespective of the choice of incision, certain caveats are universal for the safe and successful completion of a radical nephrectomy. This includes a systematic approach with careful mobilization of Gerota's fascia and early vascular control. For a flank approach, the posterior peritoneum lateral to the colon is incised along the length of the descending colon (left side) or ascending colon (right side) and reflected medially. For left-sided exposure, the lienorenal ligament is incised to mobilize the spleen cephalad. On the right side, the hepatic flexure of the colon is mobilized. The ureter is identified and encircled with a vessel loop. The gonadal vein is ligated

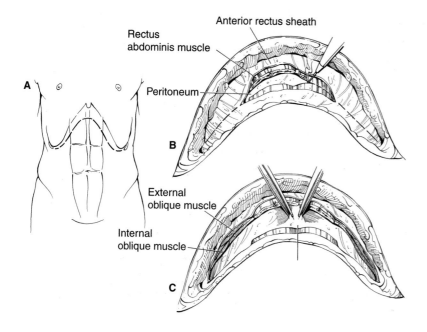

FIG. 4–5. Transabdominal chevron incision. **A:** With the patient in the supine position and slightly hyperextended, an incision is made two finger breadths below the costal margin to just below the xiphoid process and then curved gently down across to the tip of the opposite eleventh rib. **B:** Divide the subcutaneous tissue and the anterior rectus sheath bilaterally. Insinuate a Kelly or an Army–Navy retractor under the rectus muscle, and the muscle is divided with electrocautery. **C:** Divide the external oblique and internal oblique muscles and split the transversus abdominis. Enter the peritoneal cavity in the midline by tenting up on the peritoneum and incising sharply with Metzenbaum scissors.

and divided routinely on the left and when necessary on the right. The plane between the mesentery of the colon and Gerota's fascia (often referred to as the gonadal space) is then developed using a combination of sharp and blunt dissection. On the right side, kocherizing the duodenum exposes the vena cava. Using blunt dissection, the retroperitoneal fat overlying the renal vessels is separated, exposing the renal hilum. It is often helpful to ligate and divide the ureter before this to allow for mobilization and upward displacement of the lower pole of the kidney.

The dissection is then carried cephalad along the vena cava (right side) or aorta (left side). On the right side, the right renal vein is identified exiting from the vena cava, isolated, and encircled with a right-angle clamp and a 0 silk suture and tagged. After identification of the renal artery (exposure may be enhanced by the use of a vein retractor on the renal vein), the artery is dissected free and cleaned for a distance of approximately 2 to 3 cm. With a right-angle clamp, the renal artery is encircled, and 2-0 silk ties are passed (Fig. 4–6). The sutures are then separated and tied, allowing a safe distance for division of the artery and it is preferable to leave two ties on the aortic side. A right-angle clamp is placed under the artery to be divided and gently elevated, and the artery is cut with either a knife (no. 15 blade) or Metzenbaum scissors. The right

renal vein is then ligated with two 0 silk sutures and one additional 2-0 suture ligature on the side of the vena cava.

On the left, the renal vein is isolated as it courses over the aorta. The left adrenal and gonadal veins are identified emanating from the left renal vein and, if present, a posteriorly directed lumbar venous tributary is noted. A right-angle clamp is passed around the renal vein, followed by a 0 silk suture proximal to the tributaries, and tagged. The venous tributaries are then individually ligated and divided with 2-0 or 3-0 silk and small clips where necessary, leaving the 0 silk suture on the main renal vein tagged (Fig. 4–7). The left renal artery and vein are then ligated similarly to the technique described above for the right side.

Gerota's fascia is then mobilized posteriorly and superiorly using a combination of sharp and blunt dissection. Small clips placed along the superior and medial border are useful to control any potential bleeding during this portion of the procedure. The adrenal hilum is then dissected from caudal to cranial with the aid of either clips or straight clamps and ties. On the right side, the short posteriorly located right adrenal vein should be anticipated as it exits directly from the vena cava. When encountered, the right adrenal vein is isolated, ligated, and divided. The specimen is then delivered and meticulous hemostasis is achieved.

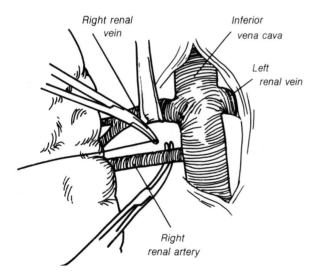

FIG. 4–6. The right renal artery is identified by palpation beneath the vein. After identification with a right-angle clamp, the artery is cleaned in the same manner as the vein. With a right-angle clamp beneath the artery, a suture is passed on a tonsil clamp to the mouth of the right-angle clamp, and the suture is passed around the artery. (From Donohue RE. Radical nephroureterectomy for carcinoma of the renal pelvis and ureter. In: Crawford ED, Borden TA, eds. *Genitourinary cancer surgery.* Philadelphia: Lea & Febiger, 1982:101, with permission.)

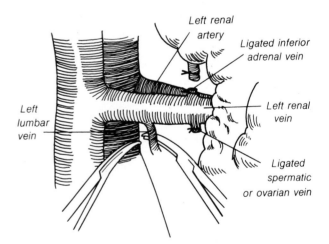

FIG. 4–7. The same technique for ligation is employed on the left side. A suture is passed around the lumbar vein proximally and distally after the vein has been cleaned, and the vein is ligated. Sutures are passed around the main renal vein but are not tied until after the branches have been ligated. The artery is identified above the vein and cleaned, isolated, and ligated, and the proximal end is sutured with a 5-0 cardiovascular silk suture. (From Donohue RE. Radical nephroureterectomy for carcinoma of the renal pelvis and ureter. In: Crawford ED, Borden TA, eds. *Genitourinary cancer surgery.* Philadelphia: Lea & Febiger, 1982:101, with permission.)

OUTCOMES

Complications

The potential for bleeding during radical nephrectomy necessitates careful patient preparation and preoperative planning to significantly reduce the chances. Any medications that interfere with platelet function or clotting should be discontinued. A preoperative hematocrit should be obtained, and a type and screen is in general recommended. In patients with significant anemia, or in those in whom significant blood loss is anticipated, a type and cross-match for possible transfusion should be performed. The patient should have either two large-bore peripheral IV lines or a central venous line to allow for rapid infusion of fluids or blood products if necessary.

Bleeding during radical nephrectomy may be from a variety of locations, including the renal hilum, collateral tumor vessels, or adjacent structures. Venous bleeding is usually the most problematic. The first maneuver is to apply direct pressure to the area of bleeding and allow for appropriate resuscitation before additional maneuvers are considered. The point of bleeding is then carefully exposed and controlled by a suture ligature. In the case of venal caval injury, an Allis or Satinsky clamp may be carefully placed, and a vascular 5-0 or 6-0 Prolene suture is used to oversew the defect. Lumbar veins should be exposed by gentle retraction of the vena cava, appropriately clamped, ligated with vascular silk suture, and divided. Renal artery bleeding may be controlled by direct pressure on the aorta proximally and distally until adequate exposure can be obtained, and the artery is then ligated. Only in rare circumstances will a pedicle clamp or mass ligature be necessary.

Adrenal tears may result in significant hemorrhage during radical nephrectomy, in particular on the right side, where the short adrenal vein enters into the vena cava directly posterior. Control of the right adrenal vein should be attempted only after control of the vena cava, adequate exposure, and proper suction. The vein is then ligated with a 2-0 or 3-0 silk tie or vascular Prolene. Venous bleeding from a torn adrenal gland can be oversewn with a running suture or stopped by placement of surgical clips. However, removal of the ipsilateral adrenal may be the most expeditious method of controlling bleeding.

Failure to recognize a rent in the pleura during flank incision will result in a pneumothorax. Filling the flank wound with sterile water or saline and administering a deep inspiratory breath may help recognize small openings in the pleura. Small tears recognized intraoperatively can be managed by closing the pleura with a 3-0 chromic pursestring suture over a 12 Fr or 14 Fr Robinson catheter. Before it is removed, all air is aspirated from the pleural cavity either by suction or by placing the Robinson catheter under water and administering a deep inspiratory breath. The air is evacuated from the pleural space and the tube is removed while the pursestring suture is simultaneously tied in place. Alternatively, the Robinson catheter can be temporarily left in place with the chromic suture secured and the fascial layers closed around the catheter, which exits from the corner of the wound. Just before skin closure, after all air has been evacuated under water seal as described above, the catheter is removed. The latter technique is helpful when the pleura is attenuated or contains multiple small holes that are not easily closed. Alternatively, a 22 Fr or 24 Fr chest tube may be placed and left to suction.

An upright end-expiratory chest x-ray is obtained after all flank incisions to ensure that no significant pneumothorax exists. A small (usually less than 15%), asymptomatic pneumothorax can be followed conservatively with serial chest x-rays and oxygen therapy. In a symptomatic or large pneumothorax, aspiration of the pleural space using a needle or a central venous catheter (Seldinger technique) introduced just over the rib in the anterior fourth or fifth interspace can be therapeutic. However, if these attempts are not successful a chest tube should be inserted and placed on suction.

Injuries to the colon during radical nephrectomy are uncommon. In locally advanced tumors, suspected of extension into either the colon or mesentery, patients should undergo a mechanical and antibiotic bowel preparation. Segmental colon resection and primary anastomosis should be possible in most cases. Inadvertent injury to the colon during radical nephrectomy can usually be repaired primarily; however, in situations where there is gross spillage of fecal contents or a devascularized segment a diverting colostomy should be considered and a general surgery consultation is advisable. Defects in the mesentery of the colon should be closed to prevent internal herniation of peritoneal contents.

Right radical nephrectomy is also associated with the potential for injury to the duodenum and liver. The duodenum must be carefully mobilized, and care must be taken to properly pad retractors to prevent injury to the bowel and adjacent structures, including the head of the pancreas. The second portion of the duodenum may be injured during a right radical nephrectomy. Duodenal hematomas should only be observed, but rapidly enlarging hematomas will require control of the bleeding and an intraoperative general surgery consultation should be obtained. Duodenal lacerations should be repaired in multiple layers with interrupted nonabsorbable sutures for the mucosal and serosal layers (7). When possible, an omental wrap may provide additional support, and all patients should be managed with a nasogastric tube during the postoperative period.

Bleeding from superficial liver lacerations may be controlled with the Bovie electrocautery or an argon beam electrocoagulator. More significant bleeding may be repaired with absorbable horizontal mattress sutures utilizing a Surgicel or Gelfoam bolster. Deep liver lacerations, which may involve the hepatic ducts, could result in bile leakage and should be drained following repair and intraoperative general surgical consultation is strongly recommended. Direct invasion of the liver by renal cell carcinoma is rare; however, resection including *en-bloc* removal is possible in selected cases. If a major lobectomy or a partial hepatectomy is to be performed because of either direct extension or major hemorrhage, a general surgeon should be present to assist in its performance.

Splenic injury is one of the most common intraoperative complications during a left nephrectomy, with an incidence as high as 10% in some series. Most superficial lacerations or tears can be managed conservatively without the need for splenectomy. Although minor tears may require only some gentle pressure and the application of a Gelfoam or Surgicel with spray thrombin, closure of a moderate splenic capsular tear is facilitated through the use of nonabsorbable sutures over bolsters of Surgicel. Major hemorrhage secondary to severe splenic lacerations may require splenectomy (7). The splenic artery and vein are controlled by compressing these structures, located in the splenic hilum near the tail of the pancreas. Initially, this can be accomplished manually by compressing the tail of the pancreas between the thumb and forefinger. Once bleeding has been temporarily controlled, the spleen is mobilized by dividing the splenocolic and splenorenal ligaments as well as taking down the peritoneal attachments to the diaphragm. The short gastric vessels are then ligated, and the hilum of the spleen is dissected free from the tail of the pancreas. The splenic artery and vein are ligated and divided. The pancreas should be inspected closely to rule out inadvertent injury. Following splenectomy, patients will have a reduced resistance to pneumococcal organisms and should receive Pneumovax and Hibtiter on a yearly basis.

Results

Surgical excision remains the only effective and potentially curative therapy for clinically localized RCC. Pathologic staging remains the best prognostic variable in terms of patient survival, and the two most commonly used staging systems are the Robson classification and the American Joint Committee on Cancer recommendations (TNM) classification (1,9). Both staging systems have demonstrated an inverse relationship between survival and increasing stage, but the TNM is in general thought to be more accurate because it more precisely defines the extent of disease (4,5).

In patients treated with radical nephrectomy and found to have tumors confined to the kidney (Robson stage I),

the 5-year survival is between 60% and 90% compared with 47% to 67% in patients whose RCC is confined to Gerota's fascia (Robson stage II). Survival for patients with distant metastases is poor, with 5-year survival of between 5% and 10% (2). Under the TNM staging system, the 5-year survival for patients with organ-confined tumors treated with radical nephrectomy for $T_1N_0M_0$ tumors is between 80% and 91%, whereas that for $T_2N_0M_0$ tumors is 68% to 92% (2,4,5). For those patients with $T_{3a}N_0M_0$ (tumor invading into the adrenal gland) and $T_{3b}N_0M_0$ (tumor invading into the renal vein) carcinomas, the 5-year survival is 77% and 59%, respectively. Finally, patients with node-positive disease ($N_{1-3}M_0$) have a 5-year survival between 5% and 30%.

Although radical nephrectomy remains the standard of care for unilateral RCC, more conservative surgical options have been proposed. Recently, excellent results have been seen in patients treated with nephron-sparing surgery, with 10-year cancer-specific survivals of greater than 90% for small (less than 4 cm), stage I tumors (10). In addition, results with laparoscopic radical nephrectomy appear equivalent to those of open techniques (8). The ultimate choice of surgical treatment in patients with clinically localized renal masses will ultimately stem from a variety of factors including patient characteristics and desires, tumor characteristics, and surgeon. Currently, open radical nephrectomy remains a gold standard in patients with clinically localized and locally advanced RCC and a benchmark by which future alternative surgical strategies will be measured.

REFERENCES

1. American Joint Committee on Cancer. *Manual for staging of cancer*, 5th ed. Philadelphia: Lippincott Williams & Wilkins, 1998.
2. Belldegrun A, deKernion JB. Renal tumors. In: Walsh PC, Retik AB, Vaughan ED Jr, Wein AJ, eds. *Campbell's urology*, 7th ed. Philadelphia: WB Saunders, 1998:2283–2326.
3. Flanigan RC, Salmon SE, Blumenstein BA, et al. Nephron sparing surgery for renal tumors: indications, techniques and outcomes. *N Engl J Med* 2001;345:1655–1659.
4. Gettman MT, Blute ML, Spotts B, et al. Pathologic staging of renal cell carcinoma: significance of tumor classification with the 1997 TNM staging system. *Cancer* 2001;91:354–361.
5. Guinan P, Saffrin R, Stuhldreher D. Renal cell carcinoma: comparison of the TNM and Robson stage groupings. *J Surg Oncol* 1995;59:186–189.
6. Jemal A, Thomas A, Murray T, Thun M. Cancer Statistics, 2002. *CA Cancer J Clin* 2002;52:23–47.
7. Naitoh J, Smith RB. Complications of renal surgery. In: Taneja SS, Smith RB, Ehrlich RM, eds. *Complications of urologic surgery: Prevention and management*, 3rd ed. Philadelphia: WB Saunders, 2001: 299–325.
8. Portis AJ, Yan Y, Landman J, et al. Long-term follow-up after laparoscopic radical nephrectomy. *J Urol* 2002;167:1257–1262.
9. Robson CJ. Staging of renal cell carcinoma. *J Urol* 1982;100:439–445.
10. Uzzo RG, Novick AC. Nephron sparing surgery for renal tumors: indications, techniques and outcomes. *J Urol* 2001;166:6–18.

CHAPTER 5

Intracaval Tumors

Thomas J. Polascik and Fray F. Marshall

Tumor thrombus extending from the renal vein into the vena cava has been reported to occur in 4% to 10% of patients with renal cell carcinoma (7). The extent of tumor thrombus involving the inferior vena cava can vary from involvement of the renal vein only to extension into the right atrium occurring in a significant number of these patients. The majority of patients with vena caval tumors have right-sided renal primaries due to the short right renal vein. In the absence of metastatic disease, numerous centers have demonstrated long-term cancer-specific survival rates comparable to early stage renal cell carcinoma following complete surgical extirpation.

Improvements in surgical technique have allowed the surgeon to safely perform a radical nephrectomy and venacavotomy. Several centers have documented reduced morbidity and mortality associated with these procedures. Technical difficulties and complications (excessive bleeding, coagulopathy, and postoperative renal failure) can accompany these procedures, especially with extensive intra- or suprahepatic caval neoplastic extension.

DIAGNOSIS

Today, the majority of patients presenting with a renal mass and intracaval tumor extension are diagnosed with computed tomography (CT). In the past, patients presenting with advanced disease had clinical signs and symptoms related to vena caval occlusion including bilateral lower-extremity edema, a recently enlarging varicocele, or dilated abdominal wall veins. Patients may also present with proteinuria, hepatic dysfunction with hepatomegaly, or pulmonary embolus.

Patients should have a thorough evaluation for metastatic disease including CT of the chest and abdomen and a bone scan if applicable. The renal vein and vena cava can be noninvasively imaged using magnetic resonance imaging (MRI). MRI can usually define the superior limit of the caval thrombus unless the distal

thrombus is mobile, thereby limiting its accuracy. MRI is also effective when total caval occlusion is present. Venacavography can be used to define a caval tumor; however, its invasive nature, false positive and negative results, and decreased ability to define the superior extent of the tumor limit its use. To fully delineate the extent of a large caval tumor, the combination of MRI and intraoperative transesophageal sonography provide the best results (11).

INDICATIONS FOR SURGERY

The primary indication for nephrectomy and venacavotomy is a renal mass with intracaval tumor extension in the absence of metastatic disease. The patient should also be medically able to tolerate an extensive surgical procedure.

ALTERNATIVE THERAPY

To date, complete surgical excision of tumor is the only curative treatment. Expectant therapy or systemic protocols may be applicable if the patient is a candidate.

SURGICAL TECHNIQUE

In addition to a general anesthetic, a thoracic epidural can be utilized and is often effective with postoperative pain management with most flank incisions. For the majority of tumors, standard intraoperative monitoring includes central venous pressure, arterial pressure tracings, electrocardiography, and urinary output. Additional monitoring is used for extensive vena caval tumors, including a Swan–Ganz catheter, esophageal and rectal temperature probes, oxygen and carbon dioxide measurements, and transesophageal sonography. A hypothermic blanket is used to maintain body temperature. Elastic stockings and sequential compression devices are placed to prevent lower-extremity venous stasis. An intravenous cephalosporin is in general sufficient as prophylactic antibiotic coverage.

The patient's body habitus and extent of both the primary and intracaval tumor direct the surgical approach. For renal tumors with neoplasm extending minimally into the inferior vena cava, a supra eleventh rib or standard thoracoabdominal approach with rib excision is ideal, especially in obese patients. For left-sided tumors and more extensive caval tumors, an anterior incision will provide good exposure. We have used a thoracoabdominal incision extending from the tip of the scapula across the costal margin to the midline halfway between the umbilicus and the xyphoid process for right-sided tumors with intrahepatic and supradiaphragmatic intracaval tumor extension. Using this approach, the patient should be positioned with the right shoulder rotated toward the contralateral side while the hips remain in the supine position and the table is slightly extended. Although this incision provides both intraabdominal and intrathoracic exposure and the dissection is easier for the urologist, cannulating the aortic arch for cardiopulmonary bypass is more difficult.

We typically use a median sternotomy extending into either a midline abdominal or a chevron incision when the intracaval neoplasm extends into or beyond the liver and cardiopulmonary bypass is considered (Fig. 5–1) (4). The chevron incision is useful in patients with a wide abdominal girth, with bulky primary tumors, and when using liver mobilization and rotation techniques to gain access to the upper retroperitoneum and chest. Although these extensive incisions provide excellent exposure allowing for additional operations to be performed, we recommend limiting the procedure to nephrectomy and caval thrombectomy.

The patient should be widely prepared with antiseptic solution and draped to approach an extensive infra- or supradiaphragmatic tumor, and consideration should be given to preparing the right axilla and left groin if venovenous bypass is considered. The operation is commenced with inspection of the abdomen and/or retroperitoneum for metastatic disease and, if discovered, the procedure is usually stopped as cancer-specific survival has not been demonstrated to be improved with surgery. In the absence of overt metastasis, the incision is extended to include a median sternotomy as this approach gives the best exposure.

The primary renal malignancy is approached first. For a right renal tumor, the right colon is mobilized along the line of Toldt and reflected medially to gain access to the retroperitoneum. For significant tumors via a midline approach, incision of the root of the mesentery up to the Treitz's ligament with placement of the bowel into an intestinal bag retracted onto the chest provides additional exposure. We use the Omni-Tract retractor (Minnesota Scientific Inc.) as it provides excellent superficial and

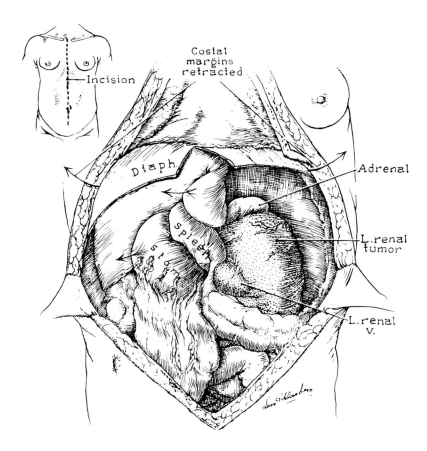

FIG. 5–1. Incision for radical nephrectomy with removal of vena caval thrombus. (From Marshall FF, Reitz BA. Radical nephrectomy with excision of vena caval tumor thrombus. In: Marshall FF, Reitz BA, eds. *Marshall's textbook of operative urology.* Philadelphia: WB Saunders, 1996, pp. 268, with permission.)

deep exposure of the surgical field. The entire kidney within Gerota's fascia is mobilized, first by a posterolateral approach developing the plane between the quadratus/psoas muscles and Gerota's fascia. After mobilizing the kidney posteriorly, the renal artery is ligated early to keep blood loss to a minimum. Anteriorly, the mesocolon is then reflected medially from the anterior surface of Gerota's fascia until the vena cava is visualized. A Kocher maneuver provides additional medial exposure near the vena cava. Superiorly, dissection above the adrenal is undertaken using ligaclips and the adrenal vein is ligated. Inferiorly, the kidney is mobilized along with ligation of the gonadal vein and ureter. Mobilization of the primary tumor is complete when the kidney remains attached to the vena cava by the renal vein.

A left-sided renal tumor with caval thrombus requires dissection on both sides of the abdomen to access both the vena cava and the left kidney. A midline or chevron incision usually provides excellent exposure. The descending colon is reflected medially by incising the line of Toldt. In a dissection similar to a right-sided tumor, the entire kidney within Gerota's fascia is mobilized until only the left renal vein remains. For large, left-sided renal tumors the pancreas and spleen can be mobilized to provide greater exposure of the left upper retroperitoneum (2,3). The ascending colon is then mobilized medially by incising the line of Toldt and the duodenum is reflected by the Kocher maneuver. Once adequate exposure to the vena cava is obtained, the remainder of the procedure is similar to a right-sided renal primary tumor.

The extent of the intracaval tumor dictates the length the vena caval needs to be isolated. Dissection should proceed directly upon the vena cava, using care to prevent potential dislodgment of caval tumor. If the intracaval tumor extends slightly beyond the ostium of the renal vein into the vena cava, a Satinsky vascular clamp can be placed on the caval sidewall beyond the tumor. This segment of caval wall can be excised with the nephrectomy specimen *en bloc*, and the cava can be oversewn with 4-0 polypropylene suture on a cardiovascular needle.

With a more extensive infra- or suprahepatic intracaval tumor, control of the vena cava must be obtained above and below the extent of the caval tumor thrombus. Often, it may be advantageous to mobilize and rotate the liver to achieve additional surgical exposure to the vena cava in the upper abdomen and lower chest. Several of these innovative descriptions of hepatic mobilization derive from liver transplantation techniques (2,3). To maximize surgical exposure, a bilateral subcostal incision is recommended that can be extended superiorly into a partial or conventional median sternotomy if additional exposure or cardiac bypass is necessary (2,3). The round ligament and the falciform ligament are ligated and divided to facilitate exposure of the coronary ligaments. The right and left coronary ligaments of the liver are incised, detaching the

liver from the diaphragm. The posterior fold between the liver and the right kidney is incised to further mobilize the right lobe of the liver. This maneuver allows the liver to rotate medially, typically providing sufficient exposure of the suprahepatic infradiaphragmatic inferior vena cava (2,3). In addition, the hepatoduodenal and hepatogastic ligaments can be incised to expose the lesser sac. One can usually appreciate a variable number of short venous branches draining the caudate lobe into the inferior vena cava. One or more of these veins may require ligation to prevent unexpected bleeding. If these veins are short, they can be controlled using suture ligatures placed into the liver parenchyma (Fig. 5–2). Often, mobilization and rotation of the liver will allow the surgeon direct access to the main hepatic vein and the porta hepatis, which may be controlled with a Rummel tourniquet (umbilical tape passed through a 16 Fr red rubber catheter) if needed. Inferiorly, a Rummel tourniquet is placed loosely below the tumor thrombus and both renal veins. For a right-sided tumor, a Rummel tourniquet is placed loosely around a segment of the left renal vein to secure control of this vessel. Cardiopulmonary bypass can be obviated when vascular control using a vascular clamp or Rummel tourniquet can be gained above the superior extent of the tumor. Division of the diaphragm may aid in gaining vascular control above the superior extent of the tumor thrombus. It must be emphasized that minimal handling of the primary tumor and intracaval neoplasm is para-

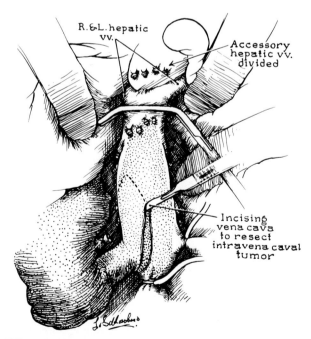

FIG. 5–2. Ligation and division of venous tributaries of the caudate lobe of the liver. (From Marshall FF, Reitz BA. Radical nephrectomy with excision of vena caval tumor thrombus. In: Marshall FF, Reitz BA, eds. *Marshall's texbook of operative urology*. Philadelphia: WB Saunders, 1996, pp. 267, with permission.)

mount to prevent inadvertent embolism. A temporary Adams–DeWeise clip can be placed above the level of the caval tumor to prevent inadvertent thromboembolism (2,3).

After adequate mobilization of the vena cava superior and inferior to the tumor thrombus with ligation of any lumbar veins, all vascular clamps or Rummel tourniquets are secured. A narrow elliptical incision circumscribing the ostium of the involved renal vein is made. If the tumor is inseparable from the caval endothelium superior to the renal veins, the involved cava is excised. The renal primary and caval tumor is removed en toto under direct vision. On occasion, we have used a dental mirror to inspect the hepatic veins or a flexible cystoscope to inspect the cava to ensure complete removal of tumor. If additional verification is necessary, transesophageal echography can be used to evaluate the superior extent of the cava or direct intraoperative sonography can be used to evaluate the extent of the cava (11).

To close the vena cava, a 4-0 or 5-0 cardiovascular polypropylene suture is used. Before completing the cavotomy closure, the inferior tourniquet is released to allow trapped air to escape through the cavotomy site. If excision of the cava decreases the vascular diameter by more than 50%, reconstruction of the vena cava is recommended to prevent caval thrombosis (Fig. 5–3). We prefer to reconstruct the vena cava using pericardium because it is less thrombogenic, although prosthetic grafts can be employed (5). Venous drainage of the right kidney must always be preserved to prevent venous infarction. In some instances, the cava has been oversewn to prevent subsequent embolism if the thrombus below

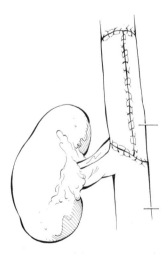

FIG. 5–3. Reconstruction of the vena cava is recommended if the cross-sectional diameter of the vena cava is reduced by mort than 50% after resection of the tumor thrombus and vena caval wall. (From Marshall FF, Dietrick DD, Baumgartner WA, Reitz BA. Surgical management of renal cell carcinoma with intracaval neoplastic extension above the hepatic veins. *J Urol* 1988;139:1166, with permission.)

the renal veins is adherent to the caval endothelium. Alternatively, an Adams–DeWeise clip can be placed on the inferior vena cava for this purpose.

Cardiopulmonary Bypass, Hypothermia, and Temporary Cardiac Arrest

Cardiopulmonary bypass, hypothermia, and temporary cardiac arrest greatly facilitate the resection of a suprahepatic caval thrombus (6). It is best to dissect as much of the kidney and the vena cava as possible prior to cardiac bypass. Following isolation of the renal tumor, the pericardium is opened and retracted with stay sutures. Typically, the right atrial appendage is cannulated with a 32 Fr venous cannula and the aorta is cannulated with a 22 Fr Bardic cannula. Heparin is then administered to maintain an activated clotting time greater than 450 seconds. The patient is placed on bypass with flow rates maintained between 2.5 and 3.5 L/minute. A core temperature of 18°C to 20°C is attained within 30 minutes while maintaining an 8°C to 10°C gradient between the perfusion and the patient's core temperature. When a rectal temperature of 20°C is reached, the aorta is cross-clamped and 500 cc of cardioplegic solution is administered. Once cardiac arrest is achieved, bypass is terminated and the patient is temporarily exsanguinated into an oxygen reservoir. The patient's brain is protected by placing ice bags around the head. At this point, there is no anesthesia, ventilation, or circulation. To reduce the incidence of complications, circulatory arrest time is best limited to 45 minutes.

An elliptical incision is made around the ostium of the renal vein and carried superiorly along the length of the vena cava. The incision can extend into the right atrium or ventricle, depending upon the superior extent of the thrombus. Using cardiopulmonary bypass and deep hypothermic circulatory arrest, the thrombus can be removed in a bloodless field and the interior of the vena cava and heart can be inspected under direct vision (Fig. 5–4). It is not uncommon to find some degree of adherence of the tumor to the endothelium. In this case, the tumor thrombus can be "endarterectomized" from the interior of the vena cava or atrium. Reconstruction of the vena cava is as previously mentioned.

Following closure of the venacavotomy, cardiopulmonary bypass is begun. The patient is slowly warmed using a 10°C gradient between the bypass machine and a warming blanket. Mannitol (12.5 g) is given along with 1 g of CaCl when core temperature reaches 25°C. Electrical defibrillation is necessary if the heart does not resume spontaneous beating. Following resumption of cardiac activity, blood is returned to the patient from the oxygen reservoir. Following the rewarming process, which can take up to 1 hour, heparin is neutralized with protamine. The patient is returned to the cardiac intensive care unit intubated.

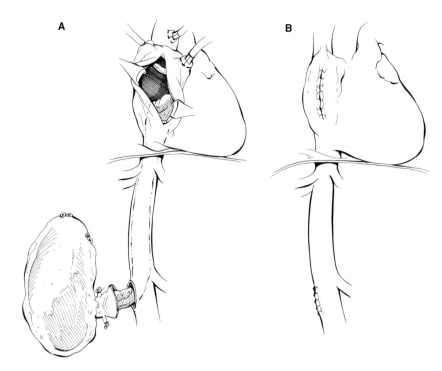

FIG. 5–4. A: The ostium of the renal vein is circumferentially incised and the right atrium is opened. **B:** Following removal of the tumor thrombus, the atriotomy and vena cavotomy incisions are closed. (From Novick AC, Montie JE. Surgery for renal cell carcinoma. In: Novick AC, Streem SB, Pontes JE, eds. *Stewart's operative urology,* vol. 1, 2nd ed. Baltimore: Williams and Wilkins, 1989, with permission.)

Recent advances in minimally invasive surgery have prompted investigators to describe alternatives to cardiopulmonary bypass with deep hypothermic cardiac arrest to minimize the risks associated with bypass and circulatory arrest and/or diminish the morbidity of the surgical incision. Venovenous bypass may be used as an alternative to cardiopulmonary bypass for patients with an infradiaphragmatic tumor and near occlusion of the vena cava who do not tolerate clamping of the vena cava (2,3). Venovenous bypass avoids the risks of cardiopulmonary bypass while ensuring adequate circulation during the venacavotomy (2,3). To establish venovenous bypass, an incision overlying the saphenofemoral junction is made and the saphenous vein is isolated. A similar incision is made in the axilla and the axillary vein is identified. The saphenous and axillary veins are incised and cannulated with a 7-mm heparinized Gott aneurysm shunt and secured with a Rummel tourniquet (2,3). Bypass is commenced with clamping of the inferior vena cava. Following completion of the procedure the shunts are removed, the axillary vein is reconstructed with 6-0 polypropylene, and the saphenous vein is ligated (2,3).

For tumors extending into the right atrium, an approach using a right parasternal incision has been described (10). This approach would enable access to the right atrium and right subclavian artery for cannulation of arterial inflow. Following isolation of the vena cava and primary renal tumor, an incision below the right clavicle is made to expose the subclavian artery. A separate incision is made from the lower segment of the third rib to the fifth rib along the right sternal border. A 3-cm segment of cartilage from the fourth and fifth ribs is resected and the right internal thoracic artery is ligated and divided. After opening the pericardium, an 8-mm collagen-coated graft is sewn to the right subclavian artery and a venous cannula is placed into the right atrium. Following cardiopulmonary bypass, circulatory arrest, tumor excision, and decannulation, a flap of periosteum, muscle, and pleura is used to close the defect associated with this minimally invasive incision (10).

OUTCOMES

Complications

Intraoperative complications include excessive bleeding and coagulopathy. Coagulopathy is more common with prolonged cardiopulmonary bypass and cardiac arrest times. Intraoperatively, red blood cells, platelets, fresh frozen plasma, and calcium chloride are routinely administered. Furosemide and/or mannitol is given if urine output remains low. Transient hypotension can occur when clamping the vena cava. This can be managed with volume expansion and is less of a problem if venous collaterals have developed with a completely occluded vena cava. Embolization of a segment of tumor thrombus can be a potentially lethal intraoperative complication and extreme care should be taken when handling the vena cava to prevent such an occurrence.

Postoperatively, several complications can occur due to the magnitude of the surgical procedure or the use of cardiopulmonary bypass. Potential complications include caval thrombosis, deep venous thrombosis, pulmonary embolus, postoperative bleeding, or coagulopathy. Patients may also develop hepatic dysfunction, renal failure, sepsis, or myocardial infarction. Although the mortality rate associated with this procedure is tolerable, most patients who die of complications within the first postoperative month succumb to multisystem organ failure.

Results

The 5-year survival rates in most reported large series vary from 14% to 68% following complete surgical removal of the renal tumor and caval extension (1,8,9). Differences in reported survival may reflect several factors, including local extension of the primary tumor, presence of lymphatic or visceral metastases, level of caval tumor extension, or invasion into the vascular wall. It is in general agreed that patients with metastatic disease and significant perinephric fat involvement tend to have a poorer prognosis. The majority of patients eventually dying of their disease succumb to metastases, which suggests that occult metastatic disease is frequently present at the time of surgery (8). Patients with good performance status who have tumors confined to the renal capsule and are without evidence of metastatic disease are ideal candidates for this surgery and have improved long-term survival.

REFERENCES

1. Glazer AA, Novick AC. Long-term follow-up after surgical treatment for renal cell carcinoma extending into the right atrium. *J Urol* 1996; 155:448.
2. Marsh CL. Application of organ transplant techniques to urologic surgery. *Urol Clin North Am* 1995;22:679–691.
3. Marsh CL, Lange PH. Application of liver transplant and organ procurement techniques to difficult upper abdominal urological cases. *J Urol* 1994;151:1652–1656.
4. Marshall FF, Dietrick DD, Baumgartner WA, Reitz BA. Surgical management of renal cell carcinoma with intracaval neoplastic extension above the hepatic veins. *J Urol* 1988;139:1166.
5. Marshall FF, Reitz BA. Supradiaphragmatic renal cell carcinoma tumor thrombus: indications for vena caval reconstruction with pericardium. *J Urol* 1985;133:266.
6. Marshall FF, Reitz BA. Technique for removal of renal cell carcinoma with suprahepatic vena caval tumor thrombus. *Urol Clin North Am* 1986;13:551–557.
7. Marshall VF, Middleton RG, Holswade GR, Goldsmith EI. Surgery for renal cell carcinoma in the vena cava. *J Urol* 1970;103:414.
8. Polascik TJ, Partin AW, Pound CR, Marshall FF. Frequent occurrence of metastatic disease in patients with renal cell carcinoma and intrahepatic or supradiaphragmatic intracaval extension treated with surgery: an outcome analysis. *Urology* 1998;52:995–999.
9. Skinner DG, Pfeister RF, Colvin R. Extension of renal cell carcinoma into the vena cava: the rationale for aggressive surgical management. *J Urol* 1972;107:711.
10. Svensson LG, Libertino J, Sorcini A, Kaushik SD, Marinko E. Minimal-access right atrial exposure for tumor extensions into the inferior vena cava. *J Thorac Cardiovasc Surg* 2001;121:589–590.
11. Treiger BFC, Humphrey LS, Peterson JCV, Oesterling JE, Mostwin JL, Reitz BA, Marshall FF. Transesophageal echocardiography in renal cell carcinoma: an accurate diagnostic technique for intracaval neoplastic extension. *J Urol* 1991;145:1138.

CHAPTER 6

Transplant Nephrectomy

Sanjaya Kumar

In the United States, renal allograft survival for all transplants is 91% at 1 year and 82% at 3 years since the introduction of cyclosporine (9,13) Notwithstanding optimal immune suppression, some allografts will fail. Failed allografts frequently result in a transplant nephrectomy in similar frequency in either cadaveric or living-related transplants. The etiology and timing of graft failure play an important role in the need for transplant nephrectomy.

DIAGNOSIS

Transplant nephrectomy is performed when the graft has failed. This may occur in the acute or chronic setting. Renal allograft rupture within days of the transplant is usually due to acute allograft rejection, renal vein thrombosis, or even acute tubular necrosis (8). Symptoms include severe allograft pain, drop in hematocrit, and hypotension. Renal scan, Doppler ultrasound, and computed tomography (CT) scan can help establish the diagnosis. Urgent transplant nephrectomy may be warranted under these circumstances.

In the chronic setting, graft function deteriorates slowly and the patient becomes azotemic and requires dialysis. Radiologic evaluation with Doppler ultrasound and renal scan are helpful. Renal biopsy is almost always performed to confirm rejection. Once it is confirmed that renal function is irreversible, immune suppression is tapered and sometimes completely withdrawn. The patient is placed on chronic dialysis and the need for graft nephrectomy is ascertained.

INDICATIONS FOR SURGERY

A renal allograft may fail for several reasons. These primarily include rejection, irreversible renal vascular compromise, or significant graft sepsis. Policy regarding graft nephrectomy varies according to the transplant institution. While most failed grafts were removed in the past, the recent trend is to remove the allograft only when necessary. Further, there is some suggestion that retaining the primary graft *in situ* may have a protective effect on the subsequent transplant (1). Over the years, the incidence of graft nephrectomy continues to trend down. The incidence varies from 4% to 8% in some recent series (5, 7,14).

Graft failure within the first few weeks following transplant is usually due to accelerated rejection or technical failure secondary to vascular compromise, and those failing within the first few months are due to irreversible acute rejection. Renal allografts rejected within the first 12 months of transplant are usually removed prophylactically regardless of the cause, even if these patients are asymptomatic (10,12,14). Significant symptoms usually develop due to the retained graft, necessitating its removal in the future. However, the policy of some centers is to remove failed transplants only when they interfere with health (7).

Graft failure that occurs 1 year after transplant is usually due to chronic rejection. Progressive withdrawal of immunosuppression may allow the patient to retain the graft in the majority (50% to 90%) of instances (4,7,10, 14). Many patients, however, will develop symptoms such as fever, malaise, gross hematuria, graft tenderness, and thrombocytopenia related to platelet consumption by the graft. It can be difficult to distinguish these symptoms from superimposed acute rejection or infection and graft nephrectomy may be the only solution. Thus, the primary indication today to remove a failed graft is graft intolerance by the host after withdrawal of immunosuppression.

Rare indications for allograft nephrectomy include the development of a renal mass (11). This may involve lesions unintentionally transmitted from the donor or lesions arising in the transplant kidney. CT scan and needle biopsy help confirm the diagnosis. Intractable urinary problems such as leaks and fistulas rarely require transplant nephrectomy today. Advances in urologic endoscopy and percutaneous techniques have virtually eliminated the need for graft nephrectomy in these patients.

ALTERNATIVE THERAPY

An alternative to graft nephrectomy is embolization of the failed allograft. The graft is embolized through femoral arterial access using coils or ethanol. The presence of multiple renal arteries is not considered a problem, although it can be technically challenging to catheterize these small arteries with thickened intimal layer and narrow ostium. Although successful embolization has been reported in 85% of patients (3), postembolization syndrome can occur in many patients including graft abscess and sepsis (6). These patients eventually require a nephrectomy. Graft embolization may thus be considered in patients with a failed renal graft and intolerable symptoms that do not improve with medical management and in whom transplant nephrectomy has a significant morbidity and risk of mortality.

SURGICAL TECHNIQUE

If available, it is important to review the previous operative notes of the transplant. This will help the surgeon understand the anatomy of the vascular anastomosis and preempt any potential catastrophe. Patients with renal failure usually have platelet dysfunction. Even though their coagulation parameters are normal, desmopressin (DDAVP) is usually given to improve platelet function. The adult dose of DDAVP is 0.3 µg/kg body weight.

The patient is placed in the supine position. An incision is made over the previous incision, which is usually is the lower quadrant (Fig. 6–1). The previous skin scar is excised. If the kidney is large and swollen, it may be necessary to extend the incision laterally. The external and internal oblique muscles and, in the lateral part of the incision, the transversalis are incised. As a result of previous surgery, rejection, or multiple renal biopsies, the kidney is stuck to the undersurface of the muscle, the pelvic side wall laterally, and the peritoneum medially. The colon may drape over the entire anterior surface of the kidney. Under these circumstances, it may be easier to extend the incision laterally and enter the retroperitoneum above the superior pole of the kidney. Once the kidney has been identified, space is created in the retroperitoneum for a self-retaining retractor (e.g., Buckwalter). The relationship of the iliac vessels, bowel, and peritoneum vis à vis the kidney is established so as not to injure them. The kidney is identified by palpation. In cases of rejection the kidney may be large, swollen, and friable.

A decision is now made on whether to perform a subcapsular nephrectomy or an extracapsular approach. Depending on the degree of reaction, one may be able to perform the entire nephrectomy staying extracapsular and removing all renal tissue. Certainly, the initial attempt can be made to perform an extracapsular nephrectomy, and as the dissection approaches the hilum or if dissection is impossible due to the inflammatory reaction resort to a subcapsular approach. Extracapsular graft nephrectomy is possible when the allograft has to be removed within a few weeks of transplant. Often, the planes of dissection may be so effaced that the only recourse may be to directly enter the renal capsule and perform a subcapsular nephrectomy from the outset. Because of the increased morbidity and mortality of the extracapsular approach, many centers routinely perform a subcapsular

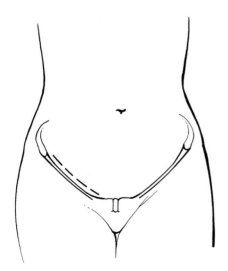

FIG. 6–1. The patient is positioned in the supine position and the incision is made over the previous lower-quadrant transplant incision.

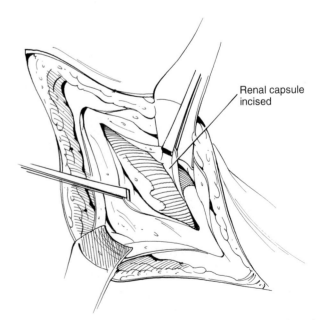

Renal capsule incised

FIG. 6–2. The incision is carried through the external and internal oblique muscles to the capsule of the kidney, where a small capsular incision is made.

proceeds toward the hilum, medially and laterally. The kidney is tethered at the hilum to the iliac vessels. Great caution is exercised here so as not to avulse the kidney. Bleeding from the cortical surface of the kidney is inevitable but can be controlled with pressure.

Once the base of the hilum is reached, the vessels are identified and ligated. This can be done entirely intracapsularly (Fig. 6–4) or extracapsularly (Fig. 6–5). The advantage of the former is that damage to the iliac vessels is minimized. One disadvantage is that donor material may be left in situ (14). To ligate the vessels outside the capsule, the reflected capsular surface is incised either posteriorly or anteriorly. The peritoneum may be adherent to the renal hilum and iliac vessels. The vessels are carefully dissected. The renal artery and vein are suture ligated individually (Fig. 6–6). It is easier to do this if the

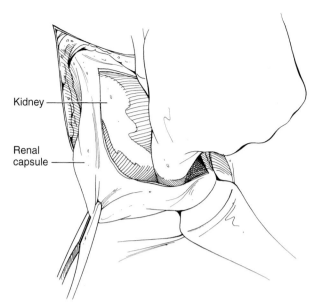

FIG. 6–3. The renal parenchyma is enucleated subcapsularly.

nephrectomy when indicated in patients with chronic rejection.

Upon identifying the kidney, the renal capsule is opened with a knife (Fig. 6–2). A plane of dissection between the renal capsule and parenchyma is developed using blunt and sharp dissection. This can usually be done bluntly with a finger (Fig. 6–3). The upper and lower poles of the kidney are mobilized, inside the capsule, and delivered into the wound. Careful dissection

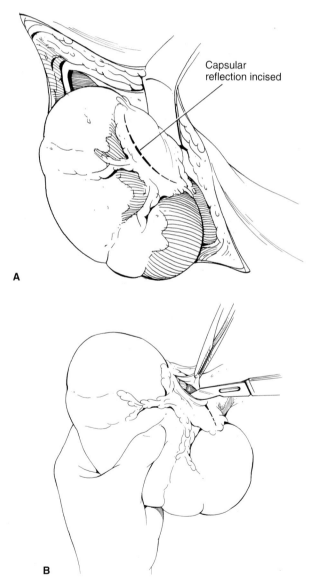

A

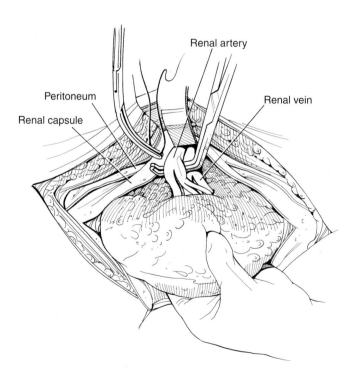

FIG. 6–4. Intracapsular ligation of renal vessels.

B

FIG. 6–5. The hilar vessels are exposed by **(A)** making an incision close to the renal parenchyma and **(B)** incising the overlying capsule.

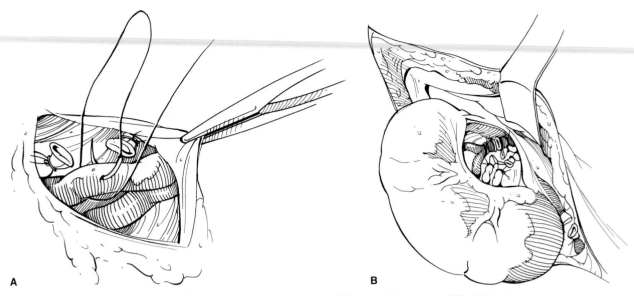

FIG. 6–6. The renal artery and vein are **(A)** suture ligated and **(B)** divided.

artery is an end-to-end hypogastric-to-renal artery anastomosis. A permanent suture such as Prolene or silk can be used for ligation. The knot is tied down to vessels. Friable vessels can tear easily. Injuries to the iliac vein can be repaired with 5-0 Prolene. While small arterial bleeding can be controlled with a fine Prolene stitch, arterial constriction must be avoided and larger defects therefore require repair with a synthetic graft (Fig. 6–7). Satinsky clamps are helpful in obtaining temporary vascular control. In the event that the hilum is plastered to the iliac vessel and the renal artery and vein are not identifiable, *en-masse* ligation of the hilum may be necessary. Satinsky clamps are placed at the base of the hilum and the kidney transected distal to the clamps. The stump is oversewn with Prolene (Fig. 6–8). When performing an

extremely difficult nephrectomy, it may be necessary to deliberately enter the peritoneum to gain proximal control of the iliac artery. The ureter is identified, dissected, and removed along with the graft. The surgeon may not be able to remove the entire ureter.

The wound is gently irrigated with antibiotic solution. Strict hemostasis is obtained and the wound is closed

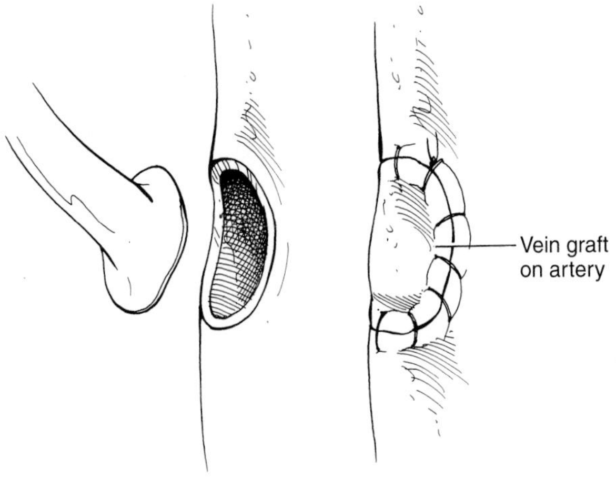

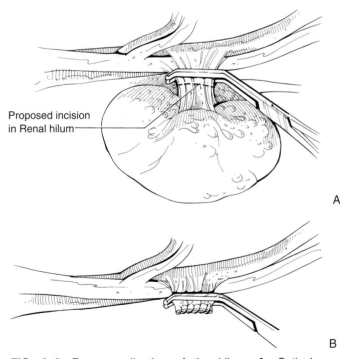

Proposed incision in Renal hilum

FIG. 6–8. *En-masse* ligation of the hilum. **A:** Satinsky clamps are placed at the base of the hilum. **B:** The kidney is transected distal to the clamps and the stump oversewn with Prolene.

Vein graft on artery

FIG. 6–7. If the renal allograft artery is completely removed, it may be necessary to cover the defect in the iliac artery with a patch graft.

without a drain. Bleeding from the capsule can be controlled with electrocautery or an argon beam coagulator. For additional security, Surgicel or Gelfoam soaked in thrombin can be placed on the surgical bed prior to closure. A drain is not used routinely because it can predispose to infection. The wound is closed in layers, if possible, with 0 Prolene. The skin is usually closed in a subcutaneous fashion.

OUTCOMES

Complications

The complication rate of transplant nephrectomy in recent series is acceptable considering the dire comorbidities in this patient population. In the past, the complication rate of transplant nephrectomy was high (24% to 60%) due to underlying uremia and immunosuppression; the mortality rate is approximately 5% (5,7). With modern immunosuppressive drugs, better control of systemic factors, and anesthetic and surgical advancements, the complication rate has been reduced considerably. The morbidity and mortality are much higher when the nephrectomy is performed under emergent circumstances. Complications usually ensue from bleeding, infection, injury to adjacent structures, and systemic causes. Today, the overall complication rate of transplant nephrectomy for chronic rejection is about 5% and mortality is less than 1% (2,10,14).

Results

Transplant nephrectomy is not necessary in all cases of transplant failure. When indicated, it can be performed successfully via an extra- or subcapsular approach. The subcapsular approach is preferred in cases of chronic rejection. Adequate preoperative patient preparation and meticulous surgical technique can minimize morbidity and mortality.

REFERENCES

1. Abouljoud MS, Deiehoi MH, Hudson SL, Diethelin AGL. Risk factors affecting second renal transplant outcome, with special reference to primary allograft nephrectomy. *Transplantation* 1995;60:138–144.
2. Bersztel A, Wahlberg J, Gannedahl G, et al. How safe is transplant nephrectomy? A retrospective study of 107 cases. *Transplant Proc* 1995;26:3461–3462.
3. Gonzalez-Satue L, Riera E, Franco E, Escalante J, et al. Percutaneous embolization of the failed renal allograft in patients with graft intolerance syndrome. *BJU Int* 2000;86:610–612.
4. Gustafsson A, Groth C, Halgrimson CG, Penn I, Starzl TE. The fate of failed renal homografts retained after retransplantation. *Surg Gynecol Obstet* 1973;137:4.
5. Koh YB, Lee IS, Moon JS, et al. Transplant nephrectomy in 927 kidney transplants. *Transplant Proc* 1996;28:1470–1476.
6. Lorenzo V, Diaz F, Perez L, et al. Ablation of irreversibly rejected renal allograft by embolization with absolute ethanol. *Am J Kidney Dis* 1993;22:592–595.
7. O'Sullivan DC, Murphy DM, McLean P, Donovan MG. Transplant nephrectomy over 20 years: Factors involved in associated morbidity and mortality. *J Urol* 1994;151;855–858.
8. Ramos M, Martins L, Henriques J, Soares J, et al. Renal allograft rupture: A clinicopathologic review. *Transplant Proc* 2000;32:2597–2598.
9. Roberts CS, Lafond J, Fitts CT, et al. New patterns of transplant nephrectomy in the cyclosporine era. *J Am Coll Surg* 1994;178:59–64.
10. Rosenthal JT, Peaster ML, Laub D. The challenge of kidney transplant nephrectomy. *J Urol* 1993;149:1395–1397.
11. Rosenthal JT. Transplant nephrectomy. In: *Glenn's urologic surgery*, 5th ed. Philadelphia: Lippincott Williams & Wilkins, 1998:79–83.
12. Sharma DK, Pandey AP, Nath V, Gopalakrishan G. Allograft nephrectomy—a 16-year experience. *Br J Urol* 1989;64;122–124.
13. United Network for Organ Sharing database. unos.org. or http://ustransplant.org/tables/K1200205-00.html.
14. Zargar MA, Kamali K. Reasons for transplant nephrectomy: A retrospective study of 60 cases. *Transplant Proc* 2001;33:2655–2656.

CHAPTER 7

Renovascular Disease

John A. Libertino

Although the true incidence of renovascular hypertension is unknown, it is estimated that between 5% and 10% of all hypertensive patients suffer from renovascular hypertension (3). During the past two decades, there have been dramatic changes in the diagnosis and treatment of renovascular hypertension. There is clearly a better understanding of the renin–angiotensin system, and newer, more potent antihypertensive medications are available. In addition, newer diagnostic radiological procedures, such as digital subtraction angiography, captopril renal scans, 3-dimensional CT scans, and balloon angioplasty, and newer surgical techniques have dramatically changed the ways in which we diagnose and treat renovascular hypertension today.

DIAGNOSIS

In the past, the clinician's task of identifying potentially curable patients in a safe, cost-effective, and reliable manner was difficult. A single-dose captopril test is reported by some investigators to be a reliable screening test and is well suited for outpatient use. In patients with a functional renal artery stenosis, angiontensin converting enzyme (ACE) inhibitors lead to a disproportionate increase in peripheral plasma renin activity although it is less reliable in patients with a degree of renal insufficiency and the test cannot be used reliably as an indicator of renal artery stenosis (1). Another test that has recently been analyzed for the detection of renal artery stenosis is the renal scintigram with isotopic nephrography following the administration of captopril (6). Using technetium DTPA (pentetic acid) scintography the sensitivity varies from 71% to 92% with a specificity of 72% to 97%. In the hipuran scintigram, the patient with renal artery stenosis showed a continual enrichment of the isotope in the renal cortex, probably related to a decreased excretion of hipuran because of the ACE inhibitor.

Digital venous subtraction angiography (DSA) remains the most definitive and reliable screening test available. It has a sensitivity and specificity of nearly 90%. Intravenous DSA is susceptible to artifacts such as crossing vessels and from intestinal motility. In these patients, digital arterial subtraction angiography achieves an excellent view of the renal circulation using less contrast dye than conventional angiography. Newer modalities include duplex Doppler ultrasound scanning and DSA in conjunction with divided renal vein renin assays, which may demonstrate contralateral suppression and remains the best screening test and predictor of treatment outcome. In those patients who have azotemia, in whom contrast is contraindicated, magnetic resonance imaging (MRI) angiography and CO_2 DSA are useful.

INDICATIONS FOR SURGERY

The surgical management of renovascular hypertension has changed dramatically in the last two decades. In the early 1970s, it was demonstrated that renal function could be preserved or restored by renal revascularization of nonfunctioning kidneys with totally occluded renal arteries. Progressive azotemia in the elderly atherosclerotic patient population is now one of the indications for renal revascularization (4).

Second, the use of alternative bypass procedures has significantly reduced the morbidity and mortality of high-risk patients undergoing renovascular surgery. The use of the hepatic artery, the gastroduodenal artery, and other alternative procedures instead of the aortorenal saphenous vein bypass graft has not only reduced the morbidity and mortality of surgery but, in doing so, has dramatically changed the nature of our patient population. Use of the thoracic aorta may also be a viable alternative on the left side because the thoracic aorta is usually less atherosclerotic than the abdominal aorta (3).

ALTERNATIVE THERAPY

Converting enzyme inhibitors prevent the conversion of angiotensin I to angiotensin II. These drugs in conjunction with calcium channel blockers have greatly improved the medical management of patients who suffer from renovascular hypertension. Unfortunately, even if adequate blood pressure control is maintained by pharmacological means progression of renal artery disease is not prevented and renal ischemia and renal damage may clearly progress (8).

When medical management fails or azotemia progresses, balloon angioplasty and surgical treatment must be considered (5). The choice between angioplasty and surgery relies on a well-defined set of criteria established by published results. Angioplasty is indicated in the treatment of fibrous dysplasia and atherosclerosis of the mid-main renal artery. Surgery is indicated for the treatment of osteal atherosclerosis and for branch lesions of the renal artery. Renal artery aneurysms are a different problem. Surgery is indicated when they are the cause of hypertension. Also, aneurysms larger than 2 cm in diameter that are noncalcified, especially in gestational women, should be repaired as they are prone to rupture during pregnancy. Patients who develop recurrent disease following balloon angioplasty are probably best subjected to surgical management, as repeat balloon angioplasty is associated with a significant complication rate.

SURGICAL TECHNIQUE

Aortorenal Bypass Graft

Bypass grafts are in particular suitable for fibrous lesions that affect long and multiple segments of the renal artery and its branches (Fig. 7–1). Dacron, autogenous artery (hypogastric and splenic), and autogenous saphenous vein may be chosen as aortorenal bypass grafts in properly selected patients. Dacron has been applied extensively in renal artery reconstruction but has been associated with a relatively high rate of early thrombosis. Excellent long-term patency rates have been reported with a segment of autogenous hypogastric artery, which matches the size of the renal artery and is sutured more simply than the Dacron prosthesis. Autogenous hypogastric artery is the most favorable graft material for children with renal artery disease but is often the first to be involved with generalized atherosclerosis and therefore is not suitable graft material in older patients. The autologous saphenous vein has emerged as our preferred graft material and is the most common source for restoration of

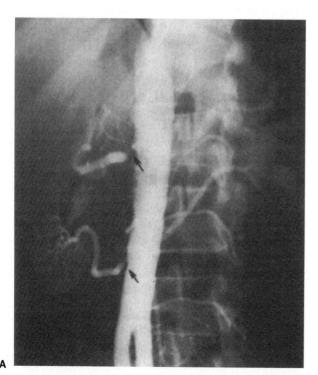

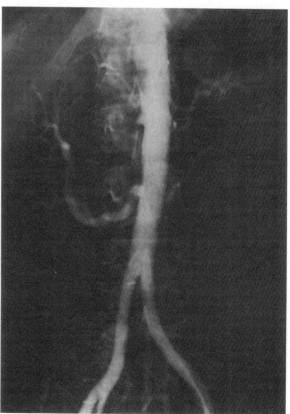

FIG. 7–1. A: An aortogram shows a double right renal artery with stenoses at the ostia of both trunks. **B:** A postoperative aortogram with the vein graft making a side-to-side anastomosis to the stenotic lower renal artery and an end-to-end anastomosis to the distal stump of the upper renal artery.

renal blood flow at our hospital. Saphenous vein is readily available, closer in size to the renal artery, and accommodates the creation of a precise contoured anastomosis with a delicate thin-walled distal renal artery and its intima is less thrombogenic than prosthetic material.

Procurement of Saphenous Vein

The saphenous vein is usually obtained from the thigh opposite the renal lesion so that two surgeons may simultaneously expose the renal vessels and mobilize the graft, shortening the operative time. The vein is mobilized through a single long incision in the upper thigh (Fig. 7–2), which begins parallel to and below the groin crease over the palpable femoral pulses and is extended toward the knee after the junction of the saphenous and femoral veins has been exposed. The incision should be made directly over the vein to avoid producing devascularized skin flaps that can result in necrotic edges and wound sepsis. Finger dissection between the trunk of the vein and the skin is helpful to ensure accurate placement of the incision and, thus, avoid development of devascularization of these flaps (see Fig. 7–2). On the day before operation, the course of the saphenous vein is outlined with an indelible pen while the patient is standing.

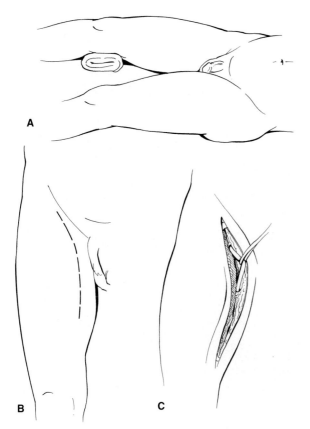

FIG. 7–2. A: Position of patient for harvesting of saphenous vein graft. **B:** Line of incision for saphenous vein graft harvest. **C:** Exposure of saphenous vein.

A 20-cm-long vein graft with an outside diameter of 4 to 6 mm is usually adequate for reconstruction of the renal artery. Excess vein should always be available for revision of any intraoperative technical problems that may occur during anastomosis. The vein is handled gently without stretching or tearing its branches. The tributaries are tied in continuity with fine silk before they are divided. The areolar tissue is dissected from the specimen, and the adventitia is left undisturbed.

To decrease transmural ischemia, the vein graft remains *in situ* until the renal vessels are mobilized and it is ready to be used. If the graft is inadvertently removed prematurely, it is placed in cold Ringer's lactate solution or autologous blood, even if only a short period of time will ensue. The distal end of the vein is transected, cannulated with a Marks needle, and secured with a silk tie (Fig. 7–3). A dilute heparinized solution of autologous blood distends the vein graft before the proximal is transected. This step helps identify any untied tributaries or unrecognized leakage and washes out any residual blood clots. The vein is distended to a minimal diameter of 5 to 6 mm by exerting gentle pressure on the syringe. The proximal end of the vein is transected, and the vein graft is now ready for use. The thigh incision is not closed until the bypass procedure has been completed to ensure that any delayed bleeding caused by the heparinized state is identified and controlled.

Insertion of Saphenous Vein Graft

Heparin is initially given systemically after the surgical dissection has been completed and approximately 30 minutes before the arteries are clamped. The saphenous vein graft should be oriented properly to avoid misalignment during implantation. Either an end-to-end or an end-to-side anastomosis can be accomplished, depending on the anatomic situation encountered. An end-to-end anastomosis is preferred under usual circumstances because it permits the best laminar flow.

The aorta, which has already been mobilized and exposed from the renal arteries to the level of the inferior mesenteric artery, is carefully palpated to determine a suitable soft location for the anastomosis that is relatively free of atherosclerotic plaque. A medium-sized DeBakey clamp is placed on the anterolateral portion of the infrarenal aorta in a tangential manner. A vertical 13- to 16-mm aortotomy is made without excising any of the aortic wall or attempting to perform a localized endarterectomy (Fig. 7–4), which may dislodge intimal plaque fragments that can form emboli to the lower extremities when the clamp is released.

Excision of the aortic wall is not necessary because intraluminal aortic pressure spreads the edge of the linear aortotomy to the appropriate dimensions when the clamp is released. The vein graft is anastomosed to the aorta with continuous 5-0 Prolene suture after it has been satisfactorily spatulated (Fig. 7–5). A microvascular Schwartz

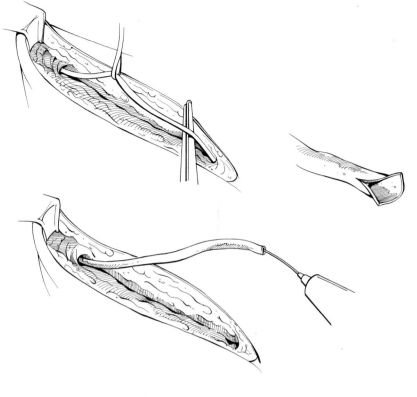

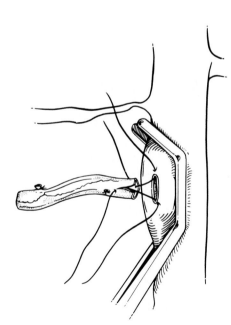

FIG. 7–3. Harvest of saphenous vein graft.

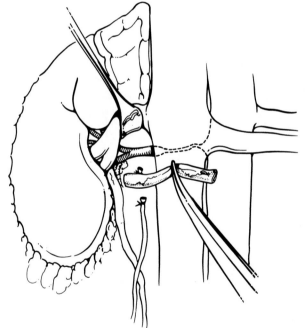

FIG. 7–4. The bypass graft is placed along the lateral aortic wall to determine the best position for its placement. (From Novick AC, Streem SB, Pontes JE, eds. *Stewart's operative urology*. Baltimore: Williams & Wilkins, 1989, with permission.)

FIG. 7–5. Following partial aortic occlusion, an oval aortotomy is made for end-to-side anastomosis with the spatulated bypass graft. (From Novick AC, Streem SB, Pontes JE, eds. *Stewart's operative urology*. Baltimore: Williams & Wilkins, 1989, with permission.)

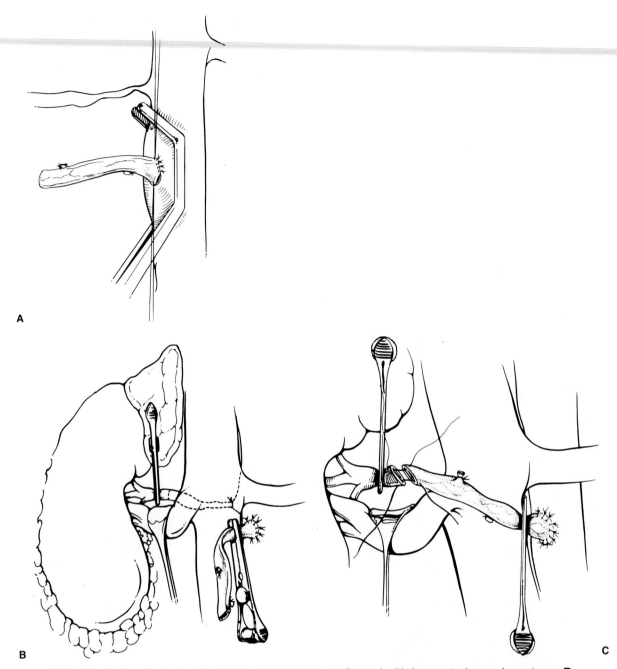

FIG. 7–6. A: Anastomosis of the graft to the aorta is performed with interrupted vascular sutures. **B:** After completion of the aortic anastomosis, the renal artery is prepared for anastomosis with the graft. **C:** A spatulated end-to-end anastomosis of the graft and distal renal artery is performed. (From Novic AC, Streem SB, Pontes JE, eds. *Stewart's operative urology*. Baltimore: Williams & Wilkins, 1989, with permission.)

clamp is placed on the end of the saphenous vein graft and the aortic clamp is released. The graft is allowed to lie anterior to the vena cava on the right side or anterior to the renal vein on the left side. Although it is preferable to leave the vein too long than too short, it should not be so long as to bend into an acute angle at any point. The renal artery is secured distally with a smooth-jawed Schwartz microvascular clamp placed on either the distal main renal artery or its branches. The proper site for the arterial anastomosis is selected. An end-to-end anastomosis is performed utilizing a continuous 6-0 Prolene suture or interrupted sutures of the same material, depending on the diameter of the anastomosis (Fig. 7–6). When the saphenous vein graft is being anastomosed with two branches 3 mm or less in size, interrupted sutures are chosen. An interrupted suture line is also selected in children to prevent a pursestring effect with growth of the vessels when the patients become older. This effect may also occur with running synthetic monofilament sutures when too much tension is applied during the creation of the anastomosis. The pursestring effect can be avoided by placing sutures at four quadrants in the arterial wall before beginning the anastomosis. Operating loupe magnification and fiberoptic headlamps are helpful at this point in the operation to allow precise placement of the sutures, in particular when exposure in the renal artery is difficult.

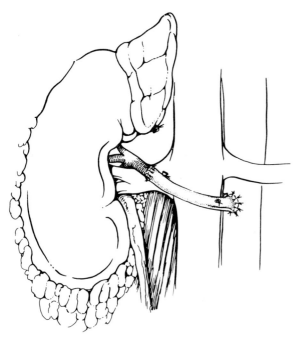

FIG. 7–7. Completed aortorenal bypass operation. (From Novic AC, Streem SB, Pontes JE, eds. *Stewart's operative urology.* Baltimore: Williams & Wilkins, 1989, with permission.)

The single most important factor responsible for long-term patency is a wide flawless anastomosis with the renal artery. After completion of the anastomosis, the microvascular bulldog clamps are removed from the distal renal circulation and the saphenous vein graft, permitting reconstitution of the renal circulation (Fig. 7–7).

Splenorenal Artery Bypass

Splenorenal arterial bypass is in particular suitable for patients who have diffuse atherosclerotic disease or thrombosis of the aortic lumen and for those who have previously undergone difficult aortic reconstructions. Carefully monitored oblique and lateral angiography of the celiac axis is required to determine the patency of this artery because atherosclerosis can affect the arterial lumen early in the patient's life. Surgical exploration and intraoperative evaluation by palpation and measurement of splenic blood flow are also helpful in establishing its suitability for renal revascularization. If the blood flow is less than 125 mL/minute, the splenic artery should probably not be utilized for renal artery bypass.

The splenic artery is exposed through a supracostal eleventh-rib flank incision (Fig. 7–8). The dissection is continued along the upper border of the rib. The overlying latissimus dorsi, the serratus posterior inferior, and the intercostal muscles are divided. Division of the intercostal ligament permits the rib to move freely. The external, internal oblique, and transversus abdominis muscles are divided, and the intercostal muscle attachments on the distal 1 in. of the rib are divided carefully until the corresponding intercostal nerve is identified. The investing fascia around the nerve is entered. Dissection in this plane allows an extrapleural approach and in general avoids entry into the pleural cavity. This approach also allows excellent exposure as the ribs are free to pivot downward in a "bucket-handle" fashion.

The plane between Gerota's fascia and the adrenal gland posteriorly and the pancreas anteriorly is entered. The splenic artery is identified at the upper border of the pancreas. Its enveloping fascia is entered, and the splenic artery is mobilized by a purely retroperitoneal approach. Several small pancreatic branches are identified, isolated, ligated, and divided. The splenic artery can usually be mobilized from the splenic hilum to the celiac axis without difficulty, and it provides sufficient length to reach the left renal artery.

After the splenic artery is mobilized, a sponge soaked with papaverine is placed on it to permit it to dilate. The artery is divided just proximal to its primary bifurcation in the hilum of the spleen after a suitable vascular clamp has been applied to the origin of the artery. If necessary,

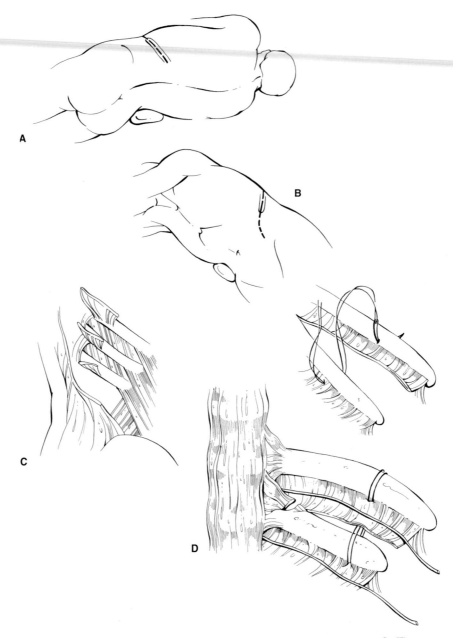

FIG. 7–8. Supracostal eleventh-rib incision. **A:** Posterior view. **B:** Anterior view. **C:** The costovertebral ligament must be divided to allow the rib to pivot inferiorly. **D:** Closure of incision, taking care to spare the intercostal nerves. The diaphragm is not incorporated in the closure.

the artery may be dilated with a Gruntzig balloon or Fogarty catheter intraoperatively to obtain maximum caliber. Removal of the spleen is not necessary because it continues to receive adequate blood flow from the short gastric arteries. The left kidney is approached posteriorly, and the left renal artery is identified and mobilized (Fig. 7–9).

The renal artery is ligated at the aorta, and an end-to-end anastomosis between the splenic artery and the distal renal artery is carried out using continuous or interrupted 6-0 Prolene sutures (Fig. 7–9). We have employed this approach in nearly 100 patients and now prefer it to the traditional transabdominal technique.

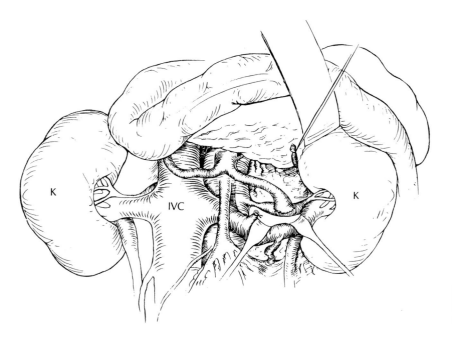

FIG. 7–9. Technique of splenorenal bypass. Note that the pancreas is lifted cephalad to expose the splenic artery.

On rare occasions, a sufficient length of splenic artery cannot be achieved. In this instance, an interposition saphenous vein graft from the splenic artery to the renal artery can be utilized. This maneuver enables the creation of a tension-free anastomosis (Fig. 7–10).

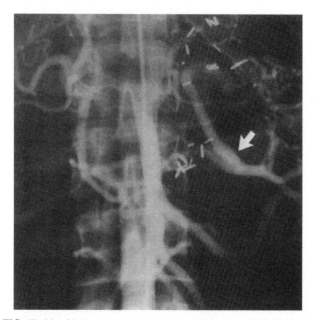

FIG. 7–10. An aortogram shows a splenorenal end-to-side bypass.

Hepatorenal Bypass Graft

Arising from the celiac axis and continuing along the upper border of the pancreas, the hepatic artery reaches the portal vein and divides into an ascending and a descending limb. The ascending limb is a continuation of the main hepatic artery upward within the lesser omentum; it lies in front of the portal vein and to the left of the biliary tree. The descending limb forms the gastroduodenal artery. In the porta hepatis, the hepatic artery ends by dividing into the right and left hepatic branches, which supply the corresponding lobes of the liver (Fig. 7–11). There are significant anatomic variations in the hepatic circulation, with the right hepatic artery being more variable than the left. Careful dissection of the porta hepatis is essential, and the common hepatic, gastroduodenal, and right and left hepatic arteries should be identified before an anastomotic procedure is attempted. Vascular elastic loops are placed about these vessels, and the common bile duct and portal vein are identified.

After careful dissection and mobilization of the renal artery, clamps are placed on the proximal portion of the common hepatic artery and its distal branches. The gastroduodenal artery is divided (Fig. 7–12). The inferior surface of the hepatic artery is mobilized from the underlying portal vein and the common bile duct. An arteriotomy, 10 to 12 mm in length, is made in the anterior inferior wall of the common hepatic artery, beginning at the ostium of the gastroduodenal artery. A reversed autogenous saphenous vein is inserted with an end-to-side anastomosis between the vein graft and the hepatic artery. This maneuver is usu-

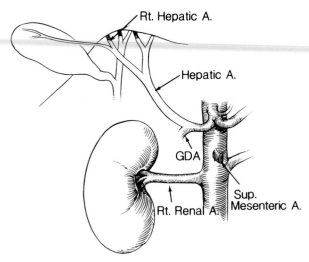

FIG. 7–11. Normal course of the main hepatic artery and its various branches. (From Novick AC. Diminished operative risk and improved results following revascularization for atherosclerotic renal artery disease. *Urol Clin North Am* 1984; 11:435, with permission.)

ally accomplished with a continuous 6-0 Prolene suture. A microvascular clamp is placed on the vein graft after it has been filled with heparin and after the proper alignment and length for the renal artery anastomosis has been determined. The clamps are removed from the hepatic circulation, and a small Schwartz microvascular clamp is placed on the distal renal artery. The vein graft is anastomosed to the right renal artery in an end-to-end fashion. When the gastroduodenal artery is used, it is divided, and an end-to-end anastomosis between the gastroduodenal artery and the renal artery is accomplished (Fig. 7–13).

We have also utilized the superior mesenteric-to-renal artery saphenous vein bypass as a "bailout procedure" as well with good results An iliac-to-renal bypass graft has been done as an alternative to the aortorenal bypass procedure in ten of our patients, again with favorable results (Fig. 7–14).

Renal Autotransplantation and *Ex Vivo* Bench Surgery

On rare occasions, kidneys with lesions of the renal artery or its branches are not amenable to *in situ* reconstruction. In these circumstances, temporary removal of the kidney, *ex vivo* preservation, microvascular repair (bench surgery), and autotransplantation may permit salvage. Autotransplantation and *ex vivo* repair should be considered in patients with traumatic arterial injuries, when disease of the major vessels extends beyond the bifurcation of the main renal artery into the segmental branches, and when multiple vessels supplying the

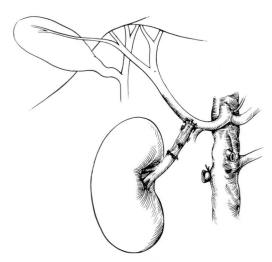

FIG. 7–12. Hepatorenal bypass performed with an interposition saphenous vein graft anastomosed end to side to the common hepatic artery and end to end to the right renal artery. (From Novick AC. Diminished operative risk and improved results following revascularization for atherosclerotic renal artery disease. *Urol Clin North Am* 1984;11:435, with permission.)

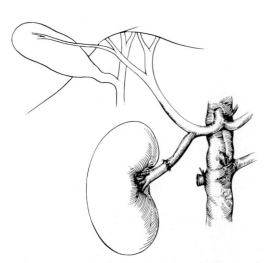

FIG. 7–13. Use of the gastroduodenal artery to perform hepatorenal revascularization through direct end-to-end anastomosis with the right renal artery. (From Novick AC, Streem SB, Pontes JE, eds. *Stewart's Operative Urology*. Baltimore: Williams & Wilkins, 1989, with permission.)

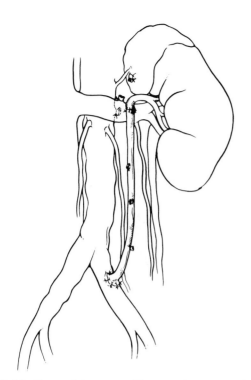

FIG. 7–14. Iliorenal bypass with a saphenous vein graft anastomosed end to side to the common iliac artery and end to end to the renal artery. (From Novick AC, Streem SB, Pontes JE, eds. *Stewart's operative urology.* Baltimore: Williams & Wilkins, 1989, with permission.)

affected kidney are involved. Bench surgery may also be required in patients who have large aneurysms, arteriovenous fistulas, dissecting aneurysms, or malformations (Fig. 7–15). Other indications for autotransplantation that usually do not require *ex vivo* repair include abdominal aortic aneurysms that involve the origin of the renal arteries and extensive atheromatous aortic disease, when an operation on the aorta itself may prove hazardous.

OUTCOMES

Complications

Complications of renal vascular surgery can be classified as early or delayed. Early complications include bleeding, thrombosis of the artery, embolization of the branch vessels, subintimal dissection, false aneurysms, and loss of the kidney. Postoperative bleeding requiring operative intervention is to some extent a technical failure but may also be a function of the structural integrity of the arterial wall in diseased segments. It is important to recognize the enlarged perihilar vessels that are seen in high-grade stenosis and be cognizant of the adrenal venous channels. Delayed bleeding may be the result of

false aneurysm formation or erosion of the graft anastomosis into the duodenum or other bowel.

Renal artery thrombosis is the most common complication of renal vascular reconstruction and is most common after either placement of a Dacron graft or endarterectomy. Predisposing factors include small Dacron grafts, renal atrophy associated with thin-walled diseased arteries and high intrarenal vascular resistance, hypotension, or hypovolemia. It has been shown that the thrombosis of both venous and synthetic grafts is partially affected by the adequacy of the peripheral runoff as well as the adequacy of resection of the endothelial plaques in atherosclerotic vessels. Embolization of plaque to the distal extremities or aortic thrombosis is rare.

Results

Balloon angioplasty is primarily used to treat patients with mural dysplasia (2,7). This modality of treatment is 80% to 85% effective in the management of these patients at our institution. Balloon angioplasty has a limited role in the management of atherosclerotic renovascular disease at our institution.

A combination of balloon angioplasty for younger, healthier patients suffering from mural dysplasia, the advent of alternative bypass procedures, and the concept of revascularization for preservation and restoration of renal function have dramatically changed the nature of the patient population being referred to our institution for renal revascularization. Most revascularizations are in elderly, higher-risk patients with diffuse atherosclerosis who have failed aggressive antihypertensive therapy to improve their renal function. We recently reported a series of more than 100 patients who have undergone renal revascularization for preservation and restoration of renal function with an 85% success rate in this high-risk patient population (4).

We recently reviewed the long-term results of patients with renal artery atherosclerotic ostial disease treated with combined percutaneous transluminal renal angioplasty (PTA) and stent placement. The mean follow-up was 40 months with a range of 14 to 66 months. Fifty-five patients were studied: 20 males and 35 females. The mean age was 56.2 years. There were 40 unilateral and 15 bilateral lesions resulting in 70 PTA and stent placements. Our short-term results (6 to 12 months) with PTA and stents were similar to the literature and were encouraging and received with enthusiasm. The long-term results revealed that 31% of patients had an improvement in blood pressure and 38% had improvement in renal function. Disturbingly, 44% of patients had failure to improve hypertension and 44% of patients failed to improve their renal function. Six of 55 patients (11%) developed chronic renal failure requiring hemodialysis.

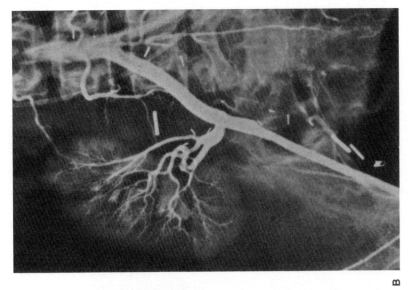

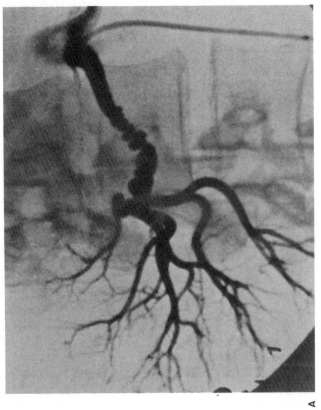

FIG. 7–15. **A:** An arteriogram shows complex involvement of the right renal artery by disease extending into the primary branches. **B:** A postoperative arteriogram shows patent anastomoses.

REFERENCES

1. Distler A, Spies KP. Diagnostic procedures in renovascular hypertension. *Clin Nephrol* 1991;36(4):174–180.
2. Englund R, Brown MA. Renal angioplasty for renovascular disease. *J Cardiovasc Surg* 1991;32:76–80.
3. Libertino JA. Surgery for renovascular hypertension. In: Walsh PC, Retik AB, Stamey TA, Vaughan ED Jr, eds. *Campbell's urology*, 6th ed. Philadelphia: WB Saunders, 1992:2521–2551.
4. Libertino JA, Bosco PJ, Ying C, et al. Renal revascularization to restore and preserve renal function. *J Urol* 1992;147:1485–1487.
5. Postma CT, van Oijen HA, Barentsz JO, et al. The value of tests predicting renovascular hypertension in patients with renal artery stenosis treated by angioplasty. *Arch Intern Med* 1991;151:1531–1535.
6. Setaro JF, Saddler MC, Chen CC, et al. Simplified captopril renography in diagnosis and treatment of renal artery stenosis. *Hypertension* 1991; 18:289–298.
7. Tegtmeyer CJ, Selby JB, Hartwell GD, et al. Results and complications of angioplasty in fibromuscular disease. *Circulation* 1991;83[Suppl 2]:1155–1161.
8. Tollefson DF, Ernst CB. Natural history of atherosclerotic renal artery stenosis associated with aortic disease. *J Vasc Surg* 1991;14:327–331.

CHAPTER 8

Anatrophic Nephrolithotomy

Elizabeth J. Anoia, Michael L. Paik, and Martin I. Resnick

The treatment of nephrolithiasis has undergone a rapid evolution over the past 25 years. The introduction and refinement of extracorporeal, endourologic, and percutaneous techniques have caused a shift in the first-line management of even complex renal stones. Anatrophic nephrolithotomy is a procedure that has been used by urologists for more than 30 years in the removal of staghorn renal calculi. The original description of anatrophic nephrolithotomy was by Smith and Boyce in 1968 (14). The operation they described was based on the principle of placing the nephrotomy incision through a plane of the kidney that was relatively avascular. This approach would avoid damage to the renal vasculature and subsequent atrophy of the renal parenchyma, hence the term *anatrophic.* Staghorn stones are often associated with urinary tract infections, and the coexistence of these two conditions makes it difficult to eradicate either. Definitive treatment of these stones is generally advocated because of the significant morbidity and mortality associated with untreated staghorn calculi. Blandy and Singh found that patient survival is reduced with untreated staghorn calculi, with a mortality rate of 28% at 10 years (3).

Anatrophic nephrolithotomy also involves reconstruction of the intrarenal collecting system to eliminate anatomic obstruction. Thus, this procedure would improve urinary drainage, thereby reducing the likelihood of urinary tract infection, which would prevent recurrent stone formation. Over the past 25 years, with the development of less invasive approaches such as extracorporeal shock wave lithotripsy (ESWL), percutaneous nephrolithotomy (PCNL), and ureteroscopic surgery, the role of anatrophic nephrolithotomy and other open stone operations has certainly diminished (2). The American Urologic Association Nephrolithiasis Clinical Guidelines Panel in 1994 recommended a percutaneous procedure with or without ESWL as an initial treatment for complex staghorn calculi. However, in specific situa-

tions anatrophic nephrolithotomy remains the best treatment option for renal calculi and thus has maintained an important, albeit smaller, role in the treatment of these large, complex stones.

DIAGNOSIS

Diagnosing nephrolithiasis is based on the patient's history, physical exam, urinalysis (UA) findings, and radiographic studies. Patients may have the typical symptoms of flank pain, fever, hematuria, and dysuria or they may be asymptomatic. Physical exam may reveal costovertebral angle tenderness. The UA may show erythrocytes, leucocytes, and nitrites or bacteria if the stone is associated with an infection. The diagnosis of chronic urinary tract infection is common in patients with staghorn stones. Urine culture is often positive, and typical organisms include urea-splitting organisms such as *Proteus, Klebsiella, Providencia,* and *Pseudomonas.*

Common radiographic studies by tradition obtained include plain abdominal radiographs, nephrotomograms, and excretory urograms to identify the stones and the collecting system and, if present, define the degree of obstruction. Retrograde pyelography is usually performed in cases of equivocal findings on excretory urography. Recently, helical nonenhanced computed tomography scanning with thin cuts of the kidneys, ureters, and bladder has become the gold standard for identifying urinary tract stones and radiolucent or poorly calcified stones. Nuclear renal scans can help determine differential renal function when such information might affect the surgical approach. Renal arteriography is usually not indicated unless there is suspicion of anomalous arterial anatomy, such as in renal fusion anomalies.

Before elective surgery, a metabolic evaluation is recommended to attempt to determine an etiology for stone formation and aid in preventing a recurrence. For instance, it is important to determine the presence of hypercalciuria, hyperuricosuria, hyperoxaluria, cystinuria, hyperparathyroidism, and renal tubular acidosis in multiple urine specimens. The measurement of serum and urine calcium, phosphorus, creatinine, uric acid, and electrolytes should be routine. A 24-hour urine collection for creatinine clearance as well as urinary calcium, phosphorus, oxalate, citrate, cystine, and uric acid is also an integral part of the workup (9).

INDICATIONS FOR SURGERY

The indications for anatrophic nephrolithotomy have changed somewhat with advances in minimally invasive methods of treating stones. However, the inability to successfully eradicate a stone with less invasive methods remains an important indication for open stone surgery. Other relative indications include select cases of complex stone disease, especially those with a dilated collecting system, stones associated with urologic anatomic abnormalities, previous renal surgery, certain features of patient anatomy, comorbid disease, and patient preference (7,8). Specific urinary tract abnormalities account for up to 24% of open stone surgeries. These include a ureteropelvic junction (UPJ) obstruction, infundibular stenosis, calyceal diverticula, ureteral stricture, or presence of a crossing vessel. By approaching these situations open, the defect can be corrected simultaneously. Patient features such as morbid obesity, limb contractures, or certain cases of transplanted kidneys may preclude proper positioning for endourologic procedures, ESWL, or percutaneous access (4). The presence of significant comorbid disease and patient preference must each be considered in choosing the best individualized treatment option.

Overall, the goals of open stone surgery should be to remove all calculi and fragments, improve urinary drainage of any obstructed intrarenal collecting system, eradicate infection, preserve and improve renal function, and prevent stone recurrence (15).

ALTERNATIVE THERAPY

As open stone surgery accounts for less than 5% of treatment modalities for staghorn and other complex stones, there are now other less invasive techniques either alone or in combination that have replaced this procedure. Most staghorn calculi can now be preferentially treated with percutaneous nephrolithotomy, with or without ESWL. The stone-free rates reported vary between 50% to 87%, whereas for anatrophic nephrolithotomy stone-free rates range from 90% to 100% (7). The advantage of the former is shorter convalescent periods; the disadvantage is the possibility of requiring multiple different procedures to accomplish a stone-free state. Endoscopic therapy with holmium:YAG laser lithotripsy is reported to have an overall stone-free

rate of 95% (10). ESWL monotherapy was found to have a 61% stone-free rate less than 10 years after its development (8). Despite impressive advances with the less invasive techniques, anatrophic nephrolithotomy remains a viable treatment option for large staghorn calculi not expected to be eliminated with a reasonable number of less invasive procedures or staghorn stones associated with anatomic abnormalities requiring open surgical correction (13).

SURGICAL TECHNIQUE

After administration of appropriate preoperative intravenous (IV) antibiotics and induction of general anesthesia, a Foley catheter is placed. The patient is then placed in the standard flank position with elevation of the kidney rest and flexion of the operating table to achieve adequate spacing between the lower costal margin and the iliac crest. Three-inch-wide adhesive tape applied at the shoulders and hips can be used to secure the patient to the table. Adequate padding should be used to protect pressure points.

A standard flank approach is used. The incision can be placed through the bed of either the eleventh or twelfth rib, depending on the estimated position of the kidney. If a previous flank incision has been made for renal surgery, it is preferable to place the incision above the old scar, ensuring that access to the kidney can be achieved through unscarred tissue. After rib resection, when access has been gained into the retroperitoneal space, Gerota's fascia is identified overlying the kidney. Gerota's fascia is incised in a cephalad–caudal direction, which facilitates returning the kidney to its fatty pouch at the end of the operation. The kidney is then fully mobilized, and the perinephric fat is carefully dissected off the renal capsule with care taken not to disrupt the capsule. Should the capsule become inadvertently incised, it can be closed at that time with chromic catgut sutures. The kidney is now free to be suspended in the operative field by utilizing a broad tape at each pole. At this point a preliminary portable plain radiograph can be obtained.

Next is the renal hilar dissection. The main renal artery and the posterior segmental branch are approached posteriorly, carefully identified, and dissected (Fig. 8–1A). The renal pelvis and ureter should be identified but not dissected. The avascular plane, or Brödel's line, can be identified by temporarily clamping the posterior segmental artery and injecting 20 mL of methylene blue intravenously. This results in the blanching of the posterior renal segment while the anterior portion turns blue, allowing identification and marking of the avascular plane (Fig. 8–1B) (6). Placing the nephrotomy incision through this plane will achieve maximal renal parenchymal preservation and minimize blood loss. The avascular plane can also be identified with the use of a Doppler

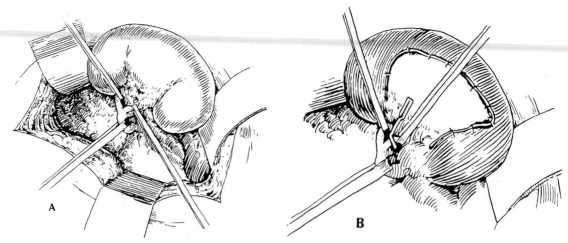

FIG. 8–1. Anatrophic nephrolithotomy. **A:** Main renal artery and branches are isolated. **B:** The posterior segmental artery is occluded and methylene blue is administered intravenously. The resulting demarcation between pale ischemic and bluish perfused parenchyma defines a relatively avascular nephrotomy plane.

stethoscope to localize the area of the kidney with minimal blood flow.

More extensive renal hilar dissection can be avoided by utilizing a modification of the original procedure described by Smith and Boyce (14). Redman and associates relied on the relatively constant segmental renal vascular supply in the identification of Brödel's line. They advocated placing the incision at the expected location of the avascular plane after clamping the renal pedicle with a Satinsky clamp in an effort to prevent vasospasm of the renal artery and warm ischemia (11). This modification can be time saving and spare extensive dissection of the renal hilum. However, we continue to advocate precise identification of the avascular plane to minimize parenchymal loss.

At this point, 25 g of IV mannitol is administered. This will promote a postischemic diuresis and prevent the formation of intratubular ice crystals by increasing the osmolarity of the glomerular filtrate. The main renal artery can now be occluded with an atraumatic bulldog vascular clamp (Fig. 8–2). A bowel bag or barrier drape is quickly placed around the kidney, and it is insulated from the body wall and peritoneal contents with dry gauze packs. Hypothermia is then initiated with iced saline slush covering the kidney. The kidney should be cooled for 10 to 15 minutes before the nephrotomy incision is made. This should allow achievement of a core renal temperature of 15°C to 20°C, which will allow safe ischemic times from 60 to 75 minutes and minimize renal parenchymal damage (5). The ice slush should be continuously reapplied as needed throughout the case.

The renal capsule is then incised sharply over the previously identified line, being careful to avoid extension into the upper and lower poles (Fig. 8–3). The renal

parenchyma can be bluntly dissected with the back of the scalpel handle. Blunt dissection minimizes injury to the intrarenal arteries that are traversed (Fig. 8–4). Small bleeding vessels can be controlled with 4-0 or 5-0 chromic catgut figure-of-eight suture ligatures. If renal backbleeding continues to be a problem despite these measures, the main renal vein can be occluded.

As the nephrotomy incision proceeds toward the renal hilum, the ideal location to enter the collecting system is at the base of the posterior infundibula. The intraoperative radiograph can be used as a guide to the pelvis and the base of the calyx. On occasion, with large posterior calyceal calculi, a dilated posterior calyx will be entered

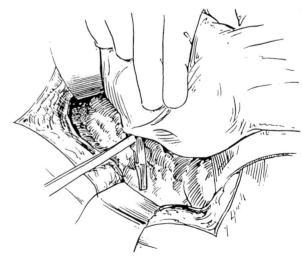

FIG. 8–2. The main renal artery is clamped and a bowel bag or rubber dam is placed around the kidney. Dry gauze packs are placed anterior to the kidney to protect the intraabdominal organs from hypothermia.

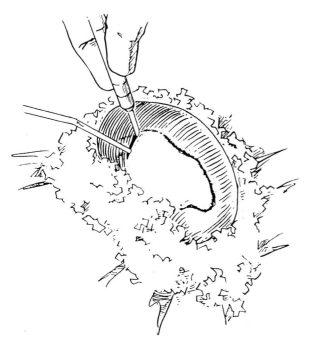

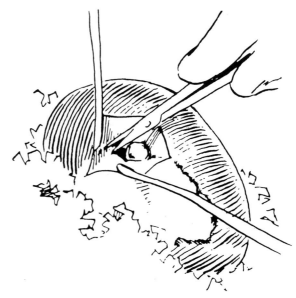

FIG. 8–5. The collecting system is carefully incised.

FIG. 8–3. A superficial incision is made in the renal capsule through the avascular plane.

initially. The remainder of the collecting system can then be identified with a probe and opened. If a posterior infundibulum is entered first, the incision is then carried toward the renal pelvis (Fig. 8–5). The stone is visualized and all ramifications of the stone are exposed by opening adjacent infundibula into the calyces. To minimize stone fragmentation and retained calculi, the stone should not be manipulated or removed until all of the calyceal and infundibular extensions are appropriately identified and incised. This allows for complete visualization and mobi-

lization of the collecting system and calculi. Ideally, the stone or stones should be removed without fragmentation; however, often it is inevitable that there will be some piecemeal extraction (Fig. 8–6). If this is necessary, a ureteral stent can be inserted to prevent stone migration during manipulation. Each calyx should be inspected for stone fragments. After removal of all stone fragments, the renal pelvis and calyces are copiously irrigated with cold saline and the irrigant is aspirated. A nephroscope can be used to look for residual fragments. A plain radiograph or

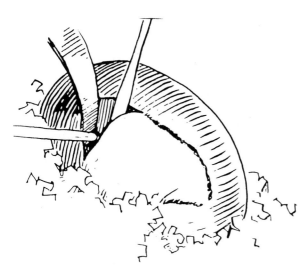

FIG. 8–4. The parenchyma is bluntly dissected with the back of a scalpel handle. The incision closely approximates the avascular plane.

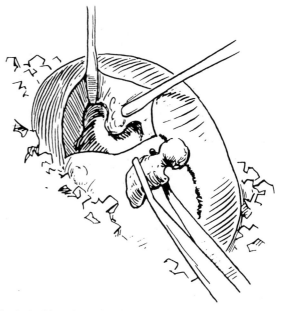

FIG. 8–6. After the collecting system is opened, calculi are extracted and total removal is confirmed radiographically.

ultrasonography are also options. At this time, a "double-J9 ureteral stent is passed from the renal pelvis into the bladder if this was not done at the time of stone manipulation (Fig. 8–7). The routine use of internal ureteral catheters is encouraged. They provide good urinary drainage, protect the freshly reconstructed collecting system, and minimize postoperative urinary extravasation. The next step in the procedure is the reconstruction of the intrarenal collecting system with correction of a coexistent anatomic abnormality if present. Infundibular stenosis or stricture, which results in obstruction promoting urinary stasis and recurrent stone formation, should be corrected with caliorrhaphy or calicoplasty. The former is the repair of a single narrowed calyx, achieved by incising the calyx along its appropriate margin (anterior margin for posterior calyces and posterior margin for anterior calyces) and suturing those margins to the renal pelvis, resulting in a shorter, wider calyx (Fig. 8–8). The infundibulum can also be incised longitudinally and then closed transversely in a Heinecke–Mickulicz fashion. Calicoplasty is the repair of adjacent stenotic calyces by suturing the adjacent walls of the neighboring calyces, thus forming a single structure (Figs. 8–9 and 8–10). All intrarenal reconstructive suturing should be accomplished with 5-0 or 6-0 chromic catgut sutures. When suturing the mucosal edges, it is important to avoid incorporation of underlying interlobular arteries, thus preventing ischemia.

The renal pelvis is then closed, first with reinforcing corner sutures and then with a running 6-0 chromic catgut suture (Fig. 8–11). The arterial clamp is briefly

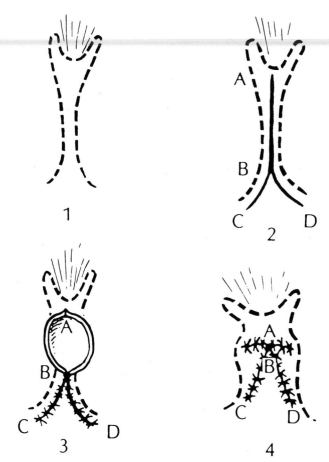

FIG. 8–8. Technique of repairing strictured infundibula. **1:** Narrowed elongated infundibulum. **2:** Incision into calyx forms an inverted Y. **3:** Pelvic flap is advanced into infundibulotomy. **4:** Incision in calyx is closed transversely.

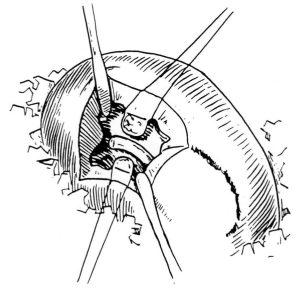

FIG. 8–7. A ureteral stent is passed in an antegrade fashion from the pelvis to the bladder. Traction sutures are placed to mark the walls of adjacent calyces before suturing them together with a running 6-0 chromic suture.

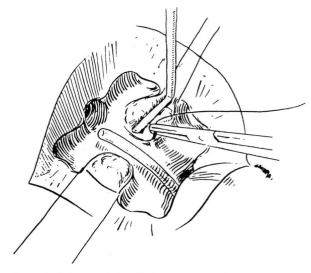

FIG. 8–9. Adjacent infundibula are sutured together starting in the renal pelvis. Peripelvic fat is depressed during this closure.

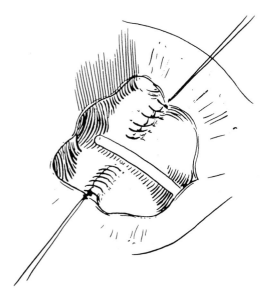

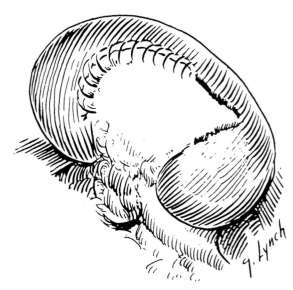

FIG. 8–10. The collecting system is completely reconstructed.

FIG. 8–12. The renal capsule is closed with a running locking 4-0 chromic suture.

released to identify parenchymal bleeding points, and hemostasis is obtained with 4-0 or 5-0 chromic catgut figure-of-eight suture ligatures before closing the renal capsule. The renal capsule is closed with a running lock stitch of 4-0 chromic catgut suture (Fig. 8–12) or mattress sutures over bolsters can be used. After the capsule is closed and adequate hemostasis has been achieved, the slush surrounding the kidney is removed and the renal artery unclamped. The kidney is observed for good hemostasis and return of pink color and good turgor after unclamping. It is then returned into Gerota's fascia, and the kidney and proximal ureter are covered with some perirenal fat to minimize the postoperative scar formation. If Gerota's fascia is unavailable because of prior

surgery, omentum can be mobilized through a peritoneal opening and wrapped around these structures. The peritoneal opening should be sutured to the omentum to prevent herniation of the abdominal viscera.

A Penrose or suction-type drain is placed within Gerota's fascia and brought out through a separate stab incision. This drain is left in place until minimal drainage occurs, usually by the third or fourth postoperative day. Nephrostomy tubes are in general avoided because of their potential for causing infection or further renal damage. The flank musculature and skin are closed in the standard fashion.

Postoperative management after anatrophic nephrolithotomy should follow the same principles that guide management after other major operations. IV fluids are maintained to achieve brisk urine output and until the patient is able to tolerate a clear liquid diet. Broad-spectrum IV antibiotics are administered perioperatively and continued postoperatively for 5 to 7 days. Antibiotic coverage is guided by preoperative urine culture and sensitivity results. The ureteral stent is removed cystoscopically at approximately 7 days postoperatively in uncomplicated cases. A urine culture is checked for persistence of infection.

OUTCOMES

Complications

Pulmonary complications are perhaps the most common following anatrophic nephrolithotomy, especially atelectasis. Patients with a history of pulmonary disease should likely undergo preoperative evaluation with pul-

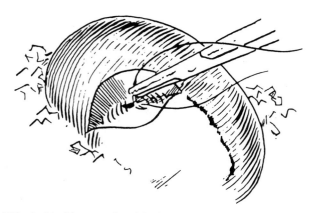

FIG. 8–11. The renal pelvis is closed with a running 6-0 chromic suture.

monary function testing and initiation of vigorous pulmonary toilet prior to surgery. Postoperatively, patients should be encouraged to breathe deeply and use of an incentive spirometer should be routine. Early ambulation will also be beneficial.

Pneumothorax should occur in fewer than 5% of patients (15). A patient with a history of pyelonephritis or previous renal surgery is at increased risk. Inadvertent opening of the pleura, usually during incision and resection of a rib, should be readily identified intraoperatively. The defect should be closed immediately with a running chromic catgut suture. The lung is hyperinflated just before the final suture is placed to ensure reexpansion of the lung. Chest tubes are not routinely used but may be necessary if any question remains regarding the reliability of the pleural closure. A chest radiograph should be obtained in the recovery room for any patient who undergoes repair of a pleural defect. Pulmonary embolism remains a potential complication of any major surgery. Routine use of elastic support hose and sequential compression stockings can lower the risk of deep venous thrombosis. Encouragement of early ambulation is also an important preventative measure. Significant postoperative renal hemorrhage should occur in fewer than 10% of patients. Assimos and associates reported an incidence of 6.4% (1). Bleeding usually occurs immediately or about 1 week postoperatively. Extensive intrarenal reconstruction, older age, worse renal function, and presence of blood dyscrasias were found to be significant risk factors. Slow bleeding will usually resolve on its own; management includes correction of any bleeding abnormalities and replacement with blood products as necessary. Oral ε-aminocaproic acid can be successful in certain cases. Bleeding that is brisk or cannot be adequately treated conservatively will require a more aggressive approach. A renal arteriogram can help identify the lesion, and an attempt at arteriographic embolization can be considered. Reexploration may be required in the remainder of the cases, with reinstitution of hypothermia and suture ligation of the bleeding vessel(s). Persistent hematuria 1 to 4 weeks postoperatively should alert the clinician to the possibility of renal arteriovenous fistula formation or a false aneurysm (1). Urinary extravasation should occur infrequently with the routine use of perinephric drains and ureteral catheter drainage. Should drainage recur or persist following removal of the drain and/or ureteral stent, replacement of the ureteral stent should be considered to decompress the system and relieve any obstruction. Other possible complications resulting from arterial clamping include renal injury and hypertension.

Results

When performed for appropriate indications and with meticulous technique, anatrophic nephrolithotomy can achieve successful removal of all calculi, preservation of renal function, improved urinary drainage, and eradication of infection. Stone-free rates greater than 90% should be achieved. Stone recurrence rates following anatrophic nephrolithotomy have been reported from 5% to 30% (15). Recurrent calculi usually form in those with persistent urinary tract infections, persistent urinary drainage impairment, and previously unidentified or refractory metabolic disturbances (12).

For large, complex staghorn calculi, especially those associated with some anatomic abnormality leading to impaired urinary drainage, anatrophic nephrolithotomy remains a first-line treatment. This modality achieves comparable or better stone-free rates and the achievement of a stone-free state with a single operative procedure. In the long term, treatment of these staghorn calculi with anatrophic nephrolithotomy should preserve renal function in the involved kidney and, in a majority of patients, eradicate stone disease and chronic urinary infection.

REFERENCES

1. Assimos DG, Boyce WH, Harrison LH, Hall JA, McCullough DL. Postoperative anatrophic nephrolithotomy bleeding. *J Urol* 1986;135:1153–1156.
2. Assimos DG, Boyce WH, Harrison LH, McCullough DL, Kroovand RL, Sweat KR. The role of open stone surgery since extracorporeal shock wave lithotripsy. *J Urol* 1989;142:263–267.
3. Blandy JP, Singh M. The case for a more aggressive approach to staghorn stones. *J Urol* 1976;115:505–506.
4. Caldwell TC, Burns JR. Current operative management of urinary calculi after renal transplantation. *J Urol* 1988;140:1360–1363.
5. McDougal WS. Renal perfusion/reperfusion injuries. *J Urol* 1988;140:1325–1330.
6. Myers RP. Brödel's line. *Surg Gynecol Obstet* 1971;132:424–426.
7. Paik ML, Resnick MI. Is there a role for open stone surgery? *Urol Clin North Am* 2000;27:323–331.
8. Paik ML, Wainstein MA, Spirnak JP, et al. Current indications for open stone surgery in the treatment of renal and ureteral calculi. *J Urol* 1998;159:374–379.
9. Parks JH, Goldfisher E, Asplin JR. A single 24-hour urine collection is inadequate for the medical evaluation of nephrolithiasis. *J Urol* 2002;167:1607–1612.
10. Razvi HA, Dendstedt JD, Chun SS, et al. Intracorporeal lithotripsy with the holmium:YAG laser. *J Urol* 1996;156:912.
11. Redman JF, Bissada NK, Harper DL. Anatrophic nephrolithotomy: experience with a simplification of the Smith and Boyce technique. *J Urol* 1979;122:595–597.
12. Russell JM, Harrison LH, Boyce WH. Recurrent urolithiasis following anatrophic nephrolithotomy. *J Urol* 1981;125:471–474.
13. Segura JW, Preminger GM, Assimos DG, et al. Nephrolithiasis Clinical Guidelines Panel summary report on the management of staghorn calculi. *J Urol* 1994;151:1648–1651.
14. Smith MJV, Boyce WH. Anatrophic nephrotomy and plastic calyorrhaphy. *J Urol* 1968;99:521–527.
15. Spirnak JP, Resnick MI. Anatrophic nephrolithotomy. *Urol Clin North Am* 1983;10:665–675.

CHAPTER 9

Renal and Retroperitoneal Abscesses

John R. Case and Anthony J. Schaeffer

Renal and retroperitoneal abscesses are uncommon clinical entities that often pose a significant diagnostic challenge. Nonspecific signs and symptoms frequently lead to a delay in diagnosis and treatment. Consequently, they are associated with significant morbidity, and mortality rates approaching 50% have been reported. An understanding of the anatomy of the retroperitoneal space is essential for classification, diagnosis, and management of renal and retroperitoneal abscesses.

CLASSIFICATION

The retroperitoneal space is bounded by the posterior parietal peritoneum and transversalis fascia (Figs. 9–1 and 9–2). It is divided into the perirenal space and the pararenal space.

The perirenal space surrounds the renal capsule and capsular artery and is bounded by the renal (Gerota's) fascia. It contains a lemon-yellow layer of fat, which is thickest posteriorly and laterally. The anterior and posterior leaves of the renal fascia fuse above the adrenal gland, becoming continuous with the diaphragmatic fascia (1). A thinner, more variable layer meets between the adrenal gland and the kidney. Laterally, the fascial layers join to form the lateroconal fascia, which becomes continuous with the posterior parietal peritoneum. Medially, the posterior layer fuses with the psoas muscle fascia and the anterior layer fuses with the connective tissue surrounding the great vessels and organs of the anterior retroperitoneum (i.e., the pancreas, duodenum, and colon). Because the perirenal space rarely crosses the midline, perirenal abscesses usually remain unilateral (20). Inferiorly, the renal fascial layers do not fuse but, rather, become continuous with the psoas and ureteral coverings (1,13). This opening inferiorly allows spread of perirenal infections to the pararenal space, pelvis, psoas muscle, and, in some cases, contralateral retroperitoneum.

The pararenal space is divided into two compartments: the anterior compartment, which is bounded by the posterior parietal peritoneum and the anterior renal fascia; and the posterior compartment, which is bounded by the posterior renal fascia and transversalis fascia. The pararenal space contains pale adipose tissue, which fills much of the retroperitoneal space. Because the anterior pararenal space extends across the midline, infection arising in one space may become bilateral. The posterior pararenal space does not cross the midline, and infection within it remains unilateral (20).

The retrofascial compartment lies posterior to the transversalis fascia. It is important only in development of the rare retrofascial abscess from abscesses of the psoas, iliacus, and quadratus muscles. The term "renal abscess" includes a wide range of abscesses arising from or around the kidney. A renal carbuncle is an abscess located on the renal capsule between the renal parenchyma and capsular artery whereas a perirenal abscess arises within Gerota's fascia external to the capsular artery. A pararenal abscess is located outside of Gerota's fascia within the pararenal space.

PATHOGENESIS

Before the advent of antimicrobial therapy, most renal abscesses occurred as a result of hematogenous spread of gram-positive organisms, usually *Staphylococcus aureus.* These abscesses, or renal carbuncles, can still be seen in intravenous drug users and in patients with dermatologic disorders. They may resolve with aggressive antimicrobial therapy if treated before frank suppuration. At present, most renal and retroperitoneal abscesses are caused by retrograde ascent of gram-negative bacteria from the bladder. The most common organisms include *Escherichia coli, Proteus, Klebsiella,* and *Pseudomonas* in descending order (8,16). Anaerobes may be isolated in abscesses associated with gastrointestinal (GI) and respiratory infections (3,6).

81

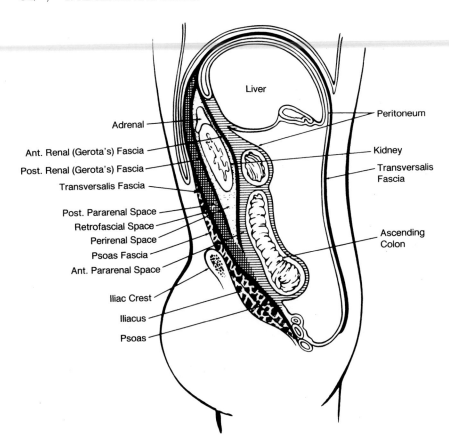

FIG. 9–1. Right sagittal view showing the anterior pararenal, perirenal, posterior pararenal, and retrofascial spaces. (From Simons GW, Sty JR, Starshak RJ. Retroperitoneal and retrofascial abscess. *J Bone Joint Surg* 1983;65A:1041, with permission.)

Abscesses caused by opportunistic organisms such as *Candida albicans, Toriolopsus glabrata,* and *Aspergillus* may occur in immunosuppressed patients (14–16). Other uncommon pathogens include *Mycobacterium tuberculosis* and *Echinococcus* (see below).

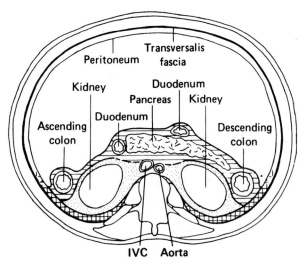

FIG. 9–2. The three retroperitoneal compartments. The striped and crosshatched areas correspond to the perirenal and posterior pararenal space, respectively. (From Meyers MA. Dynamic radiology of the abdomen. In: *Normal and pathologic anatomy*, 2nd ed. New York: Springer-Verlag, 1982:107–110, with permission.)

A renal abscess is in general preceded by pyelonephritis, which progresses to abscess formation in the presence of a virulent uropathogen, a damaged or obstructed urinary tract, or a compromised host. Renal abscesses have a predilection for the cortical medullary region and may drain spontaneously through the renal collecting system. When renal infection is complicated by obstruction, a purulent exudate collects in the renal collecting system. *Pyonephrosis* refers to infected hydronephrosis with suppurative destruction of the parenchyma of the kidney, with total or near total loss of renal function. The most frequent cause of obstruction is calculous disease (5,24). A previous history of urinary tract infection or surgery is also common.

Perirenal abscesses usually occur by erosion of abscesses or pyonephrosis into the perirenal space (18). Because of gravity, the resulting perirenal suppuration tends to localize dorsolaterally to the lower pole of the kidney. Posterior pararenal abscesses may arise from perirenal abscesses or from anterior pararenal abscesses tracking into the pelvis, where the anterior and posterior pararenal spaces communicate. On occasion, they result from hematogenous spread. Anterior pararenal abscesses are rarely urologic in origin. They arise from infection involving the organs within the anterior pararenal space, namely, the ascending and descending colon, appendix, duodenal loop, and pancreas. Abscesses arising from the

GI tract usually harbor a mixture of microorganisms, of which *E. coli* is the most prevalent. Extension of anterior pararenal abscesses into the perirenal space is uncommon.

DIAGNOSIS

The diagnosis of renal and retroperitoneal abscesses requires a high index of suspicion, as they typically present with insidious, nonspecific signs and symptoms (8,21). Presenting symptoms may include fever, chills, abdominal or flank pain, irritative voiding symptoms, nausea, vomiting, lethargy, or weight loss. Symptoms have been present for more than 5 days in the majority of patients with renal and retroperitoneal abscesses compared with 10% of patients with pyelonephritis. Over one-third of patients may be afebrile. The majority of patients diagnosed with renal and retroperitoneal abscesses have underlying, predisposing medical conditions. These include diabetes mellitus, urinary tract calculi, previous urologic surgery, urinary tract obstruction, polycystic kidney disease, malignancy, and immunosuppression.

A palpable flank or abdominal mass is present in about half of the cases. The mass may be better appreciated by examination of the patient in the knee–chest position. There may also be signs of psoas muscle irritation with flexion of the thigh.

Laboratory tests are helpful but nondiagnostic. Leukocytosis, elevated serum creatinine, and pyuria are common. Blood and urine cultures are frequently negative; when positive, they usually correlate with culture results from the abscess.

Multiple radiographic modalities may suggest the pathology including plain radiograph, excretory urography, ultrasound, and radionuclide scan, but a computer tomogram of the abdomen and pelvis remains the radiographic study of choice. Excretory urography can aid in the diagnosis of renal or retroperitoneal abscesses by showing diminished mobility on inspiratory–expiratory films. A renal abscess causes a decrease in function and enlargement of the nephrogram during the acute phase. Retroperitoneal abscesses may cause displacement of the kidneys or ureters by a mass, scoliosis of the spine, and free air or fluid in the retroperitoneal space. Computed tomography (CT) is highly sensitive for the diagnosis of renal and retroperitoneal abscesses. It precisely localizes and assesses the size of an abscess so that the type of intervention and its anatomic approach can be determined. The presence of gas within a lesion is pathognomonic for an abscess. Additional CT findings characteristic of an abscess include a mass with low attenuation, rim enhancement of the abscess wall after contrast, obliteration of tissue planes, and displacement of surrounding structures. Ultrasonography is less sensitive than CT but useful for monitoring response to therapy. Arteriography and radioisotope scanning rarely add significant information.

ALTERNATIVE THERAPY

Renal and retroperitoneal abscesses are in general lethal if untreated. Therapeutic options include antimicrobial therapy alone or in combination with percutaneous catheter drainage or open surgical drainage. Antimicrobial therapy as the sole treatment is an option with resolution of symptoms in a not insignificant percentage of renal abscesses depending on size, location, and other factors (2,4). Small renal abscesses may resolve if they are treated early at the carbuncle stage or have minimally liquified through aggressive antimicrobial therapy. Prolonged antimicrobial therapy without drainage is indicated only if favorable clinical response and radiological confirmation of abscess resolution indicate that the therapy is effective. This form of therapy has proven more successful in children when compared to adults and least successful in immunocompromised patients. If antimicrobial therapy is not effective, prompt percutaneous or open surgical drainage of the pus is mandatory. Progression of a renal abscess leads to perinephric abscess or perforation into the collecting system and results in signs and symptoms of urinary tract infection.

Antimicrobial therapy should be instituted after the urine has been Gram stained and urine and blood cultures have been obtained. Broad-spectrum coverage should be guided by the presumptive diagnosis and the presumed pathogen. An aminoglycoside for Gram-negative rods and ampicillin for Gram-positive cocci are preferred. Anaerobic coverage with a drug such as clindamycin is warranted when Gram stain reveals a polymicrobial flora or when a GI source is suspected. If the abscess may be of staphylococcal origin, a penicillinase-resistant penicillin, such as nafcillin, should be added. Antimicrobial therapy should be reevaluated when the results of culture and sensitivity tests are available. Unfortunately, urine and blood cultures are frequently sterile, and empirical therapy must be modified on the basis of clinical response and changes in imaging studies.

SURGICAL TECHNIQUE

Percutaneous Drainage

Most renal and retroperitoneal abscesses are treated with empirical antimicrobial therapy and immediate percutaneous drainage, with successful resolution of abscess at least 50% of the time (4). When successful, minimally invasive therapy minimizes operative morbidity and allows for preservation of renal tissue. The abscess must be confirmed by CT- or ultrasonography-guided needle aspiration, must not have multiple loculations, and must be drainable without injury to other organs. Immediate surgical drainage must be instituted if the procedure fails. After a multiport drainage catheter (8 to 12 Fr) is positioned, the abscess should be drained and adequate evacuation should be confirmed by CT or ultrasonography. The catheter should then be connected to low intermittent suction, and drainage outputs should be monitored daily. If drainage stops abruptly, occlusion of the catheter should be suspected and it should be irrigated gently with small amounts of normal saline. CT or ultrasonography should be performed periodically to monitor catheter position and size of the abscess. Direct instillation of contrast through the drainage tube may be helpful to confirm the catheter position or rule out a fistula. To avoid bacteremia, prophylactic antimicrobial coverage should be given, and the contrast should be instilled under gravity or by gentle injection. Instillation of 2,500 U of urokinase in 50 mL of normal saline on a daily basis may be successful in evacuating an organizing infected hematoma. Routine abscess irrigation with antimicrobials is of questionable benefit and may promote overgrowth of resistant bacteria. The catheter should be withdrawn gradually as the abscess cavity shrinks and the drainage decreases. The usual duration of drainage is 1 to 3 weeks. The catheter is removed when drainage stops and CT and ultrasonography show complete resolution.

Open Surgical Drainage

In the case of failed percutaneous therapy, deciding upon the next intervention is not always simple. Variables that must be considered in this decision include patient comorbidities and current degree of illness, functional status of both kidneys, and etiology of the renal abscess. On occasion, the decision can only be made at the time of surgical exploration. As the cure rate increases for open drainage with respect to percutaneous drainage, so does the risk of complication. Albeit rare, complications include vascular or bowel injury, new abscess formation or seeding, pneumothorax, and sepsis. Chronic fistulas might suggest residual stone, foreign body, or persistent renal obstruction. Rarely, carcinomas may predispose a kidney to abscess formation and therefore a cure would not be attained with simple drainage.

For open surgical drainage, the incision should be smaller than that used for routine nephrectomy, and usually a posterior flank muscle-splitting incision below the twelfth rib is sufficient. When the retroperitoneal abscess is entered, the pus should be cultured and the space gently but thoroughly explored to ensure that all loculated cavities are drained. Thorough irrigation of the cavity is essential. Multiple Penrose drains should be inserted into the space through separate stab wounds, and the ends of the drains should be sutured to the skin and tagged with safety pins. Fascial and muscular closure may be performed with chromic catgut suture, but skin and subcuta-neous tissue should be left open to prevent the formation of a secondary body wall abscess. The wound can be left to heal from within, or skin sutures may be placed and left untied for dermal approximation 5 to 7 days postoperatively after drainage has ceased. The wound should be packed with gauze and the packs changed daily. The drains should be left in place until purulent drainage has decreased, and then they can be removed slowly over several days.

ANCILLARY PROCEDURES

If a perinephric abscess is due to long-standing obstruction and there is no functioning renal tissue, a nephrectomy at the time of drainage is theoretically attractive. Drainage of a perinephric abscess should usually be performed as a primary procedure, however, with nephrectomy performed at a later date if necessary. Patients are frequently too ill for prolonged general anesthesia and surgical manipulation. Further, nephrectomy is usually technically difficult to accomplish and preoperative information is usually not sufficient to determine accurately the amount of functioning of salvageable renal tissue. After drainage of the abscess, removal of obstruction, and appropriate antimicrobial therapy, many kidneys may regain sufficient function to obviate future nephrectomy. Nephrectomy, if indicated, can be performed using a standard nephrectomy approach or a subcapsular nephrectomy technique outlined later.

A small renal abscess confined to one pole of the kidney may be managed by partial nephrectomy. If the infection extends beyond the apparent line of cleavage, however, it is essential to remove all infection, and the line of excision should extend through healthy tissue. If multiple abscesses are present, internal drainage is difficult and nephrectomy may be required.

Subcapsular Nephrectomy

When a kidney is so adherent to surrounding tissues that dissection is difficult and hazardous, a subcapsular nephrectomy is indicated. These conditions are usually seen after multiple or chronic infections or previous operations have caused scarring to adjacent organs. Blunt dissection results in tearing of structures such as bowel wall. Sharp dissection when there is no definable tissue plane often results in lacerations of the vena cava, aorta, duodenum, spleen, and other structures. In subcapsular nephrectomy, dissection beneath the renal capsule enables one to avoid these vital structures. Subcapsular nephrectomy should not be performed for malignant disease and is undesirable in tuberculosis.

The main difficulty with subcapsular nephrectomy is that the capsule is adherent to the vessels in the hilum, and one usually must go outside the capsule to ligate the renal pedicle. In this setting, the renal hilum usually is involved in the inflammatory reaction and separate identification of the vessels is difficult.

Kidney exposure is accomplished through the flank using a twelfth-rib incision. For low-lying kidneys, a subcostal incision may be satisfactory. When the kidney is reached, the capsule is incised and freed from the underlying cortex (Fig. 9–3). The capsule is stripped from the surface of the kidney and an incision is made carefully in the capsule where it is attached to the hilum (Fig. 9–4). The vessels may be protected by placing a finger in front of the pedicle when cutting the capsule. The dense apron of capsule can usually be incised best on the anterior aspect. Control of bleeding can be difficult in this procedure. Frequently, all landmarks are obscured and the renal artery and vein cannot be identified. Sharp dissection is usually required, and major vessels may be entered before they are recognized. Fortunately, the dense fibrous tissue tends to prevent their retraction. Frequently, several

chromic suture ligatures can be placed through the pedicle between a proximally placed pedicle clamp and the kidney. To avoid damage to the duodenum or major vessels, pieces of capsule may be left behind. However, prolonged drainage can ensue, and as much of the infected tissue should be removed as possible. After ligation and cutting of the pedicle, the ureter is identified and cut and the distal end is ligated. If distal ureteral obstruction has caused pyonephrosis, a small, 8 to 10 Fr red Robinson catheter may be placed in the distal ureter to allow postoperative antimicrobial irrigation. Multiple drains should be placed and brought through separate stab wounds.

OUTCOMES

Complications

Complications associated with percutaneous drainage include the formation of additional abscesses that communicate with the renal collecting system and may require temporary urinary diversion via percutaneous nephrostomy drainage to affect a cure. Sepsis, the most frequent complication of percutaneous drainage, occurs in fewer than 10% of patients. Other complications, such as transpleural puncture, vascular or enteric injury, and cutaneous fistula, are rare.

Additional complications to open or percutaneous drainage include prolonged purulent drainage, which may indicate a retained foreign body, calculus, or fistula.

Results

Cure rates for percutaneous drainage of renal and retroperitoneal abscesses range from 60% to 90% (10,19). Multiloculated, viscous abscesses and abscesses in immunocompromised hosts are associated with lower cure rates. Large abscesses may require more than one percutaneous access procedure to completely drain them.

In the past, mortality rates were reported to be as high as 50% in patients with retroperitoneal or perinephric abscesses. More recent reports indicate a significant improvement in mortality (approximately 10%), in large part because of more accurate diagnosis from improved imaging techniques, more effective antimicrobial therapy, and better supportive care (6,8,21).

SPECIAL CONSIDERATIONS

Renal Tuberculosis

Renal tuberculosis is caused by hematogenous dissemination from an infected source somewhere else in the body. Both kidneys are seeded with tuberculosis bacilli in 90% of cases. Clinically apparent renal tuberculosis is usually unilateral, however. The initial lesion involves the renal cortex, with multiple small granulomas in the

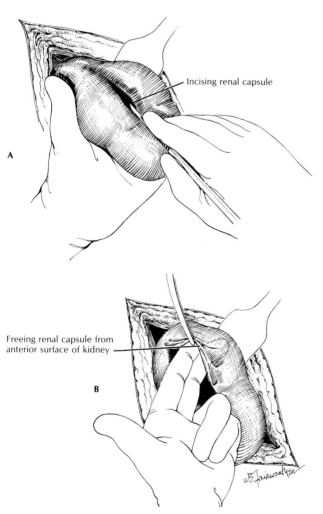

FIG. 9–3. Subcapsular secondary nephrectomy showing freeing of the capsule from anterior surfaces of the kidney.

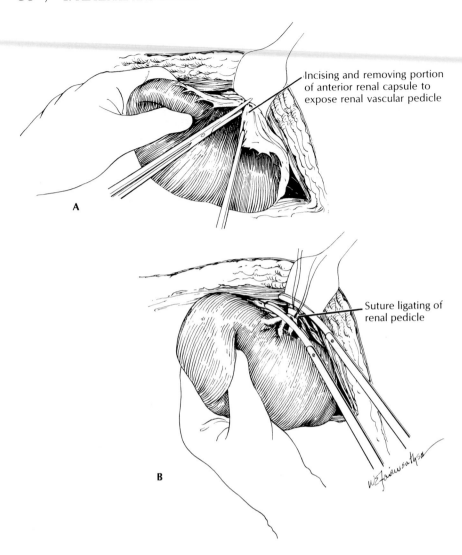

Incising and removing portion of anterior renal capsule to expose renal vascular pedicle

A

Suture ligating of renal pedicle

B

FIG. 9–4. Subcapsular secondary nephrectomy showing incision in and removal of a portion of the renal capsule to expose and ligate the renal pedicle.

glomeruli and the juxtaglomerular regions. In untreated patients who fail to heal spontaneously, the lesions may progress slowly and remain asymptomatic for variable periods, usually 10 to 40 years. As the lesions progress, they produce areas of caseous necrosis and parenchymal cavitation. Large tumor-like parenchymal lesions or tuberculomas frequently have fibrous walls and resemble solid mass lesions. Once cavities form, spontaneous healing is rare and destructive lesions result, with spread of the infection to the renal pelvis and development of a parenchymal or perinephric abscess.

Indications for Surgery

Surgery was once commonly used in the treatment of renal tuberculosis, but since the advent of effective antituberculosis chemotherapy it is reserved primarily for management of local complications, such as ureteral strictures, or for treatment of nonfunctioning kidneys. If surgery is warranted, it is wise to precede the operation with at least 3 weeks and preferably 3 months of triple-drug chemotherapy. Use of isoniazid, 300 mg per day; pyrazinamide, 25 mg per kg to a maximum of 2 g once daily; and rifampicin, 450 mg per day, is recommended. If segmental renal damage is obvious and salvage of the kidney is possible, a drainage procedure or cavernostomy can be performed (9). Removal of a nonfunctioning kidney is usually indicated for advanced unilateral disease complicated by sepsis, hemorrhage, intractable pain, newly developed severe hypertension, suspicion of malignancy, inability to sterilize the urine with drugs alone, abscess formation with development of fistula, or inability to have appropriate follow-up (11,12,17).

Alternative Therapy

Prophylactic removal of a nonfunctioning kidney to prevent complications, remove a potential source of viable organisms, and shorten the duration of convalescence and requirement for chemotherapy is advocated by some authors (7,23). Others, who followed a large series of patients treated with medical therapy alone, concluded that because the frequency of late complications is only 6% routine nephrectomy should not be performed for every nonfunctioning kidney (11). These authors, however, treated patients for at least 2 years. The merits of short-term therapy and prophylactic nephrectomy versus long-term 2-year chemotherapy and selective nephrectomy warrant further study. Modern percutaneous drainage techniques have largely replaced open cavernostomy for treatment of closed pyocalyx.

Surgical Technique

Cavernostomy

Renal tuberculosis sometimes results in caliceal infundibular scarring, causing a closed pyocalix. Unroofing of a pyocalix is called cavernostomy. If the calix still communicates with the renal pelvis, or if it is connected to significant functioning parenchyma, a cavernostomy should not be done because a urinary fistula or urinoma may result. To minimize wound contamination and tuber-

culous spread, thorough needle aspiration of purulent material and saline irrigation of the abscess cavity should be performed using a large-bore needle and syringe (Fig. 9–5). The abscess cavity is then unroofed and the edge is sutured with a running suture for hemostasis. Any unsuspected connection with the renal pelvis by an open infundibulum must be closed using 5-0 chromic catgut sutures to prevent fistula or urinoma formation. After thorough wound irrigation, multiple drains are placed and closure is undertaken. Drains are managed as previously described for perinephric abscess.

Nephrectomy

When unilateral tuberculosis causes more extensive parenchymal destruction or nonfunction, a partial or total nephrectomy, respectively, should be performed. For partial nephrectomy, a guillotine incision is made 1 cm beyond the abscess. If the renal pedicle can be freed and polar vessel located and occluded, the incision can be made at the line of demarcation of the ischemia. In partial nephrectomy, it is important to try to save the capsule (if it is not involved with the infection) to cover the raw

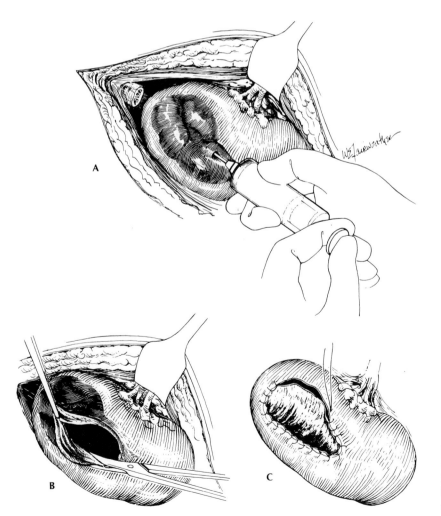

FIG. 9–5. Cavernostomy drainage of tuberculous renal abscess. (From Hanley HG. Cavernostomy and partial nephrectomy in renal tuberculosis. *Br J Urol* 1970; 42:661, with permission.)

surface for hemostasis. Alternatively, fat can be used for hemostasis. The amputated calyx is carefully ligated with a 4-0 chromic catgut suture to prevent urinary fistula or urinoma formation.

After nephrectomy, the distal ureter can be ligated and in most cases does not need to be brought to the skin because tuberculosis of the ureter in general heals with chemotherapy after nephrectomy. If renal tuberculosis is associated with severe tuberculosis cystitis, ureteral catheterization for 7 days postoperatively to minimize subsequent ureteral stump abscess formation should be considered (22).

Renal Echinococcosis

Echinococcosis is a parasitic infection caused by the canine tapeworm *E. granulosus*. Echinococcal or hydatid cysts occur in the kidney in 3% of patients with this disease. The hydatid cyst gradually develops at a rate of about 1 cm per year and is usually single and located in the cortex.

Diagnosis

The symptoms are those of a slowly growing tumor; most patients are asymptomatic or have a dull flank pain or hematuria. Excretory urography typically shows a thick-walled cystic mass that is on occasion calcified. Ultrasonography and CT usually show a multicystic or multiloculated mass. Confirmation of the diagnosis is most reliably made by diagnostic tests using partially purified hydatid antigens in a double-diffusion test (17). Complement fixation and hemagglutination are less reliable. Diagnostic needle puncture is associated with significant risk of anaphylaxis as a result of leakage of toxic cyst contents.

Indications for Surgery

Cyst removal is indicated when an enlarging cyst threatens renal function or produces obstruction.

Surgical Technique

The cyst should be removed without rupture to reduce the chance of seeding or anaphylactic-type reaction that can prove fatal in the operating room. In cases where cyst removal is impossible because of its size or involvement of adjacent organs, marsupialization is required. Initially that cyst should be isolated with sponges, the contents aspirated, and the cyst should be filled with a scolecidal

agent such as 30% sodium chloride, 2% formalin, or 1% iodide for about 5 minutes to kill the germinal portions. Complete evacuation of all hydatid tissue and thorough postmarsupialization irrigation are critical to preventing systemic effects. Penrose drains are left in the cystic cavity until drainage ceases. If large amounts of renal tissue have been damaged, partial or simple nephrectomy may be required.

REFERENCES

1. Amin M, Blandford AT, Polk HC. Renal fascia of Gerota. *Urology* 1976;7:1–3.
2. Best CD, Terris MK, Tacker JR, Reese JH. Clinical and radiological findings in patients with gas forming renal abscess treated conservatively. *J Urol* 1999;162:1273–1276.
3. Brook I. The role of anaerobic bacteria in perinephric and renal abscesses in children. *Pediatrics* 1994;93:261–264.
4. Chakroun M, Ladeb MF, Gharbi-Jemni H, Missaoui Z, M'Hiri C, Ben Salem N, Gannouni A, el May M. Non-surgical treatment of kidney abscesses. Apropos of 12 cases. *Ann Med Int* 1992;143(7):442–444.
5. Doughney KB, Dineen MK, Venable DD. Nephrobronchial colonic fistula complicating perinephric abscess. *J Urol* 1986;135:765–767.
6. Edelstein H, McCabe RE. Perinephric abscess: modern diagnosis and treatment in 47 cases. *Medicine* 1988;67:118–131.
7. Flechner SM, Gow JG. Role of nephrectomy in the treatment of nonfunctioning or very poorly functioning unilateral tuberculous kidney. *J Urol* 1980;123:822–825.
8. Fowler JE, Perkins T. Presentation, diagnosis and treatment of renal abscesses: 1972–1988. *J Urol* 1994;151:847–851.
9. Hanley HG. Cavernostomy and partial nephrectomy in renal tuberculosis. *Br J Urol* 1970;42:661–666.
10. Lambiase RE, Deyoe L, Cronan JJ, Durfman GS. Percutaneous drainage of 355 consecutive abscesses: results of primary drainage with 1-year follow-up. *Radiology* 1992;184:167–179.
11. Lattimer JK, Wechsler MW. Editorial comment: surgical management of nonfunctioning tuberculous kidneys. *J Urol* 1980;124:191.
12. Lorin MI, Hsu KHF, Jacob SC. Treatment of tuberculosis in children. *Pediatr Clin North Am* 1983;30:333–348.
13. Mitchell GAG. The renal fascia. *Br J Surg* 1950;37:257–266.
14. Noriega LM, Gonzalez P, Perez J, Canals C, Trucco C, Michaud P. [Unusual presentation of urinary tract infection in 6 cases.] *Rev Med Child* 1995;123:334–340.
15. Oda K, Inoue S, Oe H. Renal carbuncle with xanthogranulomatous change: report of a case. *Hinyokika Kiyo* 1970;16(5):211–218.
16. Patterson JE, Andriole VT. Bacterial urinary tract infections in diabetes *Infect Dis Clin North Am* 1997;11(3):735–750.
17. Schaeffer AJ. Urinary tract infections. In: Gillenwater JY, Grayhack JT, Howards SS, Duckett JW, eds. *Adult and pediatric urology*. Chicago: Year Book Medical Publishers, 1996:289–351.
18. Sheinfeld J, Ertuk E, Spataro RF, Cockett ATK. Perinephric abscess: current concepts. *J Urol* 1987;137:191–194.
19. Siegel JF, Smith A, Moldwin R. Minimally invasive treatment of renal abscess. *J Urol* 1996;155:52–55.
20. Simons GW, Sty JR, Starshak RJ. Retroperitoneal and retrofascial abscesses. *J Bone Joint Surg* 1983;65A:1041–1058.
21. Thorley JD, Jones SR, Sanford JP. Perinephric abscess. *Medicine* 1974; 53:441–451.
22. Wechsler M, Lattimer JK. An evaluation of the current therapeutic regimen for renal tuberculosis. *J Urol* 1975;13:760–761.
23. Wong SH, Lou WY. The surgical management of non-functioning tuberculous kidney. *J Urol* 1980;124:187–191.
24. Yoder JC, Pfister RC, Lindfors KK, et al. Pyonephrosis: imaging and intervention. *AJR* 1983;141:735–739.

CHAPTER 10

Renal Trauma

Daniel I. Rosenstein, Allen F. Morey, and Jack W. McAninch

Renal injuries can be some of the most complex and challenging cases faced by the urologist or trauma surgeon. The kidney is the most commonly injured genitourinary organ due to external trauma. The vast majority of renal injuries occur as a result of blunt trauma, and most of these are amenable to nonoperative management. Penetrating renal trauma usually occurs in conjunction with injuries to associated abdominal organs, which require urgent laparotomy. Systematic renal reconstruction at the time of laparotomy provides excellent functional results in the majority of cases. The goal of renal reconstruction is to preserve enough functioning nephron mass to avoid end-stage renal failure. Nephrectomy in the trauma setting should be reserved for life-threatening hemorrhage as well as kidneys that have been injured beyond repair.

DIAGNOSIS

Appropriate management of renal trauma begins with complete staging of the injury with history, physical examination, urinalysis, and radiographic imaging (if indicated). History should focus on the mechanism of trauma (blunt or penetrating), as well as the presence of significant deceleration—which should raise suspicion for significant renal injury. On physical examination, the presence of shock (defined as systolic blood pressure less than 90 mm Hg) should be recorded. The lowest recorded systolic blood pressure is critical in determining the need for radiographic imaging in adult blunt renal trauma (5). A patient in shock who cannot be resuscitated may require urgent laparotomy, thus bypassing radiographic staging of suspected renal injury. This patient will require intraoperative staging (see later). The abdomen, flank, and back should be carefully examined. Flank tenderness or ecchymosis as well as lower-rib fractures may indicate

underlying renal injury. In penetrating trauma, entry and exit wounds may point to a transrenal course.

Hematuria is the most common sign of penetrating and blunt renal trauma. However, the presence of hematuria does not correlate consistently with degree of renal injury (2). This is in particular true in penetrating injuries, where a significant percentage of patients with significant renal injuries may have no hematuria. The first voided or catheterized specimen should be analyzed because hematuria may clear rapidly. Either dipstick or microscopic analysis may be performed.

Using the clinical information outlined above, the indications for radiographic imaging may be tailored to detecting patients with a significant chance of having a major renal laceration (considered grades 3–5). Based upon our experience at San Francisco General Hospital, we recommend imaging the following categories of patients (11):

1. Penetrating trauma to the abdomen, flank, or back injury with ANY degree of hematuria, in particular when the course of the missile appears to involve the kidney or ureter.
2. Blunt trauma with either gross hematuria or microhematuria (defined as any recorded systolic blood pressure below 90 mm Hg.). Patients having sustained blunt trauma with microhematuria only can safely avoid renal imaging (6).
3. Blunt trauma in the setting of significant deceleration injury, e.g., falls from heights (1) or motor vehicle accidents. This mechanism of injury has been associated with a higher incidence of ureteropelvic junction disruption as well as renovascular trauma.
4. Pediatric penetrating injury or blunt trauma with microhematuria greater than 20 red blood cells per high power focus (7). There is mounting evidence that the adult imaging criteria outlined above will identify the majority of significant renal lacerations in children (10), but this remains a controversial topic. The clini-

The opinions expressed herein are those of the authors and are not to be construed as reflecting the views of the U.S. Armed Forces or the Department of Defense.

cian should continue to maintain a low threshold for renal imaging in the pediatric population.

The best study for assessing the injured kidney in a stable patient is a renal computed tomography (CT) scan. Renal images can be obtained in conjunction with an abdominal CT when trauma surgeons need this study to evaluate the extent of associated intraabdominal injuries. CT is noninvasive and offers accurate information regarding the depth and extent of renal lacerations, as well as the presence of two functioning kidneys. When unstable patients are taken emergently for laparotomy and renal injuries are suspected, a one-shot intraoperative intravenous pyelogram (IVP) is extremely useful. The intraoperative IVP consists of a high-dose (2 cc per kg) IV bolus injection of radiographic contrast; a single film is taken at 10 minutes. No scout film is necessary. This technique provides important information regarding the degree of injury of the kidney in question and the status of the contralateral kidney without delaying resuscitation (8). Although a one-shot IVP may be indeterminate, it has been shown to reduce the rate of unnecessary renal explorations without resulting in increased renal complications.

INDICATIONS FOR SURGERY

The decision to surgically repair the traumatized kidney is based on consideration of the patient's mechanism of injury, hemodynamic stability, associated injuries, and accurate radiographic staging of the injury (4). The vast majority of blunt traumatic renal injuries are clinically insignificant. At San Francisco General Hospital, fewer than 3% of patients with blunt renal trauma require renal exploration (Fig. 10–1). Penetrating renal injuries, on the other hand, frequently undergo laparotomy for associated injuries or hemodynamic instability. Approximately 70% of patients with penetrating renal trauma are treated surgically at our trauma center. Only when radiographic staging clearly defines a penetrating injury as minor can a nonoperative approach be used successfully (14).

The only absolute indication for renal exploration is massive and potentially life-threatening hemorrhage from a severely injured kidney. Relative indications for renal surgery include extensive urinary extravasation, nonviable renal tissue in association with a parenchymal laceration, incomplete clinical or radiographic staging, and arterial thrombosis. In the setting of a concomitant exploratory laparotomy by the trauma surgeon we will usually repair significant renal injuries at that time to prevent later complications. Nearly all renal lacerations occurring from gunshot wounds require immediate repair. In the absence of severe vascular injury or hemodynamic instability, renal reconstruction may safely be attempted. Successful reconstruction can be undertaken despite spillage from bowel injury, pancreatic injury, or other associated injuries (13).

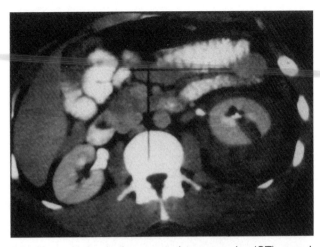

FIG. 10–1. Abdominal computed tomography (CT) reveals left renal laceration after blunt trauma (grade 3). Even major renal lacerations occurring after blunt trauma are usually amenable to nonoperative management. Renal CT provides detailed information regarding the depth of laceration, size of perirenal hematoma, tissue viability, urinary extravasation, and status of the contralateral kidney.

ALTERNATIVE THERAPY

Nephrectomy, when required after renal trauma, usually occurs when an injury is deemed irreparable (shattered kidney, avulsed renal pedicle) or in the setting of hemodynamic instability. Although nephrectomy is clearly a life-saving maneuver in these instances, it is only necessary in about 10% of cases. In general, patients requiring nephrectomy are much more seriously injured, are frequently in shock, and cannot be managed conservatively (9). In institutions where renal exploration in the trauma setting is rarely performed, nephrectomy may result from uncontrolled hemorrhage once the perinephric hematoma is released.

Renal stab wounds are successfully managed nonoperatively in about 50% of cases at San Francisco General Hospital. The types of stab wounds most amenable to an observational approach are those occurring posteriorly or in the flank, where intraabdominal organs are unlikely to be involved. For those stab-wound patients in whom conservative management is being contemplated, renal CT provides excellent information regarding the depth of laceration, extent of urinary extravasation, and size of perirenal hematoma (14). Renal stab wounds have a significant risk of delayed bleeding, so close observation with serial hematocrit measurement is prudent. Conservative management does not refer exclusively to nonoperative management. It implies that the urologist is prepared to continuously reevaluate the patient's condition and embark upon renal exploration and reconstruction if the patient's condition warrants it.

SURGICAL TECHNIQUE

Renal exploration in the trauma setting should be carried out through a standard midline abdominal incision. This approach provides complete access to the intraabdominal viscera and vasculature and also gives the greatest flexibility to assess and repair a variety of genitourinary injuries. Major bleeding noted on opening the abdominal cavity should be controlled immediately with laparotomy packs followed by surgical control and repair. Associated injuries to other abdominal organs are usually addressed before examination of the kidneys if the patient is stable. The bowel, liver, spleen, pancreas, and other organs should be inspected systematically and carefully. During this period, Gerota's fascia maintains its natural tamponade effect on the perinephric hematoma.

The renal vasculature is routinely isolated before a retroperitoneal hematoma surrounding an injured kidney is entered. This reduces the risk of uncontrolled renal bleeding and unplanned nephrectomy. To facilitate access to the retroperitoneum, the transverse colon is lifted out of the abdomen superiorly and placed on moist laparotomy packs. The small bowel is placed in a bowel bag and lifted anteriorly to the right. An incision is made in the retroperitoneum over the aorta from the level of the inferior mesenteric artery to Treitz's ligament, which can be divided for additional exposure. If a large retroperitoneal hematoma obscures the aorta, the inferior mesenteric vein is identified and the incision into the retroperitoneum is placed just medial to this important landmark. Once the aorta is identified in the lower part of the incision, it is followed superiorly to the left renal vein, which reliably crosses anteriorly. The renal arteries can be found just posterior to the left renal vein on either side of the aorta. If the right renal artery is difficult to isolate through this approach, an alternative method of exposure is to mobilize the second portion of the duodenum off the vena cava. With lateral retraction on the vena cava, the right renal artery can then be isolated in its interaortocaval location.

The ipsilateral renal artery and vein are individually isolated with vessel loops. These vessels are not occluded initially unless bleeding is heavy, which occurs in approximately 12% of cases in our experience (3). In our experience, most bleeding is successfully controlled with manual compression alone. Because the vessels are not routinely clamped, renal perfusion is continuous and warm ischemia is avoided. Patients most likely to require temporary vascular occlusion are those in shock from active, uncontrolled renal bleeding. Temporary vascular occlusion should be kept below 30 minutes to minimize warm ischemic damage.

Following proximal vascular control, the kidney is exposed by incising the retroperitoneum just lateral to the colon. The colon is reflected medially, and dissection through the hematoma allows renal exposure. After the kidney has been bluntly and sharply mobilized, the entire

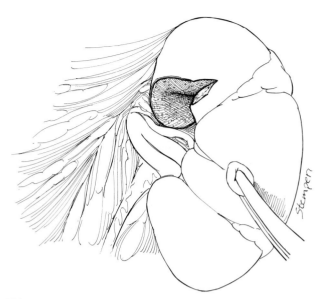

FIG. 10–2. After preliminary vascular control, the colon is reflected and the kidney explored. Here, a small gunshot entrance wound on the anterior aspect of left kidney is identified.

renal surface, renal vasculature, and upper ureter are routinely inspected for the presence of exit wounds or multiple injured areas (Figs. 10–2 and 10–3). Care is taken to maintain the integrity of the renal capsule as the kidney is mobilized to decrease hemorrhage and preserve the capsule for later closure. If heavy bleeding ensues, Rummel

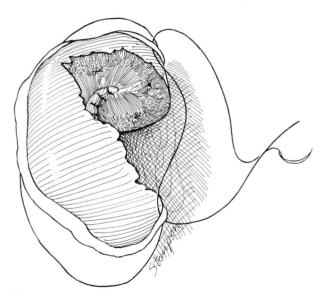

FIG. 10–3. When a renal injury is identified, the entire kidney must be examined for associated wounds. Here, a complex gaping exit wound is identified on the posterior surface of the kidney. Nonviable tissue is debrided, the collecting system is closed, and segmental vessels are individually suture ligated with 4-0 chromic sutures. Capsular sutures of 3-0 Vicryl are used to reapproximate wound edges.

tourniquets can be applied to the vessel loops for vascular occlusion. First, the renal artery alone is occluded. If bleeding persists, the renal vein is then occluded to eliminate backbleeding.

The principles that are applicable to all renal reconstructions include the following: (a) broad exposure of the entire kidney; (b) temporary vascular occlusion for bleeding not arrested by manual parenchymal compression; (c) sharp debridement of nonviable parenchyma; (d) meticulous hemostasis; (e) watertight collecting system closure; (f) primary reapproximation of the parenchymal edges or coverage of the parenchymal defect; (g) omental interposition flap placement to separate reconstructed kidney from surrounding pancreatic, colonic, or vascular injuries; and (h) retroperitoneal drain placement.

Partial nephrectomy is the most appropriate treatment for major polar injuries. The kidney should be debrided back to viable tissue. Manual compression of the adjoining normal renal parenchyma, rather than formal vascular occlusion, is extremely useful during partial nephrectomy as an adjunct during control of moderate renal hemorrhage. Arcuate arteries are individually suture ligated with 4-0 chromic sutures to control hemorrhage. The collecting system is then closed watertight with a running 4-0 Vicryl suture. Methylene blue may be injected into the renal pelvis with simultaneous compression of the ureter to elucidate any leaks in the collecting system, which may then be oversewn.

The renal parenchymal defect should be covered with thrombin-soaked Gelfoam to enhance hemostasis and then covered with renal capsule, if possible. If the capsule has been destroyed or the defect is too large to close primarily without causing ischemia, we recommend use of an omental pedicle flap for defect coverage. Its excellent vascular supply and lymphatic drainage make omentum an excellent tissue choice for coverage of renal injuries, especially in the setting of concomitant bowel or pancreatic injury. If omentum is unavailable, the defect may be closed with perinephric fat or a peritoneal free graft. In the case of multiple deep lacerations, the kidney may be placed in a Vicryl mesh envelope to stabilize the repair. A retroperitoneal drain is placed routinely. This drain should not be placed to suction, and may typically be removed after 48 to 72 hours.

Major injuries to the midportion of the kidney are best repaired by renorrhaphy. Nonviable tissue is removed sharply. Sites of bleeding are individually ligated with fine absorbable sutures, and the collecting system is closed as outlined above. Interrupted 3-0 chromic sutures placed superficially are ideal for renal capsule approximation. Capsular sutures are best placed without incorporating the underlying parenchyma, as that tissue is extremely friable. Thrombin-soaked Gelfoam bolsters are placed into the defect to enhance hemostasis, prevent urinary leakage, and stabilize capsular closure (Fig. 10–4). Again, omentum should be used if primary capsular clo-

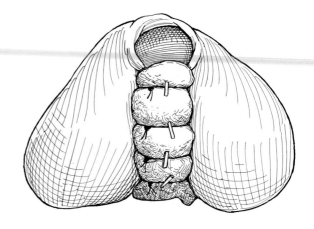

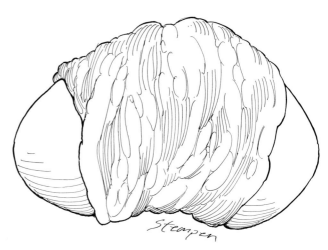

FIG. 10–4. Closure of parenchymal defect after central renal injury. Capsular sutures of 3-0 Vicryl may be used to sew gelatin foam bolsters into the repair site. Titanium clips may be placed along the repair line to identify the area of reconstruction on subsequent imaging studies. Alternatively, if primary renal closure cannot be achieved, an omental flap may be tacked over the defect using small interrupted chromic sutures.

sure cannot be achieved. We frequently place a row of small titanium staples in the renal capsule near the closure to visualize the operative site on subsequent imaging studies.

Renal stab wounds may be repaired using the same methods detailed above. As discussed, many may be amenable to nonoperative management. If laparotomy is performed for associated injuries, renal reconstruction should be done concomitantly. Tissue destruction is frequently much less than that seen with gunshot injuries. Frequently, entrance and exit wounds may be simply oversewn (Figs. 10–5 and 10–6). In the case of a deep slit-like renal stab wound, the thin parenchymal defect will not permit easy access to the collecting system. Clo-

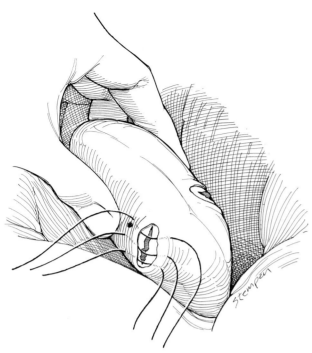

FIG. 10–5. Technique of renorrhaphy after stab wound. Gelfoam bolsters are laid into the capsular defect, and overlying 3-0 chromic sutures are placed superficially to approximate the adjoining renal capsule, thus sealing the reconstructed area.

sure of the overlying parenchyma usually rapidly seals the collecting system.

Renal vascular injuries are a major cause of renal loss and may coexist with parenchymal lacerations. Renovascular injuries are frequently irreparable and may result in

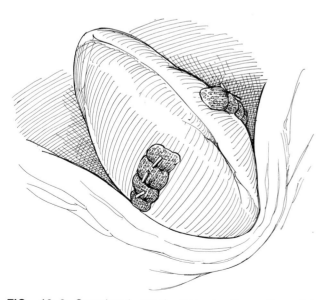

FIG. 10–6. Completed renal reconstruction after stab wound. The entire kidney has been mobilized and evaluated for associated wounds. Titanium clips along the capsular sutures denote the area of repair.

nephrectomy. Proximal control of the renal pedicle is in particular vital in these injuries to avoid significant hemorrhage. Venous injuries may occur along the main renal vein or in segmental branches. If venous reconstruction is feasible, a partially lacerated renal vein may be repaired with 5-0 Prolene following appropriate vascular clamping. Also, the left main renal vein may be ligated proximally because there is extensive collateral flow through the adrenal, lumbar, and gonadal branches. Smaller segmental veins can safely be ligated because of the internal collateral circulation of the venous system.

Outcomes of renal arterial reconstruction are time dependent because of the kidney's poor tolerance of prolonged warm ischemia. The success rate of renal arterial repair drops dramatically after 6 hours of warm ischemia. Attempts at renal arterial reconstruction should thus be reserved for the solitary kidney or bilateral renal arterial injuries. Penetrating injuries with incomplete transection may be repaired primarily with fine nonabsorbable suture, while blunt injuries typically require thrombectomy and debridement of the injured arterial segment. Segmental arterial injuries may be safely ligated, with few complications arising from the devascularized parenchyma.

Gross blood in the urine usually clears within 24 hours, and patients should be observed at bedrest during this time. Ambulation is resumed once the urine is clear. Serial hematocrits should be monitored because delayed bleeding is possible. Renal angiography and selective embolization may be considered in the event of continued hemorrhage. Retroperitoneal drains are normally removed within 48 to 72 hours. If drainage is excessive, an aliquot may be checked for creatinine; a level similar to that of serum suggests peritoneal fluid rather than urine. Blood pressure is checked before discharge. A radionuclide study is usually obtained around the time of discharge to assess function, and a renal imaging study is again obtained at about 3 months.

OUTCOMES

Complications

Small amounts of urinary extravasation are usually not clinically significant as long as they do not become infected. Large urinomas are best treated with percutaneous drainage with or without ureteral stent placement. Delayed renal hemorrhage is most likely within the first 2 weeks and is more commonly associated with stab wounds. Angiography and selective angioembolization is the treatment of choice. Hypertension occurs rarely after renal injuries, and it is usually easily controlled by medical therapy alone. Delayed nephrectomy may rarely be indicated when medical management fails to control hypertension. Arteriovenous fistula is an unusual complication of renal trauma. It is best treated with arteriography and fistula embolization.

Results

Renal reconstruction has achieved adequate preservation of function in 83% of patients at our institution (12). We have found renal salvage to be safe in the presence of concomitant bowel or pancreatic injuries (13). Early vascular control and application of reconstructive principles will help improve outcomes in the repair of the traumatically injured kidney.

REFERENCES

1. Brandes SB, McAninch JW. Urban free falls and patterns of renal injury: a 20 year experience with 396 cases. *J Trauma-Injury Infect Crit Care* 1999;47:643–649.
2. Bright TC, White K, Peters PC. Significance of hematuria after trauma. *J Urol* 1978;120:455.
3. Carroll PR, Klosterman P, McAninch JW. Early vascular control for renal trauma: a critical review. *J Urol* 1989;141:826–829.
4. McAninch JW. Surgery for renal trauma. In: Novick AC, Streem SB, Pontes JE, eds. *Stewart's operative urology*, 2nd ed. Baltimore: Williams & Wilkins, 1989:237–245.
5. Mee SL, McAninch JW, Robinson AL. Radiographic assessment of renal trauma: a 10-year prospective study of patient selection. *J Urol* 1989;141:1095–1098.
6. Miller KS, McAninch JW. Radiographic assessment of renal trauma: our 15-year experience. *J Urol* 1995;154:352–355.
7. Morey AF, Bruce JE, McAninch JW. Efficacy of radiographic imaging in pediatric blunt renal trauma. *J Urol* 1996;156:2014–2018.
8. Morey AF, McAninch JW, Tiller BK, Duckett CP, Carroll PR. Single shot interoperative excretory urography for the immediate evaluation of renal trauma. *J Urol* 1999;16(4):1088–1092.
9. Nash PA, Bruce JE, McAninch JW. Nephrectomy for traumatic renal injuries. *J Urol* 1995;153:609–611.
10. Santucci RA, et al. WHO/SIS Genitourinary Trauma Concensus Conference—Renal Trauma Subcommittee recommendations. Stockholm: S.I.U. International Conference, 2002.
11. Santucci RA, McAninch JW. Diagnosis and management of renal trauma: past, present and future. *J Am Coll Surg* 2000;191:443–451.
12. Wessels HB, Deirmenjian JM, McAninch JW. Quantitative assessment of renal function after renal reconstruction for trauma: radiographic scintigraphy results in 52 patients. *J Urol* 1997;157:1583–1586.
13. Wessels HB, McAninch JW. Effect of colon injury on the management of simultaneous renal trauma. *J Urol* 1996;155:1852–1856.
14. Wessels HB, Meyer A, McAninch JW. Criteria for conservative management of penetrating renal trauma: comparison of non-operative and surgical treatment of grade 2–4 renal lacerations due to gunshot and stab wounds. *J Urol* 1997;157:24–27.

CHAPTER 11

Renal Allotransplantation

Bruce A. Lucas

Successful transplantion of a kidney allograft and subsequent long-term immunosuppression management demand surgical precision and no tolerance for errors of judgment or technique. The devastating consequences of vascular, urologic, and infectious complications in renal transplantation, with their associated morbidity, mortality, and graft loss, are well documented. Fortunately, strict adherence to techniques and principles outlined in this chapter can reduce the incidence of these problems to low levels.

DIAGNOSIS

The diagnosis for which this procedure is performed is end-stage renal disease (ESRD). There is no specific diagnostic study that pertains to this operation.

INDICATIONS FOR SURGERY

The primary indication for renal allotransplantation is ESRD requiring chronic dialysis. Some patients with deteriorating renal function not yet requiring dialysis may also be candidates.

Active infections and malignancies are in general considered contraindications for transplantation with immunosuppressive therapy. Comorbidity in other organ systems, especially cardiovascular and pulmonary, may impose operative risks or compromise long-term prognosis significantly enough to preclude transplantation. Inadequate patient motivation, commitment, compliance, psychological stability, or social support may also be deterrents.

ALTERNATIVE THERAPY

ESRD patients may choose among the modalities of chronic dialysis for long-term life-sustaining treatment. Hemodialysis may be done at home or at a treatment center. Peritoneal dialysis is in general performed by the patient on a continuous ambulatory or overnight schedule.

SURGICAL TECHNIQUE

The prospective transplantation recipient should be in metabolic, fluid, and electrolyte balance to avoid perioperative hyperkalemia, unstable blood pressure, pulmonary edema, dehydration, or difficult operative hemostasis associated with inadequate dialysis. When dialysis can be scheduled in advance, as with living-related donor transplantation, it should be performed on the day before surgery. The patient's cardiopulmonary status needs to be well documented, and central venous pressure monitoring is routine. Swan–Ganz monitoring is often useful.

The entire abdomen to below the symphysis pubis is shaved and prepped after the induction of anesthesia and insertion of an indwelling 16 or 18 Fr Foley catheter. Any urine present in the bladder is submitted for culture. Then, the bladder is distended with 150 mL or more of an antibiotic solution, Neosporin GU Irrigant. This greatly facilitates the anterior cystotomy later in the procedure and, in addition, protects against possible wound contamination when the bladder is opened. After instillation of the antibiotic solution, the catheter is clamped. The clamp is removed only after the ureteroneocystomy and cystotomy closure are completed.

Incision and Iliac Fossa Dissection

A right or left lower-quadrant curvilinear incision is extended from the symphysis pubis passing 2 cm medial to the anterior superior iliac spine and up to about 4 to 5 cm below the lower costal margin (Fig. 11–1A). The upper half of the incision is extended through the external oblique, internal oblique, and transversus abdominis muscles; in the lower half of the incision, the anterior rectus fascia is incised. The rectus muscle can then be dissected inferiorly to its tendinous insertion on the symphysis pubis and retracted medially. In thin patients we prefer to keep the cephalad portion of the incision also within the lateral border of the rectus muscle, thereby

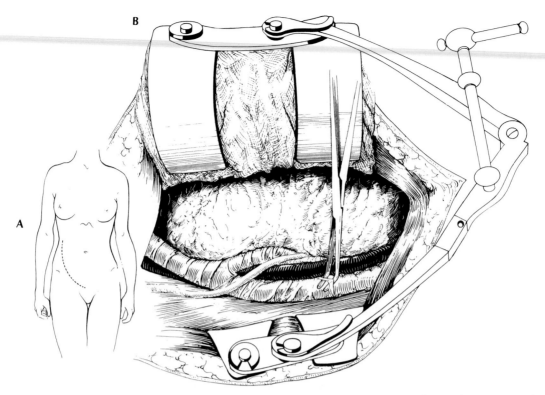

FIG. 11–1. A: The incision is depicted for the right abdomen, and subsequent illustrations represent graft implantation in the right iliac fossa. The renal transplantation, however, can be performed on either the right or left side. **B:** The iliac vessels are best exposed with a self-retaining retractor. Sequential separation, ligation, and division of perivascular tissue containing lymphatics are essential and must precede skeletonization of the iliac vessels.

obviating any transection of muscle and simplifying the closure. The inferior epigastric vessels are identified as they pass across the incision and are preserved for possible use later. Next, an anterolateral retroperitoneal fascial plane is developed, permitting extraperitoneal entry into the iliac fossa.

With medial retraction of the peritoneum, the spermatic cord in the male patient or round ligament in the female patient is easily identified. In men, some of the connective tissue around the cord is freed to permit easier retraction. Usually, cord ligation should be avoided to prevent hydrocele formation, testicular atrophy, or infertility. In women, the round ligament is divided and ligated. Further development of the extraperitoneal space in the iliac fossa is accomplished with exposure of the distal common and external iliac arteries. The insertion of a self-retaining retractor at this point assures adequate exposure for the subsequent iliac vessel dissection and vascular anastomoses.

The dissection and skeletonization of the iliac vessels must be performed in a manner that allows secure ligation of the divided lymphatics passing along and across these vessels. Usually, this process is best approached on the medial aspect of the external iliac vein, working cephalad with a right-angle clamp toward the internal

iliac artery, which crosses the vein. In some cases, especially when the donor kidney is large or has a short vein, the internal iliac artery must be sacrificed to achieve sufficient mobilization of the underlying vein. The iliac vein can be skeletonized as far cephalad as the vena cava if necessary. Posterior venous tributaries must be divided to permit maximum anterior mobility of the iliac vein. It is best to ligate all tributaries doubly with 2-0 or 3-0 silk in continuity before division because a double-clamping maneuver may sometimes result in injury or avulsion of a poorly accessible stump during ligation. Hemostasis then can be achieved only with difficulty and with risk of obturator nerve injury. Unless the internal iliac artery already has been selected for an end-to-end allograft anastomosis, right-angle clamp dissection is used to partially skeletonize the common and external iliac arteries (see Fig. 11–1B). The tissue overlying the arteries and containing the lymphatics is sequentially separated, doubly ligated with 3-0 silk, and divided, a strategy that greatly reduces the incidence of lymphocele. Again, this tissue should be doubly ligated before it is incised, in contrast with double clamping and division of the tissue. As with the vein, the anterior separation of tissue over the iliac artery is more easily performed in a cephalad direction.

At this point, palpation of the common iliac bifurcation and internal iliac artery determines the suitability of the internal iliac artery for an end-to-end anastomosis with the renal artery and the need for endarterectomy. If there is moderate or severe atherosclerosis extending into the bifurcation, or great size disparity, the internal iliac artery is usually not used. If an endarterectomy can be performed safely, or if there is little evidence of atheroma in the internal iliac vessel, skeletonization of this vessel prepares it for end-to-end anastomosis. Before skeletonization is begun, the lymphatics on the medial aspect of the iliac bifurcation should be doubly ligated and divided. If the internal iliac artery is to be used, it may be clamped proximally with a Fogarty clamp and divided distal to its bifurcation with appropriate ligation of the distal stumps deep in the pelvis. The mobilized internal iliac artery is irrigated with heparinized saline solution.

Allograft Positioning and Vascular Anastomoses

Before recipient vessel anastomotic sites are selected, visualization of the ultimate resting place for the allograft lateral or anterior to the iliac vessels should be considered, all anatomic factors being taken into account. The renal pelvis is usually positioned anterior to the renal vessels if a donor right kidney is being placed in the left iliac fossa or a donor left kidney is being placed on the right. The iliac vein is prepared for the end-to-side renal vein anastomosis by placement of clamps proximal and distal to the proposed venotomy. Fogarty clamps usually serve this purpose well. Excision of a thin ellipse of vein pro-

duces an ideal venotomy. The isolated segment of the iliac vein is irrigated with heparinized saline. After this, four 6-0 cardiovascular sutures are placed at the superior and inferior apices and at the midpoints of the medial and lateral margins of the venotomy. These sutures later are passed through corresponding points on the donor renal vein or vena cava patch for a four-quadrant end-to-side anastomosis.

If a cadaveric kidney is used, the allograft is removed from cold storage or perfusion preservation at this point. With living-related transplantation, the flushed and cooled graft is obtained from the live donor in an adjacent operating room.

The kidney is secured in a sling or a 3-in. stockinette (3) containing ice slush and held in position for the vascular anastomosis by the assistant. A clamp is used to secure the sling to relieve the assistant from holding the kidney in position with the hands, which might accelerate warming or compress the kidney during the performance of the vascular anastomoses.

The previously placed four sutures through the iliac vein are passed through the corresponding points of the donor renal vein, Carrel patch, or vena cava conduit and secured, bringing the renal vein into juxtaposition with the iliac vein (Fig. 11–2A). The medial and lateral sutures are retracted to separate the venotomy opening and facilitate rapid anastomosis without inadvertent suturing of the back wall. With the table rotated laterally, the superior suture is used as a running suture down the medial side of the renal vein to meet the inferior suture running up. The lateral suture line is then run in a similar fashion after the

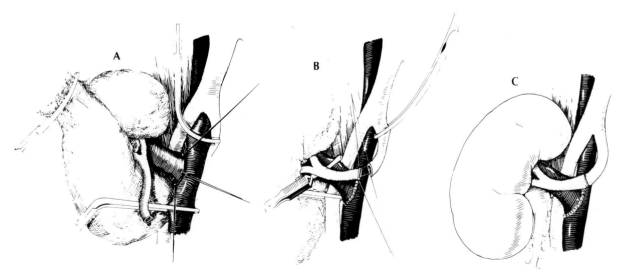

FIG. 11–2. A: The renal vein is brought into exact juxtaposition with the iliac vein phlebotomy by previously placed four-quadrant sutures. A running suture anastomosis will follow. **B:** The renal artery is positioned to the end of the internal iliac artery by superior and inferior apical sutures. Subsequent placement of interrupted sutures completes the anastomosis. Note the occluding bulldog clamp on the renal vein. **C:** The completed venous and arterial anastomoses are demonstrated.

table has been rotated medially. Although the clamps on the iliac vein may be left in place until completion of the arterial anastomosis, application of a finger Fogarty or a bulldog clamp across the renal vein at this time allows for removal of the iliac vein clamps and earlier restoration of venous return from the lower extremity.

If the internal iliac artery is to be used for the arterial anastomosis, an end-to-end anastomosis is then performed with the renal artery (see Fig. 11–2B). The two vessels are positioned to allow a gentle upward curve from the iliac bifurcation to the kidney by fixating the superior and inferior arterial apices with interrupted 6-0 cardiovascular sutures. The anastomosis is completed with continuous or interrupted sutures. With the kidney resting in the iliac fossa or suspended in a sling, the initial interrupted suture may be placed midway between the apical sutures on the anterior vessel walls facing the operator, thus allowing better approximation of the opposing arterial margins, in particular when a discrepancy exists in the size of the vessels. Subsequently, the remaining sutures are placed to approximate each anterior quadrant. Next, the previously placed apical sutures are used to rotate the arteries so that the posterior vessel walls are now in the anterior position for subsequent interrupted or running suture placement. As before, a suture placed midway between the apical sutures again divides the rotated posterior vessel walls into quadrants for subsequent suture placement. A preference for interrupted sutures instead of a running suture in this end-to-end anastomosis prevails when one needs to avoid absolutely any pursestring effect that might occur from a running suture or to achieve optimal accommodation of the two vessels to each other when a size or thickness discrepancy exists.

In most cases, the internal iliac artery is left intact to preserve potency in men as well as gluteal and pelvic blood supply in the elderly. Therefore, end-to-side anastomosis of the renal artery to the external or common iliac artery is chosen more commonly than the end-to-end procedure just described. This anastomosis usually is placed cephalad to the level of the venous anastomosis. The location of clamp placement must be carefully selected so as not to disrupt existing arteriosclerotic plaques and precipitate embolization or thrombosis. A longitudinal incision is made on the anterior or anterolateral portion of the iliac artery segment with a no. 11 blade knife, and a 4.8- or 5.6-mm aortic punch is used to prepare an ideal oval arteriotomy. After the incision is made, regional heparinization of the lower extremity may be accomplished by instilling about 80 to 100 mL of heparinized saline (1,000 U per 100 mL) into the distal iliac limb. Systemic heparinization is usually not necessary. This anastomosis is also performed with 6-0 cardiovascular continuous or interrupted sutures after initial fixation of the end of the renal artery to an apex of the

arteriotomy with sutures cinched down by the parachute technique.

The previously placed sling around the kidney is removed. The vascular clamps are released after intravenous infusion of mannitol and methylprednisolone, venous clamps before arterial. At this point, the patient should be judiciously overhydrated with saline and albumin and a dopamine drip should be ready to optimize renal blood flow if needed.

Multiple Renal Vessels

Although the Carrel patch may frequently be used with single arteries and veins, a cadaveric kidney with multiple renal arteries perfused through the aorta is especially well suited to an end-to-side anastomosis of a Carrel patch encompassing the multiple arteries (Fig. 11–3) (1). If the vessels are close to each other, a single Carrel patch is sufficient. If the vessels are more than 2 cm apart, we prefer two Carrel patches. The Carrel patch of donor aorta is fashioned to accommodate the multiple vessels, and its anastomosis to the common or external iliac artery is performed with continuous 5-0 or

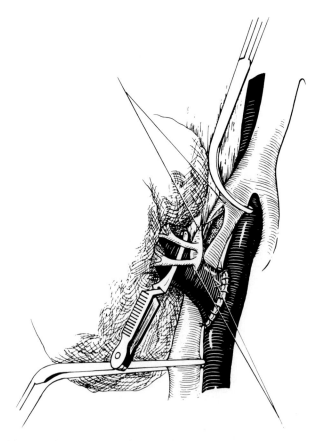

FIG. 11–3. A donor aorta Carrel patch encompassing two renal arteries is positioned by apical sutures to an iliac arteriotomy fashioned to accommodate the length and width of the patch.

6-0 cardiovascular sutures after an arteriotomy that accommodates the width and length of the Carrel patch. This anastomosis is best performed by fixating the patch at the superior and inferior apices of the arteriotomy or by the parachute technique. Each suture limb runs away from the apex.

The presence of multiple arteries in related donor transplantation is known in advance because all living-related donors have preoperative spiral computed tomography scans or arteriograms. Most donors have at least one kidney with a single artery, but, at times, a donor kidney with double or triple arteries must be used. These arteries cannot be taken with a Carrel patch because of the risk to the donor. In these instances, several strategies for arterial anastomoses are possible: (a) double end-to-side renal arteries to iliac artery, (b) end-to-end superior renal artery to internal iliac artery with end-to-side inferior renal artery to external iliac artery, and (c) implantation of an accessory artery end-to-side into the larger main renal artery, with the larger renal artery anastomosed to the internal, external, or common iliac artery. If two renal arteries are of similar diameter, the spatulation edges of the renal arteries can be joined by the "trousers technique" with a running 6-0 or 7-0 cardiovascular sutures to create a single bifurcating artery (2). An accessory artery-to-main renal artery anastomosis should be performed with *ex vivo* bench technique in cold ice slush before the renal vein anastomosis is done. Finally, some recipients have a deep inferior epigastric artery that is suitable for end-to-end 7-0 suture interrupted anastomosis of a small lower-pole artery, which may be essential for ureteral viability (7). Our experience in more than 30 cases with this technique has been excellent; no ureteral ischemia or necrosis has occurred.

Ureteral Considerations

When the recipient urinary bladder is functional, ureteroneocystostomy is the preferred technique for establishing urinary tract continuity unless the donor ureter is absent, very short, abnormal, or damaged. Ureterectasis is not a contraindication. When the donor ureter is not suitable, recipient ureter may be used for ureteroureterostomy or ureteropyelostomy (9). If recipient ureter is not available but the bladder is large, psoas hitch or Boari flap techniques may be used for ureteroneocystostomy or pyelocystostomy.

Some patients are prepared for kidney transplantation by creation of an ileal loop or isolated ileal stoma to divert urine from a dysfunctional or absent bladder. Other patients may come to transplantation with preexisting bladder augmentations or continent urinary diversions utilizing ileum and colon. The nuances of techniques in these settings are beyond the scope of this discussion.

While we have used all of the above techniques successfully, greater than 95% of all renal transplantations are performed with various modifications of the Politano–Leadbetter, Paquin, and Lich techniques for allograft ureteral implantation into the bladder. In our experience, when the bladder is very small or the donor ureter is very short an extravesical technique is best (5). Otherwise, we prefer the ease and reliability of a transvesical approach with or without a formal submucosal tunnel (6). In either case, previous filling of the bladder facilitates a longitudinal anterior cystotomy with minimal trauma to the bladder wall. In the transvesical approach, the bladder dome is packed and retracted cephalad, exposing the bas-fond. An oblique tunnel is created in the bladder floor using a tonsil clamp directed toward the trigone from outside the bladder. This maneuver prevents subsequent angulation of the ureter when the bladder is distended. An 8 Fr Robinson catheter or heavy silk is grasped by the tonsil clamp, passed through the tunnel in retrograde fashion, and secured to the donor ureter (Fig. 11–4A).

The ureter is pulled down and brought into position in the bladder by gentle traction. This maneuver avoids any handling of the ureter, which is important because the ureter of the transplanted kidney receives its blood supply exclusively from the renal vessel branches that course in its adventitia. In male patients, it is important to pass the ureter beneath the spermatic cord. Intravesically, the ureter is hemitransected about 4 cm from its entrance site into the bladder and spatulated about 1 cm.

Four sutures of 4-0 chromic catgut are usually sufficient for an anastomosis incorporating bladder mucosa and muscularis (Fig. 11–4B) as the ureteral transection is completed. When the apical stitch also catches ureteral adventitia 1 to 2 cm above the apex, a nice everted ureteral nipple may be produced. This eversion is especially desirable with patulous ureters. The ureter is not stented routinely. A no-touch technique is essential to avoid producing vascular insufficiency, ureteral necrosis, and urinary extravasation from injury to the adventitial vascular network of the ureter.

The oblique bladder tunnel and muscle hiatus must accommodate the ureter comfortably to avoid postoperative obstruction from edema, and a gentle oblique course of the ureter must be ensured so that no kinks, twists, or obstructions occur. This attention is important because the ureter of a transplanted kidney crosses the iliac vessels in a much more caudal position than the native ureter. A little redundancy of the ureter is established outside the bladder to ensure that the ureteroneocystostomy is done without tension and that postoperative allograft swelling will not unduly stretch or angulate the ureter. Patency of the ureteroneocystostomy is confirmed by gently passing a 5 Fr feeding tube or an 8 Fr or smaller soft Robinson catheter toward the renal pelvis.

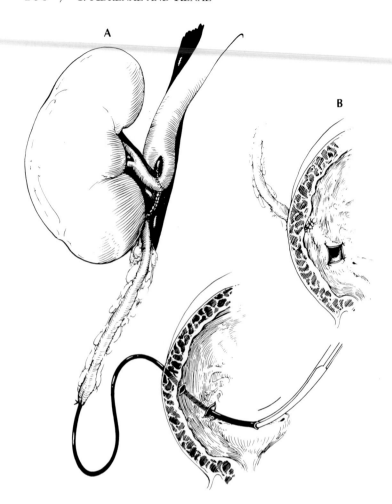

FIG. 11–4. Ureteroneocystostomy. **A:** A small Robinson catheter or heavy silk suture with donor ureter attached is brought into the bladder through an oblique hiatus. **B:** The completed transplant ureteroneocystostomy is demonstrated. Four interrupted sutures secure the spatulated ureteral orifice.

Kidneys with a double ureter can also be transplanted successfully. These ureters should be dissected *en bloc* within their common adventitial sheath and periureteral fat so that the ureteral blood supply is protected. The technique of ureteroneocystostomy is essentially the same as with a single ureter except that the ureters are brought through together side by side in a nonconstricting tunnel. The distal end of each ureter is spatulated, and the adjacent margins are approximated with 5-0 chromic catgut.

To ensure a watertight closure, the cystotomy incision is closed in three layers. The first 3-0 chromic running suture secures the full thickness of the bladder near the bladder neck and closes the mucosal layer. The second 2-0 chromic running suture is an inverting layer of muscularis. The third 2-0 chromic layer inverts the adventitia. Each layer should overlap the immediately underlying layer about 0.5 cm at each end of the cystotomy closure to avoid urinary extravasation at these two points.

Rarely, situations occur in which ureteroneocystostomy unexpectedly cannot be performed and native ureters are not available. In this setting, cutaneous ureterostomy is preferred. Alternatively, an ileal loop may be created at the time of transplantation. Ureterosigmoidostomy should be avoided.

Pediatric Kidneys

Although *en-bloc* transplantation of kidneys from very young children is often desirable (4), it is not necessary to transplant both kidneys from young children *en bloc*; each kidney can be used for a different recipient, as is the case with adult cadaveric donors, using Carrel patches of donor aorta and vena cava (Fig. 11–5) (8). A Carrel patch is mandatory in these cases because direct implantation of a small vessel into a much larger or diseased vessel may result in thrombosis or produce functional stenosis as the kidney grows. When the *en-bloc* technique is used, the two ureters are implanted separately and stented. Pediatric kidneys have proven to be excellent donor grafts for carefully selected adults and children. Avoidance of older recipients or diabetics with advanced arteriosclerosis will minimize the potential for thrombosis. Rapid growth and hypertrophy occur in the immediate posttransplantation period. If early rejection can be avoided, these allografts achieve

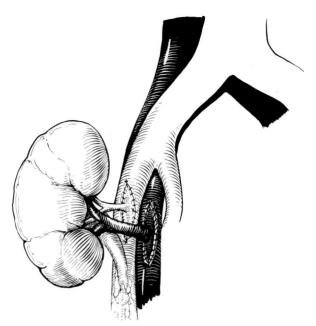

FIG. 11–5. Small pediatric cadaver renal vessels are anastomosed to larger recipient iliac vessels using Carrel patches of donor aorta and vena cava. Note donor right kidney in right iliac fossa with renal pelvis posterior to renal vessels.

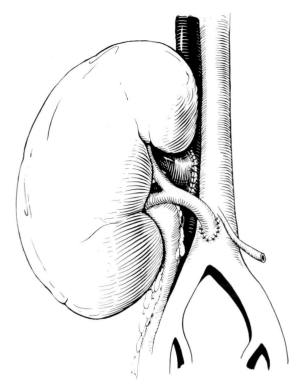

FIG. 11–6. Anatomic relationships of an adult donor kidney in a small child are shown with renal vessel anastomoses to the inferior vena cava and aorta

adult size and function in adult recipients within several weeks.

Pediatric Transplantation

In small children, the iliac fossa is not large enough to accommodate a kidney from an adult donor, and the pelvic vessels in a small child are so small that the disparity between the donor renal vessels and the recipient vessels precludes the technique described for adults. In these small children, graft implantation must use the recipient aorta and vena cava, which is best accomplished through a right-sided retroperitoneal or transperitoneal midline abdominal incision that provides ready access to the great vessels as well as the urinary bladder. After the right colon is reflected medially, the right kidney is usually removed to make room for the allograft. The vena cava is then freed from the level of the right renal vein inferiorly to its bifurcation or beyond. Posterior lumbar veins are doubly ligated with 5-0 silk and divided. Mobilization of the vena cava is important to facilitate the end-to-side anastomosis of the renal vein, which is performed with running 6-0 cardiovascular sutures, as described for the adult (Fig. 11–6). Performing the venous anastomosis superiorly allows room for an end-to-side anastomosis of the renal artery to the inferior abdominal aorta. Aortic mobilization should be limited to its distal portion, from the level of the inferior mesenteric artery, and including both common iliac arteries. The segment of the aorta to be used for the end-to-side renal artery anastomosis can

be isolated by a superior pediatric vascular clamp and by two inferior clamps or silastic loops on the common iliac arteries. The end-to-side anastomosis is performed with interrupted 6-0 cardiovascular sutures.

Important to the revascularization of an adult kidney in small children is the need to anticipate the impending consumption of several hundred milliliters of effective blood volume by the renal allograft. Initiation of blood transfusion before beginning the vascular anastomoses will avoid hypotension after release of the vascular clamps. When the vascular anastomoses are completed, the superior aortic clamp must be kept loosely in place until it is clear that hypotension is not a problem. Immediately after establishing circulation in the graft, the anesthesiologist must be continually attentive to the blood pressure until stabilization is assured. The ureteral implantation is carried out as described except that the ureter must be passed retroperitoneally behind the bladder near the midline.

Wound Closure

Except in unusual cases, the allograft ureter is not stented and the space of Retzius and iliac fossa are not drained. Jackson–Pratt suction may be employed, but Penrose drains are never used. If good hemostasis has been obtained, and if the principles of implantation as outlined in this chapter have been followed, there is no need for postoperative drainage other than a urethral catheter. The optimal period of Foley catheter drainage is debatable. We prefer to remove the catheter within 48 hours unless the patient has worrisome hematuria, large diuresis, or poor bladder function.

In preparation for closure, the wound is thoroughly irrigated with saline. A 1 or 0 Maxon running suture is used to approximate transversus abdominis and internal oblique muscles in a single-layer closure; the adjacent fascia is included inferiorly at the tendinous insertion of the rectus muscle. Next, the rectus fascia anteriorly and the fascia of the external oblique are approximated with a 1 Prolene running suture.

The subcutaneous tissue is thoroughly irrigated with saline and then may be approximated with interrupted 2-0 or 3-0 sutures. These sutures are placed about 3 cm apart and include both edges of Scarpa's fascia and the underlying fascia. In this manner, one can obliterate dead space in the subcutaneous area in which a seroma in an immunosuppressed patient might cause dehiscence and become secondarily infected. The skin is approximated with interrupted fine nylon sutures or staples.

OUTCOME

Complications

Early vascular complications of kidney transplantation include arterial thrombosis, venous thrombosis, and anastomatic bleeding. These each occur in less than 1% of cases unless the recipient or donor vessels are diseased or small caliber. Renal or iliac artery stenosis may lead to allograft ischemia or thrombosis months or years posttransplant in 2% to 10% of cases.

Urologic complications are slightly more common than vascular complications but less likely to lead to graft loss. When donor ureter and recipient bladder are normal, early ureteral necrosis, ureteral anastomotic leak, or obstruction each occur in less than 1% of cases. Compromised ureteral blood supply during donor nephrectomy or abnormal bladder are the most likely factors increasing these risks. Ureteral stenosis months or years posttransplant is most often a result of chronic rejection. Lymphocele occurring in 6% to 10% of transplants may be considered a urologic complication if it causes extrinsic ureteral obstruction or bladder compression. Lymphocele requires intervention posttransplant only if it becomes infected or causes pain, iliac vein compression, or allograft ureteropyelocaliectasis. Calyceal rupture and longitudinal allograft rupture, rarely seen in recent years, are usually associated with a combination of ureteral obstruction and the ischemia and edema produced by severe acute rejection or preservation injury.

Infectious, cardiovascular, metabolic, pharmacological, and psychosocial complications of transplantation

TABLE 11–1. *2002 annual report of the US Organ and Transplantation Network and the Scientific Registry of Transplant Recipients: Transplant data 1992 to 2001*

	Living donor	Cadaveric donor
3-mo patient survival	99.0%	97.3%
1-yr patient survival	97.7%	94.0%
3-yr patient survival	94.7%	88.4%
5-yr patient survival	89.7%	79.9%
3-mo graft survival	96.8%	93.5%
1-yr graft survival	94.4%	88.4%
3-yr graft survival	88.3%	78.5%
5-yr graft survival	76.5%	63.3%

From the Department of Health and Human Services, Health Resources and Services Administration, Office of Special Programs, Division of Transplantation, Rockville, MD; United Network for Organ Sharing, Richmond, VA; and University Renal Research and Education Association, Ann Arbor, MI, with permission.

are beyond the scope of this presentation. Acute rejection superimposed on preservation injury produced irreversible failure in more than half of all cadaver donor renal allografts in the early days of transplantation. In recent years the rate of irreversible acute rejection is less than 10% in nearly all programs. Chronic rejection, however, continues to take its toll over many years.

Results

The 2002 Annual Report of the US Organ Procurement and Transplantation Network documents 5-year allograft survival for living donor and cadaveric donor renal transplantation of 76.5% and 63.3%, respectively, as seen in Table 11–1.

REFERENCES

1. Belzer FO, Schweizer RT, Kountz SL. Management of multiple vessels in renal transplantation. *Transplant Proc* 1972;4:639–644.
2. Codd JE, Anderson CB, Graff RJ, Gregory JG, Lucas BA, Newton WT. Vascular surgical problems in renal transplantation. *Arch Surg* 1974; 108:876–878.
3. Gill IBS, Munch LC, Lucas BA. Use of a cotton stockinette to minimize warm ischemia during renal transplant vascular anastomoses. *J Urol* 1994;152:2053–2054.
4. Kinne DW, Spanos PK, DeShazo MM, Simmons RL, Najarian JS. Double renal transplants from pediatric donors to adult recipients. *Am J Surg* 1974;127:292–295.
5. Konnak JW, Herwig KR, Finkbeiner A, Turcotte JG, Freier DT. Extravesical ureteroneocystostomy in 170 renal transplant patients. *J Urol* 1975;113:299–301.
6. Lucas BA, McRoberts JW, Curtis JJ, Luke RG. Controversy in renal transplantation: Antireflux versus non-antireflux ureteroneocystostomy. *J Urol* 1979;121:156–158.
7. Merkel FK, Straus AK, Anderson O, Bannett AD. Microvascular techniques for polar artery reconstruction in kidney transplants. *Surgery* 1976;79:253–261.
8. Salvatierra O Jr, Belzer FO. Pediatric cadaver kidneys: their use in renal transplantation. *Arch Surg* 1975;110:181–183.
9. Welchel JD, Cosimi AB, Young HH, Russell PS. Pyeloureterostomy reconstruction in human renal transplantation. *Ann Surg* 1975;181: 61–66.

CHAPTER 12

Ureteral Complications Following Renal Transplantation

Rodney J. Taylor

Historically, the incidence of urologic complications following kidney transplantation, manifested primarily as ureteral leaks or obstruction, was as high as 10% (1,5). These complications often resulted in significant morbidity, graft loss, and occasional patient death. Improvements in surgical techniques, immunosuppression, and methods for diagnosing and treating the complications have led not only to a significant decline in the rate of urologic complications to the current reported incidence of 2% to 2.5% (4,7,9) but resulted in lower morbidity and rare loss of a kidney or patient to these complications. However, despite these changes, the need for diligence in diagnosing and quickly addressing them remains as true today as in the past.

The most common cause for ureteral complications following kidney transplantation is technical error (1,5,7). Damage to the ureteral blood supply during graft harvest or transplantation may result in ureteral ischemia and subsequent leak or obstruction. Additional technical errors such as excessive tension at the ureteroneocystostomy site or hematoma development within the tunnel may also cause problems (4,7). With careful attention to detail, most of these problems can be minimized, especially in the early postoperative setting. Long-term or delayed ureteral obstruction may be the result of ischemic changes secondary to chronic rejection or a continuation of the spectrum of damage associated with the organ harvest and transplantation, and although not all are preventable the incidence can be markedly reduced with good surgical technique (1,4). The types of ureteral complications can be divided into ureteral leaks and ureteral obstruction.

DIAGNOSIS

Urinary Leaks

In current practice, most surgeons utilize an extravesical ureteroneocystostomy that uses a shorter ureter, decreasing the likelihood of ureteral ischemia, and utilizes a limited cystostomy that rarely leads to leakage from the bladder (4,10). Therefore, virtually all urinary leaks seen after transplantation are ureteric. The majority of these leaks occur early after transplantation and are usually manifested by either drainage from the wound, unexplained graft dysfunction, or a pelvic fluid collection. Signs and symptoms can also include fever, graft tenderness, and lower-extremity edema (8). It is critical to differentiate a suspected urinary leak from a lymphocele, as the management is entirely different.

Urinary leaks in the early postoperative period can be divided into two types according to the timing of presentation. The first usually occurs within the first 1 to 4 days and is almost always related to technical problems with the implantation. In this case, the heel of the ureter has usually retracted out of the tunnel. This is usually caused by excessive tension at the site of the anastomosis. This complication appears to be more common with the extravesical ureteroneocystostomies and may be the result of too much shortening of the ureter and subsequent tension on the anastomosis when the kidney is positioned in the pelvis (8). Some investigators have recommended use of a ureteral stent to lessen the likelihood of this complication (4,5). We recommend placing the kidney in its eventual position before deciding how much to shorten the ureter. The old adage "measure twice and cut once" applies in this circumstance.

The second type of early ureteral leak is associated with distal ureteral ischemia, which may be a consequence of injury during the donor recovery, technical causes such as tunnel hematoma, or distal stripping of the blood supply. This type usually presents between 5 and 10 days posttransplant (7).

Urinary leaks are often suspected because of increased drainage from the wound while at the same time associated with decreased urinary output. This is especially true in patients with limited pretransplant urine production. In patients with normal pretransplant urinary output, wound drainage and graft dysfunction are the key signs. The drainage fluid should be tested for blood urea nitrogen (BUN)/creatinine to see if it is compatible with urine. The preferred radiographic tests include an abdominal ultrasound and nuclear renal scan. A renal scan demonstrating extravasation is the most sensitive method to differentiate a urine leak from other fluid collections such as lymphoceles or hematomas (2). A cystogram should be performed if a bladder leak is suspected.

Ureteral Obstruction

Ureteral obstruction can also be the result of ureteral ischemia but usually occurs later than ureteral leaks and usually presents as acute graft dysfunction. It may occur years after the transplant and in this situation may represent vascular injury associated not only with the technical complications but also with chronic rejection (1,7,8). The spectrum of ureteral ischemic injury extends from early necrosis and urinary leakage to delayed ureteral obstruction, presenting months to years after the actual transplantation.

Ureteral obstruction, usually manifested by graft dysfunction, requires evaluation, and again an ultrasound and nuclear renal scan are the most common screening studies. Additional radiographic studies such as a computed tomography (CT) scan may be of assistance in some cases. With both ureteral leak and obstruction, endourologic techniques can be both diagnostic and therapeutic.

INDICATIONS FOR SURGERY

Anything that causes graft dysfunction or results in disruption of the urinary tract in a renal transplant patient is of utmost concern and requires rapid diagnosis and treatment. In the case of ureteral leakage or obstruction, the goals of treatment include careful and accurate diagnosis of the exact cause and site. To correct the leak caused by excessive tension, it is often possible to do a repeat ureteroneocystostomy as soon as the diagnosis is made. In most other cases, especially with the current techniques of extravesical reimplantation, a different operative procedure is often more suitable (5,7).

If the graft dysfunction problem has a physical cause such as a leak or an obstruction and is not associated with an acute rejection episode, then treatment is directed at stabilization of the renal function, minimization of morbidity, and a restoration of the continuity and function of the urinary tract. If there is concomitant rejection, then definitive operative therapy is withheld pending the treatment of rejection (7,8).

ALTERNATIVE THERAPY

The need for immediate open operative surgical intervention has been replaced, to a large extent, by early endourologic intervention (1,6–8). The placement of a percutaneous nephrostomy can divert a leak or relieve obstruction and allow more definitive diagnosis. As described by Streem, endourologic management algorithms can select patients for whom the likelihood of successful nonoperative management is good. Depending on the selection criteria, the results of management of distal ureteral leaks with stenting and a nephrostomy tube show that approximately one-third of patients do well long term and require no additional treatment. For ureteral strictures or stenoses, approximately 45% of patients, carefully selected, will avoid an open operative repair (8). For the other patients, percutaneous access can allow stabilization of renal function and a more critical assessment before open surgical repair is carried out. In a few cases, percutaneous access can offer long-term treatment with chronic stent management. This choice, in my opinion, is of limited application in most patients with a well-functioning graft because of the long-term risks (i.e., stone formation, infection, etc.) and inherent costs. However, in patients who are not operative candidates and for some patients with marginal graft function chronic endourologic treatment can be an alternative to definitive repair (5).

SURGICAL TECHNIQUE

There are many procedures available to restore the continuity of the urinary tract (1–3,5–7). In our experience in dealing with a difficult ureteral stenosis or a leak from significant ureteral ischemic necrosis, we favor the use of the native ureter to replace the transplant ureter. Advantages of this repair include: The native ureter is usually nonrefluxing, the results are reliable, there is a low likelihood of recurrence of the primary problem, and a tension-free anastomosis with good blood supply is easily attained. The focus of this operative description is on that surgical choice. Other operative alternatives include reimplantation of the ureter, Boari flap ureteral replacement, pyelovesicostomy and psoas hitch with reimplantation. As with many operative procedures, having a variety of alternatives available enhances the likelihood of a successful result.

Surgical access to the transplanted kidney and ureters (transplant and native) is usually achieved by reopening the old incision. On occasion, if extensive mobilization of transplanted kidney is anticipated or access to the contralateral native ureter is planned a midline incision is another option (7). Surgical access to repair an early ureteral leak is usually simplified because dense fibrosis has not yet occurred, the fascial layers are easily opened, the peritoneum and its contents are freely mobilized medially and cephalad, and the kidney and ureter are identified without much difficulty. A primary repair can often be performed, and in most cases a repeat ureteroneocystostomy at a new site in the bladder is the best choice. Use of a mechanical retractor greatly simplifies exposure and allows excellent access to the pelvis. We also recommend the use of loupe magnification (2× to 3×) to enhance the repair.

If the repair has been delayed because of attempted endourologic management or because of delay in presentation or diagnosis, then access to the ureter and kidney can be much more challenging and hazardous. In these cases, mandatory preoperative preparation includes a review of the operative note, especially if the operation was performed by someone else. It is important to know whether the kidney to be operated on was the donor's right or left kidney. It is critical to know the position of the ureter and renal pelvis in relation to the renal vessels (below or above), and this depends on which kidney was used and into which side of the recipient's pelvis it was transplanted. Additional information to be sought includes the type of vascular anastomosis performed (end-to-end vs. end-to-side, etc.) and whether or not the iliac vessels (especially the iliac vein) were mobilized. All of this information can help determine the likely position of the kidney in relation to the transplanted and native ureter and the anticipated ease in gaining access to these structures. Figure 12–1 demonstrates the relationship of the transplanted kidney, vessels, and ureter to the recipient's iliac vessels and ureter. Note that this depicts a donor left kidney on the right side, as the renal pelvis is posterior to the renal vessels.

In terms of the recipient, it is critical to know the status of the recipient's urinary tract. This is especially true if the recipient had a history of ureteral reflux or had undergone nephroureterectomy and might not have a suitable native ureter available to use for repair. Finally, the status of the recipient's urinary bladder in terms of capacity, compliance, and function can be important in determining which other repair options are available.

Additional preoperative preparation involves stabilization of the patient and function of the graft. It is important to delay any open operative repair until concurrent rejection episodes have been adequately treated and renal function stabilized. All patients should be treated with preoperative antibiotics based on anticipated contaminants or cultures obtained from the urine. If there is a likelihood that bowel might be needed (an unusual circumstance) to repair the urinary tract, then a full bowel preparation is indicated.

The goals of surgery are to repair the ureteral defect, reestablish continuity of the urinary system, get rid of all foreign bodies as quickly as possible, and avoid graft or patient loss. With a well-planned and executed procedure, these goals should be easily obtained in essentially all cases.

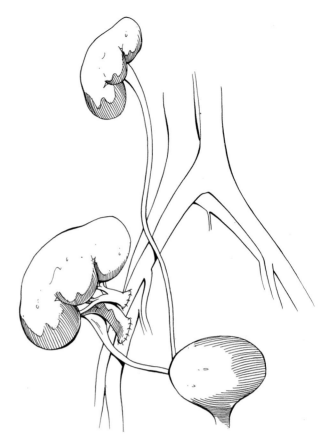

FIG. 12–1. Relationship of the transplanted kidney and its vasculature to the recipient's iliac vessels and ureter.

Delayed surgical repair because of attempted endourologic management, delayed diagnosis, or late presentation of obstruction can make surgical exposure of the kidney and ureter challenging. As noted earlier, access is almost always achieved through the old transplant incision, and cephalad extension of the incision is often needed in these cases because of perinephric fibrosis, the increased size of the kidney posttransplant, and the need to achieve access to the iliac vessels and native ureter. It is usually possible to extend the incision several centimeters cephalad. Additional exposure, if needed, can also be obtained by extending the inferior aspect of the incision across the midline, although this is rarely needed and should be delayed until the need presents itself.

With delayed repair, the normal tissue planes are obliterated and a dense fibrosis has occurred around the graft. This makes it easy to violate the "renal capsule" and get into significant bleeding. As a routine, it is preferable to operate from a position of "known to unknown" with good exposure. The surgeon should also plan to gain vascular control proximally and distally if it appears that the kidney may need to be mobilized to permit access to the renal pelvis. A three-way Foley catheter should always be placed into the bladder before the start of surgery to allow for irrigation and filling with an antibiotic solution.

To assure a safe and adequate exposure, I usually open the peritoneum early in cases where there is dense fibrosis. This allows better cephalad exposure, protects the bowel, and gives good access to the bladder.

Because the transplant ureter usually crosses the external iliac vessels below the renal vessels, one should take care to avoid these structures while gaining access to the ureter. This is a critical feature of this operative procedure because exact visualization of the renal vascular structures is often difficult, and many times one is operating based on the expected, not visualized, location of these structures. In some cases a percutaneous nephrostomy tube will be placed as well as a ureteral stent. If present, the nephrostomy tube should be accessible during a procedure as injection of saline or methylene blue may aid in identifying the ureter and renal pelvis. In some cases, because of the dense fibrosis, the ureter is identified only when it is actually cut. The routine placement of a ureteral stent is of limited value in most cases because the fibrosis is so dense that it is hard to discern the presence of the catheter. If the ureter is not in dense fibrosis, then access is usually easy.

Once access to the bony pelvis is obtained, careful dissection along the lateral wall of the bladder usually leads to the ureter. Once it is identified, care must be used in mobilizing the ureter to avoid any further vascular injury. When the site of leakage and/or obstruction has been identified, the most commonly used repairs include (a) a repeat ureteroneocystostomy, (b) use of the bladder (Boari flap or bladder hitch) to help bridge the gap, or (c) use of a native ureter to perform a ureteroureterostomy or ureteropyelostomy. Repeat ureteroneocystostomies are indicated only to repair early leaks when the problem was from tension at the anastomosis or distal ureteral ischemia and a well-vascularized minimally fibrosed ureter is present. In most circumstances, especially late, with a lot of periureteral reaction or ischemia our preferred option is the use of the ipsilateral native ureter if it is present and of adequate caliber. If not, then a Boari flap is an excellent choice.

Access to the native ureter is obtained by identifying it as it crosses the common iliac vessels. Care must be used in mobilizing the ureter down into the pelvis to the level of the superior vesical artery to avoid injury to the ureter blood supply. The ureter is divided well above the iliac vessels and the proximal end of the ureter is doubly ligated. In our experience of more than 35 cases, this has not resulted in problems of hydronephrosis with the native kidney or ureter requiring any further intervention. Figure 12–2 shows the native ureter mobilized distally and doubly ligated proximally in preparation for a ureteropyelostomy.

The operative positioning of the native ureter depends on access to the transplant ureter and/or pelvis. In addition, whether a side-to-side ureteral anastomosis or a ureteropyelostomy is to be performed may make a differ-

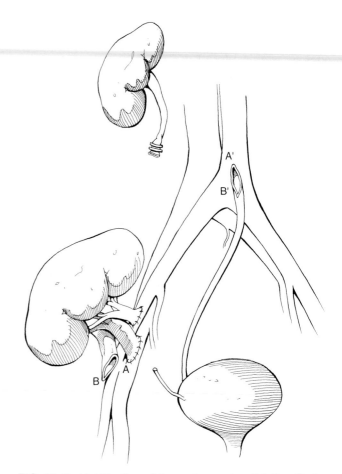

FIG. 12–2. Mobilization of the native ureter distally with the proximal segment ligated.

ence in the exact positioning of the native ureter. All of these factors relate to the extent of fibrosis and the appearance of the transplant ureter. To prevent any additional future problems, a tension-free, widely spatulated anastomosis of well-vascularized ureter to either transplant ureter or renal pelvis is critical (Fig. 12–3). The anastomosis is performed using 5-0 Maxon (Davis and Geck, Danbury, CT) or polydioxanone (PDS, Ethicon, Somerville, NJ) in a watertight single layer. The critical aspect is to obtain a mucosa-to-mucosa approximation avoiding tension, devascularization, and urinary leak. A 12-cm 4.7 double-J stent is routinely used on all anastomoses. The anastomosis may be in addition wrapped in omentum or peritoneal flap, if available, to decrease further the risk of leak. The wound is well irrigated with antibiotic solution, and if no preoperative infection was present we close the wound without a drain. If there is concern about urinary leak, lymphatic leak, or possible infection, one or two Jackson–Pratt drains are indicated. The fascia is closed in layers with a 0 or no. 1 permanent monofilament suture. The subcutaneous tissue is not closed. The skin is usually closed with staples. A nephrostomy tube, if present, is removed at day 5 to 7 after an antegrade nephrostogram has been obtained to be

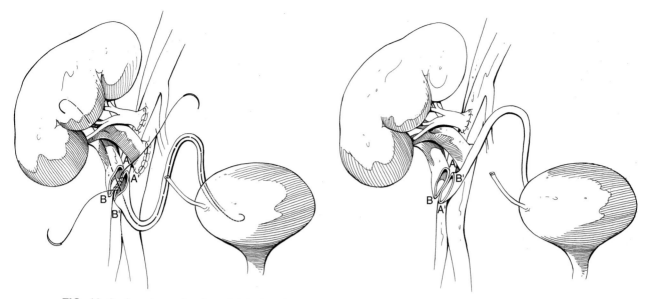

FIG. 12–3. Anastomosis of spatulated native ureter to **(A)** transplant ureter and **(B)** transplant renal pelvis.

sure that there is no leak. The ureteral catheter is left in for 4 to 6 weeks.

OUTCOMES

Complications

Complications that can occur postprocedure include infection, urinary leak, bleeding, recurrence of the stricture, and possible loss of graft. In all series, these are uncommon complications (1,7).

Results

We have performed over 35 native-to-transplant ureteroureterostomies or ureteropyelostomies to treat ureteral obstruction or ureteral leaks or deal with damaged ureters at the time of the transplant. In our experience, all kidneys involved have been "salvaged" and none lost to urologic complications. There have been no significant postoperative complications and no patient deaths. We have not had to repeat any procedures in any of the patients we have treated and have not had any recurrence of either leak or stricture. As noted earlier, we routinely tie off the proximal native ureter, do not do a nephrectomy, and have

not had any problems related to the native kidney. We feel that routine native nephrectomy is not indicated, and if one is ever subsequently indicated a laparoscopic nephrectomy would be our choice.

REFERENCES

1. Banowsky LHW. Surgical complications of renal transplantation. In: Glenn JF, ed. *Urologic surgery*, 4th ed. Philadelphia: JB Lippincott, 1991:252–266.
2. Bretan PN Jr, Hodge E, Streem SB, et al. Diagnosis of renal transplant fistulas. *Transplant Proc* 1989;21:1962–1966.
3. Gerridzen RG. Complete ureteral replacement by Boari bladder flap after cadaveric renal transplant. *Urology* 1993;41:154–156.
4. Gibbons WS, Barr JM, Hefty TR. Complications following unstented parallel incision extravesical ureteroneocystostomy in 1,000 kidney transplants. *J Urol* 1992;148:38–40.
5. Khauli RB. Surgical aspects of renal transplantation: New approaches. *Urol Clin North Am* 1994;27:321–341.
6. Martin DC, Mims MM, Kaufman JJ, Goodwin WE. The ureter in renal transplantation. *J Urol* 1969;101:680–687.
7. Rosenthal JT. Surgical management of urological complications after kidney transplantation. *Sem Urol* 1994;XII:114–122.
8. Streem SB. Endourological management of urological complications following renal transplantation. *Sem Urol* 1994;XII:123–133.
9. Taylor RJ, Rosenthal JT, Schwentker FN, et al. Factors in urologic complications in 400 cadaveric renal transplants. *J Urol* 1984;131:336A.
10. Thrasher JB, Temple DR, Spees EK. Extravesical versus Leadbetter–Politano ureteroneocystostomy: A comparison of urological complications in 320 renal transplants. *J Urol* 1990;144:1105–1109.

CHAPTER 13

Renal Autotransplantation

Ashutosh Tewari and Mani Menon

Renal autotransplantation is a safe and effective procedure to reconstruct the urinary tract. The advent of microvascular techniques and renal preservation has extended the scope of the procedure by allowing for successful extracorporeal (bench) surgery and subsequent autotransplantation. Current indications of autotransplantation include renal–vascular disease, severe ureteral damage, tumors of the kidney and ureter, complex nephrolithiasis, loin hematuria syndrome, and retroperitoneal fibrosis.

The advantages of autotransplantation include optimal surgical exposure, bloodless surgical field, and hypothermic protection of the kidney from ischemia. In cases of malignancy, with the use of bench surgery and autotransplantation there is less risk of tumor spillage and better assessment of tumor margins than by *in vivo* renal reconstruction. It is possible that this procedure may be underutilized because a good proportion of urologists are unfamiliar with the principles of renal homotransplantation.

DIAGNOSIS

Preoperative renal and pelvic arteriography should be performed to define the renal artery anatomy and ensure disease-free iliac vessels. In cases where autotransplantation is performed for the management of ureteral disease, ureteral involvement can be assessed by intravenous (IV) or retrograde pyelography. A computed tomography (CT) scan of the pelvis may be beneficial in cases of retroperitoneal fibrosis to assess pelvic extension of disease.

INDICATIONS FOR SURGERY

Renal autotransplantation is in particular attractive for a variety of vascular lesions affecting the aorta and renal artery. These include traumatic arterial injuries, renal artery stenosis with extension into the segmental branches (fibromuscular disease), large aneurysms, or arteriovenous fistulas. Other vascular indications include aortic aneurysms involving the renal arteries (Marfan's syndrome) and occlusive aortic disease.

In patients with central, intrarenal tumors or multiple tumors in a solitary kidney, renal autotransplantation with extracorporeal surgery is a useful technique. Following radical nephrectomy and extracorporeal hypothermic renal perfusion, the kidney is dissected beginning in the hilum. The vasculature to the tumor is ligated. After tumor-free margins are achieved, autotransplantation is carried out.

Renal autotransplantation allows for a direct anastomosis of the renal pelvis to the bladder. Therefore, it can be used in cases of ureteral damage or long ureteral lesions such as iatrogenic ureteral injuries, ureteral strictures, ureteral tumors, ureteral tuberculosis, failed urinary diversions, and retroperitoneal fibrosis. The procedure can also be used to facilitate stone passage in patients with complex nephrolithiasis. Renal autotransplantation has been effective in controlling the symptoms related to loin-pain hematuria syndrome.

ALTERNATIVE THERAPY

This procedure should be reserved for more serious and previously failed clinical settings. The majority of ureteral defects can be managed by conservative means or by reconstructive procedures such as ureteral reimplantation with or without a psoas hitch, Boari flap, ureteroureterostomy, transureteroureterostomy (TUU), downward renal mobilization, or a combination of these techniques. When such procedures are not possible or have failed, creation of an ileal ureter or renal autotransplantation are the only two remaining options to preserve the affected renal unit. The advantages of an ileal ureter over autotransplantation are threefold: (a) The procedure is technically less demanding; (b) vascular anastomosis is not necessary; and (c) bladder argumentation with bowel can be done simultaneously.

Disadvantages include mucus production, metabolic and electrolyte imbalance, propensity for bacteriuria, and the need for indefinite radiological surveillance of the ileal segment. Contraindications include intestinal diseases, hepatic dysfunction, and renal insufficiency (serum creatinine greater than 2.0 mg per dL).

For severe renovascular disease, the first surgical options typically include *in situ* reconstruction. This may involve endarterectomy or aortic–renal or splenorenal bypass grafting. When these techniques are not possible and microvascular reconstruction is required, autotransplantation becomes the procedure of choice.

The procedure is technically demanding and is contraindicated in the setting of severe occlusive atherosclerosis of the iliac arteries or in the presence of any active infection, which may seed the vascular anastomoses, resulting in subsequent rupture. An additional contraindication is the severe parenchymal disease or excess perivascular fibrosis in the renal hilum causing vascular spasm.

SURGICAL TECHNIQUE

Perioperatively, a brisk diuresis should be induced by IV hydration and 12.5 g mannitol given 1 hour before surgery. This will minimize ischemic injury to the kidney and hasten restoration of renal function. A broad-spectrum antibiotic is also administered 1 hour before surgery.

The surgical approach to removing the kidney is similar to that of living-donor nephrectomy. However, the particular disease process necessitating the surgery may complicate the operation. Typically, two incisions are needed: the first, either a subcostal transperitoneal or extrapleural–extraperitoneal flank to remove the kidney; the second, a lower-quadrant curvilinear or midline incision to access the iliac fossa (Fig. 13–1). In thin patients, an alternative approach is a single midline incision from the xiphoid to the symphysis pubis, although the exposure to the kidney is not optimal.

After the peritoneum and colon are reflected medially, Gerota's fascia is incised. The perinephric fat is sharply dissected off the renal capsule with minimal spreading using Metzenbaum scissors. Excessive retraction of the kidney should be avoided because that may result in subcapsular hematomas or capsular tears. The adrenal gland should be carefully separated from the upper pole of the kidney. In cases where ureteral continuity is not preserved, the distal ureter is isolated and transected before the dissection of the renal hilum. The ureteral stump can be tied with no. 0 chromic catgut suture.

The ureter should be maintained with its vascularity and the gonadal vein. To maximize ureteral viability, the tissue between the lower pole of the kidney and the ureter

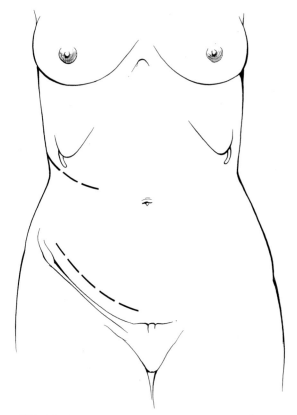

FIG. 13–1. Location of flank and inguinal incisions.

should be kept intact. Urinary output can then be assessed before the renal pedicle is approached.

On the right side, the vena cava is carefully isolated from the surrounding tissue. The gonadal vein can be ligated at its insertion on the vena cava. The renal vein should be identified anterior to the renal artery. Accessory renal veins can be ligated, but accessory renal arteries must be maintained. Careful dissection of the renal artery is performed toward the aorta by slightly retracting the vena cava with a closed forceps or vein retractor. After a further 12.5 g of mannitol has been given, a right-angle clamp is placed on the renal artery and it is transected. A Satinsky vascular clamp is then placed proximal to the renal vein ostium and the renal vein is transected. The renal artery can be tied with no. 0 silk ties or, alternatively, one no. 0 silk tie and a no. 0 silk ligature. We have found that the renal vein retracts after transection and that placement of a second, larger, Satinsky clamp behind the first allows for a less stressful closure of the renal ostium. A 5-0 Prolene suture is tied at one end, run down to the other end, back to the first, and retied. On the left side, the artery is divided at the aorta; the vein is divided anterior to the aorta and tied with two no. 0 silk sutures.

Once the kidney is removed, it is immersed in ice-cold slush at 4°C. The renal artery is flushed with either a

Collins intracellular electrolyte solution or a lactated renal solution with 10,000 U per L of heparin and 50 mEq per L of sodium bicarbonate. Flushing is continued until the effluent from the renal vein is clear. An adaptor is used to hold a good seal during flushing. Adequate flushing allows about 4 to 6 hours of renal preservation. If extracorporeal renal surgery is required, a second team can close the flank incision. In closure of the flank, strong monofilament absorbable suture such no. 1 polydioxanone suture or Maxon is used. Anteriorly, the transversus abdominis, internal oblique, and external oblique muscles are closed separately. Closure should begin after flexion is removed from the operating room table. Posteriorly, the intercostal muscles and latissimus dorsi are closed as separate layers.

The patient is placed in the supine position and draped. A Foley catheter carries 150 cc of 1% neomycin sulfate solution into the bladder and the catheter is clamped. A curvilinear incision is made, extending from the finger breadth above the pubis to two finger breadths above the anterior superior iliac spine. The incision is carried down to the rectus fascia. The rectus fascia, the external oblique, internal oblique, and transversus abdominis muscles are opened along the line of the incision. The lateral edge of the rectus muscle is transected at the pubis to get better exposure to the pelvis. The epigastric vessels are divided beneath the transversus abdominis muscle and tied with two 2-0 silk ties. The round ligament or the spermatic cord is doubly ligated. In young men, the sper-

matic cord is preserved and displaced inferomedially. The peritoneum is reflected medially to expose the iliac vessels and bladder. A Buckwalter retractor is placed into the wound to provide optimal exposure.

The iliac vessels are evaluated for potential size for anastomosis with the renal artery. If the caliber of the internal iliac artery is sufficient, and there is not significant plaque formation, then this vessel is selected. It is mobilized from the common iliac to the first branch, the superior gluteal artery. A bulldog vascular clamp is placed just beyond the origin of the internal iliac artery and a right-angle clamp is placed distally (Fig. 13–2). After transection of the vessel, the distal portion is tied with a no. 0 silk tie. The bulldog vascular clamp is opened to test for flow. The proximal portion of the vessel is flushed with 2,000 U of heparin mixed as follows: 10,000 U per 100 cc normal saline. If a plaque is discovered, it can be trimmed back, an endarterectomy can be performed, or it can be tacked down with 6-0 silk. Further dissection of the common iliac and external iliac arteries is not required. The external iliac vein is mobilized for 5 to 7 cm with special care to ligate the lymphatic vessels with 4-0 silk to prevent lymphocele formation.

When the internal iliac artery is unavailable, the external iliac artery is selected. After the external iliac artery is mobilized for 4 to 5 cm, an end-to-side anastomosis is performed between it and the renal artery (Fig. 13–3). Wide mobilization of the external iliac artery may result in kinking of the vessel. Vascular clamps are placed prox-

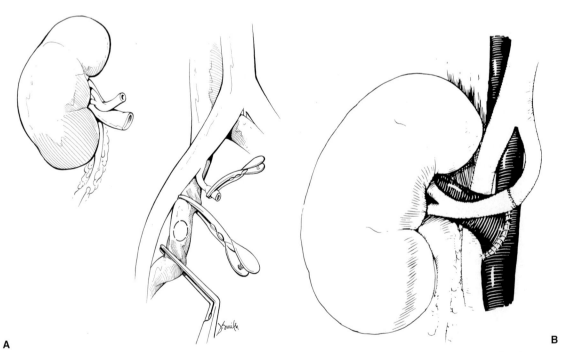

A

B

FIG. 13–2. A: Ipsilateral autotransplantation of kidney with end-to-side anastomosis of renal vein to common iliac vein and end-to-end anastomosis of hypogastric artery to renal artery. **B:** The complete venous and arterial anastomoses are demonstrated.

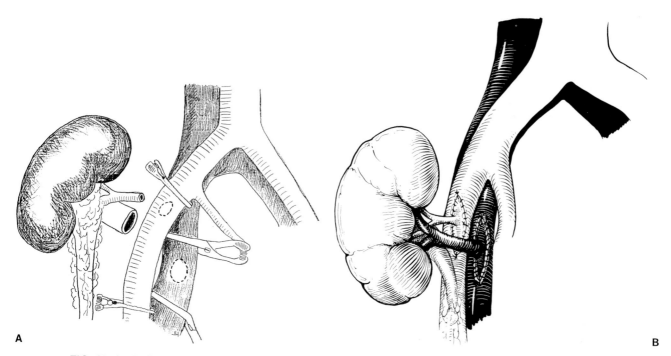

FIG. 13–3. A: Renal autotransplantation with end-to-side anastomoses of both renal and external iliac arteries and renal and external iliac veins. **B:** Small pediatric cadaver renal vessels are anastomosed to larger recipient iliac vessels using Carrel patches of donor aorta and vena cava.

imally and distally and an arteriotomy is performed. Typically, only a slit is needed and an ellipse of the anterior wall need not be removed. The distal artery is flushed with 2,000 U of dilute heparin with a red rubber catheter. A Satinsky vascular clamp is placed distally on the external iliac vein and a bulldog is placed proximal to the venotomy. The iliac vein is then carefully incised with a no. 11 blade scalpel to accommodate the renal vein. Four 5-0 Prolene sutures are placed on the external iliac vein in an outside-to-in fashion, one at each apex and one at the midpoint on each side of the venotomy.

The kidney is placed in the operative field. An assistant holds the kidney with a surgical sponge in an anatomic position with the ureter inferiorly. To minimize warm ischemia while the anastomosis is accomplished, the kidney is irrigated with cold saline. The four Prolene sutures in the external iliac vein are then brought through the renal vein in an inside-to-out fashion. The kidney is lowered into the wound and each suture is tied with the knots on the outside. The two apical sutures are used to close the venotomy. The midpoint sutures are placed with mild traction to keep the back wall from being incorporated in the running suture. The internal iliac artery is then anastomosed to the renal artery end to end with 6-0 siliconized silk sutures. The artery should be placed posterior to the renal vein to preserve anatomic relationships. The first two sutures of the arterial anastomosis are placed at either apex with double-armed needles such that the knots are on the outside. The remainders are placed

with single-armed needles. We prefer an anastomosis with interrupted sutures when the internal iliac artery is used. Sutures should be placed close enough to avoid any gaps, especially at the apex. After one side is complete, the apical sutures are rotated to give exposure to the back wall. If the external iliac artery is used, the arteriotomy should be staggered with the venotomy to avoid kinking of the vessels. The anastomosis is performed with two to four continuous 6-0 Prolene sutures. After completion of the anastomosis, oxidized cellulose is wrapped in small pieces around the arteriotomy and venotomy. The venous clamps are then removed, followed by the arterial clamps. It is important to maintain adequate intravascular volume with colloid or blood, especially when the clamps are removed, so that the kidney is well perfused. If this produces an excessively elevated central venous pressure, IV furosemide (Lasix) should be administered.

On occasion, renal autotransplantation can be performed with the ureter left intact. Although it will follow a redundant course to the bladder, normal peristalsis will provide effective drainage from the kidney. Care must be taken to avoid positioning the kidney so as to produce an obstruction of the ureter. If the ureter is transected, the urinary system can be reconstructed by a ureteroneocystostomy, ureteroureterostomy, pyeloureterostomy, or a pyelovesicostomy (Figs. 13–4 and 13–5). We prefer an extravesical ureteroneocystostomy when there is adequate length of nondiseased ureter for a tension-free anastomosis. The Buckwalter retractor is repositioned to

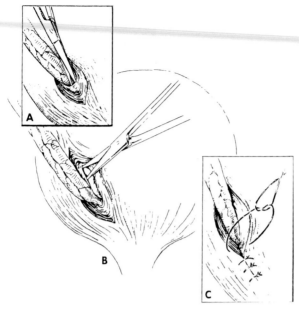

FIG. 13–4. Lich extravesical ureteroneocystostomy. Gregoir and Campos–Freire techniques are similar.

provide better exposure to the lateral wall of the bladder. A 2- to 3-cm tunnel is made in the bladder wall by incising the posterior lateral serosa and detrusor muscle. After the margins of the detrusor are retracted with 3-0 chromic stay sutures, the mucosa is mobilized and allowed to bulge. An ellipse of the mucosa is removed from the apex

of the tunnel, and the spatulated ureter is anastomosed with the bladder mucosa using a continuous 5-0 chromic catgut suture. Two sutures are used, each of which incorporates 180 degrees of the anastomosis, and are tied without tension. The anastomosis is performed over a 4.8 Fr double-J ureteric stent, which is positioned into the bladder after the bladder mucosa has been opened. The stent will be removed in the postoperative period.

The detrusor is closed over the ureter with interrupted 3-0 chromic catgut sutures. The tunnel should allow passage of a right-angle clamp between the ureter and overlying muscle. The wound is irrigated with a 1% neomycin solution. No external drains are required if the ureteral reimplantation is watertight.

In cases where the upper ureter is diseased, the area is removed and the proximal ureter or renal pelvis is anastomosed to the normal lower ureter. The ureteroureterostomy or pyeloureterostomy is performed over a ureteric double-J stent by end-to-end anastomosis of the spatulated lower ureter to either the spatulated upper ureter or the renal pelvis (Fig. 13–5). If the entire ureter is not viable, or for recurrent stone disease, a pyelovesicostomy is performed. This technique can be performed with a Boari flap and end-to-end anastomosis of the renal pelvis to tubularized bladder. The Boari flap should be secured to the psoas muscle to avoid tension on the anastomosis.

The wound is then closed in layers. The rectus muscle is approximated back to the tendinous insertion at the

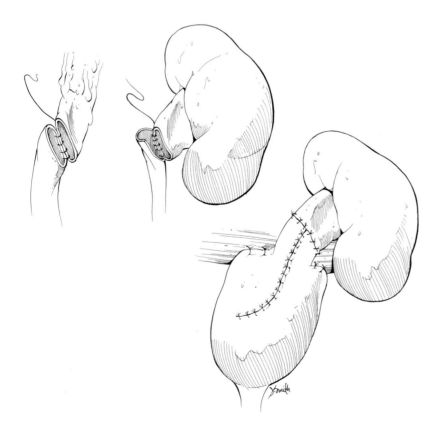

FIG. 13–5. Alternative options for reconstruction of urinary tract: ureteroureterostomy, pyeloureterostomy, or Boari flap to renal pelvis

pubic bone with a no. 0 Prolene suture. The internal oblique and transversus abdominis are closed with a no. 0 Prolene suture. The external oblique is closed with continuous no. 0 Prolene. The subcutaneous layer is closed with 3-0 Dexon and the skin is closed with 3-0 nonabsorbable sutures or clips.

For optimal renal perfusion during the immediate postoperative period, the central venous pressure should be maintained adequately and the diastolic blood pressure kept at 85 mm Hg or higher. Mild hypertension is preferred over normotension or mild hypotension. Aspirin can be started postoperatively to reduce the risks of graft thrombosis. A renal scan is obtained on the first postoperative day to document renal perfusion and again about postoperative day 7. Broad-spectrum antibiotics are administered during the immediate postoperative period to maintain sterile urine and help prevent infection of the vascular grafts. The ureteral stent is left in place for 2 to 3 weeks and is removed during outpatient cystoscopy. The Foley catheter is removed on postoperative day 5. It may be removed sooner if a ureteroureterostomy or pyeloureterostomy is performed, but it should be kept in place for 5 days following a pyelovesicostomy or ureteroneocystostomy. An IV pyelogram or a cystogram is obtained 1 to 2 weeks after surgery to evaluate ureteral integrity.

OUTCOMES

Complications

Early postoperative complications include bleeding from the vascular anastomosis, renal artery or vein thrombosis, distal extremity embolization, or urinary extravasation. Bleeding from a disrupted anastomosis is a rare event but requires immediate exploration. It is usually associated with anastomosis to diseased vessels or errors in surgical technique. Peripheral collateral vessels from the renal hilum can attain significant size if there is stenosis of the renal artery or vein and can be a source of postoperative bleeding. Renal artery or vein thrombosis occurs in fewer than 2% of cases and should be ruled out in cases of oliguria following autotransplant of a solitary kidney. The diagnosis is made by renal scan; if it is made without delay, salvage of the autotransplant should be attempted. This complication often arises due to technically imperfect anastomosis or significant hypotension or hypovolemic event in the postoperative period.

Distal extremity embolization as a result of dislodging plaque during aortic clamping or unclamping can occur, especially with diseased blood vessels. Heparinization at the time the vessels are prepared aids in preventing this problem, but the distal pulses and color of the legs should be assessed after arterial clamps are opened. Deep venous thrombosis can result in propagation of clot from the renal vein. Intimal injury, low-flow states, and venous obstruction can predispose to this condition.

Urinary extravasation is the most common complication from autotransplantation. Dissection in the renal hilum should be minimized to prevent devascularization of the renal pelvis and proximal ureter, which may produce necrosis and urine leakage. Placement of a ureteric double-J stent diminishes the mild forms of anastomotic leaks. If a leak continues for a long time, it should be treated by a percutaneous nephrostomy. On occasion, the distal ureter may become ischemic and requires reexploration and operative repair.

The most common late complications include renal artery stenosis, ureteral stricture, and ureterovesical reflux. Renal artery stenosis may be manifested by hypertension or impaired renal function. Diagnosis is made by renal scan and digital subtraction angiography. Initial management should be percutaneous angioplasty. Obstruction of the urinary system demonstrated by pain or impaired renal function can be managed by dilation and stenting.

Results

Bodie et al. reported on 24 autotransplanted kidneys in 23 patients in whom the primary indication was to place all or a major portion of the ureter (1). There was one operative death reported. Of the 24 autografts, three were ultimately lost (12.5%). The function of the remaining grafts was stable or improved postoperatively. Novick et al. reported successful outcomes in 29 of 30 patients, 10 of whom underwent autotransplantation for the management of intrarenal branch arterial lesions (4).

Reported series of patients who have undergone autotransplantation for cancer are small, although the technique does seem to offer a good alternative in some patients. van der Velden reported on six cases of renal carcinoma with 54 months follow-up and three (50%) with overall mortality (6). Zincke and Sen performed extracorporeal surgery and kidney autotransplantation in 15 patients, of whom 11 had renal cell carcinoma and four had transitional cell carcinoma (7). Three autotransplants were lost because of venous and arterial thrombosis in two and necrosis of the renal pelvis and ureter in one. The remaining patients were dialysis free with stable creatinine values. Other complications cited included a caliceal fistula requiring closure in one patient and intimal injury requiring partial replacement of external iliac artery with a Gore–Tex graft in another (7). Novick et al. observed an increased incidence of temporary and permanent renal failure for extracorporeal compared with *in situ* partial nephrectomy for renal cell carcinoma (5). Postoperative initial nonfunction occurred in five of 14 patients (36%) undergoing autotransplantation but in only two of 86 patients (2.3%) who underwent an *in situ* procedure. Permanent renal failure occurred in two of 14 (14.3%) autotransplanted patients and in one of 86 managed *in situ* (1.2%) (5).

Chin and associates (2) reviewed the long-term results of renal autotransplantation in 22 patients with the loin pain–hematuria syndrome for severe intractable flank pain and recurrent hematuria. Postoperative pain relief, narcotic use, level of function in daily activities, and status of the autograft were assessed. At a mean follow-up of 84.7 months, there were two technical failures. Overall, 18 of the 26 autotransplant procedures (69.2%) resulted in pain relief, in some cases beyond 10 years, with patients returning to normal daily activities (2).

Recently, Meraney and associates (3) reported in a pig model the feasibility of performing the entire procedure laparoscopically. The mean operating time was 6.2 hours (range, 5.3 to 7.9 hours), the venous anastomosis time was 33 minutes (range, 22 to 46 minutes), the arterial anastomosis time was 31 minutes (range, 27 to 35 minutes), and the total iliac clamping time was 77 minutes (range, 62 to 88 minutes). The total renal ischemia time was 68.7 minutes: warm ischemia, 5.1 minutes; cold ischemia, 33 minutes; and rewarming, 31 minutes. Serum creatinine concentrations remained stable: baseline, 1.3 mg per dL; after autotransplantation, 1.1 mg per dL; and after contralateral nephrectomy, 1.6 mg per dL. IV urography and aortography prior to euthanasia (N = 5) demonstrated prompt contrast uptake and excretion by the autotransplanted kidneys and patent arterial anastomoses, respectively.

REFERENCES

1. Bodie B, Novick AC, Rose M, Straffon RA. Long-term results with renal autotransplantation for ureteral replacement. *J Urol* 1986;136: 1187–1189.
2. Chin JL, Kloth D, Pautler SE, Mulligan M. Renal autotransplantation for the loin pain–hematuria syndrome: long- term followup of 26 cases. *J Urol* 1998;160:1232–1235; 1235–1236 [discussion].
3. Meraney AM, Gill IS, Kaouk JH, Skacel M, Sung GT. Laparoscopic renal autotransplantation. *J Endourol* 2001;15:143–149.
4. Novick AC, Straffon RA, Stewart BH. Experience with extracorporeal renal operations and autotransplantation in the management of complicated urologic disorders. *Surg Gynecol Obstet* 1981;153:10–18.
5. Novick AC, Streem S, Montie JE, et al. Conservative surgery for renal cell carcinoma: a single-center experience with 100 patients. 1989. *J Urol* 2002; 167:878–882; 883 [discussion].
6. van der Velden JJ, van Bockel JH, Zwartendijk J, van Krieken JH, Terpstra JL. Long-term results of surgical treatment of renal carcinoma in solitary kidneys by extracorporeal resection and autotransplantation. *Br J Urol* 1992;69:486–490.
7. Zincke H, Sen SE. Experience with extracorporeal surgery and autotransplantation for renal cell and transitional cell cancer of the kidney. *J Urol* 1988;140:25–27.

Ureter and Pelvis

SECTION EDITOR: Charles B. Brendler

Anatomy

Sam D. Graham, Jr.

The urinary collecting system begins at the calyces and includes the renal pelvis and ureter. Calyceal anatomy is a combination of a renal papilla emptying into a calyx which is invested in a cup like fashion around the tip of the papilla (Figure SII-1). The area where the calyx folds to form the cup is known as the fornix and is the weakest portion of the collecting system. In the first segment of the collecting system, calyces (either individually or as a complex calyx) empty into the renal pelvis via an infundibulum. This coalescence of infundibulae is known as a major calyceal group which is a subdivision of the renal pelvis. The renal pelvis is ordinarily a single structure, but a bifid or completely duplicated pelvis are well known variants.

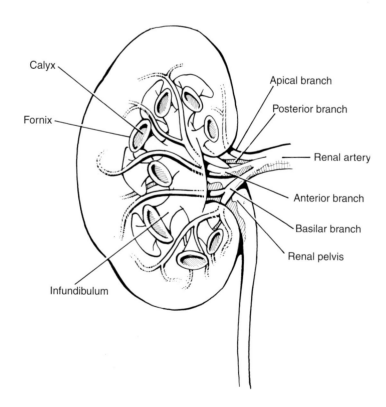

FIG. SII–1. Anatomy of the collecting system and its relationship to the renal arterial supply

TABLE SII–1. *Diameters of Ureteral Segments (2)*

Ureteral segment	Average diameter
Ureteral pelvic junction	2 mm
Abdominal ureter	10 mm
Crossing iliac vessels	4 mm
Pelvic ureter	5 mm
Uretero vesical junction	1–5 mm

The wall of the renal pelvis is composed of an adventitia, a muscular layer, and lined with transitional epithelium. The smooth muscle layer is primarily in a circular arrangement and is least prominent in the proximal regions (1).

The ureter continues from its juncture with the renal pelvis (UPJ) to the bladder extraperitoneally for 25cm to 30 cm. The exact point of transition from the renal pelvis to the upper ureter is anatomically imperceptible, but is the first of three relative anatomic constrictions of the ureter. The second area of relative constriction is where the ureter crosses the iliac vessels and the third and most constricted portion is where the ureter enters the bladder (Table SII-1).

The ureters adhere to the posterior peritoneum and therefore can be identified by elevating the peritoneum as the retroperitoneal space is entered. As the ureters cross the iliac vessels they can usually be located within 1 cm of the bifurcation of the common iliac artery. The ureters continue into the pelvis and are found posterior to the superior lateral vesical artery (the second anterior branch of the hypogastric artery) and its corresponding vein.

Histologically, the ureter has three layers including an adventitia, a muscular layer, and a layer of transitional epithelium. The adventitia glides within a sheath and distally it is continuous with the fibers of Waldeyer's sheath as it enters the bladder. The muscular layer is actually a combination of spiral and longitudinal fibers that are important for ureteral peristalsis. There are three layers of muscle, an exterior longitudinal layer, a middle circular layer, and an internal fine longitudinal layer.

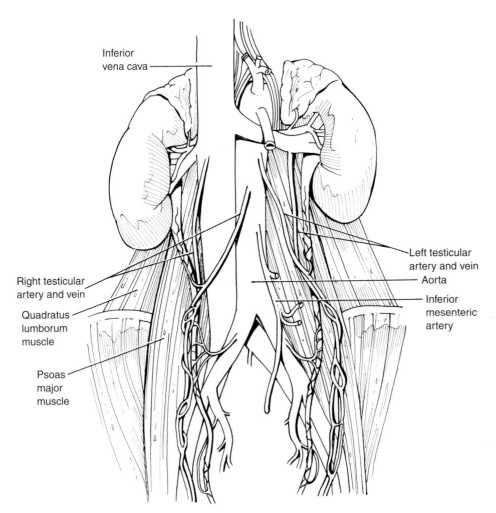

FIG. SII–2. Course of the ureters through the retroperitoneum with the relationships to the psoas muscle and the iliac vessels.

Anatomical variations in the ureteral anatomy are seen in complete and partial duplication of the ureters, as well as with renal fusion and ectopia. Retrocaval ureter and other vascular anomalies are unusual.

VASCULAR ANATOMY

The renal pelvic vascular supply is from the segmental branches of the renal vessels as well as even later branches of the renal artery and vein. The arterial branches to the ureter include a branch of the renal artery superiorly, as well as branches from the gonadal artery, the aorta, the hypogastric, vassal, and vesical arteries. In the proximal ureter, the blood supply to the ureter comes from the medial side, while the distal ureteral blood supply is from the lateral side. The ureter has a freely anastamosing network of vessels that will keep the ureter viable as long as the adventitia is intact. The adventitial network of vessels penetrates the muscle and forms a more delicate network in the subepithelial layer of the ureter. The capillaries then form a venous plexus in the subepithelial layer of the ureter and a secondary plexus in the adventitia. Venous drainage of the ureter is to the vesical, vaginal, gonadal, iliac, lumbar, and renal veins.

LYMPHATICS

The lymphatics of the ureter parallel the arterial supply.

NEURAL ANATOMY

The ureter is innervated via the autonomic nervous system via neural plexuses found between the renal artery and inferior mesenteric arteries.

CONTIGUOUS STRUCTURES

The proximal ureter course is determined by the psoas muscle (Figure SII-2). On the right, the ureter is in contact with the second portion of the duodenum proximally and the vena cava medially. The left ureter passes behind the sigmoid colon as it enters the pelvis and is lateral to the aorta. Initially, both ureters are lateral to the gonadal vessels, but prior to the bifurcation of the aorta and vena cava, the gonadal vessels cross the ureter anteriorly and remain lateral to the ureter towards the pelvis. Once in the pelvis, the ureter follows the course of the hypogastric artery. At approximately the greater sciatic foramen, the ureter angles medially to enter the bladder. In the male, the ureter then crosses anteriorly to the vas deferens before entering the bladder. In the female, the ureter crosses the the Fallopian tubes and the uterine arteries posteriorly (dorsally) and passes within 2 cm of the uterine cervix.

REFERENCES

1. Deweerd JH. Renal pelvis and ureteropelvic surgery. In: Urologic Surgery, 2nd ed., JF Glenn ed. Hagerstown: Harper and Row, 1975.
2. Stewart BH. Surgical anatomy. In: *Operative Urology.* Baltimore: Williams and Wilkins, 1975.

CHAPTER 14

Nephroureterectomy

Gary D. Steinberg

Malignant tumors of the upper urinary tract are uncommon and account for only 5% to 10% of all urothelial malignancies. The peak incidence is in the sixth and seventh decades of life with a male predominance of 2:1 (3). Most upper-tract tumors are transitional cell carcinoma (TCC, 85% to 90%), with 10% to 15% squamous cell carcinoma or mixed TCC and squamous. Adenocarcinoma of the renal pelvis is extremely rare, accounting for only 1% of upper-tract tumors.

Cigarette smoking is the major risk factor for development of TCC of the renal pelvis. It has been reported that there is a three- to sevenfold increased risk of carcinoma associated with cigarette smoking and that cessation of smoking is associated with a decreased risk.

Phenacetin abuse is also associated with an increased risk of TCC of the renal pelvis. Although the specific mechanism of tumorigenesis is unknown, the phenacetin metabolite 4-acetoaminoprophenol is thought to cause chronic inflammation and papillary necrosis. The combination of papillary necrosis and chronic inflammation has been associated with a 20-fold increased risk of cancer development (5).

Balkan nephropathy, also known as Danubian endemic familial nephropathy, is a condition strictly associated with TCC of the upper tracts. This endemic disease is confined to the Balkan states that lie on the Danube River. Cancer of the renal pelvis in these states accounts for 42% of renal tumors. The specific cause is unknown, although the drinking water has been suggested. The tumors are typically low grade, multifocal, and slow growing. Bilateral tumors occur 10% of the time. Occupational risk factors have also been correlated with TCC of the renal pelvis, including exposure to chemicals in the rubber, petroleum, plastics, and aniline dye industries. Forty percent to 80% of patients with upper-tract tumors will have urothelial carcinomas at some time elsewhere in the urinary tract, usually in the bladder. About 3% of patients with transitional cell cancer of the bladder develop upper-tract tumors; however, patients with urothelial tract tumors of the prostate or ure-

thra have approximately a 30% risk of developing upper-tract tumors (1).

DIAGNOSIS

Approximately 80% of patients present with hematuria. Some patients present with flank pain or constitutional symptoms. Intravenous pyelography (IVP) is the initial study of choice in the evaluation of a patient suspected of having a renal pelvic or ureteral tumor. Assessment of the entire urinary tract is important in evaluating patients diagnosed with a renal pelvic or ureteral tumor because the upper urinary tract has a high potential of developing multiple tumors as described by the field-change theory. Grabstald reported that approximately 50% of patients with renal tumors have coexisting tumors in the ipsilateral ureter and bladder, and 3% to 4% of those patients have tumors in the contralateral upper urinary system. A retrograde pyelogram is usually indicated if the collecting system of the affected kidney is not completely visualized or in the case of renal insufficiency or contrast allergy. Additional urothelial assessment may include renal pelvic and/or ureteral washings for cytology, brush biopsies, cystoscopy, and bladder washing for urinary cytology. The role of ureteroscopy in the diagnosis of upper-tract tumors is complementary and may confirm the findings of the IVP, retrograde pyelography, and cytology. Ureteroscopy may aid in visual identification and biopsy of tumors for grading and staging. Additional staging evaluation for the detection of metastatic disease should include a chest radiograph and/or computed tomography (CT) of the chest, abdomen, and pelvis. A bone scan may be obtained in patients with an elevated serum calcium, alkaline phosphatase, or bony abnormalities seen on CT scan.

INDICATIONS FOR SURGERY

Nephroureterectomy with excision of a cuff of bladder is the classic surgical procedure for carcinoma of the

119

renal pelvis or ureter. However, conservative surgery may be indicated in those patients diagnosed with a small, solitary, well-differentiated papillary tumor. Current staging techniques, however, may make accurate preoperative staging and grading of tumors difficult. In addition, half of all cases of ureteral tumors involve at least the musculature. Further, there is a high incidence of multiple ipsilateral tumors. Last, recurrent tumors in the remaining ureteral stump have been reported in more than 30% of patients treated by nephrectomy and partial ureterectomy. Although patients with solitary distal ureteral tumors may be successfully treated with distal ureterectomy and ureteroneocystostomy, in general, a conservative surgical approach should be reserved for the highly selected patient population in whom nephron sparing is essential, i.e., patients diagnosed with bilateral tumors, Balkan nephropathy, patients with a solitary kidney, renal insufficiency, and patients with comorbid health problems. Patients treated with a conservative approach are at increased risk of local recurrence and require frequent and careful follow-up including IVPs, retrograde pyelograms, and endoscopies (6).

ALTERNATIVE THERAPY

Alternatives to nephroureterectomy include (a) endoscopic resection and/or fulguration, in either a retrograde or antegrade fashion, (b) topical chemo- or immunotherapy via either a nephrostomy tube or ureteral stent, (c) external beam radiotherapy, or (d) laparoscopic nephroureterectomy.

Lesions in the ureter may be treated with resection of the ureteral tumor and ureteroureterostomy, replacement with ileal interposition, and ureteral reimplantation. These operations require a careful assessment of the entire urothelium and careful follow-up. Because of the field-change effect of the urothelium and multiplicity of tumors, these operations may not be appropriate in

patients with high-grade or high-stage tumors. At present, many urologists are gaining increasing experience with laparoscopic nephroureterectomy. Controversy exists as to the best method of excising the distal ureter. One approach is a hand-assisted nephroureterectomy with an incision into the bladder through the hand incision versus an endoscopic excision of the distal ureter. If using the hand "port" for the distal ureterectomy the method described in this chapter is still relevant.

SURGICAL TECHNIQUE

In performing a nephroureterectomy, technical considerations include the choice of incision, whether it is appropriate and to what extent the surgeon should perform a lymph node dissection, and excision of bladder cuff and distal ureter via an intravesical versus extravesical approach.

Two-Incision Approach

An intrathoracic, extrapleural, extraperitoneal approach, removing the kidney within Gerota's fascia without removing the adrenal gland, is our preferred procedure. To gain proper exposure, the incision can never be too high, and thus a tenth interspace or supra–eleventh-rib incision is in general utilized. The patient is placed in a modified flank position (approximately 60 degrees rotated) with the table flexed and the kidney rest elevated. The patient is taped into position with wide adhesive tape and an armrest is utilized. The patient is adequately padded with an axillary roll, pillows, and sheets and is prepped and draped from nipples to the symphysis pubis in the usual sterile fashion.

The eleventh rib and the tenth intercostal space are identified, and a supra–eleventh-rib incision is made in the tenth intercostal space. The incision extends from the edge of the erector spinae muscle and courses obliquely

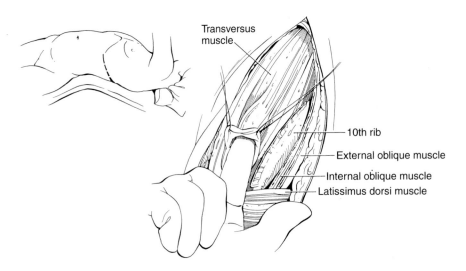

Transversus muscle

10th rib
External oblique muscle
Internal oblique muscle
Latissimus dorsi muscle

FIG. 14–1. The patient is rotated on the table and flexed in the flank position. The incision is made through the transversalis abdominis muscle off the end of the eleventh rib to avoid the pleura and peritoneum. The lower border of the pleura is shown. (From Marshall FF. Radical nephrectomy. In: Marshall FF, ed. *Operative urology*. Philadelphia: WB Saunders, 1991: 18–25, with permission.)

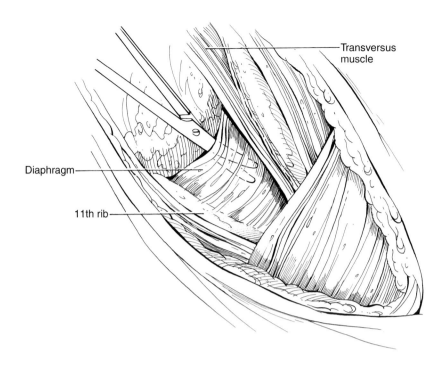

FIG. 14–2. As the left radical nephrectomy continues, Gerota's fascia is mobilized off the abdominal side of the diaphragm. The diaphragm can be seen after the transversalis muscle has been divided. Pleura is identified in the space between the transversus abdominis muscle and the diaphragm. It can then be mobilized with the Kitner dissector superiorly. (From Marshall FF. Radical nephrectomy. In: Marshall FF, ed. *Operative urology.* Philadelphia: WB Saunders, 1991: 18–25, with permission.)

and medially to the lateral border of the rectus fascia to incise the external and internal oblique muscles, exposing the transversalis fascia, and the latissimus dorsi and serratus muscles, exposing the intercostal muscles. The lumbodorsal fascia is then incised at the level of the tip of the eleventh rib to avoid inadvertent division of the peritoneum or pleura (Fig. 14–1).

The peritoneum is mobilized off the posterior aspect of the transversalis muscle, moving the peritoneum medially and inferiorly. Primarily by use of blunt dissection with minimal sharp dissection, Gerota's fascia is mobilized superiorly from the diaphragm and posteri-

orly and inferiorly from the psoas and quadratus musculature (Fig. 14–2). The intercostal muscles are then incised, carefully avoiding the pleural membrane. The plane between the pleura and chest wall is identified with careful blunt dissection along the tenth rib using a Kitner dissector. The diaphragmatic attachments to the eleventh and twelfth ribs are transected sharply down to their insertion between the quadratus and psoas muscles, avoiding the intercostal nerve and vessels. Sharp dissection is continued posteriorly until the intercostal ligament is divided, allowing the rib to hinge posteriorly (Fig. 14–3).

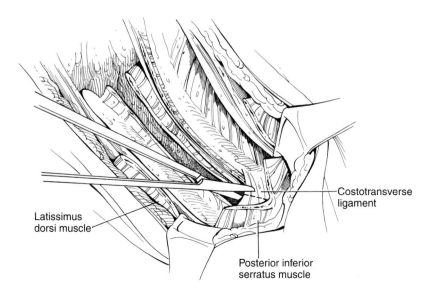

FIG. 14–3. The transverse costal (intercostal) ligament is divided after the pleura has been reflected superiorly and the diaphragm has been divided. Division of the intercostal ligament allows the eleventh rib to hinge inferiorly and improves the exposure. (From Marshall FF. Radical nephrectomy. In: Marshall FF, ed. *Operative urology.* Philadelphia: WB Saunders, 1991:18–25, with permission.)

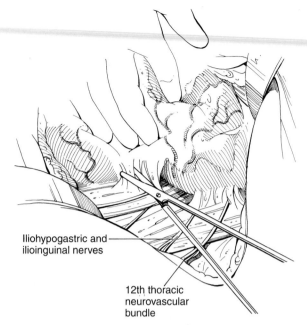

FIG. 14–4. The transversalis fascia and Gerota's fascia are mobilized from the psoas and quadratus musculature posteriorly. The iliohypogastric and ilioinguinal nerves and twelfth thoracic neurovascular bundle are seen. (From Marshall FF. Radical nephrectomy. In: Marshall FF, ed. *Operative urology*. Philadelphia: WB Saunders, 1991:18–25, with permission.)

A self-retaining retractor is placed into the wound for optimal exposure. A Balfour or Finochetto retractor may be used, but a multibladed ring retractor that is secured to the operating table, such as a Buckwalter retractor, is preferable. The renal mass within Gerota's fascia is rotated medially and the dissection is carried posteriorly off the psoas and quadratus musculature. The iliohypogastric and ilioinguinal nerves and twelfth thoracic neurovascular bundle can usually be identified (Fig. 14–4).

The colon is then held medially and superiorly, an avascular plane between the colonic mesocolon and Gerota's fascia is developed, and the renal mass is sharply separated from the peritoneum. By use of sharp and blunt dissection, the superior and inferior aspects of the kidney are dissected free of the adrenal gland and surrounding tissues, respectively. There may be several vessels between the adrenal gland and the kidney that should be ligated with ligaclips. The kidney is dissected posteriorly to the level of the renal hilum. Attention is directed to the main renal vessels. The pulsating renal artery is identified by palpation, double ligated as it exits the aorta with 0 silk ligatures, and then divided (Fig. 14–5).

On the right side, especially with a large tumor mass, the artery may be approached anteriorly or in the intera-ortocaval region, although the preferred approach to the

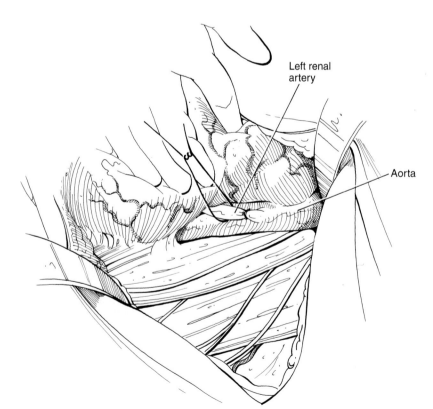

FIG. 14–5. The aorta is located and the renal artery can be identified, ligated, and divided. (From Marshall FF. Radical nephrectomy. In: Marshall FF, ed. *Operative urology*. Philadelphia: WB Saunders, 1991:18–25, with permission.)

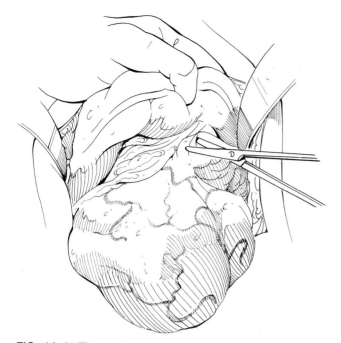

FIG. 14–6. The medial dissection includes mobilization of the colon and mesocolon from Gerota's fascia. Gerota's fascia remains with the specimen. The aorta is identified and an *en-bloc* periaortic node dissection is commenced. Care is taken not to injure the femoral branch of the genitofemoral nerve on the psoas muscle. (From Marshall FF. Radical nephrectomy. In: Marshall FF, ed. *Operative urology.* Philadelphia: WB Saunders, 1991:18–25, with permission.)

right renal artery is posteriorly. On the left side, the gonadal and adrenal veins are identified anteriorly, as is the renal vein. The gonadal and any lumbar veins are ligated before double ligating the renal vein with 2-0 silk (Figs. 14–6 and 14–7). On the right side, the inferior vena cava is identified as well as the renal vein. Careful palpation for a second renal artery is important before ligation of the renal vein. The remaining soft-tissue attachments to the kidney should be divided so that the only remaining attachment is to the ureter.

Attention is then directed to the inferior aspect of the kidney. The ureter is identified and dissected free to a level distal to the bifurcation of the iliac vessels. The ureter is ligated distally with 0 silk ligature, making sure not to include any surrounding tissue. A large, straight clip is placed proximally to prevent urine spillage and the ureter is divided. The specimen is then removed.

TCC may spread by direct extension or metastasis by hematogenous or lymphatic routes. Therefore, a regional lymphadenectomy should be performed as part of the surgical procedure. A lymph node dissection is performed by identifying the midline of the aorta for a left-sided tumor and the vena cava for a right-sided tumor. Starting from just cephalad to the renal hilum to the level of the inferior mesenteric artery, the lymphatic tissue is dissected using a "split-and-roll technique" with ligaclips placed on the lymphatics to avoid a lymphocele.

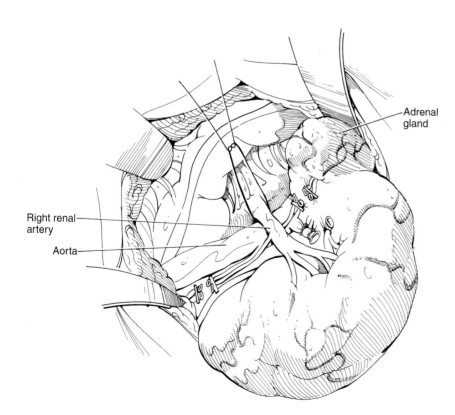

Adrenal gland

Right renal artery

Aorta

FIG. 14–7. The gonadal vessels and ureter are ligated inferiorly. The regional node dissection is carried along the aorta and the renal vein is ligated and divided. Additional vessels to the adrenal gland are ligated and divided. The adrenal gland is usually not removed with nephroureterectomy for renal pelvic or ureteral tumors. (From Marshall FF. Radical nephrectomy. In: Marshall FF, ed. *Operative urology.* Philadelphia: WB Saunders, 1991;18–25, with permission.)

Hemostasis is obtained using electrocautery. The diaphragm is not repaired if only the lateral attachments have been taken down. If a pleurotomy has been made, a red rubber catheter with additional side holes cut out is placed into the pleural space and the pleurotomy is closed with a running 3-0 chromic suture. The kidney rest is lowered, the table is taken out of flexion, and the wound is closed in two layers using a continuous suture of no. 1 permanent. The skin is closed using staples. The pleural cavity is then bubbled out with the red rubber catheter in a basin of saline. When fluid and bubbles cease to emerge from the catheter, it is removed and additional skin staples are applied. Auscultation of the chest at the apex of the lung as well as a chest x-ray should be performed postoperatively to diagnose a pneumothorax. If there are any concerns, a temporary chest tube may be placed.

The patient is taken out of flank position, placed in supine position over the break of the operating room table with the table flexed, and prepped and draped in the usual sterile fashion. A 20 Fr Foley catheter is passed into the bladder, and the bladder is then filled with 200 to 300 cc of normal saline. A lower midline abdominal incision is made and carried down through the rectus and transver-

salis fascia. A Balfour retractor is placed. The bladder is identified and opened longitudinally between two laterally placed 2-0 Vicryl stay sutures. Additional stay sutures are placed at the apex of the incision in the bladder. The ureteral orifices are identified, the bladder is packed with several sponges, and the bladder blade is placed in the dome of the bladder. A 5 Fr feeding tube is placed in the ipsilateral ureteral orifice and sewn in place with a 4-0 chromic suture. The ureteral orifice is circumscribed sharply, including a 1-cm cuff of bladder. The ureter is dissected from its orifice using a pinpoint electrocautery and sharp dissecting scissors (Fig. 14–8).

The entire distal ureter is dissected free to the level of the 0 silk tie, removed with a cuff of bladder, and passed off the table as a specimen. In most cases the remaining stump of distal ureter may be removed entirely with an intravesical approach; however, in some cases additional extravesical dissection is required in which the superior and middle vesicle pedicles are divided. A two-layer closure of the posterior bladder wall is performed using 2-0 Vicryl sutures to close the muscle and serosa and 5-0 chromic to close the bladder mucosa. A 3-0 Vicryl continuous suture and subsequently 2-0 Vicryl figure-of-eight Lembert sutures are used to close the bladder incision in two layers. A Davol drain is placed in the pelvis and secured with a 3-0 nylon suture. The abdomen is closed with a continuous no. 1 PDS suture. The skin is closed with staples.

OUTCOMES

Complications

Early complications include hemorrhage, wound infection, pneumothorax, atelectasis, and pneumonia. Meticulous dissection around the renal vessels, aorta, and vena cava will aid in decreasing intraoperative blood loss. The supra–eleventh-rib incision provides excellent exposure to the great vessels and kidney, thus reducing the chance of inadvertent injury to the vasculature. Later complications include "flank sag," which may be related to division of more than one intercostal nerve.

Results

The survival rate after nephroureterectomy is dependent on the stage and grade of the tumor. Superficial low-grade tumors rarely metastasize and when adequately treated rarely decrease life expectancy. Invasive lesions have a higher metastatic rate and are associated with a poorer prognosis. Patients with low- and high-grade tumors have approximately 80% and 20% survival at 5 years, respectively (4). Patients with pT2–3a renal pelvic and ureteral tumors have a 75% and 15% survival at 5 years, respectively, and patients with pT3b–4, N+ tumors have approximately a 5% survival at 5 years. Interest-

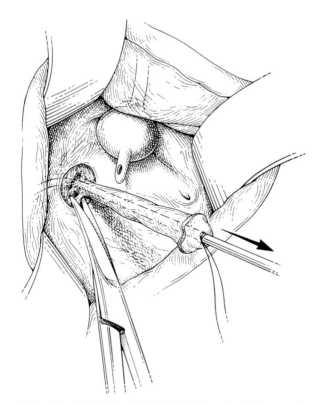

FIG. 14–8. A catheter is placed in the left ureteral orifice and sutured. A wide circumferential incision around the ureteral orifice and periureteral dissection free the intravesical ureter. (From Lange PH. Carcinoma of the renal pelvis and ureter. In: Glenn JF, ed. *Urologic Surgery*, 4th ed. Philadelphia: JB Lippincott, 1991:273, with permission.)

ingly, in patients with ureteral tumors survival may be more dependent on the stage and grade of tumor than the surgical approach (2).

REFERENCES

1. Abercrombie GF, Eardley I, Payne SR, et al. Modified nephroureterectomy: long-term follow-up with particular reference to subsequent bladder tumors. *Br J Urol* 1988;61:198.
2. Badalament RA, O'Toole RV, Kenworthy P, et al. Prognostic factors in patients with primary transitional cell carcinoma of the upper urinary tract. *J Urol* 1990;144:859.
3. Kleer E. Transitional cell carcinoma of the upper tracts. In: Soloway MS, ed. *Problems in urology*, vol. 6, no. 3. Philadelphia: JB Lippincott, 1992: 531.
4. Nielson K, Ostri P. Primary tumors of the renal pelvis: evaluation of clinical and pathological features in a consecutive series of 10 years. *J Urol* 1988;140:19.
5. Ross RK, Paganini-Hill A, Landolph J, et al. Analgesics, cigarette smoking, and other risk factors for cancer of the renal pelvis and ureter. *Cancer Res* 1989;49:1045.
6. Teffens J, Nagel R. Tumors of the renal pelvis and ureter: observations in 170 patients. *Br J Urol* 1988;61:277.

CHAPTER 15

Pyelolithotomy

John M. Fitzpatrick

Pyelolithotomy is an operation that is now uncommonly performed. The advent of percutaneous nephrolithotomy with contact lithotripsy (PCNL) and extracorporeal shock wave lithotripsy (ESWL) has reduced the indications for pyelolithotomy, which is a considerably more invasive procedure.

It is interesting to note that when surgeons were first performing pyelolithotomy there was considerable disagreement as to which was the preferred approach to stone removal. Clearly, people liked to argue even then, when one had to do so mainly by letter or book rather than by published article, conference, phone call, telefax, or Internet. Vincenz Czerny probably performed the first pyelotomy, with Sir Henry Morris performing a similar operation to remove a stone in the same year, 1880.

Further developments took place over the years, with many incisions through the thorax and abdomen being introduced, and then many incisions through the renal pelvis and renal parenchyma following. The introduction of radiological visualization of the kidney completed the picture. It is clear, however, that the landmark contributions to open surgical removal of stones from the kidney were made in recent years by Gil Vernet (5), Marshall et al. (7), Boyce and Elkins (1), and Wickham et al. (9).

DIAGNOSIS

The usual presenting symptom for renal calculi is radiating colicky flank pain, usually associated with hematuria. Larger stones, however, may be relatively asymptomatic or present with persistent infection and/or hematuria. The diagnosis of renal calculi is in general made radiographically. Currently, the most common radiological method of diagnosis is via a KUB (kidney, ureter, and bladder) and intravenous pyelography, although some centers are investigating the use of ultrasound and computed tomography.

INDICATIONS FOR SURGERY

Although surgery's use is limited because of this relative invasiveness, it sometimes has a role to play, in particular when the stone burden is large or when problems with body shape or habitus prevent percutaneous access to renal calculi or focusing on the stone by ESWL.

ALTERNATIVE THERAPY

Alternatives to pyelolithotomy include ESWL, percutaneous stone extraction/destruction, ureteroscopic stone destruction, chemolysis (uric acid or struvite stones), or anatrophic nephrolithotomy.

SURGICAL TECHNIQUE

Surgical Access to the Kidney

The urologist may consider five possible approaches to the kidney for open stone removal:

1. Flank approach.
   a. Subcostal.
   b. Costal (eleventh or twelfth rib).
   c. Intercostal (above the eleventh or twelfth rib).
2. Transabdominal.
3. Posterior lumbotomy.

The advantages of the flank approach are described after I explain why, in my opinion, the transabdominal and posterior lumbotomy incisions are rarely required in what is, after all, a relatively uncommon procedure. Transabdominal and transperitoneal access may be required if the patient has spinal deformities and on occasion after several previous surgical procedures. It is the most invasive of all the approaches, and recovery is delayed postoperatively. It should not be used as the standard approach for pyelolithotomy.

The posterior lumbotomy incision (Fig. 15–1) has its advocates, in particular because postoperative pain is minimal and recovery is quick with shortened hospital stay. The patient is placed either in the lateral decubitus position or prone, with pillows under the upper abdomen. The incision is made about 2.5 cm lateral to the erector spinae muscle from the twelfth rib down to the superior border of the iliac crest. The incision is extended through fat and fascia and then through the aponeurotic fibers of the latissimus dorsi. If further access is required, a small part of the twelfth rib can be removed or the lower end of the incision can be curved inferolaterally along the iliac crest. The advantages of this approach have been listed above, but a major disadvantage is that access to the upper pole is difficult, as is access to the ureter below its upper portion. I feel that when an open operation is being performed today for stone removal it is unlikely to be a simple procedure but rather a more complex one for which greater exposure may be required than is afforded by this incision.

Of the flank incisions, I prefer the costal route of access. The subcostal approach is usually too low for renal surgery of any complexity. In considering the incision, it is worth remembering that although it is possible to be too low, preventing complete visualization of each step of the subsequent dissection, it is never possible to be too high. For this reason, the skin incision should be made on top of or superior to one of the ribs. In this way, damage to the subcostal or infracostal nerves is prevented and the likelihood of a wound hernia is minimized. The intercostal approach requires division of the posterior costotransverse ligament to allow the rib to "bucket-handle." Otherwise, access between the ribs may be suboptimal, and, indeed, the ribs may break when spread apart by a self-retaining retractor.

When an incision is based on a rib (the costal approach), removal of the end of the rib is required. A careful review of the preoperative x-ray films and examination of the patient with the table broken will clarify whether the twelfth, eleventh, or even, on some occasions, the tenth rib should be the line of the skin incision. The patient should be placed on the table in the lateral decubitus position with the side to be operated on facing directly upward (Fig. 15–2). The patient can be stabilized by inserting three T-pieces along the sides of the table or fastening tape to the upper thorax and over the hip, thereby fixing the patient on the table. The table is broken, thus opening up the space between the ribs and the iliac crest, and then tilted 20 degrees laterally toward the surgeon. The surgeon and assistant are both positioned behind the patient, and the surgeon can sit down throughout the procedure.

The incision is made in the skin over the distal 6 cm of the rib, extending medially for another 10 to 12 cm. It

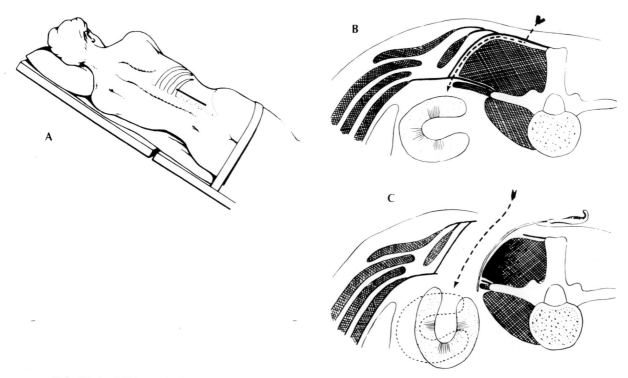

FIG. 15–1. Gil Vernet incision. **A:** Line of posterior vertical lumbotomy with patient in Murphy's position. **B:** Plane of dissection. **C:** With sacrolumbar and quadratus lumborum muscles retracted, the kidney is rotated to present the hilar surface.

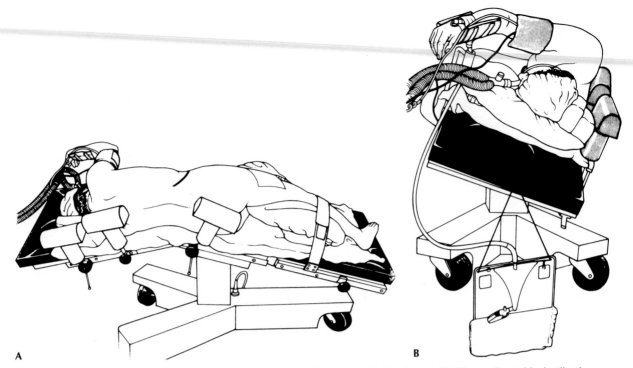

FIG. 15–2. Classic loin approach. **A:** Patient positioned and table flexed. **B:** The entire table is tilted about 20 degrees toward the surgeon, who may then be seated for the operation.

should be deepened down to the rib before any muscles are cut. Once the rib can be clearly seen, the skin, fat, and fascial layers are retracted on both sides to give a better view. The intercostal muscles are divided above the rib with a knife until the diaphragm can be seen; this is then divided with a scissors until the distal 6 cm of rib is cleared. Then, the same approach is made below the rib, with the intercostal muscles being divided if the eleventh rib is being used or the latissimus dorsi if it is the twelfth. The diaphragm will not be divided inferior to the rib, but it is advisable to identify the nerve bundle and sweep it inferiorly. Once the rib has been dissected free of the surrounding muscles, the distal 6 cm is removed with a rib shears. I do not approach the rib subperiosteally, as leaving the periosteum does not confer any advantage.

Once the rib has been removed, Gerota's fascia can be visualized and through it the kidney can be palpated. Two fingers should be introduced under the abdominal muscles through this incision and the peritoneum swept away from their under surface. The incision is then deepened through the external oblique, internal oblique, and transversus abdominus muscles using the knife or cutting diathermy. The incision should not extend as far medially as the rectus sheath.

At this stage, a body wall retractor should be inserted, preferably the Wickham retractor, which is self-retaining and shaped to the body wall. Gerota's fascia is then opened and this incision is extended upward toward the diaphragm and inferiorly toward the pelvic brim. The peritoneum can then be mobilized medially away from the ureter, which is visualized exiting from the perirenal fat, and the ureter is encircled with a loop or tape. The perirenal fat is then grasped over the lateral border of the kidney, elevated by two Babcock forceps, and incised, revealing the capsule of the kidney (Fig. 15–3). The degree of mobilization of the kidney required depends on how large the stone is. If full mobilization is required, it can be performed easily but should always be carried out by sharp dissection with a Metzenbaum scissors under direct vision. Remember that the main renal vein is always best accessed from anterior to the kidney (although there may be tributaries lying posteriorly). The main renal artery is best approached from above and posterior to the kidney, although there may be other branches, in particular an upper pole or lower pole branch directly from the aorta. The artery need not be isolated in the unusual situation that small stones are being removed unless a parenchymal incision is being contemplated. When it is isolated, a loop or tape should be put around it.

In the case of surgical access after previous surgery and after many previous surgical procedures, great care must be taken (Fig. 15–4). After incision of the muscles, the fascial and perirenal areas are likely to be greatly thickened and indurated. It is helpful to isolate the ureter first (prestented if required) and trace the ureter upward to the ureteropelvic junction. The kidney can then be dissected free from the surrounding tissues with the scissors. Care must be taken not to incise the renal capsule because considerable hemorrhage can occur under these circumstances. Because the kidney is likely to be encased in dense fibrous tissue, the perirenal anatomy will be difficult to define accurately and upper and lower pole arteries can be damaged. In addition, identification of the renal artery can be somewhat more difficult; palpation of the tissues medial to the kidney will reveal its position.

Access to the Renal Pelvis

In general terms, it is preferable to open the renal pelvis posteriorly rather than anteriorly. This approach will avoid the renal vein, which often runs along the upper part of the anterior surface of the pelvis. Damage to the renal parenchyma can be avoided if only the renal pelvis is incised. The degree of dissection around the renal pelvis will not affect renal function (2). The subparenchymal and intrasinusal pyelotomy (5) has made easier the removal of even the most complex calculi.

Simple Pyelolithotomy

This method of opening the renal pelvis would only be considered if the stone to be removed is only 1 to 2 cm in diameter in the renal pelvis or in a calyx or if there were a number of such sized calculi in several calyces.

After opening Gerota's fascia and the perirenal fat and putting a tape around the upper ureter, as described above, the amount of dissection in the region of the renal pelvis that is required is not extensive. The ureteropelvic junction and the pelvis itself should be clearly defined, but a subparenchymal dissection is not required unless the pelvis is intrarenal (Fig. 15–5). After placing two stay sutures of 4-0 polyglycolic acid or chromic catgut, make a longitudinal incision in the renal pelvis using a scalpel. The incision must not extend through or into the ureteropelvic junction because of the risk of subsequent scarring.

When the urologist is certain that all stones have been removed, the pelvis should be closed with continuous 4-0 polyglycolic acid or chromic catgut suture. The attempt is to make the closure watertight, but even making the suture continuous does not guarantee this, so the peripelvic tissues should be drained.

Extended Pyelolithotomy

In most cases, the reason for performing open pyelolithotomy will be the complexity of the stone in the renal pelvis and its multiple extensions into the calyces.

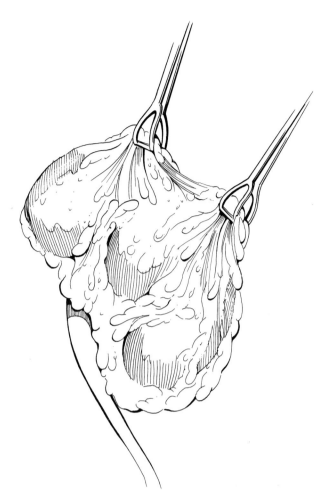

FIG. 15–3. Babcock clamps are used to grasp the perirenal fat, which is incised to reveal the renal capsule

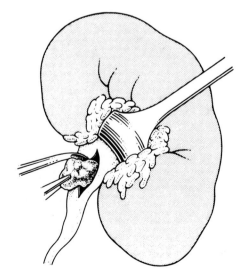

FIG. 15–4. Standard pyelothotomy with sinus retraction.

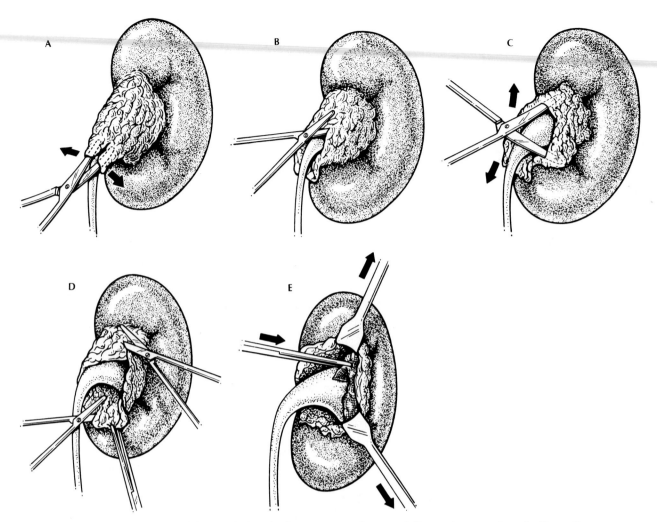

FIG. 15–5. Exposure of the renal sinus in the presence of severe inflammatory erection. **A:** Dissection begins along the upper ureter and proceeds superiorly. **B:** Peripelvic fat is mobilized and then incised. **C:** Near the hilus, peripelvic tissue is dissected bluntly. **D:** Excess adipose tissue may be excised. **E:** With hilar retractors in place, intrasinusal fat is dissected away by blunt dissection using surgical gauze.

In many cases it will be possible to remove the stone completely by extending the dissection under the parenchyma and exposing the renal pelvis and calyceal infundibula in the manner described by Gil Vernet (5). In this way, incisions into the renal parenchyma can be avoided, thus reducing the potential for renal injury.

The anatomy of the renal hilum allows for extensive exposure of the renal pelvis, but care must be taken to adhere to the correct planes of dissection. There is a thin layer of connective tissue extending from the renal capsule into the fat in the renal hilum and then onto the renal pelvis. This closes off the renal hilum, and it is this layer that must be incised to gain access to the infundibula in carrying out an extended pyelolithotomy. Once this layer of connective tissue has been incised, the dissection is continued by inserting specially designed retractors under the parenchyma. The dissection is carried out by inserting and spreading a fine scissors or by the use of a Küttner dissector. This dissection is carried out between the fatty

layer in the hilum and the pelvis itself (Fig. 15–3). If, mistakenly, the surgeon enters the layer between the fat and the parenchyma, considerable hemorrhage can be encountered because of many venous channels in this area.

Even if there is perihilar inflammation, or if there has been previous surgery, it is possible to develop this plane. Sharp dissection is required, but early insertion of Gil Vernet retractors moves the vessels in the hilum out of the way so that damage to important structures is avoided. Even if veins in this area are opened, they can be compressed by the insertion of small sponges between the retractors and the hilum, and bleeding kept to a minimum.

The subparenchymal dissection can be extended to the infundibula without damaging the superior or inferior apical branches of the renal artery. An incision is then made with a scalpel into the renal pelvis, directly down onto the main bulk of the stone. It is extended in a curved fashion with angled scissors into the necks of the superior and inferior calyces. Alternatively, a straight incision is made in the parenchyma from side to side and perpendicular extensions are made into the necks of the individual calyces (Fig. 15–6).

In general, the large central bulk of the stone is removed first. The best way to do this is to pass a stone dissector around the stone and lever it out of the pelvis. This is preferable to grasping the stone with a forceps, as the stone may break. Once the main fragment is out, fine Turner–Warwick stone forceps, either straight or curved, can be inserted into the calyces and individual fragments can be removed.

After the surgeon feels that all of the stone has been removed, it is advisable to irrigate the renal pelvis and flush smaller fragments out of the calyces. This is done by inserting a wide-bore tube into the calyces, through which a high-pressure jet of saline can be passed; the high flow of the saline is essential for effectiveness, and this is best induced by a pressure cuff around a bag of saline attached to an infusion cannula.

Contact radiography should then be performed by putting a kidney film behind the kidney. It is helpful to put the kidney into an elastic net sling and then tie the sling to the retractor or to a gantry on the retractor. Ligaclips can then be clipped onto the sling, thereby facilitating the location of even small residual fragments on the x-ray film.

The renal pelvis is then closed by using a continuous 4-0 polyglycolic acid or chromic catgut suture. Sometimes it may be easier to put one or two interrupted sutures in the apical parts of the necks of the infundibula,

and this will facilitate closure. Again, the closure may not be watertight and drainage of the area is thus required. Unless there is noticeable intrarenal hemorrhage, no nephrostomy tube is necessary.

Additional Nephrotomies

On occasion, it may not be possible to remove the entire stone through a pyelotomy and additional transparenchymal access is required; the anatrophic nephrolithotomy (1) would be excessive if the renal pelvis has been opened in the manner described above, and multiple radial paravascular nephrotomies (9) are a relatively atraumatic method of access. The method of doing this is to make a small (1 cm) radial incision over the stone, which can be localized either by palpation with a needle through the parenchyma or by intraoperative ultrasonography. The parenchyma is then separated by spreading with two MacDonald's stone dissectors until the calyx is opened and the stone removed. This can be done in a number of positions with a minimal effect on renal function (2). The nephrotomies are closed with a continuous 4-0 polyglycolic acid or chromic catgut suture, which is placed superficially, incorporating only capsule and a thin layer of parenchyma. A nephrostomy tube should be placed into the most dependent calyx opened; a 12 Fr whistle-tip catheter is satisfactory. This should be brought out through a separate stab incision in the skin.

If a radial paravascular incision is to be made, the renal artery must be located and either a silastic loop or a cotton tape passed around it to gain control. A single nephro-

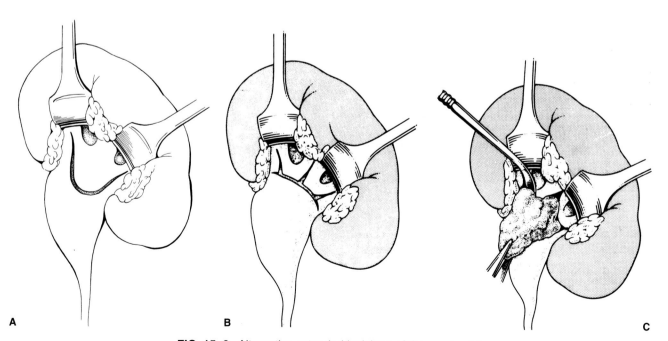

FIG. 15–6. Alternative extended incisions of the renal pelvis

tomy may not require vascular occlusion, and occlusion can be avoided altogether by the use of Doppler ultrasound, which is especially valuable in kidneys with decreased function and thinned parenchyma (4). If the renal artery must be occluded, renal function should be preserved during the period of ischemia. Renal hypothermia is achieved by surface cooling with sterile crushed ice (6) or external cooling coils (8).

A less complex method of protecting against renal ischemic damage is the use of intravenous inosine. This can be injected into a peripheral vein and is valuable in protecting renal function, in particular if the ischemic period is less than 60 minutes and overall preoperative renal function is good (3).

Wound Closure

After complete stone removal and adequate hemostasis are ensured, the wound is closed. A Robinson drain is brought out through a separate stab incision. A gravity drainage system such as this is preferable to a suction drain, which may cause a urinary fistula to develop.

The wound is closed using a series of interrupted no. 1 polyglycolic acid sutures. These are passed through all muscular layers at 2-mm intervals and are left untied until all are placed. The table is then unbroken, which brings the wound edges closer together and allows the sutures to be tied without tension. A continuous layer of no. 1 polyglycolic acid suture is then passed through the outer layer of the external oblique muscle and the fascial layers. The skin can be closed with 3-0 monofilament nylon or with skin clips.

OUTCOMES

Complications

Complications from open renal stone surgery are significant and include hemorrhage, urinary fistula, recurrent stones, and actual or functional loss of the renal unit. The risk of these complications is dependent on the associated findings of chronic infection, prior surgery, and surgeon's expertise.

There is a small chance that the pleura may be opened when a costal or intercostal incision is made, and the probability of this increases the higher the incision is made. A pleurotomy is readily identified by hearing the sound of air being sucked into the thorax and seeing the lung on inspiration. The diaphragm should be dissected free from the ribs and used to strengthen the closure of the pleura, which is itself too thin and fragile to hold a suture. The 3-0 chromic catgut suture should include the diaphragm, pleura, and intercostal muscles, and the anesthesiologist should inflate the lung before the last suture is put in. This usually prevents a pneumothorax. A postoperative chest x-ray must be performed, and, in the relatively uncommon event of a persistent pneumothorax, a chest tube should be inserted.

Results

Stone-free rates in patients undergoing pyelolithotomy are variable, depending on the number of stones, the composition of the stone, and the presence of calyceal stones or obstruction. Solitary stones have virtually a 100% stone-free rate, whereas staghorn stones (struvite) or patients with multiple stones scattered among the calyces may have an incidence of retained stones of 10% or more.

REFERENCES

1. Boyce WH, Elkins IB. Reconstructive renal surgery following anatrophic nephrolithotomy: follow-up of 100 consecutive cases. *J Urol* 1974;111:307.
2. Fitzpatrick JM, Sleight MW, Braack A, Marberger M, Wickham JEA. Intrarenal access: effects on renal function and morphology. *Br J Urol* 1980;52:409.
3. Fitzpatrick JM, Wallace DMA, Whitfield HN, Watkinson LE, Fernando AR, Wickham JEA. Inosine in ischaemic renal surgery: long-term follow-up. *Br J Urol* 1981;53:524.
4. Fitzpatrick JM, Murphy DM, Gorey TF, Alken P, Thuroff J. Doppler localization of intrarenal vessels: an experimental study. *Br J Urol* 1984;56:614.
5. Gil Vernet JM. New surgical concepts in removing renal calculi. *Urol Int* 1965;20:255.
6. Graves FT. Renal hypothermia: an aid to partial nephrectomy. *Br J Surg* 1968;50:362.
7. Marshall VF, Lavengood RW Jr, Kelly DG. Complete longitudinal nephrolithotomy and the Shorr regimen in the management of staghorn calculi. *Ann Surg* 1965;162:366.
8. Wickham JEA. A simple method for regional renal hypothermia. *J Urol* 1968;99:246.
9. Wickham JEA, Coe N, Ward JP. One hundred cases of nephrolithotomy under hypothermia. *J Urol* 1974;112:702.

CHAPTER 16

Ureterolithotomy

Michael Marberger

For centuries, "cutting for stone" was synonymous with urology, and just over a decade ago it still comprised at least one-fourth of the surgical activity in the field. The development of extracorporeal shockwave lithotripsy (SWL) and endoscopic stone surgery shattered this tradition, and the change becomes most obvious in the indications for ureterolithotomy. Once one of the most common procedures in urology, it all but vanished in the last years in spite of the fact that almost 50% of all patients with upper tract urolithiasis coming to treatment today have stones impacted in the ureter (8). Specifically, the development of ultrathin semirigid and flexible ureteroscopes with effective laser, electrohydraulic, or ballistic lithotripsy, laparoscopic ureterolithotomy, and third-generation lithotriptors with ultrasonic and fluoroscopic stone localization and small focal zones, which can be pinpointed onto ureteric stones even in infants, have closed the last gaps in the spectrum of minimally invasive therapy of ureteric calculi.

DIAGNOSIS

With less invasive methods of stone removal, a sudden change of the position of the calculus can be met without major problems, even when noticed only during the intervention. In open stone surgery, this could result in a catastrophe, with failure to remove the stone and the need for further procedures. The time-honored rule of precise delineation of the size, number, and shape of all calculi and their topography within the collecting system before an incisional procedure remains as valid as ever.

In general, ureteric stones can be located precisely with a good intravenous pyelogram with appropriate oblique, delayed, and postvoiding films. The diagnostic technique of choice today is helical computerized tomography without and with contrast dye, which will also reliably differentiate radiolucent stones from tumors, clots, or papillae. If there are any remaining questions retro-grade ureterography and, if needed, diagnostic ureteroscopy immediately before surgery will clarify the situation. Urinary infection should always be treated with appropriate antibiotics before surgery. With severe obstruction and any evidence of infection, it is prudent to first drain the kidney by percutaneous nephrostomy for about 48 hours until any pathogen is cultured and adequately treated.

A plain abdominal roentgenogram is always obtained immediately before surgery, before anesthesia is initiated. Even the largest calculus seemingly incapable of changing its position may do so, and this may necessitate a completely different surgical strategy.

INDICATIONS FOR SURGERY

In general, ureterolithotomy today becomes necessary only where extracorporeal shock wave lithotripsy (ESWL) or endoscopic techniques fail. Usually, these failures are concomitant with a complication of previous therapeutic interventions, in particular endoscopic manipulation. Urinary extravasation, an impacted ureteral basket, ureteral avulsion, and an obstructing stone are the typical scenarios. At the author's institution, incisional surgery was required in only seven of 4,201 patients subjected to a therapeutic intervention to remove ureteric stones in a 10-year period. Two patients had suffered ureteric avulsion, one patient had a basket trapped around a stone, in three patients the stones could not be reached endoscopically, and one patient, pregnant in the fourth week of gestation, required rapid removal of a large stone impacted in the lumbar ureter. Ureteric reconstruction is beyond the scope of this chapter (see Chapter 17), but the latter three cases demonstrate that there is still an occasional, anecdotal need for ureterolithotomy. Stones can, of course, also be trapped above congenital or acquired ureteric strictures. Where these require surgical correction, the stone is removed at the time of reconstructive surgery, but the underlying pathology dictates the surgical strategy and technique.

ALTERNATIVE THERAPY

Alternatives to open ureterolithotomy are observation, which is indicated in small (greater than 15 mm) stones with no signs of sepsis or extravasation, or one of many forms of minimally invasive surgeries including ESWL, endoscopic extraction (via cystoscope, nephroscope, or ureteroscope), contact lithotripsy, or percutaneous stone surgery including laparoscopic removal. The latter basically combines endoscopic, extraperitoneal exposure of the ureter with traditional ureterolithotomy techniques and represents the logical improvement of incisional surgery in the effort to reduce morbidity.

SURGICAL TECHNIQUE

In the difficult situations in which ureterolithotomy is still indicated today, ample exposure is usually needed. Many of the minimally muscle-splitting incisions designed for specific stone situations in the past, such as the Foley incision through the lumbar triangle for high ureteral stones, the gridiron incision for midureteral stones, and the transvesical or transvaginal approach for intramural stones, have become obsolete. They provide only limited access to a small segment of the ureter and should be avoided in difficult situations, especially if the surgeon has limited experience with them.

The entire proximal half of the ureter is best approached by a modified twelfth-rib supracostal incision, which is carried anterior to the tip of the rib (anterior supracostal incision). Large, firmly embedded stones in the area of the ureteropelvic junction can be removed with minimal morbidity through a posterior lumbotomy. The distal half of the ureter is best reached by a suprainguinal extraperitoneal access.

Anterior Supracostal Approach

The patient is placed in a lateral jackknife position (Fig. 16–1). The skin incision runs parallel to the upper margin of the twelfth rib and distally in the line of the rib. Its length depends on the precise nature of the procedure. For a standard ureterolithotomy in the lumbar ureter, an incision along the distal half of the rib extending 5 to 7 cm into the abdominal muscles suffices. It can be extended anteriorly as required to reach lower stones and posteriorly so that the entire kidney can be mobilized if necessary.

After the subcutaneous fat has been divided, the fibers of the abdominal musculature are incised with cutting diathermy immediately beyond the tip of the twelfth rib (Fig. 16–2). The transversus abdominis muscle blends

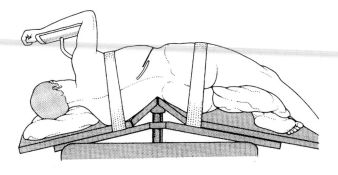
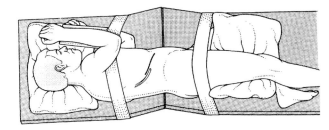

FIG. 16–1. Position of the patient for anterior twelfth-rib supracostal incision. (From Marberger M, Fitzpatrick JM, Jenkins AD, Pak CLYC. *Stone surgery*. Edinburgh: Churchill Livingstone, 1991, with permission. [8])

here with the deep leaf of the thoracolumbar fascia and should be divided along the same line. The second and third fingers of each hand are now used to sweep the peritoneum off the underside of the abdominal wall muscles before the muscle incision is extended medially as required. The incision should be kept strictly in line with the extension of the twelfth rib so as to keep well clear of subcostal vessels and nerves. Once it has been carried as far medially as needed, dissection can proceed in the opposite direction along the twelfth rib. The latissimus dorsi and intercostal muscles are divided by diathermy moving backward along the upper margin of the rib. As the rib is progressively mobilized, the insertion of the diaphragm and the pleural reflection come into view. The subcostal nerve is carefully preserved as the diaphragm is divided flush with its insertion to the abdominal wall. The pleura is pushed away by blunt finger dissection. Depending on the degree of exposure needed, dissection of the twelfth rib may proceed up to the vertebral column. After division of the costovertebral ligament, the twelfth rib can be swung outward like a door. A rib retractor or modified Wickham ring retractor permits excellent exposure. The peritoneum is retracted medially, and the ureter is exposed in the retroperitoneal space below the lower pole of the kidney, where it already lies outside of Gerota's fascia. If the stone lies higher, Gerota's fascia is incised and the ureter is followed upward to the stone, tilting the kidney anteriorly.

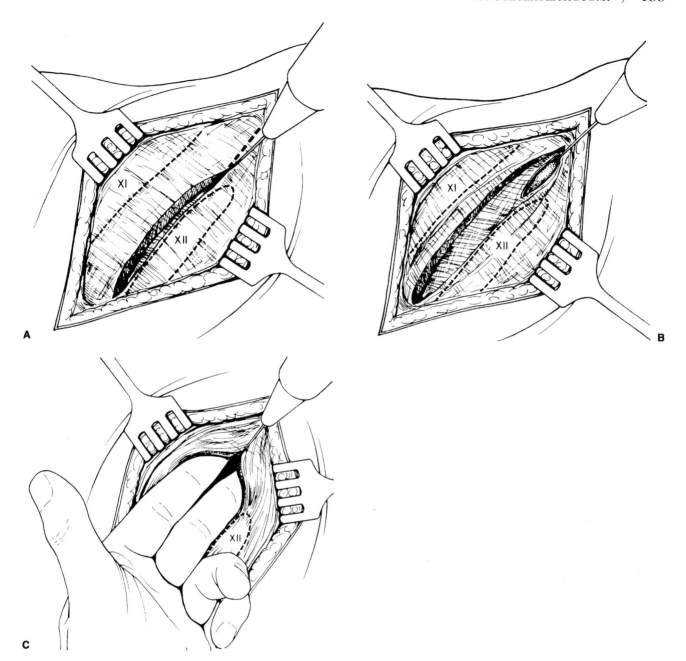

FIG. 16–2. Anterior supracostal incision. **A:** The latissimus dorsi is first incised along the upper rim of the twelfth rib. The external, internal, and transversus abdominis muscles are divided **(B)** in extension of the 12th rib as far medially as needed **(C)**. (From Marberger M, Stackl W. Surgical treatment of renal calculi. In: Schneider HJ, ed. *Urolithiasis.* Heidelberg: Springer, 1986:107, with permission. [10])

Posterior Lumbotomy

The proximal third of the ureter (and renal pelvis) can be reached with minimal muscle trauma through the thoracolumbar fascia lateral to the sacrospinalis and quadratus lumborum muscles. In terms of postoperative pain and morbidity, this incision is superior to all other lumbotomies. The twelfth rib above and the iliac crest below limit exposure of the kidney and midureter. Therefore, the ideal stone for this approach should be one that is firmly embedded in the upper third of the ureter or at the ureteropelvic junction.

The patient is placed in the lateral recumbent position, with approximately 15-degree anterior rotation, and the table is flexed at the tip of the twelfth rib. Simultaneous bilateral surgery may be performed with the patient prone (10). The most commonly used access (6) utilizes an oblique skin incision parallel and 3 cm lateral to the erec-

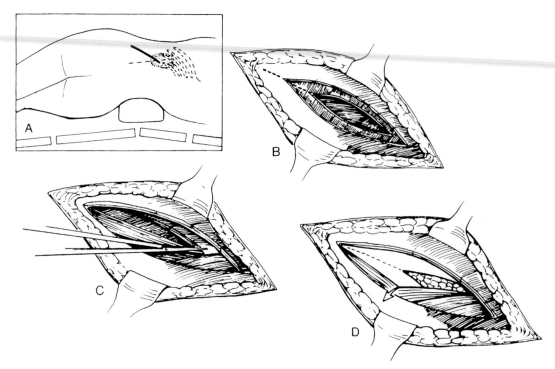

FIG. 16–3. Posterior lumbotomy. **A:** Positioning of patient with oblique and vertical incision. **B:** Oblique incision: division of latissimus dorsi and posterior inferior serratus muscle. **C:** Oblique incision: division of costovertebral ligament. **D:** Oblique incision: opening of Gerota's fascia. (From Anderson EE. Ureterolithotomy. In: Glenn JF, ed. *Urologic surgery*, 4th ed. Philadelphia: JB Lippincott, 1993:276–286, with permission. [2])

tor trunci, from the twelfth rib down to the iliac crest (Fig. 16–3). Fat and subcutaneous tissue are divided until the lateral fibers of the latissimus dorsi are exposed. The muscle is split to expose the subjacent twelfth rib. The posterior leaf of the lumbodorsal fascia is divided in the line of the skin incision, and the lateral margin of the sacrospinalis muscle so exposed is retracted medially. The middle layer of the thoracolumbar fascia is then seen and incised somewhat lateral to the fleshy belly of the sacrospinalis muscle. The lateral border of the quadratus lumborum now comes into view and may be retracted with a hook toward the vertebral column. The deep layer of the thoracolumbar fascia is exposed and opened, care being exercised to spare the twelfth subcostal nerve and the iliohypogastric nerve coursing obliquely and laterally on its deep aspect. Gerota's fascia is incised and the perirenal fat is divided by blunt dissection to expose the renal pelvis. A Finochetto rib retractor is inserted to expose the field.

Suprainguinal Approach

The distal half of the ureter is best approached by a suprainguinal extraperitoneal incision. The patient is in a prone position with the ipsilateral flank supported by a

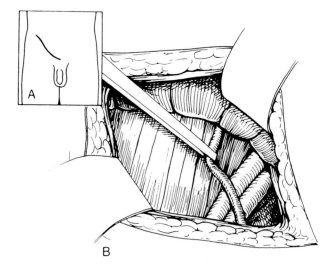

FIG. 16–4. Suprainguinal extraperitoneal approach. **A:** Incision. **B:** Exposure of ureter following incision of external and internal oblique muscles and splitting of transversalis fascia. (From Anderson EE. Ureterolithotomy. In: Glenn JF, ed. *Urologic surgery*, 4th ed. Philadelphia: JB Lippincott, 1993: 276–286, with permission. [2])

cushion. Depending on the exposure needed, the skin is incised in an oblique direction along a line from the pubic tubercle upward to a point about two finger breadths anterior to the superior iliac crest (Fig. 16–4). The external oblique abdominal muscles and the transversalis fascia are divided with cutting diathermy in the same direction. After ligation and transection of the epigastric vessels, the peritoneal fold is reflected medially to expose the ureter. It can be identified without problems either where it crosses the common iliac artery or where it runs immediately below the obliterated umbilical artery. The latter structure is routinely divided and ligated. With stones in the distal third of the ureter, a urethral catheter should routinely be placed to keep the bladder empty during the procedure.

Ureterolithotomy

Once the ureter is identified, the stone is located by palpation, carefully avoiding any milking movements that could dislocate it. Without mobilizing the ureter, it is snared with vessel loops just above and below the stone. The ureteral wall is incised with a scalpel directly onto the stone in a longitudinal direction. As soon as the mucosa is opened, the incision is enlarged with angulated scissors so that the stone can be extracted with nerve hooks. The ureter is then probed in both directions with a soft ureteral catheter to ascertain complete stone removal and is irrigated copiously.

With the slightest possibility of obstruction, extravasation, or difficult closure, a self-retaining stent is inserted, taking care to position the two ends properly in the bladder and renal pelvis. A standard double-J stent can usually be inserted from the ureterotomy. Because the distal segment of the ureter is, in general, more difficult to negotiate, especially after previous endoscopic maneuvers, it is intubated first. By reversing the stent, i.e., advancing the blunted, closed tip of the stent, which is otherwise advanced up to the kidney, down to the bladder, the ureterovesical junction can usually be passed. The guide wire is then removed and the stent is advanced further down the ureter until it almost disappears in the ureterotomy. Its upper end can now be straightened and advanced up into the renal pelvis. If the proximal corner of the ureteric incision is elevated with a nerve hook during this procedure, this rarely causes problems. It is important to note the markings on the stent for correct placement. To ascertain that the distal end of the stent is in the bladder, indigo carmine can be administered through the urethral catheter; it should reflux freely into ureter and stent. Intraoperative fluoroscopy offers a more elegant alternative.

If any problems are encountered in intubating the ureter, it should be inspected with a thin flexible ureteroscope inserted through the ureterotomy to avoid missing an additional ureteric stone. Any additional stone is either removed through a second ureterotomy or, preferably, by endoscopic lithotripsy. A guide wire is then advanced under endoscopic control down into the bladder and the stent is inserted over it. Problems in the ureter proximal to the incision are handled in a similar manner, but this segment of the ureter is usually dilated and therefore easier to engage.

Whenever self-retaining stents are used, the patient should routinely be subjected to a flexible cystoscopy at the end of the procedure to be certain the vesical end of the stent is indeed in the bladder.

The ureterotomy is closed with one to three interrupted sutures of 5-0 chromic catgut. The sutures should grasp only the superficial seromuscular layers to approximate the ureteric wall rather than achieving watertight closure. If placed too tight or too deep, they may compromise ureteric blood supply and promote leakage. Obstructing sutures have a similar effect. Whenever closure is difficult because of scarring, it is safer not to close the ureterotomy at all and to stent the ureter. The site of the ureterotomy should be covered with retroperitoneal fat or an omental flap (7).

Every ureterotomy has to be drained precisely. We routinely use an 18 Fr tube drain of silicone rubber with one or two side holes, which is brought out through all layers of the abdominal wall via a separate stab incision lateral to the lower end of the incision. The tip of the drain must be in a dependent position to the ureterotomy but not in the immediate vicinity or in contact with the ureter. If the ureter was approached transperitoneally, it should be drained through the retroperitoneum. The wound is closed in layers with absorbable suture material.

Postoperatively, patients are mobilized within 24 hours, with analgesics administered generously as needed. Antibiotics are given only with proven infection and according to appropriate sensitivity testing. The patients are well hydrated, with intravenous fluid replacement in the first two postoperative days. Especially after lumbar ureterolithotomy, bowel function may take 2 to 3 days to normalize and an enema and even cholinergic agents may be needed.

OUTCOMES

Complications

The wound drain should not be removed before the fourth or fifth postoperative day. Prolonged discharge of urine from the drain is usually caused by impaired drainage caused by a missed calculus, clot, or ureteral obstruction. On occasion, leakage results from incorrect positioning of the tip of the drain immediately adjacent to the ureterotomy. Careful retraction of the drain by 1 to 2 cm then rapidly dries up the wound. If urine leaks from the drain longer than 5 days, an indwelling ureteric stent should be inserted. Permanent urinary fistulas are extremely rare and, when present, almost always result from obstruction below the level of surgery.

Urinary extravasation may cause severe problems if the wound is improperly drained because the drain either was not placed in a dependent position or was removed too early. Urinoma formation is usually heralded by fever and flank pain but may occur inconspicuously. A high degree of suspicion should therefore be directed toward this potential complication. Any unexplained fever, flank pain, or delayed healing should be investigated immediately by ultrasonography, excretory urography with delayed films, or computerized tomography. The situation can usually be corrected by draining the kidney with an indwelling stent or a nephrostomy and draining the urinoma percutaneously.

In the pre-ESWL era, the most frustrating complication of any stone operation was the retained calculus. Although the availability of ESWL should still not be an excuse for a less careful attempt at complete stone removal once open surgery is decided on, retained stones can be treated in this manner highly successfully some days after the operation. Likewise, if a calculus below the level of surgery was overseen and resulted in obstruction and/or extravasation it can be treated endoscopically or by ESWL, just as any other ureteral stone in the immediate postoperative period.

REFERENCES

1. Adams JB. Ureteral surgery. In: Badlani G, Bagley DH, Clayman RV et al., eds. *Smith's textbook of endourology*. St. Louis: Quality Medical Publishers, 1996:962–976.
2. Anderson EE. Ureterolithotomy. In: Glenn JF, ed. *Urologic surgery*, 4th ed. Philadelphia: JB Lippincott, 1993:276–286.
3. Assimos D, Chaussy C, Clayman R, Marberger M. Predicting the future. In: Segura J, Pak C, Preminger GM, Tolley D, eds. *Proceedings of the 1st International Consultation on Stone Disease*. Paris: SCI, 2002.
4. Conlin MJ, Marberger M, Bagley D. Ureteroscopes and working instruments. In: Badlani G, Bagley DH, Clayman RV et al., eds. *Smith's textbook of endourology*. St. Louis: Quality Medical Publishers, 1996: 370–387.
5. Hofbauer J. Electrohydraulic versus pneumatic disintegration in the treatment of ureteral stones: a randomized, prospective trial. *J Urol* 1995;153:623–625.
6. Lutzeyer W. Lumbodorsal exploration. In: Glenn JF, ed. *Urologic surgery*, 2nd ed. Philadelphia: JB Lippincott, 1975:127–133.
7. Marberger M, Fitzpatrick JM, Jenkins AD, Pak CLYC. *Stone surgery*. Edinburgh: Churchill Livingstone, 1991.
8. Marberger M, Hofbauer J, Turk C, Hobarth K, Albrecht W. Management of ureteric stones. *Eur Urol* 1994;25:265–272.
9. Marberger M, Turk C, Steinkogler I. Piezoelectric extracorporeal shock wave lithotripsy in children. *J Urol* 1989;142:349–352.
10. Marberger M, Stackl W. Surgical treatment of renal calculi. In: Schneider HJ, ed. *Urolithiasis*. Heidelberg: Springer, 1986;107.

CHAPTER 17

Ureteral Reconstruction

Marc-Oliver Grimm and A. Rolf Ackermann

Partial or complete ureteral replacement remains a challenge for the urologist. The maintenance of kidney function is the primary goal of this procedure. The crucial problem with ureteral replacement is that in most cases several surgical procedures and frequently radiotherapy have been performed beforehand, and kidney function is usually already impaired at the time of intervention. Therefore, standardized procedures may not be applicable and the approach must be tailored according to the individual situation.

Several substitutes have been proposed for ureteral replacement, including blood vessels, fallopian tubes, and the appendix. Nevertheless, the use of all these tissues or organs and the corresponding procedures are associated with a significant morbidity, including recurrent infection, stone, or stricture formation, with a worsening of kidney function in many patients. Because larger series have rarely been reported, the results and morbidity of the various procedures differ significantly.

DIAGNOSIS

Partial or complete ureteral replacement with small bowel is usually a secondary treatment. Every attempt should be made to preserve as much ureteral length as possible. Antegrade and retrograde pyelography will usually provide sufficient information regarding the length and degree of the stricture, but in selected cases ureteroscopy may provide additional valuable information. A cystogram, determination of bladder capacity, and if necessary urodynamic studies are recommended in cases where psoas hitch or Boari flap reconstruction may be considered. In patients treated for malignant disease, tumor recurrence must be excluded by computed tomography scan or magnetic resonance imaging. Kidney function needs to be examined by preoperative isotope scintigraphy to ensure it is appropriate because with severely decreased function the results of ureteral recon-

struction are poor. Furthermore, preoperative isotope scintigraphy provides a baseline for follow-up examinations after surgery.

INDICATIONS FOR SURGERY

Partial or complete ureteral replacement with small bowel is indicated as a second-line treatment after failure of ureter-sparing surgery. Poor kidney function with a serum creatinine of greater than 2 mg per dl as well as bladder outlet obstruction are in general considered a contraindication.

ALTERNATIVE THERAPY

Ureteral reconstruction is most frequently required after iatrogenic and sometimes after traumatic injuries. Lesions during endoscopic urologic procedures are effectively treated by prolonged placement of ureteral stents or nephrostomies and rarely result in stricture formation (8). Ureteral injuries detected during open surgery are repaired immediately; however, 55% to 70% of injuries are recognized only postoperatively. While the traditional approach to delayed detected ureteral injuries suggests reconstruction after 6 weeks to 3 months, similar or even better results have been reported after early surgical reconstruction within 3 weeks (6).

Every attempt should be made to maintain the ureter. Depending on the length and location of the injury, preoperative evaluation should provide information about whether ureter-sparing approaches are viable alternatives to ureteral replacement (Table 17–1). The particular techniques for reconstruction do not differ from those for ureteral stricture management as described in Chapter 18.

Ureteral reconstruction of larger injuries or strictures, in particular of those located above the pelvic brim, require ureteral replacement with bowel if other attempts of reconstruction failed. Alternatively, transureter-

TABLE 17–1. *Ureter-sparing treatment options for ureteral strictures*

Location of the stricture	Possible procedure
Proximal	Pyeloplasty
	Ureterocalicostomy
Middle	Excision and reanastomosis
Distal	Psoas hitch
	Boari flap
All locations	Endoscopic procedures (endoureterotomy)
Long distance	Autotransplantation (Davis ureterotomy)

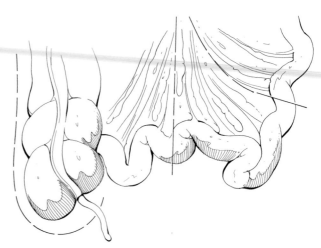

FIG. 17–1. Mobilization of cecum and ascending colon for right ureteral replacement. Selection of ileal segment.

oureterostomy has been recently reported to be safe and effective if tension on the anastomosis and kinking of the ureter can be avoided by mobilization of the affected ureter and transposition above the inferior mesenteric artery (5). However, several authors are reluctant to jeopardize the integrity of a normal upper urinary tract and put it at risk of surgical complication (1).

Autotransplantation may be another alternative of reconstruction of a long ureteral defect of patients with a solitary kidney and/or compromised renal function but carries several disadvantages and risks, especially after previous surgery and/or radiotherapy.

SURGICAL TECHNIQUE

Bladder outlet obstruction is a contraindication for ureteral replacement with small bowel and, therefore, must be excluded. If necessary, urodynamic examination of the lower urinary tract should be performed. In patients with obstructive prostatic hyperplasia, prostatectomy should be performed before ureteral replacement. Preoperative bowel preparation should be performed as in patients undergoing bowel surgery for other urologic procedures. A nephrostomy tube is already in place in most patients or should be inserted during surgery.

If both sides are affected, a midline incision or a right paramedian incision is recommended. If only one ureter is to be replaced, a lateral flank position (twist position) with the table flexed and the chest positioned at about a 60-degree angle to the table is preferable. Allow the pelvis to fall back. The incision starts between the eleventh and twelfth ribs, continues semiobliquely nearly to the midline, and ends as a paramedian incision to the os pubis. The peritoneum is opened and the small bowel packed away.

The ipsilateral colon is reflected and the diseased ureter is resected proximally to healthy tissue or, if the entire ureter is diseased, up to the renal pelvis. Mobilize the peritoneum from the bladder dome and the lateral aspect of the bladder. Carefully determine the length of intestine required for ureteral replacement.

Select an appropriate segment from the preterminal ileum (Fig. 17–1). Consider adequate vascularization of the chosen segment (see ileal conduit, Chapter 78). It is mandatory to select the sites of transection to permit a dissection deep enough for the proximal end to reach the renal pelvis and the aboral distal end to reach the bladder. The bowel is divided and the continuity restored, as described for the ileal conduit. The mesenteric defect is then closed with 4-0 Vicryl to prevent internal herniation. The excised bowel segment is irrigated with saline solution until the effluent is clear.

The mesentery of the ascending colon is incised depending on the location of the mesentery of the ileal segment and the ileum is passed into the retroperitoneal space. The ileal segment is then rotated to place the distal end near the bladder and the proximal end close to the renal pelvis or ureter. The defect in the colonic mesentery is closed using 4-0 Vicryl sutures. In this closure, it is important to avoid compression of the ileal mesenteric vessels.

Pyeloileal Anastomosis or Ileoureteral Anastomosis

In cases of partial ureteral replacement, the proximal opening of the ileal segment is closed with a running 3-0 Vicryl suture. Before the anastomosis, the ureter is stented with a 6 to 9 Fr catheter held in place with a 4-0 Vicryl rapid or chromic catgut suture. The ileoureteral anastomosis of the spatulated ureter is performed end to side with a single-layer technique with either a running suture or interrupted sutures of 4-0 or 5-0 Vicryl.

For complete ureteral replacement, the proximal opening of the ileal segment is brought to the renal pelvis. The renal pelvis is opened widely to permit end-to-end anastomosis to the ileum. In the case of a small renal pelvis, it may become necessary to taper the ileum by closing the

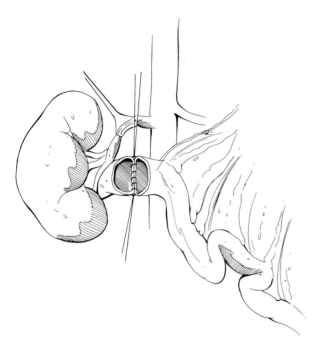

FIG. 17–2. Pyeloileal anastomosis.

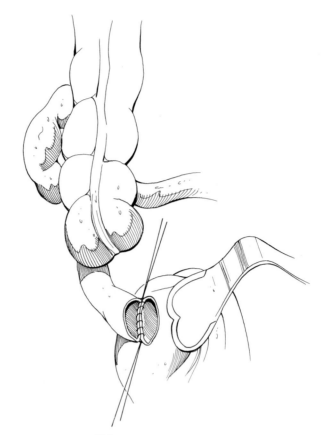

FIG. 17–3. Ileocystostomy.

proximal opening of the ileum partially on the antime-senteric side. The pyeloileal anastomosis is performed in a single layer with either a running suture or interrupted sutures of 3-0 or 4-0 Vicryl (Fig. 17–2). Because a nephrostomy tube is already in place, it is not necessary to stent the ileal ureter.

Ileocystostomy

We prefer to perform ileocystostomy on the posterior bladder wall about 1 to 2 cm craniolaterally to the native ureteral orifice to avoid extensive angulation and possible obstruction of the ileum during bladder filling. The bladder is opened anteriorly in the midline and a full-thickness segment of the bladder is removed at the site of ureterovesical anastomosis. The anastomosis is performed in a double-layered technique with a running mucosa-to-mucosa suture (4-0 Vicryl) and interrupted seromuscular–detrusor muscle sutures of 3-0 Vicryl (Fig. 17–3). Bilateral ureteral replacement can be accomplished by modifying the above technique as shown in Fig. 17–4.

OUTCOMES

Most reports on ureteral replacement with ileum are case reports including only a few patients. Because no larger contemporary series are available for review, the assessment of the outcome of this procedure is difficult.

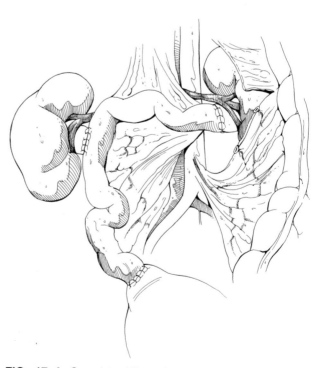

FIG. 17–4. Complete bilateral ureteral replacement with ileum.

Complications

No data are available regarding perioperative complications of ureteral replacement with ileum. It is assumed that the complications are similar to those observed after surgery for an ileal neobladder. In patients with partial replacement of the ureter, strictures at the ureteroileal anastomosis presumably occur at a similar frequency as in patients with an ileal conduit. Ileoureteral reflux is observed in 50% to 85% of patients depending on whether the bladder is filled or empty (2,4,7). The significance of this reflux is unknown.

Hyperchloremic metabolic acidosis requiring treatment has been observed in up to 50% (7). However, Mattos and Smith described metabolic acidosis in a more recent series to be a rare event, with only 3% of patients affected (4). Careful follow-up examination including routine measurements of base excess, serum bicarbonate, and pH are mandatory. Patients with ureteral replacement are certainly prone to urinary tract infections (UTIs). In 30% to 100% of patients, UTI will occur (4,7). Regular urinalysis and appropriate antibiotic treatment in cases of proven UTI are required.

Results

The results of ureteral replacement with ileum are difficult to assess because this form of surgery is rare, is not standardized, and patient selection varies considerably between the different series (4,6–8). Further, the objective goals of the procedure are not clearly defined. The values of blood urea nitrogen or serum creatinine that have been reported in some series are probably not sufficient to define the outcome in patients with bilateral kidneys. Dilation of the upper urinary tract is another parameter used in the literature. However, it is difficult to discriminate between persistent dilation despite reduction of ureteral obstruction and those cases in which dilation persists as a result of obstruction and/or reflux after surgery. To date, no reports including diuretic isotope scintigraphy have been published.

In the few studies with long-term results, a favorable outcome has been reported in up to 85% of cases (2,7). This does not include patients with impaired renal function with serum creatinine levels greater than 2.0 mg per dL. In this population, fewer than 50% will benefit from ureteral replacement.

In general, to avoid metabolic problems the length of the ileal segment should be as short as possible. Hinman and Oppenheimer, however, have shown in the dog that an ileal segment greater than 18 cm will block the transmission of 20 to 30 cm H_2O pressure (3). These experiments also form the basis for the introduction of a nontubularized ileal segment in modifications of the neobladder. Clinical reports on ureteral replacement with ileum apparently do not support this experimental observation, however, because cystoileal reflux and/or ileal–ureteral reflux can be observed in some patients at an intravesical pressure of only 3 to 8 cm H_2O (7). It is questionable whether a pressure of less than 20 cm H_2O can lead to damage to the upper urinary tract. So far, no clinical data including simultaneous measurement of intravesical and intrapelvic pressures are available. In addition, long-term results seen after ureteral replacement with ileum and experiences with the intestinal neobladder suggest that some protection of the upper urinary tract may be afforded by the ileal segment. We therefore prefer to use a bowel segment at least 15 cm in length.

In summary, ureteral replacement with ileum is a feasible technique that carries the risk of considerable perioperative and long-term morbidity and should therefore be considered only as a second-line treatment in selected patients.

REFERENCES

1. Armenakas NA. Current methods of diagnosis and management of ureteral injuries. *World J Urol* 1999;17:78–83.
2. Fritzsche P, Skinner DG, Craven JD, Cahill P, Goodwin WE. Long-term radiographic changes of the kidney following the ileal ureter operation. *J Urol* 1975;114:843.
3. Hinman F Jr, Oppenheimer R. Functional characteristics of the ileum as a valve. *J Urol* 1958;80:448.
4. Mattos RM, Smith JJ. Ileal ureter. *Urol Clin North Am* 1997;24: 813–825.
5. Noble JG, Lee KT, Mundy AR. Transureteroureterostomy: a review of 253 cases. *Br J Urol* 1997;79:20–23.
6. Png JCD, Chapple CR. Principles of ureteric reconstruction. *Curr Opin Urol* 2000;10:207–212.
7. Prout GR Jr, Stuart WT, Witus WS. Utilization of ileal segments to substitute for extensive ureteral loss. *J Urol* 1963;90:541.
8. Selzman AA, Spirnak JP. Iatrogenic ureteral injuries: a 20-year experience in treating 165 injuries. *J Urol* 1996;55:878–881.

CHAPTER 18

Ureteral Stricture

Glenn S. Gerber

The etiology of ureteral strictures includes endoscopic urologic procedures, radiation injury, open or laparoscopic surgery, passage of calculi, and penetrating traumatic injuries (5). In recent years, the incidence of ureteral strictures has increased due to a variety of factors, including the increasing use of upper urinary tract endoscopy. Ureteral strictures may occur in up to 5% to 10% of patients undergoing ureteroscopy (4,8). Several factors may contribute to an increased risk of ureteral stricture formation following endoscopic procedures, including stone impaction, ureteral injury, and direct mechanical or thermal trauma to the ureteral wall (5). Ureteral injury may also occur following a variety of surgical procedures, such as hysterectomy, repair of vascular lesions, and pelvic exploration in patients with a variety of malignancies.

In many cases, the need for surgical repair of a ureteral injury may be immediately apparent. However, other patients with ureteral obstruction and/or fistulas may not present for weeks or months following surgery. Ureteral strictures that result from endoscopic procedures or following radiation therapy may not be noted for prolonged intervals due to the slow development of ureteral fibrosis. Patients with ureteral strictures may present with acute flank pain with sepsis and pyelonephritis or an incidental finding of hydronephrosis may be noted in an asymptomatic individual. Therefore, the initial evaluation and management of patients with suspected ureteral obstruction must be handled on a case-by-case basis.

DIAGNOSIS

A number of different diagnostic modalities are available to evaluate patients who are suspected to have ureteral strictures. Those patients with acute pain and/or infection will most likely require initial decompression of the obstructed renal unit by internal (ureteral stent) or external (percutaneous nephrostomy) drainage. Further

assessment and planning of definitive repair of the stricture can then be performed in a delayed fashion once the patient's condition is stabilized. Among those patients not requiring acute drainage, a number of radiographic modalities are available for evaluating the obstructed ureter, including renal scintigraphy, intravenous or retrograde pyelography, or computerized tomography (CT) scanning. Each of these modalities offers distinct advantages and disadvantages and the choice must be tailored to the clinical situation.

INDICATIONS FOR SURGERY

The indications for surgical treatment of ureteral strictures are dependent upon the etiology of the lesion and the clinical situation. In general, injuries that are noted immediately, such as following external trauma or surgical injury, should be repaired immediately unless associated injuries or medical conditions preclude repair. In many cases, partial ureteral injuries and those presenting in a more chronic condition can initially be managed endoscopically. Ureteral strictures secondary to upper urinary tract endoscopy can often be managed successfully by balloon dilation or incision (endoureterotomy) with open surgical repair reserved for patients with recurrent obstruction.

ALTERNATIVE THERAPY

A variety of endoscopic methods are available in the management of ureteral strictures. Balloon dilation may be performed using an antegrade or retrograde approach with little risk of significant morbidity. In addition, incision of the stricture may be performed endoscopically (endoureterotomy) and this may have a higher success rate than balloon dilation, although it is associated with a greater risk of bleeding and injury to surrounding structures. In general, endourologic approaches to ureteral strictures are most appropriate in those patients with short, nonirradiated strictures of the distal ureter. Overall, endoscopic management is appropriate in most patients with ureteral strictures because the potential morbidity and recovery period is limited in most cases. In addition, a failed endoscopic repair does not preclude a subsequent successful open surgical approach. Finally, some patients with complex ureteral injuries and/or other medical problems may be best managed by nephrectomy or cutaneous ureterostomy. This approach may be considered in those with significant comorbid disease or patients in whom a urine leak could lead to serious consequences, such as those with vascular grafts in the area of the ureteral injury.

SURGICAL TECHNIQUE

Ureteroureterostomy

For patients with short ureteral strictures involving the proximal two-thirds of the ureter (superior to the bifurcation of the iliac vessels), ureteroureterostomy is the preferred surgical approach. Direct anastomosis of the ureter can also be performed in patients with intraoperative injuries, as well as those with ureteral damage secondary to external violence. When performed as a separate procedure, ureteroureterostomy can be approached through a flank, anterolateral, or midline incision. The choice of incision is based on the level of the ureteral obstruction, although an incision that allows for renal mobilization is helpful in cases in which additional ureteral length is necessary.

When performing ureteroureterostomy, the ureter is initially identified through either an intraperitoneal or extraperitoneal approach. If the ureter is difficult to locate, it can be reliably found as it crosses the bifurcation of the iliac artery. The ureter can on occasion be confused with other structures, such as the gonadal vein, and careful dissection and aspiration with a small needle may be helpful in such cases. After the ureter is identified, it should be freed by blunt and sharp dissection with as much surrounding soft tissue as possible. It is critical to avoid damage to the ureteral adventitia because this may result in ischemia and poor healing of the anastomosis. In

cases in which the ureter has been surgically transected or completely divided by a penetrating injury, both ends of the ureter must be identified.

When performing ureteroureterostomy in patients with ureteral strictures, the narrowed segment is excised after the ureter has been mobilized both proximally and distally. It is essential to perform the anastomosis with healthy, well-vascularized ureteral tissue. After removal of the strictured area, stay sutures of 4-0 or 5-0 are placed at each end of the ureter. It is important that the anastomosis be performed with absolutely no tension. If necessary, additional ureteral length can be obtained by mobilization of the kidney. The ends of the ureter should be cut obliquely to allow for a wide anastomosis. Spatulation of each end of the ureter 180 degrees apart over a length of several millimeters may also facilitate the repair. Alternatively, a fishmouth or Z-plasty repair can be performed (Fig. 18–1), although these are less common. In patients with electrocautery or penetrating high-velocity missile injuries to the ureter, extensive debridement of the ureteral ends should be performed because the degree of tissue devitalization may be underestimated at the time of surgery.

Once the ends of the ureter have been prepared, two sutures of 4-0 or 5-0 synthetic absorbable material are placed through the apex of the spatulated area on one end and out the middle of the nonspatulated area on the other end. The knots should be tied outside the ureteral lumen. The initial two sutures should be placed 180 degrees apart and are held to facilitate the completion of the repair. Running or interrupted sutures are placed on one side of the anastomosis and the holding sutures are then rotated to aid in exposure of the opposite side. Placement of a double-pigtail stent may be performed before completion of the anastomosis by initially passing the guide wire into the bladder and then passing the stent over the wire. The guide wire is then removed and passed proximally into the renal pelvis. The stent is then passed proximally over the wire, which is brought out through a side hole in the stent. To ensure proper positioning of the stent in the bladder, fill the bladder through the urethral catheter with saline mixed with indigo carmine. The appearance of blue-stained solution at the level of the anastomosis assures that the stent is in the bladder, except

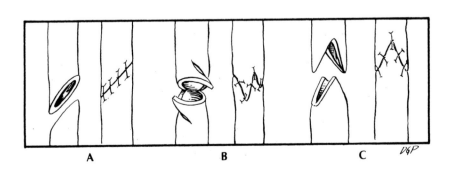

FIG. 18–1. The techniques of reanastomosis include **(A)** oblique, **(B)** Z-plasty, and **(C)** fishmouth.

A   B   C

in unusual cases of preexistent vesicoureteral reflux. Once the anastomosis is completed, it may be wrapped in omentum to facilitate healing. This may be helpful in patients with a history of radiation, abdominal vascular grafts, as well as in those with associated injuries to the bowel or pancreas. A closed suction drain is placed lateral to the anastomosis and brought out through a separate incision prior to abdominal closure. The stent may be removed 2 to 4 weeks postoperatively.

Psoas Hitch

The psoas hitch is the simplest approach to manage strictures and/or injury of the distal third of the ureter (1,7). In most cases, the bladder can be mobilized superiorly to a level above the bifurcation of the iliac vessels and the more technically difficult Boari flap (see below) can be avoided. The surgical incision may be a lower midline, Pfannenstiel, or suprapubic V approach, primarily based upon surgeon preference. In general, it is easiest to initially approach the ureter above the level of obstruction and then dissect distally. Care should be taken to avoid disrupting the ureteral adventitia and blood supply as the dissection is performed. The ureter is dissected as far distally into healthy ureter as possible to maximize available length and the distal ureteral stump is ligated with a 2-0 absorbable suture.

Adequate bladder mobilization is essential to achieving a good result with the psoas hitch. The peritoneum should be dissected off the bladder dome and the space between the rectum and bladder is developed. The superior vesical pedicles are ligated bilaterally and the bladder is opened transversely across the anterior wall at the level of its maximum diameter (7). The bladder should be adequately distended prior to selecting the site of bladder incision so that the proper location for the incision can be chosen. A common mistake is to make too small an opening in the bladder, thus limiting cephalad displacement. In general, the bladder should be opened slightly more than halfway of the entire circumference. The bladder is then brought to the psoas muscle at a point superior and lateral to the bifurcation of the iliac vessels by placing two fingers into the fundus of the bladder (Fig. 18-2). The ureter can then be gently pulled using a stay suture toward the bladder to determine if an adequate anastomosis without tension can be created. Proximal mobilization of the ureter or kidney or opening of the contralateral endopelvic fascia may be used if further ureteral length is needed. The bladder is then fixed to the psoas minor tendon or psoas major muscle using three to six 2-0 absorbable sutures. Careful placement of these sutures is important to avoid injury to the genitofemoral nerve. Femoral nerve neuropathy has also been noted after the psoas hitch and care should be taken to avoid placing the tacking sutures too deeply into the muscle (3).

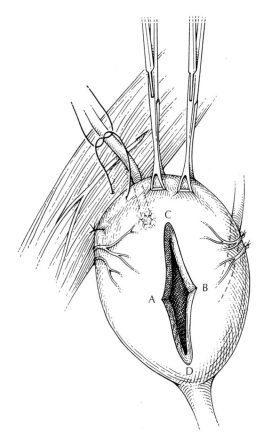

FIG. 18–2. Psoas hitch. The contralateral superior and midvesical arteries are ligated and Babcock clamps are attached to stretch bladder to the point of suture fixation. The transverse bladder incision is closed vertically.

The site of the ureteroneocystostomy is then selected prior to tying the tacking sutures between the bladder and psoas. The ureter should be anastomosed to an immobile portion of the bladder to avoid intermittent obstruction as the bladder fills to varying degrees. The ureter is pulled into the bladder using the stay suture and should be trimmed once it is clear that adequate ureteral length is present. Although a tunneled nonrefluxing anastomosis may be performed if there is adequate length, a direct, refluxing ureteroneocystostomy is acceptable in most adults. Most importantly, the anastomosis must not be under tension. The ureter is spatulated anteriorly and interrupted 4-0 or 5-0 absorbable sutures are used to complete the anastomosis. At the distal aspect of the anastomosis, two to three sutures are placed deeply into the bladder muscle and mucosa and then through the ureter. The remaining sutures should incorporate just the mucosa. The ureteral adventitia should be loosely attached to the bladder wall, where it exits using two or three 4-0 absorbable sutures placed longitudinally. An 8 Fr feeding tube or double-pigtail stent is then placed up the ureter. In general I prefer the feeding tube, which is then brought out the anterior bladder and body wall. This allows for direct monitoring of drainage and irrigation of the tube if necessary and avoids the need for cystoscopy to remove a stent. The feeding tube is loosely tied to the bladder mucosa using a 5-0 chromic suture to avoid inadvertent displacement. A suprapubic tube can be placed, although a urethral catheter is in general adequate. The bladder is closed vertically in a watertight fashion using two layers of 2-0 and 3-0 chromic sutures. A closed suction drain is positioned laterally in the perivesical space. The ureteral and bladder catheters may be removed 7 to 10 days postoperatively and a cystogram may be performed if desired prior to this to ensure adequate healing.

Boari Flap

A bladder flap is usually not needed in patients with distal ureteral strictures because a psoas hitch is adequate in most cases. If a Boari flap is necessary, the incision, ureteral dissection, and initial bladder mobilization are the same as for patients undergoing a psoas hitch. Recently, laparoscopic techniques have been used to successfully perform the Boari flap (2). The bladder flap is indicated when, despite all attempts to create adequate length, it is clear that a tension-free anastomosis cannot be created. A psoas hitch should accompany the Boari flap to help decrease the length of flap that is necessary (6).

After the bladder has been mobilized and a psoas hitch performed, the site for the base of the flap should be identified on a fixed portion of the bladder and the length of flap needed is measured. A stay suture is placed at each end of the base of the flap, which should be approximately 3 to 5 cm wide. To ensure adequate vascularity of the flap, the base should be wider when a longer flap is necessary. A stay suture is placed at each end of the apex of the flap, which should be approximately 3 cm in width. If needed, a longer flap can be created using a spiral incision in the bladder (Fig. 18–3). The flap should be developed by incising the bladder wall using electrocautery. The flap is then brought up to the ureter, which may be anastomosed to the apex using a direct or tunneled technique (Fig. 18–4). A feeding tube or stent should then be placed. The bladder is closed and the flap is rolled into a tube over the stent using a running 3-0 absorbable suture on the mucosa and interrupted 2-0 sutures on the muscularis and adventitia. A perivesical drain is placed and radiographic evaluation of the bladder and ureter should be performed prior to removal of the ureteral and urethral catheters.

OUTCOMES

Complications

The most common problem in the early postoperative period is prolonged urinary drainage. In most cases, the leak will seal as long as adequate drainage of the ureter and bladder are assured. If there is concern regarding the site of leakage, a cystogram and/or ureterogram may be performed. An intravenous pyelogram may be helpful if

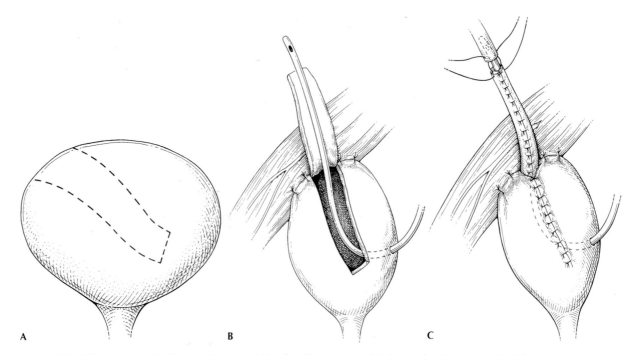

FIG. 18–3. A and B: The bladder should be fixed by a psoas hitch, a spiral transverse incision made 4 cm at the base and 3 cm at the apex. **C:** The bladder flap is tubed over a catheter and closed in two layers with a 3-0 running mucosal and 2-0 interrupted muscularis sutures.

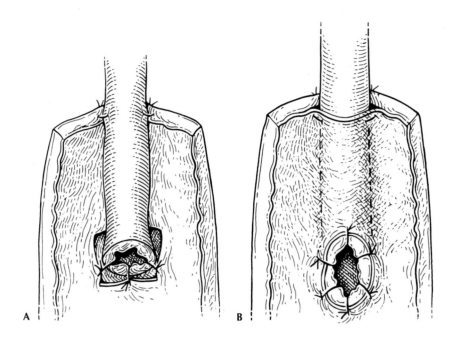

FIG. 18–4. The ureter either is **(A)** anastomosed directly to the bladder flap using additional sutures to fix the ureter to the external bladder wall and retroperitoneum or **(B)** tunneled for 3 to 5 cm to create an antirefluxing anastomosis.

an externally draining ureteral catheter is not present. Injury to the contralateral ureter may occur rarely and should be considered if unusual or complicated problems occur. When unexplained fever and/or sepsis occurs, an undrained urine collection (urinoma) should be considered and is best diagnosed by ultrasonography or CT scans. External drainage of such a collection using radiographic guidance may then be performed.

The greatest long-term risk is recurrent stricture formation at the site of the anastomosis. While some patients may present with flank pain and/or infection, others will remain asymptomatic due to the slow development of a recurrent stricture. Therefore, all patients should undergo radiographic evaluation of the upper urinary tract 6 to 12 weeks following stent removal and again 3 to 6 months following surgery. Risk factors that increase the likelihood of recurrent obstruction include previous ureteral and bladder surgery, a history of pelvic irradiation, devascularization of the ureter at the time of surgery, and an anastomosis performed under tension. If detected early, recurrent strictures may respond to endoscopic management.

Results

Excellent long-term success rates can be achieved with surgical repair of ureteral strictures. The most important factors in ureteral repair include the selection of the most appropriate surgical technique based on the site and length of the stricture. In addition, consideration of preoperative issues, such as a history of irradiation or prior surgery, is also critical in avoiding recurrent obstruction. In general, as long as a tension-free anastomosis can be performed using well-vascularized ureteral tissue the long-term success of open surgical repair of ureteral strictures should be assured in the vast majority of patients.

REFERENCES

1. Ahn M, Loughlin KR. Psoas hitch ureteral reimplantation in adults—analysis of a modified technique and timing of repair. *Urology* 2001;58:184–187.
2. Fugita OE, Dinlene C, Kavoussi L. The laparoscopic Boari flap. *J Urol* 2001;166:51–53.
3. Kowalczyk JJ, Keating MA, Ehrlich RM. Femoral nerve neuropathy after the psoas hitch procedure. *Urology* 1996;47:563–565.
4. Lytton B, Weiss RM, Green DF. Complications of ureteral endoscopy. *J Urol* 1987;137:49–53.
5. Motola JA, Smith AD. Complications of ureteroscopy: prevention and treatment. *AUA Update Ser* 1992;11:161–169.
6. Olsson CA, Norlen LJ. Combined Boari bladder flap–psoas hitch procedure in ureteral replacement. *Scand J Urol Nephrol* 1986;20:279–282.
7. Turner-Warwich R, Worth PHL. The psoas hitch procedure for the replacement of the lower third of the ureter. *Br J Urol* 1969;41:701–709.
8. Weinberg JJ, Ansong K, Smith AD. Complications of ureteroscopy in relation to experience: report of survey and author experience. *J Urol* 1987;137:384–387.

SECTION III

Bladder

SECTION EDITOR: James E. Montie.

Anatomy

Sam D. Graham, Jr.

The urinary bladder is an extraperitoneal organ that is abdominal in position in young (< 6 year old) patients and a pelvic organ after the pelvis has developed sufficiently. It is situated behind the symphisis pubis and depending upon the degree of distension may be palpated in the lower abdomen. While the body (fundus) of the bladder freely expands and contracts, the bladder neck is firmly fixed to the urethra and other ligaments in the deep pelvis.

The bladder is a hollow organ that has an inner epithelium lined with transitional epithelium (Figure SIII-1). The

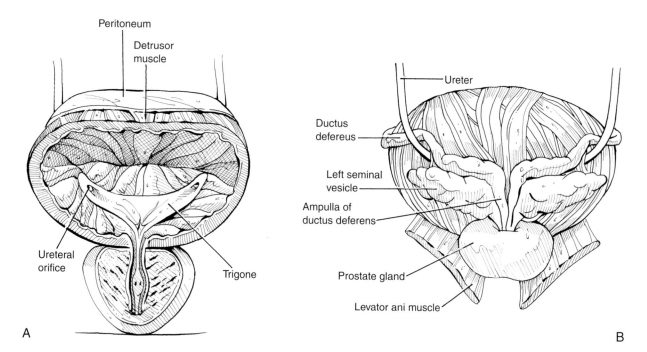

FIG. SIII–1. (A) Antertior view of the bladder of a male opened and demonstrating intravesical anatomy. Note the trigone continues into the prostatic urethra. (B) Posterior view of the bladder of a male demonstrating the relationship of the seminal vesicles, vas deferens, and ureters.

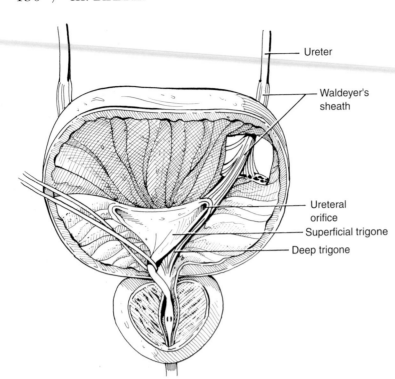

Ureter

Waldeyer's sheath

Ureteral orifice

Superficial trigone

Deep trigone

FIG. SIII–2. Lateral view of ureter as it enters the bladder via the intramural tunnel. Note Waldeyer's sheath extends from the bladder to encase the distal ureter just proximal to the bladder and fuses to the ureteral musculature. Waldeyer's sheath is a continuation of the deep trigone and connects by a few fibers to the detrusor muscle at the ureteral hiatus.

muscular wall is composed of bundles that decussate longitudinally and circularly. The musculature of the trigone is superimposed on the bladder muscle and formes the thickest and most fixed portion of the bladder. The distance between the orifices in the trigone is 3 cm to 4 cm.

The ureters enter the bladder posteriorly and inferiorly (Figure SIII-2). At the point where the ureter meets the adventitia of the bladder, it is encased in Waldeyer's

sheath which extends from the ureteral orifice to where it fuses with the musculature of the ureter. The ureteral path through the vesical wall is oblique to where it enters the bladder at the trigone.

Superiorly and, to some extent, posteriorly the bladder is covered with peritoneum. The peritoneum forms the Pouch of Douglas at its most caudal extent behind the bladder. The two leaves of the peritoneum embryologically coa-

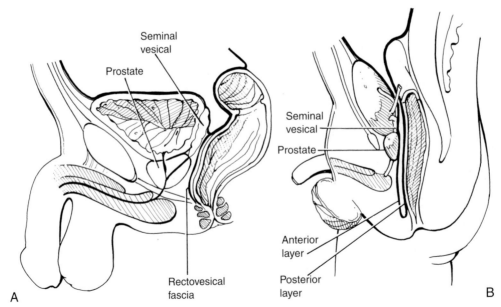

FIG. SIII–3. Lateral view of the male pelvis showing (A) the peritoneal reflection and the pouch of Douglas and (B) the formation of Denonvillier's fascia in the fetus.

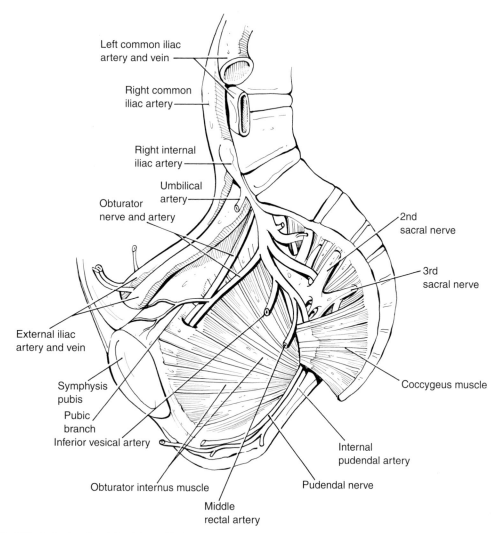

FIG. SIII–4. Lateral pelvic side wall demonstrating the vasculature and innervation of the deep pelvis. The arterial supply of the bladder is from the superior lateral vesical artery and the inferior vesical artery enclosed in the posterior pedicle.

lesce to form the anterior and posterior layers of Denonvillier's fascia (rectovesical fascia) (Figure SIII-3) (1).

The lateral vesical ligaments are a continuation of the pelvic fascia and contain the inferior and vesicodeferential arteries in the lateral extensions as well as the vasa deferentia in males, and the pudendal plexuses of nerves and vessels. Inferiorly, this blends with the fascia lining the levator ani and laterally with the fascia of the obturator internus.

Aside from the fixation of the bladder to the lateral vesical ligaments or its base to the lateral pelvic side wall and levator ani, the bladder is also fixed to the symphysis pubis by the pubovesical ligaments in females and puboprostatic ligaments in the male. Between these paired ligaments passes the dorsal vein of the clitoris or penis, respectively. These ligaments form the anteromedial protion of the space of Retzius. The space of Retzius is bound anteriorly by the transversalis fascia, the pubopro-

static (pubovesical) ligaments inferiorly, and infralaterally by the lateral ligaments of the bladder.

VASCULAR ANATOMY

The arterial supply of the bladder is from the lateral and posterior pedicles. (Figure SIII-3) The lateral pedicles are more constant and anatomically defined. The first anterior branch of the hypogastric artery is the umbilical artery. The second anterior branch is the superior vesical artery. There are usually other branches of the hypogastric artery more distally that make up the middle and inferior lateral pedicles. These arterial branches are accompanied by a complimentary vein. Posteriorly, there are paired pedicles that arise from the either the internal iliac, the pudendal, or the inferior gluteal areteries and are lateral rectum to the bladder and vagina. While some anatomists describe this as the inferior vesical artery, these vessels are less well defined and are usually smaller than the vessels of the lateral pedicles.

Venous drainage of the bladder is predominantly into lateral plexuses and then to the veins in the lateral prostatic ligaments into the internal iliac veins.

LYMPHATIC ANATOMY

The lymphatic drainage of the bladder is to the external iliac vein, the hypogastric nodes, or to the presacral promonotory.

NEURAL ANATOMY

The innervation of the bladder is primarily via the sacral nerve roots, S2, S3, and S4 which are parasympathetic.

CONTIGUOUS STRUCTURES

In the male, the bladder joins the prostate and is anterior to the seminal vesicles and ampulla of the vas deferens. In the female the bladder is in more direct contact with the pubococcygeus portion of the levator ani. Superiorly, the bladder is covered by peritoneum in both males and females. Posteriorly in females the bladder is adjacent to the uterus and vagina. In males, the posterior bladder is adjacent to the seminal vesicles and rectum.

REFERENCE

1. Weyrauch HM. Surgery of the Prostate. Philadelphia: WB Saunders, 1959.

CHAPTER 19

Simple and Partial Cystectomy

Thomas S. Lendvay and John A. Petros

SIMPLE CYSTECTOMY

Simple cystectomy, typically performed for nonmalignant diseases requiring urinary diversion, entails the removal of the urinary bladder without removing adjacent structures routinely resected during radical cystectomy. In male patients, the seminal vesicles, prostate, and urethra are left intact, thereby preserving erectile function. In female patients, the adnexa, anterior vaginal wall, uterus, and urethra are preserved. Simple cystectomy also implies that the pelvic lymph nodes are not dissected. Although this procedure is not commonly performed, a retained defunctionalized urinary bladder can lead to significant morbidity for the diverted patient.

Diagnosis

The diagnostic studies are dependent upon the underlying disease. Patients with histories of a malignancy should undergo biopsy and staging including computed tomography (CT) imaging of the pelvis and abdomen. Nonmalignant conditions resulting in simple cystectomy are usually end stage and the diagnosis is known well in advance of the proposed cystectomy.

Indications for Surgery

Supravesical diversion is indicated in patients with severe radiation or chemical (e.g., cyclophosphamide) cystitis, neurogenic bladder disease, refractory interstitial cystitis, severe incontinence, trauma, hemorrhagic cystitis, fistula, upper-tract obstruction, and uncorrectable urethral stricture disease. Supravesical diversion without cystectomy results in complication rates for the retained organ of 60% to 80%, with pyocystis being the most common (3,5). Forty-three percent require rehospitalization from sepsis, anemia, or pain,

and the salvage cystectomy rate may approach 30% (3,5). In patients who have received pelvic irradiation, the relative risk for developing urothelial carcinoma is 4.6 (5). Others advocate concurrent removal of the urinary bladder at the time of diversion for intractable inflammatory disease such as interstitial cystitis because of the increased risk of malignant degeneration in the retained inflamed bladder (4). Due to the significant morbidity of the retained bladder, we recommend supravesical diversion and concomitant simple cystectomy in those patients who will not have their diversions reversed.

Alternative Therapy

Although morbidity may be increased, radical cystoprostatectomy may be indicated in upper-tract diversion patients if there is a risk of urothelial or prostate carcinoma. Conservative management or partial cystectomy is also an alternative to open simple cystectomy. With the advances in laparoscopic surgery for urologic disease, laparoscopic simple cystectomy offers the patient the benefits of minimizing the surgical scar, hospitalization, and blood loss, but should only be practiced by an adept laparoscopic surgeon.

Surgical Technique

A male patient is prepped and draped in the standard position as for radical cystectomy, in a supine position with the legs apart with gentle hyperextension. A female patient is placed in a lithotomy position for access to the perineum. This operation can be performed entirely extraperitoneally if prior upper-tract urinary diversion has already taken place. This is preferred because it obviates the need for lysis of adhesions, which can be numerous in a patient who has had prior intraabdominal surgery and/or radiation therapy. Obviously, if urinary diversion is to take place at the same time an intraperitoneal approach is used.

In the extraperitoneal approach, we use a lower midline incision extending from the pubis to immediately lateral to the umbilicus. The space of Retzius is entered by dividing the rectus abdominis muscle in the midline. The retropubic space is developed down to the bladder using a combination of blunt and sharp dissection to separate the parietal peritoneum from the dome and posterior wall of the bladder (Fig. 19–1). It is important to repair with 3-0 or 4-0 Vicryl any tears made in the parietal peritoneum, as the parietal peritoneum provides an important boundary between the peritoneal contents and the raw surface of the pelvis after simple cystectomy. During dissection of the parietal peritoneum in the man, the vas deferens is encountered. If we are going to leave the seminal vesicles and prostate, we do not sacrifice the vasa but instead dissect them posteriorly. If the seminal vesicles and prostate are to be sacrificed, we divide the vasa. During the dissection of the parietal peritoneum posteriorly, the superior vesical pedicle is encountered. At this point it is clamped and divided between 2-0 silk ties.

After control of the superior vesical pedicles bilaterally, the ureters are identified where they enter the bladder (Fig. 19–2). In patients who have had prior upper-tract diversion, the ureters are dissected proximally to the point where they were divided previously to ensure complete excision of the distal ureters. In patients who are to undergo urinary diversion at the same time, we use an intraperitoneal approach and divide the ureters close to the bladder wall.

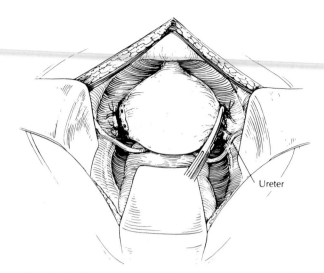

FIG. 19–2. The vesicle pedicles are clipped and divided.

The bladder is then divided from the prostate at the prostatovesical junction using electrocautery starting anteriorly at the bladder neck and working laterally on both sides until the posterior bladder neck is reached (Fig. 19–3). If the patient has significant prostatic hypertrophy, which will impede adequate closure of the bladder neck, then a suprapubic prostatectomy is performed with rigorous attention to hemostasis afterward because a Foley catheter cannot be used to help control hemorrhage. The posterior bladder wall is then divided from within using electrocautery until the ampulla of the vasa are seen. The base of the bladder is then bluntly dissected off the seminal vesicles and ampulla of the vasa (Fig. 19–4). During this dissection, the lateral vascular pedicles are identified and divided between 2-0 silk ties. The bladder is now removed from the operative

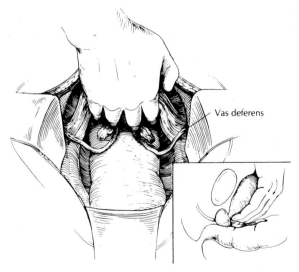

FIG. 19–1. Bladder exposed extraperitoneally with the space between the rectum and bladder developed by blunt dissection.

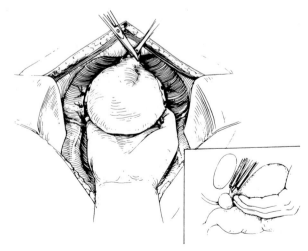

FIG. 19–3. The bladder neck is incised anteriorly.

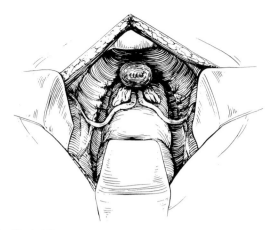

FIG. 19–4. The posterior bladder neck is divided and the bladder is removed. The distal bladder neck/urethra is oversewn.

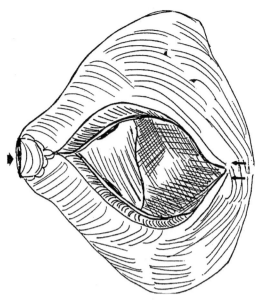

FIG. 19–5. The bladder is opened longitudinally in the midline from the bladder neck (arrow) to the bladder dome (arrows). (From Neulander EZ, Rivera I, Eisenbrown N, et al. Simple cystectomy in patients requiring urinary diversion. *J Urol* 2000;164:1169–1172.)

field. The prostate is then oversewn with a double layer of 0 silk.

In women, after development of the retropubic space the parietal peritoneum is dissected off the dome and posterior wall of the bladder until the anterior vaginal fornix is reached. The superior vesical pedicles are divided as in male patients. The ureters are handled the same way as in men, with care taken not to injure the uterine artery during their dissection. A sponge stick placed in the vagina is used for cephalad traction, and the plane between the bladder and anterior vaginal wall is developed. During dissection of this plane, the lateral bladder pedicles are divided between 2-0 silk ties as they are encountered. Once the urethra is reached, the Foley catheter is removed and the urethra is divided and oversewn with 0 silk sutures. If simple cystectomy is being performed for interstitial cystitis, it is important to remove the entire urethra and external urethral meatus because failure to do so may result in persistent symptoms.

Alternatively, some perform a bladder bivalving procedure when doing a simple cystectomy. After mobilization from the lateral pedicles, the bladder is opened longitudinally in the midline from the bladder neck through the dome and posteriorly to the trigone (Figs. 19–5 and 19–6). The peritoneum is incised horizontally as it reflects posteriorly and dissection starting at the vasa is carried out between the bladder and the seminal vesicles. The midline of the trigone is then incised along the axis of the patient to the bladder neck (Fig. 19–7). The rest of the space between the bladder and the seminal vesicles is then created, yielding a completely bivalved bladder. The bladder neck is then transected circumferentially with electrocautery. The exposed prostatic base is oversewn with 0 silk sutures (5).

If an upper-tract urinary diversion is to be performed at the same time, an intraperitoneal approach is used with an incision from the symphysis pubis to a point midway between the xyphoid process and the umbilicus. Our approach for simple cystectomy in this case is the same,

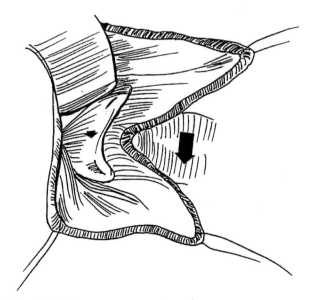

FIG. 19–6. The incision is carried further longitudinally through the bladder dome to the bladder base toward the trigone (arrow). Large arrow, vagina. (From Neulander EZ, Rivera I, Eisenbrown N, et al. Simple cystectomy in patients requiring urinary diversion. *J Urol* 2000;164: 1169–1172.)

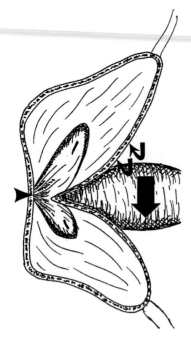

FIG. 19–7. The trigone is split in the midline toward the bladder neck (arrowhead). The bladder is completely bivalved at this point. The two bladder flaps are excised, maintaining the excision plane close to the bladder (curved arrows). Vagina, large arrow. (From Neulander EZ, Rivera I, Eisenbrown N, et al. Simple cystectomy in patients requiring urinary diversion. *J Urol* 2000;164:1169–1172.)

with the parietal peritoneum carefully preserved as a boundary between the peritoneal contents and the raw pelvic surfaces.

Postoperatively, a drain is left in the pelvic space if the operation was performed in the presence of pyocystis. We rarely find it necessary to leave this drain more than 48 hours. Otherwise, we do not routinely leave a pelvic drain unless the patient will have placement of an orthotopic bladder.

PARTIAL CYSTECTOMY

The ultimate goal of surgical intervention for malignancies is complete local excision of the tumor with an attempt at preservation of normal physiological function. Because no randomized controlled studies exist comparing partial cystectomy versus transurethral tumor resection versus radical cystectomy, it is difficult to conclude a superior technique. There are, however, tumor behaviors that make partial cystectomy a favorable option or absolutely contraindicated. In male patients who have unfavorable disease, are impotent, and can tolerate extensive surgery, radical cystoprostatectomy should be the procedure of choice. In patients who do not fall into this category, partial cystectomy is still an appealing option because full-thickness margins can be obtained with

preservation of potency, continence, and physiological bladder function while being able to sample pelvic lymph nodes.

Diagnosis

Prior to the partial cystectomy, the tumor should be biopsied or resected to perform both staging of the tumor as well as obtain histology. Mapping biopsies of the bladder should also be performed to assure that the tumor is discrete and potentially curable. CT scans of the pelvis and abdomen should be performed to assess both local stage as well as the lymph nodes, kidneys, and liver. Imaging of the upper tracts may be indicated depending upon the histology of the tumor, site of the tumor, or prior history.

Indications for Surgery

Favorable neoplastic disease amenable to partial cystectomy includes solitary lesions at or near the dome of the urinary bladder allowing for a 3-cm margin of normal tissue in the absence of any dysplastic or carcinoma in situ (CIS) field changes confirmed by random biopsies. Patients with multiple tumors, CIS, cellular atypia, prostatic or trigone invasion, prior radiation, bladder capacities risking loss of compliance if partial cystectomy attempted, extravesical extension, or a poor surgical risk are not good candidates for partial cystectomy. Patients with tumors at the bladder neck have a poorer prognosis than patients with posterior lesions. A subpopulation of urothelial tumors arising in bladder diverticuli is preferably treated with partial cystectomy over transurethral resection because the thin amuscular walls lead to a higher risk of bladder perforation and higher-stage disease than a conventional muscle-invasive lesion.

Other indications for partial cystectomy include nonurothelial malignancies, benign disease, and patient anatomy that precludes adequate transurethral tumor resection. Other bladder malignancies that have been successfully treated with partial cystectomy include osteosarcoma, rhabdomyosarcoma, paraganglioma, pheochromocytoma of the bladder, primary malignant lymphoma, leiomyosarcoma, and urachal adenocarcinoma. The urachus is a closed epithelial canal found in 30% of the population and is capable of malignant transformation. Urachal carcinoma is a unique neoplasm in that it is highly amenable to *en-bloc* excision including partial cystectomy, posterior rectus fascia, peritoneum, and umbilicus with a freedom from recurrence rate of up to 88% at 2 years (2,6). Nonurologic malignancies, such as locally invasive colorectal adenocarcinoma, are also amenable to partial cystectomy. Nonneoplastic diseases that are amenable to partial cystectomy include intractable eosinophilic cystitis, nephrogenic adenoma in children, refractory hemorrhaging hemangiomas, neurofibroma, and inflammatory pseudotumor. Large symptomatic bladder diverticuli may be treated with open or laparoscopic partial cystectomy using an Endo-GIA stapler device.

Alternative Therapy

Any tumor that can be removed with partial cystectomy can also be removed with radical cystectomy. The differences come down to recurrence risks, morbidity, and quality of life. Because transurethral techniques have advanced, the majority of lesions may be treated endoscopically. Laser tumor ablation, intravesical chemotherapy, and interstitial radiation therapy are also in the physician's armamentarium and must be discussed with the patient.

Surgical Technique

The patient is placed on the operating room table in the supine position and is sterilely prepped and draped. The sterile field includes the penis in men and vulva and vagina in women. This allows for sterile insertion of a Foley catheter into the bladder after resection of the tumor and before closure of the incision.

We prefer a lower midline incision to a transverse suprapubic incision because it allows for easier access to the peritoneal cavity if needed. We position the patient on the table such that the break in the table is at the anterior superior iliac spine, which allows for adequate flexion of the patient and elevation of the bladder into the wound. The standard incision extends from the pubic symphysis to the level of the umbilicus. The rectus abdominis muscle is divided in the midline and the space of Retzius is entered. The patient is then placed in the Trendelenburg position to elevate the abdominal contents out of the pelvis.

Depending on the location of the tumor in the bladder, we proceed with either an extraperitoneal or intraperitoneal approach. For tumors located on the dome or anterior part of the bladder, we prefer an extraperitoneal approach. For tumors located on the posterior aspect of the bladder, an intraperitoneal approach is preferred.

Extraperitoneal Partial Cystectomy

For our extraperitoneal approach, we expose the anterior surface of the bladder through the space of Retzius, mobilizing the peritoneum where it is readily separable from the bladder. A bilateral pelvic lymph node dissection is performed with the boundaries from the bifurcation of the common iliac artery superiorly to Cooper's ligament inferiorly and from the external iliac artery laterally to the internal iliac artery medially. The bladder is freed laterally and posteriorly well beyond the site of the tumor. The fat over the site of the tumor is left attached to the bladder, and the superior vesicle pedicle can be divided if necessary (Fig. 19–8).

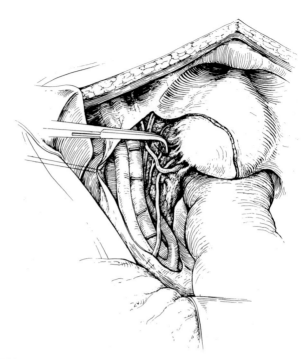

FIG. 19–8. Partial cystectomy. The peritoneum is incised over the affected portion of the bladder after a pelvic lymph node dissection has been performed.

Several stay sutures are then placed in the bladder at a site known from cystoscopy to be distant from the tumor. The wound edges are packed away from the bladder with laparotomy pads or plastic drapes, and the bladder is entered between the stay sutures using electrocautery, taking care to minimize the amount of spillage of urine to minimize the risk of tumor implantation. The incision is extended for several centimeters anteriorly and posteriorly to allow for adequate visualization of the tumor and its relationship to the ureteric orifices and bladder neck. The tumor is then excised, with care taken to leave a 3-cm margin of normal-appearing bladder surrounding the tumor (Fig. 19–9). The tumor should be removed *en bloc* with the overlying perivesical fat and peritoneum using electrocautery or sharp dissection. If the tumor lies less than 3 cm from the ureteric orifice, sacrifice the ureteric orifice and perform a ureteral reimplantation. If enough ureter remains, a Leadbetter–Politano reimplantation is preferred, although a nonrefluxing ureteroneocystostomy or simple nipple reimplantation is acceptable. If excision of the tumor involves the bladder neck, it is possible to excise the bladder neck and the surrounding prostatic capsule after enucleation of the prostate gland. We do not recommend excising any portion of the bladder neck in women to avoid incontinence.

After removal of the tumor, the bladder should be closed in two layers using a 3-0 Vicryl suture to close the urothelium and a 2-0 Vicryl suture to close the muscular

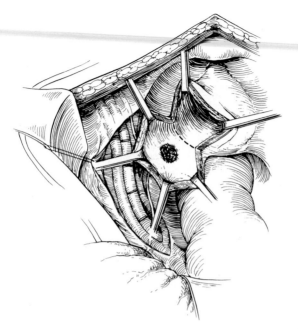

FIG. 19–9. A 3-cm margin of normal bladder is taken around the tumor.

layer (Fig. 19–10). A suprapubic cystostomy catheter is contraindicated in these patients because of the risk of tumor spillage, so it is essential that a wide-bore Foley catheter be used. We drain the perivesical space only if there is concern about the adequacy of bladder closure or a lymphadenectomy has been performed. The abdominal wall is then closed in the standard fashion.

Postoperatively, the urethral catheter should be left in place for 7 to 10 days. If there is any doubt as to the integrity of the repair, a gentle gravity cystogram may be

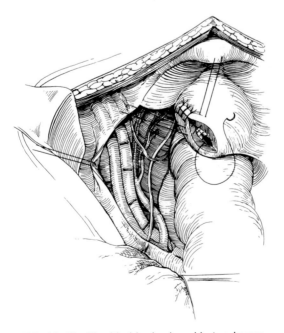

FIG. 19–10. The bladder is closed in two layers.

performed. If perivesical drains are placed, they may be removed when drainage is minimal, usually on postoperative day 3 or 4.

Intraperitoneal Partial Cystectomy

For posteriorly located tumors, we take an intraperitoneal approach. After dividing the rectus abdominis muscle in the midline, we open the peritoneum. We then put the patient in the Trendelenburg position and pack the abdominal contents out of the pelvis with laparotomy pads. The peritoneum over the iliac vessels is incised, and we proceed with our bilateral pelvic lymph node dissection as described previously. We follow the obliterated hypogastric artery to the takeoff of the superior vesical artery, which we clamp and divide.

The bladder is then freed posteriorly as needed, and stay sutures are then placed in the bladder and the bladder is opened as described previously. Removal of the bladder tumor including the perivesical fat and peritoneum, reimplantation of the ureters, closure of the bladder, management of urethral catheters and perivesical drains, and wound closure are all handled as described previously.

OUTCOMES

Complications

Perioperative death has been cited to be 0% to 10%, with all of the latest studies citing 0%. Tumor implantation of the suprapubic tract is 0% to 18%. Vesicocutaneous, vesicovaginal, and colovesical fistulas have been reported, and myocardial infarction, congestive heart failure, pulmonary embolus, upper-gastrointestinal bleed, wound hematomas/infections, and anastomotic leaks of ureteral reimplants have all been reported with an overall complication rate of 11% to 29%. Diminished bladder capacity requiring diversion or augmentation can be devastating. Some report that a functional bladder can be constructed if there is enough wall to close over an inflated Foley balloon, whereas others report that at least 50% of the bladder must remain to have tolerable physiological bladder functioning. Recurrence of disease is the most feared outcome and local rates have ranged from 38% to 78%, with half occurring in the first year. Urinary diversion is ultimately required in 4% to 15% of patients. No clear beneficial effect has been demonstrated with neoadjuvant therapy, but authors acknowledge that most studies that set out to demonstrate a survival benefit were closed prior to their completion (6).

Unique to simple cystectomy is the risk of anterior enterocele after the procedure. Because the anterior vaginal wall may be weakened by an extensive dissection, especially after treatment for interstitial cystitis, the small bowel, which deposits behind the pubis, may herniate into the anterior vaginal wall. Some suggest a colposuspension procedure at the time of cystectomy to mitigate this risk. The risk does not seen to be as high in radical surgery because of the extensive scarring (1).

Results

Simple cystectomy for benign disease and partial cystectomy for malignant disease are useful therapies for the clinician trying to balance the quality of their patients' lives with symptomatic and oncological control. Because the majority of retained bladders may ultimately cause morbidity to the patient and with minimal added morbidity a simple cystectomy can be performed, we recommend that concurrent simple cystectomy and upper-tract diversion be carried out. Partial cystectomy for superficial disease has been cited to be comparable to transurethral tumor resection, but muscle-invasive disease has superior outcomes when treated with radical cystectomy. Because perioperative morbidity from radical surgery has been minimized over the last two decades, we strongly encourage a strict use of partial cystectomy limited to small, solitary lesions at the dome.

REFERENCES

1. Anderson J, Carrion R, Ordorica R, et al. Anterior enterocele following cystectomy for intractable interstitial cystitis. *J Urol* 1998;159: 1868–1870.
2. Dandekar NP, Tongaonkar HB, Dalal AV, et al. Partial cystectomy for invasive bladder cancer. *J Surg Oncol* 1995;60:24–29.
3. Eigner EB, Freiha FS. The fate of the remaining bladder following supravesical diversion. *J Urol* 1990;144:31–33.
4. Lamm DL, Gittes RF. Inflammatory carcinoma of the bladder and interstitial cystitis. *J Urol* 1977;117:49–51.
5. Neulander EZ, Rivera I, Eisenbrown N, et al. Simple cystectomy in patients requiring urinary diversion. *J Urol* 2000;164:1169–1172.
6. Sweeney P, Kursh ED, Resnick MI. Partial cystectomy. *Urol Clin North Am* 1992;19:701–711.

CHAPTER 20

Radical Cystectomy in Men

Mohamed A. Ghonheim

One of the first detailed operative descriptions of radical cystoprostatectomy and pelvic lymphadenectomy was probably provided by Marshall and Whitmore in 1949 (2). In the 1950s and early 1960s, the operation was attended with significant mortality and morbidity. Although more complex urinary diversions are increasingly employed, contemporary cystectomy is associated with low mortality. Further, the advent of nerve-sparing cystectomy and orthotopic bladder substitution has significantly reduced functional losses and provided many patients with good locoregional control as well as a good quality of life. The technique, herein described, is based on cumulative experience of more than 20 years during which more than 1,000 cystectomies were carried out at the Department of Urology, Mansoura University, Egypt.

DIAGNOSIS

The diagnosis of transitional cell carcinoma is in general made by transurethral resection of the tumor in the bladder. Once the diagnosis has been established, it is important to know the histological stage, in particular if the tumor invades the muscularis propria. Invasion of the muscularis mucosa is not considered as constituting a muscle-invasive tumor. The clinical staging of transitional cell carcinoma can in general be performed by abdominal and pelvic computerized tomography (CT) scans. On occasion, radionuclide bone scans are indicated if there is either symptomatic bone pain, abnormalities on the CT scan, or the patient has either an elevated serum calcium or alkaline phosphatase.

INDICATIONS FOR SURGERY

The major indication for cystectomy in men is carcinoma of the bladder. In general, the operation is carried out for:

1. Patients with superficial tumors in whom endoscopic control has failed despite adjuvant intravesical chemo- and/or immunotherapy. Although these measures had proved effective in the management of such cases (less than T1), an important minority fail. High tumor grade, multifocal lesions, diffuse carcinoma *in situ*, and involvement of the prostatic urethra were all reported as high-risk factors.

2. Infiltrating tumor without evidence of distant metastasis. These include tumors infiltrating the muscle layers (P_2, P_{3a}) or the perivesical fat short of the pelvic wall (P_{3b}). Infiltration of adjacent organs (P_4) or involvement of the regional lymph nodes is not considered a contraindication for the procedure.

The extent of the radical operation in the male includes the removal of the bladder, its peritoneal covering, the perivesical fat, the lower ureters, the prostate, the seminal vesicles, and the vasa deferentia. In the standard procedure, as much as possible of the membranous urethra is also removed, and total urethrectomy is carried out only if there is involvement of the prostatic urethra (4).

ALTERNATIVE THERAPY

Alternatives to radical cystectomy include local therapy, partial cystectomy, intravenous (IV) chemotherapy, radiation therapy, or a combination of chemotherapy and radiation therapy. Local therapy in invasive disease in general results in progression of the disease and death of the patient within 5 years. Systemic chemotherapy or radiation therapy is associated with a 25% 5-year survival, although the combination of the two modalities results in significant synergy with up to 50% 5-year survival.

SURGICAL TECHNIQUE

Preparation of the Patient

In view of the extent of surgery and length of operative time, a thorough medical evaluation and anesthetic consultation are required. Bowel preparation is necessary before surgery. If it is planned to use the small bowel, oral neomycin and a low-residue diet are all that is needed. More rigorous preparation is required if the colon is utilized. This includes soapsuds enemas until the colonic contents return clear. A neomycin sulfate enema is given on the evening before the day of operation. IV fluids are also administered to maintain hydration.

Patients with histories of thromboembolic disease or varicose veins should receive a prophylactic dose of heparin (5,000 U subcutaneously) the night before the operation and every 12 hours thereafter until ambulation. A parenteral broad-spectrum antibiotic is given just before induction of anesthesia and continued postoperatively for 3 days. The region extending from the midchest to the midthigh should be cleaned and prepared on the night before surgery.

Anesthesia and Instrumentation

Full relaxation of the abdominal muscles by an appropriate anesthetic is necessary throughout the entire procedure. Hypotensive anesthesia would provide an additional advantage and would reduce blood loss.

The choice of instruments depends mainly on the surgeon's preference. Standard retractors of various sizes and curves as well as long curved and angled scissors are needed. Long curved clamps should also be available. In our practice, we prefer to retract the abdominal wall on the side where the dissection is carried out using one or two ordinary retractors. A ring retractor is applied once the lymphadenectomy is completed.

Position and Initial Exposure

The patient is put in the supine position with a Trendelenburg tilt. Slight bending of the knees would further help in the relaxation of the abdominal muscles, facilitate retraction, and provide a wider exposure. If a total urethrectomy is planned, the patient is put in a slight lithotomy position for access to the perineum.

The surgical area to be sterilized and draped extends from the lower chest down to the root of the penis. A self-retaining catheter is introduced into the bladder and kept indwelling for its evacuation throughout the procedure.

A long, vertical, right paramedian incision extending from the symphysis pubis inferiorly to a point halfway between the umbilicus and xyphoid process of the sternum superiorly is in general employed. Alternatively, a midline incision encircling the umbilicus can also be utilized. For obese patients a lower abdominal muscle-cutting transverse incision is preferred. Under such circumstances it provides wide and direct exposure of the pelvis.

Initially, the abdominal and pelvic cavities are explored. The growth is palpated, its degree of mobility determined, and its relation to the adjacent structures

assessed. The endopelvic and aortic lymph nodes are palpated and frozen sections are taken if necessary. The general peritoneal cavity, omentum, intestinal tract, kidney, spleen, and liver are thoroughly examined. If the decision is to proceed with the radical operation, the intestines are packed out of the pelvis and the retropubic space is opened by blunt dissection. Any small bleeders are coagulated. This dissection is extended inferiorly and laterally until the ventral surface of the bladder and prostate are exposed. The peritoneal incision is extended inferiorly on either side of the urachal remnant. The urachal remnant is dissected off its attachment with the umbilicus and clamped. In this manner a triangular peritoneal flap with its apex pointing superiorly is raised and will be removed later *en bloc* with the bladder.

Lymphadenectomy

The peritoneal incision, on either side, is extended posterolaterally along the lateral border of the external iliac and common iliac vessels up to the aortic bifurcation. The vas deferens is identified and ligated near the internal ring. The fascia on the iliopsoas is incised and reflected medially. Marcille's triangle is exposed by retracting the common and external iliac arteries medially and dissecting the space between these vessels and the medial border of the psoas muscle (3). Dissection of the fibrolymphatic tissues in this space will expose the obturator nerve as it emerges from the medial border of the psoas muscle (Fig. 20–1). The fibrofascial sheath covering the distal half of the common iliac and external iliac vessels is then opened and stripped medially to remove the perivascular lymphatics and lymph nodes. The vessels are gently retracted, laterally and immediately below and medial to the cleaned external iliac vein, and the obturator space is entered. By working right on the psoas and

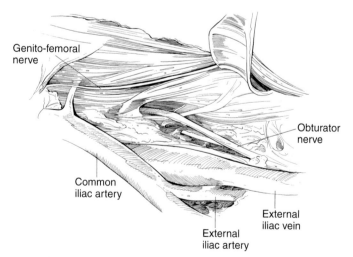

FIG. 20–1. Dissection of Marcille's triangle. The psoas muscle is retracted laterally and the iliac vessels medially. The obturator nerve is exposed in the floor of the triangle as it emerges from the medial border of the psoas muscle.

obturator muscles, one can strip all the pelvic fascia medially without difficulty. The obturator neurovascular bundle is included in the stripped mass. The obturator nerve is identified and separated from the vessels, which are divided and ligated as they leave the pelvis through the obturator foramen. Dissection is facilitated and the operating time reduced by the use of electrocoagulation to control lymphatic and small blood vessels throughout the lymphadenectomy.

Cystoprostatectomy

The fibrolymphatic mass is now reflected medially. The internal iliac artery is dissected free and its anterior division is divided and ligated. The ureter is identified where it crosses the common iliac bifurcation, dissected free for 3 to 4 cm, divided, and its distal end ligated. While traction is applied on the ligated ureteric stump of the ureter, finger dissection along its posteromedial border opens the space of Denonvilliers laterally. The step greatly helps in the definition of the plane between the bladder and rectum, which will be required at a later stage in the operation. The phases of the lateral dissection are illustrated in Fig. 20–2.

The endopelvic fascia on either side on the prostate is then opened by the tip of a blunt pair of scissors (Fig. 20–3). The optimal site for the creation of this opening is a white line marking the fusion of the parietal fascia lining the pelvic surface of the levator ani with the visceral fascia covering the lateral surface of the prostate. A right-angled clamp is used to lift the fascia from the underlying venous plexus, and it is further incised medially until the prostatic ligaments are reached. By blunt dissection, this plane is further developed posteriorly on either side of the prostate. Further anterior dissection is deferred to the final stages of the procedure to minimize the possi-

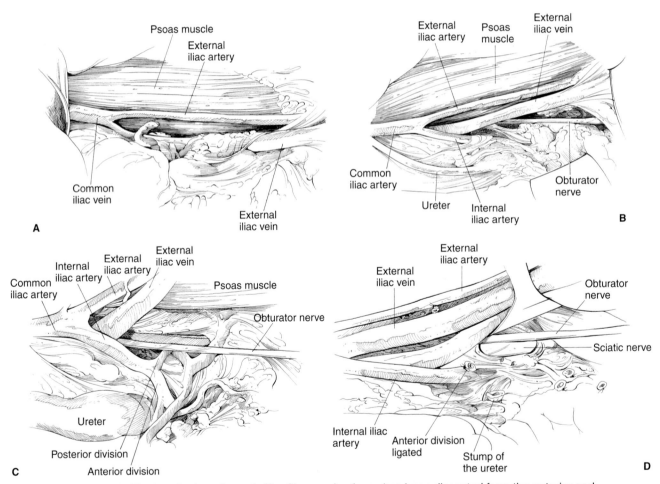

FIG. 20–2. The lymphadenectomy. **A:** The fibroareolar tissue has been dissected from the anterior and medial aspects of the psoas major muscle. The external and common iliac arteries are exposed and skeletonized. **B:** Further dissection exposes the external vein. The obturator fossa is cleared with separation of the obturator nerve. **C:** Further dissection of the internal iliac artery and its branches prior to their control. **D:** The lateral dissection is completed. The anterior division of internal iliac artery is divided with control of its parietal branches. The ureter is divided and the ligature on its stump is used for traction.

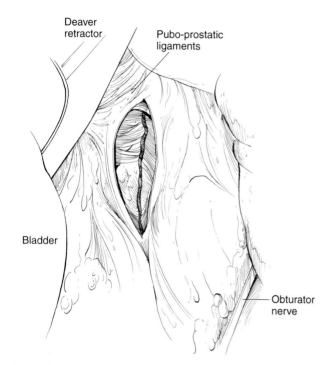

FIG. 20–3. The bladder and prostate are retracted medially by a Deaver's retractor. The reflection of the endopelvic fascia from the ventral surface of the levator ani to the prostate is opened. Blunt dissection would further develop this space and expose the lateral surface of the prostate.

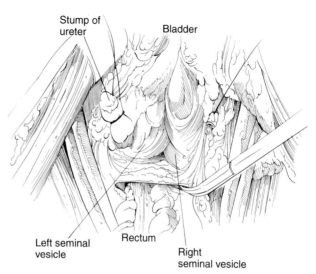

FIG. 20–4. The peritoneum of the floor of Douglas pouch is incised by diathermy. The space between the rectum posteriorly and the bladder and seminal vesicles anteriorly is dissected and opened.

bility of sudden blood losses from inadvertent injury of the prostatic venous plexus.

The specimen is now lifted ventrally by applying traction on the median umbilical ligament (urachus). The two planes developed along the posteromedial borders of the ureter on either side are easily joined together by blunt dissection. As a result, the peritoneal reflection from the anterior surface of the rectum to the back of the bladder could be stretched and safely incised by diathermy. The potential space between the rectum posteriorly and the bladder, seminal vesicles, and prostate anteriorly is opened by blunt dissection (Fig. 20–4). As the prostatic apex is reached, this space becomes obliterated as a result of fusion of the two layers of the fascia of Denonvilliers. This cul-de-sac is opened by the blunt tip of long angled scissors. Once this is completed, the tip of the surgeon's forefinger would readily feel the apex of the prostate as well as the catheter in the urethra in the midline. Alternatively, if it is directed laterally it would appear through the previously created openings on either side of the prostate (Fig. 20–5). In this manner, a thick and wide fascial band is created on either side, connecting the bladder, vesicles, and prostate anteriorly with the pararectal fascia posteriorly (the vesicoprostatopelvic fascia). This is divided piecemeal between clamps, which are underrun by 2-0 polyglactin sutures.

The bladder is now free laterally and posteriorly and the mass is left to drop in the pelvis. Attention is now focused on the anterior and final phase of the procedure. The puboprostatic ligaments are identified by applying traction on the prostate in a cephalad and posterior direction. These ligaments are carefully severed at the point of their insertion in the pubic bone. The prostatic venous plexus is controlled by one or two sutures of 3-0 polygalactic acid placed near the prostatic apex. A transverse

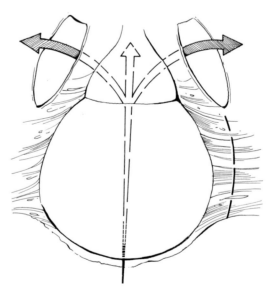

FIG. 20–5. The cul-de-sac formed by the fusion of the two layers of the fascia of Denonvilliers is opened by the tip of a blunt pair of long scissors. Thereafter, the tip of the surgeon's forefinger would feel the apex of the prostate and the catheter in the urethra. If the forefinger is directed laterally it would appear through the previously created openings on either side of the prostate. Thus, a thick, wide fascial band is defined (the vesicoprostatic pelvic fascia). It is divided piecemeal between clamps (arrow and interrupted line).

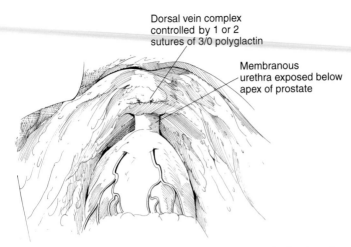

Dorsal vein complex
controlled by 1 or 2
sutures of 3/0 polyglactin

Membranous
urethra exposed below
apex of prostate

FIG. 20–6. The puboprostatic ligaments were incised and the prostatic venous complex controlled. The membranous urethra is thus exposed.

incision is made proximal to these sutures with a long scalpel and extended with sharp dissection by scissors, exposing the urethra, within which the catheter can be palpated (Fig. 20–6). The catheter is then withdrawn, the urethra is clamped and transected, the distal end is ligated, and the specimen is removed. Final hemostasis is achieved by inserting deep 2-0 polyglactin sutures between the edges of the levator ani muscles on either

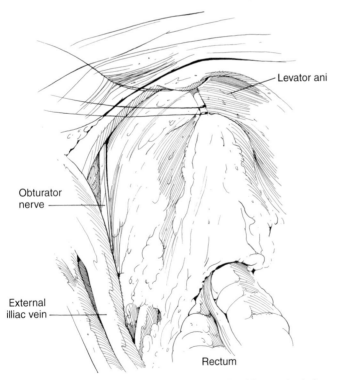

Levator ani

Obturator
nerve

External
iliac vein

Rectum

FIG. 20–7. The specimen was removed. Final hemostasis is achieved by two to three interrupted sutures of 3/0 polyglactin between the two medial borders of levator ani muscles.

side (Fig. 20–7). No attempt is made to reperitonealize the pelvis. Two tube drains are placed in the pelvic cavity and brought out through separate incisions in the abdominal wall. The wound is closed in layers with particular attention for careful closure of the anterior rectus sheath. This is closed with interrupted sutures of nylon with the knots tied to the inside.

Variations on a Theme

One-Stage Cystoprostatourethrectomy

Urethrectomy is indicated in a subpopulation of patients with multifocal tumors, diffuse carcinoma *in situ*, or tumor involving the bladder neck and/or prostate. Following incision of the puboprostatic ligaments and control of the prostatic venous plexus described, traction is applied on the cystectomy specimen in a cephalad direction. The urethra is dissected from the urogenital diaphragm with a long pair of dissecting scissors. In this manner, 2 to 3 cm of the membranous urethra can be mobilized. The pelvis is temporarily packed with gauze, and further steps are carried out perineally without urethral transaction.

A midline incision in the perineum is usually employed. The skin, subcutaneous tissue, and bulbocavernosus muscle are incised in the midline. The Foley catheter can now be palpated in the urethra. The urethra is dissected sharply from the overlying corpora cavernosus. Further dissection is carried out in the direction of the glans penis. Traction on the urethra results in inversion on the penis, allowing dissection of the urethra as far as the coronal sulcus. The penis is then allowed to restore its normal position. The urethral meatus is circumscribed sharply, and the glans penis is incised in the midline to allow dissection of the fossa navicularis. The entire penile urethra is now free. The glans penis is reconstructed by a few sutures of interrupted 3-0 chromic catgut.

Attention is now focused on dissection of the bulbar urethra. The relatively avascular tissues ventral to the bulbar urethra and beneath the symphysis pubis are dissected first. Thus, the corresponding part that had been previously dissected in the pelvis can be reached and the pelvic and perineal exposures joined. Dissection is further developed laterally and posteriorly with control of the bulbar urethral arteries. In this manner, the urethra is freed totally and the whole specimen is removed in one block.

Radical Cystoprostatectomy with Orthotopic Bladder Substitution

A standard radical cystoprostatectomy is performed except that the final stages of the operation must be done with attention to detail to avoid damage to the urethra and periurethral musculature. The integrity of these structures

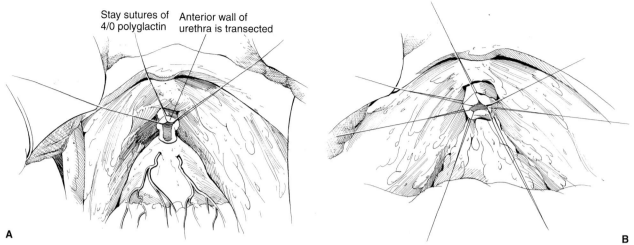

Stay sutures of 4/0 polyglactin

Anterior wall of urethra is transected

A

B

FIG. 20–8. Preparation of the urethral stump for orthotopic substitution. **A:** The anterior wall of the urethra is transected. Three stay sutures of 4/0 polyglactin are placed through the urethra at the 3-, 9-, and 12-o'clock positions. **B:** Transection of the urethra is completed and further stay sutures applied. These will prevent retraction of the urethral stump and will be later used for the urethroileal anastomosis.

has a central role in the functional success of orthotopic substitution. Following lymphadenectomy and control of the pedicles, the endopelvic fascia on either side of the prostate is opened by the tip of a blunt pair of scissors. A right-angled clamp is used to lift the fascia from the underlying venous plexus, and then it is further incised medially until the puboprostatic ligaments are reached. These ligaments are carefully severed at the point of their insertion in the pubic bone. The prostatic venous plexus is controlled by one or two suture ligatures of 3-0 polyglactin just distal to the vesicoprostatic junction. A transverse incision is made proximal to these sutures and extended by sharp dissection with scissors toward the apex of the prostate. The catheter is palpated in the urethra, the anterior wall of which is then incised just distal to the prostatic apex. The exposed Foley catheter is transected, clamped, and held for traction. At this point, three stay sutures of 4-0 polyglactin are placed through the urethra at the 3-, 9-, and 12-o'clock positions, incorporating the mucosa as well as the periurethral musculature (Fig. 20–8). These sutures prevent retraction of the urethra following its complete transection and are used later for the urethroileal anastomosis. The posterior urethral wall is then incised to expose the dorsal fibrous raphe formed by the fascia of Denonvilliers, which is lifted from the anterior surface of the rectum by a right-angled clamp and divided. The divided fascia is then included in two posterior stay sutures at the 5- and 7-o'clock positions for its later incorporation in the urethrointestinal anastomosis.

Radical Cystoprostatectomy with Nerve Sparing

This procedure was initially described by Schlegel and Walsh (5). It can be carried out in an antegrade or retrograde manner, although in our practice we prefer the antegrade approach. During radical cystectomy there are two points where the neurovascular bundle could be injured: (a) posterolateral to the prostate and (b) behind the seminal vesicles. If the extent of the pathology allows the surgeon to avoid these areas, potency could be preserved.

Bilateral lymphadenectomy with creation of the space between the rectum posteriorly and the bladder, seminal vesicles, and prostate anteriorly is carried out as previously described. By a combination of blunt and sharp dissection, the lateral surface of the seminal vesicles is freed from the medial aspect of the vesicoprostatopelvic fascia. This allows the control of these ligaments at a more ventral plane. As a result, the neurovascular pathway behind the seminal vesicles is avoided (Fig. 20–9). These pedicles are controlled by a series of simple interrupted sutures of 3-0 Vicryl. The use of heavy clamps, clips, and diathermy should be avoided. The dorsal vein complex is now controlled and the urethra isolated carefully from the adjacent fascia. The urethra is then transected and the Foley catheter is clamped and held for traction. The prostate can thus be elevated superiorly. A right-angle clamp is used to identify branches of the neurovascular bundle to the prostate. These are ligated and divided, freeing the prostate from all its lateral attachments.

Postoperative Management

IV alimentation and nasogastric suction are maintained until normal bowel activity is resumed. Systemic antibiotics are continued for 3 days postoperatively. Chest exercises and physiotherapy to the lower limbs should be carried out. Subcutaneous heparin should be administered if indicated. The tube drains are removed when drainage becomes less than 100 mL per day. It is advisable to esti-

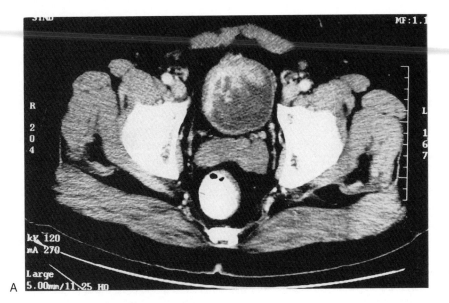

FIG. 20–9. The relationship of the neurovascular bundles to the seminal vesicles and prostate. **A:** Transverse axial scan of the pelvis at the level of the seminal vesicles. **B:** Diagrammatic representation of the same scan to demonstrate that the seminal vesicles had to be freed from the medial aspect of the vesicoprostatic pelvic fascia. **C:** This dissection would allow the control of these ligaments at a more ventral plane with preservation of the neurovascular bundle (white arrow). If this was not accomplished, the ligaments are severed at a more dorsal plain with injury to these structures.

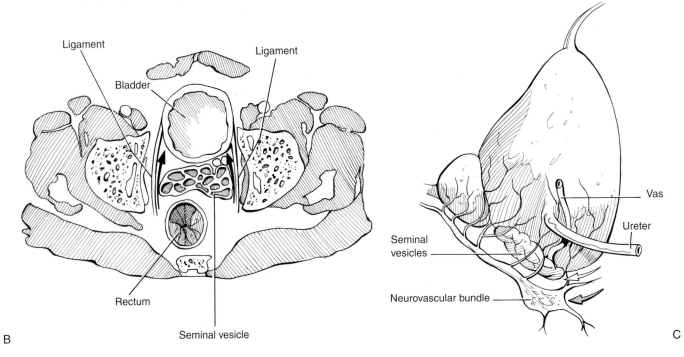

mate the creatinine content of the fluid to ensure that it is not the result of a urinary leak. Patients with an ileal conduit can be discharged on the tenth to the twelfth postoperative day. Following orthotopic substitution, patients are usually kept in the hospital for 3 weeks. Before discharge, a pouchography is carried out to make sure that there are no leaks from the neobladder or the urethroileal anastomosis.

OUTCOMES

Complications

The two most serious complications that may occur during the procedure are excessive blood loss or rectal perforation. Sudden massive bleeding is usually venous in origin, arising from tributaries of the external iliac vein during the lymphadenectomy: the deep circumflex iliac vein laterally and an abnormal obturator vein medially. Because both are located near the inguinal ligament, good retraction, illumination, and suction are needed. A laceration of the external iliac vein is then sutured with 5-0 Prolene.

Another source of bleeding is in relation to the dorsal vein complex. Dissection of this area has to be deferred to the final phase of the procedure. This venous complex is usually injured when the puboprostatic ligaments are incised. Compression of the bleeding area by a piece of gauze (4 × 8 cm.) and the tip of a long thin blade of a

Deaver's retractor are necessary until the dissection of the urethra is completed. Thereafter, bleeding is controlled by one or two interrupted 3-0 sutures of polyglactin acid placed between the two medial borders of the levator ani muscles.

However, the most serious source of bleeding is from the internal iliac vein or one of its tributaries. Sudden excessive bleeding occurs from the depth of a narrow, deep recess. Blind attempts to control the bleeding with clamps usually fail and result in more damage. In our experience, one has to achieve an initial temporary control by packing. One or two 4×8 cm. pieces of moist gauze are sufficient. The pack is tightly and constantly compressed for a few minutes and then left in place. The operator should proceed with further operative steps until the specimen is removed. Now, the working space is wide enough to allow manipulations under vision. The ipsilateral external iliac and common iliac veins as well as the main stem of the internal iliac artery are controlled by bulldog clamps. The gauze pack is then removed. There will still be some backbleeding, but with the help of a little suction the bleeding vessels are readily located and easily secured by suture ligation using 4-0 silk.

The other serious intraoperative complication is rectal perforation. This usually takes place during the final phase of the operation if the space between the prostate and rectum was not adequately and completely opened. Under such circumstances, traction on the specimen will lead to tenting of the anterior wall of the rectum. Sharp dissection with scissors or application of clamps would result in an injury of the anterior wall of the rectum well below the peritoneal reflection. If this injury is recognized, the tear is meticulously repaired. The edges are trimmed and closed in two layers using 3-0 polyglactin acid: the first through and through and the second inverting as a fascia muscular layer (Lembert technique). An omental flap is raised, brought down to the pelvis, and sutured over the repair for additional security. The pelvic cavity is then thoroughly irrigated with 1% solution of kanamycin in saline. At the end of surgery, while the patient is still under anesthesia, anal dilation is carried out up to three to four fingers to establish adequate decompression. In general, by following these principles one can avoid the need for a temporary proximal colostomy.

The postoperative mortality following contemporary cystectomy is 2% or less (6). The most common postoperative complication is prolonged ileus. This is treated by nasogastric suction, IV alimentation, and hyperalimentation if necessary. Septic complications including abdominal and/or pelvic abscesses, wound sepsis, and septicemia are not uncommon. These are treated by the appropriate antibiotics and drainage of the infected collection. This is best achieved by ultrasound-guided aspiration and/or insertion of a percutaneous tube drain. Wound dehiscence should be immediately repaired by proper closure using tension sutures. Urinary collections (urinoma) are drained under ultrasound guidance. If the source of leak is the ureterointestinal anastomosis, a percutaneous nephrostomy tube is inserted until healing is achieved and checked with an antegrade study.

Results

Radical cystectomy has evolved as the standard therapeutic modality for muscle-invasive bladder cancer. It can be accomplished with low mortality, and technical innovations with nerve-sparing and orthotopic substitution can provide many patients with a good quality of life with minimal functional losses.

All contemporary series demonstrate that radical cystectomy can result in a substantial rate of cure with overall survival ranges between 48% and 53% (1,8). For tumors with low stage (less than P_2), the survival could be as high as 75%. With further stage progression, the survival expectancy is decreased. Radical cystectomy with pelvic lymphadenectomy also provides a survival advantage for cases with nodal disease (5-year survival in the range of 20%) (7). Evidence has also been provided that adjuvant cisplatin-based polychemotherapy improves the chances of survival among patients with advanced locoregional disease (9).

REFERENCES

1. Frazier HA, Robertson JE, Dodge RK, Paulson DF. The value of pathologic factors in predicting cancer-specific survival among patients treated with radical cystectomy for transitional cell carcinoma of the bladder. *Cancer* 1993;71:3993–4001.
2. Marshall VF, Whitmore WF Jr. A technique for the extension of radical surgery in the treatment of vesical cancer. *Cancer* 1949;2:424–428.
3. McGregor AL. *A synopsis of surgical anatomy*, 9th ed. Bristol, UK: John Wright and Sons, 1963:99.
4. Schellhammer PF, Whitmore WF Jr. Transitional cell carcinoma in men having cystectomy for bladder cancer. *J Urol* 1976;115:56–60.
5. Schlegel PN, Walsh PC. Neuroanatomical approach to radical cystoprostatectomy with preservation of sexual function. *J Urol* 1987;138:1402–1406.
6. Skinner DG, Crawford ED, Kaufman JJ. Complications of radical cystectomy for carcinoma of the bladder. *J Urol* 1980;123:640–643.
7. Skinner DG. Managment of invasive bladder cancer: A meticulous pelvic node dissection can make a difference. *J Urol* 1982;128:34–36.
8. Soloway MS, Lopez AE, Patel J, Lu Y. Results of radical cystectomy for transitional cell carcinoma of the bladder and the effect of chemotherapy. *Cancer* 1994;73:1926–1931.
9. Stockle M, Meyenburg W, Wallek S, Voges GE, Rossmann M, Gertenbach U, Thuroff JW, Huber C, Hohenfellner R. Adjuvant polychemotherapy of non-organ-confined bladder cancer after radical cystectomy revisited : Long-term results of a controlled prospective study and further clinical experience. *J Urol* 1995;153:47–52.

CHAPTER 21

Radical Cystectomy in Women

Cheryl T. Lee and James E. Montie

In 2002, bladder cancer will be diagnosed in 54,500 people in the United States, including 41,500 men and 15,000 women; 12,600 will die from disease, including 8,600 men and 4,000 women (6). Thus, women account for 28% of the cases and 32% of the deaths, demonstrating the need for early and aggressive treatment. Radical cystectomy is the most effective means of cancer control of nonmetastatic high-risk transitional cell carcinoma (TCC) of the bladder and has similar indications for men and women (9). Cystectomy in women, however, may pose technical challenges for some urologists. Although the female pelvis is larger and may offer better exposure, many urologists are unfamiliar with female pelvic anatomy. Commonly, anterior pelvic exenteration is required because of high-volume disease or involvement at the trigone or posterior wall necessitating removal of neighboring pelvic structures that are at risk for direct extension. The surgeon must be prepared to proceed with total abdominal hysterectomy and anterior vaginectomy with subsequent vaginal reconstruction. Bilateral salpingo-oophorectomy is in general performed as well unless the patient is premenopausal and has grossly benign ovaries. Certainly, the age, childbearing status, and sexual function of the patient must be considered when planning such radical extirpative procedures. If the extent of disease is felt to be organ confined and located favorably, it is reasonable in young women with childbearing potential to spare the reproductive organs. Other technical concerns include (a) bleeding from the paravaginal tissues and venous plexus around the urethra, which can be brisk and tedious to control; (b) an intraoperative position change for the surgeon during urethrectomy; and (c) vaginal reconstruction, which can be complex, requiring tissue flaps to maximize organ function. Finally, as the feasibility of orthotopic diversion in women is increasingly appreciated and grows in popularity attention to urethral preparation is critical. Such preparation allows for maximum preservation of a normal voiding pattern but requires a different technique than that practiced in men. Overall, the challenges of female cystectomy are unique and may be accentuated for the surgeon who uncommonly performs cystectomy.

DIAGNOSIS

The diagnosis of TCC is covered later in this book.

INDICATIONS FOR SURGERY

The broad indication for cystectomy is a superficial, early stage, or invasive tumor that is refractory to or unlikely to be controlled by transurethral resection and intravesical therapy (3,9). The decision on when to proceed with cystectomy can be difficult for the patient and physician alike. Cystectomy may be delayed because of patient comorbidity, attempts at neoadjuvant chemotherapy, or patient and/or physician indecision. A delay in diagnosis often occurs in women presenting with hematuria as they are misdiagnosed as having a urinary tract infection. Diminished survival after cystectomy may in part be a consequence of this delay, as it is widely accepted that surgery at an earlier disease stage translates into improved outcome (9). The impact of earlier treatment on survival can be profound in view of the 30% to 40% rate of clinical understaging (4). When proceeding to definitive surgical treatment in female bladder cancer patients, the physician should consider the age, sexual function, and childbearing status of the patient in conjunction with her clinical stage. For younger female patients with carcinoma *in situ*, early invasive disease (T1), or anterior low-volume T2 disease, it may be reasonable to perform radical cystectomy with preservation of the uterus and the ovaries, thus preserving quality of life. In addition, we must consider the need to maintain body image for women by offering continent and orthotopic diversions.

168

ALTERNATIVE THERAPY

Alternatives to cystectomy include observation, systemic chemotherapy, radiation therapy, or a combination of chemotherapy and radiation. These modalities are in general offered to patients who are a poor surgical risk, refuse surgery, or are elderly. However, cystectomy is often the best option for invasive bladder cancer in the elderly who are otherwise in reasonably good health (1). Invasive bladder cancer is not an indolent disease, and death from uncontrolled TCC is high in the first 3 to 4 years. Thus, for a healthy 75-year-old woman the invasive bladder cancer is the biggest health risk. The morbidity from cystectomy in this population is historically substantial, but efforts at improved perioperative management have led to significantly improved contemporary outcomes (9). Further, the risk of radiation therapy and chemotherapy are also substantial, and elimination of the cancer is less likely (5). Unfortunately, a therapeutic strategy considered inadequate in younger patients may be employed in the healthy elderly, often with reduced doses of chemotherapy making the treatment even less likely to be successful. Improved perioperative care allows cystectomy to be done with a low operative mortality, supporting an expedient cystectomy as the overall safest and most effective approach (2,8).

SURGICAL TECHNIQUE

Female Continence

An understanding of the female continence mechanism in women is critical prior to creation of an orthotopic neobladder. There are two continence mechanisms in women (9). One is in the proximal urethra, which is innervated via the pelvic plexus that courses adjacent to the bladder neck and vagina. These nerves often are transected during a radical cystectomy. In the middle to lower third of the urethra there is an intermingling of smooth and striated muscle fibers called the rhabdosphincter muscle that is innervated via the pudendal nerves and appears to be the critical sphincter mechanism for continence in women. Because the rhabdosphincter is present in the middle to lower urethra, the entire bladder and bladder neck can be resected in a woman without compromising eventual continence. Complete resection of the bladder is necessary to minimize the transitional epithelium left *in situ* to reduce the risk of local tumor recurrence and also hypercontinence after orthotopic urinary diversion.

Access to the urethra and vagina is necessary during female cystectomy. A modified lithotomy position is used with either Allen, Lloyd–Davies, or Yellofins stirrups. Careful padding to prevent pressure points, which may cause a peroneal nerve compression or anterior compartment syndrome, is important. The vagina and

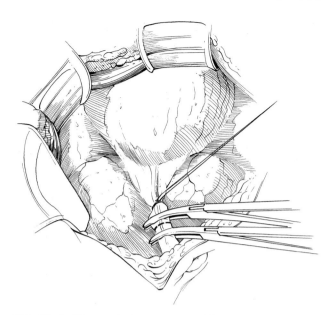

FIG. 21–1. The urachal remnant provides a convenient handle for traction on the bladder through the case and is divided between Kelly clamps and ligated.

perineum must be well prepped with an iodine or Betadine scrub. An infraumbilical vertical midline incision gives ideal exposure; however, patient habitus may necessitate an extension of this incision another 2 to 3 cm superiorly. The urachal remnant provides a convenient handle for traction on the bladder (Fig. 21–1). The peritoneum is divided along the lateral umbilical liga-

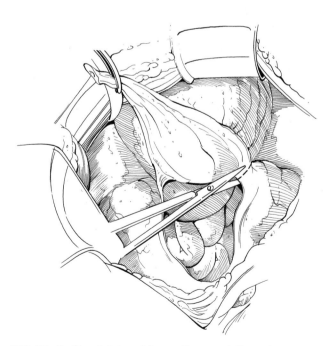

FIG. 21–2. The division of the peritoneum follows the course of the lateral umbilical ligament until the round ligament is identified, clipped, and divided.

ments (Fig. 21–2) and the round ligament is clipped and divided. A self-retaining retractor, such as the Buckwalter device, will maintain exposure. The fallopian tubes and ovaries are present and nonfunctional in this predominantly postmenopausal population and thus are ultimately removed with the uterus, cervix, and anterior vagina. The gonadal vessels and suspensory ligament are divided above the ovaries (Fig. 21–3). The ureters are mobilized with substantial periureteral adventitia to preserve optimal blood supply and later divided at the bladder hiatus (Fig. 21–4). Ligation and division of the uterine and vaginal arteries branching from the hypogastric artery is usually required to accomplish this.

Evidence continues to support the importance of complete and total pelvic lymphadenectomy in patients undergoing cystectomy (9). Although node-positive patients have a significantly shortened survival when compared to node-negative patients, 30% recurrence-free survival at 5 and 10 years is still achievable despite extravesical disease in the primary specimen. Patients with less than five nodes involved can expect a higher rate of disease—free survival than those with greater than five nodes. Total pelvic lymphadenectomy is per-

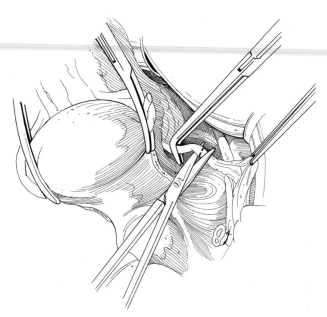

FIG. 21–4. Each ureter is mobilized with a large amount of periureteral adventitial tissue to preserve optimal blood supply. The ureter is divided a short distance above the bladder.

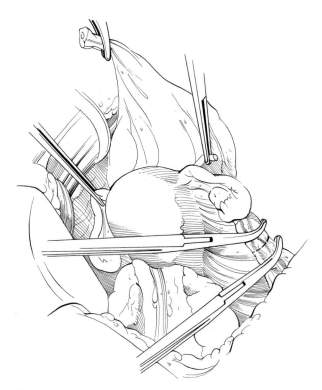

FIG. 21–3. The fallopian tubes and ovaries, if present, are commonly removed with the uterus and bladder. The gonadal vessels, surrounded by the suspensory ligament, are divided and ligated cephalad to the ovary.

formed for staging and treatment. The boundaries of dissection are the genitofemoral nerve laterally, the bifurcation of the common iliac artery superiorly, the inguinal ligament inferiorly, and the perivesical tissue medially. All tissue is removed from around the obturator nerve to the hypogastric artery, posteriorly. Specific aspects of this surgical dissection are not covered in this chapter (see Chapter 32).

The lateral blood supply to the bladder and uterus is isolated as it courses from the internal iliac artery and vein. The endopelvic fascia and the perirectal "fat pad" are exposed with medial traction on the bladder and ureter. The index finger is used to bluntly develop a plane just medial to the well-defined superior vesicle artery, aiming obliquely toward the perirectal tissue. This will isolate the superior vesicle artery, which requires ligation. Several small associated arteries and veins are controlled with ligaclips or the LigaSure device (Valley Lab, CO), thus dividing the lateral pedicle under direct vision (Fig. 21–5). Medial traction on the bladder with fingers above and below the pedicles enhances exposure.

After division of the lateral pedicles on each side, the technique is modified depending on the type of extirpative procedure to be performed. In a classic anterior pelvic exenteration, the bladder, uterus, bilateral fallopian tubes and ovaries, anterior vaginal wall, and urethra are removed *en bloc* (Fig. 21–6). This is warranted for a deeply invasive

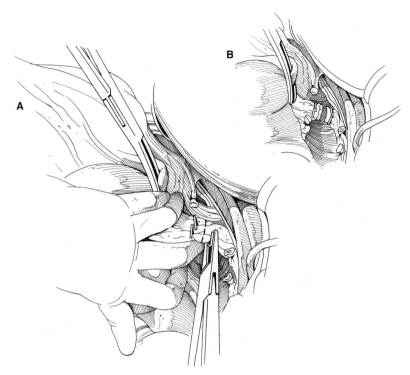

FIG. 21–5. Division of the lateral pedicle is one of the more important technical aspects of the procedure. The endopelvic fascia should be well exposed with blunt dissection. A perirectal fat pad lying adjacent to the rectum defines the lower limit of the lateral pedicle coursing from the internal iliac vessels. Medial traction on the urachal remnant and retraction of the ureter medially allow an index finger to create a plane just medial to the origin of the superior vesicle artery outlining the lateral pedicle. The caudad extent of blunt dissection is the perirectal fat tissue. **A:** The medial traction on the bladder with the surgeon's nondominant hand easily exposes the entire pedicle. **B:** The superior vesicle artery is ligated, but the remainder of the small vessels can be controlled with clips on both sides.

posterior bladder wall cancer in which orthotopic urinary diversion is not planned. Alternatively, when orthotopic diversion is planned in the sexually active woman with a tumor away from the trigore, the anterior vaginal wall and urethra are preserved. The reproductive organs should be spared if future fertility is desired.

To mobilize the anterior pelvic organs, an incision is made in the posterior peritoneum down to the rectovaginal cul-de-sac. Blunt and sharp dissection in the midline mobilizes the posterior vaginal wall; this mobility will allow the posterior vaginal wall to be rolled anteriorly away from the rectum for vaginal reconstruction

A Betadine-soaked sponge stick is placed in the vagina, elevating the apex of the vagina just posterior to the cervix. Cautery is used to open the apex of the vagina in the midline; this incision is carried laterally down the anterior vaginal wall on each side (Figs. 21–6A–C). Venous bleeding from the vaginal wall and adjacent tissue may be controlled with 2-0 Vicryl suture

ligatures. This dissection approaches the bladder neck. If orthotopic diversion is not planned, then dissection moves to the perineum after reasonable homeostasis has been ensured in the pelvis.

Urethrectomy

To perform the urethrectomy, the labia are retracted laterally with suture ligatures. Army–Navy or self-retaining retractors provide exposure to the urethral meatus. An inverted U-shaped incision is made around the urethra (Fig. 21–7) and the urethra is mobilized anteriorly and laterally. Returning to the pelvic approach, the endopelvic fascia is incised on each side. Suture ligatures are placed in the venous plexus anterior to the urethra, analogous to control of the dorsal venous plexus in men. Then, from below, the anterior vaginal wall posterolateral to the urethra is divided to connect with the pelvic dissection, which allows removal of the entire specimen.

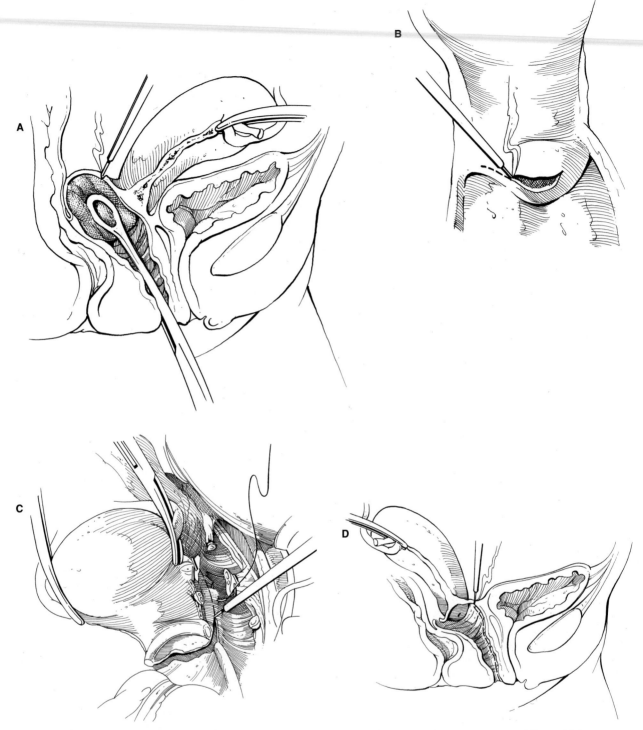

FIG. 21–6. The classic anterior pelvic exenteration includes removal of the bladder, uterus, bilateral fallopian tubes and ovaries, anterior vaginal wall, and urethra. **A and B:** An incision is made with cautery at the apex of the vagina. This is often facilitated with a Betadine-soaked sponge stick placed in the vagina on upward traction. The incision should be as close as possible to the posterior aspect of the cervix. **C:** The incision is then carried around laterally along the anterolateral aspect of the vagina. There is commonly a rich blood supply to the lateral aspect of the vagina, and this is most easily controlled with multiple suture ligatures in a stepwise fashion. The incision stops just before the endopelvic fascia. **D:** With this dissection, the entire anterior vaginal wall, posterior bladder wall, and urethra are removed *en bloc*.

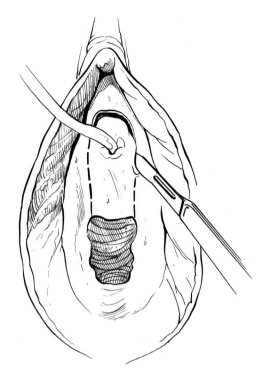

FIG. 21–7. Attention is now turned to the perineum, where an inverted U-shaped incision is made around the urethral meatus and the anterior and lateral aspects of the urethra are mobilized. Dissection returns to the pelvic exposure, where suture ligatures are placed in the venous plexus anterior to the urethra, analogous to control of the dorsal venous complex in men. The endopelvic fascia is then opened and the incisions in the anterolateral vaginal wall are connected between the perineum and the pelvic dissection. This removes the entire specimen.

Vaginal Reconstruction

The vagina is reconstructed by rotating the apex of the posterior vaginal wall anteriorly to create a foreshortened vagina that maintains the previous width (Fig. 21–8). A stay suture in the apex of the posterior vaginal wall brings the vaginal wall to the perineum; this flap of vagina is sutured to the periurethral vaginal tissue anteriorly in the midline and then sequentially on each side. After two to three interrupted sutures are placed on each side from the perineum, additional sutures higher up on the vaginal wall are more easily placed from the pelvic exposure. A watertight closure provides optimal hemostasis of the paravaginal tissue. A vaginal pack soaked in Betadine is left in the vagina for 24 hours.

In appropriately selected patients, vaginal preservation may be accomplished by establishing a plane between the posterior bladder wall and the anterior vaginal wall. Care must be taken to enter the proper plane adhering to the anterior vaginal wall. Dissection too close to either the vagina or the bladder wall can cause additional bleeding.

Urethral-Sparing Technique

In planning for orthotopic diversion, modifications in the above technique are necessary when approaching the bladder neck and urethra. It is important to maintain the integrity of the endopelvic fascia and thus preserve the support of the external sphincter. Dissection of the lateral wall of the vagina should also be avoided to prevent injury to the neurogenic innervation of the rhabdoid sphincter. Lastly, the bladder neck must be removed entirely to minimize postoperative urinary retention.

Once the bladder has been mobilized off the vagina down to the bladder neck, fine sutures are used anteriorly in the periurethral tissue as necessary for hemostasis of the venous plexus. The urethra is amputated sharply at the junction with the bladder neck, avoiding distal mobilization or dissection of the urethra (Fig. 21–9). After the bladder has been removed a sample of the urethra is circumferentially excised from the specimen or the urethral stump (if necessary) and sent for frozen section to ensure a negative urethral margin. Exposure is often ideal for the enterourethral anastomosis. The authors prefer six to ten fine absorbable sutures using 2-0 to 3-0 Monocryl taking small bites on the urethra. Mobility of the intestinal reservoir to the urethra is in general not a problem in women, although it can be in men.

In the initial experience with orthotopic diversion, the concern for stress incontinence was such that anterior urethral fixation sutures were placed to prevent hypermobility of the urethra. This maneuver is not only unnecessary (unless documented stress incontinence from hypermobility is evident preoperatively) but is counterproductive by contributing to increased urinary retention or "hypercontinence." A possible additional mechanism for postoperative urinary retention may be exacerbation of a preexisting but previously insignificant cystocele. After the cystectomy, the urethra is fixed anteriorly and the patient voids by Valsalva maneuver after relaxing the external sphincter. If a cystocele is present, the increased abdominal pressure needed for voiding across the fixed urethra and bladder neck could be blunted by the cystocele.

Postoperative Care

Establishment of a critical care pathway is useful for cystectomy patients (2). Compliance with the ideal postoperative course is difficult after cystectomy because of a high frequency of comorbid disease and complications, which may delay discharge even if they are not life-threatening. Nonetheless, the pathway provides a

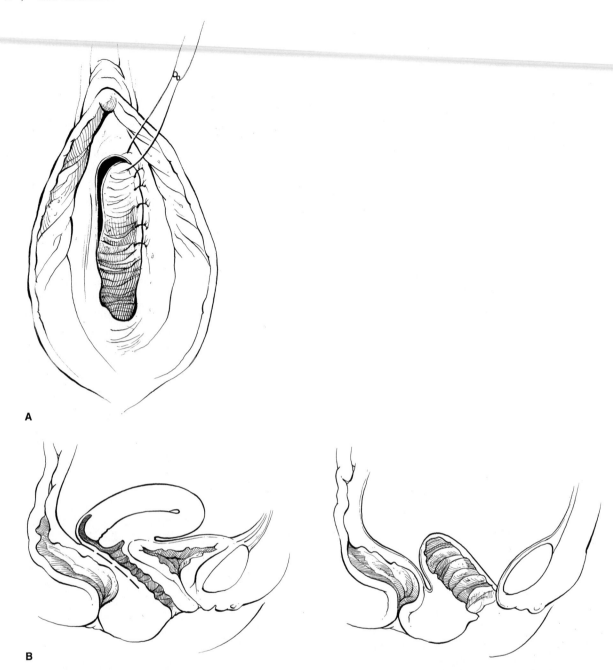

A

B

FIG. 21–8 A: Several methods of closure of the vagina are feasible. One that appears to supply strong support of the pelvis uses the posterior vaginal wall as a flap to create a neovagina. This foreshortens the vagina but does not narrow it as a side-to-side closure does and thus provides for a better return of sexual function, if appropriate. A suture is placed in the apex of the posterior vaginal wall from above; this is used to bring the posterior flap of the vagina down to the perineum. Several sutures are placed from below, incorporating a full thickness of the periurethral vaginal tissue to the posterior vaginal wall flap. Sutures closer to the apex of the vagina are more easily placed from the pelvic exposure. **B:** Diagrammatic illustration of the pelvis before and after removal of the anterior vaginal wall, bladder, and urethra. The posterior vaginal wall is then rotated anteriorly down to the perineum.

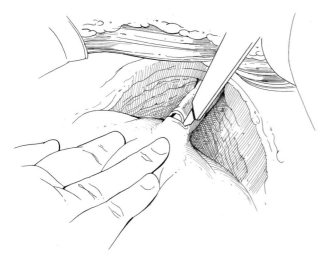

FIG. 21–9. In the situation in which an orthotopic diversion is planned, neither the endopelvic fascia nor the anterior venous plexus is disturbed. An incision is made in the anterior urethra just distal to the junction with the bladder neck. The urethra is divided completely, and the dissection of the bladder off the anterior vaginal wall can be done in either an antegrade or retrograde fashion.

target for the patient, physicians, and nursing staff for anticipated events during the hospital course. An example of the pathway currently in use at the University of Michigan Hospitals is provided in Figure 21–10. Epidural analgesia, patient-controlled analgesia, and nonsteroidal antiinflammatory agents are useful adjuncts to provide better postoperative pain control, which translates into better pulmonary hygiene, ambulation, and return of bowel function. The authors no longer routinely utilize nasogastric decompression postoperatively. This approach is long supported by the literature, which documents a less than 10% rate of nasogastric tube reinsertion in patients undergoing elective gastrointestinal surgery (7). Recognizing the impact that bowel function has on hospital stay, we recently began a phase I study to test the concept of early feeding in cystectomy patients. Eligible candidates begin an oral diet on postoperative day 1 and are advanced per protocol. Although we anticipate intolerance by some patients, we hope to delineate a cohort of individuals who can be managed aggressively with success.

Overall, excellent pain control, judicious use of diuretics to combat fluid retention, and aggressive pulmonary toilet are important strategies to prevent complications. Early ambulation and intermittent compression stockings are currently used for deep venous thrombosis prophylaxis. Routine perioperative parenteral nutrition is not necessary in the well-nourished patient; however, the clinician should institute this therapy if enteral feeding is delayed postoperatively. In our experience, approximately 10% to 15% of patients need postoperative nutritional support.

OUTCOMES

Complications

Cystectomy remains a difficult operation in men or women, with a mortality rate of 2% to 3% (9). Twenty percent to 30% of patients will have a complication delaying discharge. Many of the specific complications after cystectomy are a consequence of the urinary diversion. Complications from the cystectomy portion include bleeding with subsequent coagulation abnormalities and rectal injury. Pelvic bleeding can be more difficult to control in women. In our series, the mean estimated blood loss was 1,733 cc in women, compared to a mean of 1,211 cc in men. A rectal injury should be extremely rare in women and seen only in association with prior surgery or radiation therapy.

The postoperative care after cystectomy requires a diligence over and above that seen with other urologic procedures. Some complications are preventable. A regimented, reproducible plan for the technique of cystectomy and diversion is enormously helpful to prevent errors during a 4- to 6-hour operation. Some complications are unavoidable, but recognition early in their evolution may drastically minimize the negative consequences and a high index of suspicion is essential. Early recognition of a complication may prevent a cascade of other successive complications, which may ultimately lead to increased morbidity or mortality.

Results

From July 1990 through May 2002 we have performed 508 cystectomies; 112 (22%) patients were women. The mean age in women was 64, with a range of 35 to 86 years. Age has not been a deterrent for us to provide definitive treatment in a patient with reasonable life expectancy. Bladder cancer was the inciting disease in 91%, while 6% were treated for benign disease and 3% for other pelvic malignancies. Of 105 women with cancer, 61 (58%) had pathologically organ-confined disease and 44 (42%) had extravesical disease. Only 10 (10%) women had T4 disease with extension into neighboring pelvic organs, questioning the need for anterior pelvic exenteration in the vast majority of these cases.

Our mean operative time was 6 hours for women versus 5.5 hours for men; this time included anesthetic induction and reversal. Our mean length of stay for women undergoing cystectomy is 10 days, reflecting our willingness to offer cystectomy to an often medically complex group of patients. Urinary diversion consisted of 59% ileal conduit, 39% orthotopic neobladder, and 2% cutaneous continent diversion.

More recently we have employed a wider application of orthotopic diversion in women. In the past 2 years 23 of 37 women (62%) undergoing cystectomy received orthotopic substitution.

UNIVERSITY OF MICHIGAN·MEDICAL CENTER
CRITICAL PATHWAY RADICAL CYSTECTOMY / NEOBLADDER/ILEO LOOPS

Expected LOS: 6 days

	OP Clinic	Admit/OR Day	POD 1	POD 2	POD 3	POD 4	POD 5	POD 6
DATE:								
Expected outcomes	Pre-op tests completed/ WNL Pt./Fam. Ed. completed Consent Signed	Urine OP >160 cc over 4Hrs Urethral +/-- Suprapubic catheters freely draining Pain control thru out stay Inc C,D, & I	Temp < 101 ──────> ──────> D/c/Clamp NG (L)	Pain Controlled thru hosp. stay Inc. Clean & Dry D/C jp (L) D/c/Clamp NG (L)	D/C Drain # 1 if < 60 cc Free of Emesis + BS, +/- Flatus D/C/Clamp NG	D/C Drain # 2 if < 60 cc Passing Flatus Cont. Care Cons.	──────> Tolerates Diet D/C teaching done Plan D/C to home Cont Care completed	Plan D/C to home Return to clinic 1wk-2wks foley removal**Neobladder** E.T. or NP, D/C teach completed Bowel Function return
Consults	E.T. Therapist to mark stoma	E.T. Therapist or NP Cont. Care	──────>			Cont. Care F/U		
Tests/Labs	CBC, AB, PT, PTT, T/S, C/S, U/A, EKG, CXR	CBC, AB	CBC, AB	CBC, AB				Return to clinic in 6 wks Ileal loops for IVP, creat
Treatments	Consent Signed	SCDs/TEDs-OR IS q 1hr WA I&O VS Q4H Irr. SP tube and foley with sterile H2O or saline 30-50cc Q2H x 48 Hrs.	──────> ──────> ──────> ──────> Cont. Irrigations Q2H Ck. Drain Dsg.Change PRN	D/C SCDs ──────> ──────> Cont. Irrigations Q2H Change Abd. Dsg Change Drain dsg. PRN	TEDS ──────> ──────> VS q8H Change Irrigation to Q4H Change dsg PRN Check for Flatus or BS	TEDS ──────> ──────> ──────> ──────>	──────> ──────> ──────> Rem. Dressing Ck for flatus Check for BM	──────> ──────> ──────> Continue Irr. at home TID. Check Suture Line Check bowel fx
Drains		SP Drain DD__ Ileo loop____ Foley DD __ JP Bulb Sx __ NG LCS __if present Stent/PR	──────> ──────> ──────> ──────>	──────> ──────> ──────> ──────> DD/Clamp/Remove NG	──────> ──────> Rem. Drain # 1 NG (if used) to DD/ Clamp/Remove	──────> ──────> Rem Drain # 2 Rem. NG if not out on Day 3	──────> ──────> D/C ureteral stents if tolerating po prior to D/C	Rem. SP. Tube 2wks Home with Foley
Activity	Self Care	Bedrest Dorsiflexion exercises	Chair TID Amb. W/assist Assist with bath Dorsiflexion ex.	Amb. 6x QD Chair Ad Lib Assist with bath	──────> ──────> ──────>	──────> ──────> ──────>	──────> ──────> Shower if drains out	UAL Cont to walk at home Self bathing
Diet	Clear Liq 24 H before OR	NPO	NPO & 1 c coffee Bid* (M)	-------------→ NPO & ice limited	-------------→	Clear Liquid	Full Liquid or Reg	Regular
Medications	The DAY Prior to OR 4-6 liters PEG or til clear(S) Phospho soda PO Neomycin & E-mycin	PCA Toradolx72hrs*(M) Toradolx24hrs*(Mc)*(S) zantac till Discharge IVCefoetan x 24hrs **NEOBLADDERS*IV Cefotetan x 5 days*(M)	-------------→ Tordolx72hours(M) ──────> IV ──────>	-------------→ ──────> Dulcolax PRN IV ──────>	PCA ──────> D/C PCA start Tordol Vicodin/Darvocett IV	D/C PCA D/C Tordol --------------→ Dulcolax PRN Colace IV ──────>	Premed,gent 80mg/each stent removal --------------→ --------------→ IV D/C IV ABX - PO ABX*(M)NEOBLADDERS	Rx for Pain Med Rx for ABX PO RX for Zantac DC Hep Lock
Teaching D/C Planning	E.T. Therapist Plan of Care & D/C pamphlet Assess Support Pain Management Bowel prep instructions	Explain drains Pain Control with PCA Abd Splinting, no overhead frames IS Give D/C & Plan of care booklet Scrotal supp&meatal care	Rev. Pamphlet Reassess patient support systems	Irrigation of SP and/or foley Assess need for home supplies	Rev. Irr. with return Demo. Rev. D/C pamphlet	Teach inc. Care Pt. to irr. drains Review D/C pamphlet	Irr. cath q4H Teach leg bag if need D/C supplies to room- 2 bottles sterile H2O 2 60cc syringe Scripts written for D/C	Rev.Physician's D/C Orders & Meds Remind of return visit

A

POD 7	POD 8	F/U Clinic
D/C to home if not on Day 6 D/C teaching done	D/C to Home if not on Day 7 Return to clinic 1-2 wks for foley removal	F/U Clinic 1-2 wks(M)(S) 2wks(L) for foley rem SP2wks./**NEO** F/U Clinic 4 wks/**Ileo & Augs**
		F/U Clinic 4 wks or 6wks after foley rem. IVP, Creat.
	Continue Irr. at home TID	
		F/U Clinic 1-2 wks for foley removal

B

Variance Tracking Cystectomy / Neobladder

	Variance Description	P	S	C	None	Comments/Actions	Initials N D E
Adm Day	Date of admission _____						
Discharge	Date of discharge _____						

Code for Variance
P = Patient: Complications or other pt./family issues affecting care/achievement of outcomes (state reason)
C = Clinical: Tests, Consults, treatments & other clinical interventions not on the pathway. (state reason)
S = System: Test delays, equipment problems, interdepartmental issues affecting care/outcomes (state reason)

FIG. 21–10. Current critical pathway for radical cystectomy/neobladder at the University of Michigan Medical Center.

REFERENCES

1. Chang SS, Alberts G, Cookson MS, Smith JA Jr, et al. Radical cystectomy is safe in elderly patients at high risk. *J Urol* 2001;166:938–941.

2. Chang SS, Cookson MS, Baumgartner RG, Wells N, Smith JA Jr. Analysis of early complications after radical cystectomy: results of a collaborative care pathway. *J Urol* 2002;167:2012–2016.

3. Freeman JA, Esrig D, Stein JP, et al. Radical cystectomy for high risk patients with superficial bladder cancer in the era of orthotopic urinary reconstruction. *Cancer* 1995;76:833–839.

4. Harris RE, Chen-Backlund J, Wynder EL. Cancer of the urinary bladder in blacks and whites. *Cancer* 1990;66:2673–2680.

5. Holmiing S, Borghede G. Early complications and survival following short term palliative radiotherapy in invasive bladder carcinoma. *J Urol* 1996;155:100–102.

6. Jemal A, Thomas A, Murray T, Thun M. Cancer statistics, 2002. *CA Cancer J Clin* 2002;52:23–47.

7. MacRae HM, Fischer JD, Yakimets WW. Routine omission of nasogastric intubation after gastrointestinal surgery. *Can J Surg* 1992;35:625–628.

8. Montie JE, Pavone-Macaluso M, Tazaki H, et al. What are the risks of cystectomy and the advances in perioperative care? *Int J Urol* 1995; 2[Suppl 2]:89–104.

9. Stein JP, Lieskovsky G, Cote R, Groshen S, Reng A, Boyd S, Skinner E, Bochner B, Thangathurai D, Mikhail M, Raghavan D, Skinner DG. Radical cystectomy in the treatment of invasive bladder cancer: long-term results in 1,054 patients. *J Clin Oncol* 2001;19:666–675.

CHAPTER 22

Bladder Diverticulectomy

Michael S. Cookson and Sam S. Chang

A bladder diverticulum is the protrusion of mucosa through the detrusor muscle fibers as a result of a structural defect or chronic dysfunctional voiding. The wall of the diverticulum is composed of the following layers from inside out: mucosa, subepithelial connective tissue or lamina propria, isolated and thin muscle fibers, and adventitial tissue (Figs. 22–1 and 22–2) (7). Diverticula may be congenital or acquired, the latter developing secondary to increased intravesical pressure (5). The most frequent causes of increased bladder voiding pressure and the eventual formation of an acquired diverticulum are benign prostatic hyperplasia, urethral strictures, contracture of the bladder neck or urethral valves, and neurogenic voiding dysfunction, such as detrusor–sphincteric dyssynergy. The diverticula are located in the weakest points of the bladder, such as the ureteral hiatus (paraureteral or Hutch diverticulum) and both posterolateral walls (2,3,5).

DIAGNOSIS

Congenital diverticula are more common in males than in females, and while they may be discovered incidentally in adulthood the peak incidence is less than 10 years of age (2). In contrast, acquired diverticula have a peak incidence of greater than 60 years of age and are almost exclusively found in males (5). Acquired bladder diverticula are commonly asymptomatic, although irritative and/or obstructive voiding symptoms, pelvic pain, and hematuria may arise from complications thereof, including infection, stones, obstruction, and tumor.

Given the nonspecific nature of the presenting symptoms, diverticula are most commonly diagnosed by radiographic imaging including ultrasound, intravenous pyelogram (IVP), voiding cystourethrogram (VCUG), and contrast-enhanced computerized tomography (CT scan) (Fig. 22–3). Diverticula are also found on ultrasound of an empty and full bladder performed for the study of bladder outlet obstructive symptoms in men or repeated urinary infections in women. Cystograms obtained by IVP or through retrograde instillation of contrast medium may provide information with regard to the number, location, size, and urinary retention volume of the diverticulum. However, a VCUG with lateral, oblique, and postvoid images are important in defining the extent of the diverticulum and of particular use in congenital cases to rule out possible vesicoureteral reflux (2). A video urodynamics study can provide not only important anatomic information but also information regarding bladder function and voiding pressure, which may be of special interest in cases where neurogenic voiding dysfunction is suspected.

Cystourethroscopy should be performed to exclude urethral stricture disease and/or bladder neck contractures but is most important to rule out occult pathology such as a stone or carcinoma within the diverticulum (1). The entire surface of the diverticulum should be visualized and the relative location of the ureteral orifices should be noted to assist in planning for any potential surgical procedure. The differential diagnosis includes "pseudodiverticular" images observed in cystograms such as bladder ears, hourglass bladder, and vesical hernias. Other diagnoses include urachal cysts, prostatic utricle cysts, or müllerian duct cysts and blind-ending bifid ureters. Other less frequent congenital anomalies should also be considered, such as vesicourachal diverticulum, incomplete bladder duplication, and septation of the bladder (2).

INDICATIONS FOR SURGERY

In general, the indications for surgical intervention include chronic infections, stones, and premalignant changes such as dysplasia or carcinoma *in situ* and frank carcinoma. A large diverticulum may be the cause of deficient voiding and chronic urinary infection or obstruction of the ureter and even of the posterior urethra in children, whereas a paraureteral or hiatal diverticulum is usually associated with different degrees of reflux (4,5). In addition, spontaneous diverticular rupture or complications related to the size or location of the diverticulum are indi-

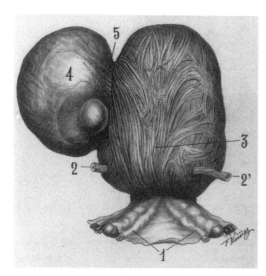

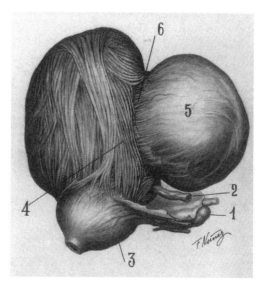

FIG. 22–1. Posterior view of bladder and diverticulum. **1:** Ampulla of vas deferens. **2 and 28:** Ureters. **3:** Posterior longitudinal bundle of the outer layer of the detrusor. **4:** Diverticulum. **5:** Circular fibers of the middle layer of the detrusor around the diverticular neck.

FIG. 22–2. Lateral view of bladder and diverticulum. **1:** Seminal vesicle. **2:** Ureter. **3:** Prostate. **4:** Anterolateral longitudinal fibers of the outer layer of the detrusor. **5:** Diverticulum. **6:** Fine, circularly oriented fibers around the diverticular neck.

cations for surgery. With the aim of improving functional voiding, we recommend the simultaneous resection of all poorly emptying bladder diverticula if the patient must undergo open prostatectomy, cystolithotomy, ureteroneocystostomy, or YV-plasty of the bladder neck. Similarly, a vesical diverticulum should never be operated on without previously or simultaneously correcting the cause, whether anatomic or functional (neurogenic bladder), of outlet obstruction that provoked it.

Although occurring in a small subset of these patients (0.8% to 10%), urothelial carcinoma can develop within

bladder diverticula at a mean age of 65 years (range, 45 to 80) (1). Approximately 75% to 80% of these tumors are urothelial carcinoma, while 20% to 25% are squamous cell carcinomas likely induced from chronic stasis of urine and infection. Because of this potential malignant risk and the fact that these tumors can be difficult to diagnose, some have advocated prophylactic diverticulectomy. Alternatively, a more conservative strategy may be offered that should include surveillance cystoscopy and urinary cytology obtained at 6- to 12-month intervals.

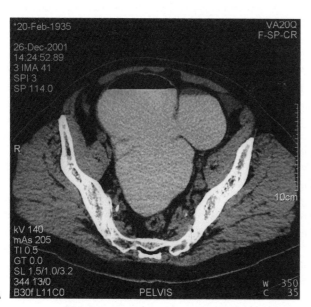

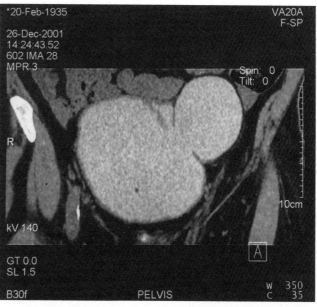

FIG. 22–3. Contrast-enhanced computerized tomography scan demonstrating a large posteriorly based bladder diverticulum seen on **(A)** transverse and **(B)** sagittal images.

ALTERNATIVE THERAPY

Many children with congenital diverticula who are asymptomatic do not require therapy and a conservative approach has been advocated (2). Saccules and small diverticula may be treated successfully by electrocoagulation of their mucosa when the primary obstructive disease is endoscopically resolved. In addition, laparoscopic approaches to bladder diverticulum may be effective as an alternative to open surgery with the distinct advantage of shortened convalescence time (6).

PREOPERATIVE ASSESSMENT

Aside from laparoscopic approach, there are essentially two methods of surgical therapy: (a) transurethral resection of the diverticular neck and (b) open diverticulectomy. In either case, infection must be adequately treated prior to surgery. If the lesion is acquired due to obstruction, the obstruction must be relieved to prevent recurrence and subsequent treatment failure or the formation of new diverticula (9). If the diverticulum is due to high detrusor pressure of neurological origin, this must also be addressed prior to surgical correction.

SURGICAL TECHNIQUE

Transurethral Resection

Transurethral resection of the neck of small to midsized diverticula in situations where the opening is not immediately impinging on the ureter is a well-recognized treatment (10). If the opening is small, a Collins knife or right angle hooked electrode can be used to open the ostium of the diverticulum to allow for subsequent inspection of the entire diverticular wall and facilitate drainage. Transurethral resection or fulguration of the mucosa with a roller ball electrode can then be used to ablate the mucosa of the inner wall.

In the case of tumor within a bladder diverticulum, caution must be exercised. Because there is no muscular backing, transurethral resection of bladder tumors within diverticula carries a high risk of perforation. Cold-cup biopsy and fulguration may be appropriate for low-grade, lowstage tumors. The holmium laser may also be of use in this unique situation because it has a small fiber and a shallow depth of penetration (only 0.3 to 0.5 mm) and would certainly lower the risk of perforation or injury to adjacent structures (8). In those patients with high-grade or large diverticular carcinomas, in particular those with narrow openings in which the risk of endoscopic perforation or inadequate resection is high, open diverticulectomy/partial cystectomy or total cystectomy has been advocated.

Open Surgical Technique

A Foley catheter is placed in the bladder on the surgically prepared field to allow for passive drainage and active filling of the bladder as needed throughout the procedure. The bladder is approached via an infraumbilical midline extraperitoneal incision, although alternatively a Gibson incision may be used. The linea of the rectus fascia is divided in the midline, along with the transversalis fascia, and the pelvis is exposed. In the case of benign bladder pathology, the dissection is carried into the space of Retzius and the anterior bladder wall and vesical neck are identified. After reflecting the peritoneum cephalad off the bladder dome, a transverse cystotomy is performed at this level. This provides better exposure of bladder contents and facilitates placement of a small self-retaining retractor and additional stay sutures. The trigone, ureteral orifices, bladder neck, and all possible diverticular orifices are clearly visualized from the bladder dome opening.

In cases of intradiverticular tumor, some have advocated the instillation of 30 mg of mitomycin C by urethral catheter before the surgery. Intraoperatively, we carefully protect the surgical field with moist, sterile towels draped around the wound to avoid possible tumor contamination during diverticulectomy. The bladder mucosa should also be thoroughly inspected to rule out papillary tumors that may have gone unnoticed on the previous endoscopic examination. The mouth of the diverticulum can also be packed with a small gauze pad to avoid or minimize potential tumor spillage.

Diverticulum excision has been described in three different approaches: extravesical (V.V. Czerny, 1896), intravesical (H.H. Young, 1906), and the intravesical and extravesical combination (G. Marion, 1913). The most commonly used procedures and the points of technique that we use are the following.

Intravesical Diverticulectomy

If the diverticulum is small (less than 2.5 cm diameter), we perform intravesicalization and eversion of its wall, grasping and tractioning its bottom gently with an Allis- or Pean-type clamp inserted through its neck. If this maneuver is performed carefully, and fibrosis secondary to infection is absent, the majority of these diverticula are rapidly and easily removed. The mucosa of the everted diverticular neck is divided using electrocautery, and the defect of the bladder wall is sutured with 3-0 chromic catgut or Vicryl using separate submucosal and muscular sutures in two separate layers. In case of a saccule, a fine ligature of the neck and resection of its everted mucosa will suffice.

If this maneuver is not feasible because of peridiverticular adhesions, we proceed to sharply split the mucosa around the diverticular orifice and dissect with scissors as far as the periadventitial space. In this way, the diverticular neck remains separated from the bladder wall and is pulled toward the vesical cavity with Allis-type clamps. At the same time, the adventitial adhesions that fix the diverticular sac are freed gently with a small moist gauze and the sac is drawn into the bladder. The bladder wall is then closed as mentioned previously (Fig. 22–4).

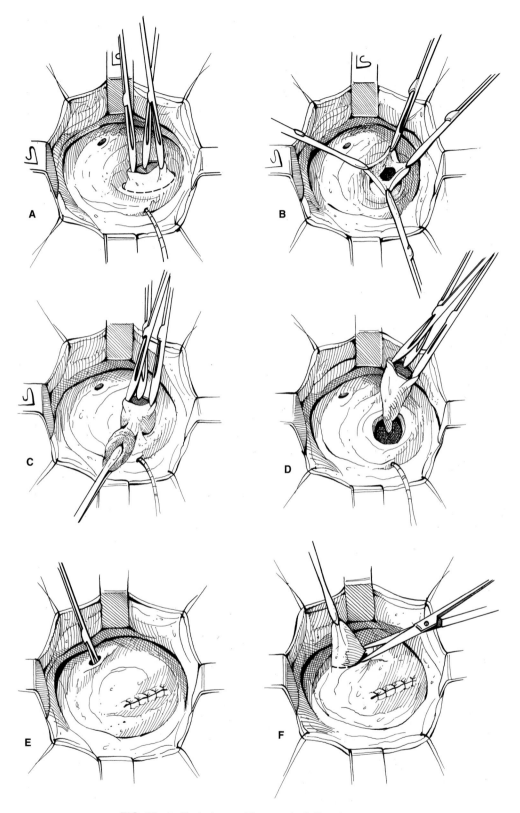

FIG. 22–4. Technique of intravesical diverticulectomy.

Combined Intravesical and Extravesical Diverticulectomy

In a large diverticulum complicated with peridiverticulitis or in a paraureteral location, it is obligatory to place a 7 or 8 Fr catheter into the ipsilateral ureter before dissection. This will allow for easy identification of the ureter and hopefully avoid inadvertent ureteral injury. If the dissection is extensive, a double-J ureteral catheter remains indwelling for a short period of time (usually 2 to 3 weeks). These diverticula must be excised by a combined intra- and extravesical approach, first identifying and dissecting the diverticular neck. For this, the maneuver of inserting the surgeon's index finger into the diverticulum and gently tractioning the upper face of its neck toward the surface is useful. We also recommend completely filling the diverticular sac with a moist gauze to unfold its wall and delimit its margins as accurately as possible. Dissection must begin at the diverticular neck, which is incised extravesically with electrocautery and separated from the bladder wall, whose orifice is sutured with 3-0 chromic catgut using extramucosal separate stitches (Figs. 22–5 and 22–6).

Tractioning the edges of the diverticular mouth toward the surface with Allis-type clamps allows the sac wall to be dissected from neighboring tissue with scissors and a small moist swab. It should always be borne in mind that the ureteral course may have been modified by the great diverticular volume, and the ureter may be closely adhered to its wall if repeated infectious processes have occurred. This dissection will be difficult if extensive peridiverticulitis is present, and it is

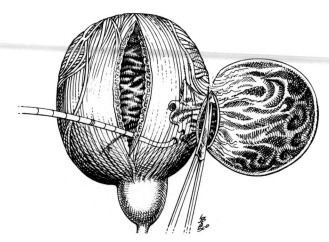

FIG. 22–6. Procedure of combined intravesical–extravesical diverticulectomy. Once the diverticulum has been dissected, the mouth of the diverticulum is excised sharply.

more advisable simply to denude it of its mucosal lining with fine scissors or with the cutting current and the ball electrode from inside the diverticular cavity and then place a suction drain within it (first described by Pousson in 1901 and Geraghty in 1922). The bladder wall is closed with absorbable 3-0 interrupted or continuous absorbable sutures, and a two-layer closure is preferable when possible. We leave a 10 Fr closed suction drain in the space of Retzius and a urethral 18 or 20 Fr Foley catheter, which may both be removed after 5 or 6 days. For more extensive cases, those requiring large cystotomies, or in situations where there is prolonged drain output, a Foley catheter may be left in place for 10 to 14 days and a cystogram may be indicated prior to catheter removal.

OUTCOMES

Complications

The most serious specific complication of excision of a bladder diverticulum is an injury to the intramural or pelvic ureter during dissection of large diverticulum. With prior placement of an ipsilateral ureteral catheter, this injury should be avoidable or at least recognizable and promptly repaired. A small ureterotomy can be easily sutured with absorbable 5-0 or 6-0 chromic or Vicryl. If the ureter has been severely damaged, or its section is complete and near the vesical hiatus, the distal ureter must be abandoned and it is preferable to carry out ureteral reimplantation following the technique of Leadbetter–Politano with or without vesical mobilization to the psoas muscle ("psoas hitch"). More extensive injuries to the ureter may require a bladder tube (Boari flap) or a transureteroureterostomy. End-to-end suture of ureteral edges must never be performed in precarious conditions because it is highly likely that it will be complicated by

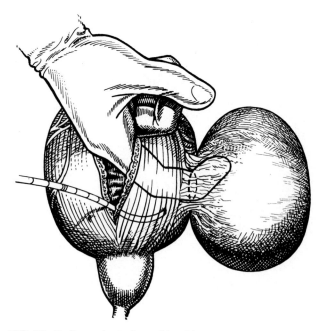

FIG. 22–5. Procedure of combined intravesical–extravesical diverticulectomy. A finger is inserted into the bladder diverticulum from within the bladder.

urinary fistula or ureteral stenosis, which will further aggravate the situation.

Other complications include urinary fistula, rectal injury, and pelvic abscess. Less serious complications include vesical urine leakage, which may cease spontaneously if the Foley catheter is maintained for additional days, providing the obstructive pathology has been resolved.

Results

With transurethral resection, approximately one-third of these lesions are cured or significantly improved. For benign disease, an open excision of the diverticulum is in general curative for that particular lesion, although correction of the underlying cause (e.g., outlet obstruction) is required to prevent formation of additional diverticulum or recurrence. In cases of diverticula involving carcinoma, the prognosis has in general been poor and attributed to the difficult and often delayed diagnosis with early escape from the confines of the bladder through the thin mucosal backing. However, more contemporary reports suggest relatively high rates of survival (~ 70% 5-year survival), attributed in part to earlier detection through improved radiographic imaging and a lower threshold for cystoscopy in the presence of hematuria coupled with early aggressive surgical treatment (1).

Nevertheless, due to the relatively paucity of cases treatment recommendations for these unique situations will continue to be based largely on patient characteristics and surgeon preferences.

REFERENCES

1. Baniel J, Vishna T. Primary transitional cell carcinoma in vesical diverticula. *Urology* 1997;50:697.
2. Canning DA, Koo HP, Duckett JW. Anomalies of the bladder and cloaca. In: Gillenwater JY, Grayhack JT, Howards SS, Duckett JW, eds. *Adult and pediatric urology*, 3rd ed. St. Louis: Mosby–Year Book, 1996:2445.
3. Hutch JA. *Anatomy and physiology of the bladder, trigone, and urethra.* New York: Appleton Century Crofts, 1972:8.
4. Jarow JP, Brendler CB. Urinary retention caused by a large bladder diverticulum: a simple method of diverticulectomy. *J Urol* 1988;139:1260.
5. Miller A. The aetiology and treatment of diverticulum of the bladder. *Br J Urol* 1958;30:43.
6. Parra RO, Jones JP, Andrus CH, Hagood PG. Laparoscopic diverticulectomy: preliminary report of a new approach for the treatment of bladder diverticulum. *J Urol* 1992;148:869.
7. Peterson LJ, Paulson DF, Glenn JF. The histopathology of vesical diverticula. *J Urol* 1973;110:62P.
8. Pietrow PK, Smith JA Jr. Laser treatment for invasive and noninvasive carcinoma of the bladder. *J Endourol* 2001;15:425.
9. Quirinia A, Hoffmann AL. Bladder diverticula in patients with prostatism. *Int Urol Nephrol* 1993;25:243.
10. Vitale PJ, Woodside JR. Management of bladder diverticula by transurethral resection: reevaluation of an old technique. *J Urol* 1979;122:744.

CHAPTER 23

Bladder Augmentation

R. Duane Cespedes and Edward J. McGuire

Bladder augmentation or augmentation cystoplasty is the addition of a segment of bowel or other suitable tissue to the *in-situ* bladder to increase capacity, improve compliance, or treat uncontrollable detrusor contractility. It is frequently used in the reconstruction of neurogenic bladders that have failed medical therapy or other conservative therapies. Augmentation cystoplasty has for practical purposes replaced cutaneous urinary diversion in this group of patients due to decreased morbidity of the procedure, decreased postoperative complications, the widespread use of clean intermittent catheterization (CIC), and improved postoperative quality of life. In addition, it has been shown that patients with cutaneous urinary diversions, draining continuously via any segment of bowel, have an inferior long-term outcome with regard to infections and upper-tract deterioration than patients with a large, low-pressure reservoir that uses the urethra as the continence mechanism. In some cases, such as chronic, intractable interstitial cystitis with a small bladder capacity and severe symptoms, a supratrigonal cystectomy may be performed and the bladder substituted with a bowel segment.

Although we prefer ileum in most cases, many different bowel segments have been used, each with its own specific advantages and disadvantages; however, no bowel segment is clearly superior in all circumstances. The most important factor is detubularization of the bowel to reduce intravesical pressure from peristalsis or mass contractions.

In most cases of neuropathic vesical dysfunction, the simplest low-pressure continent reservoir to construct involves the addition of bowel to augment the *in-situ* bladder utilizing the patient's own urethra as the continence mechanism.

The opinions contained herein are those of the authors and are not to be construed as reflecting the views of the US Air Force or the Department of Defense

DIAGNOSIS

Before consideration is given for an augmentation cystoplasty, all medical therapies and conservative treatments directed at improving detrusor compliance and increasing capacity should be exhausted. Having failed these therapies, the basic evaluation includes a cystometrogram, preferably using fluoroscopy, to evaluate bladder compliance, status of the bladder neck (open or closed at rest), and presence of vesicoureteral reflux. The bladder's functional characteristics such as capacity and compliance can sometimes dictate the type and length of bowel required.

The evaluation of urethral function is problematic, in particular in patients with poor compliance or a defunctionalized bladder, where the urethra may appear deceptively worse than it truly is. The abdominal leak point pressure (ALPP) is a good method of determining urethral resistance to abdominal pressure as an expulsive force (7). If, in addition to the augmentation cystoplasty, one of the goals of the operative procedure is to achieve continence, the abdominal pressure required to cause leakage is essential. If that pressure is very low, 0 to 60 cm H_2O, then a sling procedure, artificial urinary sphincter, or injectable agent will be required to prevent leakage. If the resistance to abdominal pressure is high, perhaps 140 to 150 cm H_2O or more, then no procedure to improve urethral function is usually necessary. In the middle range, 60 to 140 cm H_2O, any of the above treatments and perhaps a urethral suspension in females can be used to treat stress incontinence. It is important to recognize that the surgical creation of outlet resistance that completely resists intravesical pressure is inherently dangerous to the upper tracts and may contribute to rupture of the augment (8). An upright cystogram, which demonstrates that continence is maintained at the bladder neck, can be a useful adjunct to the ALPP. Even if both studies are performed and the sphincter appears functional, leakage may still occur after augmentation cystoplasty when the bladder is very full and high intraabdominal pressure is applied.

Another important sphincteric function is that it must function as a compliant voiding conduit. If the patient is neurologically normal and voiding is anticipated after augmentation cystoplasty (as in selected patients with interstitial cystitis), the sphincteric unit should open normally on a voiding urodynamic study. Voiding pressures less than 30 to 40 cm H_2O usually indicates that the sphincteric unit opens normally with voiding and CIC *may not* be required postoperatively. Voiding pressures greater than 40 cm H_2O in general indicate sphincteric obstruction or dysfunction and the patient will likely require CIC after the augmentation cystoplasty.

In general, ureteral size (or dilation) is not indicative of potential ureteral function because, in most cases, if good ureteral peristalsis is demonstrated by ultrasound, fluoroscopy, or Whitaker perfusion test the ureters will function adequately when placed into a low-pressure reservoir.

INDICATIONS FOR SURGERY

Bladder augmentation is a useful technique for the following indications:

1. Severe, medically refractory bladder instability—most commonly for multiple sclerosis, spinal cord injury, and idiopathic urge incontinence.
2. Poor bladder compliance— for neuropathic conditions, after pelvic radiation therapy, intravesical chemotherapy, prolonged catheter drainage, or from untreated obstructive uropathy.
3. Prolonged bladder defunctionalization—after long-term cutaneous vesicostomy drainage or bilateral cutaneous ureterostomy.
4. Patients previously diverted who are candidates for undiversion into a large, low-pressure reservoir.

Patient selection remains an important issue before augmentation cystoplasty. Chronic renal failure (documented by creatinine clearance) is a relative contraindication to an augmentation because both the small and large bowel resorb many urinary solutes that may cause deterioration of the metabolic status of the patient. In these patients, the use of stomach has been recommended (1).

All patients should be able to both mentally and physically perform CIC prior to a bladder augmentation even if postoperative voiding is anticipated. This is especially important at both age extremes. If any question exists, it is better to construct a cutaneous catheterizable diversion or, alternatively, a noncontinent diversion.

No bowel segment is clearly superior to another in all circumstances and the segment used is usually based on surgeon preference. In some circumstances, restrictions may exist, however. Stomach should probably not be used in patients with peptic ulcer disease and large bowel should rarely be used if a history of ulcerative colitis, previous colon cancer, or diverticulitis exists. Similarly, in cases of extensive pelvic radiation transverse colon or stomach may be preferable to small bowel. Last, consideration for preservation of the ileocecal valve should be given in patients with myelodysplasia as significant problems with diarrhea and fecal incontinence have been reported (5).

ALTERNATIVE THERAPY

Autoaugmentation of the bladder (also called partial detrusor myomectomy) in which the detrusor muscle over the dome and anterior wall is excised allows the bladder epithelium to distend outward, thereby improving storage capacity and detrusor compliance (3). The gains in bladder capacity (to a lesser degree) and compliance in patients with certain neuropathic conditions (such as myelodysplasia) are small and its routine use is not recommended in this group of patients (6). We continue to use this technique in selected patients with intractable urge incontinence with favorable results (15). In patients without neurogenic dysfunction, the advantages of this procedure include decreased operative morbidity, quicker postoperative recovery, and a uniform ability to void after the procedure.

For patients in whom a simple, low-pressure cutaneous diversion is preferable, a noncontinent ileovesicostomy (bladder "chimney") can be performed. Using similar procedures, Schwartz and colleagues (11) and subsequently Mutchnik and colleagues (9) reported excellent long-term results with few significant complications.

Nonautologous tissues (Gore-Tex, Dacron, bovine dura or pericardium, and many others) have all been utilized to augment the bladder; however, complications with the anastomosis, infections, or stone formation have precluded their routine use. More recent developments include the use of autologous bladder cell transplantation techniques and acellular collagen-based matrices, which provide a scaffolding for bladder regeneration (2). Both of these techniques remain investigational but provide much hope for future advancements in this area.

SURGICAL TECHNIQUE

Preparation of the patient is important and all patients should undergo preoperative bowel preparation. In the neuropathic patient, chronic constipation is a usually a problem and 2 to 3 days of clear liquids and a full mechanical bowel preparation the day before the procedure will be necessary to ensure removal of all solid stool. Patients with nonneurogenic conditions and the use of small bowel for the augment require a less rigorous bowel preparation. If large bowel is used, oral nonabsorbable antibiotics such as neomycin and erythromycin base should be considered. Note that intraoperatively the desired segment of bowel is sometimes found to be unsuitable and therefore a full bowel prep is recommended for the majority of cases. A preoperative dose of intravenous antibiotics is also given with special consideration given to those patients with implanted prosthetic materials such as a ventriculoperitoneal shunt or orthopedic hardware.

Other important preoperative considerations include treatment of metabolic or electrolyte disorders, documentation of sterile urine, and, in selected cases where colon will be used, a preoperative barium enema or colonoscopy.

After preparation of the skin from xiphoid to genitalia, a urethral catheter is placed and a midline (preferably) or Pfannenstiel incision is made and the retropubic space dissected until the bladder is free of adhesions. In general, if a procedure to treat incontinence is necessary it is performed first. In addition, if *low-pressure* vesicoureteral reflux has been documented preoperatively ureteral reimplantation should be considered. The ureters should be reimplanted into the bladder if possible or a colonic augment as ureteral reimplantation into the ileum is tenuous and not as favorable. We do not reimplant functional ureters that reflux due to high bladder pressures because augmentation will decrease bladder storage pressure and the reflux usually resolves. A self-retaining retractor is placed, the bladder filled with saline, and the peritoneum dissected off the bladder to the level of the trigone (Fig. 23–1). Using electrocautery, a U-shaped incision is made on the bladder starting 3 cm above the ureters, effectively creating an anteriorly based bladder flap (Fig. 23–2). This technique avoids the hourglass configuration that can develop, making the augment little more than a poorly draining bladder diverticulum. The peritoneum is opened last to minimize third-space fluid loss and urine contamination of the peritoneal cavity. A 25- to 30-cm segment

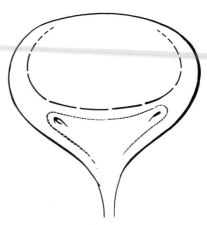

FIG. 23–2. A U-shaped incision is made on the bladder with the transverse portion just superior to the trigone and the limbs of the incision extending to the dome of the bladder.

of ileum at least 15 cm away from the ileocecal valve is selected and marked with sutures. The ileum should easily reach the bladder without tension. The mesentery is cleared from both ends to create a window and the ileum divided using a standard stapling device (Fig. 23–3). The exact amount of ileum required varies between patients but enough should be used to allow a minimum 4 hours between catheterizations after the bowel is fully "stretched" over the ensuing months. Ileal continuity is

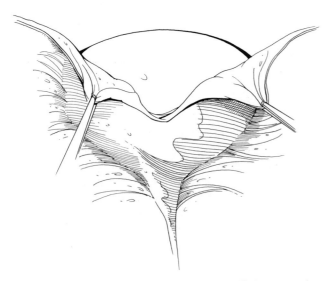

FIG. 23–1. The peritoneum is dissected off the posterior bladder to the level of the trigone and 2 to 3 cm above the level of the ureters.

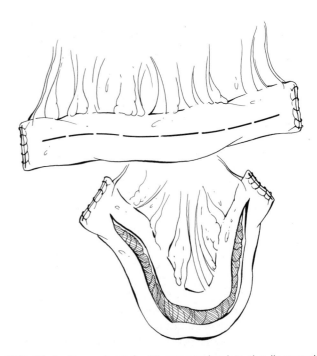

FIG. 23–3. Approximately 15 cm proximal to the ileocecal valve, a 25-cm segment of bowel is selected, the mesentery cleared, and the segment removed using standard stapling techniques. The segment of ileum is oversewn at the ends to exclude the staples and then opened along the antimesenteric border.

then achieved using one of the handsewn or stapled techniques and the mesenteric defect closed. In Figure 23–3, the ileal ends are oversewn with running 2-0 chromic catgut to exclude the staples (to prevent stone formation) and the antimesenteric surface of the bowel is opened using electrocautery. Towels should be placed under the bowel and the opened ileum irrigated into a kidney basin until clear. As seen in Figures 23–4 and 23–5, the posterior wall of the ileum is folded back on itself and sutured together using running 2-0 chromic catgut. The required size of the augmentation opening is roughly measured and the superior, anterior wall is partially closed with running 2-0 Vicryl to match this opening (Fig. 23–6). A large-bore suprapubic (SP) tube is placed through the lateral bladder wall prior to suturing the augment onto the bladder. The SP tube allows reliable postoperative drainage and irrigation of mucus until the suture lines are healed. The ileal segment is then sewn onto the opened bladder using running 2-0 Vicryl with the initial suture placement shown in Figure 23–7 and the posterior closure shown in Figure 23–8. The completed enterocystoplasty is shown in Figure 23–9. A closed-suction drain is placed near the suture line and brought through the skin on the side opposite the SP tube. The patient is closed in the usual manner. If a continence procedure has been performed, it is imperative that a urethral catheter can be easily passed; otherwise, the patient will be unable to catheterize postoperatively.

Although this is our preferred technique, other methods of performing an augmentation exist. One such method involves splitting the bladder sagittally from just

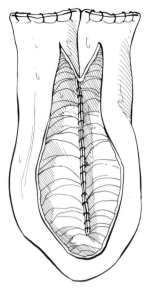

FIG. 23–5. The posterior wall of the augment is completely closed.

above the bladder neck and ending near the level of the ureters posteriorly to form a "clam" (8,14). A 25- to 30-cm segment of ileum is isolated and divided completely along the antimesenteric border (Fig. 23–10). The posterior wall of the augment is closed with running 2-0 Vicryl and then either anastomosed to the bladder as a "patch"

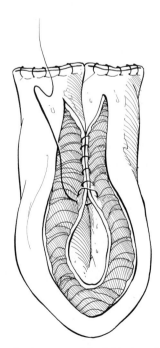

FIG. 23–4. The ileal segment is folded and closure of the posterior wall is initiated using a running absorbable suture.

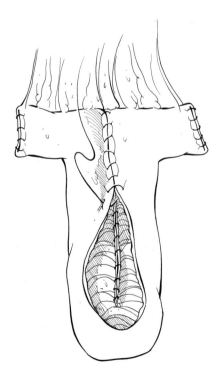

FIG. 23–6. The superior, anterior wall of the augment is partially closed. The size of the augment opening should roughly correspond to the size of the opened bladder.

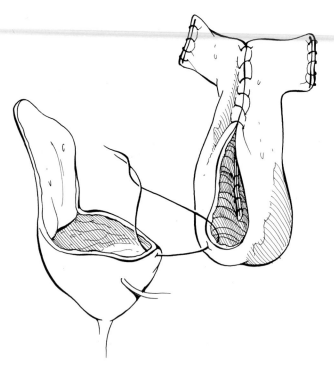

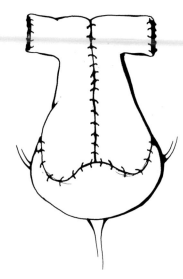

FIG. 23–9. View of the completed enterocystoplasty.

FIG. 23–7. Initial suture placement for enterocystoplasty. Note that the bladder flap opens anteriorly.

or folded again and partially closed to form a "cup." A cup is especially useful if the patient's own bladder is very small but it sometimes requires the use of up to 40 cm of bowel. In both cases, the anastomosis is started on the posterior wall until approximately one-third is closed

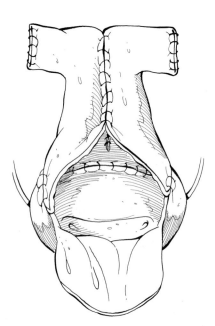

FIG. 23–8. Closure of the anterior aspect of the enterocystoplasty.

and then the anterior wall is closed. The lateral walls are closed last and any redundant bowel is closed to itself.

Postoperative care is in general straightforward. Fluid and electrolyte management is important due to large third-space losses and drainage from the nasogastric tube, which remains in place until bowel function returns. Although the recent trend is to remove the nasogastric tube early, it is important to remember that bowel function is often deranged in the neuropathic patient and recovery of bowel motility may be significantly delayed. The drain is removed after a few days when drainage tapers off. The bladder is irrigated at least three times per day with 30 to 60 mL of saline to clear mucus. In the straightforward patient, a cystogram is performed at 2 to 3 weeks and the Foley removed if no extravasation is noted. The patient begins CIC with the SP tube in place until the patient is proficient at CIC. At 3 to 4 weeks, the SP tube can usually be removed and the patient continues CIC every 2 to 3 hours during the day and twice at night. It usually takes 6 to 12 months for the augment to stretch to full capacity, during which time more frequent CIC is necessary. This may be distressing to the patient; however, liberal use of anticholinergics can help in most cases. As capacity increases, the CIC intervals can increase and, ultimately, most patients are able to wait 4 to 5 hours between catheterizations during the day and catheterize only once at night. Patients who are able to void per urethra must document consistently small postvoid residuals. In some cases, apparent early normal voiding deteriorates over time and in some cases the bowel segment can become overstretched and either rupture or stretch into an overly capacious, nonfunctional bladder. Patients who are able to void postoperatively should be followed with intermittent postvoid residuals. Daily irrigation to clear mucus is essential, especially for the first few months.

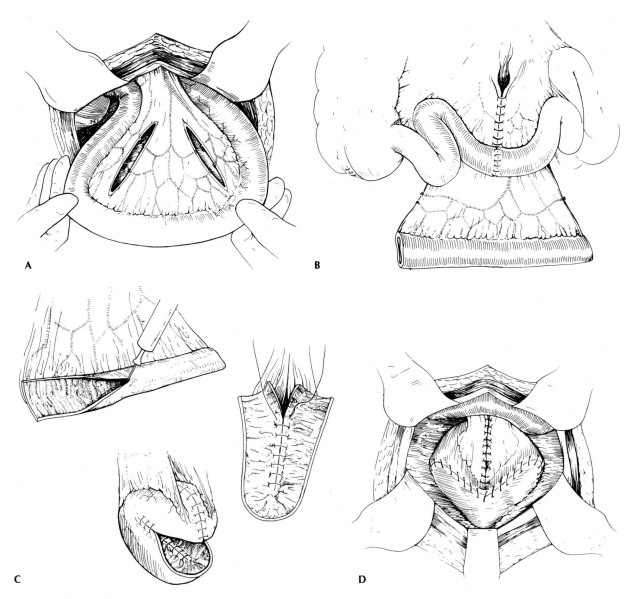

FIG. 23–10. Augmentation ileocystoplasty with formation of a cup patch. **A:** Isolation of a distal ileal segment. **B and C:** Isolated ileal segment opened on antimesenteric border and double folded to create a reservoir. **D:** Cup patch reservoir sutured to the bladder-incised sagittal plane.

Routine electrolytes, creatinine, blood urea nitrogen, and upper-tract studies should be performed at regular intervals. It is unlikely that vitamin B_{12} deficiency should develop because a short ileal segment is usually used; however, it should be kept in mind.

OUTCOMES

Complications

A comprehensive long-term study of 122 patients by Flood and colleagues reported an overall 28% early and 44% late complication rate in a difficult group of patients (4). Most of the complications were minor and involved prolonged ileus, transient urinary extravasation, or stomal problems. Surgical interventions were necessary in only 15% of patients and were mainly stomal revisions.

Small-bowel obstructions occur in approximately 3% of patients, similar to the rate reported in urinary diversions. Bladder or kidney stones vary from study to study depending on the patient population and surgical techniques used. In particular, stone formation appears to be highest in patients with continent stomas (12). Stones usually form secondary to retained mucus or exposed staples as a nidus. Routine bladder irrigation, treatment of infections, and excluding staples at the time of surgery minimize stone formation.

Reservoir perforation is perhaps the most feared complication, with reported rates of up to 6% (4,10). Perforation is a catastrophic event and the patient may quickly become septic; however, fatalities are uncommon if diagnosed early.

Metabolic problems, such as metabolic acidosis or vitamin B_{12} deficiency, that are not medically treatable are uncommon if patients are properly selected, a reasonable length of bowel is used, and appropriate labs are followed.

The development of cancer has been reported with the use of all bowel segments. Although the risk to any individual patient is small, chronic surveillance after 10 years should be considered, especially if a colonic segment is used.

If the bladder is extremely small or the bladder incision is not generous, the "augmentation" may ultimately become no more than a large, nondraining bladder diverticulum. This complication may be manifested by recurrent urinary tract infections and can easily be identified by the classic hourglass appearance on a cystogram.

Voiding dysfunction is common even in nonneurogenic patients after augmentation cystoplasty. In a review by Flood and colleagues, 89% and 67% of neurologically intact males and females, respectively, required lifelong CIC after augmentation (4). Singh and Thomas reported that 81% of patients in their series required catheterization postoperatively (13). This high incidence reinforces the need to counsel patients on the potential for lifelong CIC and preoperative demonstration of proficiency at CIC.

Results

Achieving a successful augmentation cystoplasty usually depends on three factors: the original reason for performing the procedure, proper patient selection, and a thorough preoperative urodynamic study. In selected patients with neuropathic bladders requiring improved compliance and capacity, augmentation cystoplasty has a high likelihood of improving compliance and capacity.

An augmentation is less successful in treating the symptoms of interstitial cystitis and by itself does not guarantee continence, especially in patients with high rates of intrinsic sphincter deficiency (ISD) such as myelomeningocele and radiation cystitis. A preoperative urodynamic evaluation is essential in diagnosing ISD in these patients, with concurrent continence procedures performed when necessary.

REFERENCES

1. Adams MC, Mitchell ME, Rink RC. Gastrocystoplasty: An alternative solution to the problem of urological reconstruction in the severely compromised patient. *J Urol* 1988; 140:1152–1157.
2. Atala A. New methods of bladder augmentation. *BJU Int* 2000;85 [Suppl 3]:24–34.
3. Cartwright PC, Snow BW. Bladder autoaugmentation: Early clinical experience. *J Urol* 1989;142:505–508.
4. Flood HD, Malhotra SJ, O'Connell HE, Ritchey ML, Bloom DA, McGuire EJ. Long-term results and complications using augmentation cystoplasty in reconstructive urology. *Neurourol Urodynam* 1995;14: 297–302.
5. Gonzalez R, Cabral BHP. Rectal continence after enterocystoplasty. *Dialog Pediatr Urol* 1987;10:1–3.
6. Marte A, DiMeglio D, Cotrufo AM, et al. A long term follow-up of autoaugmentation in myelodysplastic children. *BJU Int* 2002;89: 928–931.
7. McGuire EJ, Fitzpatrick CC, Wan J, et al. Clinical assessment of urethral sphincter function. *J Urol* 1993;150:1452–1456.
8. McGuire EJ, Woodside JR, Borden TA, Weiss RM. Prognostic value of urodynamic testing in myelodysplastic patients. *J Urol* 1981;126: 205–208.
9. Mutchnik SE, Hinson JL, Nickell KG, Boone TB. Ileovesicostomy as an alternative form of bladder management in tetraplegic patients. *Urology* 1997;49:353–357.
10. Rink RC, Woodbury PW, Mitchell ME. Bladder perforation following enterocystoplasty. *J Urol* 1988;139:234A(abst 285).
11. Schwartz SL, Kennelly MJ, McGuire EJ, Faerber GJ. Incontinent ileovesicostomy urinary diversion in the treatment of lower urinary tract dysfunction. *J Urol* 1994;152:99–102.
12. Shekarriz B, Upadhyay J, Demirbilek S, et al. Surgical complications of bladder augmentation: comparison between various enterocystoplasties in 133 patients. *Urology* 2000;55:123–128.
13. Singh G, Thomas DG. Enterocystoplasty in the neuropathic bladder. *Neurourol Urodynam* 1995;14:5–10.
14. Webster GD. Bladder augmentation and reconstruction. In: Glenn JF, ed. *Urologic surgery*, 4th ed. Philadelphia: JB Lippincott Co, 1991:500–502.
15. Westney OL, McGuire EJ. Surgical procedures for the treatment of urge incontinence. *Tech Urol* 2001;7:126–132.

CHAPTER 24

Management of the Distal Ureter for Nephroureterectomy

Brian D. Seifman and J. Stuart Wolf, Jr.

The traditional therapy for urothelial cell carcinoma of the renal pelvis or ureter is a radical nephroureterectomy, including a 1-cm cuff of bladder around the ureteral orifice. Performed using open surgery, this has entailed a long midline or thoracoabdominal incision or two incisions: a flank incision for the nephrectomy and a lower midline or Gibson incision for the distal ureter. Because of the morbidity associated with the extension of the incision for the distal ureterectomy, less invasive approaches such as the "pluck" and "intussusception" techniques were devised. The advent of laparoscopic nephroureterectomy, which further reduces morbidity by eliminating the large incision for the renal portion of the procedure, has stimulated the development of additional minimally invasive approaches to the distal ureter.

DIAGNOSIS

The most common presenting symptom or sign of upper-tract urothelial tumors is hematuria, which occurs in 75% of patients. Flank pain is present in 30% of patients due either to chronic obstruction or acute colic from passage of blood clots (1). The subsequent evaluation entails an upper-tract imaging study with intravenous (IV) urography, computed tomography (CT), magnetic resonance imaging, or retrograde pyelography. More than half of patients will have an irregular filling defect, consistent with a tumor. Both sides of the urinary system need to be evaluated due to the potential for bilateral tumors.

Abnormalities on the imaging studies can then be investigated with ureteroscopy and biopsy. Biopsy is helpful to determine the grade of the lesion and may determine whether or not the lesion is invasive. Urinary cytology may aid in the diagnosis. Cystoscopy is essential due to the high association with bladder tumors.

Once a urothelial malignancy is diagnosed, metastatic evaluation consists of an abdominal and pelvic CT scan and a chest radiograph. A bone scan is performed if there is bone pain, the alkaline phosphatase is elevated, or bony abnormalities are seen on other imaging studies. A complete blood count, serum electrolytes, serum creatinine, and liver function tests should also be assessed. If the creatinine is elevated, a renal scan to determine function may aid in decision making.

INDICATIONS FOR SURGERY

Radical nephroureterectomy with a 1-cm cuff of bladder is the standard therapy for upper-tract urothelial tumors. Either laparoscopic (standard or hand-assisted) or open surgical techniques are acceptable. Nephrectomy without complete ureterectomy should be avoided due to a 30% incidence of recurrence in the ureteral stump (2). Patients with a positive cytology but without an identifiable lesion on IV pyelography or ureteroscopy should be followed closely rather than undergo nephroureterectomy without a definitive diagnosis.

ALTERNATIVE THERAPY

Endoscopic resection and fulguration is acceptable for patients with low-grade, low-stage, and small tumor burdens. An alternative for a distal ureteral tumor is a distal ureterectomy with an ureteroneocystostomy or other reconstruction. Topical therapy with mitomycin C or Bacille bilié de Calmette–Guérin may be attempted for patients with carcinoma *in situ* who have limited renal function or bilateral disease.

SURGICAL TECHNIQUE

Open Surgical Techniques

Intravesical Approach

The open surgical approach can be used in conjunction with any technique used to remove the kidney. After the nephrectomy and proximal ureteral dissection is completed, the patient is placed in the supine position, with or without flexion of the table. A three-way 20 Fr Foley catheter is placed into the bladder. A lower midline incision is made, the rectus fascia divided, and the space of Retzius bluntly developed. A self-retaining retractor is placed. The bladder is filled with 300 cc of normal saline and then opened longitudinally between two stay sutures. Additional stay sutures are placed at the apex of the bladder incision. The dome of the bladder is packed with a gauze sponge and a bladder blade is used to retract the bladder dome cephalad. A ureteral catheter or feeding tube is placed in the targeted ureteral orifice and sewn in place with a 4-0 suture. The cutting current on the electrocautery device is used to incise the mucosa 1 cm around the ureteral orifice. The intramural ureter is then dissected using tenotomy scissors and pinpoint electrocautery (Fig. 24–1).

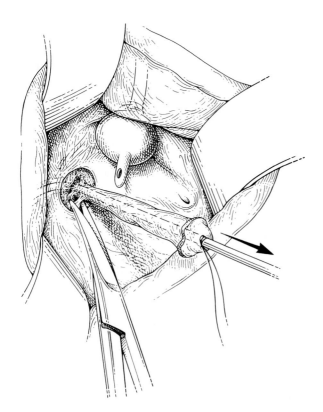

FIG. 24–1. A ureteral catheter is secured to the ureteral orifice. Tenotomy scissors and electrocautery are used to dissect free the intramural ureter. (From Lange PH. Carcinoma of the renal pelvis and ureter. In: Glenn JF, ed. *Urologic surgery*, 4th ed. Philadelphia: JB Lippincott Co, 1991:273, with permission.)

The entire distal ureter is dissected free to join the point of previous dissection completed during the nephrectomy portion of the procedure. A two-layer closure of the posterior bladder wall is completed with 2-0 absorbable sutures for the serosa and muscle and 4-0 absorbable sutures for the mucosa. The anterior bladder incision is then closed in two layers as well. A drain is inserted through a separate stab incision and placed in the pelvis. The 20 Fr Foley catheter is left for 3 days. A cystogram is performed to ensure the bladder has healed prior to removing the catheter.

At times, the dissection of the distal ureter may be difficult and the ureter may need to be dissected extravesically as well. The superior vesical artery may need to be divided to provide access to the distal ureter.

Extravesical Approach

A completely extravesical approach is best performed through a Gibson incision. After entering the retroperitoneal space and identifying the distal ureter, the bladder is retracted to the contralateral side. The superior vesical artery is divided to facilitate dissection of the distal ureter. The ureteral hiatus can then be identified. The intramural ureter is dissected free using electrocautery. Cephalad traction on the ureter will help identify the bladder mucosa. A right-angle clamp is used to secure the ureteral orifice and the ureter is divided. A 2-0 absorbable suture is tied around the right-angle clamp to close the bladder. A second layer is closed over the resection site using 2-0 absorbable sutures. Drain and catheter management are as above.

Laparoscopic Extravesical Bladder Cuff Technique (3)

This technique is similar to the open extravesical approach. The patient is placed in a modified flank position as would be for a transperitoneal laparoscopic nephrectomy. Flexible cystoscopy is performed and a ureteral catheter is placed. The laparoscopic nephrectomy is then completed and the ureter is dissected distally. Clips are placed on the ureter to prevent extravasation of tumor cells. A grasper is used to place cephalad traction on the proximal ureter. An additional 10-mm port is placed in the lower abdomen to facilitate resection of the distal ureter. An incision on the bladder just anterior to the ureter is made using electrocautery. Upon entering the bladder, the ureteral catheter identifies the ureteral orifice. The posterior portion of the bladder cuff is then excised after dividing the ureteral catheter. The bladder is suture closed using laparoscopic techniques. Drain and catheter management are similar to the above.

Endoscopic Techniques

Except for the "pluck" procedures, all of the endoscopic techniques described in this section have been developed specifically for use in conjunction with laparoscopic nephroureterectomy. The techniques are described below in the settings in which they were initially described or are in common use at this time. The hand-assisted approach to laparoscopic nephroureterectomy may be preferable with particular techniques, as indicated below, but any laparoscopic approach to nephroureterectomy can be used in conjunction with any of the following techniques with modifications. Moreover, any of these distal ureterectomy techniques can be used in conjunction with open surgical nephroureterectomy.

Transvesical Bladder Cuff Technique: Single Port (4)

After completing a hand-assisted laparoscopic nephrectomy with the patient in the lateral decubitus position, the ureter is dissected inferiorly to the bladder. Clips are placed on the ureter to prevent tumor spillage.

Without repositioning the patient, the bladder is filled with 400 cc sterile water through a three-way Foley

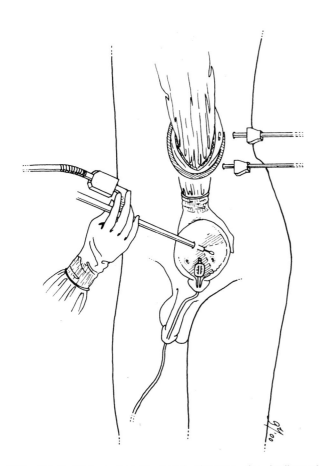

FIG. 24–2. The surgeon's hand elevates the ipsilateral hemitrigone while the Collins knife is used to incise around the ureteral orifice. (Adapted from Gonzalez CM, Batler RA, Schoor RA, et al. A novel endoscopic approach towards resection of the distal ureter with surrounding bladder cuff during hand assisted laparoscopic nephroureterectomy. *J Urol* 2001;165:484, with permission.)

catheter. A 1-cm incision is made in the midline, three finger breadths superior to the pubis. Using the surgeon's hand via the hand-assist port, the bladder is pushed upward toward the abdominal wall. A spinal needle is introduced through the incision into the bladder to ascertain proper angle and depth of entry. A 10-mm laparoscopic port is placed directly into the bladder through the extraperitoneal space. A 24 Fr resectoscope with a Collins knife is placed through the port into the bladder. The surgeon's hand alternately elevates the ipsilateral hemitrigone and retracts the ureter while the Collins knife is used to incise around the ureteral orifice and intramural ureter (Fig. 24–2). Glycine solution is used as the irrigant. During the resection, the Foley catheter is placed to drainage to minimize extravasation of urine and irrigant. Once the ureter is free, the entire specimen is removed via the hand-port incision. Note that once the bladder has been opened into the retroperitoneum it collapses completely. Therefore, care should be taken to keep the dissection at equal depth all around the orifice so that once the bladder collapses the ureter can easily be pulled free.

The bladder port is removed and the urethral catheter is placed to gravity drainage. Neither the port site nor the resection site are closed. Placement of a pelvic drain through a laparoscopic port site is optional. A cystogram is performed on postoperative day 7 prior to catheter removal.

Transurethral Bladder Cuff Technique

This technique is similar to the transvesical bladder cuff technique except that the resection is performed transurethrally, which obviates the need for placement of a transvesical port. One option is to use a flexible cystoscope with an electrocautery probe to perform the periureteral dissection. Another alternative is to position the patient in a combined lithotomy–semiflank position that allows simultaneous laparoscopic nephrectomy and transurethral access with a 24 Fr resectoscope with a Collins knife (15).

Transvesical Bladder Cuff Technique: Two Ports (6)

Prior to performing the nephrectomy portion of the procedure, the patient is placed in the lithotomy position. Cystoscopy is performed to evaluate the bladder mucosa and distend the bladder. Under cystoscopic guidance, two 5-mm balloon-tipped laparoscopic ports are placed into the bladder just above the pubic bone on both sides of the midline. Both ports are placed to wall suction to prevent extravasation and overdistention of the bladder. A 5-mm endoloop is inserted through the ipsilateral port. A 6 Fr ureteral catheter is then inserted cystoscopically into the targeted ureter. The cystoscope is exchanged for a resectoscope with a Collins knife, which is used to incise around the ureteral orifice. A grasper, inserted via the

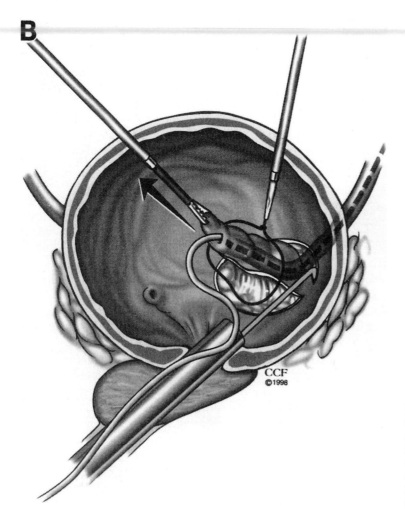

B

CCF
©1998

FIG. 24–3. The Collins knife is used transurethrally while a grasper elevates the ureter and the endoloop is around the resected orifice. (Adapted from Gill IS, Soble JJ, Miller SD, et al. A novel technique for the management of the en bloc bladder cuff and distal ureter during laparoscopic nephroureterectomy. *J Urol* 1999;161:432, with permission.)

other laparoscopic port, is passed through the endoloop and retracts the orifice anteriorly. After freeing up 3–4 cm of ureter, it is suspended from the anterior bladder wall by the grasper (Fig. 24–3). The ureteral catheter is then removed and the endoloop is tightened around the ureter to occlude the lumen.

The laparoscopic ports are removed and a urethral catheter is placed to gravity drainage. The patient is then positioned for the nephrectomy portion of the procedure. The ureter is dissected distally. With cephalad traction on the ureter, blunt and sharp dissection allows the distal ureter to be pulled into the retroperitoneal space for intact removal. The urethral catheter is left in place for 1 week and is removed after a cystogram confirms adequate bladder healing.

Ureteral Unroofing Technique (7)

Prior to performing the nephrectomy portion of the procedure, the patient is placed in the lithotomy position. Cystoscopy is performed and a ureteral dilating balloon

(5 mm diameter, 10 cm length) is placed into the targeted intramural ureter. The balloon is inflated to 1 atm pressure with dilute contrast material using fluoroscopic guidance. The cystoscope is exchanged for a resectoscope with a Collins knife. The ureteral tunnel is incised at the 12-o'clock position along the entire length of the intramural ureter. The dilating balloon is then removed and a rollerball electrode is then used to cauterize the edges and floor of the intramural ureter. A 7 Fr 11.5-mm balloon occlusion catheter is passed into the renal pelvis and inflated at the ureteropelvic junction. A urethral catheter is then placed and connected to gravity drainage, as is the balloon occlusion catheter.

The patient is then taken out of the lithotomy position and the nephrectomy is performed. Once completed, the distal ureter is mobilized laparoscopically to the ureteral hiatus. The superior vesical artery often needs to be divided. An endoscopic stapler is then used to remove the remaining distal ureter and bladder cuff (Fig. 24–4). The ureteral balloon occlusion catheter is removed just prior to engaging the stapler. The urethral

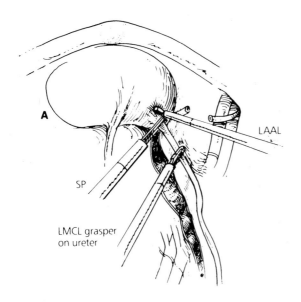

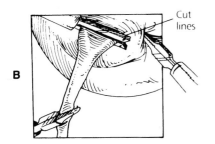

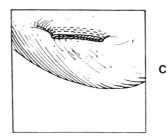

FIG. 24–4. **A:** The endoscopic stapler is placed across the ureterovesical junction. **B:** Close-up view of the stapler across the ureterovesical junction. **C:** Staples are seen securing the bladder cuff. (Adapted from Clayman RV. Laparoscopic ureteral surgery. In: Clayman RV, McDougall EM, eds. *Laparoscopic urology.* St. Louis, MO: Quality Medical Publishing, 1993:360, with permission.)

catheter is left in place for 2–3 days and removed after a cystogram demonstrates no urinary extravasation. One modification of this technique, which allows for the nephrectomy to be performed before the ureterectomy, is to address the distal ureter with a stapler as described above and then reposition the patient into the lithotomy position. Using a resectoscope and a roller-ball the intramural ureter is ablated until the staple line is visible.

Pluck Technique

The patient is placed in the lithotomy position prior to performing the nephrectomy. The targeted ureteral orifice is identified with a cystoscope. A ureteral access catheter is then placed to help identify the intramural ureter. The ureteral orifice and surrounding bladder cuff are then incised with a Collins knife on a resectoscope to the retroperitoneal fat. Alternatively, a loop resectoscope can be used to resect the orifice and intramural ureter. A 24 Fr urethral catheter is then placed to gravity drainage.

The patient is taken out of the lithotomy position and the nephrectomy is performed. The ureter is dissected distally and cephalad traction allows the ureter to be

detached from the bladder. The urethral catheter is left in place for 7 days and removed after a cystogram is performed.

A modification of this technique is to pass a 7 Fr 11.5-mm balloon occlusion catheter into the renal pelvis, snugging it down at the ureteropelvic junction, to minimize urine extravasation. Mitomycin can be instilled into the renal pelvis through this catheter (8).

Combined Open and Endoscopic Technique

Ureteral Intussusception Technique (9)

Initially, while in the lithotomy position either a stone basket or ureteral catheter is placed into the targeted proximal ureter. The patient is repositioned and nephrectomy is then performed, dissecting the ureter to the pelvic brim. The proximal end of the ureter is clipped above the basket/ureteral catheter and the ureter is divided. The stone basket is advanced into the retroperitoneum and then used to entrap the ureteral wall; alternatively, the ureter is tied with a 0 silk suture to the ureteral access catheter (Fig. 24–5). Gentle traction is then applied to the stone basket/ureteral catheter to intussuscept the ureter

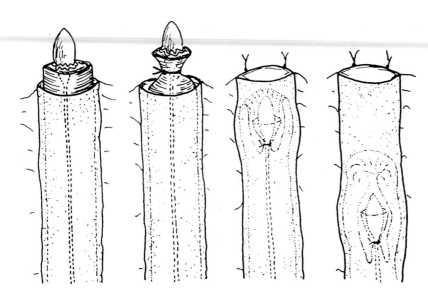

FIG. 24–5. The proximal ureter is divided and secured to the ureteral catheter. The ureter is then intussuscepted as the catheter is removed. (Adapted from Angulo JC, Hontoria J, Sanchez-Chapado M. One incision nephroureterectomy endoscopically assisted by transurethral stripping. *Urology* 1998;52: 204, with permission.)

into the bladder (Fig. 24–6). A Collins knife mounted on a resectoscope is then inserted transurethrally (after repositioning into the lithotomy position) and used to incise the bladder cuff around the ureter while exerting traction on the stone basket/ureteral catheter out of the urethra.

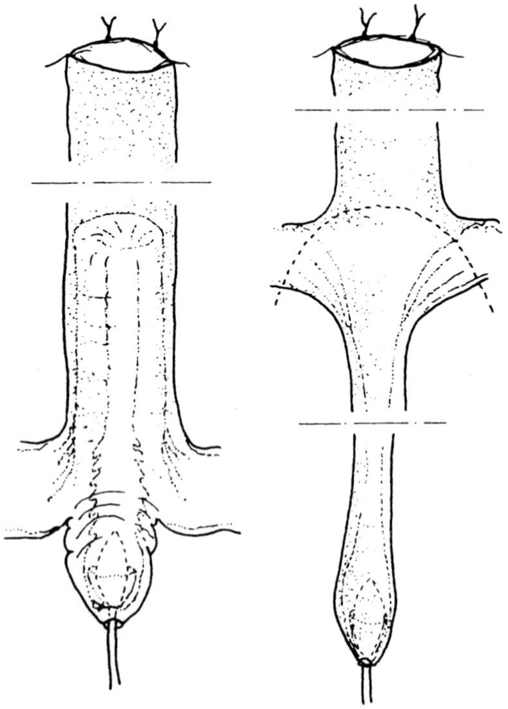

A urethral catheter is placed and removed after 7 days following a normal cystogram. This technique should not be used for distal or midureteral tumors.

OUTCOMES

Complications

Early complications include hematuria, retroperitoneal hematoma, and retroperitoneal abscess. Ureteral intussusception may be unsuccessful in 10% of patients. Prolonged urinary extravasation can in general be managed conservatively with urethral catheter drainage. Although not yet reported, there is the potential for calculi to form on the staple line when the ureteral unroofing technique is used. Other factors to be considered in the choice of technique include the risk of tumor spillage, the addition of a bladder incision, the timing of the ureterectomy relative to nephrectomy, the need for repositioning, the approach to nephrectomy that is desired, and surgeon preference. Of these, the potential for tumor cell spillage is probably the most important with regard to outcome. The technique to excise the distal ureter is probably not a factor for recurrence as long as there is no spillage of tumor cells in the retroperitoneum. Of note, isolated retrovesical recurrences following "pluck" ureterectomy have been reported. There is not yet enough reported experience with the newer endoscopic techniques to assess the relative risk of local, intra- and retroperitoneal, and port site recurrences.

Results

Survival is dependent on the grade and stage of the tumor. Five-year survival rates following a radical nephroureterectomy are for stage Tis, Ta, T1, 91%; stage

FIG. 24–6. The catheter is retracted through the bladder wall and urethra. (Adapted from Angulo JC, Hontoria J, Sanchez-Chapado M. One incision nephroureterectomy endoscopically assisted by transurethral stripping. *Urology* 1998;52: 204, with permission.)

T2, 43%; stage T3, T4 or N1, N2, 23%; and stage N3 or M1, 0% (10).

REFERENCES

1. Gonzalez CM, Batler RA, Schoor RA, et al. A novel endoscopic approach towards resection of the distal ureter with surrounding bladder cuff during hand assisted laparoscopic nephroureterectomy. *J Urol* 2001;165:483–485.
2. Bloom NA, Vidone RA, Lytton B. Primary carcinoma of the ureter: a report of 102 new cases. *J Urol* 1970;103:590–598.
3. Gill IS, Soble JJ, Miller SD, et al. A novel technique for the management of the en bloc bladder cuff and distal ureter during laparoscopic nephroureterectomy. *J Urol* 1999;161: 430–434.
4. Wong C, Leveillee RJ. Hand-assisted laparoscopic nephroureterectomy with cystoscopic en bloc excision of the distal ureter and bladder cuff. *J Endourol* 2002;16(6):329–332.
5. Messing EM, Catalona W. Urothelial tumors of the urinary tract. In: Walsh PC, Retik AB, Vaughan ED, Wein AJ, eds. *Cambell's urology*, 7th ed, vol 3. Philadelphia: WB Saunders, 1998:2383–2394.
6. McGinnis DM, Trabulsi EJ, Gomella LG, et al. Hand-assisted laparoscopic nephroureterectomy: description of technique. *Tech Urol* 2001; 7:7–11.
7. Angulo JC, Hontoria J, Sanchez-Chapado M. One incision nephroureterectomy endoscopically assisted by transurethral stripping. *Urology* 1998;52:203–207.
8. Seifman BD, Montie JE, Stuart Wolf J. Prospective comparison between hand-assisted laparoscopic and open surgical nephroureterectomy for urothelial cell carcinoma. *Urology* 2001;57: 133–137.
9. Goh M, Montie JE, Stuart Wolf J. Urothelial carcinoma of the upper urinary tract. In: Gillenwater JY, Grayhack JT, Howards SS, Mitchell ME, eds. *Adult and pediatric urology*, 4th ed, vol 1. Philadelphia: Lippincott Williams & Wilkins, 2002:641–658.
10. Shalhav AL, Elbahnasy AM, McDougall EM, et al. Laparoscopic nephroureterectomy for upper tract transitional cell cancer: technical aspects. *J Endourol* 1998;12:345–353.

CHAPTER 25

Vesicovaginal Fistula

Peter O. Kwong and O. Lenaine Westney

A vesicovaginal fistula (VVF) is an epithelialized or fibrous communication between the bladder and vagina. Physically, psychologically, and socially, it is a source of major distress for the patient contending with urine leakage from the vagina. Documentation of VVFs exists from as early as 1550 BC in the Eber papyrus of ancient Egypt (10). In 1845, James Marion Sims, considered the father of American gynecology, began his exploration into the challenges of treating the condition in Montgomery, Alabama (10). He is credited with developing the foundation of VVF repair and establishing sound surgical principles for repair of fistulae.

The causative factors leading to VVF formation can be broadly categorized into congenital and acquired (Table 25–1). The majority of cases fall into the iatrogenic and

TABLE 25–1. *Etiologies of Vesicovaginal Fistulae*

I. Congenital
  A. Cloacal Abnormality
II. Acquired
  A. Iatrogenic
    1. Post surgical
      a. Hysterectomy
      b. Cesarean Section
      c. Dilatation and Curettage
      d. Pelvic Laparoscopy
      e. Incontinence Procedure
      f. Transvaginal Biopsies
      i. Intravescial Formalin Instillation
      j. Failed Vesicovaginal Fistula Repair
    2. Radiation
  B. Noniatrogenic
    1. Obstetrical Trauma
    2. Infectious
    3. Locally Advanced Pelvic Tumor
    4. Foreign Body
    5. Pelvic trauma/fracture

Modified from Rackley RR, Appell RA. Vesicovaginal fistula: current approach. *AUA Update Series* 1998 21: 161–168.

obstetric trauma subcategories. In underdeveloped countries, the leading cause of VVFs is obstetric trauma, in which prolonged labor causes ischemic pressure necrosis of the bladder and anterior vaginal wall. In contrast, obstetric trauma accounts for only 5% of VVFs in nations where modern healthcare is present. The leading cause of VVFs in industrialized countries is iatrogenic surgical trauma, accounting for 82% to 91% of VVFs. Ninety-one percent are due to gynecologic procedures, with 80% due to abdominal hysterectomy (9). The incidence of VVF after transabdominal hysterectomy is 1.0 in 1,000, as opposed to 0.2 in 1,000 transvaginal hysterectomy. The incidence is highest (2.2 in 1,000) with laparoscopic hysterectomy (7). The most common location for a posthysterectomy VVF is the apex of the vaginal vault or "cuff" corresponding to an intravesical location just superior to the trigone (9). Theoretically, the fistula develops secondary to the unintentional inclusion of full-thickness bladder wall during closure of the vaginal cuff, an unrecognized bladder injury adjacent to the cuff suture line, or cuff abscess.

DIAGNOSIS

Classically, the postoperative VVF presents with "continuous" urine leakage from the vagina. The time of presentation peaks at 7 to 10 days after surgery but may be variable, with some patients presenting immediately after catheter removal ranging to 4 to 6 weeks after surgery (7). In the early postoperative period, there may also be associated ileus and abdominal pain due to intraperitoneal urine extravasation. VVFs due to pelvic irradiation usually have a delayed presentation, developing many months or years posttreatment due to progressive obliterative endarteritis causing tissue ischemia and necrosis.

The key to diagnosis of a VVF is a high suspicion. Often, a complete history and physical examination exposes the pathology. In the case of less obvious fistula, a dye test is utilized to more clearly visualize the passage of fluid through the fistula. In its simplest form, a saline and dye (indigo carmine or methylene blue) mixture is instilled into the bladder via a Foley catheter while inspecting the vagina for leakage or a previously placed tampon. The failure to identify any staining of the tampon may indicate a small fistula or ureterovaginal fistula. The second level of testing requires reinsertion of the vaginal gauze or tampon followed by administration of 5 mg indigo carmine intravenously to determine whether the source is ureteral. Dye from an ureterovaginal fistula may be present on the first gauze inspection prior to intravenous (IV) indigo carmine if there is vesicoureteral reflux, which can be determined with a voiding cystourethrogram (VCUG). An alternative to IV dye injection is oral phenazopyridine hydrochloride but it requires several hours of lead time before examination.

All patients should have an IV pyelogram (IVP) for upper-tract evaluation. Abnormalities to look for include extravasation into the vagina or peritoneal cavity or a displaced or partially obstructed ureter. In patients with VVF, up to 25% will have hydroureteronephrosis with 10% having a concomitant ureterovaginal fistula (6). In patients with ureteral pathology, a retrograde pyelogram is warranted to evaluate for ureterovaginal fistula if the IVP is not definitive.

Cystoscopy is performed to localize and evaluate the VVF, which often has surrounding edematous mucosa. The size and number of VVFs, their location in relation to the ureteral orifices, any lesions such as foreign bodies (i.e., sutures), tumors, and tissue quality must be noted. If there is a history of malignancy, biopsy of the VVF is indicated to rule out recurrent tumor. Vaginoscopy is performed simultaneous with cystoscopy to assess the vaginal aspect of the fistula. If IVP and retrograde pyelograms are inconclusive, then a fistulogram may be performed transvaginally.

A urodynamic study is recommended to look for other factors that may contribute to the urinary incontinence and may require surgical correction (augmentation cystoplasty, incontinence surgery) with the VVF repair simultaneously. Bladder compliance, capacity, and leak point pressure should be assessed if possible.

INDICATIONS FOR SURGERY

The issue of how long to wait before attempting surgical repair of a VVF has long been debated. By tradition, VVF repair is delayed 3 to 6 months to allow inflammation to resolve. In cases where a VVF is due to complicated operation or after obstetric trauma, this rationale holds true. However, recent studies by Blavais et al. and Blandy et al. demonstrated comparable results with early (6 to 12 weeks) repair in cases related to an uncomplicated hysterectomy (1,2). Once surgical repair is decided

upon, another issue that has to be considered is the approach: transvaginal, transvesical, or transabdominal. Often, the approach is the one that the surgeon is most experienced in performing. Advantages of the transvaginal approach are less blood loss, shorter hospital stay, avoidance of a laparotomy, and thus decreased morbidity. Many reserve the transabdominal approach for those patients requiring concomitant intraabdominal surgery (ureteral reimplantation, augmentation cystoplasty) or those patients with a narrow and deep vagina causing poor exposure to the VVF. However, Dupont and Raz reported that nearly all VVFs can be accessed and repaired transvaginally (3).

ALTERNATIVE THERAPY

Upon diagnosis, a trial of conservative therapy is started depending on fistula size. Conservative therapy consists of prolonged bladder drainage with a Foley catheter, anticholinergic agents to prevent bladder spasms, antibiotics, and estrogen if the patient is postmenopausal. Other adjunctive noninvasive treatments include attempts to destroy the epithelial lining of the VVF with fulguration (using electrocautery or laser) and use of fibrin glue. Successful closure of a VVF via conservative therapy can be expected only in those 3 mm in diameter or less.

SURGICAL TECHNIQUE

Transvaginal Approach

The patient is placed in the dorsolithotomy position. If a narrow vagina is present or the VVF site is high lying, a Schuchardt posterolateral relaxing incision at the 4-o'clock position of the vaginal introitus and distal vaginal wall may be performed to improve exposure. A suprapubic catheter may be placed with a Lowsley retractor and a urethral Foley catheter is placed. The labia minora are sutured to the inner thigh and a weighted vaginal speculum placed. The VVF is dilated to place an 8 Fr Foley catheter. Applying gentle traction to the catheter aids in exposure and dissection of the VVF.

After submucosal injection of a vasopressin mixture (10 U/100 mL normal saline), lidocaine with 1% epinephrine, or saline to elevate the anterior vaginal mucosa, the VVF is circumferentially incised. A posteriorly based inverted U-shaped incision is made with the apex continuous with the VVF incision (Fig. 25–1). If the VVF is situated deep in the vaginal vault, an anteriorly based U-shaped incision is utilized. The vaginal mucosa is dissected away from the perivesical fascia to form vaginal flaps anterior and posterior to the VVF (Fig. 25–2). Unless nonviable, the fistulous tract is not excised because excision enlarges the defect and risks injury to the intramural ureter. Left intact, the fistula tract also pro-

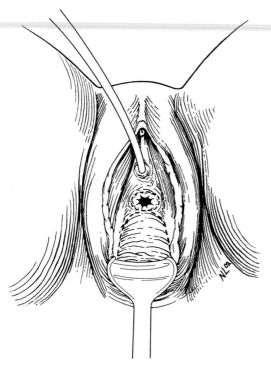

FIG. 25–1. The apex of the vaginal inverted-U incision is continuous with the circumferential fistula incision. (Modified from Raz S, Bregg KJ, Nitti VW, et al. Transvaginal repair of vesicovaginal fistula using a peritoneal flap. *J Urol* 1993;150: 56–59, with permission.)

vides strength to the VVF closure, helping decrease the risk of VVF repair disruption due to bladder spasms.

The fistula is closed in two nonoverlapping, perpendicular layers to prevent fistula recurrence. The first layer closes the fistula with interrupted 4-0 polyglycolic acid sutures, incorporating the vaginal wall overlying the VVF, the fistula tract, and the partial thickness of the bladder wall (Fig. 25–3). The second layer, using 2-0 polyglycolic acid sutures, imbricates the perivesical fascia and the deeper musculature of the bladder over the first layer in a tension-free fashion. The repair is checked for leaks by instilling indigo carmine into the bladder. The vaginal wall is advanced the over the VVF repair and closed with an interlocking, running 2-0 polyglycolic acid suture. A Betadine-soaked vaginal pack is placed.

If there is any concern about the repair, an interposing layer may be placed between the vaginal wall and bladder. The most common options are the Martius labial fat pad and the peritoneal flap. Alternative tissues include labial, vaginal wall, gluteal, and gracilis muscle flaps.

The Martius labial fat pad provides neovascularity and lymphatic drainage, fills dead space, and enhances granulation tissue formation. The flap is harvested by making a vertical incision on the labium majus; the underlying fibrofatty tissue is mobilized. The anterior portion of the graft is tied off (sacrificing the blood supply from the

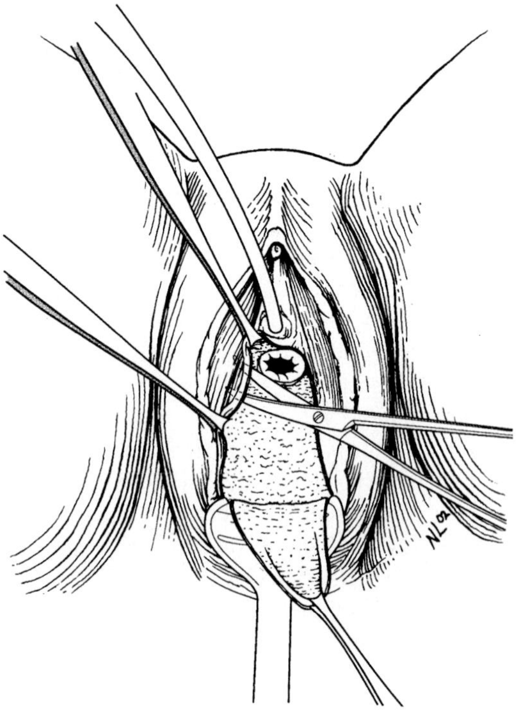

FIG. 25–2. The vaginal mucosa is dissected away from the perivesical fascia. (Modified from Raz S, Bregg KJ, Nitti VW, et al. Transvaginal repair of vesicovaginal fistula using a peritoneal flap. *J Urol* 1993;150:56–59, with permission.)

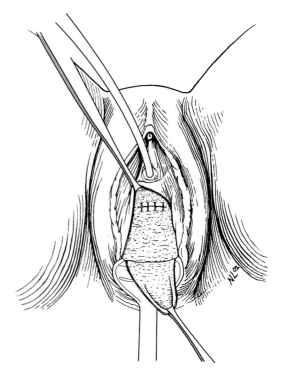

FIG. 25–3. Closure of the first layer including the fistulous tract and partial-thickness bladder wall. (Modified from Raz S, Bregg KJ, Nitti VW, et al. Transvaginal repair of vesicovaginal fistula using a peritoneal flap. *J Urol* 1993;150:56–59, with permission.)

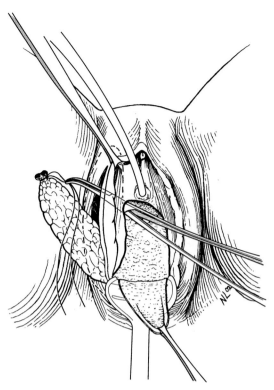

FIG. 25–4. Using a right-angle clamp, the Martius flap is passed from the labial incision to the vaginal incision.

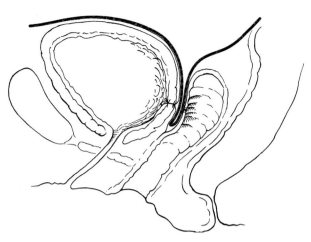

FIG. 25–6. Interposition of the peritoneum between the bladder and vagina. (Modified from Raz S, Bregg KJ, Nitti VW, et al. Transvaginal repair of vesicovaginal fistula using a peritoneal flap. *J Urol* 1993;150:56–59, with permission.)

external pudendal artery), leaving the fibrofatty pad supplied by its posterior blood source: the posterior labial artery from the internal pudendal artery. A tunnel is developed from the vaginal incision to the labium majus; the labial fat pad is transferred through the tunnel to cover the VVF repair and secured in place with interrupted 3-0 polyglycolic acid sutures (Fig. 25–4). The tunnel must be sufficiently sized to prevent constriction of the fat pad's blood supply. The labial incision is closed with a ¼-in. Penrose drain in place unless the graft bed is dry (Fig. 25–5).

Another effective method is the peritoneal interposition described by Dupont and Raz for routine use in fistula repair (3). With further posterior dissection of the anterior vaginal wall from the bladder, the glistening surface of the peritoneum in the anterior cul-de-sac is exposed. Without entering the intraperitoneal space, the peritoneum is mobilized from the posterior bladder wall to bring it down into the vagina and suture it over the VVF repair site (Fig. 25–6). The peritoneal flap has a 96% success rate when used in transvaginal VVF repair (4).

The vaginal pack is removed on postoperative day 1. The patient is given perioperative antibiotics and anticholinergics to prevent bladder spasms. Two weeks postoperatively the urethral catheter and suprapubic tube are removed if the cystogram reveals no persistent fistula or extravasation. If a fistula is still present, bladder drainage continues for another 2 to 3 weeks and the cystogram repeated at that time.

Transabdominal (Intraperitoneal) Approach

The patient is placed in a low lithotomy position. Cystoscopy is performed to visualize and cannulate the VVF with a 5 to 6 Fr ureteral catheter or guide wire. If unable

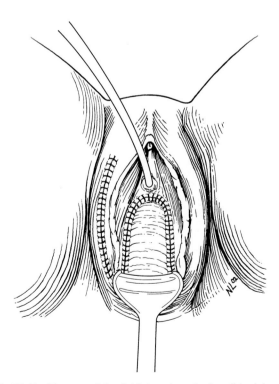

FIG. 25–5. Closure of the labial and vaginal wall incisions.

to pass the guide wire through the VVF transvesically, it is passed from the vaginal side into the bladder, grasped cystoscopically, and brought out through the urethra.

A midline infraumbilical incision is made; the rectus muscle is split midline to enter the pelvis. The bladder is opened with a midline vertical cystotomy between two stay sutures (Fig. 25–7). The VVF is identified with the guide wire exiting its opening into the bladder. The urethral end of the guide wire is pulled into the cystotomy incision. The VVF's position in relation to the ureteral orifices is noted and the ureters are cannulated with stents, if necessary. If there is any difficulty identifying the orifices due to local inflammation, IV indigo carmine may be administered.

Entering the peritoneal cavity, the dissection along the posterior bladder wall is carried out until the guide wire traversing the VVF is palpated, indicating the junction between the vagina and bladder. With a sponge stick in the vagina to help delineate the vagina, the bladder is carefully dissected away from the vagina. Wide mobilization of the bladder and vagina to allow tension-free closure of each side of the VVF is critical. The dissection bisects the fistula tract without excising the tract extending 1.5 to 2.0 cm beyond the VVF, allowing for tension-free closure (Fig. 25–8). Using interrupted 3-0 polyglycolic acid sutures, the vaginal defect is closed in two nonoverlapping layers. The bladder defect is also closed in two nonoverlapping layers with running 4-0 polyglycolic acid and 3-0 interrupted sutures.

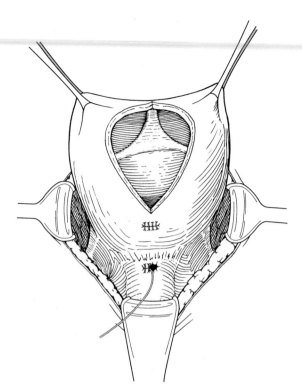

FIG. 25–8. After dissecting between the bladder and vaginal, both defects are closed in two layers.

After the bladder and vaginal fistulous defects are closed, attention is turned to developing an omental pedicle flap to interpose between the bladder and vagina. A recent study recommended routine use of an interposition flap during intraabdominal VVF repair, noting a success rate of 100% with a flap versus 63% to 67% without a flap (5). Not only does the interposition flap add an extra layer to the VVF repair to prevent recurrence, it also increases lymphatic drainage and decreases the risk of infected fluid collection. Alternatives to omentum include lateral pelvic peritoneum, pericolic or mesenteric fat, and free bladder mucosal graft.

The omentum is identified and an omental flap based on the more reliable right gastroepiploic artery is developed (Fig. 25–9). The flap is brought down to the pelvis and placed between the bladder and vagina, covering the fistula repair (Fig. 25–10). The graft is secured in place with interrupted 3-0 polyglycolic acid sutures.

With the VVF repair completed, a suprapubic catheter and urethral Foley catheter are placed with 5-mL balloon inflation each. In patients with prolonged large fistula, the bladder capacity is reduced due to the constant drainage. Therefore, the placement of two fully inflated balloons in combination with irritation from the incisions may lead to intensification of bladder spasms. The vertical bladder incision is closed in two layers with 2-0 polyglycolic acid sutures. A closed pelvic drain is also placed. Postoperative care is similar to that after transvaginal VVF repair.

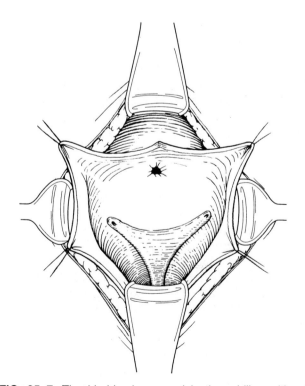

FIG. 25–7. The bladder is opened in the midline without extending the cystotomy to the fistula.

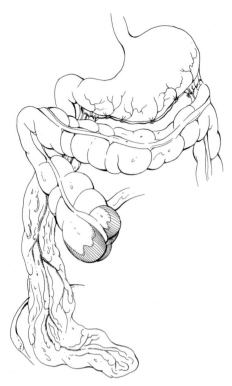

FIG.25–9. Development of an omental pedical flap based on the right gastroepiploic artery.

An alternative to the above intraabdominal technique above is the standard O'Conor technique. The bladder is bivalved posteriorly from the dome to the level of the VVF. Then, the VVF is excised entirely (Figs. 25–11 through 25–13). After further dissection of the bladder

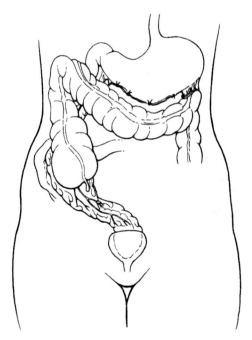

FIG. 25–10. Placement of the distal end of the omental graft posterior to the detrusor covering the repairs.

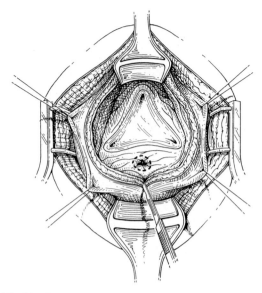

FIG. 25–11. Cystotomy extended down to the fistula site.

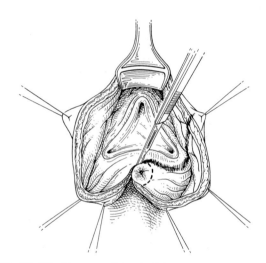

FIG. 25–12. Circumscribing incision around the fistula.

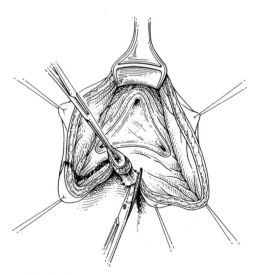

FIG. 25–13. Sharp excision of the fistula tract.

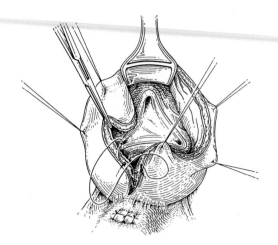

FIG. 25–14. Relation of the cystotomy to the vaginal closure.

from the vagina, the vaginal defect is closed in two nonopposing layers with interrupted absorbable sutures (Fig. 25–14). An interposition flap is tacked over the vaginal closure and the bladder is closed. The first technique is slightly more difficult in that the fistula is approached posteriorly and transected between the bladder and vagina. However, the advantages are that the smaller cystotomy is separated from the repair.

Transvesical (Extraperitoneal) Approach

The advantage of this approach is the avoidance of entering the peritoneal cavity. Through a midline infra-

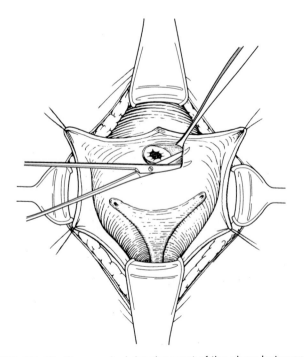

FIG. 25–15. Transvesical development of the plane between the bladder and vaginal walls.

umbilical incision, the bladder is identified and opened with a midline vertical incision. The VVF is located and the ureteral orifices are cannulated with stents. The fistulous opening is circumscribed carefully with a scalpel, incising only the thickness of the bladder mucosa and staying out of the vagina. This is performed to leave the fistula tract intact along with a 2- to 3-mm ring of bladder mucosa. With sharp dissection directed radially away from the VVF for 1 to 2 cm, the bladder is mobilized away from the vagina (Fig. 25–15). To help with exposure, a Foley catheter may be placed transvesically in the VVF for upward traction.

With interrupted 3-0 polyglycolic acid sutures, the fistula and vagina are closed together. Next, the bladder muscle is closed perpendicular to the fistula and vaginal closure, also with 3-0 polyglycolic acid sutures. Finally, the bladder mucosa is closed with running 4-0 polyglycolic acid sutures. A suprapubic cystotomy catheter and a urethral Foley catheter are placed and the bladder is closed in two layers with 2-0 polyglycolic acid sutures. Postoperative care is similar to that previously described.

OUTCOMES

Complications

Clearly, the most problematic complication is recurrent or persistent fistula. The catheter is replaced for several weeks and the cystogram repeated. If the fistula fails to resolve or improve, then endoscopic evaluation—vesical and vaginal—is performed in preparation for a second procedure. For recurrent fistulas complicated by prior pelvic irradiation, a conservative approach is wise, waiting 6 to 12 months before attempting repair. Frequency, urgency, and urge incontinence in the early preoperative period are treated symptomatically with anticholinergic therapy. These, however, are expected due to bladder decompensation and trigonal/suture line irritation. Residual incontinence must be evaluated with physical examination and fluoroscopic urodynamics. Occult or *de novo* stress urinary incontinence occurring in 10% to 12% of patients requires separate treatment after recovery from the VVF repair. Ureteral obstruction, prolonged ileus, and bowel obstruction are uncommon.

Results

A review of the VVF series from the last two decades demonstrates the success rate of transvaginal and transabdominal repairs to be 92.5% to 96% and 85% to 100%, respectively (1,2,4,8). Therefore, when the appropriate approach is selected based on the etiology, location, concomitant pathologies, and surgeon experience excellent results can be expected in the great majority of patients. However, in those who have failed multiple repairs due to severe tissue compromise secondary to radiation or who have developed the end-stage detrusor diversion may be the only alternative.

REFERENCES

1. Blaivas JG, Heritz DM, Romanzi LJ. Early versus late repair of vesicovaginal fistulas: vaginal and abdominal approaches. *J Urol* 1995; 153:1110–1113.
2. Blandy JP, Badenoch DF, Fowler CG, et al. Early repair of iatrogenic injury to the ureter or bladder after gynecological surgery. *J Urol* 1991; 146:761–765.
3. Dupont MC, Raz S. Vaginal approach to vesicovaginal fistula repair. *Urology* 1996;48:7–9.
4. Eilber KS, Rosenblum N, Rodriguez LV, et al. 10-Year experience of transvaginal vesicovaginal fistula repair utilizing a peritoneal flap. *J Urol* 2002;167[Suppl]:202 (abst 814).
5. Evans DH, Madjar S, Politano VA, et al. Interposition flaps in transabdominal vesicovaginal fistula repairs: are they really necessary? *Urology* 2001;57:670–674.
6. Goodwin WE, Scardino PT. Vesicovaginal and ureterovaginal fistulas: a summary of 25 years of experience. *J Urol* 1980;123:370–374.
7. Harkki-Siren P, Sjoberg J, Tiitinen A. Urinary tract injuries after hysterectomy. *Obstet Gynecol* 1998;92:113–118.
8. Mondet F, Chartier-Kastler EJ, Conort P, et al. Anatomic and functional results of transperitoneal–transvesical vesicovaginal fistula repair. *Urology* 2001;58:882–886.
9. Tancer ML. Observations on prevention and management of vesicovaginal fistula after total hysterectomy. *Surg Gynecol Obstet* 1992;175: 501–506.
10. Zacharin RF. A history of obstetric vesicovaginal fistula. *Aust NZ J Surg*. 2000; 70:851–854.

CHAPTER 26

Enterovesical and Rectourethral Fistulae

Aaron J. Milbank, Kenneth W. Angermeier, and Eric A. Klein

An enterovesical fistula is an extraanatomic, epithelialized connection between the intestines and the bladder. This chapter will describe the etiology, evaluation, and management of enterovesical fistulae and the less common rectourethral/rectovesical fistulae. The last half-century has seen a dramatic change in the management of enterovesical fistulae with a reduction in morbidity and mortality.

ENTEROVESICAL FISTULAE

In unselected series, the most common etiology of enterovesical fistulae is diverticulitis. In seven series of patients with enterovesical fistulae, the etiology was diverticulitis in 53% (range, 39% to 77%). Moreover, it has been reported that 10% of surgically treated cases of diverticulitis are associated with a colovesical fistula. There is a significant male predominance, a finding that has been attributed to a "protective barrier" provided by the uterus and broad ligament (13).

Other common causes of enterovesical fistula are pelvic malignancy (21%) and Crohn's disease (15%). Crohn's disease patients tend to present at a younger age than those patients with diverticular or malignant etiologies. Radiation injury is an infrequent cause of enterovesical fistulae. Most enterovesical fistulae following pelvic radiotherapy are secondary to recurrent disease. The etiologies of enterovesical fistulae are listed in Table 26–1.

Diagnosis

Although enterovesical fistulae are almost always secondary to extravesical pathology, the presenting symptoms are in general urinary in nature. The most common presenting symptom is pneumaturia, reported in 50% to 85% of patients, although some series report irritative voiding symptoms in as many as 71% to 93%. Fecaluria

is reported in 21% to 68% of patients with enterovesical fistulae and tends to be more common with diverticular and malignant fistulae. Other symptoms include hematuria, abdominal pain, diarrhea, urinary retention, perineal pain, hematochezia, and fever. Urine in the stool is rarely reported with enterovesical fistulae; these fistulae tend to be unidirectional with flow from the high-pressure intestinal tract to the low-pressure urinary tract.

TABLE 26–1. *Specific causes of vesicoenteric fistulas*

Inflammatory
  Diverticulitis
  Crohn's Disease
  Ulcerative Colitis
  Appendiceal/Pelvic Abscess
  Meckel's Diverticulum
  Tuberculosis
  Actinomycosis
  Bladder Malakoplakia
  Colonic duplication
Neoplastic
  Carcinoma of Sigmoid Colon and Rectum
  Lymphomas
  AIDS-Related Lymphomas
  Carcinoma of Cervix
  Leiomyosarcoma of Bladder
Traumatic
  Gunshot Wounds
  Penetrating Injuries
  Pelvic Fractures
  Transurethral or Open Prostatectomy
  Vesical Formalization
  Pelvic External Beam Radiation
  Prostatic Brachytherapy
  Cryoablation of the Prostate
  Transurethral Microwave Thermotherapy
Pelvic
  Gynecologic Cancer
Foreign Body

AIDS, acquired immunodeficiency syndrome.

Physical signs of enterovesical fistulae are subtle or absent. Abdominal tenderness and a palpable mass may be reported in as many as 35% and 27% of patients, respectively, and is not specific. In patients with rectal disease, a rectal mass or rectal tenderness may be present. Rarely, an enterovesical fistula may present as epididymitis. In general, physical findings are most commonly seen in patients with Crohn's disease.

Urinalysis discloses pyuria and cultures are positive in 80% to 100% of cases of enterovesical fistula. *Escherichia coli* is the most commonly identified organism and approximately one- to two-thirds of cultures show polymicrobial growth.

The diagnosis of an enterovesical fistula is clinical and in some instances, despite numerous radiographic studies, the first objective demonstration of the fistula is at laparotomy. Nonetheless, numerous studies have been described to aid in the diagnosis and/or localization of fistulae. Functional studies include the charcoal test, administration of visible dyes (methylene blue, indigo carmine), and the Bourne test, in which urine voided after a barium enema is radiographed for the presence of barium. The charcoal test involves the ingestion of nonabsorbable charcoal followed by the observation of charcoaluria. Although these tests have been reported to have sensitivities of 80% to 100%, they are rarely performed because they provide no localizing anatomic information and the information they do provide is usually evident from the patient's history.

Cystoscopy is the most commonly abnormal investigation in patients with enterovesical fistulae, although direct observation of a fistula is relatively unlikely. Approximately 90% of cystoscopies show at least indirect evidence of the fistula, most commonly bullous edema, and in 33% to 46% of cystoscopies the fistulous opening is identified.

Barium enema has been a commonly utilized study in the evaluation of enterovesical fistulae, with some series reporting 100% abnormal studies and fistula identification in as many as 16% to 63% of patients. Colonoscopy rarely demonstrates a fistulous tract, but the study is important in the evaluation of potentially malignant fistulae.

Computed tomography (CT) has supplanted most of the older imaging studies in the evaluation of suspected enterovesical fistulae. Although the fistula tract may be identified in some cases, indirect evidence of the fistula, including air in the bladder, focal bladder and bowel wall thickening and closely apposed bowel and bladder, may be present in 85% to 100% of cases. CT also provides important information in the evaluation of patients with Crohn's disease and colorectal carcinoma. CT cystography in our institution has replaced many other studies, including standard cystography, intravenous pyelography (IVP), and magnetic resonance imaging (MRI).

Indications for Surgery

Given the symptomatic nature of enterovesical fistulae and their association with recurrent urinary tract infections and sepsis, most fistulae should be addressed surgically. Over the course of the past 30 years, a one-stage operation has become the favored procedure because of reports of fewer complications and lower mortality. It has been demonstrated that a one-stage procedure may be safely performed in the setting of an abscess or purulent peritonitis provided that the inflammatory focus can be removed and the bowel anastomosis can be "quarantined from any inflammatory nest" (13). In general, diverticular disease is in particularly well suited to one-stage procedures because the fistulous process is either chronic or, if acute, controllable with antibiotics.

A two-stage procedure should be considered in patients who have an obstructed bowel, have residual significant intraabdominal inflammation, are significantly ill, and in whom a healthy anastomosis is unlikely (due to poor blood supply or tension at the anastomosis). The two stages (for colovesical fistulae) may consist of resection with Hartmann's pouch and end colostomy followed by reanastomosis or resection, anastomosis, and transverse colostomy followed by reversal of the colostomy. Fistulae secondary to radiation injury in general require multiple staged repairs and, frequently, permanent bladder and bowel diversion (8).

Alternative Therapy

Nonoperative management may be considered in patients who are extremely debilitated. There are a few reports of spontaneous closure of fistulae with medical management. This spontaneous resolution has been reported with traumatic fistulae and in a subset of fistulae secondary to Crohn's disease. Placement of bowel stents and endoscopic clipping of the colonic terminus of the fistula have also been reported for patients who are too ill to undergo open surgical procedures. Experimental evidence suggests that enterovesical fistulae, when chronic, are physiologically well tolerated (5). Amin et al. followed a cohort of four patients with diverticular colovesical fistulae who refused surgery; with 3 to 14 years of follow-up, there were no significant complications (1).

Surgical Technique

One-Stage Surgery (Fig. 26–1)

On the day prior to the operation, a mechanical bowel preparation is administered and the patient is maintained on a clear liquid diet. Gram negative and anaerobic coverage is provided by administering a third-generation cephalosporin (ceftizoxime) and metronidazole 1 hour prior to the surgical procedure.

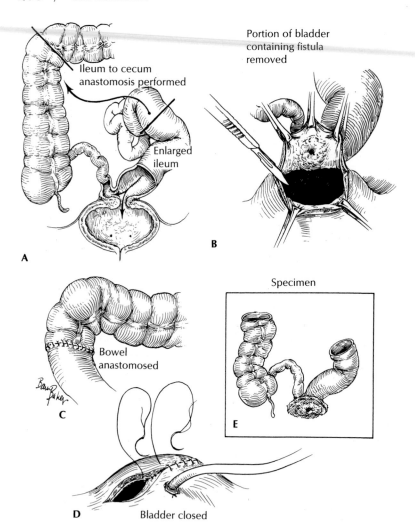

FIG. 26–1. Management of an enterovesical fistula using bowel resection and restitution with primary bladder closure.

Most fistulae are best approached via a midline incision extending from the pubic ramus to the umbilicus. This incision may be extended cranially as needed. Some authors prefer an infraumbilical transverse incision. The peritoneal cavity is entered and adhesiolysis is performed. The point of the fistula is identified. The remainder of the procedure is determined by the disease causing the fistula and intraoperative findings. In the setting of diverticular fistulae, the diseased colon is resected and an anastomosis is performed suturing normal bowel to normal bowel without tension and with adequate blood supply. Patients with Crohn's disease often have multiple fistulae not involving the urinary tract and require multiple resections or stricturoplasties. With diverticular disease, the fistula may often be "pinched off" from the bladder with curettage of the fistula tract. For malignant fistulae, the requisite oncological procedure is performed and the malignant fistula tract is excised. Partial cystectomy may be required for large or malignant fistulae; radical cystectomy is in general not required.

Closure of small bladder fistulae is not essential. Large defects should be closed in two layers using absorbable sutures. In the setting of ureteral involvement, ureteroneocystostomy may be required. Ideally, an omental flap should be interposed between the anastomosed bowel and the bladder. When an omental flap is not constructable, a peritoneal flap may be used. Suprapubic catheters and drainage of the extraperitoneal space are optional. In general, a urethral catheter is maintained until 1 week after surgery. Complete healing of the bladder defect may be confirmed with a cystogram prior to removal of the catheter. The aforementioned procedure has also been performed laparoscopically with good results.

Outcomes

Complications

Major complications of operative repair of enterovesical fistulae include death (0% to 5%), myocardial infarction (2% to 6%), anastomotic leak (0% to 5%), enterocutaneous fistula (0% to 1%), wound infection (0% to 21%), wound dehiscence (0% to 2%), pulmonary embolus (0% to 1%), deep vein thrombosis (0% to 1%), prolonged ileus (0% to 5%) and urine leak (0% to 3%) (4,9,12,13). One of the largest surgical series (104 patients) reported a 6.4% overall complication rate with no operative mortality (7). Significantly greater morbidity is observed in series focusing on radiation-induced and malignant fistulae (6,8).

Results

The results of the one-stage procedure for enterovesical fistulae are very much dependent upon the etiology of the fistula. Fistula recurrence following colonic resection in patients with diverticular fistulae is virtually nonexistent (13). Following surgical intervention for Crohn's disease with enterovesical fistulae, recurrent enterovesical fistulae are observed in 0% to 13% of patients (4,9). In a surgical series of 13 patients with malignant fistulae, 2 (15%) patients developed recurrent fistulae (6). In a surgical series of 13 patients with radiation-induced fistulae, 5 (39%) failed to resolve or recurred (8). It should be noted that seven of these operations were diversions or isolations; of the six patients who underwent resections, only one developed a recurrent fistula.

RECTOURETHRAL FISTULAE

Rectourethral fistulae are rare clinical entities. The most common cause is iatrogenesis, usually incurred during prostatic or rectal surgery or following radiation. Other etiologies include congenital, infectious, and neoplastic fistulae.

Diagnosis

Diagnosis of a rectourethral fistula is usually straightforward and suggested by the medical history. Preoperatively, antegrade and retrograde studies of the urinary tract, cystoscopy, proctoscopy, and, if indicated, anal manometry are performed to delineate the site and extent of the fistula as well as rule out distal obstruction or sphincteric incompetence. If there is clinical suspicion of disease recurrence, a biopsy should be performed.

Indications for Surgery

Many different approaches have been proposed for the management of rectourethral fistulae. It is imperative to individualize management. There are five key factors that must be considered prior to determining the ideal approach:

1. *Sphincteric function.* In the setting of anal sphincteric incompetence, complex anal sphincter-spar-

ing procedures should be deferred and consideration given to permanent fecal diversion. Similarly, in the setting of failure of the urinary sphincter supravesical diversion is a valid consideration if placement of an artificial urinary sphincter is not feasible.

2. *Presence of urethral stricture or vesical neck contracture.* Coexisting urethral disease may be present in patients with rectourethral fistulae, in particular iatrogenic fistulae (surgical or radiation-induced). Distal obstruction will compromise a technically adequate repair and should be treated prior to fistula repair.

3. *Status of adjacent tissue.* Pelvic radiation induces both delayed endothelial cell damage and damage to the connective tissue stroma of blood vessels (10). This arteritis may result in atrophy, fibrosis, and necrosis. As a result, radiation-induced fistulae in general require more extensive repairs involving interposition of omentum or muscle flaps, have high failure rates, and on occasion require permanent diversion.

4. *Size and location of the fistula.* Whereas small distal fistulae may be effectively repaired via a transanal approach, large fistulae often require the greater exposure provided by transsphincteric, abdominal, or combined approaches. Moreover, large defects may require the interposition of vascularized tissue (omentum or muscle flaps).

5. *Overall condition and life expectancy of the patient.*

Our preferred approach is either the transanal approach and the posterior sagittal or York–Mason approach.

Alternative Therapy

Initial treatment of iatrogenic fistulae in general consists of colostomy, prolonged urinary drainage with a suprapubic catheter, and broad-spectrum antibiotics although some authors have advocated the selective use of elemental or parenteral nutrition in lieu of bowel diversion (3). Approximately 25% of iatrogenic fistulae will resolve with conservative management (2). For those fistulae that do not close, numerous surgical repairs have been proposed (2). Transabdominal repairs allow for a colonic pull-through if necessary and also allow for the interposition of omentum or a gracilis or rectus abdominis muscle flap. They are limited, however, by an increased risk of fecal incontinence, the morbidity of an abdominal operation, and the simultaneous need for a perineal approach to the posterior urethra. A perineal approach may be effective but will in general be complicated by scarring induced by the original procedure. There may also be an increased risk of erectile dysfunction using the perineal approach. The anterior transanorectal approach (sphincter divided) and the

Kraske laterosacral (sphincter not divided) approach both provide excellent exposure of the fistula; however, the former may be associated with erectile dysfunction if the plane of dissection strays from the midline and the latter procedure risks fecal incontinence associated with denervation.

Surgical Technique

Transanal Approach

The procedure is performed in the prone jackknife position. A speculum is introduced into the anus and the fistula is exposed. Two alternative procedures may be performed: The fistula may be circumscribed with mobilization of the rectal mucosa in a circumferential fashion; the fistula is excised and the underlying rectal wall muscle and mucosa are closed separately. Alternatively, the mucosal dissection may be limited to the rectal wall lateral and distal to the fistula. The proximal rectal wall is then mobilized for 4 cm, thereby creating a full-thickness U-shaped flap that is pulled down over the fistula and sutured to the edge of the rectal mucosa (Fig. 26–2). A catheter is maintained for 2 to 3 weeks. The main limita-

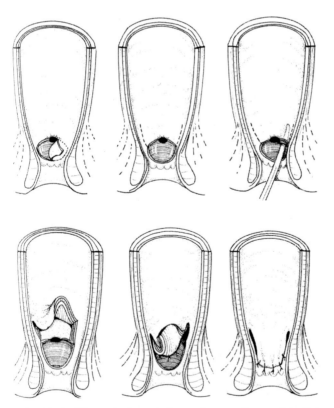

FIG. 26–2. Through the anal canal, an ellipse of rectal mucosa is removed. A full-thickness U-shaped flap of rectal wall is elevated above the fistula. The full-thickness flap of rectal wall is brought down over the fistula and sutured in two layers to the rectal wall. (From Tiptaft RC, Motson RW, et al. Fistulae involving rectum and urethra: the place of Parks' operations. *Br J Urol* 1983;55:711–715, with permission.)

tion of this approach is the limited exposure and it is best suited for small distal fistulae.

York–Mason Approach

The York–Mason procedure is performed in a prone jackknife position with the buttocks taped laterally (11) (Fig. 26–3). A midline incision is made from the sacrococcygeal articulation to the anal verge. Prior to dividing the muscular layers of the posterior anus, matching sutures are placed on either side of the intended incision so as to allow for subsequent precise reapproximation. Each layer is marked separately and then divided. Once the sphincter is divided, the mucosa of the posterior anus and the entire posterior rectal wall are divided in midline, thereby providing excellent exposure of the fistula. The fistula is then entirely excised and any inflammatory tissue is removed. The plane between the anterior rectal wall and the urethra/bladder may then be dissected to allow sufficient mobility for closure of the rectal defect. The urethra (or bladder) is closed with absorbable sutures in either one or two layers. The rectum is closed in two layers. The posterior rectal wall and anal mucosa are then reapproximated. Finally, using the previously placed marking sutures, the anal sphincter is reapproximated in layers. Drainage of the presacral space is optional. A Foley catheter is placed and maintained for 2 to 3 weeks, at which point the absence of a leak is confirmed radiographically.

Outcomes

Complications

Specific complications include recurrent fistula formation, urinary and/or fecal incontinence, and erectile dysfunction.

Results

Based upon literature reports, the York–Mason approach has become the favored repair for rectourethral fistulae not amenable to a transanal approach. There have been two relatively large series reported recently. Fengler and Abcarian performed eight York–Mason repairs for rectourethral fistulae with no recurrences and no fecal incontinence (3). Fecal diversion was performed in three of the eight patients. Stephenson and Middleton reported on 16 York–Mason repairs for rectourinary fistulae (rectovesical in 8, rectourethral in 7), with 1 recurrence and no fecal incontinence (11). The one recurrence was treated successfully with a second York–Mason procedure. In this series, four patients with urinary incontinence prior to the repair subsequently underwent artificial urinary sphincter placement; no patients developed urinary incontinence as a result of the repair. A diverting colostomy was used in nine of the patients.

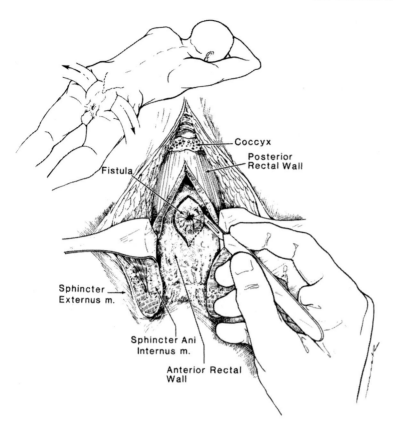

Coccyx

Posterior Rectal Wall

Fistula

Sphincter Externus m.

Sphincter Ani Internus m.

Anterior Rectal Wall

FIG. 26–3. Posterior sagittal, transrectal (York–Mason) approach for repair of rectourinary fistulae. The patient is placed in the prone jackknife position with tape used to displace the buttocks laterally. After division of the posterior anus and rectum, the fistula is easily identified with ample room for excision and repair. [From Stephenson RA, Middleton RG. Repair of rectourinary fistulas using a posterior sagittal transanal transrectal (modified York–Mason) approach: An update. *J Urol* 1996; 155:1989–1991, with permission.]

REFERENCES

1. Amin M, Nallinger R, et al. Conservative treatment of selected patients with colovesical fistula due to diverticulitis. *Surg Gynecol Obstet* 1984;159:442–444.
2. Elmajian DA. Surgical approaches to repair of rectourinary fistulas. *AUA Update Series* 2000;XIX(6):41–48.
3. Fengler SA, Abcarian H. The York Mason approach to repair of iatrogenic rectourinary fistulae. *Am J Surg* 1997;173:213–217.
4. Greenstein AJ, Sachar DB, et al. Course of enterovesical fistulas in Crohn's disease. *Am J Surg* 1984;147:788–792.
5. Heiskell CA, Vjiki GT, et al. A study of experimental colovesical fistula. *Am J Surg* 1975;129(3):316–318.
6. Holmes SA, Christmas TJ, et al. Management of colovesical fistulae associated with pelvic malignancy. *Br J Surg* 1992;79:432–434.
7. King RM, Beart RW Jr, et al. Colovesical and rectovesical fistulas. *Arch Surg* 1982;117:680–683.
8. Levenback C, Gershenson DM, et al. Enterovesical fistula following radiotherapy for gynecologic cancer. *Gynecol Oncol* 1994;52:296–300.
9. McNamara MJ, Fazio VW, et al. Surgical treatment of enterovesical fistulas in Crohn's disease. *Dis Colon Rectum* 1990;33:271–276.
10. Mundy AR. Pelvic surgery after radiotherapy. *Br J Urol* 1997;80[Suppl 1]:66–68.
11. Stephenson RA, Middleton RG. Repair of rectourinary fistulas using a posterior sagittal transanal transrectal (modified York–Mason) approach: an update. *J Urol* 1996;155:1989–1991.
12. Vasilevsky CA, Belliveau P, et al. Fistulas complicating diverticulitis. *Int J Colorectal Dis* 1998;13(2):57–60.
13. Woods RJ, Lavery IC, et al. Internal fistulas in diverticular disease. *Dis Colon Rectum* 1988;31:591–596.

CHAPTER 27

Vesical Trauma and Hemorrhage

Badrinath R. Konety, Michael P. Federle, and Robert R. Bahnson

VESICAL TRAUMA

Vesical injury can occur as a result of blunt or penetrating trauma to the lower abdomen and pelvis. It is more commonly associated with blunt trauma such as that sustained from motor vehicle accidents, falls, blows, and during contact sports. Penetrating trauma resulting in vesical injury occurs from gunshot wounds and knife wounds. Bladder injuries can also be iatrogenic from transurethral surgery, gynecologic procedures, laparoscopy, and other intraabdominal surgery. Bladder injury, in particular bladder rupture, is associated with pelvic fractures in 75% to 83% of patients (5). However, only 5% to 10% of patients with pelvic fractures will have associated bladder rupture (2,4). There is also a high incidence (less than 185%) of injuries to other organs in patients with bladder rupture (4). Concomitant bladder rupture is found in 10% to 29% of patients who present with rupture of the posterior urethra, and this is the most common injury to the genitourinary tract associated with bladder rupture (4,5). The mortality rate in patients with bladder rupture ranges from 11% to 44% and is mainly attributable to other associated organ injuries.

Anatomy

In children, the bladder is mainly an abdominal organ located behind the anterior abdominal wall. Growth of the bony pelvis allows the bladder to assume its position behind the pubic symphysis by the end of the sixth year of life (2). In its extraperitoneal location, the bladder is protected by the bony ring of the pelvis. It is attached to the pelvic bones and the lateral pelvic wall by means of various ligaments. The superior surface (dome) of the bladder in women and the dome and a portion of the base of the bladder in men are covered by parietal peritoneum. A fibrous cord, the median umbilical ligament, extends from the apex of the bladder to the umbilicus and is a remnant of the urachus. The dorsolateral ligamentous attachments of the bladder contain the nerves and vascular supply to the bladder. The fascial attachments between the bladder and the pubic bones are termed the pubovesical ligaments in women and the puboprostatic ligaments in men. Ligamentous attachments also connect the bladder anteriorly and laterally to the pelvic side wall.

The arterial supply to the bladder is derived from the superior, middle, and inferior vesical arteries, which are branches of the anterior division of the internal iliac (hypogastric) artery. The vesical venous plexus drains into the internal iliac veins. The sympathetic nerve supply to the bladder originates in the thoracolumbar sympathetic trunks and is via the superior hypogastric plexus to the pelvic plexus, where it joins with the parasympathetic nerves. The parasympathetic nerve supply is from the sacral parasympathetic outflow to the pelvic plexus and then to the bladder.

Mechanism of Injury

Bladder injury occurs as three predominant types: contusion with only intramural injury and extraperitoneal or intraperitoneal bladder rupture. The exact incidence of bladder contusion is not known because of the lack of large studies involving this type of bladder injury. It is a partial-thickness tear of the bladder mucosa with ecchymosis of the bladder wall. It is often associated with a "teardrop" bladder, which occurs as a result of the presence of compressive pelvic hematomas from pelvic fractures (17). It is usually self-limiting and rarely requires treatment. Extraperitoneal bladder rupture occurs less frequently than intraperitoneal rupture (34% versus 58% of cases). Combined intra- and extraperitoneal rupture is seen in 8% of cases (16). It was initially believed that bladder rupture, especially extraperitoneal rupture, resulted from the traumatic dislodgement of the bladder from its points of attachment. Penetration of the bladder wall by fragments of the fractured pelvic bones was also thought to be another possible etiologic mechanism (2). However, Carroll and McAninch noted that only 35% of bladder ruptures in their series were accompanied by ipsilateral pelvic fractures (3). Hence, it is likely that the bladder may sustain an extraperitoneal rupture when it suffers from a bursting-type injury. In intraperitoneal rupture, the dome of the bladder, which is the weakest portion of the wall, usually gives way, resulting most often in a horizontal tear (2).

Diagnosis

Patients with bladder injury usually complain of lower abdominal pain and tenderness. Such an injury should be suspected in any patient with a pelvic fracture. Most patients with bladder trauma, including those with bladder contusions, will have gross or microscopic hematuria. Patients with contusion alone are usually able to void, whereas those with a ruptured bladder are often unable to void spontaneously. Acidosis with prerenal azotemia and elevated blood urea nitrogen is sometimes noticeable when there is a delay in diagnosis (16).

Presence of blood at the urethral meatus mandates performing a retrograde urethrogram. This is performed to rule out urethral injury before catheterization or instrumentation. If the retrograde urethrogram is normal, a urethral catheter is placed and a retrograde cystogram is obtained. This is performed by instilling at least 250 to 400 cc of water-soluble contrast (Cystografin) in the bladder under gravity to ensure adequate distension and visualization of possible areas of rupture (5,16). One of the principal reasons for false-negative cystograms is instillation of an inadequate amount of contrast in the bladder. Static anteroposterior, oblique, or lateral films are obtained with the bladder full, and a washout film is obtained after drainage of the contrast material from the bladder. These additional films are useful in evaluating patients with posterior wall ruptures, which may be obscured in the anteroposterior view by a contrast-filled bladder. The drainage film also helps detect residual extravasation.

The cystogram is usually normal in the presence of a bladder contusion. Intraperitoneal rupture results in ill-defined spillage of contrast into the peritoneum (Fig. 27–1). The extravasated contrast may outline loops of bowel or accumulate in the paracolic gutters, beneath the diaphragm or over the bladder, in an hourglass pattern. Extraperitoneal rupture is seen as streak-like extravasation of contrast confined to the pelvis on retrograde cystogram (Fig. 27–2). Corriere and Sandler (6) further distinguished extraperitoneal ruptures as simple (confined to the perivesical space) or complex (extravasation into the scrotum, retroperitoneum, abdominal wall, etc.). Displacement of the bladder by a pelvic hematoma can result in a teardrop-shaped bladder on cystogram (6).

Recently, examination of a contrast-filled bladder during computed tomography (CT) scan has been used as a

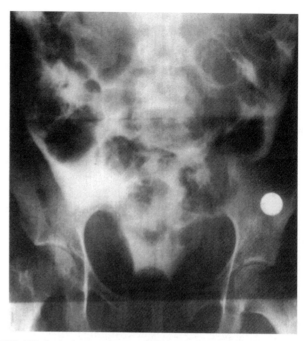

FIG. 27–1. In intraperitoneal rupture of the bladder, free contrast within the peritoneal cavity outlines bowel loops.

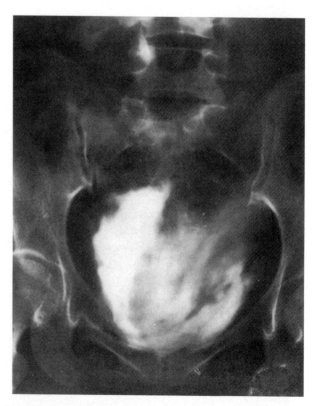

FIG. 27–2. In extraperitoneal rupture of the bladder, contrast fills the pelvic cavity around the bladder.

method of assessing injury. This is in particular applicable in patients who first undergo abdominal CT scans to rule out suspected visceral injuries. In these situations, the ability to simultaneously evaluate the bladder would obviate the need for an additional plain-film cystogram. However, during routine abdominopelvic CT scan the bladder may not be adequately distended to allow evaluation for rupture. Mee et al. (12) reported on two patients who were evaluated for bladder rupture on CT scan. Both patients received intravenous (IV) and oral contrast, and their Foley catheters were clamped to allow bladder filling. Despite this, one of the patients had a false-negative result. The bladder rupture was subsequently visualized on plain-film cystography in both cases. The results of CT cystography are better when the bladder is filled in a retrograde fashion with large volumes of contrast (250–500 cc) (11). Intraperitoneal bladder rupture can be distinguished from extraperitoneal rupture on CT scan. Presence of contrast around the bladder (Fig. 27–3A) and in the paracolic gutters on either side (Fig. 27–3B) and around abdominal viscera such as the liver (Fig. 27–3C) indicates intraperitoneal rupture. In the case of extraperitoneal rupture, contrast extravasation is usually seen around the bladder, in the presacral space (Fig. 27–4A)

and in the retroperitoneum anterior to the great vessels (Fig. 27–4B). Bladder contusions may be seen on CT scan as intramural hematomas. Despite the improved accuracy of CT scans, plain-film cystography is still the diagnostic modality of choice for detecting bladder ruptures. The accuracy of CT cystography may be significantly improved if retrograde bladder filling with adequate amounts of contrast is employed. In these situations, its accuracy may even approach that of plain-film cystography. CT cystography may be in particular useful in the select group of patients who undergo a CT scan as their initial radiological evaluation and are unable to undergo routine cystography because of the nature of their injuries or time constraints.

Intraoperatively, bladder rupture can be diagnosed by extravasation of saline, sterile milk, methylene blue, or indigo carmine, which is instilled in the bladder through a Foley catheter. In some situations, an IV pyelogram may be required to rule out other ureteral or renal injuries.

Indications for Surgery

1. Intraperitoneal bladder rupture.

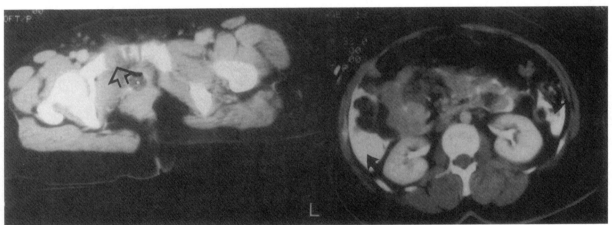

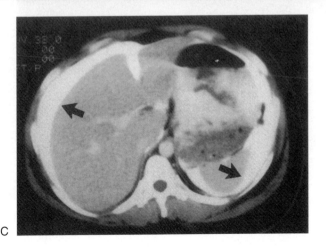

FIG. 27–3. A computed tomography cystogram showing evidence of intraperitoneal rupture of the bladder with extravasation around the (**A**) bladder (*arrow*), (**B**) paracolic space (*solid arrows*), and (**C**) abdominal viscera (*solid arrows*).

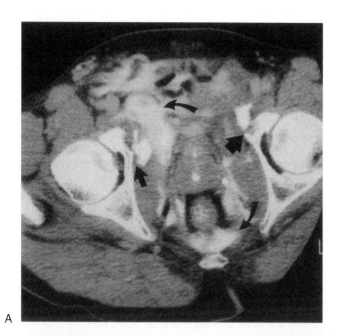

A

FIG. 27–4. Extraperitoneal rupture showing contrast in the (**A**) presacral space (*curved arrow*), prevesicle space (open arrow), and (**B**) retroperitoneum (*solid arrow*). B, bladder.

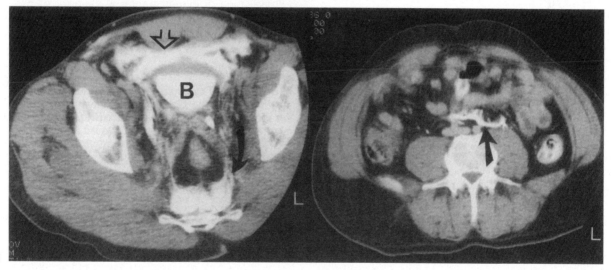

B

2. Bladder rupture or perforation sustained during another surgical procedure.
3. Extraperitoneal bladder rupture in the presence of other intraabdominal injuries requiring surgical intervention.
4. Extraperitoneal bladder rupture with the bladder being inadequately drained by urethral catheter drainage.

Alternative Therapy

Alternative treatments of bladder trauma are predominantly Foley catheter drainage, which is indicated in patients with bladder contusions and extraperitoneal extravasation. Injuries occurring during other procedures such as laparoscopic surgery may be repaired laparoscopically.

Surgical Technique

Intraperitoneal Bladder Rupture

Intraperitoneal bladder rupture requires immediate surgical repair. The abdomen is opened through a vertical lower midline incision, which affords better exposure and is extendable in case a laparotomy is required. The rupture, which is usually placed horizontally on the dome of the bladder, is identified. In some situations, this may require instillation of saline or dye in the bladder through a previously placed urethral catheter. In cases where additional extraperitoneal ruptures are suspected, the opening in the bladder wall can be extended to allow better visualization of the interior and bladder neck. These extraperitoneal tears can be closed from inside the bladder in one or two layers using running absorbable suture (3-0 chromic or polyglycolic/polygalactic acid). The intraperitoneal rupture(s) are closed in at least two layers using running 3-0 chromic or polyglycolic/polygalactic acid suture. The mucosa, muscle, and peritoneum are all closed in separate layers. The bladder is filled with saline after completion of the closure to evaluate for leaks. If any leaks are detected, they can be closed using interrupted figure-of-eight sutures.

In some situations, bony spicules that have penetrated the bladder wall may need to be removed before closure of the bladder. In cases of penetrating trauma or erosion of the bladder wall by pelvic abscess, nonviable tissue must be debrided and the edges of the perforation freshened prior to closure. In these cases, the tissue may be extremely friable and a single-layer closure may need to be performed. The ureteral orifices should be identified and observed to ensure normal efflux of urine. This may be done after administration of IV indigo carmine to facilitate visualization. If efflux of urine is not seen, proximal ureteral obstruction, especially by fractured bony fragments, should be ruled out. This can be done by performing a retrograde or IV pyelogram on the operating table.

An 8 Fr Malecot suprapubic catheter is placed through a separate cystotomy to drain the bladder. Care must be taken not to disturb the pelvic hematoma that is invariably present. Disruption of the pelvic hematoma may give rise to significant bleeding. This can be controlled by packing the area with Gelfoam, Surgicel, or laparotomy tapes. The abdomen can be temporarily closed with the packing in place for about 24 hours; the packing is removed at the time of reexploration. In extreme cases, angiographic embolization of the pelvic vessels may be necessary.

A 0.5-in. Penrose drain is placed adjacent to the bladder and left in place for 48 hours. In some cases, if the pelvic hematoma has not been disturbed and the bladder closure is truly watertight, drains can be omitted altogether. The abdominal fascia and skin are closed in the usual fashion.

In patients with small bladder ruptures, we have opted to drain the bladder postoperatively via a urethral catheter and have noted no significant adverse effects. The catheter is left in place for 7 to 10 days. A gravity cystogram is obtained at the end of this time to ensure absence of extravasation. The catheter is then removed if no extravasation is evident on cystogram.

Iatrogenic bladder injury, if suspected to have occurred during other operative procedures, should be documented by instillation of methylene blue or indigo carmine in the bladder and noting any extravasation. The rupture or tear can be closed primarily in two or three layers using absorbable suture as in other cases of rupture. Bladder perforations sustained during laparoscopic procedures can be diagnosed by noting distention of the urethral catheter drainage bag with gas (18). These injuries can be repaired as described previously by laparotomy or even laparoscopically (14).

Extraperitoneal Bladder Rupture

Until the 1970s, extraperitoneal bladder rupture was managed as an intraperitoneal rupture. Since then several studies have demonstrated that these injuries can be managed nonoperatively (5,6). Corriere and Sandler successfully managed 41 patients with extraperitoneal bladder rupture by prolonged urethral catheterization alone. All patients healed the bladder injury spontaneously without complications (6). Since then, other studies have duplicated these results.

Isolated extraperitoneal rupture can be treated by simple urethral catheter drainage. Once urethral injury has been ruled out by means of a retrograde urethrogram, a urethral catheter is placed. The catheter is left in place for 10 to 14 days. Repeat cystograms are performed at the end of this period. If no extravasation is observed, the catheter can be removed. If any contrast extravasation is evident on the cystogram, catheter drainage is continued. Cystograms are repeated at weekly intervals until no extravasation is demonstrable. A majority of extraperitoneal ruptures treated in this manner will heal by 2 weeks, and almost all will show healing within 3 weeks.

Severe bleeding with clots or sepsis should prompt surgical exploration even in cases of extraperitoneal rupture. If patients are undergoing laparotomy for other intraabdominal injuries, it is reasonable to repair extraperitoneal ruptures surgically.

Outcomes

Complications

Some patients may notice persistent urgency and increased frequency of micturition after repair of bladder ruptures. These symptoms are usually temporary and tend to subside with time. Vesical neck injuries increase the risk of subsequent incontinence, and attention should be paid to careful repair of these injuries. Infection of pelvic hematomas can result in abscess formation requiring prolonged drainage and antibiotic treatment. This can be prevented to some extent by taking care to avoid disrupting the hematoma intraoperatively. Unrecognized injury to adjacent structures can lead to subsequent vesicovaginal or vesicoenteric fistula formation. Otherwise, this complication is uncommon.

Complications such as clot retention and pseudodiverticulum formation are seen in fewer than 10% of patients treated with catheter drainage alone for extraperitoneal rupture (4,5). Significant sepsis, delayed healing, formation of bladder calculi, and vesicocutaneous fistula formation have been noted to occur in patients treated with urethral or suprapubic catheter drainage for extraperitoneal rupture (9). These patients most often had poorly functioning catheters or did not receive prophylactic antibiotics. Hence, it is important to ensure that urethral catheters are functioning adequately when used in these situations. Use of larger catheters and resorting to immediate open repair if catheters remain nonfunctional after 24 to 48 hours will help avoid these complications. Prophylactic antibiotics with gram-negative coverage, when administered for the duration of catheterization, will help prevent urinary tract infections.

Results

Open repair with adequate closure of the rupture is almost uniformly successful in all patients treated in this manner, and 74% to 87% of patients managed with urethral catheter drainage for extraperitoneal rupture will show evidence of healing by 10 to 14 days (5,9). The remainder will heal with an additional 7 to 10 days of catheter drainage.

VESICAL HEMORRHAGE

Significant bleeding from the bladder in the absence of trauma is usually associated with hemorrhagic cystitis. This can result from a variety of infectious and noninfectious etiologies. Sports hematuria or stress hematuria is a well-known cause of vesical hemorrhage seen mainly in marathon runners and other athletes. It is believed to be caused by the repeated impact of the posterior wall and base of the bladder, which results in mucosal contusions (1). An empty bladder at the time of running facilitates this process. Maintaining a partially full bladder in which the urine acts as a hydrostatic cushion will help prevent it.

Infections with various viruses such as the BK virus, adenovirus, and the influenza A virus can result in hemorrhagic cystitis. Bacterial infections, most often with *Escherichia coli,* can also result in hemorrhagic cystitis. Fungal infections seen frequently after treatment with broad-spectrum antibiotics can also result in this condition. Parasitic infections with organisms such as *Schistosoma hematobium* are known to be associated with this form of cystitis. Possible etiologic factors for hemorrhagic cystitis are listed in Table 27–1. This indicates that hemorrhagic cystitis is a symptom of an underlying condition rather than a disease in itself. Infection-related hemorrhagic cystitis is usually treatable by addressing the underlying cause.

Radiation therapy to the prostate, bladder, or other pelvic organs can result in hemorrhagic cystitis. Initially, there is mucosal edema with submucosal hemorrhage. Chronically, radiation causes obliterative endarteritis with subsequent urothelial ischemia. Various measures such as steroids, vitamin E, and trypsin have proved futile in treating radiation-induced cystitis, which can manifest many years after exposure. Coating the bladder mucosa with synthetic agents such as sodium pentosanpolysulfate has some beneficial effect (15). Hyperbaric oxygen therapy has also proved effective (13).

Amyloidosis of the bladder, which tends to occur in patients with rheumatoid arthritis and Crohn's disease, can also result in hemorrhagic cystitis. The hemorrhage can be in particular severe after instrumentation or biopsy of the bladder. This hemorrhage may require aggressive treatment measures including angiographic vessel occlusion or cystectomy.

Urothelial malignancies can also cause significant bleeding, which can be controlled by transurethral resection of tumor and fulguration with electrocautery in most cases. In patients with metastatic or unresectable bladder tumors and severe hematuria, local radiation can be used to palliate the symptoms. In some cases, cystectomy or urinary diversion by means of percutaneous nephrostomy or conduit urinary diversion may be the only viable option.

A wide range of drugs and industrial toxins can also give rise to hemorrhagic cystitis. Aniline and toluidine dyes are well known to be associated with this side effect. Treatment is largely conservative as the cystitis is self-limiting and resolves after removal of the offending agent. Antibiotics such as nitrofurantoin, ether, and accidental insertion of spermicidal contraceptives into the urethra can also result in severe hemorrhage from the bladder. Conservative treatment with adequate hydration, bladder irrigation, and discontinuing the causative agent would suffice as treatment for most cases.

Chemotherapeutic agents are a major cause of hemorrhagic cystitis. Busulfan, commonly used for treatment of leukemia, can give rise to hemorrhagic cystitis. Administration of *N*-acetylcysteine (Mucomist), used to treat some other forms of chemically induced cystitis, would only worsen the condition. Most other measures are also ineffec-

TABLE 27–1. *Etiologic agents for hemorrhagic cystitis*

Infectious causes	Noninfectious causes
Viral: BK virus, Adenovirus, JC Virus, Influenza Virus	Amyloidosis
Bacterial: Escherichia Coli, Staph Saprophyticus, Proteus mirabilis, Klebsiella	Radiation
Fungal: Candida Albicans, Aspergillus Furmigatus, Cryptococcus Neoformans, Torulopsis Glabrata	Chemicals: Anilines and Toluidines, Pesticides (Chlordimeform), Ether, Gentian Violet, Spermicidal Suppositories, Turpentine
Parasitic: Schistosoma Hematobium, Echinococcus granulosus	Drugs: Penicillins (Carbenicillin, Penicillin G, K, Ticarcillin, Methicillin, Piperacillin), Methenamine Mandelate, Danazol
	Chemotherapeutic Agents: Busulfan, Thiotepa, Cyclophosphamide, Isophosphamide

tive in this situation. Intravesical administration of thiotepa can result in this complication, which can occur up to 6 months after cessation of therapy. Alkylating agents such as cyclophosphamide and isophosphamide, which are employed in chemotherapeutic regimens for various solid tumors and lymphoproliferative disorders, are common culprits for hemorrhagic cystitis. The incidence ranges from 2% to 40%, and significant mortality rates have also been reported (10). It is dose dependent and related to the route of administration of the chemotherapeutic agent (higher with IV administration). It is more severe in dehydrated patients. Acrolein, which is a liver metabolite of cyclophosphamide, is the principal inciting agent and acts by direct contact with the bladder mucosa. Histological changes that occur in the bladder are similar to those seen with radiation and include edema, ulceration, neovascularization, hemorrhage, and necrosis. Prophylactic hydration and the use of protective agents such as Mucomist or 2-mercaptoethane sulfonate (Mesna) can reduce the incidence of this complication. Systemic administration of Mucomist can decrease the antineoplastic effect of cyclophosphamide.

Treatment of Hemorrhagic Cystitis

A practical algorithm for the management of hemorrhagic cystitis is outlined in Figure 27–5. Mild hematuria can be managed by vigorous hydration and oral adminis-

tration of agents such as aminocaproic acid or conjugated estrogens, which inhibit fibrinolysis and promote coagulation.

Moderate hematuria can be treated with continuous saline irrigation through a Foley catheter after all clots have been evacuated. In some situations such as with radiation cystitis, irrigation with cold saline for 24 to 48 hours may prove more effective. If hematuria persists, continuous bladder irrigation with 1% alum (potassium or ammonium aluminum sulfate) is helpful. The alum acts as an astringent and precipitates the surface proteins. Aluminum levels must be monitored, in particular in patients with renal insufficiency. Severe acidosis and encephalopathy can occur in such patients as a result of high aluminum levels. Periodic intravesical instillation of prostaglandins (PGE_2, $PGF_{2\alpha}$) and $PGF_{2\alpha}$ analogs (carboprost) have also proved effective. They decrease the inflammatory response and reduce the hemorrhage. They can be used prophylactically or therapeutically. Prostaglandin E_2 has been used in a dose of 0.75 mg in 200 cc of normal saline instilled for 4 hours. The effective dose of $PGF_{2\alpha}$ has been 1.4 mg in 200 cc of normal saline. Carboprost has been used in a dose of 0.8 mg per dL diluted in normal saline instilled for 1 hour at 6-hour intervals with good results in 62% of patients according to one study (8). Instillation of silver nitrate (0.5% to 1% solution) for short periods of time followed by saline irri-

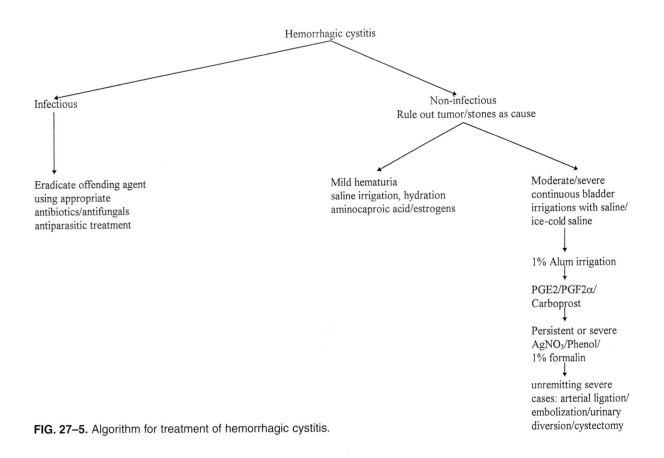

FIG. 27–5. Algorithm for treatment of hemorrhagic cystitis.

gation of the bladder to remove residual silver nitrate is also an effective technique.

Persistent severe hemorrhage that has not subsided despite the above-mentioned measures can be treated with intravesical instillation of carbolic acid (phenol) or 1% formalin. This requires general anesthesia. Phenol is instilled in a dose of 30 cc of a 100% solution mixed with an equal volume of glycine for 1 minute. This is washed out with 95% ethanol (60 cc) and saline to prevent methemoglobinemia. It is necessary to rule out vesicoureteral reflux by performing a voiding cystourethrogram before using formalin as it can cause fibrosis and scarring of the ureters and renal pelvis. If need be, the ureters can be occluded with Fogarty balloon catheters to prevent reflux while formalin is instilled. Fifty milliliters of 1% formalin (0.37% formaldehyde) diluted with saline should be instilled for 4 to 10 minutes. This should then be washed out with saline and the saline irrigation continued for 24 hours. The external genitalia are covered with towels or Vaseline to prevent irritation.

In recalcitrant cases, use of medical antishock trousers and cryotherapy have been reported (7). Embolization of the hypogastric arteries with autologous clot, Gelfoam, coils, or ethanol can also be resorted to in such cases. This may result in temporary gluteal claudication. Open ligation of the hypogastric artery can also be performed. Supravesical urinary diversion by means of percutaneous nephrostomy tubes or ileal or sigmoid conduit urinary diversion with or without cystectomy remains as a final but viable option.

REFERENCES

1. Blacklock NJ. Bladder trauma in the long-distance runner. 910,000 meters hematuria.9 *Br J Urol* 1977;49:129.
2. Bodner DR, Selzman AA, Spirnak JP. Evaluation and treatment of bladder rupture. *Sem Urol* 1995;13:62.
3. Carroll PR, McAninch JW. Major bladder trauma: mechanisms of injury and a unified method of diagnosis and repair. *J Urol* 1984;132:254.
4. Cass AS. Diagnostic studies in bladder rupture. Indications and techniques. *Urol Clin North Am* 1989;16:267.
5. Cass AS, Luxenberg M. Features of 164 bladder ruptures. *J Urol* 1987;138:743.
6. Corriere JN, Sandler CM. Mechanisms of injury, patterns of extravasation and management of extraperitoneal bladder rupture due to blunt trauma. *J Urol* 1988;139:43.
7. deVries CR, Freiha FS. Hemorrhagic cystitis: A review. *J Urol* 1990;143:1.
8. Ippoliti C, Przepiorka D, Mehra R, et al. Intravesicular carboprost for the treatment of hemorrhagic cystitis after marrow transplantation. *Urology* 1995;46:811.
9. Kotkin L, Koch MO. Morbidity associated with non-operative management of extraperitoneal bladder injuries. *J Trauma* 1995;38:895.
10. Krane DM. Hemorrhagic cystitis. *AUA Update* 1992;XI;lesson 31.
11. Lis LE, Cohen AJ. CT cystography in the evaluation of bladder trauma. *J Comput Assist Tomogr* 1990;14:386.
12. Me SL, McAninch JW, Federle MP. Computerized tomography in bladder rupture: diagnostic limitations. *J Urol* 1987;137:207.
13. Norkool DM, Hampson NB, Gibbons RP, Weisman RM. Hyperbaric oxygen therapy for radiation induced hemorrhagic cystitis. *J Urol* 1993;150:332.
14. Parra RO. Laparoscopic repair of intraperitoneal bladder perforation. *J Urol* 1994;151:1003–1005.
15. Parsons CL. Successful management of radiation cystitis with sodium pentosanpolysulfate. *J Urol* 1986;136:813.
16. Peters PC. Intraperitoneal rupture of the bladder. *Urol Clin North Am* 1989;16:279.
17. Sandler CM. Bladder trauma. In: Pollack HM, ed. *Clinical urography.* Philadelphia: WB Saunders, 1990:1505–1521.
18. Schanbacher PD, Rossi LJ, Salem MR, Joseph NJ. Detection of urinary bladder perforation during laparoscopy by distension of the collection bag with carbon dioxide. *Anesthesiology* 1994;80:680–681.

CHAPTER 28

Interstitial Cystitis

Kenneth M. Peters and Ananias C. Diokno

Interstitial cystitis (IC) was first described greater than 80 years ago and is one of the most common missed diagnoses in urology (2). The presentation may be variable; however, the key symptoms are urinary frequency, urgency, and pelvic pain. Until recently, IC has been thought to be a disease predominantly of women; however, more men are now being diagnosed with this disease. Men presenting with symptoms of genital pain, perineal pain, frequency, or dysuria are often labeled as having chronic, abacterial prostatitis; in fact, many of them suffer from IC.

DIAGNOSIS

One can often suspect IC on history alone after ruling out other causes that can mimic the disease such as documented bacterial cystitis, overactive bladder, endometriosis, bladder cancer, and urethral diverticulum. In 1987 and 1988 the National Institute of Diabetes and Digestive and Kidney Diseases (NIDDK) developed a research definition for IC, but these criteria were found to be far too restrictive to be used as a clinical diagnosis for IC (1).

IC is a disease that may present as mild irritative symptoms to severe symptoms refractory to all standard therapies. Treating the disease early often leads to rapid improvement in symptoms; thus, it is important to recognize IC early so that therapy can be initiated.

A physical exam including a good pelvic and neurological exam should be performed. A postvoid residual should be obtained to rule out urinary retention. Urethral fullness, tenderness, or expression of pus may suggest a urethral diverticulum requiring further workup. The pelvic examination should include evaluation for tenderness of the anterior vaginal wall and levator muscles, ability to contract and relax the pelvic floor muscles, and the degree of pelvic relaxation. A rectal examination can rule out any rectal abnormalities or masses, and in men the prostate should be palpated.

A urinalysis, urine culture, and cytology should be performed to exclude active infection or evidence of carcinoma *in situ*. Sterile pyuria should prompt urine tuberculosis cultures. If microscopic hematuria is present, a workup including upper-tract imaging, cystoscopy, and cytology should be performed to rule out bladder cancer or stone disease. A voiding diary with both fluid intake (amount and kind) and urine output, including voided volumes, daytime frequency, and nocturia, should be completed. Sequential voiding diaries and symptom questionnaires allows one to determine the impact of various treatments for IC.

A cystometrogram may be performed to rule out uninhibited contractions and determine the functional bladder capacity. Another test more specific to IC is the potassium sensitivity test, based on the hypothesis that there is increased epithelial permeability in the bladder of IC patients (4).

INDICATIONS FOR SURGERY

Any patient with unexplained urinary urgency, frequency, and pelvic pain would be a candidate for an operative hydrodistension to aid in the diagnosis and possibly improve symptoms. Patients with ulcerative disease may benefit from ablation of the ulcers with cautery or laser.

Radical surgery for IC is rarely indicated and should be used as a last resort. A magnetic resonance imaging (MRI) of the pelvis may demonstrate a thickened, end-stage bladder that may be amendable to radical surgery (Fig. 28–1). Patients who undergo bladder augmentation or replacement need to be willing and able to perform clean intermittent catheterization and accept that their frequency may improve but their pain may not resolve. Diverting the urine without removing the diseased bladder is not sufficient to relieve the symptoms of IC and should not be used to treat this disease.

Sacral nerve modulation has been effective in treating refractory urinary urgency and frequency. IC is a syn-

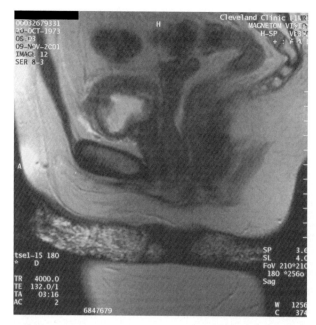

FIG. 28–1. Magnetic resonance imaging scan of pelvis of 28-year-old female with end-stage interstitial cystitis demonstrating a small, thickened, contracted bladder. (Courtesy of Raymond Rackley, Cleveland Clinic Foundation, with permission.)

drome of urgency, frequency, and pain and patients refractory to standard therapies would be candidates for sacral nerve stimulation.

ALTERNATIVE THERAPY

Justifying a patient's symptoms by making a diagnosis of IC and educating the patient about this disease is usually therapeutic. A multimodality approach is the most effective means of treating IC. Behavioral therapies must be stressed such as fluid management, pelvic floor exercises, dietary restrictions, and relaxation therapy. Many IC patients suffer from pelvic floor spasm causing pelvic pain, dyspareunia, and urinary hesitancy. Treatment by a therapist knowledgeable in myofascial release techniques may be of benefit. Once behavioral therapy is optimized, oral medication is a reasonable first-line treatment for IC.

The only US Food and Drug Administration (FDA)-approved oral therapy for IC is pentosan polysulfate sodium (Elmiron), a glycosaminoglycan that binds tightly to the bladder mucosa. Pentosan polysulfate should be considered a first-line therapy for IC; however, because it may require several months before any clinical improvement is seen it should not be used as a single agent for the treatment of IC. Other oral medications used in selected patients are hydroxyzine, antidepressants, muscle relaxants such as diazepam or low-dose baclofen, urinary analgesics, anticholinergics, and pain medications. Chronic pain is recognized as a legitimate complaint and

should be treated aggressively. Various narcotics and anti-inflammatories can be tried, along with nerve blocks or implantable pain pumps, to treat the severe pain that can be associated with IC.

Intravesical therapies for IC have been a mainstay in treatment for many years. Dimethylsulfoxide (DMSO) is the only FDA-approved intravesical therapy for this disease, although other agents such as Bacillus Calmette-Guérin (BCG), heparin, sodium oxychlorosene, and silver nitrate have been used.

SURGICAL TECHNIQUE

Bladder Hydrodistension

A complete cystoscopy is performed to assess the urethra and bladder (Fig. 28–2). After careful inspection, the bladder is filled by gravity drainage at 100 cm per H_2O pressure to its capacity. Upward pressure along each side of the urethra is often needed to maximally distend the bladder to prevent leakage around the cystoscope. The bladder is distended until no further water will run into the bladder and this is allowed to dwell for

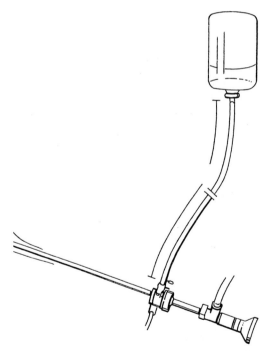

FIG. 28–2. Hydrodistension is carried out with the irrigation bag hung 100 cm above the level of the bladder. Bladder capacity is reached when irrigant flow stops. During filling, the bladder mucosa is typically normal appearing. After 2 minutes of distention, the bladder is drained and the capacity is measured. At the termination of bladder emptying, the irrigant fluid is often blood tinged or grossly hemorrhagic in patients with interstitial cystitis (IC). Repeat cystoscopy will demonstrate diffuse glomerulations in all sectors of the bladder consistent with IC. Repeat hydrodistension is performed to maximally distend the bladder.

2 minutes. The bladder is drained and the volume measured. The procedure is then repeated a second time. Typically with IC there is terminal hematuria noted when the bladder is drained. Upon reinspecting the bladder, the vast majority of patients will have glomerulations seen in all sectors of the bladder, suggestive of interstitial cystitis. Approximately 15% of IC patients will have focal deep cracks or ulcers in their bladder called Hunner's ulcers, which are associated with more severe symptoms (Fig. 28–3).

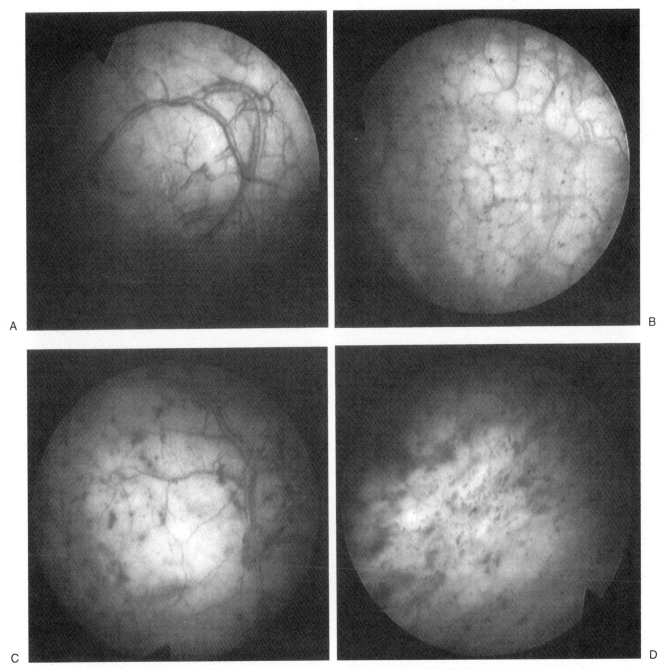

FIG. 28–3. A: Normal appearance of the bladder urothelium before hydrodistension in a patient with symptoms consistent with interstitial cystitis. **B:** Same patient following hydrodistension. The urothelium is abnormal, revealing minimal to moderate glomerulation. **C:** Cystoscopic appearance of a patient with moderate glomerulations and submucosal hemorrhage. **D:** Hunner's ulcer with marked hemorrhage surrounding the ulcer. This patient was successfully treated with neodymium:YAG laser ablation therapy.

Endoscopic Resection or Fulguration of Ulcers

Approximately 15% to 20% of IC patients have ulcerative lesions within their bladder that often are associated with worse pain and frequency symptoms. A loop resectoscope can be used to resect these lesions and the base cauterized. Alternatively, the involved areas can be cauterized with a Bugbee electrode, ball electrode, or neodymium:YAG laser. The laser is set at 15 W with a firing duration of 1 to 3 seconds. The laser fiber is maintained in con-

stant motion over the target and the procedure is completed when the ulcer is completely blanched (6).

Augmentation Cystoplasty

Simple augmentation of the bladder should only be performed if one has an operative bladder capacity with hydrodistension of less than 300 cc. The bladder is isolated and a posterior-based U-shaped incision is created on the anterior bladder (Fig. 28–4). A 30-cm segment of

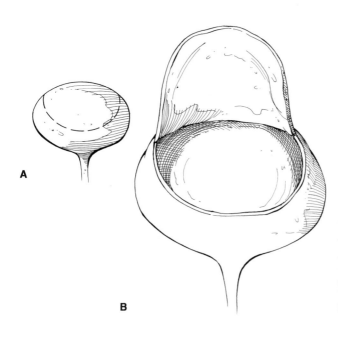

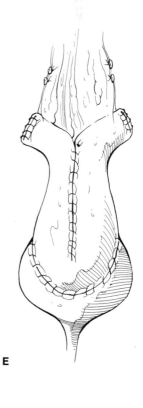

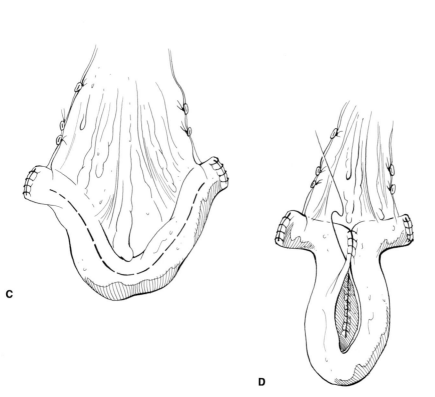

FIG. 28–4. Ileal augmentation cystoplasty. **A:** Posterior-based U-shaped incision is created on the anterior bladder. **B:** Completion of the posterior-based bladder flap. **C:** A 30-cm segment of the distal ileum is isolated and divided along the antimesenteric border. **D:** The ileal segment is then folded and the posterior surface is closed completely with a running absorbable suture. The anterior segment is partially closed. **E:** Completed ileal bladder anastomosis.

distal ileum is isolated in the standard fashion and opened along its antimesenteric border. The ileal segment is folded to create a nonperistaltic ileal patch. This is secured to the anterior bladder with running absorbable suture, effectively increasing the functional capacity of the bladder. Patients undergoing an augmentation must understand that their pelvic pain symptoms may not resolve and they may need to perform intermittent straight catheterization to effectively empty their bladder.

Partial Cystectomy and Substitution Cystoplasty

Supratrigonal cystectomy with enterocystoplasty is preferred over simple augmentation cystoplasty because the majority of the diseased bladder is removed (Fig. 28–5). This technique should be reserved for patients

with small bladder capacity under an anesthetic (less than 300 cc). Patients with a primary pain complaint are not good candidates for supratrigonal cystectomy, in particular if the pain is urethral in nature. In addition, patients should be able to perform intermittent straight catheterization and bladder irrigation.

The patient is placed in a supine position and a Foley catheter is placed sterilely in the bladder. The peritoneal cavity is entered through a vertical midline incision and an appropriate segment of either large or small bowel with a mesentery long enough to reach down to the bladder is selected. The preferred bowel segments are the cecum, sigmoid colon, or ileum. The bladder is filled via the Foley and divided using a clamshell technique, exposing the trigone. Ureteral catheters are placed before resection of the bladder to avoid injury to the ureters.

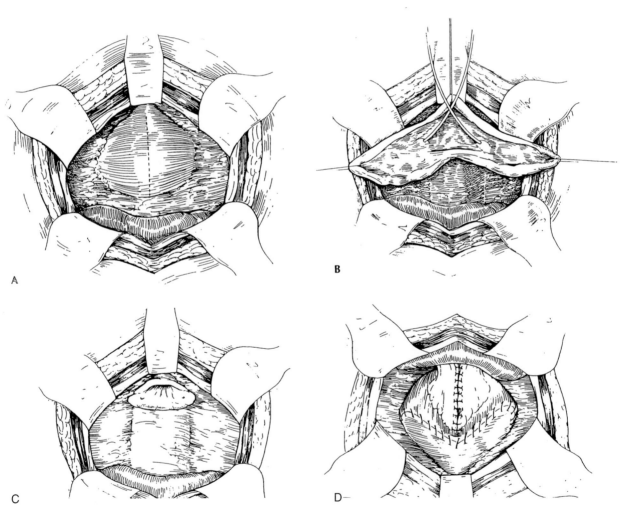

FIG. 28–5. Technique of subtotal cystectomy and substitution cystoplasty. **A:** The bladder is being bivalved with electrocautery. **B:** View of the bladder with both ureteral orifices cannulated with ureteral catheters to avoid injury to ureters during bladder resection. **C:** Completion of subtotal cystectomy with only a small cuff of bladder remaining, which consists of the urethra, bladder neck, and trigone. **D:** Completed anastomosis of the bowel onto the bladder cuff. A Foley catheter (not shown) and a suprapubic tube are placed to ensure adequate drainage during the immediate postoperative period.

Using electrocautery, a supratrigonal cystectomy is performed, resecting all but a 1- to 2-cm cuff of bladder that includes the trigone and bladder neck. Placing Allis clamps on the edges of the remaining bladder controls hemostasis. The vesicoenteric anastomosis is completed using a single-layer running closure of 3-0 Vicryl suture. A 22 Fr Foley catheter is placed through the bowel segment and used as a suprapubic tube. Both tubes are kept to dependent drainage for 21 days, when a cystogram is performed to assure integrity of the anastomosis. The patient is then started on intermittent catheterization.

Total Cystectomy with Orthotopic Neobladder or Urinary Diversion

A total cystectomy has the benefit of removing the entire diseased bladder and may be the treatment of choice for the IC patient with an "end-stage" bladder. The choice of performing a continent versus incontinent diversion is based mainly on patient preference. If a patient has significant urethral symptoms, an orthotopic neobladder may not be the preferred conduit. The benefits of continent diversions are obvious; however, there have been reports of IC developing in the continent bowel segments. An informed and motivated patient would be the best candidate for a continent diversion. The techniques of cystectomy and urinary diversion, including complications, are described in detail in Section III.

Cytolysis

Bladder denervation procedures have been reported in the treatment of patients with intractable bladder pain and urinary frequency and urgency (3). Division of the posterior sacral roots, posterior rhizotomy, or division of the inferior vesical neurovascular pedicle has resulted in temporary improvement in urinary frequency, urgency, and pain. Ingelmann-Sundberg described a more selective denervation in which a transvaginal approach is used to resect the inferior hypogastric plexus, dividing both the sympathetic and parasympathetic fibers (Fig. 28–6). Candidates for the transvaginal denervation are selected by first performing a subtrigonal injection of bupivacaine, resulting in significant relief of their irritative symptoms.

The patient is placed in a lithotomy position, ureteral stents are placed, and the location of the bladder neck and trigone are located by palpation of the Foley catheter balloon. A posterior-based U-shaped incision is made in the anterior vagina and the vaginal epithelium is sharply dissected off the underlying proximal urethra, bladder neck, and distal trigone. The vaginal epithelium is then reapproximated using a running suture of 2-0 or 3-0 Vicryl. The ureteral stents are removed and the Foley catheter is left indwelling for 24 hours.

Sacral Nerve Stimulation

Chronic inflammation in a pelvic organ may lead to nerve upregulation to the spinal cord, affecting all pelvic structures. Sacral nerve modulation (InterStim Medtronic, Inc) is approved by the FDA for urinary urgency, frequency, urge incontinence, and idiopathic urinary retention. Preoperatively, the efficacy of sacral nerve stimulation is determined by a test performed prior to placing a permanent generator. If a patient experiences at least a 50% improvement in their symptoms and desires a permanent implant, the neurogenerator can be placed permanently in a subcutaneous pocket in the upper buttocks. Patients have an external programmer to control the degree of stimulation.

InterStim therapy has evolved since its approval in the United States in 1997. Initially, a percutaneous lead was placed in the sacral foramen under local anesthetic in the office and the lead was taped to the skin. The patient was discharged to home with an external stimulating box and the lead was stimulated for 3 to 5 days while voiding diaries were kept. The lead was then removed and patients responding to the test were candidates for a permanent implant that was performed in the operating room under a general anesthetic. The permanent implant was relatively complicated because it required exposing the periosteum of the sacrum, dissecting the foramen, and securing the permanent lead to the bone after testing for muscle response. This lead was then connected to an implantable pulse generator placed in a subcutaneous pocket under the upper buttocks.

Several problems were identified with the percutaneous testing/implant technique. These include migration of the percutaneous lead resulting in an inadequate test period, uncomfortable sensory response when the permanent lead was placed under a general anesthetic, the morbid nature of placing the permanent lead, and the inability to duplicate placement of the permanent lead in the identical location of the temporary percutaneous lead, resulting in a poor clinical response. The most significant advance with InterStim therapy is the introduction of a tined permanent quadripolar lead, allowing for percutaneous placement of the permanent lead for the test period. The most common procedure for InterStim therapy is a "staged implant."

Staged Implant

The patient is given broad-spectrum antibiotic coverage, lightly sedated, and placed in the prone position on the operating room table. The lower back and buttocks are prepped and draped. Fluoroscopy is used to mark the midline of the sacrum and the sacral iliac junction. This intersection corresponds to the area of the S3 foramen. A mark is made 2 cm lateral and superior to this intersection, the area is infiltrated with lidocaine, and the foramen needle is

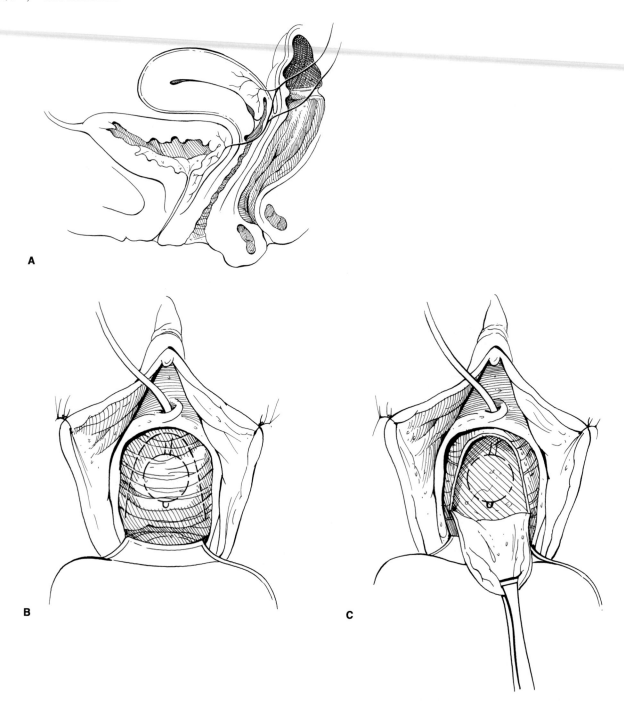

FIG. 28–6. Ingelmann-Sundberg transvaginal denervation. **A:** Diagram depicting the position of the nerves innervating the bladder and their position relative to the trigone and bladder neck. **B:** Outline of the posterior-based inverted-U-shaped incision. The Foley balloon depicts the location of the trigone. **C:** Completed sharp dissection of the vaginal epithelial flap exposing the bladder neck and trigone. After completion of the dissection, the vaginal epithelium is reapproximated with running 2-0 or 3-0 absorbable sutures.

advanced at a 60-degree angle into the S3 foramen with fluoroscopic guidance (Fig. 28–7). Current is applied to the needle and the motor and sensory response is assessed. An ideal motor response is good anal bellows, sacral flattening, and minimal dorsiflexion of the greater toe. The patient should report a gentle tapping or pulsating sensa-

tion in the rectal, vaginal, or perineal region. If the stimulation is painful, the lead should be readjusted in the operating room. To confirm S3 placement, a needle is always passed into the foramen superior to the first. Stimulation of this lead results in leg rotation consistent with S2 placement and this ensures S3 placement of the final electrode.

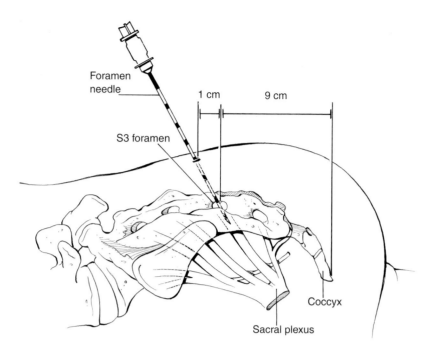

FIG. 28–7. Insertion of a foramen needle through the S3 foramen in preparation for testing the motor and sensory responses.

Next, a small skin nick is made alongside the needle, through the dermis of the skin. A directional guide wire is passed through the foramen needle and the needle is removed. The lead introducer is advanced over the guide wire, through the dorsolumbar fascia and the foramen, and below the bone plate. The trocar is removed and the permanent quadripolar lead (Medtronic no. 3889) is advanced through the lead introducer (Fig. 28–8). Fluoroscopy is used to confirm that all four stimulation points lie beneath the sacral bone plate. The patient is awakened and sensory and motor responses are assessed with stimulation of each electrode. After confirming good lead placement, the lead introducer is removed under fluoroscopy, deploying the tines to secure the lead. A site on the ipsilateral upper buttocks is chosen where a future permanent generator would be placed if the patient responded to therapy. A small (2

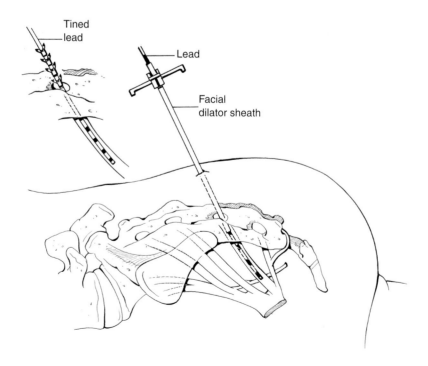

FIG. 28–8. Stage I implant. Advancement of permanent tined lead through the lead introducer parallel to the nerve (see inset). Motor and sensory response tested and lead introducer removed, deploying the tines and securing the lead.

cm) transverse incision is made and a subcutaneous pocket created. The proximal end of the lead is then tunneled to this pocket using the lead introducer. The permanent lead is then connected to a temporary extension wire and the distal end of the wire is tunneled to the contralateral upper buttocks and externalized (Fig. 28–9).

One of four electrodes is chosen for initial outpatient stimulation and the patient is discharged wearing the standard external generator for 2 weeks. The permanent lead allows for four different points of stimulation along the nerve and a multitude of variables such as rate, pulse width, and voltage can be adjusted by the patient with guidance from the clinician over the phone. The patient monitors voids per day, voided volume, urge scores, incontinence episodes, and pelvic pain during the 2-week test period. Responders are considered those with at least a 50% improvement in symptoms and the desire for a permanent implant based on improvement in quality of life. Nonresponders have the leads removed while responders have a permanent generator placed. Permanent generator placement in the staged technique involves extending the incision and subcutaneous pocket in the ipsilateral but-

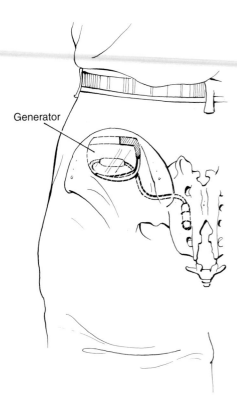

FIG. 28–10. Stage II implant. Patients not responding to the therapy have the lead removed. Responders have the extension lead removed, the ipsilateral subcutaneous pocket extended, and the generator placed. The generator is then programmed to the settings that gave a good clinical response during the test phase.

tocks, removing the temporary extension lead, and connecting the permanent generator (Fig. 28–10). At the end of the procedure, the generator is programmed to the settings to which the patient responded during the test stimulation so that there is no interruption in therapy.

OUTCOMES

Complications

Complications of hydrodistension with or without fulguration are listed in Table 28–1. The most serious complication is bladder rupture, which should be considered

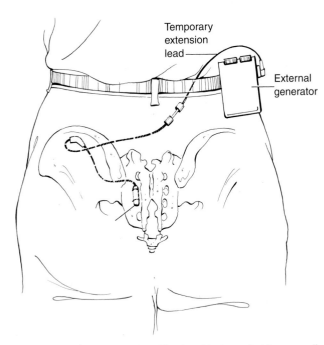

FIG. 28–9. Stage I implant. The lead is tunneled to a small, subcutaneous pocket on the ipsilateral side. The lead is then connected to a temporary extension lead, which is tunneled to the contralateral side and externalized. The external generator is then connected to the extension lead. The patient is discharged to home and sacral nerve stimulation is tested over a 14- to 21-day period. Voiding logs and pain scores are maintained and the program is changed as needed to maximize the clinical response.

TABLE 28–1. *Complications of bladder hydrodistension and fulguration of ulcers*

Gross Hematuria
Bladder Rupture of Perforation
Urinary Tract Infection
Exacerbation of Bladder Symptoms
Bowel Perforation

if there is resumption of fluid inflow after maximally distending the bladder, return of significantly less fluid than what was instilled upon bladder draining, or severe suprapubic or abdominal pain or distension. If a bladder rupture is suspected, an immediate cystogram should be performed. Prolonged Foley catheter drainage is usually all that is needed to allow the rupture to heal spontaneously.

Early and late complications secondary to major bladder reconstruction are listed in Table 28–2. Persistence of IC symptoms is probably the most common and disheartening outcome for both the patient and surgeon.

The major risk of selective denervation cytolysis is ureteral injury during the vaginal dissection and is avoidable by placing ureteral catheters.

No serious, irreversible adverse events have been reported with sacral nerve stimulation. Infection of the device requiring explantation occurs infrequently. Perioperative, broad-spectrum antibiotic coverage during implantation of the lead and generator should be administered to decrease the rate of infection. Reoperation occurs in 10% to 40% of patients undergoing sacral nerve implantation. Causes for reoperation include sensory discomfort, lead migration, device failure, pocket revision, and infection.

Results

Symptoms of IC may worsen for 2 to 3 weeks after a hydrodistension. Approximately 40% to 50% of IC patients undergoing a hydrodistension will have prolonged symptom improvement. If symptoms improve significantly for at least 4 to 6 months, repeat bladder hydrodistension may be indicated. Fulguration of Hunner's ulcers improves greater than 80% of patients undergoing this therapy. The improvement in pain is usually seen in the first 2 to 3 days and may be long-lasting. For those who relapse, repeat fulguration of ulcers usually yield a similar response.

The more aggressive, open surgical approaches have shown good results in carefully selected patients. Relief of symptoms in patients undergoing reconstructive surgery ranges between 60% to 90%. Patients with classic ulcerative IC have been reported to have better results. Although a significant percentage of this highly select group of patients who undergo cystectomy will experience significant relief, there are reports of patients having persistent pelvic pain despite having no pelvic organs.

Recently, we reviewed our experience with sacral nerve modulation for refractory IC (5). When a traditional test was performed with a temporary lead, we had a test-to-implant rate of 52% versus a 94% test-to-implant rate in the staged approach. The benefit of the staged test is that the permanent lead is more programmable and can be tested for an extended period of time. If a response is found, the lead does not need to be removed prior to placing the generator and the settings that worked on the temporary generator can be programmed into the permanent implanted neurostimulator so that there is no interruption in therapy. Twenty-six patients with refractory IC who have failed six previous treatments for their disease were implanted with a permanent generator. With a mean follow-up of 5.6 months, 96% of patients said they would undergo the implant again and would recommend the therapy to a friend. Significant improvements were seen in the number of day voids (47%) and nocturia (60%). The majority of patients reported at least a 50% improvement in frequency (72%), urgency (68%), pelvic pain (71%), pelvic pressure (67%), quality of life (76%), incontinence (69%) and vaginal pain (60%). No patients showed a greater than 50% worsening in any symptom. The overall reoperation rate was 11.5% (3 of 26). An objective measurement of pain improvement was reported. Twenty IC patients with pelvic pain had a permanent implant placed with a median follow-up of 272 days. Seventeen of 20 (85%) used chronic narcotics prior to implant. Nineteen of 20 (95%) reported moderate or marked improvement in pain after implantation of permanent generator. Morphine dose equivalents (MDEs) decreased from 86 mg per day to 56 mg per day (34%) (P = 0.015) after implant and 24% stopped all narcotics.

TABLE 28–2. *Complications of major bladder reconstructive surgery*

Early
 Ileus
 Intraperitoneal Abscess
 Upper-Tract Obstruction
 Thromboembolic Events
 Pneumonia
 Wound Infection
 Cardiac Events
 Difficulty with Catheterization
Late
 Persistence of Interstitial Cystitis Symptoms
 Upper-Tract Deterioration
 Urolithiasis
 Metabolic Abnormalities
 Spontaneous Rupture of Bowel Conduit
 Difficulty with Catheterization
 Ureteral Stenosis
 Ureteral Reflux
 Neoplasia
 Bladder Neck Contracture
 Urinary Incontinence
 Pyelonephritis/Urinary Tract Infection

REFERENCES

1. Hanno PM, Landis JR, Matthews-Cook Y, et al. The diagnosis of interstitial cystitis: Lessons learned from the National Institutes of Health interstitial cystitis database study. *J Urol* 1999;161:553–557.

2. Hunner GL. A rare type of bladder ulcer in women: Report of cases. *Boston Med Surg J* 1915;172:660–664.
3. Ingelmann-Sundberg A. Partial bladder denervation in the treatment of interstitial cystitis in women. In: Hanno PM, Staskin DR, Krane RJ, Wein AJ, eds. *Interstitial cystitis*. London: Springer-Verlag, 1990;189.
4. Parsons CL. Potassium sensitivity test. *Tech Urol* 1996;2:171–173.
5. Peters KM, Carey JM, Karstardt DB. Sacral neuromodulation for the treatment of refractary interstitial cystitis: outcomes based on technique. *Int Urogynecol* 2003;14:223–228.
6. Rofeim O, Hom D, Freid RM, Moldwin RM. Use of the neodymium:YAG laser for interstitial cystitis: a prospective study. *J Urol* 2001;166:134–136.

SECTION IV

Prostate

SECTION EDITOR: Randall G. Rowland

Anatomy

Sam D. Graham, Jr.

The normal prostate is a firm, elastic organ located immediately below the bladder and resting on the superior layer of the urogenital diaphragm to which it is firmly attached. The normal adult prostate is approximately 4 cm in length and 4cm to 5 cm in width. It is traversed throughout its length by the urethra and ejaculatory ducts entering at the base and terminating in the posterior prostatic urethra.

In the past the prostate has been divided into three to seven lobes. Most commonly, these segments are the two lateral lobes, a median lobe, a posterior lobe, and an anterior lobe. With the advent of ultrasound, the anatomy is now defined as a transition zone comprised of periurethral glands and a peripheral zone or true prostate. Anatomically, no true lobar anatomy exists and the prostate has been shown to have the two concentric areas seen on ultrasound. The peripheral zone is mostly posteriorly located and is comprised of long, branched glands from which most carcinomas are thought to arrive. The central zone is comprised of submucosal glanduloductal units and short glands from which prostatic hypertrophy is thought to arise. Scattered throughout the prostate are smooth muscle fibers that are thought to be involved in ejaculation.

The prostate has a tough capsule of fibrous tissue and muscular elements completely enveloping the prostate and is densely adherent to it. This capsule is actually aglandular prostatic tissue that is connected to the acini and inseparable from the parenchyma. This is surrounded by a periprostatic fascia.

There are significant fascial investments around the prostate. The endopelvic fascia is a continuation of the endoabdominal fascia. In the pelvis, there are three parts of this fascial plane (1). The parietal layer covers the muscles lining the pelvic wall (pyriformis, and obturator internus) and continues superiorly to connect with the transversalis and iliopsoas fascias. All somatic nerves except for the obturator nerve are beneath this fascial layer. A thickening of this fascia extending from the pubis to the ischial spine is known as the arcus tendineus. The second portion of the endopelvic fascia (diaphragmatic portion) covers the two muscles on each side of the pelvis whicdh makes up the pelvis diaphragm (coccygeus and levator ani). A third (visceral) portion of the endopelvic fascia is continuous with the diaphragmatic fascia and extends upon the pelvic organs for a variable distance, blending into their fibrous coats. Anteriorly, the endopelvic fascia coalesces into the medial puboprostatic ligaments connecting the pubis to the prostatic capsule. The lateral puboprostatic ligaments extend from the superior diaphragmatic layer of the endopelvic fascia to the prostate.

Posteriorly, the prostate is invested by the two layers of Denonvillier's fascia which embryologically is derived from the peritoneum. The posterior layer exists as the rectal fascia, while the anterior layer fuses laterally to the endopelvic and periprostatic fascia.

The urethra runs completely through the prostate though the path is angled approximately 45° at the veru montanum. The veru montanum represents the terminal end of the ejaculatory ducts as they course through the prostate from the seminal vesicles/vas deferens (Figure SIV-1). The opening in the apex of the veru montanum is known as the prostatic utricle. In addition, there are a series of ductal openings directly into the prostatic urethra from the prostatic glands. The urethra exits the

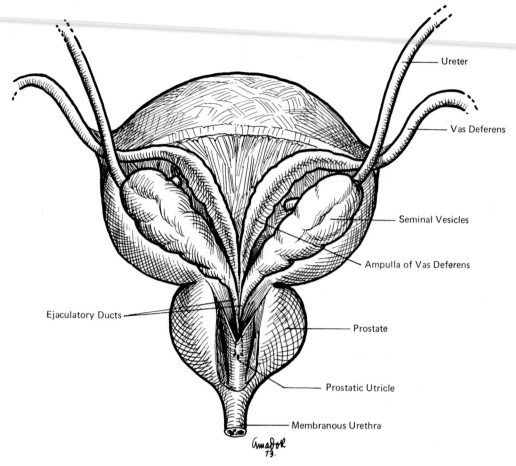

FIG. SIV–1. Relationship of the prostate and the seminal vesicles.

prostate at the apex and while the anatomical drawings traditionally show the apex directly on the pelvic floor, dissections during radical prostatectomies show that there is approximately a 1 cm gap from the apex to the pelvic floor.

VASCULAR ANATOMY

The prostatic blood supply comes predominantly from the internal iliac artery and is a series of lateral pedicles, the most prominent and constant of which is the pedicle at the base of the prostate (superior prostatic artery) Additional branches may also exist most usually at the apex of the prostate (Figure SIV-2). The superior prostatic artery enters just below the bladder neck and forms two branches, one to the capsule and the other to the urethra. As patients age, the latter becomes more prominent with prostatic enlargement (2). Other sites of origin for the prostatic artery are the internal pudendal, the superior vesical, or the obturator artery.

The past 20 years have emphasized the "nerve sparing" technique for both prostatectomy and cystectomy. This operation is actually a neurovascular sparing technique which involves separating the neurovascular bundle from the prostate. The neurovascular bundle can be located along the posterior lateral prostate at the base of the prostate beneath the anterior layer of Denonvillier's fascia. More distally, the neurovascular bundle crosses the apex of the prostate and enters the pelvic diaphragm posteriorlaterlly to the membranous urethra.

The venous drainage of the prostate is via the anterior venous plexus (Santorini) which is found on the anterior and lateral prostate. This plexus receives blood from the dorsal vein of the penis and empties into the hypogastric vein.

LYMPHATIC ANATOMY

The lymphatic drainage of the prostate is predominantly along the path of the prostatic artery with the primary nodal drop site being the obturator nodes. Other potential sites of nodal metastases include the external iliac and presacral nodes.

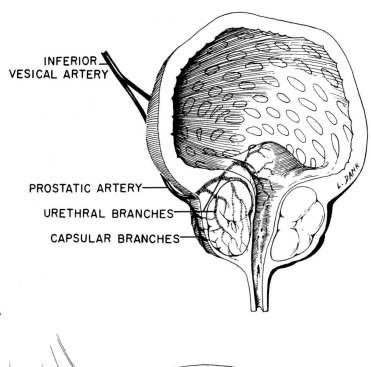

INFERIOR
VESICAL ARTERY

PROSTATIC ARTERY

URETHRAL BRANCHES

CAPSULAR BRANCHES

A

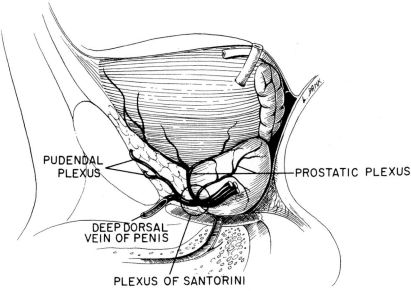

PUDENDAL
PLEXUS

PROSTATIC PLEXUS

DEEP DORSAL
VEIN OF PENIS

PLEXUS OF SANTORINI

B

FIG. SIV–2. Vascular anatomy of the prostate. **(A)** Arterial anatomy. **(B)** Venous anatomy.

NEUROANATOMY

The prostate has sympathetic, parasympathetic, and somatic innervation. The sympathetic innervation is from L1 and L2 via the superior hypogastric plexus. The parasympathetic and somatic innervation is from S2,3,4 via the inferior hypogastric plexus and pudendal nerves respectively.

CONTIGUOUS STRUCTURES

The prostate is inferior to the bladder and anterior to the rectum (Figure SIV-3). The perineal anatomy is a complex of muscles and tendons that comprise the pelvic floor. Beginning from the skin of the perineum, the superficial (Camper's) and deep (Colle's) fascia. The latter is attached to the ischiopubic rami and the border of the urogenital diaphragm and is continuous with Scarpa's fascia. The most superficial pelvic musculature is the ischiocavernosus, the bulbocavernosus, the superficial transverse perineal muscles, and the external anal sphincter (Figure SIV-4). These muscles are united in the midline as a central tendon (perineal body) and function as a single muscle. This central tendon is attached to the bulb of the rectum by fibrous

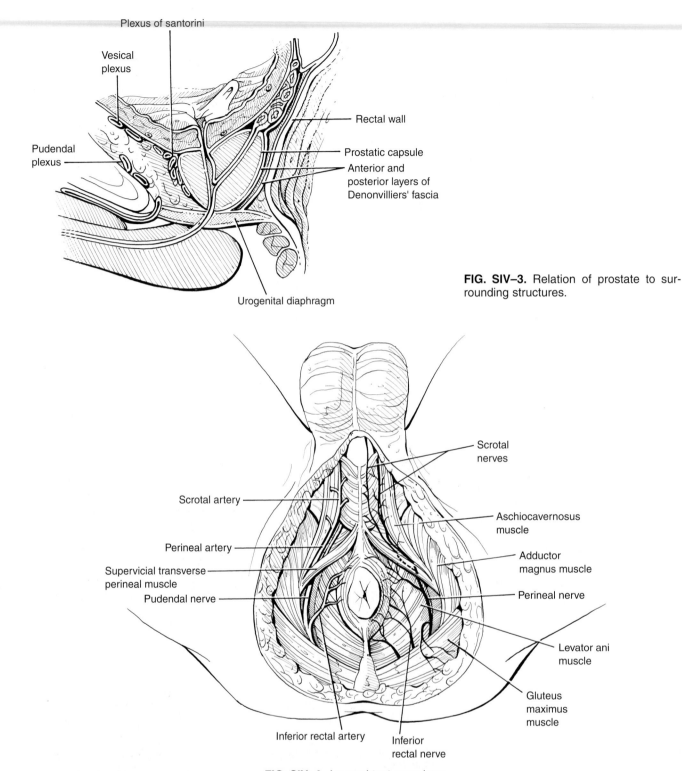

FIG. SIV–3. Relation of prostate to surrounding structures.

FIG. SIV–4. Legend text goes here.

bands of muscle known as the rectus urethralis (3). Beneath this layer of muscles is the deep perineal compartment which is predominantly the urogenital diaphragm which is attached to the inferior rami of the ischia and pubis.

REFERENCES

1. Healey JE. *A Synopsis of Clinical Anatomy.* Philadelphia: WB Saunders, 1969.
2. Brendler H. Prostatic hypertrophy and perineal surgery. In: Urologic Surgery, JF Glenn, ed. Hagerstown: Harper and Row, 1975.
3. Weyrauch HM. *Surgery of the Prostate.* Philadelphia: WB Saunders, 1959.

CHAPTER 29

Open Prostatectomy

Ray E. Stutzman

Open prostatectomy is the enucleation of the hyperplastic adenomatous growth of the prostate. This procedure does not involve total removal of the prostate. A tissue plane exists between the adenoma and the compressed true prostate, which is left intact. Three surgical approaches to the prostate are described in this chapter: suprapubic, retropubic, and perineal.

DIAGNOSIS

Over 90% of prostatectomies for benign prostatic hyperplasia are performed by transurethral resection of the prostate (TURP). When the obstructing tissue is estimated to weigh more than 50 g, serious consideration should be given to an open procedure. Digital examination, prostatic ultrasound, and cystourethroscopic measurement of the prostatic length may aid in estimation of the size of the gland. Findings on cystourethroscopy may indicate an open procedure, such as sizable bladder diverticuli, which justify removal, or large bladder calculi, which are not amenable to easy fragmentation. The association of an inguinal hernia with an enlarged prostate may lead to a suprapubic or retropubic procedure because the hernia may be repaired by way of the same lower-abdominal incision (12).

INDICATIONS FOR SURGERY

The indications for prostatectomy include the following symptoms or findings secondary to prostatic obstruction: acute urinary retention; recurrent or persistent urinary tract infections (UTIs); recurrent gross hematuria; documented significant residual urine after voiding with or without overflow incontinence; pathophysiological changes of the kidneys, ureters, or bladder; abnormally low urinary flow rate; and normal flow rate with abnormally high intravesical voiding pressure and intractable symptoms such as nocturia, frequency, and urgency.

Contraindications to an open prostatectomy include a small, fibrous gland, carcinoma of the prostate, or prior prostatectomy in which most of the prostate has previously been resected or removed and the planes are obliterated.

ALTERNATIVE THERAPY

Alternative therapies to open prostatectomy include TURP, endoscopic procedures including incision of the prostate, laser ablation, vaporization techniques, thermotherapy, and medical management. Most of these therapies are effective for moderate (medical management) to severe symptoms in prostates less than 60 g (alternative surgical techniques) and are therefore not indicated in the majority of patients who are candidates for open prostatectomy. The patient's bladder outlet symptoms could also be managed alternatively by intermittent catheterization, an indwelling catheter, or a suprapubic cystostomy. None of these are good alternatives if the patient is a reasonable surgical risk.

SURGICAL TECHNIQUE

Preoperative Management

The average age of patients is about 70. Many patients have histories of cardiovascular disease, chronic obstructive pulmonary disease, diabetes, or hypertension. It is preferable to evaluate the upper urinary tract with either an intravenous (IV) pyelogram and a postvoid film if the patient's renal function is normal or an abdominal radiograph and a renal sonogram. Cystourethroscopic examination should be performed to rule out unexpected bladder pathology. This can be done just before surgery under the same anesthetic. If the patient has a documented UTI, it should be treated before planned elective surgery and may necessitate indwelling catheter drainage before the procedure.

Transfusion of blood may be required in about 15% of patients undergoing open prostatectomy. It is prudent to have 2 or 3 U of blood available when contemplating the procedure. The safest transfusion is autologous blood, and individual units can be drawn 1 week apart while the patient is on oral iron medication.

Spinal or epidural anesthesia is preferred in all prostatectomy procedures. If regional anesthesia is contraindicated, a general anesthetic with adequate relaxation may be used.

Informed consent is necessary. The patient must be made aware of the risks and complications. Most patients can be evaluated as an outpatient and then admitted to the hospital on the day of surgery. This is cost effective and reduces hospitalization.

Suprapubic Prostatectomy

Suprapubic prostatectomy or transvesical prostatectomy is the enucleation of the hyperplastic adenomatous growth of the prostate performed through an extraperitoneal incision of the anterior bladder wall (9). Eugene Fuller of New York is credited with performing the first complete suprapubic removal of a prostatic adenoma in 1894. This was a blind procedure with digital enucleation of the gland. Suprapubic and perineal drainage tubes were placed to wash out clots and control bleeding. Peter Freyer of London popularized the operation and subsequently published his results of over 1,600 cases with a mortality rate of just over 5%. The entire operation was usually a 15-minute procedure. A 5- to 8-cm midline suprapubic incision was made, and the bladder was opened without opening the lateral tissue spaces or entering the space of Retzius. Digital enucleation of the prostate was then performed. One or two fingers were placed in the rectum for counterpressure while the suprapubic enucleation was accomplished. The prostatic fossa was left alone because Freyer thought that the capsule and surrounding tissues at the bladder neck would contract down enough to control bleeding, somewhat like a parturient uterus immediately after childbirth. He left an indwelling urethral catheter and a large suprapubic tube to evacuate clots. His low mortality and morbidity rates are remarkable considering that no blood transfusions or antibiotics were available at that time. This blind enucleation remained popular for over 50 years. The low transvesical suprapubic prostatectomy with visualization of the bladder neck and prostatic fossa and placement of hemostatic sutures has supplanted the blind procedure (4). This operation is presented in more detail.

The patient is placed in the supine position with the umbilicus positioned over the kidney rest; the table is slightly hyperextended and in a mild Trendelenburg position. A catheter is introduced into the urinary bladder; the bladder is irrigated and then filled with 200 to 250 mL of water or saline and the catheter is then removed. The abdomen and genitalia are prepped from nipple line to midthigh. A vertical midline suprapubic incision is made through the skin and linea alba with the incision extending from below the umbilicus to the symphysis (Fig. 29–1). The rectus muscles are retracted laterally and the prevesical space is developed, with the peritoneum swept superiorly. It is not necessary or desirable to expose the retropubic or lateral vesical spaces. For more adequate exposure, a self-retaining retractor is used.

Two sutures are placed in the anterior bladder wall below the peritoneal reflection. A vertical cystotomy is then made and the incision is opened down to within 1 cm of the bladder neck, allowing visualization of the bladder neck and prostate. A medium Deaver retractor is placed into the open bladder, retracting superiorly. A narrow Deaver retractor is then placed over the bladder neck just distal to the trigone. The curved end of the Deaver retractor provides an excellent semilunar line for incising the mucosa around the posterior bladder neck just distal to the trigone (Fig. 29–2). By this method, the ureteral orifices are well visualized and are not compromised. Metzenbaum scissors are introduced at the 6-o'clock position and, by gentle dissection, the plane between the adenoma, bladder neck, and the capsule of the prostate is developed.

The remainder of the procedure is done by digital dissection, freeing the posterior lobes down to the apex of the prostate and then circumferentially sweeping anteriorly (Fig. 29–3). The urethra is firmly attached at the

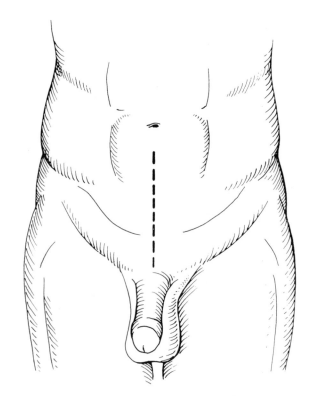

FIG. 29–1. Midline vertical incision.

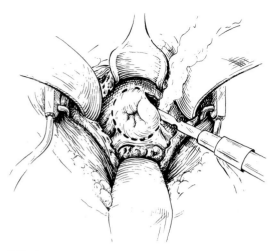

FIG. 29–2. Incision of mucosa over the adenoma.

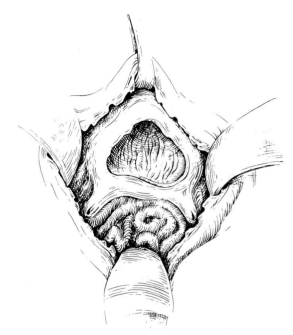

FIG. 29–4. View of the empty prostatic fossa.

apex. It is preferable to use scissors to sharply incise the urethra, keeping close to the prostatic adenoma so as not to cause injury to the sphincter and subsequent incontinence. With large glands it is often preferable to remove one lobe at a time, or if there is a large intravesical protrusion of the middle lobe this may be removed separately.

After removal of the adenoma, the prostatic fossa is inspected and a digital sweep is made to ascertain if there is any remaining nodular adenomatous tissue (Fig. 29–4). There is usually minimal bleeding; however, bleeding is frequently seen in the 5- and 7-o'clock positions. The prostatic arteries enter the capsule and prostate at this level near the bladder neck. Suture ligature of these vessels is done even if there is no active bleeding (Fig. 29–5). Figure-of-eight sutures of 2-0 chromic on a ⅝ circle needle provide good hemostasis.

A 22 Fr, 30-mL balloon, three-way Foley catheter is passed through the urethra. A 26 or 28 Fr Malecot suprapubic tube is passed through a separate stab wound in the anterior bladder wall and brought out through a stab

wound in the lower abdominal wall (Fig. 29–6). A watertight, single-layer, interrupted closure of the bladder with either 2-0 chromic catgut or Vicryl is done, just missing the mucosa but including full thickness of the muscularis and serosa. The balloon of the Foley catheter is inflated to 45 mL and placed on no traction. A 4-0 chromic catgut suture is placed as a pursestring around the suprapubic tube; this prevents any leakage and helps hold the suprapubic tube gently in position during wound closure. A

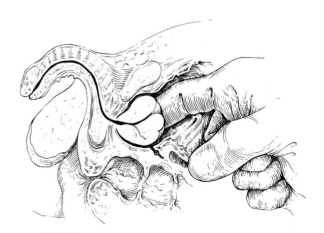

FIG. 29–3. Digital enucleation of the adenoma.

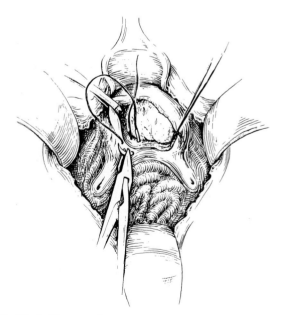

FIG. 29–5. Hemostatic suture ligatures at the 5- and 7-o'clock positions.

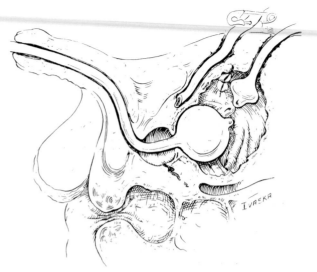

FIG. 29–6. Foley catheter snug at the bladder neck: prevesical drain and Malecot catheter.

Penrose drain is placed down to the cystotomy site and brought out through a separate stab wound. The bladder is irrigated until clear and checked for significant leakage.

The wound is irrigated and the linea alba is closed with a running no. 2 nylon or no. 1 PDS suture. The skin is approximated with skin staples. The drain and suprapubic tube are sutured to the skin with nylon sutures and a dressing is applied (11).

Postoperatively, excessive blood loss is the most common immediate complication encountered; about 15% of

patients require a blood transfusion. If excessive bleeding from the prostatic fossa is noted intraoperatively, two techniques are effective in stopping the bleeding. Malament described the placement of a no. 1 or no. 2 nylon pursestring suture around the vesical neck; the suture was brought out through the skin and tied snugly (7). This effectively closes the bladder neck and tamponades the prostatic fossa with control of bleeding (Fig. 29–7). Between 24 and 48 hours after placement, the suture is cut on one side and removed. O'Conor (10) described placation of the posterior capsule using 0 chromic catgut on a ⅝ curved needle. This placation narrows the fossa and results in effective hemostasis (Fig. 29–8). Point fulguration of bleeders in the fossa may also provide hemostasis.

Antibiotics are not indicated for elective prostatectomy in patients who have had no UTIs and have sterile urine. If there has been a long-term indwelling catheter or preoperative infection, appropriate perioperative antibiotics, a cephalosporin and an aminoglycoside or a fluoroquinolone, are indicated.

The patient is usually limited to IV fluids the day of surgery, but the following day he can usually tolerate oral nutrition, often having a full diet. A stool softener or mild laxative is given to prevent straining with bowel movements or fecal impaction. Continuous bladder irrigation by way of the three-way Foley catheter is maintained for 12 to 24 hours. The Foley catheter usually is removed after 3 days, although one can remove the suprapubic catheter first. If the Foley catheter is removed first, the suprapubic tube is clamped at 5 days to give the patient a trial at voiding. It is removed the following day if voiding

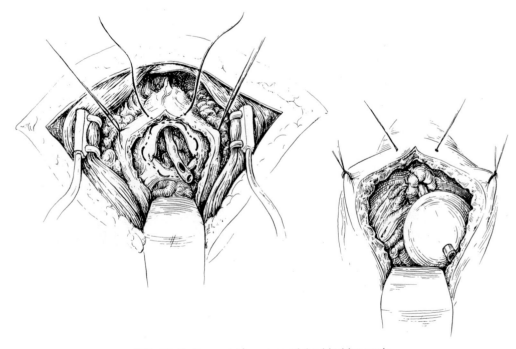

FIG. 29–7. Pursestring suture of the bladder neck.

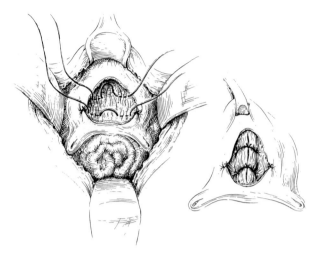

FIG. 29–8. Plicating sutures in the posterior capsule.

is satisfactory with little residual. The drain is removed a few hours after removal of the suprapubic tube if there is no drainage. The skin staples are removed on the postoperative day 7 and the skin is covered with sterile strips. On discharge from the hospital, the patient is encouraged to increase his activity gradually and should be able to resume full activity 4 to 6 weeks postoperatively, with outpatient visits at 3 and 6 weeks.

Retropubic Prostatectomy

Simple retropubic prostatectomy is the removal of the hyperplastic prostatic adenoma by way of a prostatic capsule incision. Van Stockum is credited with performing the first retropubic prostatectomy, which he called "extravesical suprapubic prostatectomy" (14). A longitudinal capsular incision was made on one side of the midline. Millin (8) reported his operative technique and results in 1945. His procedure gained wide acceptance, and he is credited with popularizing retropubic prostatectomy. Various modifications have subsequently been described (1,3,13).

The patient is placed in the supine position with the umbilicus positioned over the kidney rest; the table is slightly hyperextended and in a mild Trendelenburg position. The lower abdomen and suprapubic area are shaved and the entire operative field from nipple line to midthigh is scrubbed with surgical solution. A Pfannenstiel incision (Fig. 29–9) may be used, but I prefer a vertical midline incision extending from below the umbilicus to the symphysis (see Fig. 29–1). The linea alba is opened and the rectus muscles are retracted laterally.

The prevesical and retropubic space is developed, with the peritoneum and extraperitoneal fat swept superiorly. A self-retaining retractor is placed in the incision to obtain maximal exposure. There are several large veins in the loose areolar tissue and fat over the anterior capsule

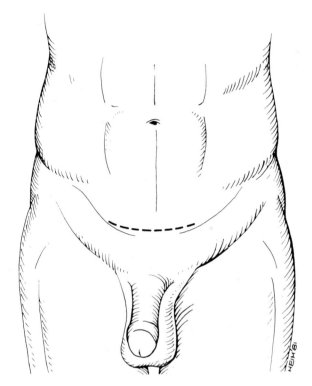

FIG. 29–9. Modified Pfannenstiel incision.

of the prostate. These should be suture ligated and divided; smaller vessels may be fulgurated to avoid troublesome bleeding (Fig. 29–10).

The vesical neck can be visualized and palpated. Two traction sutures are placed in the prostatic capsule above and below the planned site of the capsular incision, which is made about 1 cm distal to the bladder neck (Fig. 29–11). As the capsule is opened, one can recognize the

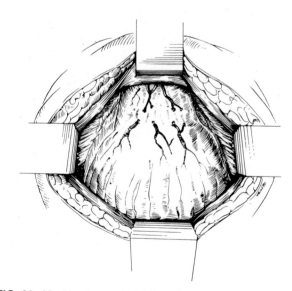

FIG. 29–10. Ligation and division of periprostatic veins over the prostatic capsule anteriorly.

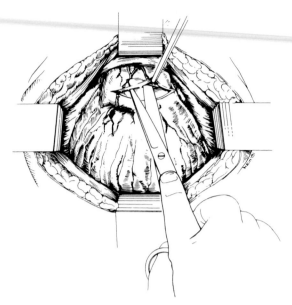

FIG. 29–11. Transfixion sutures placed on the capsule anteriorly with an incision made transversely in the prostatic capsule.

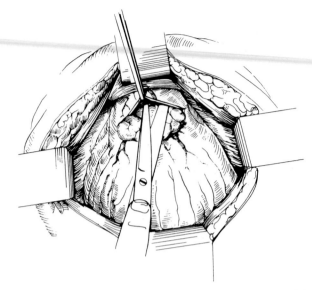

FIG. 29–13. Continuing the dissection of the prostate of the adenoma from the prostatic capsule using Metzenbaum scissors.

white outer part of the adenoma. The length of the incision depends on the size of the gland and should be sufficient to dissect the adenoma.

The cleavage plane between the prostatic adenoma and the surgical capsule or true prostate is developed using Metzenbaum scissors (Figs. 29–12 and 29–13). The dissection may be completed with scissors; in large adenomas, digital enucleation can easily be performed. The urethra is firmly attached at the apex. It is preferable to use scissors to incise the urethra sharply, keeping close to

the prostatic adenoma to avoid causing injury to the sphincter and subsequent incontinence.

After removal of the prostatic adenoma, the fossa is inspected for any remaining nodules of adenoma and for sites of bleeding. The main sources of bleeding are the arteries at the 5- and 7-o'clock positions, which lie just distal to the bladder neck. Figure-of-eight suture ligatures of 2-0 chromic catgut are placed to secure hemostasis (Fig. 29–14). Bleeding vessels in the prostatic fossa can be fulgurated under direct visualization. If the surgeon wears a headlight for illumination, visualization is much improved.

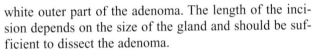

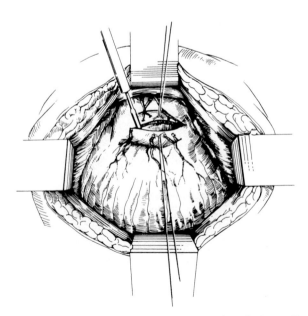

FIG. 29–12. Identification of the cleavage plane between the prostatic adenoma and the surgical capsule of the prostate.

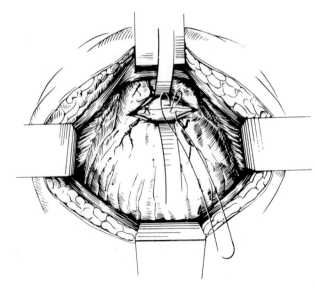

FIG. 29–14. Figure-of-eight sutures are applied at the vesicle neck at the 5- and 7-o'clock positions to secure hemostasis.

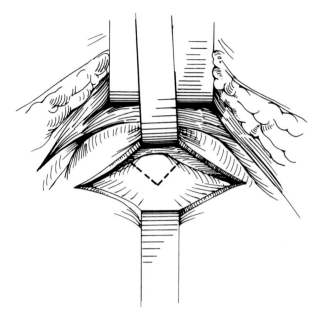

FIG. 29–15. Wedge resection of the vesical neck posteriorly.

In some patients, the posterior lip of the vesical neck is prominent and protrudes into the lumen. This can be removed by wedge resection by grasping the midline with an Allis clamp and, with either scissors or a knife, the wedge can be excised (Fig. 29–15). A running suture may be placed for hemostasis.

A 22 Fr Silastic-coated three-way irrigating Foley catheter with a 30-cc retention balloon is inserted through the urethra into the bladder. The transverse incision of the prostatic capsule is then closed with a continuous suture of 2-0 chromic catgut or Vicryl, ensuring a watertight closure (Fig. 29–16). Slight catheter traction is applied and

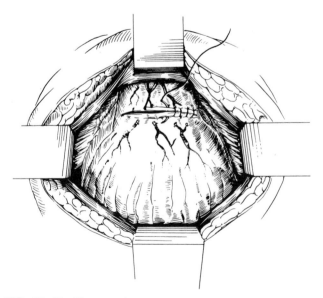

FIG. 29–16. Closure of the incision of the prostate capsule anteriorly with interrupted chromic sutures.

continuous bladder irrigation is instituted. If excessive bleeding from the prostatic fossa is noted, the source should be sought before wound closure. Suture placation of the prostatic fossa may be helpful (see Fig. 29–8). A suprapubic catheter is used only if there is significant bleeding.

A Penrose drain is placed into the space of Retzius and brought out through a stab wound lateral to the incision and sutured to the skin. The wound is irrigated and the linea alba is closed with a running no. 2 nylon or no. 1 PDS suture (11). The skin is approximated with skin staples. A wound and drain dressing is applied.

Postoperatively, the Foley catheter is irrigated until it runs clear and continuous bladder irrigation with saline is used for several hours. The catheter is usually removed on postoperative day 5 or 6. The Penrose drain is moved partially outward on that day and is removed the following day if no drainage occurs. The skin clips are removed and sterile strips are applied.

Perineal Prostatectomy

The first operations for relief of urinary retention from prostatic enlargement were probably done through the perineum, and early medical writings contain references to division of the bladder neck through the perineum for this purpose. Covillard, in 1639, was apparently the first to remove a hypertrophied middle lobe by tearing it away with forceps after perineal lithotomy. In 1848, Sir William Fergusson exhibited specimens of hypertrophied prostates he had enucleated through the perineum after removal of bladder calculi. Kuchler, in 1866, formulated the first systematic technique for radical perineal prostatectomy, but his operations were done only in the cadaver. In 1867, Billroth used Kuchler's method to carry out the first two intentional prostatectomies in living subjects. Apparently, however, the lobes were not entirely removed in these patients.

In 1873, Gouley advocated systematic enucleation of the lateral lobes and excision of the median lobe through the perineum. Goodfellow is credited (4) as the first to perform a perineal prostatectomy successfully on a routine basis. His method involved the use of a midline vertical incision from the base of the scrotum to the anal margin, followed by incision of the membranous urethra, extension of the opening into the bladder, and complete enucleation of the prostatic lobes. His technique, although differing in certain respects from that used today, nevertheless forms the basis of current methods.

During the next decade, a number of technical modifications were suggested by Nicoll, Alexander, Albarran, Proust, dePezzer, Legueu, and others. For the most part, those changes were concerned with improving delivery of the prostatic lobes into the perineal incision for enucleation. In 1903, Young described his operative technique developed at the Johns Hopkins Hospital; this is still the approach most widely used. In 1939, Belt and colleagues introduced an important modification in the perineal approach to the prostate that did much to reduce the risk of rectal injury inherent in the operations of Young and earlier surgeons. Belt's method of closure also was a great improvement over earlier methods and shortened convalescence considerably (2).

Either spinal or general anesthesia can be used. Caudal block is also acceptable. With general anesthesia, tracheal intubation ensures adequate respiratory exchange.

Preoperatively, the patient should self-administer an enema to clean the lower bowel and rectum and receive appropriate antibiotics for a 1-day bowel prep. The genitalia are cleansed thoroughly, after which cystoscopy is performed. The entire operative area, from costal margins to midthigh, is then prepped. Bilateral vas ligation is now rarely performed.

Perfect positioning is essential for the perineal operation. The patient is placed in the exaggerated lithotomy position on any ordinary operating table (Fig. 29–17). Sandbags are placed beneath the sacrum to position the perineum as close to horizontal as possible. The table is then elevated to bring the operative area up to the level of the operator's chest. This makes the operation a good deal easier and improves visualization considerably. The perineum can usually be positioned adequately without resort to the Trendelenburg position, but on occasion a slight Trendelenburg position may be necessary. Under no circumstances should shoulder braces be used for fear of causing postoperative brachial palsy. All other points

where pressure is likely (e.g., popliteal areas) are carefully padded.

The curved Lowsley tractor is passed through the urethra and held upright with blades unopened (Fig. 29–18). A curved skin incision is made about 1 cm from the anal margin. The anus is excluded from the operative field by being covered with a towel secured by three Allis clamps to the posterior edge of the incision. With the index fingers, the ischiorectal fossae are developed perpendicular to the plane of tile perineum. The central tendon is gently separated from the underlying rectum and cut across distal to the external anal sphincter, with care taken not to disturb that structure (Fig. 29–19). A bifid posterior retractor is placed in the ischiorectal fossae and gentle traction is exerted. The lateral fossae are developed next and held with two small lateral retractors. The rectourethralis muscle is identified and cut (Fig. 29–20).

By carefully incising the pararectal fascia (posterior layer of Denonvillier's fascia), the rectum can be gently peeled posteriorly off the apex of the prostate. The Lowsley tractor is passed fully into the bladder and the blades are opened. The bifid posterior retractor is replaced by a plain posterior one (the lipped Richardson is useful here), with a moistened pad used to protect the rectum. The posterior layer of Denonvillier's fascia is progressively incised and retracted posteriorly until a window appears through which the anterior layer of

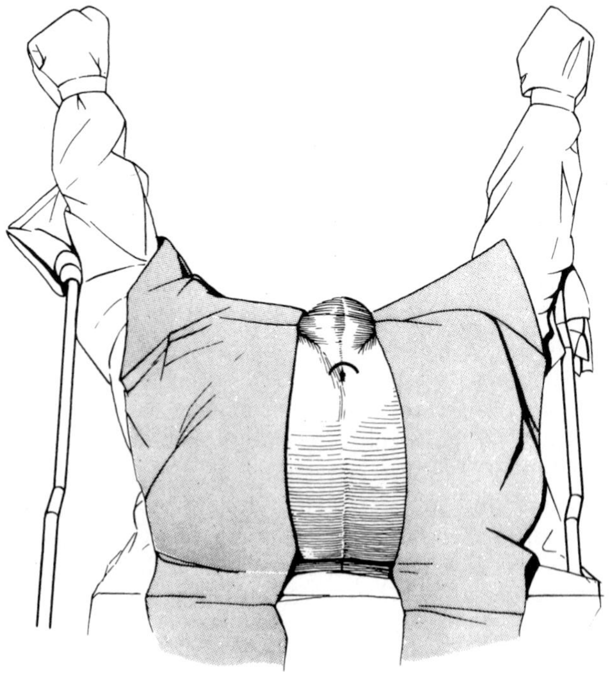

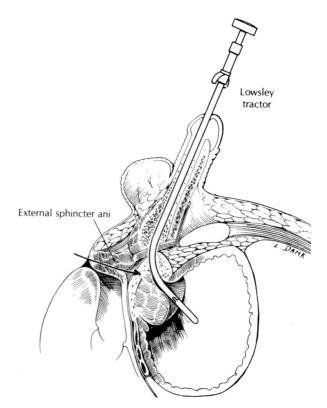

FIG. 29–17. Perineal prostatectomy. A standard operating table is used for the exaggerated lithotomy position. A classic inverted-U incision is shown.

FIG. 29–18. Perineal prostatectomy. A curved Lowsley tractor is in place at the outset of the operation.

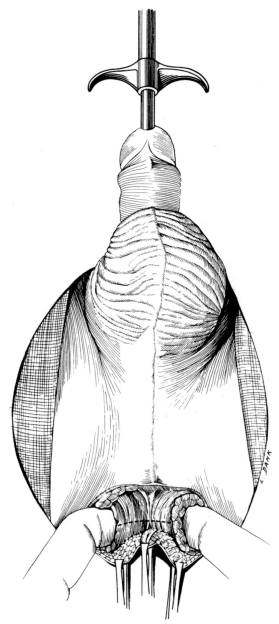

FIG. 29–19. Perineal prostatectomy. After the perineal incision, ischiorectal fossae are developed by blunt dissection. The central tendon of the perineum is isolated. The line of incision is shown.

Denonvillier's fascia—the "pearly gates"—can be seen clearly.

At this point, the operator simultaneously depresses the handle of the Lowsley tractor toward the abdominal wall and exerts firm downward traction on the posterior Richardson retractor (Fig. 29–21). The remaining posterior fascial layer is thereby stripped away from the prostate, which comes clearly into view, covered only by the glistening anterior layer of Denonvillier's fascia. This is a most effective maneuver, but it should not be done before dissection of the posterior fascial layer has been completed at the apex.

An inverted-V or curved prostatotomy is made (Fig. 29–22) and a plane of cleavage is established with the dissecting scissors (Fig. 29–23A). Care is taken to peel back and preserve the posterior flap for subsequent closure of the prostatotomy. The urethra is incised, the curved Lowsley tractor is removed, and the regular Young prostatic tractor is inserted gently into the bladder through the prostatotomy, using a rotary motion. The blades of the tractor are then opened, the prostate is drawn down, and enucleation is begun.

As soon as possible, the urethra at the apex of the adenoma is cut across with the scissors, thereby facilitating enucleation distally and minimizing the danger of damage to the external urethral sphincter (see Fig. 29–23B). Enucleation is carried out essentially under direct vision, using the scissors and the finger. Enucleation can sometimes be facilitated by removing the Young tractor and grasping the lobes with forceps especially designed for this purpose. The lobes can then be drawn progressively into the operative field. The hypertrophied lobes are cut away sharply from the bladder neck under direct vision (Fig. 29–24). With care, the bladder neck can be preserved intact, even after removal of a large adenoma.

After enucleation has been completed, the bladder neck is grasped with Millin T-clamps, which were originally designed for the retropubic operation. These have the advantage of being offset so that one can obtain an unimpeded view of the bladder neck (Fig. 29–25). A careful search is made for bleeding vessels (especially at the 5- and 7-o'clock positions). Smaller ones are controlled effectively by electrocoagulation. Larger arteries require mattress sutures of 2-0 plain catgut. The interior of the bladder is explored with the finger and any blood clots are removed. The entire prostatic fossa is inspected carefully for residual adenomatous tissue. Remaining tags of tissue are trimmed away from the bladder neck.

A 22 Fr Foley catheter is passed through the urethra and into the bladder, where the balloon is inflated with 30 to 45 mL of water. The bladder neck, which feels like a soft cervical os dilated to about two finger widths, retains the balloon nicely. Wedge resection of the posterior lip is in general unnecessary. If desired, a three-way Foley catheter may be used to permit through-and-through irrigations postoperatively.

Closure is simple. The edges of the prostatotomy are approximated with interrupted 2-0 chromic catgut sutures (Fig. 29–26). The rectum is inspected for possible injury. No effort is made to bring the levator ani fibers together. A Penrose drain is left in the retroprostatic space. Skin edges are approximated with interrupted Dexon or Vicryl sutures (Fig. 29–27). A simple dressing is applied to the wound using a split-T binder. The lower extremities are brought down simultaneously and gradually. Too rapid depositioning may result in hypotension because of the sudden rush of blood into the legs, in particular if they have not been wrapped preoperatively.

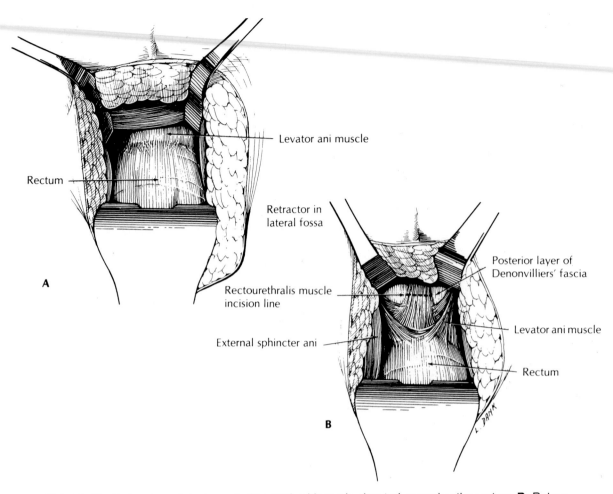

FIG. 29–20. Perineal prostatectomy. **A:** The anal sphincter is elevated, exposing the rectum. **B:** Retractors in the lateral fossae. The rectourethralis muscle has been developed.

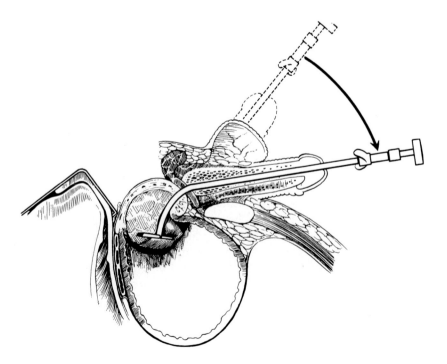

FIG. 29–21. Perineal prostatectomy. The sagittal view shows exposure of the posterior capsule of the prostate.

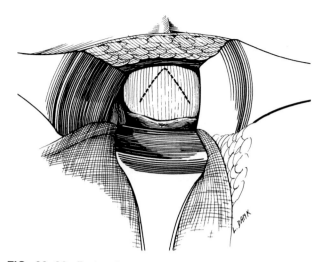

FIG. 29–22. Perineal prostatectomy. The usual inverted-V capsulotomy is used in perineal enucleation.

Excessive bleeding is seldom encountered during perineal prostatectomy. If care is taken to obtain adequate exposure, bleeding vessels can usually be identified and secured without difficulty. The only other complication that may occur during the operation is laceration of the rectum, which is readily recognized from the characteristic appearance of the rectal mucosa. The injury should be completely mobilized and repaired with interrupted 4-0 chromic catgut sutures placed so that the mucosal edges are inverted. The muscularis should be closed in two additional layers, again using interrupted sutures of 4-0 chromic catgut.

If the injury is recognized before the urinary tract is opened, it is best to close the perineal incision and enucleate the gland through a suprapubic incision. If the rectal injury is not appreciated until after the urinary tract has been entered, the laceration should be repaired metic-

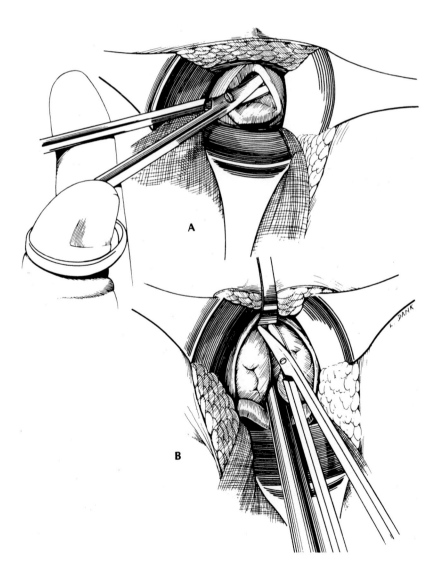

FIG. 29–23. Perineal prostatectomy. **A:** Enucleation of an adenoma is initiated by developing a cleavage plane between the capsule and adenoma. **B:** An incision is made into the prostatic urethra. A Young's tractor is placed into the bladder, enabling mobilization of the adenoma and amputation of the urethra at the apex.

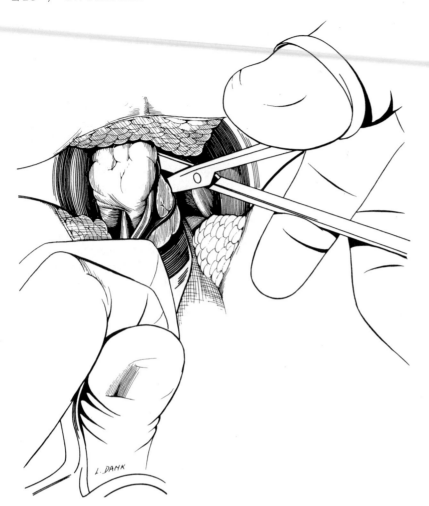

FIG. 29–24. Perineal prostatectomy. The adenoma is freed from the bladder neck by blunt and sharp dissection.

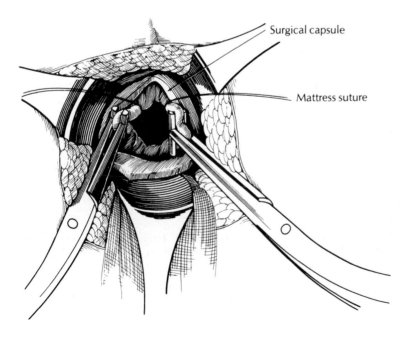

Surgical capsule

Mattress suture

FIG. 29–25. Perineal prostatectomy. The vesical neck is grasped and drawn down with Millin T-clamps, enabling hemostatic mattress sutures to be placed.

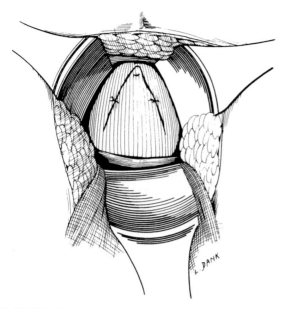

FIG. 29–26. Perineal prostatectomy. The surgical capsule is closed with interrupted sutures.

ulously, as just outlined. Postoperatively, the patient should be maintained on a low-residue diet and bowel activity should be completely suppressed with paregoric for 7 days.

After removal of the hypertrophied lobes, the raw surfaces of the prostatic fossa soon reepithelialize. The compressed outer prostate (prostate proper, or surgical capsule) eventually reexpands to normal size. Scattered areas of induration usually persist indefinitely and can be detected by rectal palpation.

Postoperatively, if a regular Foley catheter has been used it is simply attached to straight bedside drainage. From time to time, gentle manual irrigation may be carried out to keep the system free of clots. The catheter is secured to the thigh, but no traction is necessary. If a three-way catheter has been used, it is attached to a through-and-through irrigating system containing sterile saline solution, which is run in just rapidly enough to keep the efflux reasonably clear. The patient is given appropriate antibiotics. Fluids may be given by mouth during the first day, and they are customarily supplemented by IV infusions to maintain a satisfactory intake.

The perineal Penrose drain is usually removed on postoperative day 1. At this time, the patient may be placed on a soft or regular diet and allowed out of bed. Early ambulation is encouraged.

Usually the perineal wound heals benignly, but sometimes partial separation of the skin edges may occur. Healing may be promoted by removal of the dressing and exposure to a heat lamp. Warm sitz baths are also effective.

The urethral catheter is removed between postoperative days 7 and 10. Not infrequently, urinary leakage may occur from the wound for a day or two after the catheter has been taken out. If it continues longer than this, an 18 Fr, 5-mL Foley catheter may be reinserted for a day or two. Care must be taken in passing the catheter to be certain it does not curl up in the prostatic fossa. Sometimes a stylet is helpful, with the aid of a finger in the rectum.

During the immediate postoperative period, it is important that no rectal instrumentation be performed. No thermometers or rectal tubes should be inserted; this must be made clear to the nursing staff.

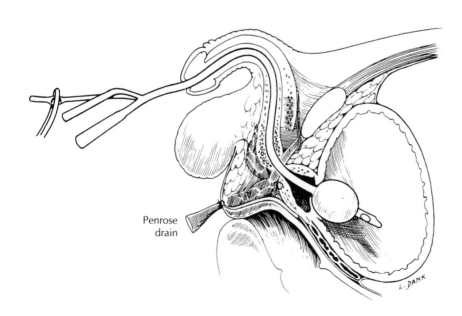

Penrose drain

FIG. 29–27. Perineal prostatectomy: closure of muscles and subcutaneous fat of perineum. Penrose drain is left indwelling and skin edges are approximated with interrupted sutures.

OUTCOMES

Complications

Hemorrhage

Delayed bleeding as occasionally seen after TURP is uncommon after open prostatectomy.

Infections

Wound infections occur in fewer than 5% of patients and are usually limited to the skin and subcutaneous tissue. Postoperative epididymoorchitis is uncommon and may occur early or late. This complication is most commonly seen in patients who have had a long-term indwelling catheter or UTI.

Incontinence

Incontinence of urine is an uncommon complication of open prostatectomies and usually results from perforation and partial avulsion of the prostatic capsule or avulsion of the urethra at the apex of the prostate. With careful enucleation of the adenoma, the capsule is not perforated. With sharp excision of the urethra at the apex rather than avulsion, incontinence should not occur. Some patients may experience stress incontinence or urge incontinence, and detrusor instability may be the cause. In perineal prostatectomies, about 10% of patients experience some urinary incontinence for a few days after removal of the catheter. This disappears rapidly in the vast majority, but up to 6 months may be required for complete cessation of leakage in the occasional patient. Permanent incontinence is highly uncommon after an uneventful perineal prostatectomy.

Other Urologic Complications

In suprapubic and retropubic prostatectomies, urinary fistulas have been reported. Persistent perineal urinary fistula has been feared by those unfamiliar with perineal surgery; in actuality, this complication is rarely seen. Its occurrence should lead one to suspect some form of urethral obstruction, e.g., a postoperative stricture.

Urethral stricture and bladder neck contracture occur most commonly as complications of transurethral resection and are uncommon after suprapubic prostatectomy. A single, gentle dilation with a urethral sound usually suffices to take care of this. Erectile dysfunction after prostatectomy should not occur unless the capsule has been violated. Retrograde ejaculation is common.

Other Complications

Rectal injury is a rare occurrence. Osteitis pubis is rarely seen but can be disabling. The condition is usually self-limited. Analgesics and antiinflammatory drugs provide symptomatic relief.

Surgical mortality for open prostatectomy should be less than 1%; myocardial infarction, pneumonia, and pulmonary embolus are the most common causes. Early ambulation, leg movement in bed, and breathing exercises decrease morbidity.

Results

Enucleation of the enlarged prostatic adenoma by an open procedure is applicable in 5% to 10% of patients presenting with significant bladder outlet obstruction. The operative mortality and morbidity are minimal.

REFERENCES

1. Blue GD, Campbell JM. A clinical review of one thousand consecutive cases of retropubic prostatectomy. *J Urol* 1958;80:257–259.
2. Brendler H. Perineal prostatectomy. In: Glenn JF, ed. *Urologic surgery*, 3rd ed. Philadelphia: JB Lippincott Co, 1983:867–878.
3. Dittmar H. Modification of technique for retropubic prostatectomy: report of 100 cases. *J Urol* 1959;81:558–561.
4. Freyer PJ. One thousand cases of total enucleation of the prostate for radical cure of enlargement of that organ. *Br Med J* 1912;2:868.
5. Gibson TE. George E. Goodfellow (1855–1910). *Invest Urol* 1969;7:107–109.
6. Harvard BM. Low transvesical suprapubic prostatectomy with primary closure. In: Campbell MF, ed. *Urology*. Philadelphia: WB Saunders, 1954:1965–1968.
7. Malament M. Maximal hemostasis in suprapubic prostatectomy. *Surg Gynecol Obstet* 1965;120:1307–1312.
8. Millin T. Retropubic prostatectomy: new extravesical technique: report on 20 cases. *Lancet* 1945;2:693–696.
9. Nanninga JE, O'Conor VJ Jr. Suprapubic and retropubic prostatectomy. In: Walsh PC, Gittes RF, Perlmutter AD, Stamey TA, eds. *Campbell's urology*, 5th ed. Philadelphia: WB Saunders, 1986:2739–2744.
10. O'Conor VJ Jr. An aid for hemostasis in open prostatectomy: capsular plication. *J Urol* 1982;127:448.
11. Poole GV Jr. Mechanical factors in abdominal wound closure: the prevention of fascial dehiscence. *Surgery* 1985;97:631–640.
12. Schlegel PN, Walsh PC. Simultaneous preperitoneal hernia repair during radical pelvic surgery. *J Urol* 1987;137:1180–1183.
13. Straffon RA. Retropubic prostatectomy. In: Glenn JF, ed. *Urologic surgery*, 3rd ed. Philadelphia: JB Lippincott Co, 1983:861–866.
14. Weyrauch HM. *Surgery of the prostate*. Philadelphia: WB Saunders, 1959.

CHAPTER 30

Prostatic Ultrasound and Needle Biopsy

William T. Conner and Randall G. Rowland

Adenocarcinoma of the prostate (PC) is the most common cancer of men in the United States and Europe. Concomitant development of prostatic-specific antigen (PSA) assays and transrectal ultrasound (TRUS) provided the tools for diagnosis of PC at an earlier, and presumably more curable, stage. The transvaginal ultrasound probe was adapted to transrectal use and the spring-loaded Biopty gun with a disposable 18-gauge needle was invented to permit ultrasound-guided biopsies (USBs) with TRUS guidance. PSA, TRUS, and USB are now the standard methods for diagnosis of PC. TRUS is an adjunct for staging PC, while PSA is the most sensitive method of evaluating response to therapy. Methods to enhance the TRUS images with an intravenous microbubble agent, Doppler ultrasound (US), or three-dimensional TRUS are being actively explored and may become standard (2).

DIAGNOSIS

Screening PSA tests are in general performed between ages 50 and 75, starting 5 years earlier in African-American men. Values up to 4 ng/mL are considered to be normal below age 60, although increased PSA velocity greater than 0.75 ng/mL per year is an indication for careful surveillance and possible biopsy. A value of greater than 0.75 ng/mL per year requires three PSA values over a 2-year period to be statistically valid (6). PSA levels increase with age. The formula for calculating the "age-adjusted normal" is age minus 20 divided by 10. Thus, a 50-year-old man would have an age-adjusted normal of 3.0 ng/mL while the value for a 70-year-old man would be 5.0 ng/mL. There is controversy concerning the use of the age-adjusted values, although it seems clear that this technique improves the sensitivity for cancer detection in men below age 60 (5).

Both benign and malignant prostatic cells produce PSA. Infection, trauma, and ejaculation are some of the benign conditions that may cause a PSA elevation. After excluding other causes for an increased PSA, TRUS and USB are scheduled.

INDICATIONS FOR SURGERY

The most common reasons for TRUS and USB are an elevated screening PSA or an abnormal digital rectal exam (DRE). Prior to the mid-1980s PC was usually suspected because of an abnormal DRE. Biopsies were typically performed under spinal or general anesthesia using a digitally guided transperineal approach. With the development of PSA and TRUS with USB, the procedure became simpler, safer, more precise, and more economic.

Other indications for TRUS and USB are a suspicious prostatic nodule, asymmetry of the prostate, and, rarely, unexplained metastatic malignancy. TRUS without USB is used for evaluation of ejaculatory duct cysts, prostatic stones, unexplained urinary tract infection (UTI), and suspected prostatic abscess. Prostatic biopsy without TRUS is on occasion performed for very ill patients with highly suspicious prostate glands, for whom the procedure is performed at the bedside. Confirmation of the diagnosis allows prompt hormonal ablation, often with improvement in hematuria or pain. An Iowa Trumpet (©V. Mueller) allows access for the digitally guided transrectal biopsy while protecting the finger of the operator.

ALTERNATIVE THERAPY

Not everyone who has an elevated PSA or abnormal DRE should have a prostatic biopsy. Patients should be counseled concerning the risks and benefits of both the biopsy and possible treatment. Thus, an 85-year-old man with Alzheimer's disease and no significant urinary symptoms who has an ill-advised PSA test with a result of 8 ng/mL should not have a biopsy unless there is an unusual reason. He should have another PSA in 6 months. If there is no significant change, PSA testing should be stopped.

General medical evaluation should detect anticoagulation, medications, significant cardiovascular disease, diabetes mellitus, and excessive apprehension. Any of these factors may require a change of plans for USB.

SURGICAL TECHNIQUE

Anticoagulation must be stopped before USB. Consultation with the patient's physician will determine if it is safe to stop oral anticoagulation 5 days in advance. If not, he is changed to a form of heparin, which is stopped for 6 to 12 hours for the biopsy. Gross hematuria requiring a Foley catheter is more common in this group.

Antibiotics are commonly given before and after the biopsy. Regimens vary, but the usual protocol in the United States includes a full dose of a fluoroquinolone before the biopsy and for 2 to 3 days after. Routine use of antibiotics can lead to resistant organisms. Simpler regimens are being evaluated to reduce this risk. Patients with artificial heart valves, total joint prostheses, or implanted devices are routinely treated using standard American Heart Association guidelines. Most American urologists use cleansing rectal enemas, although there is some controversy concerning their need (8).

Some patients require monitored anesthesia care. These include those with anal stenosis, excessive apprehension, or serious cardiac arrhythmias and patients without a rectum. Oral sedatives and analgesics may be given, provided the patient has a driver to take him home.

The patient is placed in the left lateral recumbent position on the table in the US suite. The operator sits at a comfortable level beside the table and again explains the procedure as it is being performed. A gentle, thorough rectal examination is performed, noting significant external hemorrhoids, anal sphincter diameter and tone, and lesions in the rectum. Examination of the prostate includes specific notes concerning size, texture, tenderness, borders, fixation or mobility of the apex, symmetry, location of the midline sulcus, and the seminal vesicles. Any prostatic nodules or abnormal areas are noted.

We use similar B&K Medical (Wilmington, MA) US systems with either a 7.0- or 7.5-MHz endorectal probe. For the rare instances of TRUS for patients without a rectum, a 3.5- or 4.0-MHz probe is used. The TRUS probe has been prepared in advance by decontamination with glutaraldehyde solution or heated 35% peroxyacetic acid solution (Steris) sterilization. A finger cot is placed snugly over the inflation port and inflated to exclude air bubbles, which interfere with the US image. Finally, a condom containing about 15 cc of US gel is placed over the rectal end of the probe. The US gel reduces artifacts during TRUS. The probe is lubricated and gently inserted into the rectum. Inflation of the finger cot with 25 to 40 mL of water produces an acoustic window, which allows better definition of the rectal wall and prostate.

Local anesthesia has become a frequent adjunct to TRUS and USB (4). Periprostatic nerves can be blocked by injecting 5 to 10 cc of 1% lidocaine without epinephrine just lateral to the junction of the seminal vesicle and prostate on each side (Fig. 30–1). After guiding a 22-gauge, 7-in. spinal needle (Becton/Dickinson, Franklin Lakes, NJ) to the correct spot with US, and aspirating to be sure a vein has not been entered, the anesthetic is slowly injected. The area of injection expands and produces a hypoechoic image that confirms the proper location of the drug. Local anesthesia allows multiple biopsies to be taken with little discomfort for most patients. As with all procedures with conscious patients, each

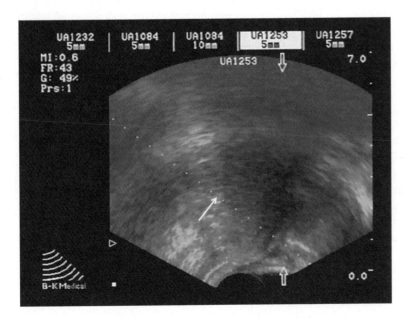

FIG. 30–1. Prostate ultrasound. Dotted line indicates path of biopsy needle on sagittal view.

event must be announced in advance. Lidocaine causes the same stinging sensation in the periprostatic area that occurs with dental or other local injections. Neutralizing the lidocaine solution with alkali can prevent this, but the shelf life of the drug is significantly reduced.

The prostate is then imaged in transverse and longitudinal planes, noting areas of abnormal echogenicity, cysts, calcifications, indistinct borders, lesions of the seminal vesicles or ejaculatory ducts, and other abnormalities. Tiny corpora amylacea are easily visible and usually define the border of the transitional and peripheral zones. Bladder US can be performed if desired but is best accomplished as a suprapubic exam with a 3.5- to 4-MHz probe.

Prostatic volume is calculated using the greatest transverse, anterior–posterior, and longitudinal dimensions. Most modern TRUS machines have computer programs for computing the volume. One formula for calculating the volume of a prolate ellipse by US is: height × width × length divided by 0.52. Images are recorded to show anatomy of the prostate and seminal vesicles, abnormalities, and prostatic volume. Digital recording of the procedure is possible. The volume of suspicious hypoechoic lesions is measured and recorded. The TRUS procedure takes several minutes, enough time for the lidocaine to anesthetize the periprostatic nerves.

Biopsies are obtained with a sharp, disposable spring-loaded 18-gauge needle, which produces a 17-mm specimen with little crush artifact. Several such needles are available. Some are completely disposable devices while others use a permanent biopsy gun and disposable needles. Most brands of needles have a slightly abraded tip that makes them echogenic and easier to see. We currently use either a Bard Magnum Biopty Needle Gun with a disposable needle or a Microvasive Topnotch disposable gun and needle. The device is fired before the biopsy to familiarize the patient with the sound.

We routinely obtain 10 biopsies: lateral and medial at each base, lateral and medial at the midgland on each side, and one biopsy at each apex, as described by Gore et al. (1) and others. Patients who need a second biopsy because of a high suspicion of cancer will have 12 to 20 biopsies, including specimens from the transition zones (TZs) and far lateral peripheral zone. "Saturation" biopsy under anesthesia obtains up to 45 cores of tissue, although this technique is reserved for the patient who has had multiple negative biopsies and still has a suspicious PSA or rectal exam (7). The great value of TRUS is to be able to precisely sample specific areas of the prostate. Anesthetizing the urethra with lidocaine reduces the additional urethral pain with TZ biopsies but does not decrease the additional urethral bleeding. Bleeding usually stops without treatment within 24 hours.

After all biopsies are obtained and carefully labeled, the US probe is removed. A useful technique to control rectal bleeding is to roll a handtowel into a tight roll about 6 in. long and 3 in. in diameter, then have the patient sit with the towel between his ischial tuberosities for 10 minutes. This places pressure on the perineum, compressing the prostate against the symphysis pubis. Blood pressure, pulse, and R are again recorded. The patient sits on the table for about 10 minutes, then voids. The urine usually contains blood, especially if TZ biopsies have been obtained.

When the patient is stable and voiding well, he is given his postbiopsy instructions and allowed to leave, with a return appointment for 1 to 2 weeks depending upon the response time of the pathology department.

Instructions include:

1. Expect blood with urination and bowel movements for 1 to 7 days.
2. Expect blood with ejaculate for up to 6 weeks.
3. Take medications as prescribed.
4. Report temperature over 101 degrees, passage of clots after 24 hours, persistent rectal bleeding, difficulty with urination, pain, or any other symptom that concerns him.
5. Return for discussion of the biopsy as scheduled.
6. Resume all other medications, with special instructions for anticoagulants.
7. Resume preoperative activities after 24 hours, avoiding heavy lifting for 72 hours.

OUTCOMES

Complications

Hematuria, hematochezia, and hematospermia are expected, as mentioned above. Excessive bleeding requires evaluation and treatment. Rarely, patients require admission for bladder irrigation for urinary bleeding. Patients who are on anticoagulants on occasion require cystoscopy with fulguration of bleeding vessels. Rectal bleeding is usually minor and self-limited. If rectal bleeding is persistent or causes the hematocrit to fall, proctoscopic examination is indicated. The urologist, a general surgeon, or a gastroenterologist, depending upon the time of occurrence and the training of the physician, may perform this. Arterial or venous bleeding may be controlled with direct suture ligation or injection of epinephrine around the vessel. Hematospermia requires reassurance only. Urinary retention usually resolves unless the patient has bladder outlet obstruction.

Bacteriuria and bacteremia are fairly common but usually asymptomatic and resolve without further complications (3). Isolated reports of perirectal abscess, septic shock, disseminated intravascular coagulation, and osteomyelitis are in the literature. Seeding of the biopsy tract with implantation of cancer is a theoretical complication that has been rarely reported. The biopsy technique does not interfere with radical prostatectomy, external radiation, or brachytherapy.

REFERENCES

1. Gore JL, Shariat SF, Miles BJ, et al. Optimal combinations of systematic sextant and laterally directed biopsies for the detection of prostate cancer. *J Urol* 2001;165:1554–1559.
2. Halpern EJ, Frauscher F, Rosenberg M, et al. Directed biopsy during contrast-enhanced sonography of the prostate. *AJR* 2002;178: 915–919.
3. Lindert KA, Kabalin JN, Terris MK. Bacteremia and bacteriuria after transrectal ultrasound guided prostate biopsy. *J Urol* 2000;164:76–80.
4. Pareek G, Armenkadas NA, Fracchia JA. Periprostatic nerve blockade for transrectal ultrasound guided biopsy of the prostate: a randomized, double-blind, placebo controlled study. *J Urol* 2001;166:894–897.
5. Polascik TJ, Oesterling JE, Partin AW. Prostate specific antigen: a decade of discovery—what have we learned and where are we going. *J Urol* 1999;162:293–306.
6. Potter SR, Carter HB. The role of prostate-specific antigen velocity in prostate cancer early detection. *Curr Urol Rep* 2000;1:15–9.
7. Stewart CS, Leibovich BC, Waver AL, et al. Prostate cancer diagnosis using a saturation needle biopsy technique after previous negative sextant biopsies. *J Urol* 2001;166:86–91.
8. Terris MK. Letter to the Editor. *J Urol* 2002;167:2145–2146.

CHAPTER 31

Pelvic Lymphadenectomy

Ralph W. deVere-White

The pelvic lymph nodes are the initial site of spread of prostatic, bladder, and proximal urethral cancers. Tumors of the penis, scrotum, and distal urethra spread primarily to the inguinal lymph nodes but can involve the pelvic lymph nodes at a later stage. Testicular tumors rarely involve the pelvic lymph nodes unless there is massive retroperitoneal disease (retrograde spread) or a history of orchidopexy or prior pelvic procedures.

The standard practice has been that all patients undergoing radical prostatectomy undergo a pelvic lymph node dissection. A pelvic lymph node dissection is performed currently only if a patient is at significant risk for metastasis. Risk factors such as preoperative prostate-specific antigen (PSA), biopsy Gleason score, and clinical stage define those patients at risk for nodal metastasis. Knowing the nodal status of a patient aids in determining prognosis; however, the therapeutic value of removing positive lymph nodes remains controversial at best. When a cystectomy is indicated for bladder cancer, the standard of practice is still to perform an extended bilateral pelvic lymphadenectomy.

DIAGNOSIS

Lymphadenectomy carries great significance for tumor staging and when performed in a consistent manner allows not only the optimal selection of additional therapies but the comparison of benefit or otherwise lack of such therapies among institutions. The diagnostic modalities for these entities are discussed in Chapters 23, 24, 33, 34, and 111.

INDICATIONS FOR SURGERY

Prostate

Pelvic lymphadenectomy adds modest additional operating room time, cost, and complication risk to radical prostatectomy and when performed independently requires a separate anesthetic and exposes the patient to the cardiopulmonary, thromboembolic, and wound complications associated with a pelvic surgical procedure. Several investigators have, therefore, attempted to identify groups of prostate cancer patients in which pelvic lymphadenectomy can be omitted with an acceptable risk for failing to identify metastatic disease. By combining these criteria, patients can be grouped as low (2% to 5%), moderate (20%), and high (40%) risk categories for lymph node metastases (2,7). Patients at highest risk for lymph node metastases include those with a Gleason score of 7 and PSA 20 ng per mL, Gleason score of 8 and PSA 10 ng per mL, or PSA 50 ng per mL (Table 31–1). Using a decision analysis, Meng and associates have shown that lymph node dissection is unnecessary in those with less than 18% risk for lymph node involvement (1).

Analogous to the drop in the number of preoperative bone scans with the widespread PSA screening, application of the selection criteria (Table 31–1) may decrease the total number of lymph node dissections performed, although it is unlikely to eliminate lymphadenectomies completely.

We currently perform pelvic lymph node dissection concomitantly with a retropubic prostatectomy except in those with T1 cancer, PSA 15 ng per mL, and/or those with high-grade tumors (biopsy Gleason score less than 7). Due to the stage migration, we feel that performance of lymphadenectomy as a separate procedure, i.e., laparoscopically, is not cost effective. The yield of cancerous nodes for clinical stage T1c tumor of a Gleason sum less than 7 and a preoperative PSA 10 ng per mL is well within the 5% to 10% margin of error of a false-negative diagnosis at frozen section, which also supports the notion that routine pelvic node dissection in such patients is not cost effective whatever may be the technique and subjects the patient to an unnecessary procedure with possible morbidity. We no longer perform lymph node dissection prior to radiation therapy.

TABLE 31–1. *Selection criteria for pelvic lymphadenectomy*

Procedure	Criteria	% of all patients	% with positive lymph nodes
No Lymphadenectomy[a]	PSA <10, Gleason Score <7, and Clinical Stage <T2	~50%	~2%
Intended Retropubic Prostatectomy; No Laparoscopic Pelvic Lymphadenectomy, but Open Lymphadenectomy May be Performed at the Time of Prostatectomy	PSA ≥10 or Gleason Score ≥7 or Clinical Stage ≥T2c	~50%	~2%
Intended Perineal Prostatectomy; Laparoscopic Pelvic Lymphadenectomy May be Considered[b]			
Intended Retropubic Prostatectomy; Laparoscopic Pelvic Lymphadenectomy May be Considered	PSA ≥50 or (PSA ≥20 and Gleason Score ≥7) or (PSA ≥10 and Gleason Score ≥8)	~10%	~40%

Modified from Wolf JS. Indications, technique, and results of laparoscopic pelvic lymphadenectomy. *J Endourol* 2001;15(4):427–435, with permission.

PSA, prostate-specific antigen.

[a]Staging lymphadenectomy does not affect outcome (PSA recurrence at 2 years). From ElGalley RES, Keane TE, Petros JA, Sanders WH, Clarke HS, Cotsonis GA, Graham SD. Evaluation of staging lymphadenectomy in prostate cancer. *Urology* 1998;52:663–667, with permission.

[b]Pelvic lymphadenectomy has not been shown to affect the intermediate outcome. From Salomon L, Hoznek A, Lefrere-Belda MA, Bellot J, Chopin DK, Abbou CC. Nondissection of the pelvic lymph nodes does not influence the results of perineal radical prostatectomy in selected patients. *Eur Urol* 2000;37:297–300, with permission.

Bladder Cancer

Most urologists perform an extended bilateral pelvic lymphadenectomy (to include lymphatics as far lateral as the genitofemoral nerve) in bladder cancer based on Skinner's early 1980s data that such a dissection can improve 5-year survival by up to 36% (5), which suggests that lymphadenectomy may have some curative potential in bladder cancer patients with limited nodal disease. Survival rates have been shown to be similar (55%) in those with minimal (N1) and those without pelvic lymph node involvement if the primary cancer is organ confined (P0 to P3a).

The presence of positive lymph nodes in bladder cancer has therapeutic implications. Some urologists would, whereas others favor debulking the tumor with cystectomy followed by postoperative chemotherapy.

If we find grossly enlarged lymph nodes with histological evidence of metastasis, we treat with chemotherapy and reevaluate the bladder rather than proceeding with radical cystectomy. However, if the lymph nodes are grossly normal we proceed with the radical cystectomy without sending the nodes for frozen section evaluation.

ALTERNATIVE THERAPY

Pelvic lymph node dissection is currently the only definitive means of evaluating lymph node status. Enlarged lymph nodes suspicious for metastases may be identified by ultrasound, cross-sectional imaging with thin-cut computed tomography (CT) scans, magnetic res-

onance imaging (MRI), and pedal lymphangiography, all of which have low sensitivity. Unless bulky disease is seen on a CT scan (1 cm), a tissue sample (e.g., by CT-guided needle aspiration core biopsy) is required for validation of a suspicious scan finding. Drawbacks with CT scan include size limitation, random sampling error, disruption of nodal architecture, low cellular yield, and need for an expert cytopathologist.

The use of PSA alone is not a good predictor of pathologic stage, as there can be significant overlap between PSA and the pathologic stage. Costly alternatives such as radioisotopic metabolic imaging using positron emission tomography scans and tumor-directed imaging by labeled antibody scans (^{111}In-capromab pendetide, the *ProstaScint* scan, Cytogen Corp., Princeton, NJ) are currently being investigated to identify low-volume disease in low-risk patients with clinical T1 disease. Results obtained with reverse transcriptase polymerase chain reaction (RT-PCR) have shown inconsistent results.

SURGICAL TECHNIQUE

Prostate Cancer

The boundaries of the traditional pelvic lymph node dissection were those used in radical cystectomies for bladder cancer and include the pelvic sidewall laterally, the paravesical fascia and peritoneum medially, the genitofemoral nerve superiorly, the obturator nerve inferiorly, and the femoral canal distally (Fig. 31–1). Proximally, the dissection is carried varying distances up the

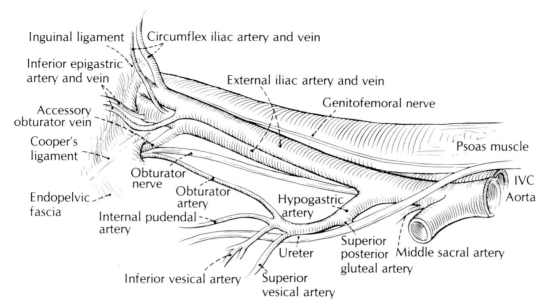

FIG. 31–1. Right lateral pelvic wall. Anatomy of pelvic blood vessels and nerves encountered in a pelvic lymph node dissection is depicted.

common iliac artery (Figs. 31–2 and 31–3). Most urologists feel that only the obturator nodal packet need be removed for three reasons:

1. The obturator nodes are involved in 87% of cases when lymphatic metastases are found.

2. The procedure is for staging and not therapy, so a more extensive dissection is of little benefit.

3. If radiation therapy is used for local control following surgery, patients who had an extensive lymphadenectomy have a higher incidence of scrotal or lower-limb edema.

Preoperatively, pneumatic compression devices (PCDs) are placed and patients are given subcutaneous heparin as prophylaxis against deep venous thrombosis. The supine or lithotomy position may be used, although we recommend the low lithotomy position. The sacrum is positioned over the table break or a roll to allow for hyperextension of and better vision into the pelvis. The bladder is emptied using a Foley catheter. A midline incision is made from below the umbilicus to the symphysis pubis down through the anterior rectus sheath. The posterior rectus sheath is incised for 2 to 3 cm above the linea semilunaris to aid in lateral retraction of the wound. An extraperitoneal lymph node dissection is usually performed. If the peritoneum is entered during this incision, the defect is closed with absorbable sutures.

The transversalis fascia is sharply divided in the midline to allow lateral dissection superficial to the peritoneum, which helps avoid injury to the inferior epigastric vessels. The iliac vessels are exposed by bluntly sweeping the peritoneum superomedially. The vasa deferentia are encountered during this maneuver and may be divided. The table is tilted toward the first side for evaluation. If the prostate cancer is confined to one lobe, the dissection is begun on that side. A self-retaining retractor is applied, with care taken not to injure the inferior epigastric vessels. We use the Bookwalter retractor without

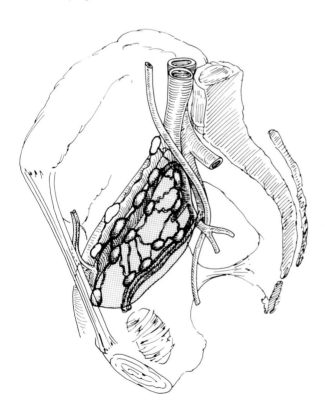

FIG. 31–2. Shaded area shows the iliac and obturator nodes that are to be removed.

the post, as it can be more quickly applied and the post can interfere with the surgeon. Other self-retaining retractors may be used.

We place the Bookwalter retractor on top of sterile towels, one on each thigh and one on the abdomen. A bladder blade and moist lap sponge are used to retract the wound laterally on the side of the dissection. A malleable retractor and moist lap sponge are placed on the bladder and used to retract the bladder toward the contralateral side. A third retractor is placed at the apex of the wound. With these three retractors, excellent visibility can be obtained.

The nodal packet is palpated to detect grossly enlarged lymph nodes. If such nodes are found, they are sent for frozen section evaluation following removal. If no enlarged nodes are palpated, we continue with the lymphadenectomy and prostatectomy and do not send the lymph nodes for frozen section.

The external iliac artery is identified and dissection of the lymph node packet is begun over its anteromedial aspect. The correct plane of dissection is easily found here and there are no other structures in this area to be damaged (Fig. 31–4). The dissection is brought proximally to the bifurcation of the common iliac vessels and distally to the femoral canal. The lymph node of Cloquet is the most distal aspect of the dissection. Lymphatic channels into this node and surrounding the external iliac vein are carefully clipped and divided. We place a right-angle clamp around the lymph node packet and ligate it with a 2-0 Vicryl tie. A large right-angle clip is placed below the tie. As the nodal packet is divided and swept superiorly, an accessory obturator vein may be found medial to the internal iliac artery and should be ligated (rather than clipped) and divided to avoid avulsion. Identification of this vein is necessary as damage can cause extensive bleeding.

With gentle lateral retraction of the external iliac vein, the lymph node packet is dissected off the pelvic sidewall laterally. Although a vein retractor is usually used for this

maneuver, we use a peanut/Kitner dissector. Identification of the obturator nerve is essential as the dissection is carried into the pelvic fossa to avoid injuring it. The packet is freed from the obturator nerve and vessels. The obturator vessels are spared if they are in their usual location below the nerve. If the vessels are above the nerve or involved with the lymph node packet, it is best to ligate and divide them to prevent avulsion and bleeding. This is especially true near the femoral canal. The superior attachment of the packet is now near the internal iliac artery. Previously we used to identify and dissect out the ureter, but, in most cases, we no longer do this. To ensure the ureter is not damaged by a clip, the specimen is split over the obturator nerve and a right-angle clip is placed over either limb of the split packet on each side of the nerve so that the ureter cannot accidentally be included in the clip. Additional loose attachments to the proximal hypogastric vessels are clipped and divided. The entire packet is sent to pathology as the two portions divided over the obturator nerve. The obturator fossa is irrigated with sterile saline. It had been our routine to leave a gauze sponge in the fossa for hemostasis; however, we now do this only for minimal oozing. The same dissection is then performed on the contralateral side to complete the lymph node dissection. We place one or two Jackson–Pratt drains in the pelvis postoperatively.

Bladder Cancer

The dissection is similar to the one described above for prostate cancer with some differences. The incision is carried to just above the umbilicus and down to the pubic bone. We palpate the pelvic lymph nodes while remaining extraperitoneal. If no grossly enlarged nodes are felt, the dissection becomes intraperitoneal. The peritoneum is entered in midline and inspection is performed of the intraabdominal organs for signs of metastases. If none are found, dissection is continued by mobilizing the cecum and ascending colon. The peritoneum is incised along the

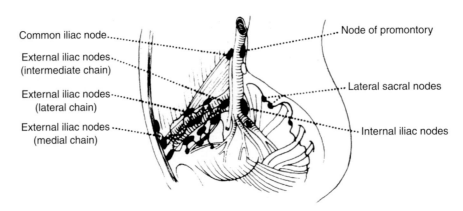

Common iliac node

External iliac nodes
(intermediate chain)

External iliac nodes
(lateral chain)

External iliac nodes
(medial chain)

Node of promontory

Lateral sacral nodes

Internal iliac nodes

FIG. 31–3. Incision of fibroareolar tissue loosely adherent to adventitia of the iliac artery and vein. This allows a portion of the areolar tissue to pass lateral to the iliac vessels into the obturator fossa.

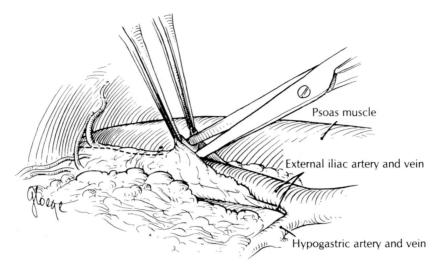

Psoas muscle

External iliac artery and vein

Hypogastric artery and vein

FIG. 31–4. Correct plane of dissection is shown.

white line of Toldt and the right hemicolon is rolled medially. The right ureter is identified and freed superiorly and inferiorly. Inferiorly, this leads to the bifurcation of the iliac vessels. In freeing the peritoneum, we routinely divide the vas deferens. On the left the peritoneum is incised lateral to the sigmoid colon, and it is reflected medially. The left ureter is identified and freed as on the right. Mobilization is aided by dividing the vas deferens.

The self-retaining retractor may be placed as described above. The bowel can easily be retracted into the upper abdomen, as it has been mobilized. The node dissection begins over either common iliac artery just proximal to the bifurcation. It is carried down the hypogastric artery to the superior vesical artery, which is identified and divided. The remainder of the lymph node dissection is similar to that for prostate cancer.

Limited Versus Extensive Lymph Node Dissection

Variation in reported 5-year survival rates (5% to 30%) in lymph node-positive cases treated with radical cystectomy and pelvic lymph node dissection may be partly explained by the extent to which the lymph node dissection was performed. Internal iliac lymph node dissection is an important prognostic factor with respect to cancer-specific survival. Vieweg and associates advocate deep and extensive lymph node dissection medial to the internal iliac vessels including ligation and division of these vessels and obturator vessels to facilitate the removal of as much lymphatic tissue as possible (6). Poulsen and associates in a retrospective analysis have shown that extending the limits of pelvic lymph node dissection from the common iliac bifurcation to the bifurcation of the aorta along with removal of the perivesical fat containing paravesical lymph node improves the recurrence-free sur-

vival rate following radical cystectomy for bladder cancer confined to the bladder wall (pT3a) (85% for less than pT3a vs. 64% for those with pT3b) (4).

OUTCOMES

Complications

Although pelvic lymph node dissection is usually a relatively short procedure with little morbidity, it has a potential for significant complications. These can be divided into intra- and postoperative (early and late) complications (Table 31–2). Paul and associates reported an

TABLE 31–2. *Complications of pelvic lymphadenectomy*

Intraoperative Complications
  Vascular Injury
  Ureteral Injury
  Obturator Nerve Injury
Postoperative Complications
  Wound-Related
    Hematoma
    Seroma
    Wound Infection
    Wound Dehiscence
  Non–Wound-Related
    Pulmonary Atelectasis
    Pneumonia
    Myocardial Infarction
    Congestive Cardiac Failure
    Prolonged Lymph Drainage
    Lymphocele Formation
    Deep Venous Thrombosis/Pulmonary Embolism
    Epididymoorchitis
    Urinary Tract Infection
    Prolonged Ileus
    Urinary Retention
    Chronic Lymphedema

8.6% incidence of intraoperative complications, an 8.7% immediate postoperative wound complication incidence, and an additional 31.4% immediate non–wound-related complication rate (3). They also reviewed the complication rates reported in multiple studies. These ranged from 4% to 53% with a mean rate of 26.6% (3). Intraoperative complications can be minimized by familiarity with the pelvic anatomy and careful dissection to identify vulnerable structures. The most common vascular injury is to the accessory obturator vein. Care should be taken not to avulse the obturator vessels as they enter the pelvic foramina because they will retract caudally and ligation will be difficult. If this occurs, bone wax can be used. Significant injuries to the external iliac vessels require repair, sometimes with the aid of a vascular surgeon. Transection or avulsion of the obturator nerve leads to difficulties with adduction of the ipsilateral leg and is usually irreparable. Splitting the nodal packet as described reduces the chance of inadvertent nerve injury.

Ureteral injuries are uncommon and require repair when encountered. A problem with ureteral injuries is that they are not always identified at the time of surgery. These are often the result of a clip inadvertently being placed across the ureter. Therefore, as we now dissect out the lymph node packet we no longer specifically look for the ureter. However, we always place a clip on the upper end of the nodal packet after splitting it over the obturator nerve in a cranial-to-caudal direction to avoid ureteral injury, identified or not. If there is any concern for ureteral injury, the ureter must be dissected out and fully visualized.

Postoperative complications include those related and unrelated to the wound. Wound infections are uncommon, especially when prophylactic antibiotics are given. Dehiscence is similarly uncommon. Seroma and hematoma formation are more common and may require drainage and local wound care.

Prolonged lymph drainage and lymphocele formation may occur in 3% to 12% of patients. Prolonged drainage is treated by instilling autologous blood or Betadine solution through the preexisting drains as sclerosing agents. If Jackson–Pratt or similar drains are used, tissue will eventually grow into the drains. This has occurred twice in our experience, and in both cases a general anesthetic was required for drain removal. We now remove all drains or treat them as described above for prolonged drainage at the end of 2 weeks. Although it has been reported that the use of subcutaneous heparin increases the incidence of prolonged lymph drainage, this has not been our experience. Our rate of prolonged lymph drainage and/or symptomatic lymphocele formation is less than 3%. Treatment of symptomatic lymphoceles varies from percutaneous drainage under radiological guidance and sclerotherapy to laparoscopic or open marsupialization into the peritoneal cavity. Although some lymphatic drainage is expected, careful dissection and meticulous ligation of lymphatic channels help minimize the risk of prolonged drainage.

Any patient with prolonged or excessive lymph drainage must be evaluated for a urinary leak. This may be done by sending a sample of the fluid for creatinine testing. If a urine leak is found, this may be from either the anastomosis or an unrecognized ureteral injury. If the latter is suspected, it should be immediately investigated.

Thrombophlebitis and deep venous thrombosis are recognized complications of pelvic lymph node dissection. Although the studies are conflicting, most have shown that some method of anticoagulation, low-dose heparin or pneumatic compression stockings, are beneficial in reducing the risk of these complications. We routinely administer subcutaneous heparin preoperatively and every 8 to 12 hours postoperatively as well as use pneumatic compression stockings until the patient is discharged.

Chronic lymphedema of the lower extremities and external genitalia may occur, and these may be worsened by radiotherapy. Although extended dissections have been reported to result in improved survival rates in retrospective studies, they may be associated with increased incidence of lymphedema. Poor macrophage function and relative tissue hypoxia may result in pain, risk of local infection, hyperkeratosis, decreased motor function, and paresthesias. The modified pelvic lymph node dissection has been a reliable way of preventing chronic lymphedema.

REFERENCES

1. Meng MV, Carroll PR. When is pelvic lymph node dissection necessary before radical prostatectomy? A decision analysis. *J Urol* 2000;164:1235–1240.
2. Partin AW, Kattan MW, Subong EN, et al. Combination of prostate-specific antigen, clinical stage, and Gleason score to predict pathological stage of localized prostate cancer: A multi-institutional update. *JAMA* 1997;227:1445–1451.
3. Paul DB, Loening SA, Narayan AS, Culp DA. Morbidity from pelvic lymphadenectomy in staging carcinoma of the prostate. *J Urol* 1983;129:1141.
4. Poulsen AL, Horn T, Steven K. Radical cystectomy: extending the limits of pelvic lymph node dissection improves survival for patients with bladder cancer confined to the bladder wall. *J Urol* 1998;160:2015.
5. Skinner DG. Management of invasive bladder cancer: a meticulous pelvic node dissection can make a difference. *J Urol* 1982;128:34.
6. Vieweg J, Gschwend JE, Herr HW, et al. Pelvic lymph node dissection can be curative in patients with node positive bladder cancer. *J Urol* 1999;161:449.
7. Wolf JS. Indications, technique, and results of laparoscopic pelvic lymphadenectomy. *J Endourol* 2001;15:427–435.

CHAPTER 32

Radical Retropubic Prostatectomy

Joseph A. Smith, Jr.

Despite the continued development of alternative treatments, surgical removal of the prostate by radical prostatectomy remains the preferred treatment for most men with clinically localized carcinoma of the prostate and at least a 10-year life expectancy (1). With greater experience and refinement in surgical technique, perioperative morbidity with radical prostatectomy has diminished markedly compared to historical series (8). Further, selection of patients most likely to be cured by surgery has improved while the benefit of local control is recognized even in those who may develop recurrent disease. Long-term follow-up after surgery has shown radical prostatectomy to be the most proven definitive therapy for men with clinically confined prostate cancer.

INDICATIONS FOR SURGERY

Radical prostatectomy is indicated in patients with carcinoma of the prostate seemingly confined within the surgical capsule of the gland who, in general, would otherwise have a life expectancy of at least 10 years.

Despite its well-recognized limitations, digital rectal examination (DRE) remains a standard method for assessing tumor extent within the prostate, although it frequently understages palpable tumors. Large, palpable tumors frequently are found to have histological evidence of extracapsular extension. Transrectal ultrasonography (TRUS) likewise is not sufficiently accurate for staging and prospective studies have not shown the superiority of TRUS compared to DRE for staging the local extent of prostate cancer (9). Further, other imaging modalities such as magnetic resonance imaging (MRI) are being explored.

Algorithms to predict the likelihood of extracapsular tumor extension have been developed and validated. These may take multiple factors into account but the most commonly used are DRE, serum prostate-specific antigen (PSA), and tumor grade using the Gleason scoring

system (2). As an independent variable, a PSA level of greater than 20 ng per mL predicts a high probability of extracapsular disease. Likewise, clinically confined disease is unlikely with a Gleason score of 8 or more.

Capsular penetration or extracapsular extension do not necessarily imply the inability to remove the tumor completely by surgery. Almost one-half of patients with positive surgical margins remain free of clinical or biochemical evidence of disease recurrence. Further, the debulking effect of surgery and the local control provided may be of benefit even in men not completely cured by radical prostatectomy.

Radical prostatectomy usually is not indicated in patients who otherwise have a less than 10-year life expectancy. Although carcinoma of the prostate is a progressive disease, the rate of tumor growth is such that competing causes of death dominate in elderly patients or those with poor overall health. Both chronological as well as physiological age must be taken into account (3). Life table analysis indicates that most men less than 70 to 75 years of age with good overall health can anticipate at least 10 years of additional life.

ALTERNATIVE THERAPY

Alternatives to radical retropubic prostatectomy include nonsurgical approaches such as observation, hormonal deprivation, or radiation therapy. Alternative surgical approaches are the perineal prostatectomy and laparoscopic prostatectomy.

SURGICAL TECHNIQUE

Same-day admission is routine and patients report to the hospital 2 hours before the scheduled surgery time. Blood is obtained for a type and screen. Autologous blood donation is not used as our requirement for homologous blood transfusion, even in the absence of autolo-

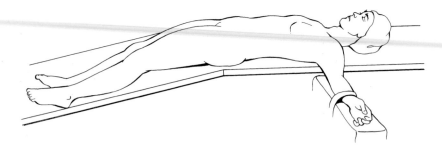

FIG. 32–1. Position of the patient for a radical retropubic prostatectomy with the table flexed at the hips and the kidney rest elevated to enhance visualization and dissection.

gous donation, is less than 1% of our patients (4). Low-molecular-weight heparin (enoxaparin 30 mg subcutaneous) is administered just prior to the surgical incision in patients at increased risk for deep venous thrombosis such as those with obesity or a prior history of thromboembolic problems. Pneumatic intermittent calf compression devices are used routinely.

The patient is placed in a supine position with the kidney rest elevated and the table slightly flexed (Fig. 32–1). The legs are not separated. The surgical field is prepped and draped sterilely and an 18 Fr Foley catheter is inserted into the bladder.

A midline incision is made from below the umbilicus to the pubis. It is not necessary to extend the incision all the way to the umbilicus, and the entire length of the incision is only 10 cm (7). The anterior rectus fascia is incised and then the rectus muscles are retracted laterally (Fig. 32–2). Blunt and sharp dissection is used to mobilize the peritoneal envelope superiorly. Blunt finger dissection can help create a pocket directly over the psoas muscle and just lateral to the common iliac artery, which facilitates superior retraction of the peritoneum. The vas deferens is retracted along with the peritoneum. Care

should be taken to make certain that the epigastric vessels are not injured beneath the belly of the rectus muscle during this maneuver.

We use a Bookwalter self-retaining retractor (Fig. 32–3). An oval ring is used and short Richardson blades retract the skin and rectus muscle at the inferior and lateral aspect of the incision. Deeper retractors at this point can result in femoral neuropathy or compression of the iliac vein. At the superior and lateral portion of the incision, additional Richardson blades are used to retract the peritoneum. Placement of the retractors in this manner provides excellent exposure of the operative field.

We continue to prefer bilateral pelvic lymph node dissection. Even though the incidence of nodal metastases in patients with favorable features of the primary tumor is low, node dissection adds minimal time or morbidity to the procedure. In a prospective comparative study, we found that a limited dissection identified nodal metastasis as often as a more extended dissection. Accordingly, the boundaries of the dissection are the external iliac artery laterally, the bifurcation of the common iliac artery superiorly, and the bladder wall medially. Distally, dissection is carried to the node of Cloquet, identified at the

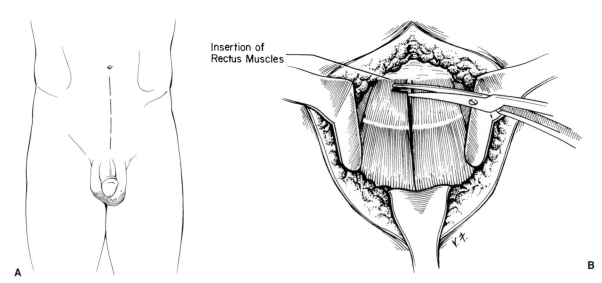

Insertion of Rectus Muscles

A **B**

FIG. 32–2. A: A midline incision is made from 5 cm below the symphysis pubis to the umbilicus. **B:** Division of the midline of the rectus abdomini.

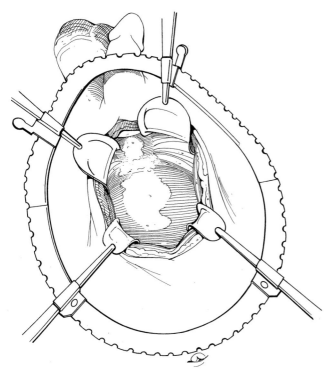

FIG. 32–3. A Bookwalter retractor is placed to aid in dissection.

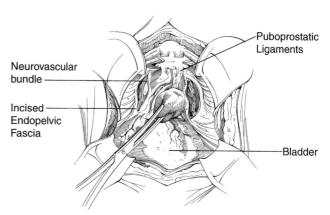

FIG. 32–4. The endopelvic fascia is incised and the neurovascular bundles are exposed.

point where the superficial epigastric vein crosses the external iliac artery. The dissection is carried into the obturator fossa along the anterior surface of the obturator nerve. Even though this is a limited dissection, it is important to remove the nodes along the proximal obturator nerve and hypogastric artery. Clips are used on lymphatic channels, especially at the distal part of the dissection where the lymphatics enter the pelvis from the leg.

A sponge stick is used to displace the prostate and bladder medially. A Kitner dissector is used to remove some of the loose fat overlying the endopelvic fascia and expose the junction between the lateral prostate and the levator ani muscle. Electrocautery is used to incise the endopelvic fascia overlying this space (Fig. 32–4). A Kitner dissector then separates the levator muscle from the lateral margin of the prostate. If the incision is made too close to the prostate, bleeding from the overlying venous plexus can occur on the lateral margin of the prostate. Under these circumstances, it is best to place a suture of 3.0 Vicryl along the lateral prostate to gain hemostasis.

After the endopelvic fascia has been incised bilaterally, a sponge stick is used to depress the bladder posteriorly. The fatty tissue overlying the anterior prostate is carefully teased away using forceps and the sucker tip. This exposes the superficial dorsal vein (Fig. 32–5). We prefer to control this vein separate from the deep dorsal vein complex using electrocautery. Even though the superficial dorsal vein may be large, it does not require a liga-

ture and can easily be avulsed in attempting to tie a suture. The vein is freed of surrounding fat and lifted from the surface of the prostate with a right-angle clamp. It is grasped with forceps and cauterized proximally and distally and then divided.

After the superficial dorsal vein is divided, a Kitner dissector is used to define the puboprostatic ligaments. These usually are evident as a distinct white ligamentous structure. Often, there is some adherent levator muscular tissue just lateral to the puboprostatic ligament. Sometimes, there is a small vein within this tissue. A right-angle clamp passed just lateral to the puboprostatic ligament can define this tissue well and allow it to be dissected off of the lateral prostatic apex using Bovie electrocautery.

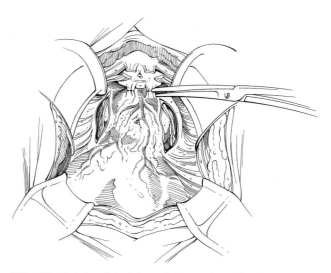

FIG. 32–5. Lateral incision of the endopelvic fascia up to puboprostatic ligaments after division of the superficial dorsal vein.

It is important to define the puboprostatic ligaments precisely as described above. This allows accurate placement of a ligature that will incorporate the dorsal vein complex. The deep dorsal vein complex runs parallel to the urethra at the prostatic apex and then fans out over the anterior prostate. We feel that it is important to control these vessels preemptively rather than simply to incise them and place sutures afterward. A McDougal clamp is useful for this purpose (Fig. 32–6). Using the thumb and forefinger of the left hand, the dorsal vein complex can be pinched partially off of the anterior urethra and the jaws of the McDougal clamp passed just anterior to the urethra. Bleeding is rare during this maneuver if the anatomic structures are carefully dissected and defined. Spreading the jaws of the clamp should be avoided so as not to injure the anterior sphincter mechanism. A 1 Vicryl ligature is then tied around the dorsal vein complex. The McDougal clamp is then passed through the same space

again and held in position while a 0 Vicryl suture on a CT-1 needle is passed through the center of the dorsal vein complex just distal to the previous ligature. After the anterior portion of this stick suture is tied, the McDougal clamp is used to pull the end of the suture around the posterior aspect of the dorsal vein complex, which is then controlled further by tying the two suture ends. Back-bleeding is prevented by placing a 0 Vicryl suture on a CT-1 through the veins of the dorsal vein complex where they fan out over the anterior prostate. Grasping the lateral margins of the veins with an Allis clamp helps bunch them in the middle and facilitates placement of this hemostatic suture (Fig. 32–7). The McDougal clamp is again passed through the previously defined space. Electrocautery is then used to divide the dorsal vein complex just proximal to the 0 Vicryl ligature placed earlier. Sometimes, this ligature becomes displaced during this process, but the backup 0 Vicryl fixed suture maintains

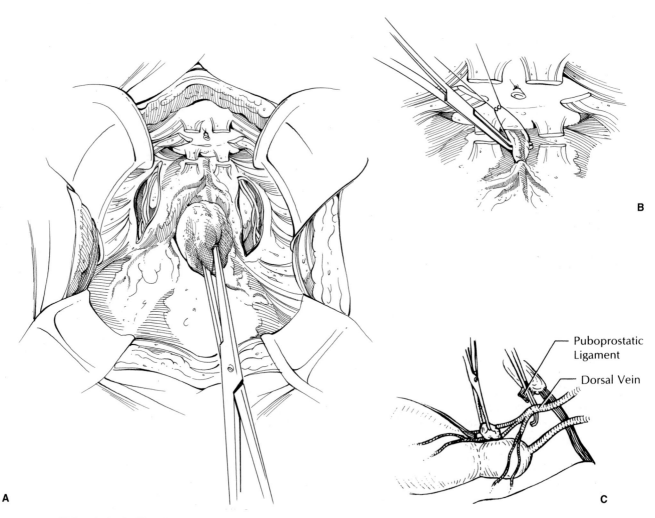

FIG. 32–6. A: The deep dorsal venous complex is identified. **B:** A McDougal clamp is placed around the dorsal vein and it is ligated proximally. **C:** Lateral view of the plane between the prostate and the dorsal vein showing how posterior depression of the superior prostate aids in the dissection.

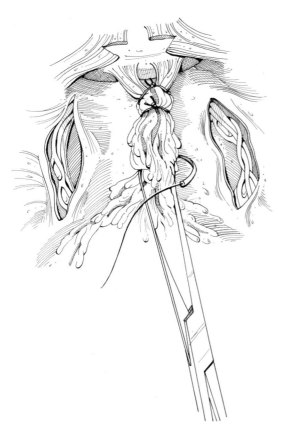

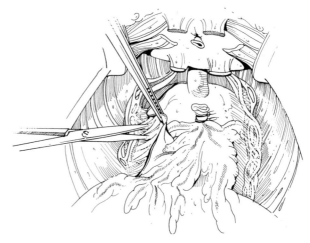

FIG. 32–8. Dissection of the lateral fascia off of the prostate to release the neurovascular bundle before dividing the urethra.

FIG. 32–7. Suture ligation of the proximal dorsal venous complex with an Allis clamp aiding in identification of the bundle.

hemostasis. The McDougal clamp is gently lifted as the electrocautery is used to displace the electrical energy away from the sphincter muscle.

This entire technique usually allows total hemostasis during division of the dorsal vein complex and no additional hemostatic sutures in general are required. When bleeding occurs, it is usually from a vein that is located posterolaterally and just at the surface of the prostate. If the prostate is depressed with a sponge stick, this vein can be identified for precise placement of a 4.0 Vicryl suture on an RB-1 needle.

At this point, the anterior sphincter muscle should be untouched and the prostatic apex and membranous urethra visible. Attention is now turned toward dissection of the neurovascular bundle off of the prostate. To accomplish this, the lateral fascia overlying the prostate is gently lifted with forceps. Metzenbaum scissors are used to dissect the fascial layer of the lateral prostate and, in doing so, carry the neurovascular bundle posterolaterally (Fig. 32–8). Some bleeding occurs during this maneuver but it is not usually enough that any directed hemostatic efforts are required. The most important part of this aspect of the dissection is at the apex and just lateral to the urethra. The bundle is gently separated from the lateral margin of the urethra. Performing the dissection in

this manner facilitates not only preservation of the neurovascular bundle but also identification of the urethra.

The urethra is divided sharply just at the prostatic apex (Fig. 32–9). The Foley catheter is identified and withdrawn through the partially severed urethra after cutting off the injection port and connector end. The Foley catheter is not used for traction as this can injure the sphincter muscle or cavernous nerve. The posterior portion of the urethra is divided under direct division using Metzenbaum scissors.

With dissection of the neurovascular bundle prior to division of the urethra, the prostatorectal fascia or rectourethralis muscle is readily identifiable. This is incised sharply at the posterior lip of the prostate (Fig. 32–10).

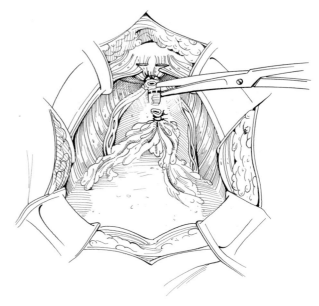

FIG. 32–9. Division of the membranous urethra.

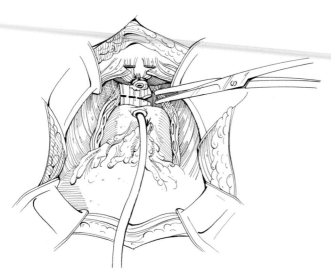

FIG. 32–10. Division of the rectourethralis, taking care to avoid the neurovascular bundles.

The entire prostatic apex must be well visualized at this point to make certain that all apical tissue is excised. Excellent hemostasis is necessary to perform this maneuver under direct vision.

The appropriate plane of dissection along the anterior rectal wall is visible and can be developed partly with sharp dissection. Blunt finger dissection can also be used but blunt dissection should not be used to break into this plane (Fig. 32–11). This risks rectal injury. Once the proper plane has been entered, the prostate can be gently lifted anteriorly. This allows a right-angle clamp to be passed between the posterior lateral prostate and the neurovascular bundle. We use small hemoclips to secure perforating vessels from the bundle to the prostate. The bundle is gently dissected from the prostate all the way up to the level of the prostatic pedicle.

At this point, the table is placed in the partial Trendelenburg position to allow better visualization of the posterior prostate, the seminal vesicles, and the prostatic pedicle. An incision is made through the posterior layer of Denonvillier's fascia (Fig. 32–12). This exposes the seminal vesicles and ampulla of the vas deferens. It also facilitates identification of the prostatic pedicle. A right-angle clamp placed just lateral to the seminal vesicle can encircle the vascular pedicle (Fig. 32–13). A 2.0 Vicryl suture is used to ligate the prostatic pedicle. It is important to ligate the pedicle sufficiently distant from the prostate that an adequate incision can be made through the pedicle without incising into the prostatic capsule. Some backbleeding from the prostate occurs but this is readily controlled with pressure or electrocautery.

Complete division of the prostatic pedicle greatly facilitates visualization and dissection of the seminal vesicles (Fig. 32–14). A right-angle clamp is passed around the ampulla of the vas deferens just medial to the seminal vesicle. The ampulla is divided with electrocautery. The seminal vesicle is then dissected free. The neurovascular bundle lies just lateral to the seminal vesicle so minimal

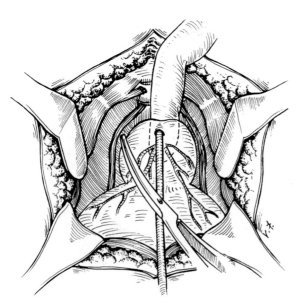

FIG. 32–11. The prostate is mobilized off the rectum in the midline and the lateral pelvic fascia is incised carefully between the posteriolateral surface of the prostate and the neurovascular bundle. (Modified from Catalona WJ. *Prostate cancer*. Orlando, FL: Grune & Stratton, 1984:107, with permission.)

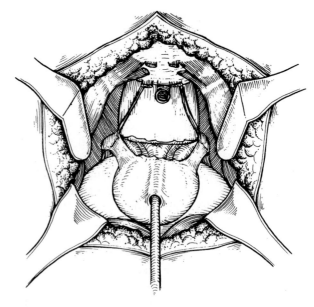

FIG. 32–12. Denonvillier's fascia is incised between the base of the prostate and the anterior rectal wall, exposing the ampullary portions of the vasa deferentia and the medial wall of the seminal vesicles. The proper plane of dissection for the prostatic vascular pedicles is just lateral to the seminal vesicles.

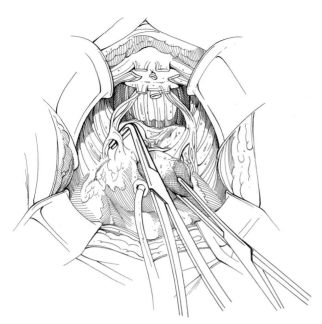

FIG. 32–13. A right-angle clamp is used to dissect out the superior vascular pedicle, taking care to divide the pedicle close to the prostate and avoiding injury of the neurovascular bundles.

electrocautery is used at this point. When a nerve-sparing approach is used, we often do not excise the very tip of the seminal vesicle. This adds nothing in terms of tumor control and avoids dissection near the neurovascular bundle. The artery to the seminal vesicle tip is identifiable and can be clipped.

After both seminal vesicles have been divided, they are lifted superiorly to expose the junction between the pos-

terior prostate and the bladder neck. This is developed with electrocautery and any lateral attachments are also taken down with electrocautery. This should provide good definition of the bladder neck. A bladder neck-sparing procedure is used. We do not believe that this helps with continence but it does allow a complete anatomic section with excision of all prostatic tissue. Further, avoidance of sutures at the bladder neck may help decrease the risk of bladder neck contracture postoperatively. The bladder neck is incised and the surgical specimen is removed (Fig. 32–15). The bladder neck is usually fingertip size at this point (Fig. 32–16). If the bladder neck has been well defined in this manner, identification of the ureteral orifices is not necessary before completing the removal of the surgical specimen. However, if there is a question of tumor encroachment toward the bladder neck wider margins should be taken. Under these circumstances, it is best to visualize the bladder trigone before incising the posterior bladder neck.

After the surgical specimen is removed, careful hemostasis is obtained. There are usually a number of bleeding vessels around the bladder neck and on the pedicle that can be controlled with electrocautery. Larger bleeding vessels along the neurovascular bundle are controlled with individual sutures of 4.0 Vicryl.

We have found a grooved urethral sound useful for placement of the urethral anastomotic sutures. External perineal compression has been unnecessary as the urethral stump in general is readily visible and suture placement not difficult. The operating surgeon uses his left hand to manipulate the urethral sound and the right hand to place the anastomotic sutures. We use five sutures spaced proportionately around the urethral circumference

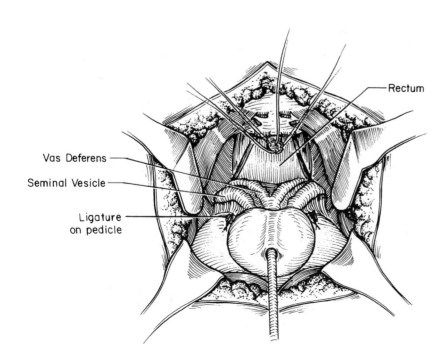

FIG. 32–14. The prostatic vascular pedicles have been divided to a point cephalad to the seminal vesicles, exposing the ampullae and the seminal vesicles and mobilizing the prostate. (Modified from Catalona WJ. *Prostate cancer.* Orlando, FL: Grune & Stratton, 1984:110, with permission.)

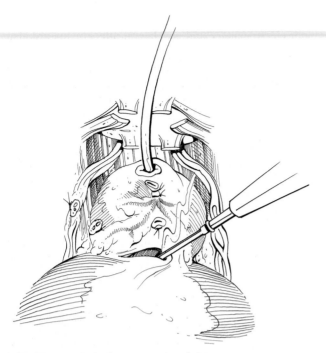

FIG. 32–15. Division of the anterior bladder neck with the cautery.

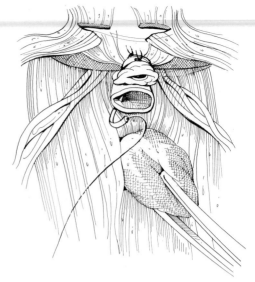

FIG. 32–17. Initial sutures placed in the urethra.

(Fig. 32–17). The sutures on the patient's left side are most easily placed outside to in and incorporate only the urethra. Care should be taken to avoid the neurovascular bundle. We use 2.0 Vicryl for the anastomosis and have a double-armed needle that allows inside-out placement of the sutures on the patient's right side. The sutures are then placed in a corresponding position in the bladder neck (Fig. 32–18). We do not place mucosal eversion sutures prior to the anastomosis, but an Allis clamp placed anteriorly on the bladder neck can nicely evert the mucosa. An 18 Fr Foley catheter with a 5-cc balloon is passed through the anastomosis prior to placement of the most anterior suture to prevent any tangling of the sutures that

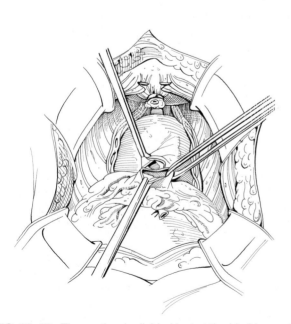

FIG. 32–16. The urethra is divided just at the bladder neck.

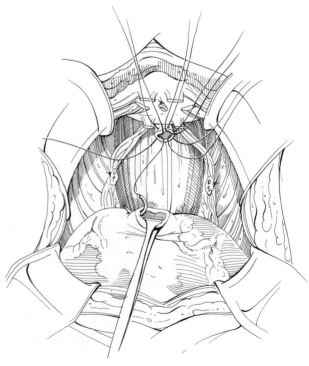

FIG. 32–18. Urethral sutures are placed close together.

could result in catheter entrapment. The same style of clamps is always used to tag these sutures and avoid any confusion. For example, straight hemostats are used for the two most posterior sutures, curved hemostats for the two paired anterolateral sutures, and a Kocher clamp for the most anterior suture.

The Foley catheter balloon is inflated with 12 cc of water and the table flexion is released. A sponge stick is used to displace the bladder medially so that the anastomotic sutures can be tied. After all of the sutures have been tied, the anastomosis is inspected both visually and manually to make certain that all of the ties have gone down completely and that there is no portion of the catheter either visible or palpable. Rarely, the anastomosis is not felt to be completely secure. Under these circumstances, we take down the anastomosis and redo it. Although this is painstaking, a secure anastomosis can help avoid long-term complications after the procedure.

We insert a single Jackson–Pratt drain through a right lower-quadrant stab wound and place this directly over the anastomosis. The incision is closed with a running 1 Vicryl suture. The skin is closed with a subcuticular 4.0 Vicryl suture.

POSTOPERATIVE CARE

We have designed and implemented a collaborative care pathway for patients undergoing radical retropubic prostatectomy (6). The target date for hospital discharge is postoperative day 1. Ninety-four percent of our patients are discharged by postoperative day 2.

Early ambulation is performed and patients are walking in the hallways on the evening of the surgical procedure. They are kept NPO until the following morning. Patients are usually thirsty postoperatively and may take copious amounts of clear liquids, which can lead to early problems with ileus. We have preferred to wait until the morning after surgery to begin a full liquid diet and then advance the patient immediately to a regular diet. Our goal is to have the patient taking a regular diet without problems by the afternoon of postoperative day 1. We do use Dulcolax suppositories as needed. We have not had a rectal injury in over 1,000 consecutive patients and so are not concerned about gentle placement of a suppository.

Postoperative analgesia is provided by use of ketorolac, 30 mg administered intravenously in the operating room and then every 8 hours for three consecutive doses. With short-term use of this drug, we have not observed any apparent drug-related bleeding complications or gastrointestinal side effects. Few patients require supplementary oral narcotics and we have found parenteral narcotics via patient-controlled analgesia unnecessary. Do not use epidural catheters postoperatively. These are unnecessary for analgesia in patients undergoing radical prostatec-

tomy and can lead to prolonged ileus and decreased ambulation.

The Foley catheter is removed 1 week postoperatively unless the patient has had prolonged drainage. In leaving the catheter for 1 week, we do not need to perform a cystogram prior to catheter removal. Urinary retention requiring reinsertion of a catheter is exceedingly rare.

OUTCOMES

Complications

Using the aforementioned technique, intraoperative bleeding complications are unusual. Our median blood loss is less than 500 cc. We do not ask patients to donate autologous blood preoperatively as our transfusion requirement for homologous blood is less than 1%.

Thromboembolic complications remain the most frequent cause of serious morbidity and occasional mortality after radical prostatectomy. Clinically recognized deep venous thrombosis occurs in 3% to 5% and pulmonary embolus in 1% to 3% of patients. Our use of perioperative low-dose heparin in patients at a high risk for thrombolic complications helps decrease this risk (5).

The most common problem leading to prolonged hospitalization is ileus. Around 4% of our patients are not able to be discharged by the second postoperative day and this is usually because of abdominal distension from ileus. Minimizing use of parenteral narcotics diminishes postoperative ileus.

Results

Radical prostatectomy has maintained a cardinal role in the management of patients with carcinoma of the prostate. If the tumor is completely confined within the prostatic capsule, nearly 90% of patients have an undetectable PSA postoperatively. As with any surgical procedure, the success of radical prostatectomy depends upon appropriate patient selection and careful attention to anatomic detail and surgical technique.

REFERENCES

1. Gerber GS, Thisted RA, Scardino PT, et al. Results of radical prostatectomy in men with clinically localized prostate cancer. *JAMA* 1996; 276:615–619.
2. Hoenig DM, Chi S, Porter C, et al. Risk of nodal metastases at laparoscopic pelvic lymphadenectomy using PSA, Gleason score and clinical stage in men with localized prostate cancer. *J Endourol* 1997;11: 263–265.
3. Koch MO, Miller DA, Butler R, Lebos L, Collings D, Smith JA Jr. Are we selecting the right patients for treatment of localized prostate cancer? Results of an actuarial analysis. *Urology* 1998;51:197–202.
4. Koch MO, Smith JA Jr. Blood loss during radical retropubic prostatectomy: Is preoperative autologous blood donation indicated? *J Urol* 1996;156:1077–1079.
5. Koch MO, Smith JA Jr. Low molecular weight heparin and radical prostatectomy: a prospective analysis of safety and side effects. *Prostate Cancer Prostatic Dis* 1997;1:101–104.

6. Koch MO, Smith JA Jr, Hodge EM, Brandell RA. Prospective development of a cost-efficient program for radical retropubic prostatectomy. *Urology* 1994;44:311–318.

7. Smith JA Jr. Techniques to decrease morbidity with radical prostatectomy. *AUA Update Ser* 2000;19:273–280.

8. Smith JA Jr, Koch MO. Collaborative care pathways: impact on treatment costs and quality of care after radical prostatectomy. *J Managed Care* 1997;1:36–38.

9. Smith JA Jr, Scardino PT, Resnick MI, Hernandez AD, Rose SC, Egger MJ. Transrectal ultrasound versus digital rectal examination for the staging of carcinoma of the prostate: results of a prospective, multi-institutional trial. *J Urol* 1997;157:902–906.

CHAPTER 33

Radical Perineal Prostatectomy

Sam D. Graham, Jr.

Radical perineal prostatectomy was first introduced in 1869 by Buchler and popularized in the United States by Young in 1903. It remained the primary surgical approach to carcinoma of the prostate the mid-1970s. With the recognition of the importance of assessing pelvic lymph nodes preoperatively and the advantage that retropubic prostatectomy offered with the concomitant pelvic node dissection, perineal prostatectomy declined in popularity for the treatment of prostate cancer. The perineal approach, however, saw a resurgence in the 1990s for several reasons: (a) the trend toward minimally invasive surgery with a focus on reducing the morbidity and therefore hospital stay of patients, (b) the advent of laparoscopic surgery for lymph node assessment, (c) the introduction of prostate-specific antigen (PSA) for screening for prostate cancer with reduction in the numbers of patients with node-positive disease, and (d) algorithms that may predict patients at high risk for positive lymph nodes. The procedure is also associated with reduced blood loss and low morbidity and can be modified to incorporate the neurovascular-sparing techniques for preservation of potency.

DIAGNOSIS

All potential candidates for radical perineal prostatectomy should undergo preoperative staging to ensure that they are operable candidates. Methods of differentiating local versus advanced disease include digital rectal examination, transrectal ultrasonography, radionuclide bone scan, assessment of pelvic lymph nodes, as well as pathologic indicators of progression such as Gleason sum and other markers.

Since the late 1980s, PSA has made a significant impact on the preoperative stage of patients with prostate cancer. Patients presenting for surgery are in general younger, healthier, and more likely to have organ-con-

fined prostate cancer than the population treated only a decade earlier; this in many ways attributes to the large increase in the number of radical prostatectomies done in the United States in the past decade.

Digital rectal examination has a limited role in the assessment of the clinical staging of prostate cancer. Its primary attribute is to crudely estimate the volume of the cancer. Transrectal ultrasonography is another modality that has limitations in assessing local disease but combined with digital rectal examination at least gives some gross assessment of likelihood of extracapsular disease. Other modalities such as transrectal magnetic resonance imaging (MRI), computed tomography (CT) scan, and pelvic MRI have been shown to have limited usefulness. Radionuclide bone scans are useful in assessing advanced bony disease but in general are not positive in patients under 20 and with no other sign of advanced disease.

For the past 16 years we prospectively applied an algorithm to the preoperative assessment of patients with prostate cancer based upon the evaluation of more than 400 patients who had undergone pelvic node dissection. The current algorithm includes patients with a Gleason sum of 6 or less (or a Gleason 7, providing the predominant pattern is 3), a low-volume cancer (T_{1b-1c}, T_{2a}), normal acid phosphatase, and PSA of less than 10 ng per mL. Patients meeting all of these criteria have a less than 5% chance of positive lymph nodes and, therefore, we do not perform pelvic lymph node dissections (1). Patients exceeding any one of the above criteria are considered to be in the high-risk group and have undergone pelvic lymph node dissections. Using this method of assessment, our overall PSA recurrence rate from 1986 to 1993 was 24%. This compares favorably to other series of retropubic prostatectomies, which have shown PSA recurrence rates between 24% and 28%. Comparative studies have shown no difference in recurrence rates between perineal and retropubic prostatectomy (3–5).

INDICATIONS FOR SURGERY

Patients who are candidates for radical prostatectomy must have clinically organ-confined prostate cancer (T_{1-2}). In addition to having organ-confined disease, other factors needing to be taken into consideration are the patient's life expectancy, other comorbidities, or any other factors that may affect the patient's choice. We in general would not offer a radical prostatectomy to patients who have a less than 10-year life expectancy. Over the age of 70, we would offer a radical prostatectomy only in selected cases where we feel that the benefits that can be obtained outweigh the potential risks, in particular when compared to alternative therapies.

ALTERNATIVE THERAPY

Alternatives to perineal prostatectomy include retropubic and laparoscopic prostatectomies. The retropubic approach allows simultaneous node dissection and removal of larger prostate glands, although the length of hospitalization and immediate postoperative morbidity are higher at our institution. The laparoscopic approach allows some improvement in visualization due to the magnification but has yet to show any advantages in terms of operative morbidity, length of stay, or reduction in long-term morbidity. In addition, it requires two surgeons and is a considerably longer operation than either the retropubic or perineal approach.

Alternatives to radical prostatectomy include observation, hormonal deprivation, and radiation therapy. We do not consider either observation or hormonal deprivation to be curative and the patients for whom this is a good option are those with less than 5 years of life expectancy, patients who are > 70 years old with a well-differentiated cancer, or patients who are a high risk for surgery and refuse radiation. Radiation therapy, however, may be definitive and has an equivalent 5- and 10-year survival. The recurrence rates with radiation therapy are bimodal, with initial recurrences within 1 to 2 years of treatment and a delayed peak at 5 to 7 years after treatment. If the patient is young and has a 15-year or longer outlook, our results would favor radical prostatectomy.

SURGICAL TECHNIQUE

The patient is placed in an exaggerated lithotomy position (Fig. 33–1). It is important that the patient's perineum be parallel to the floor as this directly affects exposure. We use a standard operating room table with folded sheets under the patient's sacrum supporting the patient's entire weight. We do not use shoulder braces, and if a patient tends to slide off of the sheets we will place the table in a slight reverse Trendelenburg position. The patient's legs are stabilized using candy-cane stirrups, again taking precautions to prevent stretching the ham-

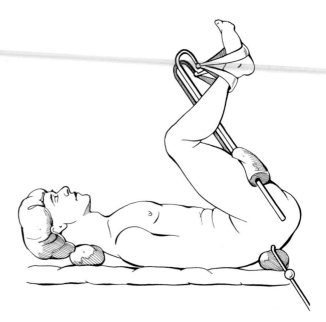

FIG. 33–1. Positioning of the patient requires the perineum to be parallel to the floor. The sacrum supports the patient's weight and the legs are positioned with no traction on the hamstrings. No shoulder braces are indicated.

string or causing pressure on the legs. Prior to putting the patient in position, the legs are wrapped with Ace bandages.

Five instruments are significant in assisting the surgeon for this operation. These include the Lowsley curve tractor, the Young straight prostatic tractor, a halogen headlamp, a harmonic scalpel, and an Omni-Tract miniwishbone retractor system. The curved Lowsley tractor is used to bring the prostate up into the perineum to allow the section against the prostate while operating the rectum from the prostate. The straight Young tractor is used to manipulate the prostate laterally as well as cephalad and caudad after the membranous urethra has been divided. The halogen headlamp is important in that it allows the surgeon to aim a strong light into the operative field, which may be deep and narrow, preventing standard operating lights to adequately illuminate the structures. The harmonic scalpel allows coagulation and closure of vessels without transmission of electrical current, thereby reducing the risks to the neurovascular bundles. The Omni-Tract miniwishbone allows virtually unlimited retraction in any direction.

Note that in manipulation of the prostate the pelvis should be viewed as a cone, with the apex of the cone being the incision (Fig. 33–2). To get better visualization at times, it is necessary to actually push the prostate further into the pelvis. Also note that traction is not placed directly on the bulb or membranous urethra as this will decrease the likelihood of restoration of potency and potentially affect the patient's continence postoperatively.

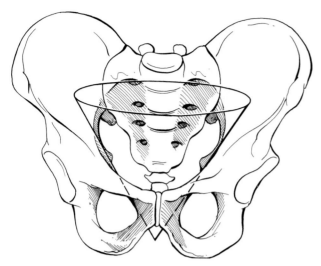

FIG. 33–2. The bony pelvis is a cone with the apex at the incision. Better visualization can be obtained in many cases by actually pushing the prostate deeper into the pelvis.

The incision is made from the ischial tuberosity crossing the midline at the juncture between the squamous epithelium and mucocutaneous border of the rectum (Fig. 33–3). The incision posteriorly extends to a line equal to the posterior portion of the anus. Using sharp dissection and electrocautery, the ischiorectal fossa are entered and using blunt dissection the central perineal tendon is identified and transected with an electrocautery. At this point, we employ the Belt approach and dissect down to the white fascia of the rectum and proceed subsphincterically (Fig. 33–4). Using predominantly blunt dissection with an index finger in the rectum, the rectal sphincter and levator ani can be dissected free of the rectum with minimal bleeding (Fig. 33–5). The blades from the miniwishbone retractor are then used to retract these muscles anteriorly and laterally. With tension on these muscle and tension on the rectum, the rectourethralis is identified and divided, allowing the surgeon to dissect the rectum free of the apex of the prostate (Fig. 33–6).

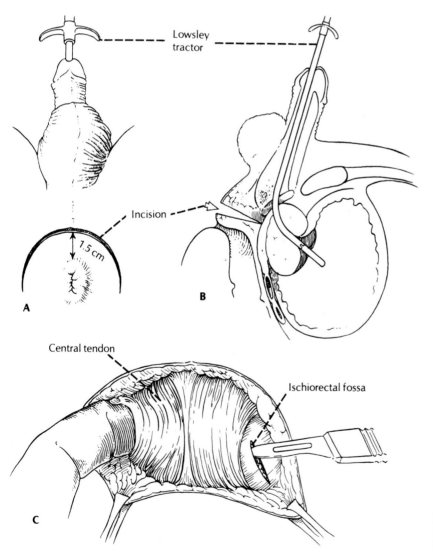

FIG. 33–3. An inverted U-shaped incision is made in the perineum extending from ischial tuberosity to ischial tuberosity.

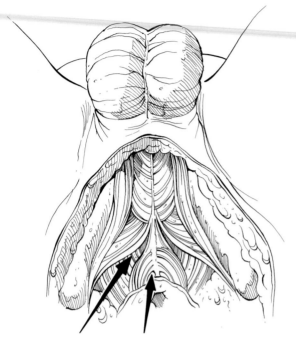

FIG. 33–4. The dissection is carried along the rectal fascia, sparing the anal sphincter.

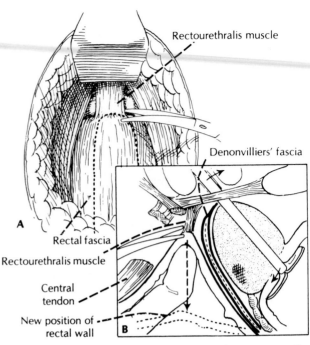

FIG. 33–6. Dissection of the rectum from the prostate after division of the rectourethralis is facilitated with the surgeon's finger in the rectum.

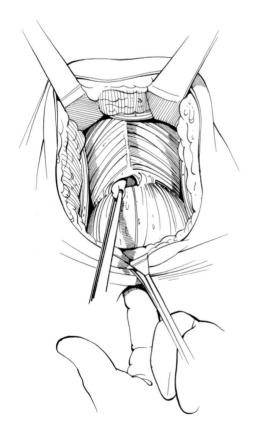

FIG. 33–5. Levator ani and anal sphincter retracted to expose the rectourethralis.

If this is to be a nerve-sparing technique, the dissection is carried down to approximately 1.5 to 2 cm from the apex, at which point the external layer of Denonvillier's fascia is divided and dissection is carried between the two layers of Denonvillier's fascia (Fig. 33–7). Care is taken to not damage the neurovascular bundles that course along the lateral posterior prostate on either side (Fig. 33–8).

The distal portion of Denonvillier's fascia is then incised in the midline with scissors, the tag is then used to facilitate dissection of the neurovascular bundle from the prostate (Fig. 33–9), and the inferior pedicle, if present, is ligated and divided (Fig. 33–10). If the dissection is any way impaired by fibrosis such that there is a potential for prostatic tissue to be left behind, the neurovascular bundle is sacrificed on that side. Note that during this dissection the neurovascular bundle actually courses across the posterior surface of the prostate at the apex and enters the urogenital diaphragm just posterior to the membranous urethra. This proximity should be noted in that the vesicourethral anastomosis may incorporate the neurovascular bundle if the surgeon is not precise with the placement of sutures in the posterior urethra. The retraction of the neurovascular bundle on either side thereby exposes the proximal membranous urethra.

A right-angled clamp is placed around the membranous urethra and in general meets little resistance if one stays posterior to the endopelvic fascia (Fig. 33–11). The Lowsley tractor is removed and the membranous urethra divided. The Young tractor is then placed into the bladder

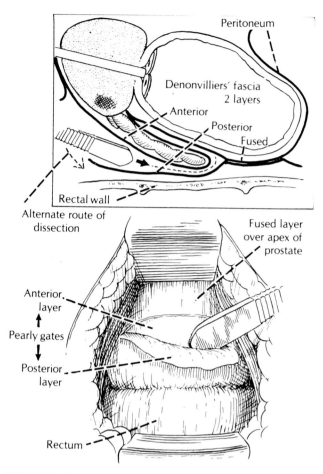

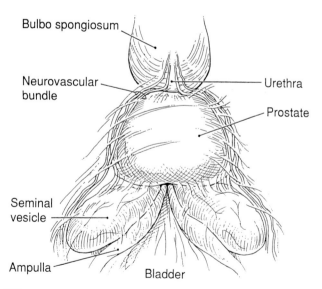

FIG. 33–7. An incision into the posterior layer of Denonvillier's fascia allows the dissection to continue between the two layers. For a nerve-sparing technique, this incision is made transversely 1 to 2 cm proximal to the apex of the prostate, avoiding carrying the incision into the neurovascular bundles.

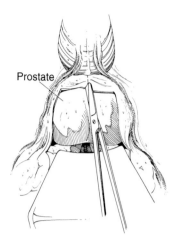

FIG. 33–9. Incision of the distal posterior layer of Denonvillier's fascia in the midline. This is best done *without* electrocautery if a nerve-sparing technique is planned.

via the severed prostatic urethra, and the endopelvic fascia divided with the harmonic scalpel.

The anterior prostate is dissected free of the bladder. Note that there are in general two small arteries that enter the prostate along the anterior bladder at the 10- and 2-o'clock positions that should be cauterized and divided. The groove between the prostate and bladder is identified and, either with sharp or blunt dissection, the prostate and bladder can be separated. If there is any resistance to blunt dissection, this should be performed sharply and biopsies taken of the bladder neck to ensure that this is not secondary to bladder neck invasion by the cancer. Patients who have had prior transurethral resections may have an obliteration of the plane between the prostate and bladder; the blades of the Young tractor can be used to aid in this identification.

In most cases, there is insignificant bleeding from the dorsal venous complex in the endopelvic fascia. How-

FIG. 33–8. Anatomic view of the neurovascular bundles from the posterior view of the prostate. The vessels course along the lateral and posterior prostate and cross the apex to enter the urogenital diaphragm posterior to the membranous urethra.

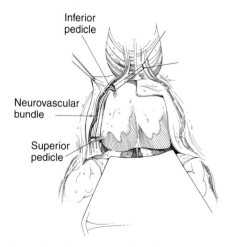

FIG. 33–10. Using the wings of the distal posterior layer of Denonvillier's fascia to aid in dissection, the inferior branch from the neurovascular is isolated and divided.

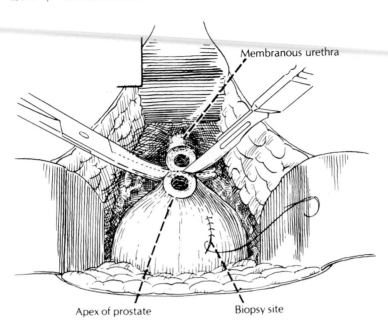

FIG. 33–11. Division of the membranous urethra at the apex of the prostate.

ever, if there should be communicating veins they should be suture ligated using 3-0 Vicryl. The prostate is dissected from the bladder anteriorly to the 5- and 7-o'clock positions, respectively, on the patient's left and right, the bladder neck is divided over the Young tractor, and the Young tractor is removed (Fig. 33–12). The bladder is evacuated of any urine and the posterior bladder neck is divided with the cautery. The prostate is then dissected free from the posterior bladder.

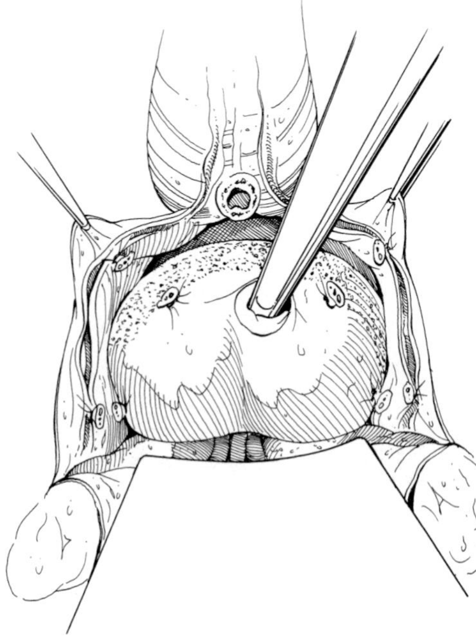

Attention is then directed to the posterior surface of the prostate. The rectum is swept free of the neurovascular bundles, allowing identification of the superior pedicles of the prostate as well as the seminal structures. The superior pedicles are divided with the harmonic scalpel. The seminal vesicles are dissected to their tips with blunt dissection, and the artery from the seminal vesical is either cauterized or ligated while the vas deferens are divided with the harmonic scalpel. Any remaining fibrolymphatic tissue is then divided, allowing removal of the prostate.

After ensuring complete hemostasis, the bladder neck is reconstructed using 3-0 Vicryl on an SH needle beginning posteriorly to anteriorly (Fig. 33–13). This direction of the closure, beginning in the posterior bladder, is done

FIG. 33–12. A Young prostatic tractor is used to manipulate the prostate and identify the vesical neck.

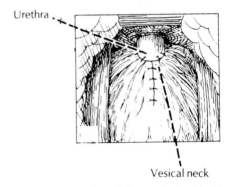

FIG. 33–13. Reconstruction of the posterior bladder neck is carried from posterior to anterior, leaving an opening of approximately 22 Fr.

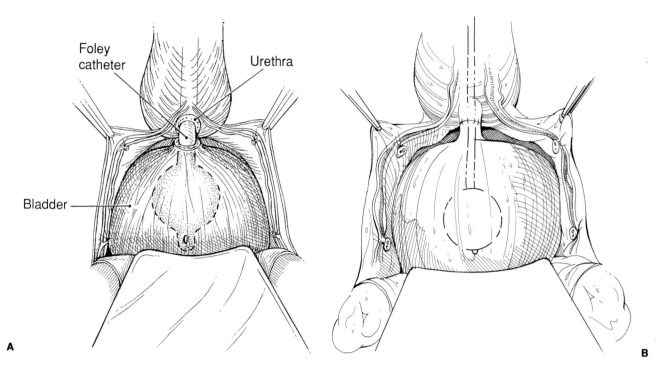

FIG. 33–14. Anastomosis of the urethra to the bladder is performed over a 22 Fr Foley catheter.

to facilitate the closure without injury to the ureters and also to take advantage of the anatomic relationship between the bladder neck and the membranous urethra with a closer distance being anteriorly. The anastomosis is performed using 3-0 Vicryl simple sutures using an RB-1 controlled-release needle (Fig. 33–14). The anastomosis is performed around a No. 22 Fr 5-cc Foley catheter and in general seven to eight sutures are used for this anastomosis. Care should be taken that small portions of the membranous urethra are incorporated in the anastomosis such that the continence mechanism is left undisturbed, as well as the neurovascular bundles that contribute to potency.

The rectum is then inspected, a Foley balloon inflated, and a Penrose drain placed through the left ischiorectal fossa and a separate stab incision. The incision is closed with a 3-0 chromic gut closure. One suture is placed to reapproximate the central tendon and the remainder of the sutures are used to close the skin in a horizontal mattress fashion (Fig. 33–15).

Postoperatively, patients have low requirements for pain medication. Most patients either do not require parenteral pain medication or are off the parenteral medications within 12 to 24 hours. Average time to discharge is approximately 48 hours from the time of surgery (Table 33–1). The patient's catheter is removed

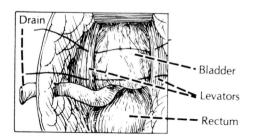

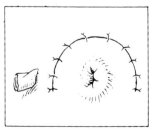

FIG. 33–15. Closure of the incision.

TABLE 33–1. *Post Op Orders*

Lab
- CBC, Basic Metabolic Panel in AM

Interventions/Treatments
- Vital signs q4h
- I & O q shift
- Urinary catheter to bedside bag
- Leg bag at bedside upon admission to unit. Post Op day 1, staff nurse to begin leg bag teaching. Ensure that catheter remains secure at all times using catheter holder (Cath Secure)
- Dressing Changes prn
- Ace wraps to lower extremities until patient ambulatory

Activity
- Dangle at bedside evening of surgery, may get out of bed to chair
- Starting post op day 1, out of bed to chair for meals and ambulate in hall

Diet
- Clear liquids immediately post op, regular diet as tolerated

IV Fluids
- RL at 125cc/hr
- convert to heparin lock in AM

Medications
- Cefazolin 1 gram IV q 8h x 4 doses
- Gentamicin 80mg IV q 8h x 3 doses
- Morphine Sulphate 2-4 mg IV q 3h prn severe pain
- Percocet 5/325 q 3h prn pain

Respiratory
- Incentive Spirometry q2h while awake

Patient and Family Teaching
- Review discharge instructions with patient and family on day of surgery and reinforce daily
- Instruct patient on leg bag usage, catheter care, and diet^

on postoperative day 12. The Penrose drain is removed prior to discharge.

OUTCOMES

Complications

Perioperative complications include hemorrhage, wound infection, cardiovascular complications, and rectal injury. The instance of rectal injury is less than 2%. With current techniques and antibiotics, preoperative bowel preparation (Go-Lytely), and antibiotics, these are closed primarily in two layers without the need to perform a diverting colostomy. Wound infection rates are less than 1% and cardiovascular complications are approximately 1%. The average blood loss in these patients is approximately 450 cc, and our transfusion rate is less than 2%.

Long-term complications include incontinence and impotence. Incontinence requiring intervention such as pads, clamps, or inflatable devices occurs in 2.8% of the patients. We have found that incontinence in general occurs in patients who are older, obese, and have had prior radiation therapy. Potency following nerve-sparing perineal prostatectomy is dependent upon the patient's age and preoperative status. Patients under the age of 60 who are fully potent and have both neurovascular bundles spared have approximately a 50% potency rate. Patients who are over the age of 60 have a reduced rate of potency,

and we have not yet had a patient over the age of 70 who has spontaneously regained his potency. Patients who are having difficulties with potency prior to surgery and patients in whom the neurovascular bundles could not be spared will likely be impotent. We in general advocate early use of pharmacotherapy or other means of assistance in these patients.

Results

Following radical prostatectomy, recurrence can be measured using PSA, which is exquisitely sensitive. Any patient who undergoes a radical prostatectomy can expect their PSA to fall below detectable levels. Failure to do so in general means that the patient has significant residual disease, either locally or distantly. Another group of patients will have an initial drop of their PSA to undetectable levels and then a return to measurable levels. These patients may have local and/or distant recurrence of their disease or possibly residual malignancy. Patients who develop recurrence based upon PSA will in general manifest a clinical progression within 18 months. In addition, if the PSA is going to rise it will do so within 2 years in 90% of patients and within 4 years in virtually every patient. Based upon PSA, we can now predict disease recurrence earlier, allowing assessment of the outcome of radical prostatectomy within 5 years as opposed to the older data, which required a 7- to 10-year follow-up (3).

Using a clinical care pathway, we have seen better pain control, earlier ambulation, quicker short-term recovery, and earlier discharge than in patients undergoing radical retropubic prostatectomy. This has been confirmed in other studies and will lead to a lower cost of care (2,6).

REFERENCES

1. El-Galley RE, Keane TE, Petros JA, Sanders WH, Clarke HS, Cotsonis GA, Graham SD Jr. Evaluation of staging lymphadenectomy in prostate cancer. *Urology* 1998;52:663–667.
2. Harris MJ. Radical perineal prostatectomy: cost efficient, outcome effective, minimally invasive prostate cancer management. *Eur Urol* 2003;44:303–308; discussion 308.
3. Iselin CE, Robertson JE, Paulson DF. Radical perineal prostatectomy: oncological outcome during a 20-year period. *J Urol* 1999;161: 163–168.
4. Lance RS, Freidrichs PA, Kane C, Powell CR, Pulos E, Moul JW, McLeod DG, Cornum RL, Brantley Thrasher J. A comparison of radical retropubic with perineal prostatectomy for localized prostate cancer within the Uniformed Services Urology Research Group. *BJU Int* 2001; 87:61–65.
5. Sullivan LD, Weir MJ, Kinahan JF, Taylor DL. A comparison of the relative merits of radical perineal and radical retropubic prostatectomy. *BJU Int* 2000;85:95–100.
6. Weizer AZ, Silverstein AD, Young MD, Vieweg J, Paulson DF, Dahm P. Prospective evaluation of pain medication requirements and recovery after radical perineal prostatectomy. *Urology* 2003;62:693–697.

CHAPTER 34

Brachytherapy for Localized Prostate Cancer

Haakon Ragde and William A. Cavanagh

"Brachy"(therapy), meaning "short" in Greek, describes treatment with radioactive sources or materials placed into, or at a short distance from, the tissue to be radiated. Brachytherapy stands in contrast to "tele"(therapy)—Greek for "long"—which refers to external radiation delivered at a distance from the patient and the tumor. The 1990s witnessed a remarkable growth in prostate brachytherapy and increasingly the procedure plays a major role in the treatment of clinically localized prostate cancer.

Brachytherapy offers several advantages over radical prostatectomy, which include patient convenience, no surgical incision, ability to treat patients who are considered at risk for general anesthesia complications, minimal blood loss, and rapid recovery. The spatially controlled radiation resultant from the modern permanent brachytherapy implant has measurable advantages over external beam radiation therapy (EBRT). These advantages include the low-energy (less than 30 keV) radiation sources penetrate tissue in the millimeter range; this manifests as a sharp "dropoff" at the edge of the gland that limits exposure to adjacent, normal tissue. Other advantages are that brachytherapy is not affected by prostate gland movement, the convenience of a single session versus 7-week outpatient treatment, and the precision and conformal nature of brachytherapy allows for the administration of a radiation dose 50% to 100% greater than that which can safely be delivered by EBRT. This last point is especially significant as evidence mounts that local tumor control improves with the dose of radiation delivered.

Today, the great majority of prostate implants are performed in a cost-effective outpatient setting using ^{125}I and ^{103}Pd, both of which are low-energy, short-range sources. They are referred to as *permanent implants* as the sources are left in the patient to decay to an inert state. Another form of brachytherapy that has been employed to treat prostate cancer is high dose rate (HDR) brachytherapy

employing highly radioactive ^{192}Ir as a source; HDR is usually performed in combination with a course of EBRT. A robot assists in moving the radioactive sources through plastic catheters inserted in the prostate. It is not possible to deliver an adequate radiation dose in a single setting, so several administrations are usually required. Because the radioactive source is removed from the patient at the end of each HDR treatment, the procedure is also known as *temporary* brachytherapy.

DIAGNOSIS

Diagnosis of prostate cancer is by a biopsy following either an abnormal prostate-specific antigen (PSA) or digital rectal examination.

INDICATIONS FOR SURGERY

Patients selected for seed implant must exhibit strong clinical evidence of organ-confined disease. Clinical stage, Gleason score, and serum PSA—assembled into predictive algorithms such as the Partin tables—may be helpful in objectively identifying those patients at high risk for extraprostatic disease (10). Patients presenting with T1 or T2a tumors with Gleason scores of 6 or less and serum PSAs of 10 ng per mL or less have an approximate 80% probability of organ-confined disease. As such, we in general recommend seeds alone for patients meeting these criteria. Patients with clinically localized disease who exceed any of these three boundaries may benefit from a course of EBRT designed to ensure coverage of locoregional disease. In addition to stage, Gleason score, and PSA level, other factors such as patient age, the number of positive biopsy cores, amount of tumor in each core, as well as the presence or absence of perineural invasion and positive prostatic base biopsy may be added to the available evidence used to decide whether a patient should opt for brachytherapy alone (monother-

TABLE 34–1. *Patient selection factors*

	Monotherapy	Combination therapy
Nodule	None or small	Large or Multiple
Gleason Sum	2–6	7–10
PSA	≤10 ng/mL	≥10 ng/mL
Biopsy	Unilateral Disease	Bilateral or locally extensive disease

PSA, prostate-specific antigen.

apy) or combined modality treatment. For patients with several high-risk factors, neoadjuvant/adjuvant androgen ablation therapy may be added. Commonly used patient selection factors are listed in Table 34–1.

ALTERNATIVE THERAPY

The advantage of accurate localized doses observed with brachytherapy is also a potential drawback for patients who may present with microscopic disease spread outside the effective implantation volume. External beam therapy can encompass a safety margin outside the prostate to provide treatment to potential areas of microscopic spread. Other alternatives include observation, hormonal deprivation, or radical prostatectomy.

SURGICAL TECHNIQUE

Treatment Planning

The treatment planning process has three components: patient selection, isotope selection, and seed mapping (Fig. 34–1). In the past, prostate brachytherapy was con-

sidered a three-step process: treatment planning, operative seed insertion, and a postprocedure evaluation of implant to verify that the radiation delivered was acceptable. Both the preliminary workup and postoperative evaluation were performed in the physician's office. In recent years, some centers have begun to perform the ultrasound volume study and treatment plan creation at the time of the operative implant. It is also possible to calculate the postimplant dosimetry in the same operating room session at the end of the implant process. This approach has been termed "intraoperative" or "real-time" dosimetry. The superiority of either the "preplanned" or the conventional real-time method remains to be demonstrated.

Planning begins with a transrectal ultrasound (TRUS) volume study with the patient in a dorsal lithotomy position and the ultrasound probe positioned in the rectum as it will be at the actual implant (Fig. 34–2). It is critically important that the position of the probe be identical for the planning study and the implant. The volume study provides serial transverse images of the gland at 5-mm increments (Fig. 34–3). The target domain is determined on each of the transverse images by inscribing a 5-mm margin onto the periphery of the prostate except at the posterior boundary. The volume study also helps determine the presence of pubic arch overlay, i.e., those cases where needle access to the anterior and anterolateral aspects of the prostate is blocked by the pubic bone. In most instances this obstruction can be overcome by positioning the patient in an exaggerated lithotomy position or angling the probe in a vertical direction. For patients with significant pubic arch overlay [shown on computed tomography (CT) in Fig. 34–4], a 3-month course of

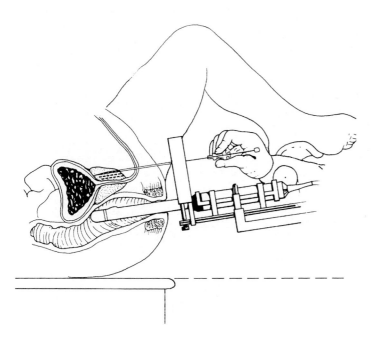

FIG. 34–1. Schematic of the closed, ultrasound-guided implantation technique.

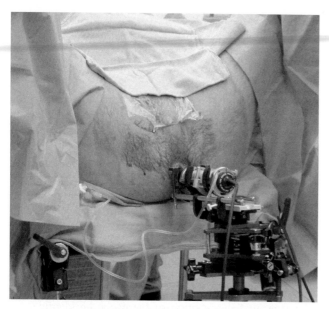

FIG. 34–2. Patient positioned for volume study.

androgen suppression therapy may be used to reduce the size of the gland and thereby the degree of arch blockage.

The transverse images are then entered into a treatment planning computer that will determine the optimal seed configuration and seed activity that will deliver a minimum prescribed dose to the periphery of the prostate while sparing adjacent uninvolved structures. The software is interactive and allows for virtual placement of seeds within the prostate with instant display of resultant isodose curves over transverse, sagittal, and coronal image planes. Dose prescription is in general based on the minimum peripheral dose (MPD), defined as the lowest dose that covers the periphery of the gland: 144 Gy for ^{125}I monotherapy and 129 Gy for [103]Pd. The conventional approach for evaluating a treatment plan involves visual inspection of the isodose surfaces (Fig. 34–5) of the different plans. With this approach, the radiation oncologist and physicist judge which isodose level best covers the target yet spares the neighboring structures. The dose–volume histogram may further be used to evaluate several brachytherapy treatment options before selecting a final plan. Figure 34–6 shows a relative dose–volume histogram for a permanent prostate implant with the curves for the prostate, bladder, and rectum. The graph displays the dose delivered on the abscissa and the vol-

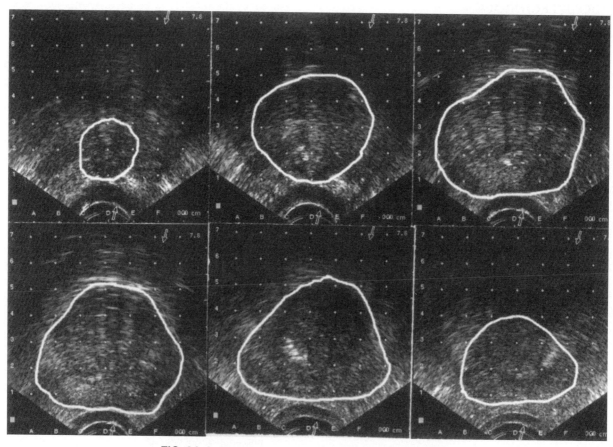

FIG. 34–3. Ultrasound images obtained at volume study.

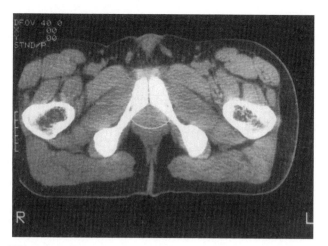

FIG. 34–4. Computed tomography image of a patient with significant interference to the prostate presented by the pubic arch.

ume receiving "at least" that dose on the ordinate. As expected, the curve shows large volumes receiving low doses and small volumes receiving high doses.

Selection of Isotope

The seeds of ¹²⁵I and ¹⁰³Pd are physically similar and both produce low levels of radiation with short penetrance. The differences between them are the half-lives and the dose rates at the time of implantation (Table 34–2). In treating poorly differentiated and presumably

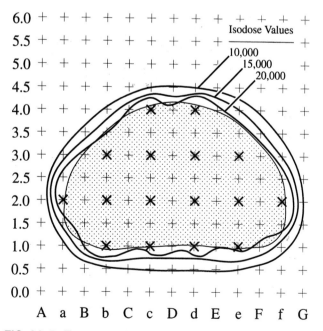

FIG. 34–5. Treatment planning transverse image of the mid-prostate showing isodose lines for a uniform seed distribution.

rapidly proliferating tumors, some investigators hold that the 7- to 10-cGy per hour initial dose rate of ¹²⁵I may be less effective than the 20- to 25-cGy per hour initial dose rate of ¹⁰³Pd. The higher dose-rate concept is supported by mathematical models employing cell lines, but to date there is no clinical evidence from human trials to document tumoricidal differences between the two isotopes (8). Typical seed activities for patients treated with ¹²⁵I alone are 0.34 to 0.5 mCi, with 144 Gy given as the prescribed MPD. Typical seed activities for ¹⁰³Pd implants are 1.4 mCi, with an MPD of 115 Gy. The currently recommended doses for the two isotopes in monotherapy and in combination with external beam therapy are shown in Table 34–3.

Source Loading Approaches

Several loading methods are available. The Manchester system, also known as the Paterson–Parker system, and the Quimby system, or some derivative of these, are the ones in general employed for prostate brachytherapy. In the Manchester system the majority of the seeds are kept toward the periphery of the gland with the goal of delivering a *uniform* dose to the implant volume, the *uniformity* meaning the prescribed dose ± 10%. In the Quimby system, the seeds are distributed in a uniform fashion throughout the prostate. The uniform loading results in an inhomogenous dose distribution, delivering a higher dose to the center of the implant than to the periphery. Regions of high dose, as long as they remain small and isolated, have no clinical significance in the intact prostate; however, recent practice leans toward minimizing urinary morbidity by deleting seeds adjacent to the urethra. One should, however, keep in mind that a recent study showed that 17% of prostate cancers abutted the urethra.

Intraoperative Seed Implantation

The implant procedure can in general be completed in 30 to 45 minutes. The anesthetized patient is placed in the dorsal lithotomy position with the hips flexed as much as possible. A Foley catheter is inserted and left indwelling and the bladder is filled with dilute contrast media. This demarcates the prostate base, allows visualization of the urethra—reducing needle insertion and inadvertent seed placement into the urethra, and helps restrict prostate gland movement.

The perineum is prepped and draped and the scrotum elevated onto the abdominal wall with a plastic adhesive (Fig. 34–2). A C-arm fluoroscope is centered over the prostate to visualize the area from the lower part of the bladder to the apical gold seed marker at the apex. A biplanar multifrequency ultrasound probe is inserted into the rectum perpendicular to the perineum and at a slightly downward angle to best approach the posterior margin of the prostate. The probe is supported by a table-mounted,

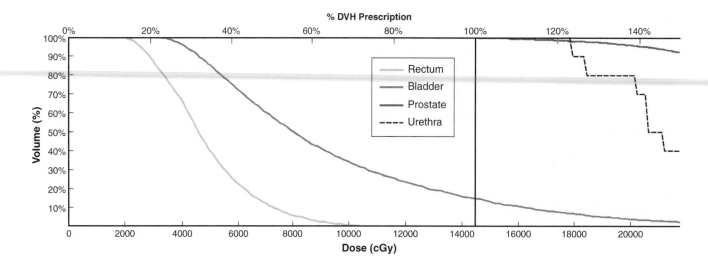

DVH Prescription: 14500.0 cGy   **Isotope:** I125-3631AM-99 (Permanent)
Dose Level: **14500.0 cGy**   **Activity:** 0.390 U (802.2 U-hrs)
Bin Size: 100 cGy   **Number of Bins:** 218

Volume Name	Volume Total (cc)	Dose Level Volume (cc)	Dose Level Volume (%)	V150 (cc)	V150 (%)	V100 (cc)	V100 (%)	V90 (cc)	V90 (%)
— Prostate	27.2	27.1	99.8	25.0	92.1	27.1	99.8	27.2	100.0
— Bladder	4.5	0.7	14.9	0.1	2.6	0.7	14.9	0.9	19.4
— Rectum	12.1	0.0	0.0	0.0	0.0	0.0	0.0	0.0	0.0
-- Urethra	0.0	0.0	100.0	0.0	40.0	0.0	100.0	0.0	100.0

Volume Name	D100 (cGy)	D90 (cGy)	D80 (cGy)	Min Dose	Max Dose	Mean Dose	Median Dose	Modal Dose
— Prostate	12500.0	21797.5	21786.7	12497.1	114029.7	21557.6	21750.0	21750.0
— Bladder	3100.0	4517.9	5318.3	3034.3	104771.2	9284.1	7950.0	21750.0
— Rectum	1900.0	2868.5	3364.6	1837.7	11465.7	4864.7	4550.0	4450.0
-- Urethra	17900.0	18400.0	20200.0	17811.8	25903.1	20560.0	20550.0	21750.0

FIG. 34–6. Dose–volume histogram for an implanted prostate depicting percentage of prescribed dose to the prostate, bladder, rectum, and urethra.

TABLE 34–2. *Characteristics for the two most commonly used permanent sources*

	^{103}Pd	^{125}I
Half-Life	17 d	60 d
Dose Rate (Initial)	20 cGy/h	8 cGy/h
Average Energy	21 keV	29 keV
Typical Activity	1.3–1.8 mCi	0.3–0.9 mCi

TABLE 34–3. *Typically prescribed minimum peripheral doses for Pd-103 and I-125*

	^{103}Pd	^{125}I
Monotherapy	124 Gy (NIST-99)	144 Gy (TG-4)
Combined Therapy[a]	90–120 Gy	60–113 Gy

[a]In addition to 40–50 Gy External Beam Radiation Therapy.

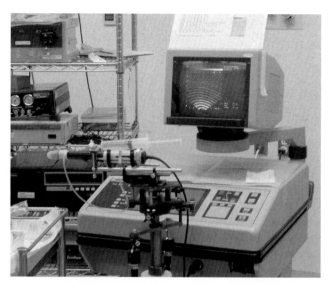

FIG. 34–7. Ultrasound monitor and probe in ratcheting cradle.

multipositional cradle system (Fig. 34–7) containing a stepper unit that allows advancement and retraction of the ultrasound probe in 5-mm increments. A template is then attached to the cradle system. There should be a space between the template and perineum to facilitate manual manipulation of the implant needles when this is required. The template is aligned to ensure that a vertical line through the midplane apertures bisects the gland and the posterior row of apertures runs along the inferior border of the prostate. The volume study is repeated to make certain no significant changes in prostate volume and shape have occurred since the original volume study was performed.

An inactive gold seed marker is placed at the prostate apex (Fig. 34–8). The marker seed is readily visualized on fluoroscopy and is the most accurate means of identifying the inferior margin of the gland. This marker allows the operator a means of avoiding the placement of seeds inferiorly, where radiation might affect structures such as the penile bulb and membranous urethra. Excessive irradiation to these structures has been implicated in posttreatment impotency and urethral stricture formation.

The prostate is a mobile and pliable organ, and real-time ultrasound and fluoroscopic monitoring of the needle insertion and seed placement are critical. Any deviation or internal distortion of the gland should be recognized and corrected. Glandular movements can be minimized using stabilizing needles. The implant needles are inserted to the base of the gland while imaging the largest transverse image, typically one row at a time using a 1-cm square grid within the prostate volume. It is important that parallel needle paths be maintained at all time. In general, four to five rows will cover the prostate. Within rows, central needles are inserted first. Subsequent placements are made in an alternating left to right pattern. This technique helps prevent lateral or rotational movements of the prostate.

The implant begins with the most anterior row and ends with the most posterior row. Implanting the most posterior rows, seeds are also routinely placed into the medial sections of both seminal vesicles. After satisfactory placement of a row of needles, as checked with a combination of transverse and sagittal (Fig. 34–9) ultrasound views and fluoroscopy, the seeds are inserted into the gland using a Mick applicator. The Mick applicator [Mick Radionuclear Instruments (Fig. 34–10)] gives the physician the flexibility to fine-tune the seed positions, something not possible when using preloaded needles. Typically, the seeds are spaced 1 cm apart, but may end up closer depending on the individual row. The first seed should be placed at the junction between the bladder and the prostate and the last seed in the capsule at the apex.

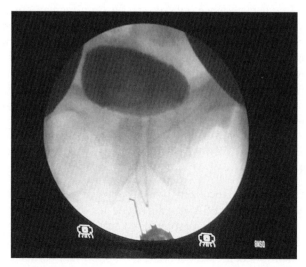

FIG. 34–8. Fluoroscopic image of a gold seed marker being extruded from the implant needle at the prostate apex.

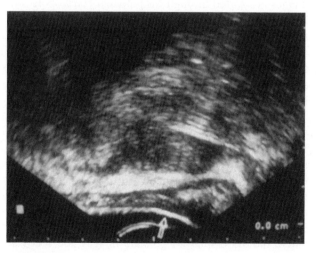

FIG. 34–9. Sagittal ultrasound image of implant needle in the prostate.

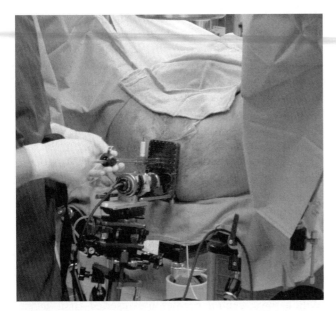

FIG. 34–10. Operator implanting seeds via the Mick applicator at surgery.

For small glands, lower-activity seeds are used and in general placed with the ends abutting one another. As each seed is placed it is visualized using real-time fluoroscopy to ensure distribution and spacing in accordance with the treatment plan.

Attention to the fluoroscopic and ultrasound images during needle insertion is critical. The physician must recognize and immediately adjust for the effects of cephalad movement, internal distortion, and rotation of the prostate. Sometimes the Mick applicator will fail to inject a seed at its intended site or a seed will move laterally after leaving the rigid confines of a needle. The aberration is readily detected on fluoroscopy, allowing for immediate correction and adjustments of the seed array.

At completion of the implant, the resultant ultrasound images are sorted through for potential "cold spots" that have developed because of unavoidable prostate movement or distortions to needle insertions. Additional seeds may be placed at this time. The Foley catheter is removed and the patient is typically discharged within 2 hours after the procedure. Discharge medication in general includes an alpha-blocker and an oral antibiotic.

Dosimetric evaluation of the implant is performed on every patient within 24 hours postimplant using 3D CT-based analysis. Three-millimeter transverse CT images of the prostate are taken through the implant volume, with the target volume identified on each image. This will verify that the prostate has been implanted and that normal tissue structures are out of the high-dose radiation volume. The images are entered into a planning computer where the 3D display of prostate images and seeds are computer analyzed and overlaid with isodose contour margins for construction of a dose–volume histogram.

The dose–volume histogram permits detailed and accurate evaluation of the implant quality and is in particular valuable in detecting consistent errors in implantation.

OUTCOMES

Complications

Most patients experience some degree of irritative and/or obstructive urinary tract symptoms following treatment. The symptoms usually begin 1 to 2 weeks after implant and persist in varying degrees for 2 weeks to several months. These symptoms, due to ongoing radiation, are usually mild and short-lasting. Symptoms manifesting immediately following the implant procedure are often due to the mechanical trauma from the implant needles. Patients with large glands, which require a greater number of needle punctures and seeds, may experience a greater degree of postimplant discomfort than those with small glands.

Approximately 10% to 15% of cases require intermittent or indwelling catheterization to relieve urinary outlet obstruction. It is our experience that even protracted urinary retention will improve over time. Acute proctitis, manifesting as frequent blood-tinged bowel movements, is infrequent in our experience. When it occurs it is in general mild and does not require treatment. Where treatment is necessary, local treatment with steroids is normally sufficient. Long-term symptoms of proctitis are in general mild and characterized by intermittent rectal bleeding.

Significant urinary incontinence is rare in patients who have not had a prior transurethral resection of the prostate (TURP), although over 20% of patients with a history of TURP and a uniform type implant may experience incontinence, mainly of the stress type. A TURP postimplant in such cases may raise the incontinence rate to nearly 80% and should therefore be avoided.

In our experience, erectile dysfunction increases with age and averages 30% for all ages. Patients younger than 60 years of age, who claimed adequate potency prior to the implant, for the most part maintain potency after the procedure. Some patients experience temporary difficulties, and at least some significant proportion of patients experiencing erectile dysfunction will benefit from treatment with sildenafil.

Results

Monitoring localized prostate cancer outcome post-treatment using PSA as a surrogate for disease-free survival has become widespread and accepted. On the basis of biochemical (PSA) outcomes, several reports published in recent years support the notion that permanent brachytherapy for prostate cancer results in outcomes comparable to radical surgery and external beam radia-

TABLE 34–4. *Summarized biochemical (PSA) outcomes: brachytherapy only*

Study	N	Actuarial time (yr)	Median follow-up (yr)	BRFS* (%)
Merrick et al. (10)	425	5	3	94
Potters et al. (12)	493	5	3.5	82
Grado et al. (5)	392	5	2.5	80
Zelefsky et al. (14)	248	5	4	71
Blasko et al. (2)	231	9	5	84
Grimm et al. (6)	125	10	7	85
Ragde et al. (13)	147	10	10	66

PSA, prostate-specific antigen.
*

TABLE 34–5. *Summarized biochemical (PSA) outcomes: EBRT + brachytherapy*

Study	N	Actuarial time (yr)	Median follow-up (yr)	BRFS* (%)
Lederman et al. (8)	348	6	4	77
Critz (3)	689	6	4	88
Dattoli (4)	124	4	3.8	79

PSA, prostate-specific antigen.
*

tion therapy. Table 34–4 summarizes six series reporting intermediate to long-term follow-up following brachytherapy as the sole intervention for localized prostate cancer. Table 34–5 contains results from series in which 4500 cGy EBRT was delivered in tandem with the permanent brachytherapy implant. It bears mentioning that while all reported results describe biochemical, i.e., serum PSA, endpoints controversy surrounds the nature of the most appropriate biochemical endpoint for radiation-treated localized prostate cancer series. On the basis of a symposium called by the American Society for Therapeutic Radiology and Oncology (ASTRO) in the mid-1990s, a failure definition for use in actuarial analysis was agreed upon, by which biochemical failure was defined as three consecutive rises in serum PSA, with the time of treatment failure defined as the midpoint between the lowest value obtained and the first of the three rises (1).

REFERENCES

1. American Society of Therapeutic Radiology and Oncology. Consensus statement: Guidelines for PSA following radiation therapy. *Int J Radiat Oncol Biol Phys* 1997;37:1035–1041.
2. Blasko JC, et al. Palladium-103 brachytherapy for prostate carcinoma. *Int J Radiat Oncol Biol Phys* 2000;46:839–850.
3. Critz FA. A standard definition of disease freedom is needed for prostate cancer: undetectable prostate specific antigen compared with the American Society of Therapeutic Radiology and Oncology consensus definition. *J Urol* 2002;167:1310–1313.
4. Dattoli M. Prognostic role of serum prostatic acid phosphatase for 103Pd-based radiation for prostatic carcinoma. *Int J Radiat Oncol Biol Phys* 1999;45:853–856.
5. Grado GL, et al. Actuarial disease-free survival after prostate cancer brachytherapy using interactive techniques with biplane ultrasound and fluoroscopic guidance. *Int J Radiat Oncol Biol Phys* 1998;42:289–298.
6. Grimm P, et al. 10-year biochemical (prostate-specific antigen) control of prostate cancer with 125-I brachytherapy. *Int J Radiat Oncol Biol Phys* 2001;51:31–40.
7. Lederman GS, et al. Retrospective stratification of a consecutive cohort of prostate cancer patients treated with a combined regimen of external-beam radiotherapy and brachytherapy. *Int J Radiat Oncol Biol Phys* 2001;49:1297–3003.
8. Ling CC. Permanent implants using Au-198, Pd-103 and [125]I: radiobiological considerations based on the linear quadratic model. *Int J Radiat Oncol Biol Phys* 1992;23:81–87.
9. Merrick GS, et al., Five-year biochemical outcome following permanent interstitial brachytherapy for clinical T1–T3 prostate cancer. *Int J Radiat Oncol Biol Phys* 2001;51:41–48.
10. Partin AW, et al. Combination of prostate-specific antigen, clinical stage, and Gleason score to predict pathological stage of localized prostate cancer. A multi-institutional update [see comments]. *JAMA* 1997;277:1445–1451; erratum *JAMA* 1997;278:118.
11. Potters L, et al. Risk profiles to predict PSA relapse-free survival for patients undergoing permanent prostate brachytherapy. *Cancer J Sci Am* 1999;5:301–306.
12. Ragde H, et al. 12-year follow-up after transperineal brachytherapy of localized prostate cancer. *J Urol* 2000;163[Suppl 4]:336–337(abst 1493).
13. Zelefsky MJ, et al. Five-year biochemical outcome and toxicity with transperineal CT-planned permanent ^{125}I prostate implantation for patients with localized prostate cancer. *Int J Radiat Oncol Biol Phys* 2000;47:1261–1266.

Urethra

FEMALE URETHRA

The female urethra extends from the bladder neck to the external urethral meatus and varies in length from 3 cm to 5 cm. The urethra is a fibromuscular tube composed of a mucosal lining, a submucosal layer, and a muscle layer. Proximally the transitional cell mucosa is continuous with the bladder epithelium. Distally the mucosa is nonkeratinized stratified squamous epithelium (Figure SV-1). The submucosa consists of abundant longitudinal and circular elastic fibers and contains a prominent venous system. The mucosa and submucosa act as a washer producing a seal that contributes to urethral closure pressure (1). These tissues are estrogen dependent and in hypoestrogenic states thinning of the tissue may result in incontinence (2). The smooth muscle layer consists of a thick sheet of longitudinally oriented fibers and a thin outer layer of circular fibers. These muscles are continuous with the bladder neck proximally and terminate distally in the subcutaneous tissue surrounding the external urethral meatus. Colleselli and others have shown in the cranial and most of the middle third of the urethra that there are three smooth muscle layers (3).

In the distal two-thirds of the urethra a circular layer of striated muscle, the rhabdosphincter, surrounds the smooth muscle layer. The rhabdosphincter is composed of delicate Type I (slow twitch) fibers and consists of three distinct muscles. Proximally the muscle forms a ring (*sphincter urethrae*) that encircles the urethra. Distally the muscle (*compressor urethra*) fans out laterally along the curve of the inferior border of the pubic rami to compress the urethra against the anterior vaginal wall. At the vestibule the muscle completely surrounds the urethra and vagina to form a *urethrovaginal sphincter.* (Figure SV-2) (4). The three muscles work together to provide constant urethral tone (Figure SV-3)(5). Normally the striated sphincter plays a minimal role in resisting abdominal pressure. However preservation of the rhabdosphincter is necessary for continence after creation of a female neobladder (3).

Paired periurethral (Skene's) glands drain on either side of the midline just posterior to the urethral meatus. There are also numerous small periurethral mucous glands that open into small recesses in the mucosa.

Vascular Anatomy

The arterial supply to the female urethra is from the urethral artery, a branch of the internal pudendal artery,

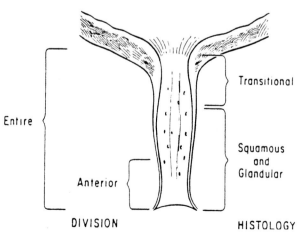

FIG. SV–1. The female urethra.

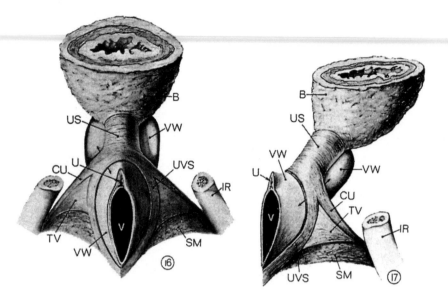

FIG. SV–2. Striated urogenital sphincter muscle seen from below after removal of the perineal membrane and pubic bones. US, urethral sphincter; UVS, urethrovaginal sphincter; CU, compressor urethrae; B, bladder; IR, ischiopubic ramus; TV, transverse vaginae muscle; SM, smooth muscle; U, urethra; V, vagina; VW, vaginal wall. (From Oelrich TM. Anat Rec 1983; 205:223, with permission.)

which in turn is a branch of the internal iliac artery (8). The venous drainage is via the pelvic venous plexus.

Innervation

The smooth muscle of the urethra is innervated by parasympathetic nerves. The predominant sympathetic receptors are alpha- adrenergic (9). These receptors are responsible for urethral smooth muscle contraction and possibly engorgement of the submucosal vasculature to create a watertight seal of the urethral mucosa (10). The

striated muscle fibers of the external intrinsic sphincter receive innervation from the pudendal and pelvic somatic nerves (11). Both somatic and autonomic nerves to the urethra travel on the lateral walls of the vagina near the urethra. Dissection in this area should be avoided during transvaginal surgery to prevent development of type III urinary incontinence (12,13).

Lymphatics

The lymphatic drainage of the proximal urethra is to the deep pelvic nodes. The drainage of the distal portion of the urethra is to the inguinal nodes.

Contiguous Structures

A "hammock" of vaginal tissue supports the urethra (6). The urethral supports, also termed pubourethral ligaments, include fascial and muscular attachments to the arcus tendineus fascia pelvis and levator ani muscles. These supports are only present in the distal third of the urethra and fix the urethra to the pubic bone. The pubovesical muscle is a separate structure that is an extension of the smooth muscle of the bladder, which extends from the detrusor muscle to the arcus tendineus fascia pelvis and pubic bone (Figure SV-4) (7).

Posteriorly the urethra is intimately related to the anterior surface of the vagina. The periurethral fascia is located immediately beneath the vaginal epithelium and is seen as the glistening white layer that surrounds the urethra when an incision is made in the anterior wall of the vagina. The fascia extends from the meatus to the bladder neck and laterally to where it fuses with the endopelvic fascia at the pubic bone (Figure SV-5).

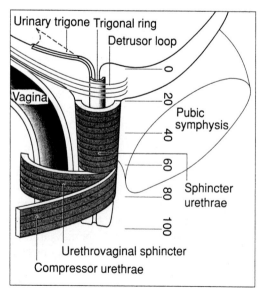

FIG. SV–3. Location of various structures along the urethra. Note the three parts of the rhabdospincter (Copyright University of Michigan, 1989, with permission)

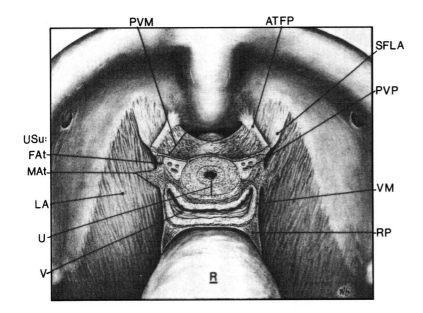

FIG. SV–4. Cross section of the urethra (U), vagina (V), arcus tendineus fasciae pelvis (ATFP), and superior fascia of levator ani (SFLA) just below the vesical neck (drawn from cadaver dissection). Pubovesical muscles (PVM) lie anterior to urethra and anterior and superior to para urethral vascular plexus (PVP). The urethral supports (Usu) (the pubourethral ligaments) attatch the vagina and vaginal surface of the urethra to the levator ani muscles (MAt, muscular attachment) and to the superior fascia of the levator ani (Fat, fascial attachment). R, Rectum; RP, rectal pillar; VM, vaginal wall muscularis. (From DeLancey JOL. Neurol Urody 1989;8:53, with permission.)

MALE URETHRA

Gross/Microscopic

The posterior urethra is the portion of the urethra extending from the bladder neck through the prostate and through the urogenital diaphragm. It is divided into the prostatic urethra and the membranous urethra that traverses the urogenital diaphragm just prior to entering the corpora spongiosa. The anterior urethra runs from the urogential diaphragm to the tip of the glans penis and may be further divided into the bulbous urethra extending from the root of the penis to the convergence of the corpora cavernosa and the pendulous or penile urethra that traverses the pendulous portion of the penis. There is a dilation of the urethra in the area of the glans penis called the fossa navicularis (Figure SV-6).

A number of ducts empty into the lumen of the urethra. Two to three cm distal to the membranous urethra the paired orifices of Cowpers glands (bulbourethral glands) are noted on the floor. On the roof of the pendulous urethra there are openings for the glands of Littre or the submucosal urethral glands and small recesses termed urethral lacunae. The lacuna magna is a larger lacuna in the midportion of the anterior aspect of the fossa navicularis.

The urethral epithelium varies along the length of the urethra. In the prostatic urethra the cells are transitional whereas in the membranous urethra they are stratified columnar. The epithelium of the penile urethra is composed of pseudostratified and columnar cells. In the fossa navicularis, the epithelium is composed of stratified squamous cells.

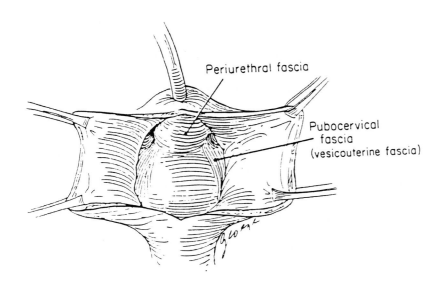

FIG. SV–5. View of the anterior vaginal fascial support, which is found beneath the vaginal wall (shown retracted). The periurethral fascia, which forms the vaginal layer of the urethropelvic ligaments, is continuous with the pubocervical fascia proximally.

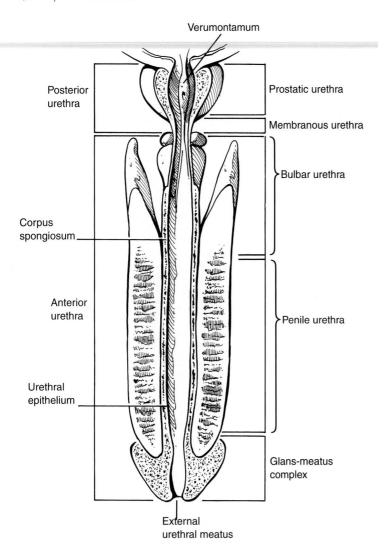

FIG. SV–6. The male urethra and its divisions with associated histology.

Vascular Anatomy

Paired bulbourethral arteries, which arise as the first of three penile branches of the internal pudendal artery, supply the urethra. The venous drainage is via the emissary veins, which drain to the circumflex branches of the deep dorsal vein of the penis.

Innervation

The urethra mucosa is innervated via the urethrobulbar nerve. It is a branch of the nerve to the bulbocavernosus, which is a branch of the perineal nerve, which is derived from the pudendal nerve. A branch of the bulbocavernosus nerve at the 3 and 9 o'clock positions penetrates the striated urethral sphincter (15). The pudendal nerve consisting of fibers from the second, third and fourth sacral spinal nerves, is thus both motor to the urethral sphincter and sensory to the urethra and glans penis.

Lymphatics

The lymphatic drainage of the anterior urethra is into the superficial and deep inguinal node and ultimately to the external iliac nodes. The lymphatics of the posterior (the bulbous, membranous and prostatic) urethra can take three routes: to the external iliac nodes, to the obturator and internal iliac nodes or to the presacral nodes.

Contiguous Structures

The membranous urethra is covered by the fibers of the striated urethral sphincter (rhabdosphincter). Brooks used computer generated, three-dimensional reconstruction of the male pelvis from the Visible Human data set to show that the striated urethral sphincter is circular with abundant tissue posteriorly. Anteriorly the sphincter is approximately twice as long as it is posteriorly. An intrinsic smooth muscle lies between the urethral mucosa and the striated urethral sphincter. This muscle begins above the striated sphincter and then gradually thins distal to the striated sphincter (14).

The remainder of the anterior urethra lies within the corpus spongiosum lying in the ventral groove of the corpora cavernosa of the penis. Cowper's glands (bulbourethral glands) lie within the urogenital diaphragm posterior and lateral to the membranous urethra.

REFERENCES

1. Raz S, Caine M, Zeigler M. The vascular component in the production of intraurethral pressure. *J Urol* 1972;108:93–96.
2. Klutke JJ, Bergman A. Nonsurgical management of stress urinary incontinence. In: Ostergard DR, Bent AE, eds. *Urogynecology and Urodynamics,* 4th ed. Baltimore: Williams and Wilkins, 1996: 505–516.
3. Colleselli K, Stenzl A, Eder R, Strasser H, Poisel S, Bartsch G. The female urethral sphincter: a morphological and topographical study. *J Urol* 1998;160:49–54.
4. Oelrich TM, The striated urogenital sphincter muscle in the female. *Anat Rec* 1983;205:223–232.
5. DeLancey JOL. Functional anatomy of the female pelvis. In: Kursh ED, McGuire EJ, ed. *Female Urology.* Philadelphia: JP Lippincott. 1994:3–16.
6. DeLancey JOL. Structural support of the urethra as it relates to stress urinary incontinence: the hammock hypothesis. *Am J Obstet Gynecol* 1994;170:1713–1723.
7. Strohbehn K. Normal pelvic floor anatomy. *Obstet Gynecol Clin North Am* 1998;25:683–705.
8. Ferner H, Staubesand J, eds: *Sobatta Atlas of Human Anatomy,* 10th ed. Munich/Baltimore: Urban & Schwartzenberg, 1982.
9. Ek A. Innervation and receptor functions of the human urethra. *Scan J Urol Nephrol* 1997;S45:1–50.
10. Huisman AB. Aspects on the anatomy of the female urethra with special relation to urinary incontinence. *Contrib Gynecol Obstet* 1983;10:1–31.
11. Borirakchanyavat S, Aboseif SR, Carroll PR, Tanagoho EA, Lue TF. Continence mechanism of the isolated female urethra: an anatomical study of the intrapelvic somatic nerves. *J Urol* 1997;158:822.
12. Ball TP Jr., Teichman JHM, Sharkey FE, Rogenes VJ, Adrian EK Jr. Terminal nerve distribution to the urethra and bladder neck: considerations in the management of stress urinary incontinence. *J Urol* 1997; 158:827.
13. Raz S, Sussman EM, Erickson DB, Bregg KJ, Nitti VW. The Raz bladder neck suspension: results in 206 patients. *J Urol* 1992;148:845.
14. Brooks JD, Chao W, Kerr J. Male pelvic anatomy reconstructed from the visible human data set. *J Urol* 1998;159:868–872.
15. Shafik A, Doss S. Surgical anatomy of the somatic terminal innervation to the anal and urethral sphincters: role in anal and urethral surgery. *J Urol* 1999;161:85–89.

CHAPTER 35

Abdominal Retropubic Approaches for Female Incontinence

Toby C. Chai

Kelly published the first description of a successful transvaginal repair for stress urinary incontinence (SUI) in 1914 where sutures were applied to the anterior vaginal wall at the level of the bladder neck ("Kelly plication") (14). Marshall, Marchetti, and Krantz ("the MMK") in 1949 (19) reported the first successful retropubic approach for correction of SUI. This repair was accomplished by placement of sutures in the periurethral tissue and elevation of this area to the periosteum of pubis symphysis. The MMK was further modified by Burch in 1961 to reduce the tendency of the periosteal sutures from pulling out and utilized more lateral placement of the periurethral sutures that were anchored to Cooper's ligament (2). Through the years, the Burch procedure and its subsequent modifications (24) have become the gold standard transabdominal approach for the surgical correction of SUI.

The intent of surgical procedures for SUI is to ameliorate the symptom of incontinence, but whether these procedures actually reverse or correct the pathophysiological defect is unknown because the current understanding of the pathophysiology is still evolving (4). The decision to perform one type of procedure over another may depend on the bias of the surgeon as to which pathophysiological theory is believed to be the cause of SUI. Often, the choice of surgery is totally empirical and based on experience, knowledge, and comfort level of the surgeon for a particular surgical approach.

An early theory for the cause of SUI was proximal urethral hypermobility. As proposed by Einhorning, a normally continent woman has a well-supported proximal urethra located in a retropubic, intraabdominal position that does not change position during stress (e.g., it is not hypermobile) (Fig. 35–1A) (8). During increased abdominal pressures, there is equal pressure transmission to the bladder and the proximal urethra, thus preventing SUI. In a patient with SUI, the proximal urethra is hypermobile and traverses from its intraabdominal retropubic position during increased abdominal pressures. Thus, the proximal urethra loses its mechanical advantage and incontinence occurs (Fig. 35–1B). This theory is probably not correct because incidence of urethral hypermobility is equivalent in both continent and stress-incontinent females (9). Also, the observation that the midurethral placement of a tension-free polypropylene sling that does not correct hypermobility, yet does correct the symptom of SUI (15), argues against hypermobility as a distinct pathophysiological entity for SUI.

Another theory for the etiology of SUI is intrinsic sphincteric deficiency (ISD) as proposed by McGuire (20). He based this theory on urodynamic observations of females with recurrent SUI after previous failed antiincontinence surgeries. McGuire surmised that these patients had something intrinsically deficient (anatomic or physiological) in their urethra as a result of the multiple surgeries in the urethral area. In fact, these patients were classically described to have SUI in the setting of a nonmobile, retropubically fixed urethra. He further advanced this theory by developing the Valsalva leak point pressure (VLPP) test as a urodynamic tool for assessing the competence of the urethra to resist loss of urine during a sudden increase in abdominal pressures. The VLPP was important at the time of its development because it purportedly provided an ability to discriminate between those females with SUI due to hypermobility versus those with ISD. This was based on the observation that those with SUI due to hypermobility had significantly higher VLPP compared to those with ISD (23). However, the simple dichotomy of SUI into hypermobility and ISD is probably overly simplistic in that ISD can exist even in SUI patients who have *not* had prior surgical repair and can coexist with a hypermobile urethra

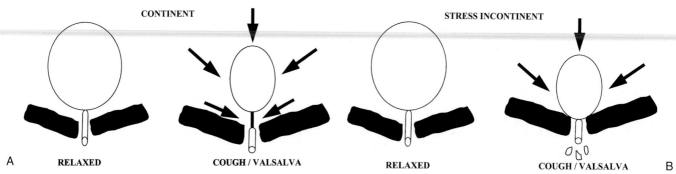

FIG. 35–1. A: Concept of well-supported intrapelvic proximal urethra and its ability to prevent SUI during cough because of equal pressure transmission. **B:** Hypermobility of the urethra is due to anatomic defects in the support of the urethra. The urethra will drop below the level of the symphysis, thus allowing a pressure differential between the bladder and urethra.

(13,16). While the technique of the VLPP test has not been standardized, its clinical usefulness, ease of use, and reliability has been demonstrated (1). In addition, use of urethral pressures [such as urethral pressure profiles (UPPs) and maximal urethral closure pressure (MUCP)] to classify SUI has also been proposed, although there is debate as to whether urethral pressures correspond to VLPP during the evaluation of incontinent females (1,21,22).

A third theory, advanced by DeLancey, is the "hammock" or "backboard" concept, where the tissues below the bladder neck and proximal urethra provide a strong hammock or backboard to allow occlusion of these structures during increased abdominal pressures, thus preventing SUI (Fig. 35–2A) (3). If the strength of this area was deficient, then during stress maneuvers the bladder neck and proximal urethra would not be adequately compressed and development of SUI would ensue (Fig. 35–2B). The fact that urethral hypermobility exists in a population of continent women does not necessarily argue against the hammock theory. As long as there is

sufficient compressive effect even with hypermobility of the urethra, continence can be maintained (Fig. 35–2C).

These different theories have led to the development and utilization of both abdominal and transvaginal surgical procedures to ameliorate SUI. It is important to realize that correction of the symptom of SUI does not necessarily imply the reversal of the pathophysiological defect that gave rise to SUI. In fact, the treatment of SUI is still empirical even today. Further refinements in the understanding of the precise mechanisms that lead to the symptom of SUI will help improve both surgical and medical approaches to the treatment of SUI.

DIAGNOSIS

In the strictest sense, it is not possible to diagnose SUI because it is a symptom and not a disease. When we acquire further knowledge of the precise pathophysiological pathways leading to the symptom of SUI, we can then perhaps diagnose the different etiologies that cause SUI. Therefore, the various clinical tests currently used

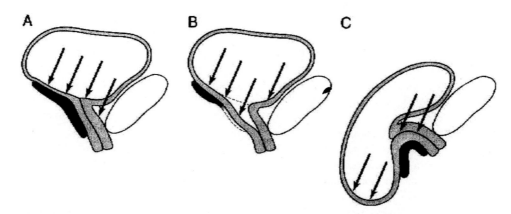

FIG. 35–2. A: Normal continent female with normal hammock support of the bladder neck and proximal urethra. **B:** Stress-incontinent female with deficient hammock support. **C:** Hypermobility of the urethra and bladder base (cystocele) does not necessarily result in stress incontinence.

are not truly diagnostic tests but rather tests to confirm the presence of the symptom of SUI in a controlled clinical setting.

A thorough and detailed patient history should elicit symptoms of SUI significant enough to justify further testing. Various questionnaires have been developed to help differentiate stress from urge incontinence because the treatments of these two conditions are very different. One validated questionnaire is the Medical, Epidemiologic, and Social Aspects of Aging Urinary Incontinence Questionnaire (MESA) (5,6), in which the scores for stress and urge components can be calculated.

During the physical examination, a hypermobile urethra can be measured by performing a Q-tip test. A Q-tip, inserted transurethrally to the proximal urethra, when deflected greater than 30 degrees from the resting angle during Valsalva is considered to be hypermobile. As previously presented, the presence of urethral hypermobility is not pathognomonic for SUI as continent women may have the same finding. A stress test should also be performed during the physical exam to confirm the symptom of SUI. The bladder is filled with sterile water or saline to 250 to 300 cc via a urethral catheter and then the catheter is removed. The patient then is asked to increase abdominal pressures either with strain (Valsalva) or cough and observation of leakage of fluid through the urethral meatus constitutes a positive stress test.

Urodynamics represent a combination of several tests that are commonly performed in the evaluation of SUI. The measurement of the pressure–volume relationship of the bladder during filling and emptying summarizes the main goal of urodynamics. The abdominal pressure at which SUI occurs during a slow voluntary increase in abdominal pressure (asking the patient to strain) is the VLPP. Decision to perform one type of surgery over another based on VLPP has been empirically advocated although there have been no large prospective trials validating the prognostic significance of VLPP. However, as discussed previously, the actual pathophysiological mechanism leading to the symptom of SUI is unknown and VLPP is not a pathophysiological test but rather a method to quantitate the resistance of the urethra to urinary leakage during increases in abdominal pressures. A cough leak point pressure (CLPP) is the abdominal pressure induced by coughing at which fluid leaks out the urethral meatus. The CLPP can be difficult to reliably measure as the changes in abdominal pressure are much more rapid than in the VLPP. However, some patients will only leak with cough as they cannot generate high enough pressures with Valsalva.

INDICATIONS FOR SURGERY

The indications for a transabdominal surgical approach include the presence of symptomatic SUI that adversely affects quality of life. In addition, the patient must be suf-

ficiently healthy to undergo regional or general anesthesia, be able to be placed in dorsal lithotomy position, and have a habitus allowing a suprapubic incision.

ALTERNATIVE THERAPY

Conservative therapies for SUI may involve use of pessaries, urethral inserts, or physical therapy for pelvic floor muscle rehabilitation. Currently, there is no US Food and Drug Administration (FDA)-approved oral medication for SUI although duloxetine has recently completed phase III clinical trials and is awaiting FDA approval for use in SUI. Use of vaginal topical estrogen in the periurethral area and bladder neck has been used also to decrease SUI presumably through increased coaptibility of the urethra by increased vascularity. Other surgical procedures for SUI utilizing other approaches include transvaginal and laparoscopic techniques, which are covered in other chapters.

SURGICAL TECHNIQUE

MMK Procedure

The patient is placed in the low dorsal lithotomy position and the vagina and abdominal are prepped. A 16 Fr Foley is inserted into the bladder. A Pfannenstiel or low transverse incision is made. Self-retaining retractors are used to retract the rectus muscle. The retropubic space is dissected out. Using a finger in the vagina, the urethral balloon is palpated to delineate the position of the vesicourethral junction. Using 0 chromic or other similar absorbable sutures, the periurethral vaginal tissue is sutured as shown in Figure 35–3. Typically, 3 chromic sutures are placed on either side of the urethra at the level of the proximal urethra and vesicourethral junction. A finger in the vagina can help with the dissection as well as the suture placement such that the sutures traverse the vaginal tissue and not the urethra (Fig. 35–4). The sutures

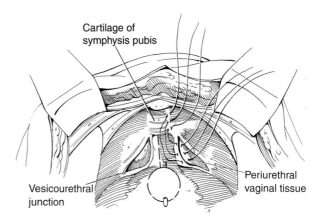

FIG. 35–3. MMK procedure. Sutures are placed through the periurethral vaginal tissue at the level of the vesicourethral junction and passed through the cartilage of the symphysis pubis. Three sutures are used on the right side.

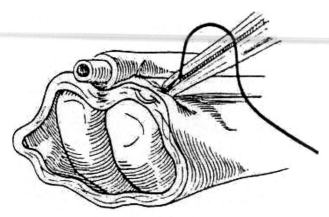

FIG. 35–4. MMK procedure. Fingers in the vagina guide placement of sutures excluding the vaginal epithelium.

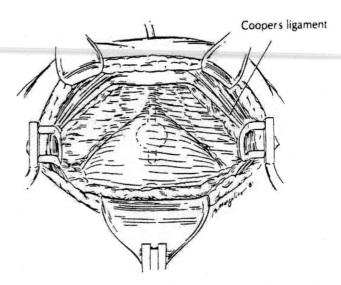

Coopers ligament

FIG. 35–7. Burch procedure. Retropubic space showing the bladder neck, Foley balloon, and Cooper's ligament.

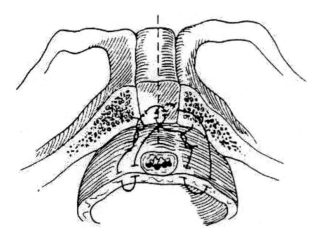

FIG. 35–5. MMK procedure. Sutures connect the periurethral vaginal tissue and periosteum and cartilage of the symphysis pubis.

are then attached to the symphysis pubis either at the cartilaginous midline in the symphysis pubis or to the periosteum just lateral to the midline (Figs. 35–3 and 35–5). The sutures are then tied without any slack, thus tenting the urethra to the back of the symphysis pubis (Fig. 35–6).

Because absorbable sutures are used, a cystoscopy is usually not performed. Drains are not typically used. The Foley catheter is left in usually 24 hours and removed and voiding trial initiated. Patients should be instructed that temporary intermittent self-catheterizations may be required and that spontaneous voiding may be delayed.

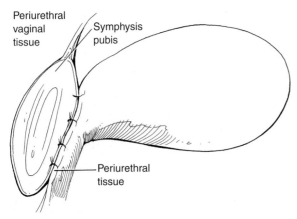

Periurethral vaginal tissue

Symphysis pubis

Periurethral tissue

FIG. 35–6. MMK procedure. Lateral view of the periurethral vaginal tissue tented to the symphysis pubis.

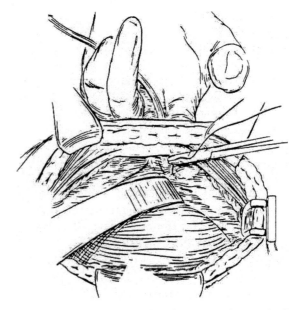

FIG. 35–8. Burch procedure. The first suture bite at the level of the vesicourethral junction/proximal urethra with a finger in the vagina helps exclude the suture from the vaginal epithelium.

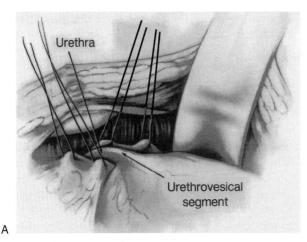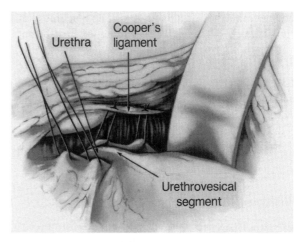

A   B

FIG. 35–9. Burch procedure. **A:** A total of four sutures are placed at the urethrovesical junction; lifting helps cystoscopic imaging make sure no sutures violated the bladder or ureteral orifices. **B:** The two right-sided sutures are passed through Cooper's ligament and tied; note that there is a gap in the sutures giving a banjo string appearance.

Burch Colposuspension

The patient is placed in a low dorsal lithotomy position and the vagina and abdomen are prepped and draped. A 16 Fr Foley catheter is placed and a Pfannenstiel or low transverse incision is made. Dissection of the space of Retzius is performed and self-retaining retractors are placed. Cooper's ligament can be identified (Fig. 35–7). The left and right perivaginal fascia lateral to the vesicourethral junction under the symphysis is dissected using a sponge stick or Metzenbaum scissors with fingers in the vagina as a guide. Care must be used as vaginal and pelvic veins are often encountered in this area. Palpation of the Foley balloon will help delineate the vesicourethral junction. It is critical to be sufficiently underneath the symphysis to ensure that the vaginal suspension sutures are placed at the level of the proximal urethra (Fig. 35–8). Failure to place the sutures appropriately beneath the symphysis may result in an inadequate hammock or backboard support of the bladder neck and proximal urethra. The suture bite should encompass vaginal tissue without perforating the vaginal epithelium. For each suture, a double bite of the vaginal tissue is taken to ensure strength and durability. Placement of the sutures into the vagina is aided by elevation of the anterior vaginal wall with a sponge stick or hand in the vagina, similar to that performed for the MMK procedure (Fig. 35–4). Another suture is placed more proximally at the level of the urethrovesical junction. A total of four permanent, nonabsorbable sutures such as no. 0 or no. 1 polypropylene or Gore-Tex sutures are placed (two on each side; Fig. 35–9A).

A cystoscopy is performed next to ensure that the sutures did not perforate the bladder and that the ureteral orifices are intact. Methylene blue can be used to help identify efflux of urine from the ureteral orifices. Lifting of these sutures during cystoscopy will help delineate their location. If there is violation of either the bladder or the ureteral orifices, the suture(s) is (are) removed and repassed.

These four sutures are then placed through Cooper's ligament on both sides and tied. It is imperative that the sutures are tied so there is distance (space) between the Cooper's ligament and the vaginal tissue (Fig. 35–9B). This prevents overcompression of the urethra, which can cause obstruction (Fig. 35–10). Sutures after tying should

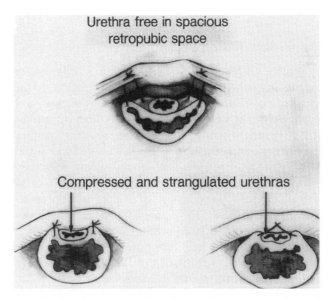

FIG. 35–10. Burch procedure. Once all four sutures are tied, there should be a space between the symphysis and urethra; the urethra should not be compressed nor strangulated.

have the appearance of "banjo strings." The placement of these sutures and how tight they are tightened is different from the initial description of Burch (2), where the sutures were tied down with complete approximation of the perivaginal tissue onto Cooper's ligament. After tying these sutures, cystoscopy is performed again to examine for efflux of urine from the orifices to ensure that the tied sutures did not occlude the ureteral orifices.

OUTCOMES

Complications

Complications from abdominal approaches for correction of SUI can occur. A metaanalysis of the literature comparing abdominal to transvaginal approaches for SUI revealed no significant differences in the complication rates (17). Besides the standard complications including bleeding, retropubic hematoma, and infections (wound, urinary tract), the following complications should be considered when counseling a patient on abdominal approaches to correcting SUI.

Urinary Retention

Patients may not return to spontaneous voiding when the Foley is removed postoperatively. These patients should be taught intermittent self-catheterization. The majority of these patients will return to spontaneous voiding within several weeks; however, if spontaneous voiding does not occur urethral obstruction must be ruled out. The incidence of urinary retention lasting greater than 4 weeks postoperatively was 5% (17). In cases of persistent urinary retention, urethrolysis may be necessary.

Postoperative Voiding Dysfunction

Surgical correction of SUI does not necessarily reverse the precise pathophysiological defect(s) giving rise to the symptom of SUI. Because of this reason, patients postoperatively may develop lower urinary tract symptoms (LUTSs) such as urinary frequency and urgency that they did not have preoperatively (e.g., de novo detrusor instability). One must rule out urethral obstruction secondary to overcompression of the urethra as the cause of LUTS, although the absolute diagnosis of bladder outlet obstruction may be difficult. The combination of history, physical exam showing a fixed urethral position, and urodynamic testing may help diagnose obstruction. These patients may need urethrolysis to relieve LUTS. In a large series of almost 400 Burch colposuspensions, the risk of developing de novo detrusor instability was 17% (25).

Patients with LUTS not having evidence of bladder outlet obstruction should be treated with behavioral mod-

ification (such as fluid restriction) and antimuscarinic therapy. In difficult cases, augmentation cystoplasty, autoaugmentation (detrusor myectomy), or sacral neuromodulation may be required.

Bladder and/or Ureteral Injury

The risk of this complication, while rare, can damage involved renal units. Cystoscopy performed routinely intraoperatively should reduce this risk. Prompt recognition of this complication will allow the surgeon to remove these sutures and repass them so that bladder and ureteral integrity is maintained. A review of suture injury to the urinary tract revealed that even with intraoperative cystoscopy delayed erosions of sutures can occur (7).

Pelvic Organ Prolapse

The MMK cannot correct a cystocele because of the location of the suspending sutures. While the Burch procedure can correct a cystocele, manifestation of other compartment defects may occur after the Burch procedure. These include development of enterocele (apical vaginal compartment) and rectocele (posterior vaginal compartment). The likely reason for this is that because the Burch procedure sufficiently corrected the anterior compartment (cystocele) any laxity in other compartments can be unmasked. Recurrent cystoceles can occur because the Burch procedure does not correct central deficit cystoceles, which require a transvaginal approach to repair. The incidence of pelvic organ prolapse of any type was up to 27% (26) in a large series of patients undergoing Burch colposuspension.

Osteitis Pubis and Osteomyelitis

The MMK because of the nature of the suture placement through the periosteum of the symphysis pubis may be complicated by osteitis pubis or osteomyelitis of the pubic bone. Osteitis pubis refers to a noninfectious inflammatory condition that occurs after surgical or obstetric trauma to the pubic symphysis. This complication is said to occur in 2% to 3% of MMK patients (18). The patients typically complain of difficulty in ambulation and have a characteristic "waddling gait." A low-grade fever, elevated sedimentation rate, and mild leukocytosis may be encountered. Radiographic findings of the symphysis pubis, which lag about 4 weeks behind symptoms, may show reactive sclerosis, rarefaction, and osteolytic changes. Treatments for this inflammatory condition include rest, nonsteroidal antiinflammatory agents, and/or corticosteroids (localized injections or systemic) (10,11).

An infection of the pubic bone is termed osteomyelitis, which is a distinctly separate entity from osteitis pubis. It is usually difficult to confirm the diagnosis of infectious osteomyelitis because bone cultures would be required. A contemporary review of over 2,000 MMK procedures showed that while the incidence of osteitis pubis symptoms was very low, 0.74%, in those patients from whom bone cultures were available, 71% were positive for microorganisms, suggesting that perhaps osteomyelitis occurs more frequently than previously thought. Early aggressive use of antibiotics should be instituted if osteomyelitis is suspected (12).

Results

The surgical approaches to SUI, both abdominal and transvaginal, have not been subject to rigorous large randomized clinical trials with long-term follow-up to determine which of these many procedures are superior. While ample retrospective and prospective single-cohort studies exist, typically showing an "80% to 90% success rate" in the short term (less than 2 years follow-up) for many different anti-SUI procedures, it is apparent that durability is a critical issue. Failure rates for antiincontinence procedures may not be detected until 2 to 3 years postoperatively, so long-term follow-up is critical. Further, many new technological advances in surgical approaches to SUI are rapidly incorporated into clinical practice without adequate evidence-based data. Part of the reason for the lack of high-quality clinical data is the traditional manner in which SUI surgical data has been collected—namely, without standardization of preoperative evaluation, intraoperative methods, and postoperative outcome measures. Another reason for the rapid development of these techniques is the drive to minimize surgical morbidity and increase operative efficiency, which often supercedes other considerations. Last, perhaps the lack of mortality and minimal morbidity from SUI are reasons why there is not a demand for high-quality outcomes data afforded by well-conducted randomized trials. However, it is precisely for these reasons that randomized trials should be performed: Because of the low mortality and morbidity from surgical approaches to SUI, there should be randomized trials to compare the different approaches. In short, the "cart is ahead of the horse" phenomenon has occurred in the arena of surgical treatment for SUI. It may be difficult to acquire evidence-based data as many of different types of anti-SUI surgical procedures are already in widespread clinical use.

Therefore, the future for surgery to correct SUI will require the critical assessment of parameters such as how we define SUI, how we define cure of SUI, how we define voiding dysfunction, and how we define quality of life issues. While changes in techniques come and go, we must scientifically evaluate, by using the best clinical science available, which of the surgical procedures are most effective in alleviating the symptom of SUI.

REFERENCES

1. Bump RC, Coates KW, Cundiff GW, Harris RL, Weidner AC. Diagnosing intrinsic sphincteric deficiency: comparing urethral closure pressure, urethral axis, and Valsalva leak point pressures. *Am J Obstet Gynecol* 1997;177:303–310.
2. Burch JC. Urethrovaginal fixation to Cooper's ligament for correctoin of stress incontinence, cystocele and prolapse. *Am J Obstet Gynecol* 1961;81:281–290.
3. DeLancey JO. Structural support of the urethra as it relates to stress urinary incontinence: the hammock hypothesis. *Am J Obstet Gynecol* 1994;170:1713–1720.
4. DeLancey JO. Stress urinary incontinence: where are we now, where should we go? *Am J Obstet Gynecol* 1996;175:311–319.
5. Diokno AC, Catipay JR, Steinert BW. Office assessment of patient outcome of pharmacologic therapy for urge incontinence. *Int Urogynecol J Pelvic Floor Dysfunct* 2002;13:334–338.
6. Diokno AC, Dimaculangan RR, Lim EU, Steinert BW. Office based criteria for predicting type II stress incontinence without further evaluation studies. *J Urol* 1999;161:1263–1267.
7. Dwyer PL, Carey MP, Rosamilia A. Suture injury to the urinary tract in urethral suspension procedures for stress incontinence. *Int Urogynecol J Pelvic Floor Dysfunct* 1999;10:15–21.
8. Einhorning G. Simultaneous recording of intravesical and intraurethral pressure. *Acta Chir Scand* 1961;276:1–6.
9. Fleischmann N, Flisser AJ, Blaivas JG, Panagopoulos G. Sphincteric urinary incontinence: relationship to vesical leak point pressure, urethral mobility and severity of incontinence. *J Urol* 2003;169:999–1002.
10. Garcia-Porrua C, Gonzalez-Gay MA, Picallo JA. Rapid response to intravenous corticosteroids in osteitis pubis after Marshall–Marchetti–Krantz urethropexy. *Rheumatology* 2000;39:1048–1049.
11. Holt MA, Keene JS, Graf BK, Helwig DC. Treatment of osteitis pubis in athletes. Results of corticosteroid injections. *Am J Sports Med* 1995; 25:601–606.
12. Kammerer-Doak DN, Cornella JL, Magrina JF, Stanhope CR, Smilack J. Osteitis pubis after Marshall–Marchetti–Krantz urethropexy: a pubic osteomyelitis. *Am J Obstet Gynecol* 1998;179(3, Pt 1):586–590.
13. Kayigil O, Iftekhar Ahmed S, Metin A. The coexistence of intrinsic sphincter deficiency with type II stress incontinence. *J Urol* 1999;162: 1365–1366.
14. Kelly HA, Dunn WM. Urinary incontinence in women without manifest injury to the bladder. *Am Coll Surg* 1914;18:444–450.
15. Klutke JJ, Carlin BI, Klutke CG. The tension-free vaginal tape procedure: correction of stress incontinence with minimal alteration in proximal urethral mobility. *Urology* 2000;55:512–514.
16. Kreder KJ, Austin JC. Treatment of stress urinary incontinence in women with urethral hypermobility and intrinsic sphincter deficiency. *J Urol* 1996;156:1995–1998.
17. Leach GE, Dmochowski RR, Appell RA, et al. Female Stress Urinary Incontinence Clinical Guidelines Panel summary report on surgical management of female stress urinary incontinence. The American Urological Association. *J Urol* 1997;158(3, Pt 1):875–880.
18. Lentz SS. Osteitis pubis: a review [Review]. *Obstet Gynecol Surv* 1995;50:310–315.
19. Marshall FV, Marchetti AA, Krantz KE. The correction of stress incontinence by simple vesicourethral suspension. *Surg Gynecol Obstet* 1949;88:509–518.
20. McGuire EJ. Urodynamic findings in patients after failure of stress incontinence operations. *Progr Clin Biol Res* 1981;78:351–360.
21. McGuire EJ, Fitzpatrick CC, Wan J, et al. Clinical assessment of urethral sphincter function. *J Urol* 1993;150(5, Pt 1):1452–1454.
22. Panhoncini C, Constantini E, Guercini F, Porena M. Intrinsic sphincter deficiency: do the maximum urethral closure pressure and the Valsalva leak-point pressure identify different pathogenic mechanisms? *Int Urogynecol J Pelvic Floor Dysfunct* 2002;13:30–35.
23. Petrou SP, Wan J. VLPP in the evaluation of the female with stress urinary incontinence. *Int Urogynecol J Pelvic Floor Dysfunct* 1999;10:254–259.
24. Tanagho EA. Colpocystourethropexy: the way we do it. *J Urol* 1976; 116:751–753.
25. Vierhout ME, Mulder AF. De novo detrusor instability after Burch colposuspension. *Acta Obstet Gynecol Scand* 1992;71:414–416.
26. Wiskind AK, Creighton SM, Stanton SL. The incidence of genital prolapse after the Burch colposuspension. *Am J Obstet Gynecol* 1992;167: 399–404; discussion 404–405.

CHAPTER 36

Vaginal Approaches for Stress Urinary Incontinence

Lynn Stothers

This chapter describes the four most commonly performed procedures for stress incontinence that use a vaginal approach but do not require a harvested graft or synthetic sling. The four procedures are the Stamey bladder neck suspension, the Gittes no-incision urethropexy, the buried (also known as "*in situ*" or "island") vaginal wall sling, and the Raz anterior vaginal wall sling. Vaginal and abdominal approaches to correct stress incontinence have evolved concurrently (Fig. 36–1), and modifications continue to be made to increase simplicity and/or improve outcome.

DIAGNOSIS

The diagnosis of stress urinary incontinence is made by a combination of a detailed history, physical examination, and urodynamics.

INDICATIONS FOR SURGERY

Stamey, Gittes, and buried vaginal wall sling procedures are indicated for clinically significant stress incontinence with little or no cystocele. The Raz anterior vagi-

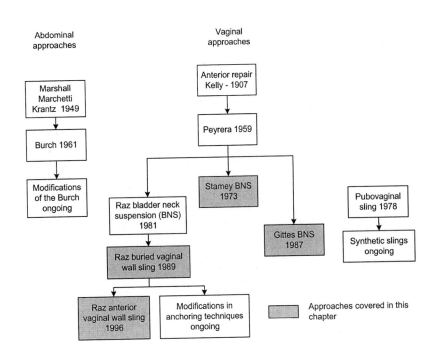

FIG. 36–1. The evolution of surgical approaches for the treatment of stress incontinence.

300

nal wall sling is indicated for clinically significant stress incontinence secondary to bladder neck hypermobility [anatomic incontinence (AI)] or intrinsic sphincter dysfunction (ISD) with little (grade 1) or no cystocele. This procedure can be modified to treat incontinence associated with grade 2 or 3 cystocele (six-corner suspension). In grade 4 cystocele, the sling is incorporated into a more extensive procedure that repairs both central and lateral defects (grade 4 cystocele repair).

ALTERNATIVE THERAPY

Alternatives to the vaginal approach are either periurethral injections of bulking agents or transabdominal approaches.

SURGICAL TECHNIQUE

Preparation for All Vaginal Approaches

Following general or spinal anesthesia, the patient is placed in the lithotomy position with the buttocks just overhanging the edge of the operating table. This allows the weighted vaginal speculum to hang freely without contacting the operating table. The feet are adequately padded in protective boots and placed in leg-supporting stirrups. Slight Trendelenburg positioning of the table helps expose the suprapubic region.

To obtain maximum exposure, a 30-degree weighted vaginal speculum is placed in the vagina. To enhance exposure, two single 3-0 silk labial retraction sutures are placed into the labia minora, anchoring the labia both laterally and superiorly to expose the urethra and bladder neck region of the anterior vaginal wall. Retraction sutures are applied only after the vaginal speculum is in place to avoid unnecessary tension or suture pullout.

Stamey Bladder Neck Suspension

Following standard preparation, a no. 14 Fr Foley catheter is placed per urethra. A T-shaped incision is made in the anterior vaginal wall. The surgeon dissects down to the glistening periurethral fascia and then laterally until the bladder neck is exposed sufficiently for placement of the Dacron grafts. The balloon can be palpated against the bladder neck to help identify the bladder neck vaginally.

Two suprapubic stab-wound incisions are made, one on each side of the lower abdomen, and dissection is carried out down to the level of the rectus fascia. The appropriate single prolonged Stamey needle (0-, 15-, or 30-degree angle at the distal end) is selected based on the patient's body habitus. The surgeon passes the Stamey needle through the rectus fascia adjacent to the periosteum, alongside the bladder neck, and out through the periurethral fascia under fingertip control (Fig. 36–2). After

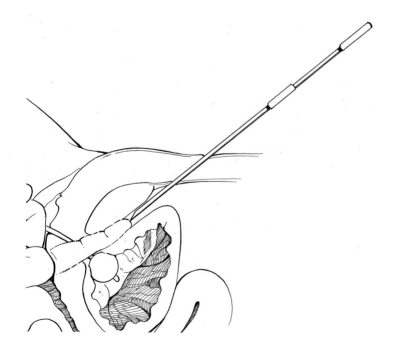

FIG. 36–2. The needle is guided along the posterior surface of the pubic symphysis under fingertip control to avoid injury to the bladder. (From Shortliffe LMD, Stamey TA. In: McDougal WS, ed. *Operative urology.* Kent, UK: Butterworth, 1985, with permission.)

passage of each needle, the Foley catheter is removed and cystoscopy performed to ensure that the needle has not perforated the bladder wall. If perforation is found, the needle is removed and repassed in the correct position.

Once the needle is placed, one end of a no. 2 nylon suture is threaded through the needle, and retraction of the needle transfers the suture through the suprapubic incision. A second pass of the Stamey needle is completed 1 cm lateral to the first pass. The vaginal ends of the nylon sutures are threaded through a 10-mm × 5-mm Dacron arterial graft and the free vaginal end of the nylon sutures is placed in the needle holder and transferred suprapubically (Fig. 36–3). During the transfer of the second end of the suture, the Dacron graft is guided into appropriate position at the urethrovesical junction. When suture placement is completed on one side, it is repeated on the contralateral side. After both sutures and their respective grafts are in position, cystoscopy is performed with gentle elevation of the sutures to ensure that there is adequate elevation of the bladder neck.

The vaginal wound is irrigated with copious amounts of antibiotic solution and the position of the graft is checked before closure to ensure that it is adequately buried beneath the vaginal wall to prevent graft erosion through the vaginal incision. The vaginal incision is closed with a running, locking 2-0 polyglycolic acid suture. The vagina is then packed with antibiotic-soaked gauze, the nylon sutures are tied in place, and the stab wounds are closed with a 4-0-polyglycolic acid subcuticular closure. A suprapubic catheter is then placed using standard technique.

The vaginal pack and Foley catheter are removed within 24 hours of surgery (as early as several hours postoperatively if the patient is ambulating well) and the suprapubic catheter is clamped. The patient is discharged with the suprapubic catheter in place and instructed to record residual volumes at home. The suprapubic catheter is removed in the office once the postvoid residual urine is consistently low.

Gittes Bladder Neck Suspension

Following standard preparation, a no. 14 Fr Foley catheter is placed per urethra. Two suprapubic stab-wound incisions are made in the lower abdomen approximately 5 cm lateral to the midline at the upper margin of the symphysis pubis. Dissection is carried out with a small forceps until the rectus fascia is exposed. A single-pronged Stamey needle is inserted into the medial edge of one of the suprapubic wounds. The surgeon should be able to feel the back of the needle in contact with the posterior aspect of the pubic bone as the needle is passing. By palpating the Foley catheter balloon, the anterior vaginal wall is identified and elevated with the surgeon's sec-

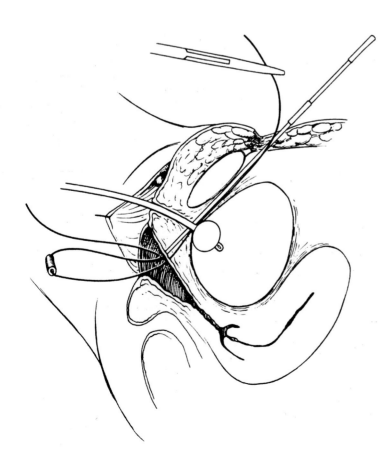

FIG. 36–3. The Stamey needle is passed a second time after the suture is passed through the Dacron graft. (From Shortliffe LMD, Stamey TA. In: McDougal WS, ed. *Operative urology.* Kent, UK: Butterworth, 1985, with permission.)

ond hand. The needle is directed toward the fingertip in the vagina and, when palpable, advanced through the anterior vaginal wall and out through the introitus (Fig. 36–4). Correct positioning of the needle is confirmed by removing the Foley catheter and performing a cystoscopy after each needle passage. If the needle is appropriately positioned, it will indent the ipsilateral bladder neck when moved medially but will not have perforated the bladder wall.

One end of a no. 2 Prolene suture is threaded through the needle and the needle is retracted superiorly out of the vagina, thereby transferring the end of the suture out through the lower abdominal stab wound. The Stamey needle is passed again through the same ipsilateral abdominal incision 1 cm lateral to the first pass. Under fingertip guidance, the needle should be directed to perforate into the vagina 1 cm lateral to the initial pass to avoid tenting up a large amount of vaginal tissue at the completion of the procedure (Fig. 36–5). The free vaginal

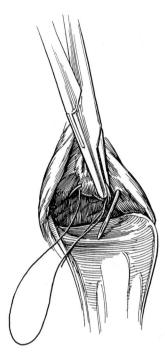

FIG. 36–5. After the second pass of the Stamey needle, the vaginal end of the suture is threaded onto a Mayo needle. Several deep bites of vaginal mucosa are taken before threading the free end of the suture into the eye of the Stamey needle and delivering it to the suprapubic area. (From Kursh and McGuire. *Female urology*, with permission.)

end of the suture is threaded through a Mayo needle and two or three helical bites of vaginal tissue are taken between the first and second vaginal perforations. After unthreading the Mayo needle, the free end of the Prolene suture is threaded through the Stamey needle, which is withdrawn from the abdominal incision, transferring the other end of the Prolene suture. The two ends of the Prolene are held with a hemostat for later tying. Needle passage and suture transfers are completed in a similar fashion on the contralateral side.

When suture placement is complete, cystoscopy is performed again to demonstrate adequate elevation of the bladder neck when the sutures are gently elevated through the abdominal incisions. The vagina is packed with an antibiotic-impregnated vaginal pack prepared as for the Stamey procedure. Each Prolene suture is tied to itself and the abdominal stab wounds are closed with a 4-0 subcuticular closure and steristrips. If desired, a suprapubic catheter is placed in the standard fashion and connected to straight drainage along with the Foley catheter. The vaginal packing may be removed 2 hours after surgery. With healing, the vaginal suture cuts through the vaginal wall and a curtain of scar tissue is left to provide support for the bladder neck (Fig. 36–6).

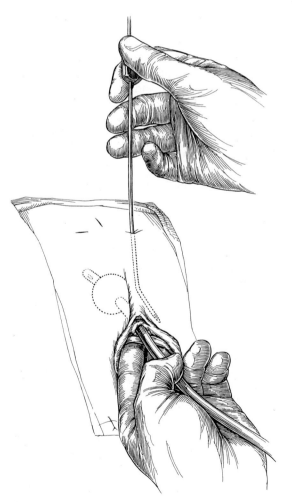

FIG. 36–4. The Stamey needle is advanced through the supporting urethral fascia and vaginal mucosa between the index and long fingers. (From Kursh and McGuire. *Female urology*, with permission.)

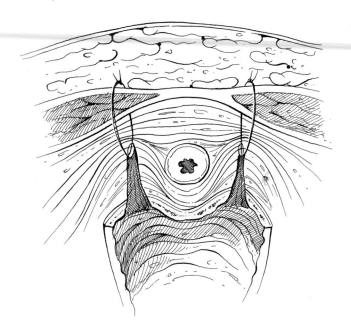

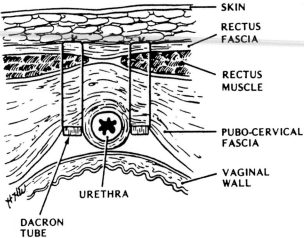

FIG. 36–6. Diagrammatic representation of no-incision urethropexy approximately 1 month after surgery. As the suture slowly cuts through the vaginal wall and fascia, a curtain of scar tissue is left and provides support to the vesical neck.

Buried (*In Situ* or Island) Vaginal Wall Sling

Following standard preparation, a no. 14 Fr Foley catheter is placed per urethra and a suprapubic catheter is inserted. The anterior vaginal wall is infiltrated with saline in the region of the planned incision to facilitate the dissection. An inverted U-shaped incision is made in the anterior vaginal wall with its apex just proximal to the urethral meatus. The arms of the incision are extended to create the base of the U 2 to 3 cm proximal to the bladder neck, and a cross incision is made to allow isolation of an island of vaginal wall. A transverse incision is made at the level of the bladder neck to join the lateral borders of the original inverted U, creating the rectangular island. The island retains its own vascular supply and will function as the *in situ* sling (Fig. 36–7). The size of the island can be tailored to the length and caliber of the urethra.

Using Allis clamps to aid in exposure, dissection is carried out laterally along the glistening surface of the periurethral fascia. Lateral dissection continues on both sides, and the retropubic space is entered using curved Mayo scissors. With a finger in the retropubic space, the urethra is mobilized. Any adhesions are taken down with a combination of sharp and blunt dissection to free the retropubic space and allow for easy passage of the double-pronged needle carrier.

To create the anterior vaginal wall flap that will be advanced to cover the island, the vaginal wall is dissected in the inferior portion of the inverted U. The four corners of the rectangle that will form the buried sling are anchored with individual no. 1 Prolene sutures applied in a helical fashion.

A small suprapubic stab incision is made in the midline and the sutures are transferred from the vagina to the suprapubic incision in the standard fashion. Cystoscopy is performed following indigo carmine injection to ensure that no sutures have entered the bladder and that there is blue efflux from each ureteral orifice.

The anterior vaginal wall flap is then advanced over the sling to provide an epithelial cover and restore the integrity of the vagina using a running locking 2-0 Vicryl suture. A vaginal pack is placed and the Prolene sutures are tied. Each suture is tied to itself and then to its mate on the contralateral side. The Prolene sutures are buried in the suprapubic fat and the suprapubic stab wound is closed with intradermic 4-0 absorbable sutures and steristrips. Postoperative care is the same as for the anterior vaginal wall sling.

Modifications to this procedure include the used of bone anchors placed via a prepubic incision into the pubic tubercles. The suspending sutures are anchored to the island of vaginal wall and tied to the anchors in the prepubic area. Another modification is to use the *in situ* sling but not bury it, keeping the urethropelvic ligaments intact. Using blunt and sharp dissection, the urethropelvic ligament is dissected to the level of the tendinous arc at the pelvic sidewall, without entering the retropubic space. Each corner of the sling is anchored with a no. 1 Prolene suture incorporating the vaginal wall, pubocervical fascia, and the urethropelvic ligaments at the level of the bladder neck. The suture is continued cephalad in a helical fashion, incorporating the periurethral fascia, medial edge of the urethropelvic ligament, and the vaginal wall distally (Fig. 36–8). The vaginal sutures are transferred to the suprapubic area through a 1- to 2-cm incision using the double-pronged needle.

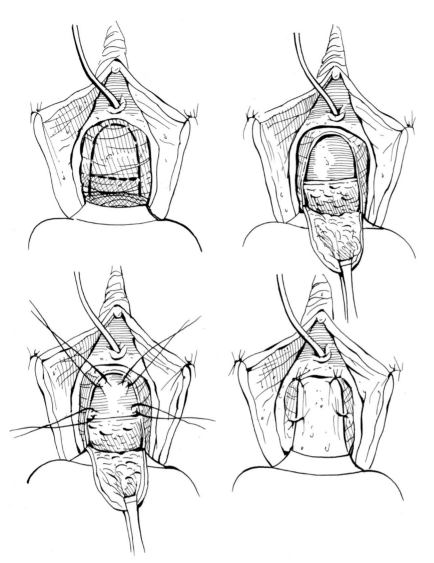

FIG. 36–7. Inverted U vaginal incision with transverse incision at the level of the vesical neck to an create island. Undermining of the vaginal wall proximal to island to create flap. Anchoring of four corners of island with individual polypropylene sutures applied to helical fashion. Proximal vaginal wall flap advanced over island to cover sling. (Redrawn from Raz S, et al. *J Urol* 1989;141:44, with permission.)

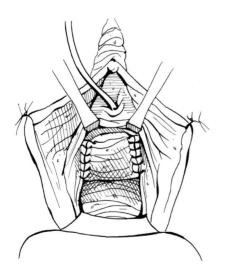

FIG. 36–8. Rectangular vaginal sling. Running polypropylene suture on either side incorporates vaginal wall and surrounding paravaginal tissue. (Redrawn from Kaplan et al. *J Urol* 2000;164:1623–1627, with permission.)

Raz Anterior Vaginal Wall Sling

Following standard preparation, a no. 14 Fr Foley catheter is used for suprapubic drainage and a second no. 14 Fr Foley catheter is inserted into the bladder per urethra to help identify the bladder neck vaginally. Three Allis clamps are placed at the level of the midurethra (midway between the bladder neck and external meatus) on the anterior vaginal wall and retracted upward, exposing the anterior vaginal wall. To facilitate dissection, 10 cc of saline are injected just beneath the vaginal wall along the anticipated suture lines. Two oblique incisions are made in the anterior vaginal wall, extending from the level of the midurethra to 2 cm below the bladder neck (Fig. 36–9). Dissection is carried out laterally using Metzenbaum scissors to expose the vaginal side of the urethropelvic ligament bilaterally. This dissection should be kept superficial because deep dissection with perforation of the ligament can result in excessive bleeding. The sur-

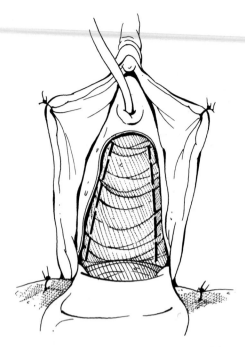

FIG. 36–9. The patient is in the lithotomy position with the weighted vaginal speculum in place along with labial retraction sutures. The positions of the two oblique incisions in the anterior vaginal wall are shown by the dotted lines. Note that the incisions do not cross or meet in the midline.

geon can feel the attachment of the urethropelvic ligament to the tendinous arc by placing a finger, pointed toward the ipsilateral shoulder of the patient, into the incision. With gentle pressure, the curved Mayo scissors are placed into each wound against the tendinous arc and

advanced until the retropubic space is entered. The blades of the scissors are opened to help detach the urethropelvic ligament from the tendinous arc. A finger is inserted through the wound into the retropubic space, and blunt finger dissection is used to detach any adhesions from either side. The space should feel freely open and the urethra should be easily palpable in the midline (Fig. 36–10).

Two pairs of no. 1 Prolene suture on a half-circle, tapered MO-5 needle are used to complete the sling. The proximal pair of Prolene sutures is placed first. A long forceps is placed into the retropubic space and the urethra and bladder are retracted medially. A no. 1 Prolene suture is placed in a helical fashion into the urethropelvic ligament, taking several passes. With the needle kept parallel to the plane of the vagina, the suture is passed in the vaginal wall (excluding the epithelium) to incorporate a large surface area of the underlying vesicopelvic fascia. The same procedure is carried out on the contralateral side.

To place the second, more distal pair of Prolene sutures, the long forceps are placed into the open retropubic space. The jaws of the forceps are opened parallel to the floor and retracted inferiorly to create an open triangle in the retropubic space. The apex of the triangle is formed by the levator muscle as it inserts into the pubic symphysis and the midurethral segment. The medial side of the triangle is formed by the urethropelvic ligament as it inserts into the urethra. The lateral side of the triangle is formed by the pelvic sidewall, and the cardinal ligaments run parallel to the base.

Several passes of no. 1 Prolene suture are run through the levator muscle and the edge of the urethropelvic ligament. To obtain an adequate amount of levator tissue, the

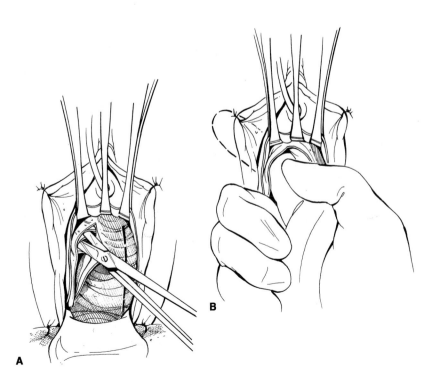

FIG. 36–10. A: Dissection is carried out over the glistening periurethral fascia. The curved Mayo scissors are shown entering the retropubic space. The scissors are pointed toward the shoulder of the patient. Misdirecting the scissors too far medially could result in bladder perforation. **B:** The surgeon's finger is inserted into the open retropubic space through each vaginal incision and adhesions are taken down. The inside of the pubic ramus is easily palpated. In patients with prior surgery, a Deaver retractor may be placed in the retropubic space, and sharp dissection under vision can be used to safely incise any dense urethral adhesions from the pubic bone.

needle must be placed deep into the retropubic space. The levator should be visualized on the arc of the needle. The forceps are repositioned to put downward traction on the anterior vaginal wall in the area of the midurethra. Suturing continues with several helical bites of the underlying periurethral fascia, incorporating tissue up to but not across the midline. As in placing sutures into the vesicopelvic fascia, it is important to keep the needle parallel to the vaginal wall to prevent suture material from entering the spongy tissue of the urethra itself. Once all four Prolene sutures are in place, a rectangle of support for the bladder neck and midurethra can be visualized (Fig. 36–11).

A small incision, the width of a double-pronged needle carrier, is made in the midline just above the superior margin of the pubic bone down to, but not through, the rectus fascia. If the incision is made too high, the sutures will be transferred over a mobile area of the anterior abdominal wall fascia, which can result in pain or incomplete support. With a finger in the retropubic space serving as a guide, the double-pronged needle carrier is advanced through the suprapubic incision into the retropubic space and out through the vaginal incision (Fig. 36–12). The free ends of one of the ipsilateral Prolene sutures are placed through the needle holes in the double-pronged ligature carrier. The needle carrier is retracted to deliver both ends of the sutures out through the suprapubic incision. A total of four passes are made. The sutures should be transferred one at a time to avoid tangling or knotting with other Prolene sutures.

Indigo carmine is injected intravenously, the urethral Foley is removed, and a cystoscopy is performed to ensure that (a) the suprapubic catheter is in good position, (b) blue efflux is noted from both ureteral orifices, (c) no Prolene suture material has entered the bladder, and (d) upward retraction on the suprapubic Prolene sutures provides support to the bladder neck and midurethra.

The two oblique vaginal incisions are closed with a running, locking, absorbable suture of 2-0 polyglycolic acid on a tapered UR-5 needle. An antibiotic-impregnated vaginal pack is inserted and the weighted vaginal speculum is then removed. Last, the Prolene sutures are

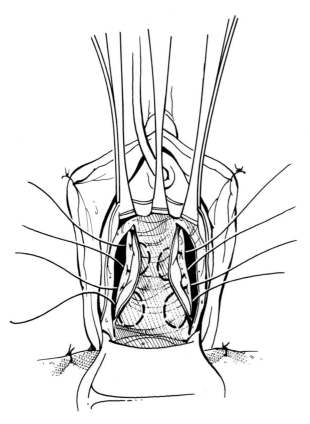

FIG. 36–11. The second more distal pair of Proline sutures is placed at the level of the midurethra. These sutures include the levator muscle, the edge of the urethropelvic ligament, and the underlying periurethral fascia. Once the four Proline sutures are in place, one can visualize the rectangle of support that will be given to the underlying urethra and bladder neck.

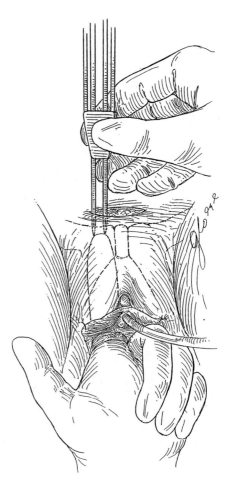

FIG. 36–12. Double-pronged ligature carrier being passed with finger guidance. (From Kursh and McGuire. *Female urology*, with permission.)

tied independently to their ipsilateral mates on the rectus fascia, creating the hammock of support. The Prolene sutures are buried in the suprapubic fat and the suprapubic stab wound is closed with intradermic 4-0 absorbable sutures and steristrips. The urethral catheter and vaginal pack are removed within 24 hours and the suprapubic catheter is plugged once the patient begins to move freely.

Six-Corner Suspension: Modification for Grades 2 and 3 Cystocele

Following standard preparation, a no. 14 Fr Foley urethral catheter and a suprapubic catheter are placed using the technique described for the Raz anterior vaginal wall sling. The same incision as for the Raz anterior vaginal wall sling is made but extended in the vagina 2 cm more toward the top of the vault (Fig. 36–13). Using Metzenbaum scissors, the lateral dissection is carried out distally to expose the urethropelvic ligament and proximally to expose the cardinal ligaments. The retropubic space is opened in the standard fashion using curved Mayo scissors and adhesions are taken down in the retropubic space, leaving the urethra freely mobile.

Three sutures of no. 1 Prolene are placed on each side. The proximal suture is passed parallel to the plane of the vagina into the perivesical fascia, incorporating the area of the cardinal ligaments at the apex of the vagina. The middle suture is first placed at the level of the bladder neck and is passed with helical bites through the perivesical fascia parallel to the anterior vaginal wall excluding the epithelium. The bladder neck is then held medially and the suture is placed through the freed proximal edge of the urethropelvic ligament. The third and most distal suture is passed just the same as for the anterior vaginal wall sling, incorporating the levator, the edge of the urethropelvic ligament, and the anterior vaginal wall without epithelium, which overlies the region of the midurethra. The sutures are transferred through a single midline suprapubic stab incision using the double-pronged needle carrier as previously described. Cystoscopy, closure of the vaginal wall, packing of the vagina, and finally tying of the suspension sutures and closure of the suprapubic wound are completed.

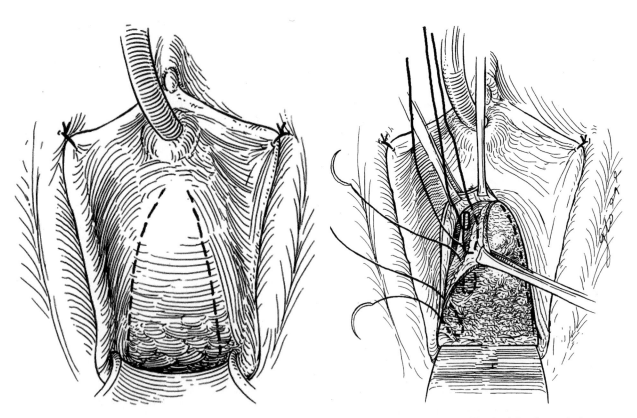

FIG. 36–13. A: Oblique vaginal incisions used for six-corner bladder suspension. The incision is carried from the midurethra to the apex of the vagina. (Adapted from Raz S, Stothers L, Chopra A. Raz techniques for anterior vaginal wall repair. In: Raz S, ed. *Female urology*, 2nd ed. Philadelphia: WB Saunders, 1996, with permission.) **B:** Location of the polypropylene sutures used in the six-corner suspension prior to transfer. (Adapted from Raz S, Stothers L, Chopra A. Raz techniques for anterior vaginal wall repair. In: Raz S, ed. *Female urology*, 2nd ed. Philadelphia: WB Saunders, 1996, with permission.)

Grade 4 Cystocele Repair

The vagina is exposed using stay sutures and a weighted vaginal speculum using the technique described for the vaginal wall sling. A Scott ring is placed with hooks at the 1-, 3-, 9-, and 11-o'clock positions to add further lateral and superior exposure. If the vagina is narrow, a right-angle Heaney retractor can be used in place of the weighted vaginal speculum.

A suprapubic catheter inserted and a no. 14 Fr Foley catheter is placed per urethra. If there is significant uterine prolapse, a hysterectomy is performed before proceeding with the bladder repair and the *cul-de-sac* is closed completely. If the patient has no uterus but has a significant enterocele, the enterocele is repaired and culdoplasty is performed before proceeding with the bladder repair.

An Allis clamp is placed in the midline at the level of the midurethra and retracted upward to aid exposure. A "goalpost" incision is made with the "posts" 2 cm in length on either side of the urethra, beginning at the midurethra and ending 1 cm proximal to the bladder neck. Connecting the proximal ends of the posts creates the "crossbar" incision. To create the "base" of the goalpost, the midline incision is extended from the center of the crossbar to the base of the cystocele or to the vaginal cuff following hysterectomy (Fig. 36–14a).

To expose the central defect of the cystocele over the base of the bladder, the edges of one side of the midline incision are grasped with Allis clamps and dissection is carried out laterally in the plane just deep enough to reach the vaginal wall. Dissection continues laterally to expose the central defect of the vesicopelvic fascia and inferiorly to expose the separated cardinal ligaments. The procedure is repeated on the contralateral side until the cystocele is seen bulging in the midline. If, during dissection, an enterocele sac is seen protruding between the separated cardinal ligaments, the edges of the sac are grasped and the peritoneal cavity opened. The hernia is closed with a pair of 2-0 polyglycolic acid sutures placed in a pursestring fashion. If the enterocele is large and the peritoneal contents protrude, the enterocele sac is opened in a similar manner but closed by performing a culdoplasty as described in Chapter xx.

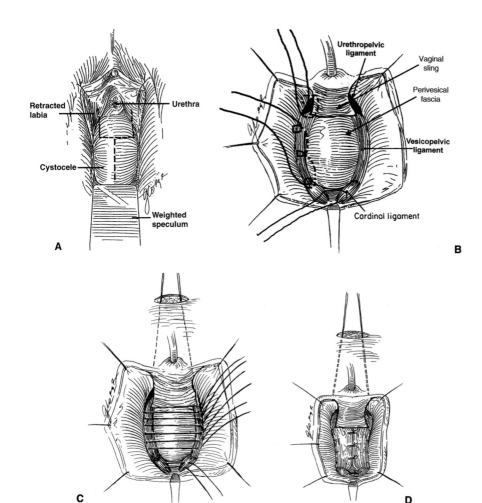

FIG. 36–14. A: The incision for the combined lateral and central fascial defect repair. The distal limbs extend to the midurethra and are connected across the midline proximal to the bladder neck. The midline incision is carried to the level of the vaginal cuff. (Adapted from Raz S, Stothers L, Chopra A. Raz techniques for anterior vaginal wall repair. In: Raz S, ed. *Female urology*, 2nd ed. Philadelphia: WB Saunders, 1996, with permission.) **B:** Location of sutures for repair of the lateral defect and vaginal wall sling. (Adapted from Raz S, Stothers L, Chopra A. Raz techniques for anterior vaginal wall repair. In: Raz S, ed. *Female urology*, 2nd ed. Philadelphia: WB Saunders, 1996, with permission.) **C:** Location of sutures for repair of the central defect. The mesh is not depicted. The suspension sutures have already been passed and are not seen here. (Adapted from Raz S, Stothers L, Chopra A. Raz techniques for anterior vaginal wall repair. In: Raz S, ed. *Female urology*, 2nd ed. Philadelphia: WB Saunders, 1996, with permission.) **D:** After cystoscopy, the sutures closing the central defect are tied.

To facilitate entry into the retropubic space, the lateral edges of the posts of the goalpost incision are grasped and dissection is carried out toward the ipsilateral shoulder of the patient, as in the dissection for the anterior vaginal wall sling. The retropubic space is entered, the urethropelvic ligament is separated from the tendinous arc of the obturator, and all adhesions in the retropubic space are taken down.

A povidone/iodine-soaked gauze is folded and placed over the center of the cystocele. Gentle cephalad retraction using a Heaney retractor over the gauze reduces the central defect of the cystocele. Two 1-0 suspensory Prolene sutures on an MO-5 needle are placed on each side. The proximal sutures are placed first, incorporating helical bites of three structures: the urethropelvic ligament at the level of the bladder neck, the perivesical fascia along the lateral reflected margin of the vaginal wall, and the ipsilateral cardinal ligament. The distal sutures are placed to incorporate the levator, the edge of the urethropelvic ligament as it enters the midurethra, and the anterior vaginal wall below the depth of the epithelium (Fig. 36–14b). The two pairs of Prolene sutures are transferred through a midline stab wound using a double-pronged needle. These sutures provide urethral and bladder neck supports and correct the lateral defect.

The final stage of the reconstruction involves repairing the central defect. The Heaney retractor and the gauze over the central portion of the cystocele are removed to reveal the cystocele's bulging surface. A 4- × 8-cm rectangle of polyglycolic acid mesh is folded and placed over the center of the cystocele to reduce the central hernia and aid in exposure of the lateral margins of the central defect. To close the central defect, several midline plication sutures of 2-0 polyglycolic horizontal mattress sutures are placed. The number of sutures needed depends on the extent of the cystocele. The first suture is placed just inferior to the crossbar, with the remaining sutures progressing 6 mm apart toward the base of the cystocele (Fig. 36–14c). The horizontal mattress sutures must not be placed too deep or they may enter the bladder or injure a ureter. Cystoscopy is performed following indigo carmine injection to ensure that no sutures have entered the bladder and that there is clear efflux from both ureteral orifices. The first step in closing the repair is to tie the horizontal mattress sutures. The mesh is buried beneath them and maintains reduction of the central hernia during healing (Fig. 36–14d). The vaginal goalpost incision is then closed with a running and locking 2-0 Vicryl suture in the standard fashion. A vaginal pack is placed. Finally, the four Prolene sutures are tied without tension in the suprapubic incision. The knots are buried and the suprapubic stab wound is closed in the standard fashion described for the vaginal wall sling.

OUTCOMES

Complications

Potential complications of vaginal approaches for stress incontinence are listed in Table 36–1. The majority are preventable by (a) proper positioning of the patient, (b) careful dissection and correct identification of important anatomic landmarks, and (c) routine performance of intraoperative cystoscopy for early identification and correction of potential problems. Patients at increased risk for complications include those with a history of prior bladder or pelvic surgery, endometriosis, pelvic infection, pelvic fracture, or significant pelvic prolapse. These factors may alter the anatomy by scarring or, in the case of prolapse, distort the usual position of structures.

Minor bleeding is the most frequent intraoperative complication. Sources of hemorrhage include arterial vessels within the vaginal wall (rare), dissection in the wrong fascial plane, or following opening of the retropubic space. In addition, the patient may notice vaginal

TABLE 36–1. *Classification of potential complications related to vaginal approaches for stress urinary incontinence in the female*

Intraoperative
  Hemorrhage
  Misplacement of Suture Material
  Urethral injury
  Ureteral Injury
    Ligation
    Incision
    Crush or Clamp
    Cautery Burn
  Bladder Injury
    Incision or Perforation
    Suture Related
    Cautery Burn
  Neurological Injury Related to Positioning
    Peroneal Nerve Palsy
    Femoral Neuropraxia
    Lower-Limb Compartment Syndromes
Postoperative
  Early
    Vaginal Bleeding or Discharge
    Urinary Tract Infection
    Pain
      Suprapubic
      Vaginal
    Voiding Dysfunction
    Urinary Retention
    Recurrent Stress Urinary Incontinence
    De Novo Urgency Incontinence
    Pelvic/Suture Infection
    Exposure of Permanent Sutures Vaginally
  Late
    Vaginal Shortening or Stenosis
    Dyspareunia
    Secondary Genital Prolapse

spotting during the first 3 weeks postoperatively. If vaginal bleeding persists or increases in amount, a vaginal examination should be performed to identify the site of bleeding and a temporary vaginal pack should be placed if necessary.

Misplacement of the Prolene sutures can occur when the anatomic landmarks are not clearly exposed and identified, and has the potential to cause ureteral or bladder perforation or injury. Both of these complications can be diagnosed with the use of intraoperative indigo carmine and careful cystoscopy. If suture material is identified within the bladder, the offending suture is immediately removed and the ureters are checked to ensure they are intact. If necessary, retrograde pyelograms should be performed.

Postoperative suprapubic pain over the site of suspension sutures may occur and is often activity related, subsiding with several weeks of decreased physical activity. Muscle entrapment of the sutures can occur when suture placement is lateral and superior to the pubic margin and may present as activity-related suprapubic pain. This problem can be prevented by passing the suture-transferring needle as close to the pubic bone as possible, avoiding tying sutures under tension, and carefully burying the sutures under the subcutaneous fat during closing.

Infection is strongly suggested by pain in the suprapubic area accompanied by redness. If this occurs, the suprapubic wound should be opened, cultured, and packed to allow healing by secondary intention. The need to remove Prolene sutures due to infection is extremely rare. Although graft rejection can lead to infection, the Dacron pledget used in the Stamey needle suspension has been shown to have a very low rejection rate.

Vaginal stenosis or shortening may result from excessive plication of the vaginal epithelium during closure or from secondary scarring. A history of new onset of dyspareunia or pelvic or vaginal pain and the finding of foreshortening on physical examination confirm the diagnosis. Mild shortening or stenosis may be treated with longitudinal relaxing incisions in the lateral vaginal wall with transverse closure.

Voiding dysfunction in the early postoperative period is common following surgery for stress incontinence. Urinary retention in the immediate postoperative period resolves in the majority of patients with the use of a suprapubic catheter or intermittent self-catheterization. Permanent retention is extremely rare. Urgency and frequency of urination should be evaluated with physical examination, urinalysis, and measurement of residual urine.

Results

A number of factors influence the cure rate for stress incontinence with vaginal procedures. Patient factors that may influence outcome include obesity, presence of respiratory distress, severity of incontinence initially (number of pads or as determined by the leak point pressure at urodynamics), and hormonal status. The definition of "cure" also influences the results. Cure rates for stress incontinence are always the highest at short-term follow-up and decrease with time.

Cure/improved rates for the Stamey needle suspension were initially reported as 90%. In retrospective case series over the last 10 years, cure rates have ranged from 52% to 80% (1,4,5,8). Mills et al. (12) reported that cure rates declined to 33% at 10-year follow-up. Conrad et al. (2) reported that, although only 50% of women were completely dry 5 years following surgery, over two-thirds reported a substantial improvement in quality of life. Retrospective case series of the Gittes no-incision urethropexy report short-term cure/improved rates between 81% and 94% (9–11,15). Elkabir and Mee (3) reported that while initial results were encouraging only 38.5% of patients were considered cured at 2 years, decreasing to 23.1% at 4 to 5 years follow-up. One combined long-term follow-up comparing Stamey and Gittes procedures (13) showed a decline in continence from 93% at 3 months to 38% (Stamey) and 14% (Gittes) at 5 years and to 28% (Stamey) at 9 years. The authors concluded that the procedures are not durable, Gittes procedures have an earlier failure rate than Stamey procedures, and repeat procedures are not worthwhile. In a longer follow-up study (7), 71.5% of patients who had undergone Stamey procedures were continent 14 years postoperatively, compared to only 37% for the Gittes at 6 years follow-up ($p < 0.0001$). The authors concluded that the Stamey procedure is superior to the Gittes procedure and that women with type III incontinence should not undergo either procedure.

Long-term data for the buried (*in situ*) vaginal wall sling procedure and the Raz procedure are not available. With the buried sling procedure, 94% of women with stress incontinence were reported as cured at 24 months (6). The Raz anterior vaginal wall sling has similar results. In a prospective cohort study, 152 of 163 patients with a median 17-month follow-up were cured of stress incontinence (14).

REFERENCES

1. Ashken MH. Followup results with the Stamey operation for stress urinary incontinence of urine. *Br J Urol* 1990;65:168.
2. Conrad S, Pieper A, De la Maza SF, Busch R, Huland H. Long-term results of the Stamey bladder neck suspension procedure: a patient questionnaire based outcome analysis. *J Urol* 1997;157:1672–1677.
3. Elkabir JJ, Mee AD. Long-term evaluation of the Gittes procedure for urinary stress incontinence. *J Urol* 1998;159:1203–1205.
4. Gofrit ON, Landau EH, Shapiro A, Pode D. The Stamey procedure for stress incontinence: long-term results. *Eur Urol* 1998;34:339–343.
5. Hilton P, Mayne CJ. The Stamey endoscopic bladder neck suspension; a clinical and urodynamic investigation, including actuarial follow-up over four years. *Br J Obstet Gynaecol* 1991;98:1141.
6. Juma S, Little NA, Raz S. Vaginal wall sling; four years later. *Urology* 1992;39:424.

7. Kondo A, Kato K, Gotoh M, Narushima M, Saito M. The Stamey and Gittes procedures: long-term followup in relation to incontinence types and patient age. *J Urol* 1998;160(3, Pt 1):756–758.

8. Kuczyk MA, Klein S, Grunewald V, Machtens S, Denil J, Hofner K, Wagner T, Jonas U. A questionnaire-based outcome analysis of the Stamey bladder neck suspension procedure for the treatment of urinary stress incontinence: the Hannover experience. *Br J Urol* 1998;82: 174–180.

9. Kursh ED. Factors influencing the outcome of a no incision endoscopic urethropexy. *Surg Gynecol Obstet* 1992;175:254.

10. Kursh ED, Angeli AH, Resnick MI. Evolution of endoscopic urethropexy; seven-year experience with various techniques. *Urology* 1991;37:428.

11. Loughlin KR, Whitmore WF III, Gittes RF, Richie JP. Review of an 8 year experience with modifications of endoscopic suspension of the bladder neck for female stress urinary incontinence. *J Urol* 1990; 143:44.

12. Mills R, Persad R, Ashken MH. Long-term follow-up results with the Stamey operation for stress incontinence of urine. *Br J Urol* 1996; 77:86.

13. Nigam AK, Otite U, Badenoch DF. Endoscopic bladder neck suspension revisited: long-term results of Stamey and Gittes procedures. *Eur Urol* 2000;38:677–680.

14. Raz S, Stothers L, Young G, et al. Vaginal wall sling for anatomic incontinence and intrinsic sphincter damage—efficacy and outcome analysis. *J Urol* 1996;156:166–170.

15. Theodorou C, Floratos D, Katsifotis C, Moutzouris G, Mertziotis N, Thermogianni H. Transvaginal incisionless bladder neck suspension. A simplified technique for female genuine stress incontinence. *Int Urol Nephrol* 1998;30:273–278.

CHAPTER 37

Pubovaginal Fascial Slings

R. Duane Cespedes and Edward J. McGuire

The first urethral sling procedure was described by Von Giordano in 1907; however, even after numerous technical improvements and application of many different materials the pubovaginal sling (PVS) was rarely used until repopularized by McGuire and Lytton in 1978 (6). The pubovaginal sling has by tradition been used only when other incontinence procedures such as a bladder neck suspension or retropubic urethropexy have failed. Currently, the preoperative diagnosis of intrinsic sphincter deficiency (ISD) can be determined by use of the Valsalva (VLPP) or abdominal leak point pressure (ALPP) during incontinence evaluations (5). Accordingly, the diagnosis of ISD can be made before surgery and a PVS performed as the primary incontinence procedure to reduce the rate of procedural failures.

Stress urinary incontinence (SUI) in females is classified by the presence and degree of urethral mobility and functional status of the urethra. In types I and II SUI, the urethral sphincter functions normally; however, abdominal pressure can drive the sphincter into a position where it does not function normally. This type of stress incontinence is due to urethral hypermobility and can be successfully treated by a procedure that immobilizes the bladder neck, such as a bladder neck suspension, retropubic urethropexy, or one of the sling procedures. Type III SUI, now called ISD, is usually characterized by a minimally mobile urethra and incompetence of the urethral sphincter during increases in abdominal pressure. It is important to note that the severity of urethral hypermobility and sphincteric incompetence are on a continuum and exist to some degree in many patients. Therefore, it is likely that some patients will have incontinence due to coexisting ISD and urethral hypermobility. All patients with ISD are effectively treated with a PVS; therefore, many urologists use a PVS routinely because it will treat incontinence due to both hypermobility and ISD.

DIAGNOSIS

The preoperative evaluation is directed toward identifying ISD. The history can be helpful becauase patients with ISD usually have severe leakage with minimal activity or have a history of radiation to the pelvis, a prior incontinence procedure, or are elderly (especially new-onset incontinence in patients over 70). The incidence of ISD increases after each failed incontinence procedure: 9% if no previous surgery, 25% after one failed procedure, and 75% after two failed procedures (4).

The physical exam is directed toward demonstrating leakage, urethral hypermobility, and pelvic prolapse. Urinary leakage without significant hypermobility constitutes presumptive evidence of ISD. A careful evaluation for associated cystocele, rectocele, enterocele, and uterine prolapse is important for ALPP interpretation and in planning the appropriate operative procedures. Failure to repair associated pelvic prolapse conditions will put undue stress on any incontinence procedure, including a pubovaginal sling, which may increase the failure rate.

After the postvoid residual is determined, a cystometrogram is performed to exclude poor detrusor compliance and overt detrusor instability. To diagnose ISD, an ALPP is indispensable. The bladder is filled to a standard volume of 200 mL (children to one-half functional bladder capacity) and a slow Valsalva maneuver is performed with the patient in the upright position until leakage is noted. Performing this several times and determining an average improves accuracy. If a well-performed Valsalva maneuver fails to induce leakage, vigorous coughing may be required. If coughing is required, the ALPP is almost always greater than 100 cm H_2O. If the ALPP is below 60 cm H_2O, ISD is present. If the ALPP is greater than 90 cm H_2O and minimal pelvic prolapse exists, pure urethral hypermobility is usually present. Patients with significant pelvic prolapse conditions may not demonstrate stress incontinence unless the prolapse is reduced with a vaginal pack. This type of leakage is called occult inconti-

The opinions contained herein are those of the authors and are not to be construed as reflecting the views of the US Air Force or the Department of Defense.

nence (1,3). In addition, even if the patient complains of stress incontinence, reduction with a vaginal pack will usually demonstrate a greatly reduced ALPP, which may change the incontinence procedure contemplated (3). ALPP values between 60 to 90 cm H_2O form a gray area in which hypermobility and ISD coexist.

INDICATIONS FOR SURGERY

The most common indications for a PVS are urodynamically documented ISD with or without urethral hypermobility and prior failed incontinence procedures. In addition, because of the long-term success and durability of PVS, many patients with SUI due to urethral hypermobility may be better served with a sling procedure. These include females who engage in vigorous athletic activities, are significantly obese, or who cough frequently due to pulmonary disease.

ALTERNATIVE THERAPY

In selected female patients with ISD and minimal urethral hypermobility, collagen can be injected at the bladder neck with a success rate of 63% using a mean 9.1 mL and 1.5 treatments (8). Winters and colleagues found similar results, with 79% dry or socially continent using a mean 1.9 injections and 14.6 mL of collagen (12).

Other types of slings also exist that utilize synthetic mesh for the sling and are minimally invasive procedures. These procedures—including tension-free vaginal tape (TVT), which utilizes a transvaginal approach, and a SPARC procedure that utilizes a suprapubic approach—are relatively new and long-term results have not yet been published. These procedures will be outlined in other chapters in this book.

SURGICAL TECHNIQUE

Patients with atrophic vaginitis should be treated with topical estrogens for 2 weeks before the procedure. It is helpful to teach the patient clean intermittent catheterization before the procedure because incomplete emptying is common for a few days postoperatively. One dose of intravenous antibiotics should be given preoperatively. General or regional anesthesia may be used without particular advantage to either technique.

The procedure is performed in the low lithotomy position using Allen stirrups with feet squarely in the stirrups to avoid pressure on the calf areas. The legs should only be moderately flexed at the hips to allow simultaneous exposure to the vagina and the lower abdomen. A 16 Fr Foley catheter is placed and the balloon inflated with 10 mL to allow palpation of the bladder neck and urethra. A weighted vaginal speculum is placed. The labia may be sewn laterally if the view is obstructed.

Autologous Fascial Slings

The rectus fascia is usually harvested first to minimize vaginal bleeding. In adults, an 8- to 10-cm Pfannenstiel incision is made approximately 2 to 3 cm above the pubis (Fig. 37–1). The subcutaneous tissue is cleared from the rectus fascia and a relatively scar-free area is selected. Even the most scarred and thickened rectus fascia is usually suitable as a sling. Incising parallel to the fibers, obtain a fascial sling approximately 8 to 10 cm in length with a center portion 1.5 to 2.0 cm wide, tapering the ends to 1 cm wide (Fig. 37–1 inset). Free the upper and lower fascial leaf from the recti muscles superiorly and inferiorly for approximately 1 to 2 cm to allow a tension-free fascial closure. The sling sutures may be placed before or after transection. We place the sutures off the field. The size and type of suture used is a matter of personal preference but we currently use 1-0 polyglactin absorbable sutures, which decrease postoperative suture pain (as compared to nonabsorbable sutures) and does not compromise durability. The distal 1 cm of the sling ends are folded over and the sutures are placed perpendicular to the direction of the fibers approximately 0.5 cm from the ends incorporating all of the fibers in the bites.

The vaginal procedure begins by placing an Allis clamp midway between the bladder neck and the urethral meatus with traction placed superiorly. It is very important to maintain this traction throughout the vaginal procedure. Injectable saline is infiltrated beneath the vaginal epithelium over the proximal urethra to facilitate the dissection. A 3-cm midline incision or inverted "U" incision is made over the proximal urethra and the initial vaginal dissection is performed with a scalpel or Church scissors, which allows one to quickly find the proper plane superficial to the white periurethral fascia. Damage to the underlying urethra and bladder is minimized when dis-

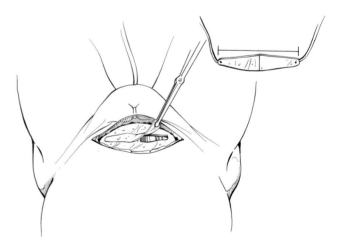

FIG. 37–1. Harvesting of the rectus abdominis fascial sling. The sling should be at least 8 to 10 cm long and 1.5 to 2.0 cm wide in the center. The sling ends are folded and then sutured with 1-0 absorbable sutures incorporating all of the fibers.

section proceeds in this plane. The dissection is facilitated by maintaining outward traction (toward the operator) on the developing vaginal flap and maintaining the tips of the scissors on the vaginal flap at all times. Carry the dissection laterally to the endopelvic fascia and repeat this procedure on the other side. Perforation of the endopelvic fascia is performed last to minimize blood loss. Enter the retropubic space inferior to the ischium, at the level of the bladder neck, by perforating the endopelvic fascia using curved Metzenbaum or Mayo scissors with tips pointed laterally and slightly superiorly (Fig. 37–2). The bladder neck can be localized by pulling on the Foley balloon. Blunt finger dissection should not be used to perforate the endopelvic fascia as bladder injury may occur. Once the endopelvic fascia is entered, gently advance the closed scissors laterally and slightly upward for 1 to 2 cm before opening widely. Gentle blunt finger dissection of the retropubic space superiorly to the rectus muscle is performed (Fig. 37–3). Through the abdominal incision, the lateral border of the rectus muscle is retracted medially to expose a defect just lateral to where the rectus muscle inserts onto the symphysis (Fig. 37–4). Gentle dissection in this area allows safe and easy access into the retropubic space. If finger dissection of the retropubic space is difficult, as it sometimes is after prior incontinence procedures, place the tips of Metzenbaum scissors directly on the posterior pubis and slowly advance them with constant pressure against the pubic periosteum. After this is completed, no tissue should be palpable between fingers inserted into the retropubic space from above and the vaginal incision below. If some intervening tissue is found at the level of the pelvic floor,

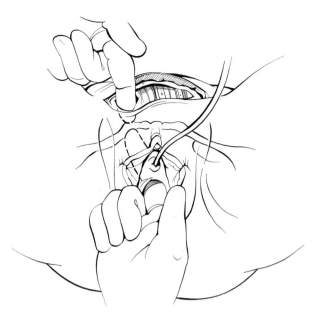

FIG. 37–3. Blunt finger dissection creates a tunnel to the rectus muscles above. Wide dissection is unnecessary and may cause significant bleeding or bladder injury.

penetration of that tissue is safe. If the tissue is higher than the pelvic floor, it is often the bladder attached to the posterior pubis. The bladder can be carefully dissected off the pubis by keeping the scissors on the back of the pubis at all times. A similar procedure is performed on the other

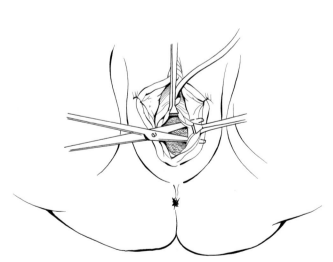

FIG. 37–2. The vaginal dissection is performed superficially to the white periurethral fascia. With the scissors parallel to the plane of the perineum and tips pointing superiorly and laterally, the retropubic space is entered and subsequently enlarged by further advancing the scissors 1 to 2 cm and then opening them.

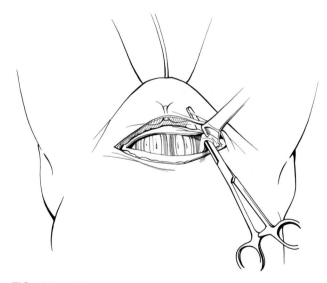

FIG. 37–4. The approach to the retropubic space from above is located below the rectus fascia and lateral to where the rectus muscles attach to the pubic symphysis. Minimal dissection in this area allows safe and easy access to the retropubic space previously dissected by the vaginal operator.

side. Extensive retropubic space dissection is unnecessary and may lead to excessive bleeding or bladder injury. A Sarot or Crawford clamp is placed into the retropubic space from above and directed into the vaginal incision using manual guidance (Fig. 37–5). The tip of the clamp should remain in contact with the pubic periosteum and under the vaginal operator's finger at all times. After clamps have been passed bilaterally, cystoscopy is performed to ensure there has been no damage to the urethra or bladder. Each sling suture is pulled into the abdominal incision placing the sling under the urethra. Proper function and longevity of the sling does not depend on the sutures to hold tension indefinitely (because the sutures are absorbable) and thus it is critical that a good portion of the sling extend into the retropubic space to allow good fixation. One or two 3-0 absorbable sutures are placed through the edge of the sling and superficially through the periurethral fascia to secure it in place (Fig. 37–6). The sling sutures are passed through the rectus fascia, directly above the retropubic "tunnels," using a right-angle clamp before the rectus fascia is closed. It is important not to tether the sutures in the fascial closure. If a suprapubic tube needs to be placed, it is done under direct vision at this time. The vagina is closed with a running, locking 2-0 absorbable suture. The weighted speculum, packing, and all other instruments should be removed from the vagina. The sling sutures are gently pulled up to remove any slack and tied over the rectus (Fig. 37–7). A shodded clamp can be used to hold tension on the untied

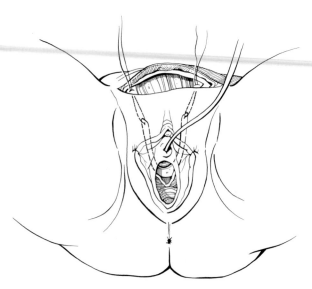

FIG. 37–6. The sling ends are pulled well into the retropubic space to allow good fixation. The sling is seated at the proximal urethra and sutured to the periurethral fascia using 3-0 absorbable sutures.

sutures until the appropriate tension is obtained and the sutures tied down (Fig. 37–8). The appropriate tension is the minimum amount required to stop urethral motion, which is tested by pulling on the urethral catheter. The bladder neck should descend only 0.5 or 1.0 cm when pulled on to ensure that the sling is "tight enough." Also, two fingers should easily slide under the suture knot to ensure that the sling is "loose enough." If in doubt, it is

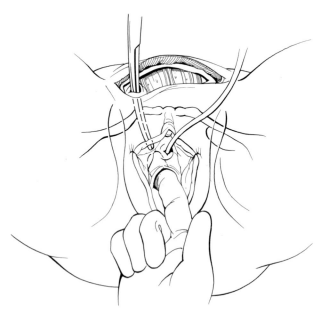

FIG. 37–5. Using manual guidance, a Crawford clamp is passed from above toward the vaginal incision with the tip of the clamp in contact with the pubic periosteum and the vaginal operator's finger. After the passage of clamps bilaterally, cystoscopy is performed to ensure no injury to the bladder has occurred.

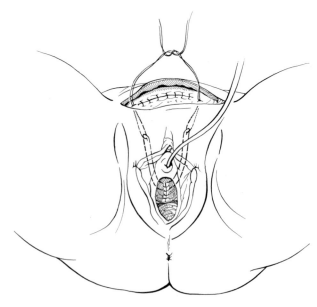

FIG. 37–7. The sling sutures are passed through the rectus fascia before the fascia is closed. The vaginal mucosa is closed, the weighted speculum removed, and the sling sutures tied down over the rectus fascia under minimal tension.

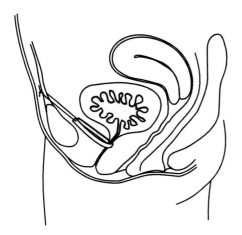

FIG. 37–8. A lateral view of the completed pubovaginal sling procedure.

better to err on the side of too little tension. We do not place a vaginal pack to support the urethra before tying the sutures. We have not found it useful to judge how tight to pull the sling by visual assessment during cystoscopy nor by tightening the sling until leakage cannot be produced by compressing the bladder. In addition, there is no evidence that attaching the sling directly to the pubis using either sutures or bone anchors improves results or reduces morbidity. In the situation where the patient does not void and permanent urinary retention is desired, increased tension can be applied. The skin is closed and a vaginal pack placed. When the abdominal and vaginal components are performed synchronously, the average operating time is 40 minutes with 150-mL average blood loss.

Allograft/Xenograft/Mesh Sling Procedures

These procedures utilize "off-the-shelf" materials as the sling material. Currently, there are numerous choices including human fascia and dermis, porcine dermis, and bovine products. Human cadaveric fascia is the most commonly used and appears to have results similar to autologous fascia (13). If mesh is utilized, Prolene mesh appears to be the most appropriate choice based on non-reactivity and the "openness" of the weave (11). A discussion of the relative merits of the various materials is beyond the scope of this chapter.

The sling procedures using these materials are typically less morbid, requiring a much smaller suprapubic incision. The vaginal incision and preparation of the graft is similar to the previous description. The only major change is the size of the suprapubic incision and the passage of the suture needles. Because there are no fascial incisions, a suitable suture passer such as a Pereyra or Stamey needle is used to perforate the rectus fascia and bring the sling sutures from the vagina into the abdominal incision. We make a 3-cm long abdominal incision approximately 1 cm above the pubis. Tensioning of the

sling is the same as previously described. If bone anchors are placed from below without using an abdominal incision, tensioning of the sling is more difficult; however, if the sling ends are within the retropubic space results similar to the standard pubovaginal sling should be obtained.

On postoperative day 1, the vaginal pack is removed and, if the patient is ambulating well, the Foley catheter is removed. Patients are discharged within 24 hours. Oral antibiotics are not routinely prescribed postoperatively. The patient performs clean intermittent catheterization after each void, or a minimum of every 4 hours if unable to void, until the postvoid residual is less than 60 mL for 24 hours. Patients should refrain from vigorous activities and sexual intercourse for 4 to 6 weeks to allow proper fixation of the sling.

OUTCOMES

Complications

When rectus fascia is used for the urethral sling, the most common complications include detrusor instability and urinary retention. Approximately 15% to 25% of patients will have residual urgency symptoms with less than one-half demonstrating occasional urge incontinence. Less than 10% will develop new onset detrusor instability. In a recent report by Morgan and colleagues, 26% of patients had residual urgency symptoms (74% had resolved their symptoms), 7% developed *de novo* urge incontinence, and 2% required urethrolysis for obstructive symptoms (9). In most cases, urgency symptoms respond well to anticholinergic medications and subside over a period of 3 to 6 months. Persistent postoperative urinary retention, although believed to be a common complication, is not statistically more common after pubovaginal slings than after suspension procedures when equivalent patient groups are compared (2).

Superficial wound infections and pelvic hematomas are uncommon and significant blood loss occurs in approximately 1% to 2%. Of note, wound infections rarely result in sling failure. Persistent postoperative pain is rare when absorbable suture is used. McGuire and O'Connell reported that no patient had to take analgesics chronically and no patient had a procedure to relieve pain (7).

Results

In a recent series involving 257 patients with a mean follow-up of 51 months, 88% of patients were cured of stress incontinence (9). A recent quality of life study reported a 97% objective long-term cure rate in 57 patients who underwent a PVS. In this study, 88% felt the procedure had improved their quality of life, 84% believed the procedure had cured their incontinence, and 82% would have the procedure again (10). Other long-term series have documented a greater than 80% cure and over 90% significantly improved rate. In addition, mild residual stress incontinence usually responds well to injectable agents such as collagen because the sling provides a strong backing for the periurethral fascia.

The pubovaginal fascial sling is the procedure of choice for treatment of females with urinary incontinence due to ISD. Even though many patients are prior surgical failures, excellent results can be obtained with minimal morbidity but is dependent upon an accurate preoperative evaluation and careful placement of the sling at the proximal urethra without undue tension. Newer procedures utilizing synthetic and allograft sling materials may one day replace the traditional autologous pubovaginal; however, these newer procedures will require more experience with their use and long-term results.

REFERENCES

1. Chaikin DC, Groutz A, Blaivas JG. Predicting the need for anti-incontinence surgery in continent women undergoing repair of severe urogenital prolapse. *J Urol* 2000; 163:531–534.
2. Demirci F, Yucel O. Comparison of pubovaginal sling and Burch colposuspension procedures in type I/II genuine stress incontinence. *Arch Gynecol Obstet* 2001;265:190–194.
3. Gallentine MJ, Cespedes RD. Occult stress urinary incontinence and the effect of vaginal vault prolapse on abdominal leak point pressures. *Urology* 2001;57:40–44.
4. McGuire EJ. Urodynamic findings in patients after failure of stress incontinence operations. In: Zinner NR, Sterling AM, eds. *Female incontinence*. New York: Alan R. Liss, 1981:351–360.
5. McGuire EJ, Fitzpatrick CC, Wan J, et al. Clinical assessment of urethral sphincter function. *J Urol* 1993;150:1452–1455.
6. McGuire EJ, Lytton B. The pubovaginal sling for stress urinary incontinence. *J Urol* 1978;119:82–85.
7. McGuire EJ, O'Connell HE. Surgical treatment of intrinsic urethral dysfunction: Slings. *Urol Clin North Am* 1995;22:657–664.
8. O'Connell HE, McGuire EJ, Aboseif S. Transurethral collagen injection therapy in women. *J Urol* 1995;154:1463–1465.
9. Morgan TO, Westney OL, McGuire EJ. Pubovaginal sling: 4-year outcome analysis and quality of life assessment. *J Urol* 2000;163:1845–1848.
10. Richter HE, Varner RE, Sanders E, et al. Effects of pubovaginal sling procedure on patients with urethral hypermobility and intrinsic sphincteric deficiency: would they do it again? *Am J Obstet Gynecol* 2001; 184:14–19.
11. Rodriguez LV, Raz S. Polypropylene sling for the treatment of stress urinary incontinence. *Urology* 2001;58:783–785.
12. Winters JC, Chiverton A, Scarpero HM, Prats LJ. Collagen injection therapy in elderly women: long-term results and patient satisfaction. *Urology* 2000;55:856–861.
13. Wright EJ. Current status of fascia lata allograft slings treating urinary incontinence: effective or ephemeral? *Tech Urol* 2001;7:81–86.

CHAPTER 38

Injectable Therapies for Incontinence in Women and Men

Richard T. Kershen, Randy A. Fralick, and Rodney A. Appell

Since their introduction, injectables have been an attractive form of urinary incontinence therapy for patients and physicians alike. Effective, minimally invasive, cost effective, and adeptly administered under local anesthesia, these agents offer significant tangible advantages over alternative invasive surgical therapies. As newer and more durable agents are developed and approved for use by the US Food and Drug Administration (FDA), injectables could well emerge as the treatment of choice for stress urinary incontinence (SUI) in the future. At present two injectables are currently approved for human use in the United States: bovine gluteraldehyde-cross-linked (GAX) collagen (Contigen; Bard, Inc.) and pyrolytic carbon-coated zirconium beads (Durasphere; Carbon Medical Technologies, Inc.). As with any therapy, optimal patient selection guided by proper evaluation to determine suitability for intraurethral injections is essential to predict treatment success. The cause(s) of incontinence must be identified to recommend appropriate therapy. Intraurethral injections benefit patients with incontinence occurring at the level of the bladder outlet. Incontinence occurring at this level may be caused by anatomic displacement of a normally functioning urethra (anatomic genuine SUI) in women or intrinsic incompetence of the urethral closure mechanism [intrinsic sphincteric dysfunction (ISD)] in women or men. Patients with ISD commonly have had a previous surgical procedure on or near the urethra, a sympathetic neurological injury, or myelodysplasia. Female patients with genuine SUI have adequate urethral function but hypermobility of the bladder neck and proximal urethra resulting from a deficiency in pelvic support. These patients benefit from bladder neck elevation and stabilization. Patients with ISD have poor urethral function and require procedures to increase outflow resistance. Patients with a fixed, well-supported urethra in association with ISD are excellent candidates for periurethral injection. In men this is most commonly encountered following radical prostatectomy, whereas in women the primary cause of ISD is a residual effect of multiple surgical resuspension procedures for genuine SUI (1).

DIAGNOSIS

A directed urogynecologic and neurological history as well as physical examination is performed on every patient who presents with complaints of SUI. All patients are asked to empty their bladders completely prior to examination. We then begin with urethral catheterization for assessment of postvoid residual volume. A lubricated cotton swab may be carefully inserted into the urethral meatus and advanced into the bladder. After pulling the swab back to the bladder neck the resting urethral angle is then determined. The patient is then asked to perform a Valsalva maneuver; a Q-tip deflection angle greater than 30 degrees from the horizontal plane is suggestive of significant urethral hypermobility. A pelvic examination utilizing a half-blade of a vaginal speculum is then performed to assess for the presence of pelvic prolapse. A digital rectal exam is performed for elicitation of the bulbocavernosus reflex to assess pelvic floor innervation. Vaginal and perineal sensation is then assessed to rule out occult sensory neuropathy.

We favor a complete fluorourodynamic evaluation of all of our incontinent patients to determine the precise urodynamic diagnosis, directing appropriate choice of therapy. Patients with ISD fluorourodynamically display an open bladder outlet at rest in the absence of a detrusor contraction. However, standardization of a methodology to determine ISD has not yet been accepted. We determine the Valsalva or abdominal leak point pressure (LPP_{abd}) by direct measurement of the abdominal pressure required to overcome urethral resistance and pro-

319

duce leakage. This determination may be considered an indirect method of measuring the closure forces of the urethra during straining maneuvers. It is used primarily in women with SUI to differentiate between anatomic displacement of a normal-functioning urethra (SUI caused by hypermobility) from poor outlet function (ISD). Patients with ISD demonstrate minimal urethral resistance to straining and therefore the urethral opening pressure is very low, whereas patients with an anatomic displacement of a normally functioning urethra have high urethral opening pressures and therefore the LPP_{abd} will be higher. As a general rule in regard to leak point pressures, until a universally accepted technique is established a single mode with which the physician is comfortable should be used in the same manner on every patient whether for a preoperative evaluation or for the evaluation of a patient with an unsatisfactory result.

An alternative method to evaluate outlet function is the determination of maximum urethral closure pressure (UCP_{max}) obtained during urethral pressure profilometry. Women with $UCP_{max} = 20$ cm H_2O have a "low-pressure urethra" or ISD, and these patients failed standard bladder neck suspension procedures that fail to provide suburethral or intrinsic urethral support (16).

INDICATIONS FOR SURGERY

It is clear that the ideal patient for injectable therapy will have pure ISD with a nonmobile urethra. In the past, injectable therapy has been performed on patients with a poorly functioning urethra (ISD) and good anatomic support. More recent data, however, suggest that injectables may be used for selected female patients with anatomic SUI. In all patients, male or female, a suitable recipient site for injection is an absolute prerequisite for this form of therapy, as dense urethral scarring will preclude entrance into the correct plane and inhibit bleb formation. Also, the presence of detrusor instability and poor bladder compliance should be detected prior to injection therapy as these conditions will severely limit treatment success.

ALTERNATIVE THERAPY

In recent years, the surgical armamentarium available for the treatment of urinary incontinence related to the incompetent urethra has rapidly expanded. Pubovaginal slings made of autologous, synthetic, or cadaveric materials have become the gold standard to which all other therapies are compared. Minimally invasive approaches to slings have been developed including the use of bone anchors, transvaginal tape (TVT), and the SPARC system. Bulbourethral slings have been employed for males with neurogenic and postprostatectomy incontinence. In addition, the implantable artificial urinary sphincter remains a viable therapy for both men and women with urethral incompetence.

SURGICAL TECHNIQUE

Although the techniques involved with injectable therapy are not difficult, meticulous and precise placement of the material is essential to ensure an optimal result. The equipment required for injection depends on the bulk-enhancing agent injected. The injection can be performed either suburothelially through a needle placed directly through the mucosa via a cystoscopic needle (transurethral injection; antegrade injection) or periurethrally with a needle inserted percutaneously and positioned in the urethral tissues in the suburothelial space, with the manipulation observed by cystourethroscopy (1). Men are injected predominantly by the transurethral or antegrade approach and women are injected by either the transurethral or periurethral approach. The periurethral approach, although considered more technically challenging, is advantageous through minimization of intraurethral bleeding and extravasation of the injectable substance. There is certainly a learning curve with any technique chosen, which ultimately results in using less injectable material to attain the desired result of continence. We perform all injections in females under local anesthesia only, while males are injected under local anesthesia with or without monitored sedation. Patients receiving GAX collagen must undergo a skin test 1 month prior to their first injection to exclude allergy to the material. Injection techniques using both bovine GAX collagen and Durasphere are presented.

Injection in the Female Patient

Women may be injected by way of a transcystoscopic (transurethral) technique or by a periurethral approach (1). We prefer the transurethral approach for GAX collagen injection, while we use the periurethral approach for Durasphere. Both agents, however, may be injected by either technique. In general, we give the patient a single oral dose of a fluoroquinolone antibiotic 1 hour prior to the procedure; the antibiotic is continued for 3 days postprocedure.

The patient is placed in the lithotomy position and prepped and draped in the usual fashion. The introitus and vestibule are anesthetized with 20% topical benzocaine ointment and the urethra is anesthetized with 10 mL of 2% lidocaine jelly. Following this, a painless injection of 1% plain lidocaine is performed periurethrally at the 3- and 9-o'clock positions using 2 to 4 mL on each side. Complete urethral sensory blockade is achieved.

Periurethral Approach

Bovine GAX Collagen

Panendoscopy is performed with a 0- or 30-degree lens, and a 20- or 22-gauge spinal needle is positioned periurethrally at the 4- or 8-o'clock position with the bevel of the needle directed toward the lumen (Fig. 38–1).

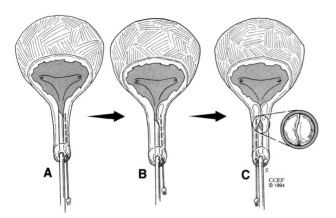

FIG. 38–1. Transurethral injection in a male patient.

The needle is then advanced through the urethral musculature into the lamina propria in an entirely suburothelial plane. Once the needle is positioned in the lamina propria, it usually advances with little force. The needle may also be introduced between the urethral fascia and vaginal epithelium at the 6-o'clock position and, again, needle placement is fully observed endoscopically. Bulging of the tip of the needle against the mucosa of the urethra is observed during advancement of the needle to ensure its proper placement. When the needle tip is properly positioned 0.5 cm below the bladder neck, the material is injected until swelling is visible on each side, creating the appearance of occlusion of the urethral lumen. Once the urethra is approximately 50% occluded, the needle is removed and reinserted on the opposite side and additional material is injected until the urethral mucosa coapts in the midline, creating the endoscopic appearance of two lateral prostatic lobes.

A useful "trick" described by Neal et al. is to add methylene blue to the injectable lidocaine to aid in the location of the needle tip before injecting the bulking agent (14). Once the needle is located at the bladder neck position, the syringe of anesthetic/methylene blue is removed and the syringe containing the bulking agent is engaged. When the desired appearance of the coapted mucosa is attained, have the patient stand and cough to see if there is any leakage; if there is, reposition the patient and reinject.

Durasphere

Durasphere was approved by the FDA in 1999 for the treatment of SUI. A radiopaque, synthetic, nonantigenic, nonbiodegradable material with large particle size, it has been promoted as possessing the potential for a more durable treatment result than bovine collagen. Due to its larger particle size, it requires injection through a larger needle delivery device than collagen (18 gauge vs. 23 gauge). Practical experience has shown that there is some difficulty injecting the material due to resistance to flow

of the irregularly shaped beads through the delivery needle. Because of this, we prefer the periurethral approach, which allows the use of a shorter needle. In addition to facilitating the injection, this method prevents extrusion of the material through what would be a large-bore puncture site in the mucosa created by the transurethral needle.

Practical experience has shown that if resistance to injection is encountered the best approach is to avoid increasing injection pressure, which will result in needle obstruction. Rather, the needle should be gently repositioned into the proper suburothelial plane. Lightner et al., in their initial study evaluating the safety and effectiveness of Durasphere, recommended slightly withdrawing the needle during injection to ease delivery, avoiding bead compression and carrier gel extrusion (12).

Recently, the manufacturer has made available a specially designed angled needle that aids in proper placement into the suburothelial plane during the periurethral approach. This has been termed the "bent needle" technique (Fig. 38–2). In this technique, the bent needle is advanced periurethrally with the bevel toward the urethral lumen until the tip of the needle is cystoscopically identified in the suburothelial plane at the bladder neck. Gentle hydrodissection with normal saline is then performed through the needle under cystoscopic guidance, raising a mucosal bleb, mimicking the desired shape of the implant. The Durasphere implant is then injected with minimal resistance into the potential suburothelial space created by the hydrodissection. The Durasphere implant displaces the normal saline that is dispelled around the needle tip. This technique facilitates precise implant placement, minimizing extrusion of the material and ultimately the amount of implant required for urethral coaptation.

Transurethral Approach

The transurethral approach is nearly identical for GAX collagen or Durasphere, notwithstanding the aforementioned modifications in injection technique required for injection of the more viscous Durasphere implant. A standard 21 Fr to 24 Fr cystoscope or hysteroscope that can accommodate a 5 Fr working element with a 0-, 12-, or 30-degree lens is used to perform cystourethroscopy. The region of injection just distal to the bladder neck is identified and a needle delivery system with or without external sheath is advanced through the working channel. The needle with bevel facing toward the lumen then punctures the mucosa and is advanced proximally into the submucosal space, typically at the 4- or 8-o'clock position. The bulking material is slowly injected until a mucosal bleb of sufficient size is achieved. The process is repeated on the opposite side and at any other site necessary to achieve total mucosal apposition (Fig. 38–3). Care must be taken to avoid puncturing the mucosa at previously injected

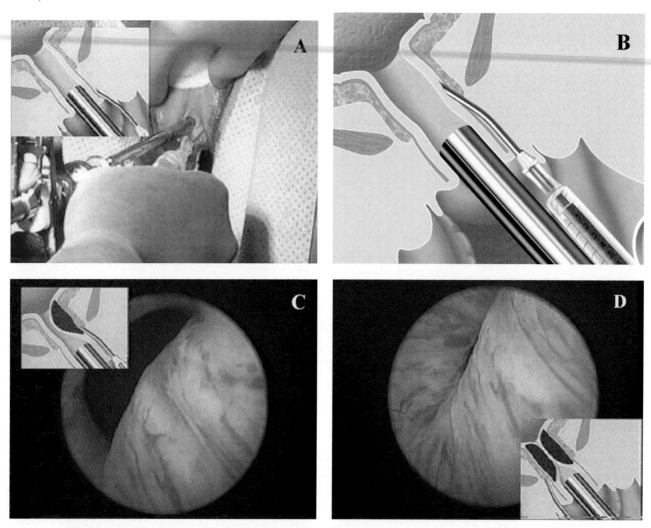

FIG. 38–2. Bent needle periurethral injection technique of Durasphere in a female patient. **A:** Bent needle is advanced into the suburothelial plane toward the bladder neck. **B:** Hydrodissection with normal saline is gently performed, creating a submucosal space. **C:** The Durasphere implant is injected with minimal resistance into the created space. **D:** Appearance after completion of bilateral injections.

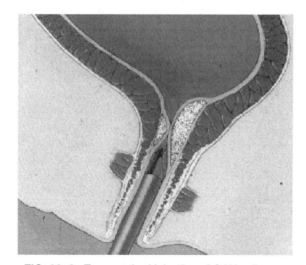

FIG. 38–3. Transurethral injection of GAX collagen.

sites as this may result in extrusion of the bulking material. When using Durasphere, the injection needle should be removed slowly to avoid extrusion of the material through the large-bore injection site.

Injection in the Male Patient

Transurethral Approach

The patient is positioned in the semilithotomy position and prepped and draped in the usual fashion. Ten milliliters of 2% lidocaine jelly is inserted intraurethrally and left in place for 10 minutes before instrumentation. Cystourethroscopy with a 0-degree lens is employed. The injectable material is then delivered suburothelially by way of a transcystoscopic injection needle under direct vision. The needle is advanced under the mucosa with the

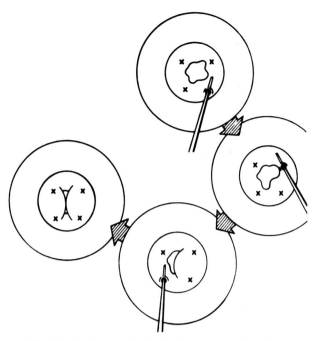

FIG. 38–4. Transurethral injection in a male patient.

beveled portion of the needle facing the lumen of the urethra. This is performed in a circumferential matter, employing four quadrant needle placements (Fig. 38–4). The material is injected until a mucosal bleb is created in each quadrant. Gradually, after the circumferential injections, the urethral mucosa meets in the midline, although additional needle placements may be required for completion.

In cases of ISD following a radical prostatectomy, a short segment of urethra remains above the external sphincter. If visualization of this segment of the urethra is difficult, the needle may be placed at the level of the external sphincter and advanced to ensure deposition of the material proximal to the external sphincter. To be effective, any injectable material must be injected in the urethra superior to the external sphincter, even if this means injecting into the actual bladder neck on the proximal side of the anastomosis. It is important to note that the material should not be injected directly into the external sphincter, as this can cause pudendal nerve irritation with resultant sphincter spasm and discomfort. The depth of injection is also critical. The materials must deform the urethral mucosa so that it closes the urethral lumen. Too deep an injection site is a waste of the material and is not effective.

Antegrade Approach

Injection is more difficult in patients with postradical prostatectomy incontinence resulting from the short segment of urethra above the level of the external sphincter and extensive scarring, which usually occurs in this area following surgery. This problem can be circumvented by using an antegrade approach. The technique is performed by passing a cystoscope with a 5 Fr working port through a small suprapubic cystotomy tract. The vesical neck and proximal urethra are then visualized, and subepithelial injections are performed until the bladder outlet is coapted (Fig. 38–5). Frequently, there is less scar tissue in this location, which results in better tissue coaptation. In early clinical trials, this technique seems to facilitate more precise injection of material, generating improved results with the use of less material (5). In the authors' opinion this technique should be considered in any post-prostatectomy man not achieving adequate success by

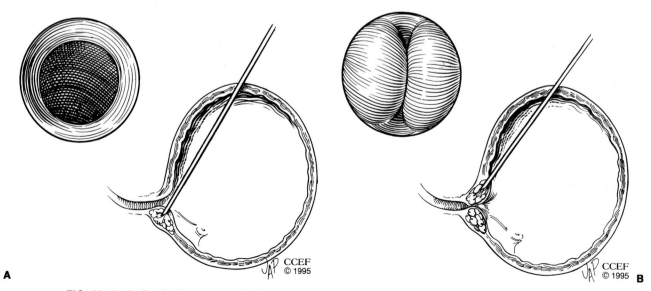

FIG. 38–5. A: Beginning antegrade injection in a male patient. **B:** Completion of antegrade injection.

way of the standard transurethral approach. Postradical prostatectomy urothelium covers scar, and there is migration of any injectable substance distally along the urethra. Once this stops, there is a "wall" to abut the freshly injected material at the bladder neck. Therefore, this additional technique is not recommended as the primary method for an initial injection.

A small subset of patients continues to have some degree of incontinence after the placement of a bulbous urethral artificial urinary sphincter. To date the only options to address this problem have been to place a more distal second (tandem) cuff around the bulbous urethra or place a higher-pressure regulating balloon. Injectable agents have in general been avoided in this setting because of fear of damaging the sphincter cuff. The antegrade approach can be used for this situation without fear of damaging the cuff, although it remains important to know the location of the pressure-regulating balloon before performing the punch cystotomy.

In cases of ISD following transurethral prostatic resection, a short segment of urethra remains below the verumontanum and yet is still proximal to the external sphincter. The injections should be made in this position circumferentially until urethral coaptation is visible. Extrusion of material into the urethral lumen from the needle holes may occur but can be minimized by not traversing the injected area with the distal end of the cystoscope once the material has been injected. In other words, do not enter the bladder.

OUTCOMES

Complications

Complications associated with the use of injectables for the treatment of SUI are uncommon. Most patients are able to void without difficulty following the procedure; however, if retention does develop clean intermittent catheterization is begun with a 10 Fr to 14 Fr soft catheter. An indwelling urethral catheter is to be avoided in patients, as this promotes molding of the material around the catheter. Although it is usually unnecessary, if longer-term catheterization is needed suprapubic cystotomy may be performed in these patients. Patients are contacted 2 weeks postprocedure to determine their continence status. Repeat injections are scheduled as necessary and at a time interval appropriate for the injectable substance.

In the multicenter clinical trial using Contigen injections, transient retention developed in approximately 15% of patients, but only 1% of patients experienced irritative voiding symptoms, and 5% developed a urinary tract infection (6). Other authors have reported *de novo* urgency and urinary retention rates at 13% and 2%, respectively (19). In all cases, urinary retention is short lived as a rule, resolving spontaneously.

Hypersensitivity responses with Contigen are not a problem as the possibility is assessed by skin testing (wheal and flare) with the more immunogenic and sensitizing non–cross-linked collagen prior to treatment. Those with a positive skin test are excluded from treatment. Although local complications with Contigen such as sterile abscess formation have been observed in a few patients, there have been no reports of complications related to distant migration or embolization of the material (20).

In their initial study evaluating Durasphere, Lightner et al found nearly a 1.5-fold increased incidence of acute urinary retention in the group of patients who received Durasphere relative to collagen (12). As with collagen, however, all cases resolved spontaneously by 1 week postimplant. There was no evidence of adverse immunologic response or particle migration in any of the patients who received Durasphere.

It should be noted that a group from Germany recently reported what they considered to be radiological evidence of particle migration of the Durasphere implant into regional and distant lymph nodes in two patients (15). These were incidentally discovered on pelvic radiographs and neither of the patients had any clinically evident adverse sequelae. This would be a highly unusual situation given the large particulate size of Durasphere. As the suspected migratory particles were visualized by plain radiograph only, and were not confirmed histologically, it remains unproven whether these were indeed Durasphere implants. There were no preoperative radiographs presented in this report to confirm that the visualized abnormality was not present prior to implantation. Until other reports surface to confirm this migratory phenomenon we cannot draw any definitive conclusions from this isolated report.

Regardless of the material, the use of periurethral injections has proven to be safe, eliciting only minor complications. All complications resolve rapidly, and a serious long-term complications from the use of periurethral GAX collagen or Durasphere injections have yet to be reported.

Results

There are no controlled, long-term reports available on any injectable. In fact, it is difficult to glean information from any group reported as to etiology of the incontinence. For example, in women results of injectables are reported without differentiating among patients with hypermobility, those with ISD, and those with both; and, men with prostatic resection for benign disease are not separated from those having had a radical prostatectomy. Thus, results have been a combination of anecdotal reporting mixed with conjecture, speculation, and the hope that the truth is involved. Having stated this, it appears that injectables are helpful for some incontinent patients, especially selected women. There are three major disadvantages to the use of injectables: (a) the inability to determine the quantity of material needed for an individual patient; (b) the safety of nonautologous products for injection with respect to migration, foreign body reaction, and immunologic effects; and (c) the transient therapeutic responsiveness and need for repeated injections over time. At this point in time only Contigen and Durasphere have been approved for use as injectable agents for incontinence in the United States, and results presented are confined to these approved substances.

Results in Females

There have been more studies evaluating the efficacy of collagen for the treatment of female SUI than any other injectable agent. Studies having a minimum of 1 year mean follow-up report cured or improved rates from 26% to 95%. Results of the North American Contigen Study Group of 127 women demonstrated 46% dry and 34% socially continent (patients requiring a single mini-pad per day) with 77% remaining dry once continence had been attained (4). This was confirmed in a study with longer (50 month) follow-up where the efficacy was 30% cured and 40% improved (7). In this group 33% of patients required more than one injection session to achieve treatment success. The average volume of collagen injected to achieve cure in their cohort was 8.8 cc. As with most injectables to date, a loss of treatment efficacy over time and need for reinjection has been observed with collagen. Studies have shown that 12% to 40% of patients who achieve initial success will need reinjection within 2 years.

Success rates in women with type III SUI (ISD) have been reported as high as 95% (2). During the multicenter investigation of collagen in the treatment of ISD, the patients selected with anatomic (type II vesicourethral hypermobility) incontinence did not fare well (13). Only 60% to 65% of women with type II SUI were cured or improved after variable follow-up and these results have been corroborated (7). The degree of hypermobility may have a bearing on the degree of efficacy as Faerber demonstrated that 83% of elderly women with type I SUI could be cured by collagen injection alone (9). Several investigators have found that results in patients with ISD and concomitant hypermobility may be achieved that are similar to patients with ISD alone (10,17,18). It may be correct to think of the performance of normal urethral function (continence) as a dynamic continuum of anatomic support of the proximal urethra working in concert with an intact, mucosally coapting intrinsic urethral sphincter. In the case of hypermobility, incontinence may be cured by enhancement of mucosal coaptation in a previously noncompensating urethra (10).

In summary, patients with no anatomic hypermobility and ISD appear to be the most satisfactory candidates for intraurethral collagen injections. In selected elderly and less mobile female patients with anatomic incontinence, recent data suggest that collagen may also be useful in this patient population (9).

Lightner et al. performed the first study evaluating the safety and effectiveness of Durasphere compared to bovine collagen for the treatment of ISD (12). A total of 355 women with ISD were randomized to receive either Durasphere or bovine collagen. At 12 months follow-up from baseline, patients who received Durasphere were shown to have a similar mean reduction in pad weight as patients who received bovine collagen (27.9 g and 26.4 g, respectively) and similar improvement in Stamey continence grades (66.1% vs. 65.8% of the patients who received bovine collagen). When evaluated at 1 year following the date of the last injection, 80.3% of women who were treated with Durasphere were improved relative to 69.1% of the women who received collagen. The mean number of injections were similar for both groups (Durasphere, 1.69; bovine collagen 1.55), but the total volume of material injected was lower in the Durasphere group (7.55 mL vs. 9.58 mL).

A recent report of long-term follow-up (average, 24.2 months) in 50 of these patients who received Durasphere found that, subjectively, 86% had experienced leakage since their injections were performed (8). Durasphere had a transient effect lasting an average of 7.7 months in 38% of patients. Only 24% of patients felt that Durasphere had a durable effect and was still working at an average time since last injection of 21.9 months (range, 12.1 to 52.8 months). This follow-up study reveals that, despite initial enthusiasm for Durasphere as a more durable bulking agent, its long-term results are no better than GAX collagen, with the majority of patients experiencing recurrent or persistent leakage within 8 months after treatment, even after initial apparent success.

Results in Males

Results of the North American Contigen Study Group of 134 postprostatectomy patients (17 postresection; 117 postradical prostatectomy) and 17 postradiation incontinent men demonstrated that only 22 men (16.5%) regained continence following injections of collagen but 78.7% were dry or significantly improved at 1 year of follow-up and 67% at 2 years following injections (3,13). Use of the antegrade injection technique in men failing the standard retrograde, cystoscopic approach increased the "cured" rate at 1 year by another 37.5% (5). Klutke et al. reported long-term follow-up in men with postradical prostatectomy incontinence who underwent a single antegrade collagen injection and found a 45% cured or improved rate with mean follow-up of 28 months (11). To date, there have been no studies of Durasphere for the treatment of male postprostatectomy urinary incontinence.

Clinical experience with both GAX collagen and Durasphere has demonstrated that the endoscopic correction of female SUI is both possible and effective. It is clear, however, that durability remains a primary concern when implementing this approach to treatment. Injectables are still in the developmental stages and their roles in the management of incontinence still need to be defined more precisely. Results with currently available injectable agents throughout the world are presented (Table 38–1). Careful review and critical analysis of new bulking agents will soon reveal which materials approach the therapeutic ideal. Because the methods are less invasive and in general performed on an outpatient basis, medical costs should be reduced and there should also be a more rapid return to the patient's normal activities. The ideal material is still sought and should combine ease of administration with minimal tissue reaction, lack of migration, and persistence over time. The physician considering injectables for his or her patient should consider that there is a learning curve in patient selection as well as method of delivery of the bulking agents to attain optimal results.

REFERENCES

1. Appell RA. Collagen injection therapy for urinary incontinence. *Urol Clin North Am* 1994;21:177.
2. Appell RA. Injectables for urethral incompetence. *World J Urol* 1990; 8:208–211.
3. Appell RA, McGuire EJ, DeRidder PA, et al. Summary of effectiveness and safety in the prospective, open, multicenter investigation of Contigen implant for incontinence due to intrinsic sphincteric deficiency in males. *J Urol* 1994;151:271A.
4. Appell RA, McGuire EJ, DeRidder PA, et al. Summary of effectiveness and safety in the prospective, open, multicenter investigation of Contigen implant for incontinence due to intrinsic sphincteric deficiency in females. *J Urol* 1994;151:418A.
5. Appell RA, Vasavada SP, Rackley RR, et al. Percutaneous antegrade collagen injection therapy for urinary incontinence following radical prostatectomy. *Urology* 1996;48:769.
6. Bard CR. PMAA submission to US Food and Drug Administration for IDE G850010. 1990.
7. Corcos J, Fournier C. Periurethral collagen injection for the treatment of female stress urinary incontinence: 4-year follow-up results. *Urology* 1999;54:815–818.
8. Chrouser KL, Lightner DJ, Fick F, et al. Durasphere injection for intrinsic sphincter deficiency: Long-term assessment of patient continence and satisfaction. *J Urol* 2002;167[Suppl 4]:420A.
9. Faerber G. Endoscopic collagen injection therapy in elderly women with type I stress urinary incontinence. *J Urol* 1996;155:512–514.
10. Herschorn S, Radomski SB. Collagen injections for genuine stress urinary incontinence: patient selection and durability. *Int Urogynecol J Pelvic Floor Dysfunct* 1997;8:18–24.
11. Klutke, JJ, Subir C, Andriole G, et al. Long term results after antegrade collagen injection for stress urinary incontinence following radical retropubic prostatectomy. *Urology* 1999;53:974–977.
12. Lightner D, Calvosa C, Andersen R, et al. A new injectable bulking agent for treatment of stress urinary incontinence: results of a multicenter, randomized, controlled, double-blind study of Durasphere. *Urology* 2001;58:12–15.
13. McGuire EJ, Appell RA. Transurethral collagen injection for urinary incontinence. *Urology* 1994;43:413–415.
14. Neal D Jr, Lahaye K, Lowe D. Improved needle placement technique in periurethral collagen injection. *Urology* 1995;45:865–866.
15. Pannek J, Brands FH, Senge T. Particle migration after transurethral injection of carbon coated beads for stress urinary incontinence. *J Urol* 2001;350–1353.
16. Sand PK, Bowen LW, Panganiban R, et al. The low-pressure urethra as a factor in failed retropubic urethropexy. *Obstet Gynecol* 1987;69:399.
17. Swami S, Batista JE, Abrams P. Collagen for female genuine stress incontinence after a minimum 2-year follow-up. *Br J Urol* 1997;80: 757–761.
18. Steele AC, Kohli N, Karram MM. Periurethral collagen injection for stress incontinence with and without urethral hypermobility. *Obstet Gynecol* 2000;95:327–331.
19. Stothers L, Goldenberg SL, Leone EF. Complications of periurethral collagen injection for stress urinary incontinence. *J Urol* 1998;159: 806–807.
20. Sweat SD, Lightner DJ. Complications of sterile abscess formation and pulmonary embolism following periurethral bulking agents. *J Urol* 1999;161:93–96.

CHAPTER 39

Synthetic Sling

Darshan K. Shah, Omid Rofeim, and Gopal Badlani

The pubovaginal sling has become the treatment of choice for urethral incontinence in the past decade. According the "integral theory" of female stress urinary incontinence (SUI) (10), laxity in the pubourethral ligaments, which normally act as a fulcrum, leads to funneling of the bladder neck at the time of increased intraabdominal pressure. The aim of the pubovaginal sling is to reinforce the "functional" pubourethral ligaments and fixation of the midurethra to pubic bone and provide continence by kinking the urethra during active movement of the urethra with Valsalva maneuver or stress.

Autologous tissue has been the traditional material since Von Giordano first introduced the sling concept using gracilis muscle, yet autologous and homologous materials have certain drawbacks (Table 39–1). The basis for choosing synthetic material is twofold. First, it provides a nondegradable, readily available, consistent, and disease-free material for a minimally invasive approach. As it is nonabsorbable, the tensile strength of the sling does not decrease with time and may even increase with tissue ingrowth through the interstices of the graft (7).

Second, there may be a biochemical basis for SUI in that women with SUI have higher plasma proteolytic activity than their age and parity match controls. This suggests that the host tissue, used primarily or as ingrowth on a platform of absorbable material, has a higher chance of early proteolytic degradation and subsequent failure (4). These advantages have to be balanced with the reported incidence of infection and erosion with synthetic materials. Based on our experience we believe that patient selection, preoperative preparation, surgical technique, choice of sling material, and finally surgeon's experience in vaginal surgery can play a significant role in the outcome.

A number of synthetic materials are available (Table 39–2) (6). The experience with different types of synthetic sling materials is mainly from hernia repairs. While information regarding tissue reaction is pertinent, extrapolation of data from other surgical disciplines to vaginal use is misleading. The absolute requirement for tensile strength, load, and displacement are unknown for vaginal use with these materials. To our knowledge, none of the materials have failed in this regard. Thus, the choice depends on pore size, tissue reaction, bacterial adherence, and cost.

We have tested polypropylene, ProteGen, and Gore-Tex along with cadaveric fascia *in vivo* and *in vitro* for cell growth, tissue reaction, and effect on load and displacement. We have further tested various materials for

TABLE 39.1. *Pitfalls using organic material*

Autologous fascia	Introduces another incision and increases the operative time and morbidity.
	Quality of harvested tissue is also variable, depending on the patient's age and associated medical or previous surgical conditions.
	Sometimes difficult to obtain adequate tissue length.
Allogenic and homologous grafts	Theoretical risk of disease transmission and graft rejection.
	Strength of the fascia is variable depending on the source.
	Fascia is primarily collagen types I and III, therefore it can be resorbed. The strength of the reconstruction will then depend entirely upon the scar tissue left from the operation.

TABLE 39.2. *Synthetic sling materials used for suburethral sling procedures*

Material	Composition
Mersilene	Polyethylene terephthalate
Marlex, prolene	Polypropylene
Silastic	Silicone rubber reinforced with polyethylene terephthalate
Teflon	PTFE*
Gore-tex	Expanded PTFE

*Polytetrafluoroethylene

bacterial adherence *in vitro*. Based on the above, polypropylene—with its large pore size, low bacterial adherence, easy availability, and relative low cost—is our material of choice (8).

DIAGNOSIS

Evaluation of patients who are potential candidates for pubovaginal slings should include a complete physical examination and urodynamics. Patients with intrinsic sphincteric deficiency (ISD), hypermobility, and leak point pressure (LPP) less than 60 cm H_2O are candidates for a standard pubovaginal sling with synthetic material. Patients with hypermobility, LPP greater than 60 cm H_2O (mild to moderate ISD), and no significant prolapse are candidates for midurethral synthetic slings (11).

INDICATIONS FOR SURGERY

Pubovaginal slings are indicated in patients with SUI secondary to hypermobility, ISD, or combination of the two are candidates for a pubovaginal sling. The choice of technique depends on (a) associated degree of bladder prolapse, (b) concomitant uterine or vaginal vault prolapse, (c) degree of previous vaginal scarring, and (d) associated metabolic condition that may prevent healing (immune suppression, chronic steroid use).

Prior anterior vaginal wall surgery is not an absolute contraindication but requires a higher degree of skills and prior experience with vaginal surgery. The shape, size, and fixation techniques are chosen based on the degree of any associated cystocele. We prefer not to use synthetic material when associated procedures such as vaginal hysterectomy or vault suspension are performed as the duration of surgery, length of incision, larger mesh requirement, and direct adherence of the vault to the mesh increase the risk of vaginal erosion. Severe ISD at rest with or without hypermobility, previous urethral surgery or injury, and hypersensitivity to the synthetic material are contraindications to tension-free vaginal tapes (TVTs) or percutaneous vaginal tapes (PVTs).

ALTERNATIVE THERAPY

Surgical alternative therapies to pubovaginal sling are covered in the other chapters within this section. Nonsurgical alternatives include pessaries, indwelling catheters, pads, and medical therapy including alpha-adrenergics and hormonal replacement therapy. Most of these nonsurgical therapies are not efficacious in the treatment of moderate SUI.

SURGICAL TECHNIQUE

If there is no contraindication, vaginal estrogen cream is prescribed 4 to 6 weeks preceding surgery. The patient is asked to discontinue the use of pessary at least 2 weeks prior to surgery. Aspirin is discontinued 5 to 7 days preoperatively. A fluoroquinolone is started 48 hours prior to surgery and patient receives routine preanesthetic instructions for the night preceding the surgery. No food or liquids are allowed 8 to 10 hours prior to the procedure. Laxatives are prescribed for patients who suffer from constipation. Complete blood count, serum electrolytes, coagulation studies, urinalysis, and urine culture are obtained. The procedure should be postponed in the presence of urinary tract infection or coagulopathy.

On the day of surgery, a parenteral antibiotic, such as a first-generation cephalosporin or a fluoroquinolone, is administered and continued for 24 to 48 hours. The choice of general or regional anesthesia depends on the anesthesiologist and patient preferences. A sequential compression device is used on the lower extremities prior to the induction of anesthesia. The procedure is performed in the lithotomy position using Allen stirrups. The lower abdominal and pubic areas are shaved, prepped, and draped using a Lingeman Gyn surgery drape (Microtek Medical, Isolyser Healthcare, Columbus, MS).

To retract the labia, a Lone Star surgical retractor (Medical Products Inc, Houston, TX) is used. Alternatively, the labia can be sutured laterally. Weighted vaginal speculums are avoided not to distort the anatomy by pulling downward. A 16 Fr urethral catheter is placed and the balloon is palpated at the bladder neck.

An Allis clamp is placed between the bladder neck and the meatus and pulled anteriorly. Injectable saline is infiltrated into the anterior vaginal wall to facilitate the dissection. A 3- to 4-cm midline incision is made over the bladder neck to avoid injury to the somatic and autonomic neurons that travel laterally through the anterior vaginal wall to the urethra and supply the urethral sphincter. With sharp scissors thick flaps of the anterior vaginal wall are developed bilaterally. Traction is applied on the vaginal wall with Allis clamps to facilitate flap dissection. Minimal bleeding is noted if the correct depth of dissection is reached.

The bladder and urethra can be peeled away from the flaps with the rolling action of gauze wrapped around the index finger. The urethropelvic ligament is identified and preserved. The retropubic space is entered anterior to the urethropelvic ligament using curved Metzenbaum scissors pointing toward the ipsilateral shoulder. The endopelvic fascia is carefully perforated with scissors or blunt finger dissection (Fig. 39–1).

At this time a 2.5-cm horizontal incision is made over the pubic symphysis. The dissection is carried with electrocautery to the level of periosteum. A flat surface of the bone is chosen and two Vesica bone anchors (Microvasive, Boston Scientific Corp, Watertown, MA) are placed, one on either side of the midline, with the Vesica bone locator (Microvasive, Boston Scientific). The anchors are pre-attached to no. 1 monofilament nonabsorbable

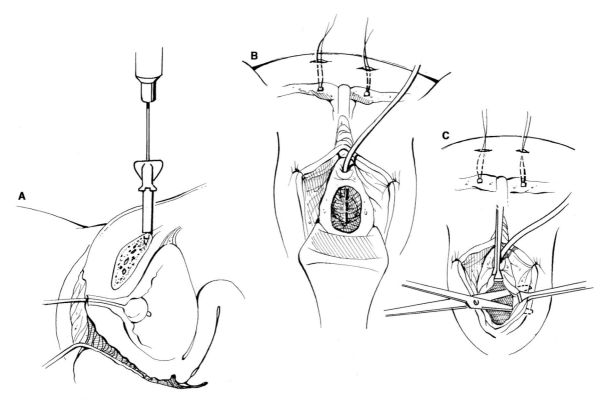

FIG. 39–1. The endopelvic fascia is carefully perforated with scissors or blunt finger dissection.

sutures. The anchors should not be palpable over the bone. Alternatively, anchors can be placed transvaginally in a retrograde fashion and secured to the inner surface of the pubis.

The bladder must be empty prior to the passage of the Stamey needles to decrease the possibility of bladder injury. One end of the anchoring suture is placed through a single-eye Stamey needle. With the dominant hand, the Stamey needle is passed through the incision behind the pubic bone pointing 5 to 10 degrees laterally. The nondominant index finger is placed through the vaginal incision in the endopelvic fascia to guide the Stamey needle through the retropubic space and deliver it via the vaginal incision. The anchoring suture is removed from the Stamey needle, leaving the needle in place, and then placed through the end of a 2×8-cm piece of polypropylene mesh soaked in antibiotic solution. The anchoring suture is placed back into the Stamey needle and pulled back up through the retropubic space. This is performed bilaterally (Fig. 39–2).

The urethral catheter is removed and cystoscopy is performed to assess for bladder injury. A 14 Fr suprapubic catheter is inserted under direct vision with the cystoscope. The urethral catheter is replaced. The sling is placed against the bladder neck without any tension by pulling on the anchoring sutures. Absorbable 3-0 monofilament sutures, such as polydioxanone (PDS), are

used to secure the sling on the periurethral tissue to prevent rolling of the sling. The anterior vaginal wall is closed from distal to proximal end using a running 3-0 absorbable monofilament suture. The anchoring sutures are tied in an "air-knot" fashion at the skin level. The suprapubic incision is closed with a running 3-0 absorbable monofilament suture and skin staples. Vaginal packing is placed. Both urethral and suprapubic catheters are placed for drainage.

The urethral catheter and the vaginal packing are removed and the suprapubic catheter is capped on postoperative day 1. The patient is instructed to uncap the suprapubic catheter every 4 hours and/or after each void to record the residual volume. Most patients are discharged on postoperative day 1. Intercourse and heavy lifting are avoided for 4 to 6 weeks. The suprapubic catheter is removed in less than 1 week if the postvoid residual volume is less than 50 mL.

Technique Modifications with Cystocele

The anterior vaginal incision is made longer proximally over the cystocele. The flaps are developed in a similar manner as above on both sides of the cystocele. If the prolapse is mild to moderate, the midportion of the sling is made wider to cover the cystocele. The prolapse is reduced using 2-0 absorbable interrupted Lembert

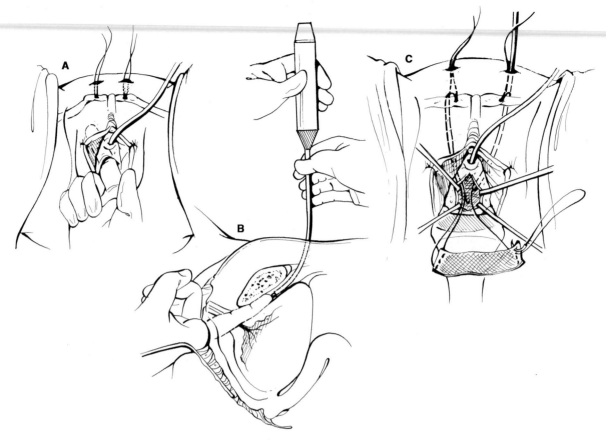

FIG. 39–2. The anchoring suture is placed back into the Stamey needle and pulled back up through the retropubic space. This is performed bilaterally.

sutures. Sutures are placed through the perivesical fascia and outer layer of the detrusor muscle, avoiding the vaginal flaps. If the cystocele is large, the sling is fashioned similar to the letter "T" extending proximally from the bladder neck to cover the cystocele. The broad base of the sling is sutured to the levator muscle. Excess vaginal flaps may need to be excised prior to closure. During cystoscopy indigo carmine (Taylor Pharmaceuticals, Decatur, IL) is given parenterally to assess efflux of urine from the ureteral orifices.

Midurethral Slings

Midurethral synthetic sling are gaining increased attention in patients with urethral hypermobility and without significant pelvic organ prolapse. TVTs (Gynecare, Johnson and Johnson, Somerville, NJ) and PVTs (SPARC, American Medical System, Minnetonka, MN) are two potential choices for placement of synthetic sling material at the midurethra. Polypropylene mesh, a nonabsorbable synthetic material, is used in both.

The preoperative preparation is similar to other synthetic slings. The aim of the TVT and PVT procedures is to place the tape at the midurethra. A midline anterior vaginal wall incision is made about 1 cm from the exter-

nal urethral meatus. Minimal paraurethral dissection is performed on both sides of the urethra. The bladder is drained using a urethral catheter.

The TVT, covered by a plastic sheath, is introduced with the help of the trocars (Fig. 39–3). A straight

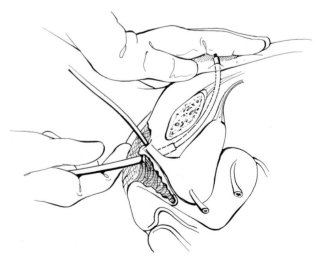

FIG. 39–3. The TVT, covered by a plastic sheath, is introduced with the help of the trocars.

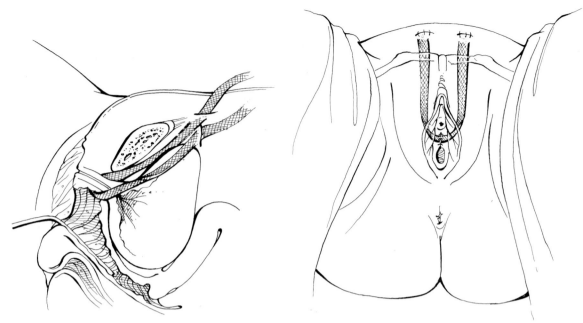

FIG. 39–4. The tape is positioned properly so that it lies in a U-shape around the urethra.

catheter introducer placed inside of the urethral catheter facilitates positioning of the urethra and bladder neck away from the trocar. Through the vaginal incision, each trocar perforates the urogenital diaphragm and is then moved through the retropubic space to emerge through two separate stab incisions on the abdominal wall.

In the PVT procedure, after loading appropriate suture material, percutaneous ligature carriers are introduced in antegrade fashion though two suprapubic stab incisions overlying the top of the symphysis on either side of a finger placed in the midline. It is necessary to stay on the posterior or back side of the symphysis to prevent entering the rectus muscle and fascia too far cephalad from its insertion on the symphysis (11). Cystoscopy is done after introducing each trocar or needle to rule out any bladder or urethral perforation. The tape is positioned properly so that it lies in a U-shape around the urethra (Fig. 39–4) (11).

If the procedure is done under local anesthesia, the patient is asked to cough or an assistant applies suprapubic pressure to simulate cough to adjust the position of the tape. Polypropylene tape is self-retaining and does not require any fixation. In the PVT procedure a suture running through the mesh allows adjustment of the sling if needed. The incisions are sutured with appropriate material.

OUTCOMES

Complications

Intraoperative complications such as significant bladder injury and hemorrhage are rare and are avoided by correct plane of dissection. With midurethral slings (TVT), the incidence of bladder perforation is 5.4% (0% to 23%), being higher in patients who have undergone prior retropubic procedures (2). If a bladder perforation is noted with the TVT trocar or Stamey needle, the needle or trocar is removed and repositioned. The procedure is completed by placing the synthetic sling. In such cases urethral catheter drainage is continued for 1 week. Hemorrhage is often controlled by placing the sling and the vaginal packing. The incidence of intraoperative ureteral injuries is low, yet the surgeon needs to be more aware of increased risk of ureteral injuries in the presence of large prolapsing cystoceles.

The primary reason for sling failure is applying too much tension on the sling, which can result in significant obstruction, urinary retention, and/or detrusor instability. Postoperative urinary retention is noted in 5% of those undergoing the pubovaginal sling procedure and is usually managed by clean intermittent self-catheterization. Retention is usually of relatively short duration and urodynamics are not performed unless retention persists at least 6 weeks to 3 months following surgery. Long-term management of retention is by intermittent catheterization or surgical incision of the mesh. Appell (1) reported that only 2% of women required long-term self-catheterization with fascial slings placed under minimal tension.

De novo urinary urgency occurs in up to 12% of patients (3). Most patients respond to anticholinergic medications and are cured after 3 to 6 months. Intractable postsling detrusor instability may benefit from neuromodulation.

Failure or delay of healing of the vaginal incision is initially treated conservatively with antibiotics and hormonal cream. Persistent delay in vaginal incisional healing is treated by operative intervention. The synthetic sling is removed and may be replaced by autologous fascial sling and the vaginal flaps are sutured with interposition of Martius flap.

The most serious delayed complication of all synthetic slings is erosion. Earlier studies of synthetic slings reported a high rate of synthetic sling erosion, infection, and sling explant (9). Contemporary series show no erosions or infections and transient to no retention using polypropylene mesh (12).

Most erosions occur within 6 months of placement and are associated with significant voiding dysfunction or urinary retention. Urethral erosion mandates removal of the mesh. Urethral erosion can be prevented by tying the anchoring sutures loosely at the skin level. This maneuver also reduces the possibility of postoperative retention and urgency.

Isolated bladder erosion is rare and often represents inadvertently placed sutures in the bladder and missed by cystoscopy at the time of surgery. It is treated by cystoscopic removal of that suture.

Delayed vaginal erosion may be related to subclinical infection. Therefore, removal of vaginal packing in less than 24 hours, soaking the mesh in antibiotic solution, and sterile urine are important. Using monofilament sutures, such as polypropylene or PDS, can be beneficial in reduction of infection. It cannot be overemphasized that thin vaginal flaps must be avoided because flap ischemia can easily lead to erosion. Vaginally eroded mesh is removed and the defect is covered with a thicker flap of the anterior vaginal wall and reinforced by Martius flap interposition.

Results

Few long-term results of sling surgery are available and most of the reports are only subjective cure rates. Jarvis (5) reported an objective cure rate of 85.3% and subjective cure rate of 82.4% following sling surgery using synthetic material.

REFERENCES

1. Appell R. Primary slings for everyone with genuine stress incontinence. *Int Urogynaecol J Pelvic Floor Dysfunct* 1998;9:249.
2. Boustead G. The tension free vaginal tape for treatment of female stress urinary incontinence. *BJU Int* 2002;89:687.
3. Choe J, Ogan K, Battio B. Antimicrobial mesh versus vaginal wall sling: a comparative analysis. *J Urol* 2000;163:1843.
4. Corujo M, Badlani G. The use of synthetic material in the treatment of women with SUI lends strength and disability. *Contemp Urol* 1999;11:76.
5. Jarvis G. Stress incontinence. In: Mundy A, Stephenson T, Wein A, eds. *Urodynamics: Principles, practice and application*, 2nd ed. New York: Churchill Livingstone, 1994:299–326.
6. Jensen J, Rufford H. Sling procedures—artificial. In: Cardozo L, Staskin D, eds. *Textbook of female urology and urogynaecology*. London: ISIS Medical Media, 2002.
7. Law N, Ellis H. A comparison of polypropylene mesh and expanded polytetrafluoroethylene patch for the repair of contaminated abdominal wall defects—an experimental study. *Surgery* 1991;109:652.
8. Marinkovic S, Youssefzadeh D, Badlani G. Bone anchored pubovaginal sings: Vaginal wall slings vs. modified pubovaginal slings using polypropylene mesh. Success, complications and quality of life analysis. *J Endourol* 1999;13:127.
9. Morgan JE. A sling operation using Marlex proplene mesh for treatment of recurrent stress incontinence. *Am J Obstet Gynecol* 1970;106:369.
10. Petros P, Ulmsten U. An integral theory on female urinary incontinence. Experimental and clinical considerations. *Acta Obstet Gynecol Scand* 1990;69:153.
11. Rackley RR, Abdelmalak JB, Tchetgen MB, et al. Tension free vaginal tape and percutaneous vaginal tape ling procedures. *Tech Urol* 2001;7:90.
12. Rodriguez L, Berman J, Raz S. Polypropylene sling for treatment of stress urinary incontinence: an alternative to tension free vaginal tape. *Tech Urol* 2001;7:87.

CHAPTER 40

Combined Abdominal and Vaginal Bladder Neck Suspension with Mesh Bolsters for Female Stress Incontinence

Hunter A. McKay

Bladder neck suspension surgery for pelvic relaxation and stress urinary incontinence is successful most often when the bladder neck and proximal urethra can be elevated and stabilized in a retropubic location with supporting sutures from above. The evolution from retropubic operations such as the Marshall–Marchetti–Krantz (3) and its variants, like the Burch (1) operation, to combined retropubic and vaginal operations (4–6) has been driven by the hope for an improved cure rate of the incontinence. The advantage of an endoscopic confirmation of needle and suture placement has proven to be a valuable benefit of those operations collectively known as needle suspensions. However, the long-term success rates of various stress incontinence operations are not as high as the short-term results, are quite variable, and have been disappointing to many researchers (2,7,8). Because of the concern for the increasingly large numbers of failures reported with the retropubic and needle suspension operations, a combined technique using monofilament flat bolsters to gently distribute suture load forces was devised in the mid-1980s.

The weak link in stress incontinence surgery appears to be at the endopelvic fascia. Adequate support for the suspensory sutures used in bladder neck suspensions is essential for a long-lasting repair. However, traditional retropubic repairs utilize a series of endopelvic fascia sutures, which are placed adjacent to the urethral axis and then attached to structurally sound tissues of the pelvis. These individual retropubic sutures are tied with varying degrees of tension, and thus the pressure of the sutures on the endopelvic fascia is variable and one of these individual sutures will be most vulnerable to pulling through the fascia. Pressures of 360 psi per suture have been calculated to occur when traditional retropubic repairs are performed.* After any one of the sutures has pulled through, the next suture with the highest pressure will be most vulnerable to fail. After all sutures have pulled through, only retropubic scarring will be available to maintain the repair. Perhaps scarring alone in this area is sufficient to maintain the desired anatomic correction for a while, and this scarring concept is what justifies the use of absorbable suture materials for these repairs. Also, absorbable suture material is less likely to be problematic should the sutures inadvertently penetrate the bladder or urethra, but most pelvic surgeons would prefer the reliability of a permanent suture for the repair, if possible. The advent of the endoscopic correction of stress incontinence, as popularized by Stamey in the 1970s, allowed the urologist to confirm the safe placement of suspensory sutures outside the urothelium. Permanent sutures have become standard, and the reliance on retropubic scarring became less important in the 1980s. To decrease the pressure of the suspensory sutures on the fragile endopelvic fascia, Stamey used an "off-the-shelf" bolster material of Dacron tube graft. This easily procured material was unfortunately prone to bacterial contamination, as evidenced by a high incidence of bolster rejection or erosion. To avoid infection-prone materials, and to use an off-the-shelf product, polypropylene mesh was selected as the bolster material for the combined bladder neck suspension operation to be described.

This bolster material exhibits a flat geometry without a dead space and is of loosely knitted monofilament construction, with wide interstices. These properties are

---

*Pressures were calculated using finite element modeling with ANSYS v.5.3 and LS-Nike3D software programs.

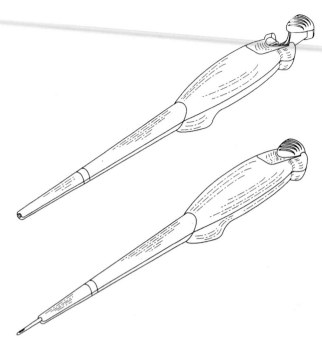

FIG. 40–1. The ND-1 single-point instrument with needle retracted and extruded (Island Biosurgical/Torpent Technologies).

important in reducing the risk of infection as compared to Dacron arterial tube graft, which is tightly knitted and has a large, circular dead space. In an attempt to lessen the pressure of any single suture on the endopelvic fascia, a pair of monofilament sutures woven into a fabric mesh bolster appeared to have great potential. This multiple-suture philosophy is similar to that of most retropubic operations, except that no bolster is used in those procedures. A 1.5-cm × 2.0-cm segment of monofilament polypropylene mesh with a no. 2 monofilament suture woven along each of the long edges has become our bolster material of choice. To avoid confusion when tying these sutures down, two different suture colors (blue polypropylene and black nylon) are used. When eventually positioned between the endopelvic fascia and the vaginal epithelium, these flat mesh bolsters, with parallel and fully integrated sutures separated by about 10 mm of mesh, are able to distribute the load onto the endopelvic fascia with much less pressure (about 90 psi per bolster*) than can any single suture, be it bolstered or unbolstered. Two new suture-carrying instruments were designed to aid in the accurate positioning of the bolsters. The first of these was an instrument that could both aid in the blunt dissection of retropubic adhesions from prior surgeries and also carry sutures back from the vaginotomy area. This "needle dissector" (ND-1) instrument was designed in 1986 and has a 0.9-cm × 20-cm shaft, with a 2-cm ×

10-cm handle (Fig. 40–1). A 35-cm long obturator with tapered 0.3-cm diameter pointed tip slides through the hollow handle and shaft. Four detents allow for accurate control of the sliding obturator as it is extruded from within the shaft. Thus, the instrument can act as a dissector when the needle is retracted and the pointed obturator can controllably and accurately penetrate the endopelvic fascia when the blunt end with its protected needle point is properly positioned. The eye-hole in the needle portion allows for sequential capture of several suture ends. A needle dissector with four points (ND-4) was developed in 1989 and allows for the capture of all four suture ends of the bolster at a single pass.

DIAGNOSIS

The diagnosis of stress urinary incontinence is made by a combination of history, physical examination, and urodynamics. The initial patient group undergoing this mesh bladder neck suspension was evaluated by means of a questionnaire, physical examination, urinalysis and urine culture, urodynamics with stress testing, occasional cystoscopy, and the Stamey incontinence criteria.

INDICATIONS FOR SURGERY

Indications for surgery are stress urinary incontinence types 2 and 3. Patients with mixed incontinence are not excluded from surgical correction but are advised that their urgency and urge incontinence symptomatology may remain unchanged, worsen, or improve. Anticholinergic medications may be needed postoperatively if the unstable bladder symptoms are troublesome.

ALTERNATIVE THERAPY

Alternative therapies to this and other operations for incontinence include conservative therapy such as Kegel exercises, biofeedback training, and estrogen replacement. Other surgical options for these types of patients might include open bladder suspensions, endoscopic and percutaneous suspension procedures, and various slings.

SURGICAL TECHNIQUE

The typical patient is prepared for combined abdominal and vaginal surgery in the low lithotomy position. Two short transverse skin incisions are made at the pubic tubercle regions to allow for access to the rectus fascia on each side. The fascia is entered sharply with a 1-cm incision, which allows limited entry into the space of Retzius and permits blunt dissection alongside the previously filled bladder and bladder neck. Sharp dissection with heavy Mayo scissors and/or electrocautery is also usually necessary if the patient has had prior retropubic surgery.

Pressures were calculated with NSYS v.5.3 and LS-Nike3D software programs.

Filling the bladder to capacity facilitates the dissection and prevents inadvertent entry into the bladder in most instances. A calibrated 20 Fr Malecot catheter is used transurethrally for the several bladder fillings between cystoscopies. Unlike the Pereyra (4), Stamey (6), or other slender suture-carrying needles, the ND-1 is of substantial diameter and rigidity and aids in bluntly pushing the endopelvic fascial adhesions from previous surgeries away from the undersurface of the pubis and thus frees the bladder neck and urethra for the subsequent suture and bolster placement. A to-and-fro motion of the handle of the ND-1 is used to gently dissect those adhesions that lie in the depths of the perivesical area at the level of the endopelvic fascia. Only a limited exposure is necessary, as the dissection is done mostly by tactile means. After completion of this urethrolysis, the surgeon can confidently place the blunt end of the distal portion of the ND-1 precisely at one side of the bladder neck as defined by the filled bladder and the large-caliber urethral catheter. This tip of the ND-1 rests on top of the flat endopelvic fascia as confirmed by palpation transvaginally. Again, the filled bladder facilitates the accurate placement of the instrument. The needle of the ND-1 is subsequently extruded precisely at the bladder neck, through the endopelvic fascia, and into a 3-cm vaginotomy (Fig. 40–2). The mesh bolster apparatus is brought near the introitus and the medial end of the blue suture is passed through the eye of the needle of the ND-1. The needle is withdrawn into the hub of the ND-1 (which remains above the endopelvic fascia), and the blue suture is captured within the shaft of the ND-1. The blunt tip of the instrument, with its captured suture, is moved atraumatically about 1.5 cm lateral to the initial endopelvic fascia penetration. The needle is extruded again through the endopelvic fascia and then directed into the vaginotomy. The second end (lateral portion) of the blue suture is

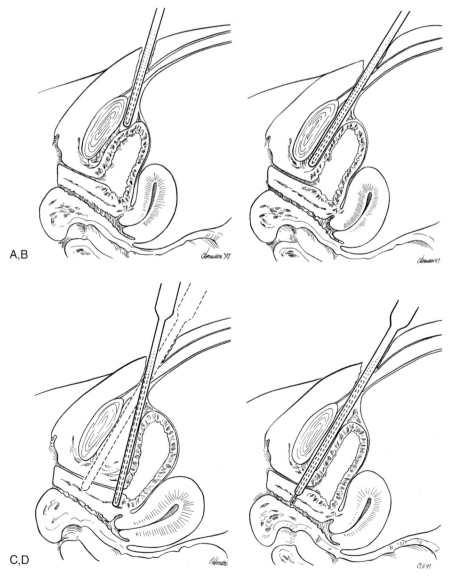

A,B

C,D

FIG. 40–2. The ND-1 shown in sequential blunt dissection and then with needle penetration of the endopelvic fascia.

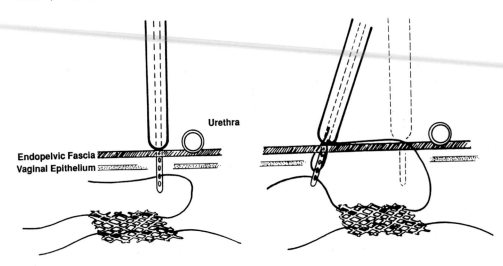

Endopelvic Fascia
Vaginal Epithelium
Urethra

FIG. 40–3. Suture capture sequence of the proximal (blue) suture of the right bolster.

picked up (Fig. 40–3). When the entire ND-1 is withdrawn with a cephalad maneuver, the two blue suture ends are delivered into the suprapubic area. A similar procedure is used to position the black suture about 1.5 cm distally along the urethra. The blue and black sutures on the contralateral side are retrieved in a similar fashion. It is important that the needle penetrate into the vaginotomy without epithelial entrapment and that the sutures not be tangled so as to avoid folding the bolster (Fig. 40–4). No significant disruption of the endopelvic fascia occurs, and blood loss is minimal. Cystoscopic confirmation is usually delayed until after suture delivery but can be done

earlier if there is concern about possible penetration of the bladder. If a penetration is observed, the offending suture should be withdrawn and then repositioned with the ND-1. Assessment of the positions of the suspensory sutures with respect to the ureteral orifices is also accomplished during the cystoscopic examination. When traction is applied to the individual sutures, no encroachment on the orifices should occur. The intravenous injection of indigo carmine has not been necessary. A physiological test is performed by using the Credé maneuver to reproduce the leakage. The leakage should disappear with mild traction on right, left, and both groups of sutures. Failure to demonstrate this correction usually means that there are still significant adhesions preventing full mobility of the proximal urethra or that the sutures have been placed too far from the urethra. Copious irrigation is followed by closure of the vaginotomies with 3-0 Vicryl sutures. The pubic tubercle or Cooper's ligament may be used for the placement of the right and left suture groups. The blue sutures (which had been positioned along the cephalad aspect of the bolster) are passed in the more lateral position on the pubic bone location and will have moderate tension applied when tied. These blue sutures are more important than the black sutures because of their position closer to the bladder neck. The black (more distal) sutures are passed through a somewhat more medial position on the pubic bone. After the blue sutures have been tied, the black sutures are tied with minimal tension to avoid kinking the urethra. The wound is closed in routine fashion. Parenteral antibiotics are essential.

With further experience with the technique and the availability (in 1989) of the somewhat larger ND-4, that instrument can be used if a larger (6 cm) midline fascial incision is made. After preliminary dissection with the ND-1, the ND-4 is positioned precisely at the right side of the bladder neck (Fig. 40–5) and then its four points are extruded into the endopelvic fascia only. The filled bladder facilitates the accurate placement of the instrument. A 3-cm longitudinal vaginotomy is made directly

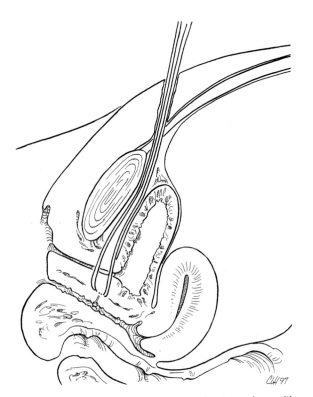

FIG. 40–4. Left suspensory bolster and sutures in position, sagittal view.

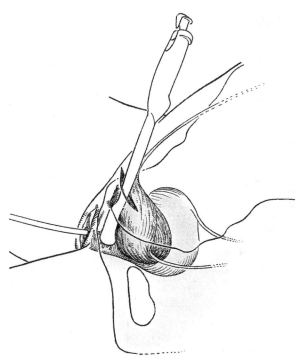

FIG. 40–5. The ND-4 has been passed retropubically, oblique view. The four needle points are shown penetrating the endopelvic fascia only.

between the four points of the ND-4, and these points are delivered into the vaginotomy without epithelial entrapment (Fig. 40–6). The advantage of the four-point instrument is that the 1.3-cm distance between the needle points ensures that a good web of supporting endopelvic fascia will be available for the suspension. Also, all four suture ends of the bolster can be retrieved with a single pass of the instrument, without the risk of entanglement. As with the ND-1, the previously fashioned flat bolster is to be located between the vaginal epithelium and the endopelvic fascia. After placing all four suture ends through the eyes of the ND-4, the instrument is withdrawn in a cephalad maneuver, delivering the two black and two blue suture ends into the suprapubic area. An identical procedure is performed on the opposite side. The bolsters are "seated" into their positions beneath the endopelvic fascia and the vaginal incisions are closed. The remainder of the procedure is performed in a fashion similar to that where the ND-1 alone is used; however, because of the 6-cm abdominal incision Cooper's ligament is more easily available as the anchoring location.

OUTCOMES

Complications

Complications have included an epithelial "erosion" rate of less than 2% and a long-term retention rate of less than 0.5% in 600 cases.

Results

The patient satisfaction questionnaire as advocated by Walker and Texter (8) has become our preferred method of assessing the outcome of surgical procedures. Seventy-two patients underwent a modified retropubic suspension using the ND-1 instrument and flat fabric mesh as a bolster on each side of the bladder neck. Seventy-nine percent of these patients were satisfied with the results of their procedure at 10 years postoperatively (Fig. 40–7). The clinical results of an additional 169 patients who

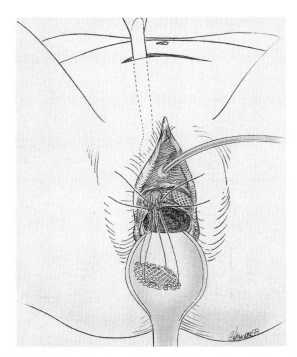

FIG. 40–6. Introital view of the ND-4 positioned alongside the right bladder neck area with right bolster sutures engaged. The previously placed left bolster is seen faintly through the vaginal epithelium.

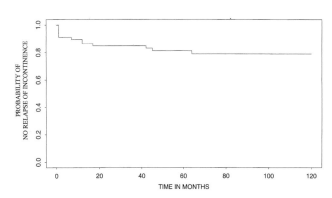

FIG. 40–7. Long-term success rate for the fabric mesh bolster repair procedure.

underwent their bladder neck suspension with the ND-4 from 1989 to 1994 are similar to those undergoing the ND-1 procedure. Forty-five percent of the patients undergoing this mesh repair had had a previous failed incontinence procedure.

The ND instruments allow for percutaneous or open dissection of the scarred retropubic space and then precise needle placement with subsequent exact suture and bolster placement. The suture-carrying instruments are blunt rather than sharp and thus the bladder can be filled enough to define the urethrovesical junction. This definition permits the more accurate positioning of the sutures than is possible with the Stamey needle or during a Marshall–Marchetti–Krantz procedure, and with a minimal risk of bladder perforation. Because the endopelvic fascia is penetrated only by needle points, it remains a major anatomic strength area for this repair. That portion of the fascia that lies underneath the bladder neck and proximal urethra becomes the sling portion of the repair and has considerable elasticity (thus, it is more forgiving than a strip of polypropylene going completely under the urethra). The flat monofilament mesh bolsters have wide interstices and no appreciable dead space as compared to Dacron tube graft material; the incidence of bolster problems is thereby reduced when polypropylene mesh is used. Pelvic surgeons realize that the principle of tension-free closure when tissues are approximated is crucial in bladder neck suspension surgery. The "cheese cutter" effect, which occurs when solitary sutures are used to elevate the endopelvic fascia, results in tissue laceration and eventual failure of the repair. When the suspensory sutures have cut through the tissues, the only mechanism for continued support of the repair will be the residual and unreliable retropubic adhesions. When these adhesions fail, the repair breaks down. Many authors (2,7,8) have shown the decrease in long-term success rates of various bladder neck operations as their patients are followed over time.

The technical assistance of Darrell Tubb, Anita Rocha, Cheryl Herndon, Mario Tapia, and William Cliber is gratefully acknowledged.

REFERENCES

1. Burch JC. Urethrovaginal fixation to Cooper's ligament for correction of stress incontinence, cystocele, and prolapse. *Am J Obstet Gynecol* 1961; 81:281–290.
2. Korman HJ, Sirls LT, Kirkemo AK. Success rate of modified Pereyra bladder neck suspension determined by outcomes analysis. *J Urol* 1994; 152:1453–1457.
3. Marshall VF, Marchetti AA, Krantz KE. The correction of stress incontinence by simple vesicourethral suspension. *Surg Gynecol Obstet* 1949; 88:509–518.
4. Pereyra AJ, Lebherz TB. Combined urethrovesical suspension and vaginourethroplasty for correction of urinary stress incontinence. *Obstet Gynecol* 1967;30:537–546.
5. Raz S. Modified bladder neck suspension for female stress incontinence. *Urology* 1981;17:82–84.
6. Stamey TA. Endoscopic suspension of the vesical neck for urinary incontinence. *Surg Gynecol Obstet* 1973;136:547–554.
7. Trockman BA, Leach GE, Hamilton J, Sakamoto M, Santiago L, Zimmern PE. Modified Pereyra bladder neck suspension: 10-year mean followup using outcomes analysis in 125 patients. *J Urol* 1995;154:1841–1847.
8. Walker GT, Texter JH. Success and patient satisfaction following the Stamey procedure for stress urinary incontinence. *J Urol* 1992;147: 1521–1523.

CHAPTER 41

Cystocele and Anterior Vaginal Prolapse

Roger R. Dmochowski and Alexander Gomelsky

Anterior compartment vaginal prolapse, cystocele, is one of numerous types of pelvic floor relaxations that arise from weakening of the endopelvic fascia and herniation of pelvic viscera through the potential space of the vagina. Weakness of the levator fascia results in loss of pelvic floor support and subsequent formation of anterior compartment defects (the preferable term according to International Continence Society terminology) (1) or cystoceles.

The fascia of the levator floor has a primary supportive role function for not only the anterior vaginal wall but also the bladder and urethra in composite. The abdominal aspect of this fascia is referred to as the endopelvic fascia, while the vaginal side is referred to as the perivesical fascia (at the level of the bladder base) and the periurethral fascia at the level of the bladder neck. The term pubocervical often refers to the combined periurethral and perivesical fascia complex. The vaginal and abdominal components of these fascial sheets fuse laterally at their insertion into the tendinous arch of the obturator internus [arcus tendineus fasciae pelvis (ATFP)], which forms the pelvic side wall anchor for these structures.

When viewing vaginal support from cephalad to caudad, the cardinal ligaments support the upper vagina and cervix and anchor them to the pelvic sidewall (Fig. 41–1). In the midvagina, the vesical pelvic ligament extends from the pelvic sidewall to the bladder base and supports it and the anterior vaginal wall. Finally, the urethropelvic ligaments support the urethra from urethral meatus to bladder neck. The arcuate line (arcus tendineus) of the pelvis, which is the condensation of the obturator internus fascia and endopelvic fascia, provides the lateral support insertion for all these structures. This strong insertion provides a stabilization point for the entire pelvic floor hammock (2). Cystocele defects are commonly associated with other forms of pelvic relaxation, including loss of support of the uterus and vaginal apex (enterocele vault prolapse in uterine) and loss of posterior compartment support, including perineum (perineal relaxation and rectocele).

Defects of the anterior compartment may result in either isolated urethral or bladder support defects or a combination of support defects of both structures (Fig. 41–2). Loss of support of the urethra may result in urethral hypermobility without a concomitant cystocele defect being identified. Cystocele defects are more complex and may involve either defects termed central or lateral or a combination of both. Lateral defect cystoceles result from disruption or separation of the condensation of the vesical pelvic ligament to the arcus tendineous on either lateral side of the vagina. Central defect cystoceles result from attenuation of the perivesical (pubocervical) fascia without compromise of the urethral pelvic and vesical pelvic ligaments. Central defect cystoceles are often associated with attenuation of upper vaginal support as well, including loss of cardinal ligament support (with a concomitant enterocele). The most common form of cystocele is a combination cystocele. Isolated central defects comprise less than 10% of diagnosed cystoceles. Isolated lateral defects are more common and are often

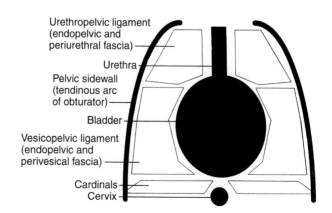

FIG. 41–1. The cardinal ligaments support the upper vagina and cervix and anchor them to the pelvic sidewall.

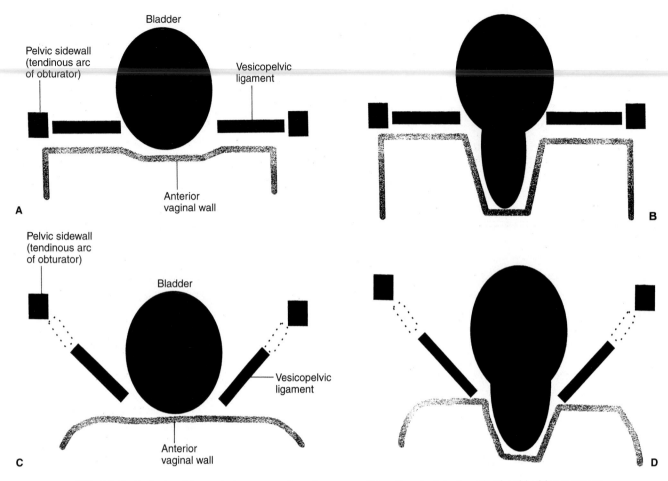

FIG. 41–2. Defects of the anterior compartment may result in either isolated urethral or bladder support defects or a combination of support defects of both structures.

associated with urethral hypermobility. When combined central and lateral defects are present, more severe degrees of prolapse often result.

DIAGNOSIS

Cystocele defects produce a variety of symptoms, including: "mass effect" symptoms (perineal or intravaginal bulge or sensation of mass effect in vagina), stress urinary incontinence, dyspareunia, vaginal irritation or bleeding (due to excoriation of exposed vaginal mucosa), and, if large enough, defecatory symptoms. Surprisingly, even large cystoceles may also be totally asymptomatic. Large cystocele defects may be associated with a kinking effect of the proximal urethra by the bladder base, resulting in concomitant incomplete emptying, obstructive voiding symptoms, and, rarely, urinary retention. Severe cystoceles may also result in upper urinary tract changes, including hydronephrosis and, rarely, renal failure due to urethral or ureteral obstruction or a combination of both. Smaller degree cystoceles may be responsible for dyspareunia or incontinence only during sexual activity and

may be a reason for early presentation prior to the onset of pelvic descensus symptoms in certain individuals.

Physical examination of the vagina will demonstrate a mass occupying the anterior vaginal wall from the vaginal apex (or cervix, if hysterectomy has not been performed) to the bladder neck and/or urethra. If significant pelvic relaxation is present, this cystocele defect may actually protrude from the vaginal introitus with activity or may present exteriorized at rest. Supine vaginal examination is aided by a half Grave's speculum with the woman at rest and straining. The examination should be repeated in the standing position to identify more subtle defects. This method of examination is important to grade a cystocele and also to identify concomitant prolapse defects such as an enterocele and/or large-degree rectocele.

Cystocele grading uses several different taxonomies, with the Baden–Walker being the simplest and most reproducible and the Pelvic Organ Prolapse Quantification System (POP-Q) providing the most descriptive method (Table 41–1). Vaginal apical examination is crucial to locate the vaginal cuff and other forms of prolapse

TABLE 41–1A. *Classification of cystocele*

Grade	Definition
I	Bladder Neck Hypermobility
II	Bladder Base Reaching Introitus with Strain
III	Bladder Base Bulging Through Introitus with Strain
IV	Bladder Base Outside Introitus at Rest

Adapted from Stothers L, Chopra A, Raz S. Vaginal reconstructive surgery for female incontinence and anterior vagina-wall prolapse. *Urol Clin North Am* 1995;22:644, with permission.

TABLE 41–1B. *Classification of cystocele*

Point Aa: Anterior Wall Genital Hiatus	Point Bb: Anterior Wall Perineal Body (pb)	Point Cc: Cervix or Cuff Total Vaginal Length (TVL)
Point Ap: Posterior Wall	Point Bp: Posterior Wall	Point D: Posterior Fornix

International Continence Society assessment of prolapse: (a) points of measurement—gh, genital hiatus; pb, perineal body; tvl, total vaginal length; and (b) method of notation on the measurements.

present posterior or behind the cuff (enterocele and/or high rectocele). The location of the cuff establishes the usual limit of surgical dissection for the vaginal cystocele repair and recognition of the cuff position allows identification of a concomitant enterocele.

Examination should focus on the integrity of the bladder base and presence or absence of the lateral vaginal fornices. Isolated central defect cystoceles will present with a large anterior vaginal wall bulge with preservation of the lateral fornices on either side of this bulge. Often, however, central defects are associated with lateral defects and the preservation of these lateral fornices is not noted. With isolated central defects, urethral hypermobility is often not noted; however, this finding is not universal. Lateral cystocele defects are associated with combined anterior vaginal wall and urethral hypermobility.

During pelvic examination, it is important to determine the presence or absence of urinary incontinence. With significant anterior compartment defects, urinary urgency and urge incontinence from detrusor instability may also be identified. The possibility of bladder outlet obstruction should also be considered in patients who have undergone a prior incontinence procedure and developed *de novo* anterior prolapse. In those patients, a hyperangulated or nonmobile urethra with increased urinary residuals and symptoms compatible with outlet obstruction should warrant consideration of urethrolysis at the time of cystocele correction. Videourodynamic evaluation may be indicated for these patients to best identify any contributing obstructive voiding component. This patient may be at risk for persistent outlet obstruction postoperatively and should be alerted to the risk of long-term catheterization.

INDICATIONS FOR SURGERY

Surgical intervention is predicated by several symptomatic factors. Symptoms arising from the cystocele (incomplete emptying, vaginal mass, or perineal prolapse symptomatology) and the presence of urinary incontinence form the cornerstone indications for repair. The presence of dyspareunia should be carefully considered as this symptom often coexists with other associated cystocele mass effect complaints. Dyspareunia as an isolated indication for surgery, however, must be judiciously considered as the complaint may or may not respond to anatomic correction.

The appropriate operation is based upon the degree and severity of the patient's incontinence, the magnitude of the cystocele (grade), the underlying nature of the fascial defect (central/lateral), and the patient's ability to empty her bladder. Comprehensive surgical planning also includes identification of associated prolapse elements (and their symptoms) including enterocele, rectocele, and apical prolapse defects.

The type of anterior compartment repair is indicated by the preoperatively defined fascial defect. Central fascial defects may be managed with either a plication type of repair and/or an interposition graft repair with or without concomitant sling dependent upon the presence of incontinence. Isolated central defect repair is rare in the absence of a concomitant stress incontinence procedure.

Lateral defect repairs may be performed with a variety of techniques, including multiple-point repairs (four- or six-corner bladder suspensions) as well as vaginal–paravaginal repairs or abdominal–paravaginal repairs with combined incontinence intervention. Severe cystoceles with combined central and lateral defects require concomitant stress procedures as well as interpositional graft placement to compensate for complete disruption of the supportive pelvic floor structures.

ALTERNATIVE THERAPY

Optional management for small, relatively minor, degrees of pelvic floor descensus includes pelvic floor physiotherapy using biofeedback and behavioral modification. The utilization of topical estrogens may augment the symptomatic response to this intervention in those patients who demonstrate poor vaginal estrogen support and have a component of associated urinary irritative symptoms. A patient with an asymptomatic small cystocele with adequate vesical emptying and no incontinence does not require surgical intervention.

Smaller-grade cystoceles (grades 1 or 2) often are repaired by outlet procedures performed at the level of the bladder neck, including pubovaginal slings and earlier forms of suspensions such as needle suspensions. Large defects may often be managed effectively with pessary placement. This option should be discussed with all women who experience symptoms of anterior compartment mass effect, as substantive clinical improvement may result. In some women, the use of a pessary may actually unmask occult incontinence and nullify any symptomatic benefit that the device has conveyed.

SURGICAL TECHNIQUE

Combination Repair of Defects With Mesh/Interposition Graft and Vaginal Sling

Associated urethral hypermobility and lateral and central defects may be addressed by a combined mesh inlay and pubovaginal sling procedure (Fig. 41–3). The choices for mesh interposition include synthetic, xenograft, autograft (free full-thickness vaginal wall), and allograft materials. Long-term data are not yet available to support one material as preferential; however, some evidence exists from experience with alternative slings that may be extrapolated to these inlays. If a synthetic is chosen, polydioxanone is a viable choice (6). This material is conformal, modestly rigid, and, most importantly, eventually degraded (and hopefully replaced by host fibrosis). Allografts that are fresh frozen appear to have poor durability, whereas those that are solvent deactivated or radiated maintain structural integrity, which has translated to increased durability. Xenografts (dermis) are the most

conformal to underlying tissues, less rigid, and relatively less expensive. The authors favor the latter based on experience with more than 60 women receiving these materials as graft inlays.

Defect repair may be addressed either with a single-component interposition that serves as both bladder base and urethral support (CAPPS) (3) or with a two-component interposition with a separate material strip providing the sling and another for the anterior compartment repair. The authors favor the two-component method.

At the time of repair, the vaginal apex should be stabilized with cardinal ligament plication sutures and/or some other form or vaginal apical fixation such as the ileococcygeal- or sacrospinalis-type suspensions. Inlay repairs address both central and lateral defects. Further lateral defect correction may also be created by suture placement through the vesicopelvic ligaments and subsequent suspension to the anterior rectus fascia.

The woman is placed in the dorsal lithotomy position and, utilizing hydraulic stirrups, placed in the lithotomy position with no extremity flexed at greater than 90 degrees. After prepping the abdomen, perineum, and vagina, the posterior compartment is draped away from the surgical field; however, it can be accessed under an adherent drape should access be necessary. A weighted speculum and a ring retractor are used for vaginal exposure.

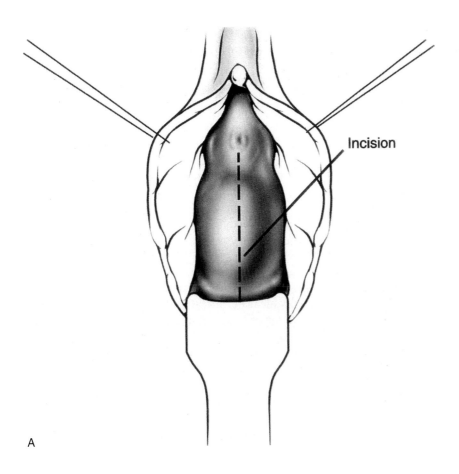

FIG. 41–3. A: The incision for the interposition graph is made in the midline from the midurethra to vaginal apex.

A

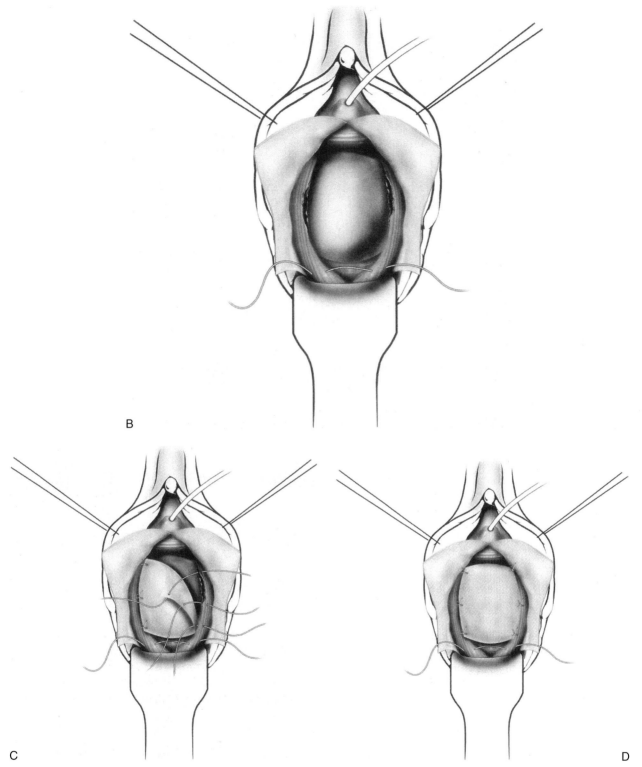

B

C

D

FIG. 41–3 *Continued.* **B:** After completion of dissection and entry into the retropubic space, identification of the cardinal ligament complex and the obturator internus is completed. The area of the cardinal ligament complex on either side is identified and the ligaments are reapproximated to reconstruct the vaginal apex. **C:** The interpositional graft is inlaid in the defect. Sutures are placed sequentially in the obturator internus fascia and through the inlay material. **D:** Final repair demonstrating placement of the free graft from the bladder neck to vaginal apex. Closure is accomplished after this.

A Foley catheter is placed and dissection begun with a midline incision from the midurethra to vaginal apex. The anterior vaginal wall, overlying the cystocele, is infiltrated with either normal saline or dilute vasoconstrictor and dissected away from the underlying attenuated pubocervical fascia. The dissection plane is identified by the glistening white pubocervical fascia and the vaginal wall itself is very thin in this dissection plane. Dissection in the wrong plane is usually associated with significant bleeding and inability to identify the underlying fascia.

Once the dissection of the vaginal wall has been completed to the fornix on either side of the bladder neck, sharp dissection is utilized to enter the retropubic space immediately under the arch of the pubis. This plane is in general avascular and should separate well from the underlying fascial components. In previously operated cases, this space may be difficult to identify and it is important to utilize sharp, shallow dissection (immediate proximity to the arch of the symphysis pubis) to avoid inadvertent entry into the pelvic viscera, including bladder and urethra.

After entry into the retropubic space, lateral and anterior dissection is carried out to mobilize the bladder and urethra. Subsequently, dissection is performed to the vaginal cuff in a line parallel to the orientation of the vaginal vault. During this dissection in women who are posthysterectomy, the stump of the uterine arterial complex is commonly encountered and bleeding may occur due to disruption of this structure. Suture ligature with 4-0 polydioxanone of these vessels should be contemplated to avoid persistent blood loss during the reconstructive segment of the operation. Cautery should be minimized to avoid devascularization of the underlying tissues.

Apical dissection should be meticulous so as to identify any enterocele component and, if found, excise and close the defect. Apical enteroceles may be small and somewhat obscured by the bladder base descensus. The cardinal ligaments can often be identified at this level of the dissection, and when found plication with a 0 or 2-0 synthetic absorbable suture (SAS) can be performed. If indicated (high-grade cystocele—grade 4, concomitant cystocele), placement of sutures posteriorly in the coccygeus region will also provide further support and stability to the anterior compartment repair. These sutures are then brought through the vaginal apex to be tied at the completion of the procedure, after the vaginal wall has been closed.

Once dissection of the retropubic space is completed and it is freely mobile, a sling is placed. The sling may either be autologous tissue harvested through a separate abdominal incision or may be any of a variety of tissues, including bovine, porcine, or allograft. Ligature passage needles are directed from suprapubic to vaginal incisions on either side of the proximal urethra and bladder neck with digital guidance. Once placed, cystoscopy is performed to exclude needle entry into the bladder or urethra. Suspending sutures of 0 or no. 1 polypropylene (PPS) or SASs are placed through either end of the sling material and the suspending suture is then transposed from vaginal to suprapubic incisions using the ligature carrier. The sling is then affixed to the underlying periurethral fascia with 4-0 SASs.

Following these steps, either absorbable or nonabsorbable 0 or 2-0 sutures are placed in the obturator internus fascia at the level of the arcuate line in an interrupted manner from the bladder neck to vaginal apex. This step usually requires from two to four sutures in sequence. A separate sheet of graft material, either 6 × 8 cm or 8 × 8 cm dependent upon the dimensions of the defect, is suitably sized and affixed to the preplaced sutures in the arcuate internus fascia. The material should be placed loosely under the bladder base from the bladder neck to vaginal apex. The vaginal wall is then closed with a running 2-0 SAS. Apical relocation sutures (if placed) are tied at this juncture.

After completion of the above steps, cystoscopy is again performed to ensure that no penetration of the bladder has occurred, that there is bilateral efflux from both ureteral orifices, and that the bladder base has been corrected with the inlay material. Sling tension is then set and the suprapubic incision closed.

The vaginal pack is removed 12 to 24 hours postoperatively and the patient performs a voiding trial. If this is not successful, the Foley catheter is reinserted or intermittent catheterization may begin. Alternatively, if a suprapubic tube has been placed at the time of surgery the patient cycles the suprapubic tube during at-home convalescence. Lifting (greater than 5 lb) is avoided for 6 weeks.

Alternative Methods for Suspension

Vaginal /Paravaginal Repair

This procedure does not use inlay material and instead utilizes the APTF as the strong anchoring point for sutures placed through the anterior vaginal wall on either side of the bladder base (7). The surgical field is prepared as above with dissection of the retropubic space, which frees the base of the bladder from the pelvic floor. Once the dissection is complete, the bladder base is retracted medially with curved retractors and the ischial spine is palpated. A 1-0 permanent suture is placed into the white line just distal to the spine. A series of 1-0 sutures are then placed in sequence to the urethrovesical junction (usually four to six). These sutures are then passed through the pubocervical fascia and vaginal wall beneath the bladder base from the bladder neck to apex of vagina. These steps are repeated on the contralateral side and then all are tied to reduce the cystocele. Subsequent placating sutures of 1-0 delayed absorbable material may be used to plicate the vaginal muscularis prior to closure. Postoperative care is similar to the inlay procedure.

Needle Suspension

These procedures rely on a sequence of sutures placed through the pubocervical fascia that are then secured to the anterior rectus muscle. Preparation is as similar to the previously described inlay repair. Two parallel anterior vaginal wall incisions that extend from the bladder neck to vaginal apex are created. These incisions are on either side of the midline in an oblique fashion so as to be able to reflect the lateral wall off the underlying anterior vaginal wall. Once the incisions are completed, sharp dissection is carried out laterally to enter the retropubic space and identify the attenuated edge of the pubocervical fascia. In addition, the location of the cardinal ligament complex at the apex of the vagina is identified on either side.

After vaginal dissection has been completed, four (four-corner suspension) or six (six-point suspension) suspending sutures in pairs, two proximal (at the vaginal apex), two midvaginal, and two distal (level of the bladder neck), of no. 1 polypropylene are placed that incorporate the pubocervical fascia and, at the vaginal apex, the cardinal ligaments. The distal sutures are placed in the midurethral complex. These sutures are then transferred from the vaginal to the suprapubic incision using needle carriers placed as previously described. This repair may be augmented with SAS mesh or other inlay materials affixed to the pubocervical fascia with 0 or 2-0 SASs or PPS sutures. The vaginal wall is then closed with a 2-0 absorbable suture and then the suprapubic incision is irrigated and closed (5).

Repair of Isolated Central Defect Cystoceles

Repair of isolated defects with a well-supported, nonobstructive urethra may be performed with plication of the pubocervical fascia or with interposition grafts (Fig. 41–4). Urethral sphincteric function should be eval-

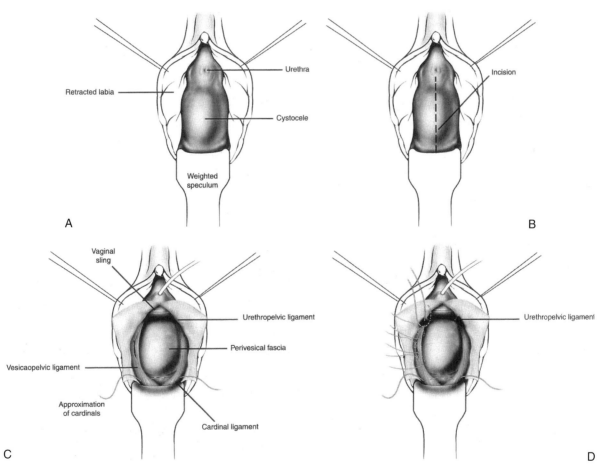

FIG. 41–4. A: Demonstration of the central cystocele defect with preservation of the lateral vaginal sulci. **B:** A midline incision is created from the midurethra to vaginal apex in the vaginal wall. The retropubic space is developed on either side of the urethra and bladder. **C:** The vesicopelvic ligaments are identified as are the cardinal ligaments. The cardinal ligament complex is reconstituted in the midline with sutures so as to provide apical support for the repair. **D:** For those repairs involving suture suspension techniques, sutures may be placed throughout the vesical pelvic ligament and transposed from the vaginal to suprapubic area for subsequent stabilization (the six-point repair). These steps are repeated on the contralateral side. *Continued on next page*

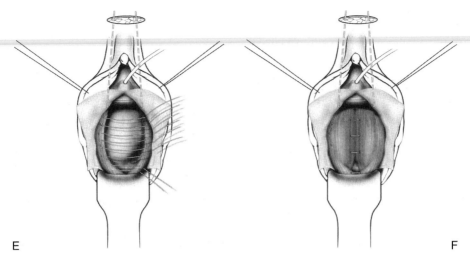

FIG. 41–4 *Continued*. E: In those circumstances where plication alone is performed, sutures are placed across the base of the bladder from the vesicopelvic ligament on one side to the vesicopelvic ligament on the contralateral side and the two structures are reapproximated. **F:** Completion of combined plication repair with needle suspension of the proximal urethra and bladder neck.

uated to determine if a concurrent sling is indicated. Patient preparation, positioning, and placement are similar to the previously described procedure. The anterior vaginal wall is infiltrated with injectable saline and a single midline incision is formed from the bladder neck to vaginal apex. The anterior vaginal wall is then dissected off the underlying attenuated pubocervical fascia utilizing countertraction with Allis clamps facilitated by the operative finger of the nondominant hand. This technique splays and flattens the tissue, easing dissection and identification of the correct surgical plane. The dissection is continued to the level of perivesical fascia. Once this is reached, the retropubic space is entered and the defect is defined from the introitus to vaginal apex.

Repair commences with reapproximation of the pubocervical fascia with 2-0 interrupted SASs along the base of the bladder from the bladder neck to vaginal apex. This effectively relocates the cystocele behind the reconstituted pelvic floor. This repair may be bolstered with mesh to further strengthen the fascial reapproximation. The cardinal ligaments should also be reapproximated in the midline to secure the apex of the repair. The cardinal ligaments are then corrected with interrupted 2-0 absorbable sutures.

Cystoscopy is performed to ensure that the bladder is intact and there is ureteral efflux. Vaginal closure is then carried out utilizing a running 2-0 absorbable suture.

Abdominal Repairs

The abdominal approach for cystocele repairs is exclusively for lateral defects (Fig. 41–5). This approach yields superb visualization of the lateral defect and surrounding structures. Also, retropubic incontinence procedures or slings may both be performed with this approach. Prepa-

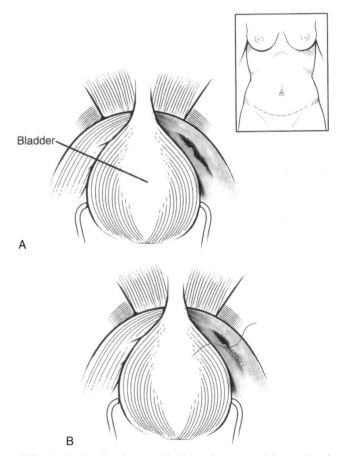

FIG. 41–5. Positioning and incision for retropubic repair of lateral cystocele defects. A Pfannenstiel incision is made in the lower abdomen to expose the retropubic space. The dissection exposes the obturator internus fascia, and the fascial defect is identified as seen in the right aspect of the diagram. Using interrupted delayed absorbable or permanent sutures the disrupted fascial edges are reapproximated. The sutures are placed from the ischial spine to the level of urethrovesical angle as noted.

ration includes positioning the patient in the low lithotomy or frog-legged position so as to have sterile access to the vagina during the procedure. A lower-abdominal incision is made, which can either be horizontal or transverse.

The retropubic space is entered and developed on either side of the bladder and urethra so as to identify the obturator internus fascia. This is best performed bluntly, with the suction tip or a sponge stick, so as to sweep the overlying adipose tissue from the underlying structures. The ischial spine is identified and the white line traced from its origin at the ischial spine to the urethrovesical angle. The fascial defect will often be easily identifiable once this dissection is complete. The operating surgeon may also place a sponge stick or the nondominant hand in the vagina to displace the vaginal wall superiorly and better demonstrate the edges of the fascial defect.

Once dissection is complete, interrupted sutures (four to six) are placed in the disrupted edges of the defect so as to reappose the obturator internus fascia and the medially displaced pubocervical fascia. After all sutures are placed they are tied sequentially. Prior to closure of the abdomen, cystoscopy is performed to exclude suture distortion or entry into the bladder and confirm ureteral efflux.

OUTCOMES

Complications

The most common complication associated with repair of a cystocele is injury to the underlying structures such as the urethra, bladder, or, in rare occurrences, other pelvic viscera including the small or large bowel. Incidental cystostomy may be repaired with layered closure, nonopposing suture lines, and maximization of urinary drainage. Although rarely caused by this procedure, uretero- or vesicovaginal fistulas represent the most severe complication. Injury to the bowel should be closed with layered SASs and silk. Large-bowel injury necessitates prolongation of antibiotic coverage and change in the postoperative diet.

Cystoscopic evaluation intraoperatively should indicate the possibility of ureteral obstruction with nonreflux from one side. Sutures may be removed at this time prior to completion of the procedure. Stenting should only be considered in the case of significant disruption or trauma to the ureteric orifice. Nonabsorbable suture present in the bladder may result in stone formation or recurrent infections and should be removed and relocated.

Postoperative voiding dysfunction may be caused by detrusor instability, urethral obstruction, or recurrence of the cystocele. Resolution of preoperative urgency will occur in up to 70% of patients; however, *de novo* detrusor instability will occur in approximately 5%. Urinary retention may occur in up to 20% of patients on a short-term

basis (less than 4 weeks). Long-term obstruction should occur in less than 1% of patients. Poor or inadequate detrusor contractility may be a reason for incomplete emptying and should be predictable on the basis of preoperative urodynamic evaluation. Long-term catheterization may be indicated in these patients.

Long-term dyspareunia, pelvic pain, or vaginal stenosis may ensue from aggressive plication and/or excision of vaginal mucosa. However, the majority of women appear to have improved dyspareunia after surgery, largely due to resolution or improvement of stress urinary incontinence. In those women who had deterioration of sexual functioning, the majority appear to have this associated with simultaneous posterior colporrhaphy (approximately 10%). Vaginal shortening from inadequate apical reconstruction also may contribute to dyspareunia. Finally, late-onset apical prolapse and enterocele formation may occur due to alterations of the vaginal axis and insufficient repair of the apex. Meticulous attention to apical reconstruction should avert this consequence.

Results

Long-term results for these procedures are still undergoing evaluation. Results should reflect cure of prolapse and remediation of incontinence. Risk factors for operative failure may include advanced age, hormonal depletion, inadequate preoperative identification of all anatomic defects, incomplete surgical reconstruction, or technical failure. In addition, obesity, chronic pulmonary disease, bowel dysmotility (chronic constipation), and genetic predisposition have also been implicated in surgical failure. Interpositional grafts appear to convey a significant reduction in prolapse recurrence (to approximately 10% to 20%). Plication repairs have rates of recurrence (for incontinence) ranging from 20% to 50% and from 9% to 66% for incontinence. A recent pooled analysis of anterior repair procedures for incontinence demonstrated a cure rate of 65% (31% to 91%) and a complication rate of 14% (4).

Vaginal paravaginal repairs have reported failure rates of 3% to 14% at 1 year. The six-corner bladder suspension has shown reasonable results at 2 years. Combined repairs have an associated risk of cystocele (5%) and enterocele (8%) formation, but have been reported to have a 94% success rate for cure of incontinence (8).

REFERENCES

1. Bump RC, Mattiasson A, Bo K, et al. The standardization of terminology of pelvic organ prolapse and pelvic floor dysfunction. *Am J Obstet Gyneol* 1996;175:10–17.
2. Delancey JOL. Anatomic aspects of vaginal eversion after hysterectomy. *Am J Obstet Gynecol* 1992;166:1717–1728.
3. Kobashi KC, Mee SL, Leach GE. A new technique for cystocele repair and transvaginal sling: the cadaveric prolapse repair and sling (CAPS). *Urology* 2000;56:9–14.
4. Kohli N, Karram MM. Surgery for genuine stress incontinence: vaginal

procedures, injections, and the artificial urinary sphincter. In: Walter MD, Karram MM, eds. *Urogynecology and reconstructive pelvic surgery*, 2nd ed. St Louis, MO: Mosby, 1999:171–196.

5. Raz S, Stothers L, Young GP, et al. Vaginal wall sling for anatomical incontinence and intrinsic sphincter dysfunction: Efficacy and outcome analysis. *J Urol* 1996;156:166–170.

6. Sand PK, Koduri S, Lobel RW, Winkler HA, Tomesko J, Culligan PJ, Goldberg R. Prospective randomized trial of polyglactin 910 mesh to prevent recurrence of cystoceles and rectoceles. *Am J Obstet Gynecol* 2001;184:1357–1362.

7. Shull BL, Benn SJ, Kuehl TJ. Surgical management of prolapse of the anterior vaginal segment: an analysis of support defects, operative morbidity, and anatomic outcome. *Am J Obstet Gynecol* 1994;171: 1429–1439.

8. Weber AM, Walters MD. Anterior vaginal prolapse: review of anatomy and techniques of surgical repair. *Obstet Gynecol* 1997;89:311–318.

CHAPTER 42

Transvaginal Enterocele Repair

Harriette M. Scarpero and Victor W. Nitti

An enterocele is a hernia of the peritoneal Douglas' pouch extending caudally between the vagina and rectum. It usually contains small bowel with or without omentum. Nichols described four types of enteroceles: congenital, pulsion, traction, and iatrogenic (7). The two types of enteroceles that urologists most often encounter are traction enterocele associated with anterior vaginal wall prolapse such as cystocele and iatrogenic enterocele that follows surgery on the anterior vaginal wall. The true prevalence of enterocele is not known but is estimated to be 0.1% to 17%. Women who present with pelvic prolapse have a combination of pelvic floor support defects including cystocele, rectocele enterocele, and uterine prolapse.

To understand the pathophysiology of an enterocele one must first consider normal pelvic anatomy. After hysterectomy, the apical portion of the vagina is supported by sheet-like extensions of the endopelvic fascia that attach it to the pelvic side wall and levator ani fascia, referred to as the paracolpium (Fig. 42–1), which provides two levels of support (4). Level I, or upper support, "suspends" the vagina, attaching it to the pelvic side wall. Level II, or midvaginal support, which includes the pubocervical fascia, "attaches" the midvagina more directly to the pelvic walls, including the levator fascia and arcus tendineous. Damage to midlevel support usually results in cystocele and rectocele, while damage to upper-level support results in vaginal (or uterine) prolapse, including enterocele. As a result of this support, the distal vagina forms an approximately 45-degree angle with the vertical line while the proximal vagina forms a 110-degree angle and sits almost horizontally over the levator plate (Fig. 42–2) (8). When there is an alteration anatomy, for example after incontinence surgery, fascial supports may be compromised, predisposing the patient to an enterocele (Fig. 42–3) (8).

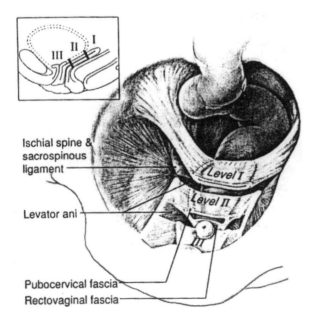

Ischial spine & sacrospinous ligament

Levator ani

Pubocervical fascia
Rectovaginal fascia

FIG. 42–1. Level I (suspension) and level II (attachment). In level I the paracolpium suspends the vagina from the lateral pelvic walls. Fibers of level I extend both vertically and also posteriorly toward the sacrum. In level II the vagina is attached to the arcus tendineus fasciae pelvis and superior fascia of levator ani. (From DeLancey JOL. Anatomic aspects of vaginal eversion after hysterectomy. *Am J Obstet Gynecol* 1992;166:1717–1728, with permission.)

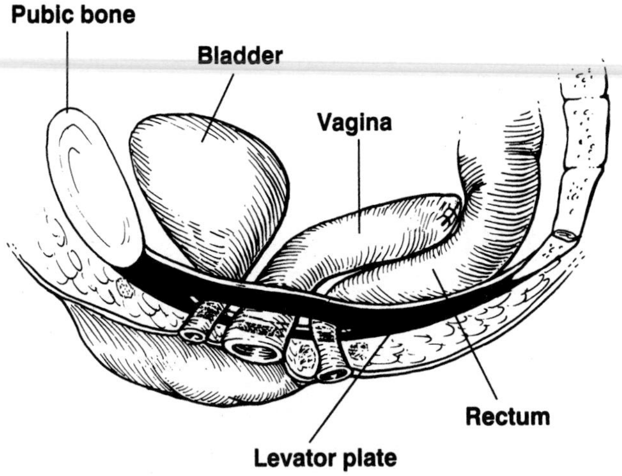

Pubic bone

Bladder

Vagina

Rectum

Levator plate

FIG. 42–2. Normal pelvic anatomy and support after hysterectomy. The horizontal levator plate supports the rectum and vagina proximally and posteriorly before opening at the levator hiatus. The bladder and urethra are located anteriorly. Note the axis of the proximal vagina, which is approximately 110 degrees with the vertical. (From Nitti VW. Transvaginal enterocele repair with variations. *Contemp Urol* 1994;6: 50–64, with permission.)

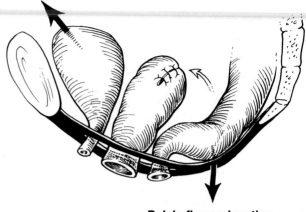

Bladder-neck suspension

Pelvic floor relaxation

FIG. 42–3. The effect of anterior vaginal wall surgery (e.g., bladder neck suspension, culposuspension) in the face of uncorrected posterior pelvic floor relaxation. The anterior vaginal wall is now well supported while the lax levator plate sags downward. The result is an altered vaginal axis with the posterior vaginal wall and vault no longer supported by the levator plate. These areas are now subject to increases in abdominal pressure and are predisposed to further prolapse (i.e., enterocele and rectocele). (From Nitti VW. Transvaginal enterocele repair with variations. *Contemp Urol* 1994;6: 50–64, with permission.)

DIAGNOSIS

Prolapse is described in terms of anterior, apical, and posterior as opposed to "cystocele, enterocele (or uterine prolapse), and rectocele." This is because most prolapse is multicompartment and the support of one pelvic structure is dependent on the support of other structures. Second, it is sometimes difficult to tell on physical exam exactly what organs are prolapsed. An enterocele may present as anterior prolapse (usually in conjunction with a cystocele), apical prolapse, posterior prolapse, or a combination depending on where the break in support is. It is also important to ascertain if the vaginal vault is prolapsed as this will affect the type of enterocele repair performed.

The extent of prolapse is first evaluated with the patient in the lithotomy position. The presence of urethral mobility, stress incontinence, and anterior, apical, and posterior prolapse should be assessed. The patient should be instructed to cough and perform a Valsalva maneuver to assess the effect of increased abdominal pressure on the prolapse. With the prolapse reduced (manually or with a ring forceps, packing, or pessary), the patient should be asked to cough and perform a Valsalva maneuver to evaluate for occult stress incontinence. To ascertain the full extent of the prolapse, the patient should also be examined in the standing position with one foot elevated on a stool. The degree of prolapse of the various compartments may be quantified using a variety of systems. Currently, the Pelvic Organ Prolapse Quantification System (POP-Q) is the most comprehensive (1). Imaging studies including cystogram, defecography, ultrasound, computed tomography (CT) scan, and magnetic reso-

nance imaging (MRI) may also be used to help define pelvic anatomy.

INDICATIONS FOR SURGERY

In general, the degree of pelvic prolapse (including enterocele) and the severity of the symptoms it causes are the main indications for treatment. Small enteroceles are often asymptomatic and need not be treated. In general, treatment is driven by the patient's symptoms, which include an uncomfortable feeling of prolapse that may limit activity, obstructive voiding, and constipation. Often, enteroceles are associated with other forms of prolapse and stress incontinence, which may ultimately drive the patient toward treatment. The patient's age, general health, performance status, degree of sexual activity, and expectations from treatment will play a role in the type of treatment or surgical procedure performed. Finally, some patients may suffer serious sequela of prolapse such as hydronephrosis from ureteral obstruction or urinary retention from urethral obstruction.

ALTERNATIVE THERAPY

Nonsurgical treatment involves supporting the pelvic floor with a device such as a pessary. Pessaries come in a variety of shapes and sizes and are fit depending of the patient's size, anatomy, and the components of the prolapse. Many women find pessaries a satisfying alternative to surgery that can comfortably control the symptoms of pelvic prolapse, while others are unable to hold a pessary due to their specific anatomy or other symptoms such as discomfort, bothersome discharge, or bleeding. For those women who do not remove the pessary, regular follow-up (every 1 to 3 months) is necessary so the pessary can be removed, cleaned, and replaced and the patient examined.

SURGICAL TECHNIQUE

There are several surgical treatments of enterocele. Prolapse can be approached vaginally or abdominally depending on its degree, patient characteristics, and desired outcomes. While the focus of this chapter is on transvaginal repair, there are situations where the abdominal approach (either open or laparoscopic) is preferred, such as in young women with vaginal vault prolapse or those with failed transvaginal procedures (11). In the frail elderly population, colpocleisis, in which the entire vagina is closed, may be considered. We believe that the vaginal approach to prolapse repair is appropriate for many of the enteroceles encountered in urologic practice.

Transvaginal Enterocele Repair

Transvaginal enterocele repair may be performed either intraperitoneally or extraperitoneally. In most cases, we prefer the intraperitoneal approach; however, in cases where the enterocele is small or difficult to find an extraperitoneal approach may be appropriate. There are several variations of the repair depending on the degree of prolapse and whether or not a vault suspension is necessary, yet all variations start with the basic intraperitoneal repair.

The patient is placed in the dorsal lithotomy position and prepped, with attention to adequately scrub the inside of the vagina in preparation for surgery. The labia are retracted with silk sutures. If an antiincontinence surgery such as a pubovaginal sling is to be performed concomitantly, a suprapubic tube may be placed at the beginning of surgery either by the Lowsley tractor technique or percutaneously. A Scott ring retractor (Lone Star Medical Corp.) is useful in exposing the operative field.

The first step is to isolate, repair, and remove the enterocele sac. This is begun by grasping the enterocele with two Allis clamps and bringing it outside of the vaginal introitus. A longitudinal incision is made in the vaginal wall along the entire length of the enterocele (Fig. 42–4). The vaginal wall is then carefully dissected away from the underlying pubocervical fascia and enterocele sac. In the initial dissection, care must be taken to stay very superficial and develop the proper plane. This is best accomplished by placing the curve of the Metzenbaum scissors against the vaginal wall. A finger can be placed on the outside of the vaginal wall to stabilize the initial dissection. Once the proper plane is entered, it is usually easy to

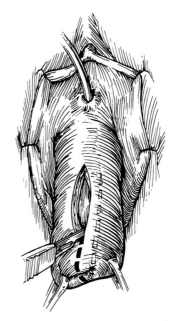

FIG. 42–4. The vaginal wall is grasped with two Allis clamps and brought outside the vaginal introitus. A midline incision is made. (From Nitti VW. Transvaginal enterocele repair with variations. *Contemp Urol* 1994;6:50–64, with permission.)

dissect the vaginal wall away from the underlying enterocele sac. Care taken here will prevent early entry into the peritoneal cavity. The dissection of the enterocele is continued all the way to the neck of the enterocele sac (Fig. 42–5). After the enterocele has been completely isolated,

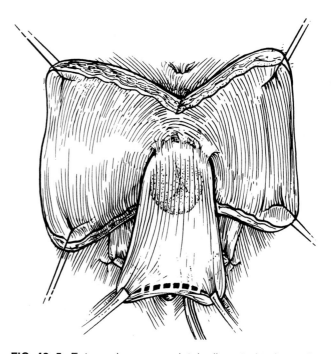

FIG. 42–5. Enterocele sac completely dissected to its neck. (From Nitti VW. Transvaginal enterocele repair with variations. *Contemp Urol* 1994;6:50–64, with permission.)

the sac is opened and the peritoneal cavity is entered. At this time, one may see small bowel, omentum, or ovary and fallopian tube in cases where previous hysterectomy without oophorectomy has been performed (Fig. 42–6).

The next step is closure of the enterocele defect or Douglas' pouch. Retraction of the peritoneal contents is best performed using a moist pediatric lap pad and a narrow Deaver retractor. Placing the patient in the Trendelenburg position so that abdominal organs fall slightly cephalad assists this. The enterocele repair begins posteriorly while the abdominal contents are retracted anteriorly using the Deaver. A no. 1 polyglactic acid (PGA) suture is first placed through the peritoneum and into the prerectal fascia that overlies the rectum (Fig. 42–7). A circumferential closure of the defect is then performed by placing the pursestring suture laterally in the right uterosacral–cardinal ligament complex, anteriorly in the peritoneum, overlying the base of the bladder, laterally on the left in the uterosacral–cardinal ligament complex, and finally again posteriorly in the prerectal fascia (Fig. 42–8). After this pursestring suture has been placed, a second one is placed in the identical structures in close proximity to the first. Care should be taken to place these sutures deep enough to ensure that adequate vaginal depth can be achieved. After the second pursestring suture has been placed, a third no. 1 PGA suture is placed from the right to the left uterosacral–cardinal ligament complex. This suture helps reinforce the repair and also will be left tagged to help identify this complex later, for

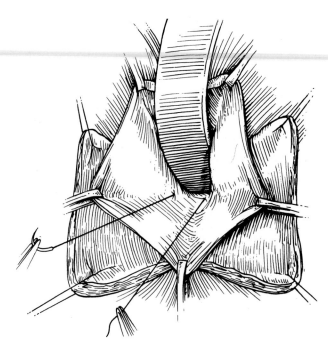

FIG. 42–7. A Deaver retractor is used to retract abdominal contents so that pursestring sutures can be placed. (From Nitti VW. Transvaginal enterocele repair with variations. *Contemp Urol* 1994;6:50–64, with permission.)

example, if a uterosacral ligament suspension is performed. After all sutures are placed, the assistant cinches down and places tension on one of the pursestrings while the surgeon ties the other. After this has been tied, the second pursestring is tied in a similar manner, followed by the uterosacral–cardinal ligament suture. The two pursestring sutures may now be cut while the third is left tagged. The excess enterocele sac may be excised and the ends oversewn with a 2-0 PGA suture (Fig. 42–9). If only a simple enterocele repair is performed, the tagged suture may now be cut.

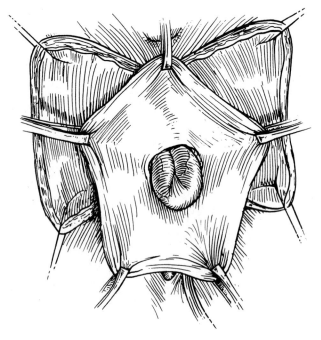

FIG. 42–6. The enterocele sac is opened, exposing intraabdominal contents. (From Nitti VW. Transvaginal enterocele repair with variations. *Contemp Urol* 1994;6:50–64, with permission.)

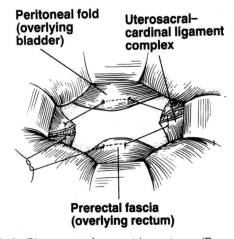

Peritoneal fold (overlying bladder)

Uterosacral–cardinal ligament complex

Prerectal fascia (overlying rectum)

FIG. 42–8. Placement of pursestring sutures. (From Nitti VW. Transvaginal enterocele repair with variations. *Contemp Urol* 1994;6:50–64, with permission.)

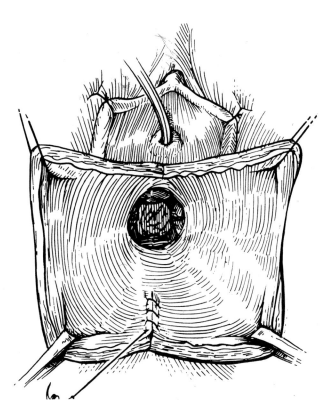

FIG. 42–9. Completed closure of enterocele with excision of excess sac. (From Nitti VW. Transvaginal enterocele repair with variations. *Contemp Urol* 1994;6:50–64, with permission.)

Cystoscopy is performed to document that there has been no injury to the bladder and that the bladder neck and proximal urethra elevate and coapt nicely. Ureteral injury is ruled out by intravenous indigo carmine. Excess vaginal wall is then excised, and the vaginal wall is closed with a 2-0 PGA suture incorporating deep tissue to obliterate any dead space. Antibiotic-impregnated vaginal packing is placed for 24 hours.

In some cases of suspected enterocele, the enterocele sac may be very small and difficult to dissect from the bladder or rectum. An extraperitoneal closure of the cul-de-sac may be performed in these cases. In this method the peritoneum over the bladder is sutured to that overlying the rectum with no. 1 PGA sutures placed in an anterior to posterior orientation as in the Halban technique. The placement of these sutures obliterates the space between the bladder and the rectum and will prevent the recurrence of the enterocele.

Enterocele Repair with Vault Suspension

Transvaginal vault suspension procedures may be used with enterocele repair when the vaginal vault has prolapsed to correct all of the fascial defects from a vaginal approach. There are several techniques commonly used to accomplish a transvaginal vault suspension, and the best technique is still debated. We will review the uterosacral ligament suspension, sacrospinous ligament fixation, our preferred method of transvaginal vault suspension, as well as other common methods.

Uterosacral Ligament Suspension

Suspension of the vaginal vault to the uterosacral ligaments preserves a more natural vaginal axis than the sacrospinous ligament fixation. Without the posterior deflection of the vagina caused by fixation to the sacrospinous ligament, the risk of prolapse of the anterior vaginal compartment is reduced. Identification of the uterosacral ligaments posthysterectomy can be difficult. Their origin is at the sacrum, and they reflect anteromedially toward insertion at the cervix. After the uterus and cervix are removed, these ligaments meld into the surrounding connective tissue. The optimum site of fixation to the uterosacral ligament is in the intermediate portion of the ligament, which has fewer vital adjacent structures, is a strong fixation site, and tension has little effect on the nearby ureter. The ischial spine can be used to reliably identify the intermediate portion of the uterosacral ligament. Sutures should be placed at the level of the ischial spine, 1 cm posterior to the anterior most palpable margin of the uterosacral ligament on tension. The uterosacral ligament is very close to the intrapelvic ureter and the ureter can be injured if incorporated by one of the sutures or kinked by traction from a suture. The intraperitoneal approach, however, allows for better visualization and thus better suture placement as compared to the visualization in the narrow, deep pararectal space.

Using the enterocele repair technique described above, the uterosacral plicating suture that was left tagged can be fixed to the vaginal apex. In either case, the vagina can be foreshortened. The uterosacral ligaments are attached to the ipsilateral vaginal cuff, thereby increasing vaginal depth, obliterating the cul-de-sac, supporting the vaginal cuff, and restoring the normal proximal vaginal anatomy above the levator plate.

Sacrospinous Ligament Fixation

This technique is used to correct vault prolapse in cases in which the anterior vaginal wall is well supported. In this case, vaginal depth and axis are restored by posterior fixation of the vaginal vault to the sacrospinous ligaments. The sacrospinous ligament stretches from the ischial spine to the sacrum and is covered by the coccygeus muscle.

As the enterocele repair is completed, the posterior vaginal wall must be opened far enough distally to facilitate dissection to the sacrospinous ligament. When a simultaneous rectocele repair is to be performed, the entire posterior vaginal wall is opened through the perineum. After the posterior vaginal wall is incised in the midline, it is gently dissected laterally from the underlying prerectal fascia for a short distance. Next, the sacrospinous ligament must be identified. This is done by penetrating the right or left rectal pillar (pararectal fascia) sharply and entering the pararectal space (Fig. 42–10). Blunt dissection of the pararectal space can be performed with a combination of finger dissection and the use of deep Breisky–Navratil retractors. This dissection is performed until the sacrospinous ligament is palpated and overlying coccygeus muscle is seen. The Breisky–Navratil retractors will help expose the ligament. Once the ligament is identified, a no. 1 permanent braided suture is placed through the ligament and coccygeus muscle complex 2 cm medial to the ischial spine, which is also identified by palpation. It is important to place the suture in this position to avoid injury to the pudendal nerve and vessels, which run just below the ischial spine. It is also important to include the strong ligament in addition to the overlying coccygeus muscle. These tasks can be made easier by carefully dissecting over the ligament with a spreading motion of the Metzenbaum scissors and with the aid of a Kitner dissector. Visualization of the ligament itself helps avoid incorrect placement of the sutures. Another helpful tool is the Capio CL transvaginal suture-capturing device (Boston Scientific). This tool allows for placement of the suture and retrieval of the needle in this deep and narrow space with just the depression of a lever on the instrument's end. It has greatly simplified suture placement in our procedures. Tension should be placed on the suture to make certain that it is in the strong ligament. A second suture should be placed adjacent to the first. Each of these sutures is then placed through the vaginal wall, excluding the epithelial layer at the level of the dome, approximately 1 cm apart, and left untied. If a rectocele is present, it is repaired at this time. The dome of the vagina can be directed under finger guidance to the deepest possible portion, where it will be fixed. The vaginal wall is then closed with a running interlocking 2-0 PGA suture, and then the previously placed sacrospinous ligament fixation sutures are individually tied. Antibiotic-impregnated vaginal packing is then placed.

After sacrospinous ligament fixation, recurrences usually occur in the anterior vaginal compartment. This observation has led some investigators to try a modification of the sacrospinous ligament fixation meant to reduce recurrences in the anterior compartment by avoiding the downward deflection of the vagina. The anterior approach to sacrospinous ligament fixation approaches the ligament from the retropubic space and dissection of the ipsilateral paravaginal space from the level of the bladder neck to the ischial spine. Theoretically this approach should reduce postoperative vaginal narrowing and posterolateral deviation of the upper vagina, resulting in improved functional outcome. An additional modification is the bilateral anterior sacrospinous ligament fixation. Bilateral fixation should provide additional support and longevity over a single fixation point and may also increase the area of the vagina over the pelvic floor, improving its ability to withstand increases in intraabdominal pressure. A limitation of this technique is that not all women have vaginal anatomy that is able to stretch to bilateral ligaments.

Iliococcygeus (Prespinous) Fixation

Iliococcygeus or prespinous fixation for vaginal vault prolapse is yet another method to suspend the vaginal vault created to address what was considered to be a high rate of anterior compartment prolapse after sacrospinous ligament fixation and damage to the pudendal neurovascular bundle. In an iliococcygeus fixation the vaginal apex is fixed bilaterally to the iliococcygeus fascia using one no. 1 polydioxanone suture. The incision and dissection are carried out posteriorly. The rectovaginal fascia is dissected off the posterior vaginal wall laterally all the way to the pelvic sidewall. The ischial spine and sacrospinous ligament are identified as a landmark for the iliococcygeus fascia, which will be found anterior to them.

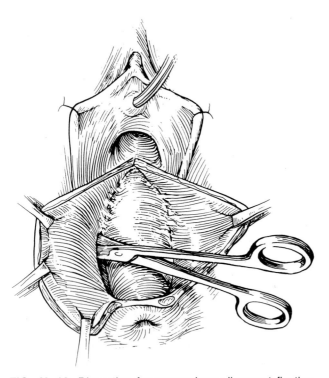

FIG. 42–10. Dissection for sacrospinous ligament fixation. The rectal pillars are sharply penetrated and the pararectal space entered. The space is widened with blunt dissection to expose the superior surface of the pelvic diaphragm. The sacrospinous ligament can then be palpated and the coccygeus muscle overlying it can be seen. (From Nitti VW. Transvaginal enterocele repair with variations. *Contemp Urol* 1994;6:50–64, with permission.)

Levator Myorraphy

Proponents of this technique argue that it avoids possible damage to the pudendal nerve and vessels that can occur with a sacrospinous ligament fixation. The basic goal is to use the levator shelf to recreate the pelvic floor and anchor the upper vagina. As described, cystoscopy is performed at the start of the procedure and for large prolapses a suprapubic tube is placed with the aid of a Lowsley retractor. Incision and dissection are carried out as described for enterocele repair. Once the peritoneum is opened, the levator musculature is identified bilaterally along the pelvic sidewall and lateral to the rectum. The preferred suture is a no. 1 absorbable suture. It is placed deeply into the levator muscle starting 3 cm above the junction of the levator with the rectum. The same suture is used to secure the levator muscle on the contralateral side. With placement of these sutures, there is a possible risk of ligating or kinking one or both ureters.

A second suture is positioned into the body of the levator 1 cm proximal to the previous one. They will be tied across the midline to accomplish the levator myorraphy after closure of the enterocele sac and cystoscopy to confirm ureteral patency. Cystoscopy should be performed again after tying the levator sutures to confirm efflux. If there is any doubt of ureteral patency, the levator sutures may need to be cut and replaced. It is also important to assess the caliber of the upper vagina after tying the levator sutures. The upper vaginal cavity should be able to accept two or three fingers with ease. If not, the more distal of the levator sutures should be removed.

Next, the vaginal apex is affixed to the newly rebuilt levator plate. A no. 6 curved Mayo needle is used to suture the levator myorraphy sutures to the new vaginal apex from inside out, one end of the suture at a time. The proximal and distal suture sets are kept 1 cm apart on the vaginal apex. Finally, the ends of the levator sutures are

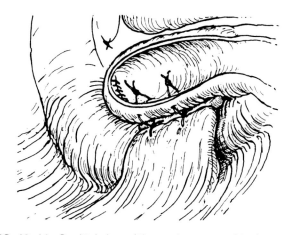

FIG. 42–11. Sagittal view of the vagina secured to the recreated levator plate at the conclusion of levator myorraphy procedure. (From Lemack GE, Zimmern PE, Blander DS. The levator myorraphy repair for vaginal vault prolapse. *Urology* 2000;56[Suppl 6A]:50–54, with permission.)

secured to each other, anchoring the upper vagina to the levator plate (Fig. 42–11).

After completion of the vaginal surgical procedure, the antibiotic-soaked vaginal packing is left in the vagina until the next morning. Patients receive two to three postoperative doses of intravenous antibiotics before they are switched to broad-spectrum oral antibiotic for 7 days. In cases where a suprapubic tube is left indwelling, antibiotics may be continued until normal voiding resumes and all tubes are removed. Patients are usually hospitalized for 24 to 48 hours. They may resume light activity upon discharge but should refrain from intercourse for 6 weeks and heavy lifting and strenuous exercise for up to 12 weeks. Patients should be careful to avoid constipation during the healing process.

OUTCOMES

Complications

In all the above procedures, the major risks are bleeding due to vascular injury, nerve entrapment, ureteral injury or kinking, bowel injury, wound infection, and persistent or recurrent prolapse. During placement of the pursestring sutures of an enterocele repair, one must take care to not disturb the ovarian vessels, which lie near the uterosacral–cardinal complexes. The pudendal vessels and nerve, which lie beneath the sacrospinous ligament, are at high risk of injury during sacrospinous ligament fixation. Pudendal entrapment may occur if sutures are placed too laterally, whereas the sciatic nerve is at risk if the sutures are placed too cephalad. Pelvic and gluteal pain, although usually transient, can occur as a result of injury to the pudendal and sciatic nerves. The intrapelvic ureter is intimately associated with the uterosacral ligaments but can be injured or kinked by any of the transvaginal vault suspensions. Ureteral injury or kinking in cases of vault suspension has a reported rate of 1% to 11% (5). The anterior vaginal compartment is at highest risk for persistent or recurrent prolapse, but in many cases this prolapse may be asymptomatic and does not require reoperation.

Results

Enterocele repair alone is not as common as enterocele repair performed with repair of other support defects and vault prolapse. Success rates for enterocele repair are in general reported with outcomes of concomitant procedures. The recurrence rate of enterocele after repair and culdoplasty is 0% to 4% (2,3). The reported success rates of transvaginal sacrospinous ligament fixation vary from 81% to 100% (6,9). At follow-up of the sacrospinous ligament fixation at 4.8 years, 119 of 123 patients had no sign of urinary incontinence or prolapse. Four patients (3.25%) showed recurrent vaginal vault prolapse (6,9).

The anterior approach offers a statistically significant anatomic outcome advantage versus the posterior approach in regard to mean total vaginal length and lower rates of anterior vaginal wall relaxation. Rates of postoperative dyspareunia were equivalent in both groups.

Uterosacral ligament fixation has been shown to be effective and durable in several recent studies (5). In 289 patients 87% had no persistent or recurrent prolapse at any site. Five percent had grade-2 or greater persistent or recurrent prolapse of the anterior compartment, which was the site of most postoperative support defects (10). Another study that provided assessment by quality of life instruments Urogenital Distress Inventory (UDI)-6 and IIQ-7, as well as by exam, found that 89% of patients were satisfied with their surgical outcome and showed improvement in all aspects of daily living (5). There was a 5.5% reoperation rate for prolapse in one or more segments, however.

REFERENCES

1. Bump RC, Mattiasson A, Bo K, et al. The standardization of terminology of female pelvic organ prolapse and pelvic floor dysfunction. *Am J Obstet Gynecol* 1996; 175:10–17.
2. Comiter CV, Vasavada SP, Raz S. Transvaginal culdosuspension: technique and results. *Urology* 1999;54:819–822.
3. Cruikshank SH, Kovac SR. Randomized comparison of 3 surgical methods used at the time of vaginal hysterectomy to prevent posterior enterocele. *Am J Obstet Gynecol* 1999;180:859–865.
4. Delancey JOL Anatomic aspects of vaginal eversion after hysterectomy. *Am J Obstet Gynecol* 1992;166:1717–1728.
5. Karram M, Goldwasser S, Kleeman S, et al. High uterosacral vaginal vault suspension with fascial reconstruction for vaginal repair of enterocele and vaginal vault prolapse. *Am J Obstet Gynecol* 2001;185:1339–1342.
6. Lantzsch T, Goepel C, Wolters M, et al. Sacrospinous ligament fixation for vaginal vault prolapse. *Arch Gynecol Obstet* 2001;265:21–25.
7. Nichols DH. Types of enterocele and principles underlying choice of operation for repair. *Obstet Gynecol* 1972;40:257.
8. Nitti VW. Transvaginal enterocele repair, with variations. *Contemp Urol* 1994;6:50–64.
9. Paraiso MF, Ballard LA, Walters MD, et al. Pelvic support defects and visceral and sexual function in women treated with sacrospinous ligament suspension and pelvic reconstruction. *Am J Obstet Gynecol* 1996;175:1423–1431.
10. Shull BL, Bachofen C, Coates KW, et al. A transvaginal approach to repair of apical and other associated sites of pelvic organ prolapse with uterosacral ligaments. *Am J Obstet Gynecol* 2000;183:1365–1373.
11. Sze EH, Kohli N, Miklos JR, et al. A retrospective comparison of abdominal sacrocolpopexy with Burch colposuspension versus sacrospinous fixation with transvaginal needle suspension for the management of vaginal vault prolapse and coexisting stress incontinence. *Int Urogynecol J Pelvic Floor Dysfunct* 1999;10:390–393.

CHAPTER 43

Anatomy of the Female Pelvic Floor

Nirit Rosenblum, Karyn S. Eilber, and Shlomo Raz

Female pelvic anatomy is a complex combination of muscles, ligaments, nerves, and blood vessels that act dynamically to provide support for the urethra, bladder, uterus, and rectum. An understanding of normal mechanisms of pelvic support are essential in the evaluation of women with voiding complaints, urinary incontinence, and bowel dysfunction related to pelvic floor relaxation. This chapter will focus on normal female pelvic anatomy, including the supporting structures relevant to voiding dysfunction and incontinence, as well as the pathophysiology of pelvic floor relaxation, with a description of the various components of pelvic organ prolapse.

PELVIC SUPPORTING STRUCTURES

Bone

Passive support of the pelvic floor is provided by the bony structures, which act as anchors for the important muscular and fascial structures comprising the pelvic floor. The pubic rami, ischial spines, and sacrum represent the anchoring points of the true bony pelvis, which is made up of pubis, ilium, ischium, sacrum, and coccyx (4). The pelvic floor is diamond shaped with the pubic symphysis and sacrum at the anterior and posterior apices while the ischial spines serve as lateral anchors. The pelvic floor can be further subdivided into anterior and posterior compartments by drawing a line between the two ischial spines.

Ligaments

The sacrospinous ligaments span the posterior portion of the pelvic floor, from the ischial spines to the anterolateral aspect of the sacrum and coccyx. The coccygeus muscle is found between the ischial spines and the lateral aspect of the sacrum and coccyx, overlying the sacrospinous ligament, and is an important landmark in vaginal surgery. Above the coccygeus muscle lies the sci-

atic nerve and its plexus, while the pudendal nerve and vessels lie lateral (Alcock's canal). Medially, the sacrospinous ligament fuses with the sacrotuberous ligament (2). Anteriorly, the tendinous arc, a curvilinear condensation of pelvic fascia arising from the obturator internus muscle, runs between the ischial spines and the lower portion of the pubic symphysis. This crucial structure provides a musculofascial origin for the majority of the anterior pelvic diaphragm, allowing its attachment to the bony pelvis. The tendinous arc flanks the urethra and bladder neck anteriorly and rectum posteriorly, providing lateral attachment of the pelvic diaphragm and its ligaments (4).

The perineal body is a tendinous structure located in the midline of the perineum between the anus and the vaginal introitus that provides a central point of fixation for the transverse perineal musculature (7). This anchoring site provides a second level of pelvic support to the posterior vaginal wall and rectum, incorporating the levator ani and transverse perineal musculature as well as the external anal sphincter.

Musculature

The striated musculature comprising the pelvic floor acts as a supporting structure for the visceral contents of the abdominopelvic cavity as well as a dynamic organ involved in maintenance of urinary and fecal continence. The pelvic diaphragm is composed of the levator ani and coccygeus muscles. The levator ani muscle group and its fascia provide the most critical support for the pelvic viscera, acting as the true muscular pelvic floor. The levator ani group is composed of the pubococcygeus, ischiococcygeus, and iliococcygeus, named according to their origin from the pelvic sidewall (6). This broad sheet of muscular tissue extends from the undersurface of the pubic symphysis to the pelvic surface of the ischial spines, taking origin from the tendinous arc laterally. The anterior

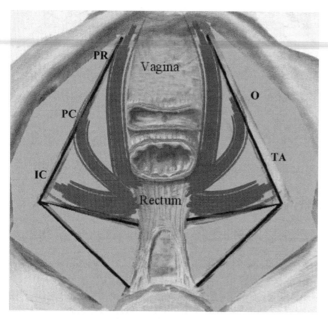

FIG. 43–1. Schematic diagram of the striated musculature of the pelvic floor. PR, puborectalis; PC, pubococcygeus; IC, iliococcygeus; O, obturator muscle; TA, tendinous arc of the obturator muscle.

muscle group, primarily made up of pubococcygeus (puborectalis) with its overlying endopelvic fascia, directly attaches to the bladder, urethra, vagina, uterus, and rectum, actively contributing to visceral control (Fig. 43–1). This important muscular support mechanism is crucial during times of suddenly increased intraabdominal pressure (4).

The posterior muscle group consists of the posterior portion of the levator ani and the coccygeus muscle. Their points of origin include the more posterior portions of the tendinous arc and the ischial spines. The two sides fuse in the midline posterior to the rectum and attach to the coccyx. This plate of horizontal musculature spans from the rectal hiatus to the coccyx and allows maintenance of the

normal vaginal and uterine axis. The upper vagina and uterine cervix lie on this horizontal plane created by the levator plate. This posterior muscle group is active at rest and contracts further during rectus abdominis contraction, maintaining proper vaginal axis (4).

Midline apertures in the levator ani group, collectively referred to as the levator hiatus, allow passage of the urethra, vagina, and rectum. Adjacent fascial attachments provide support to these pelvic viscera as they exit the pelvis, fashioning a "hammock" of horizontal support (5). The bladder, proximal vagina, and rectum rest on the levator floor and become coapted against it during periods of increased intraabdominal pressure. Resting tone of the levator muscle, as well as reflex and voluntary contraction, acts to pull the vagina and rectum forward, thereby preventing incontinence of both urine and stool. These active mechanisms of pelvic floor support maintain both urinary and fecal continence.

ANTERIOR VAGINAL SUPPORT

The fascia overlying the pelvic floor musculature plays a critical role in pelvic support. The abdominal portion of the fascia is referred to as the *endopelvic fascia* and represents a continuation of the abdominal transversalis fascia (4). The levator ani muscle is covered superiorly and inferiorly by a fascial layer (Fig. 43–2). The two fascial layers split at the levator hiatus to cover the pelvic organs that traverse it. The superior or intraabdominal segment (endopelvic fascia) and the inferior or vaginal side of the levator fascia together constitute the pubocervical fascia in the classic anatomic descriptions. This levator fascia is divided into discrete areas of specialization, depending on the associated organ it supports. The specialization of levator fascia around the urethra, the pubourethral ligament, represents a fusion of the periurethral fascia and endopelvic fascia attaching to the tendinous arc. The levator fascia associated with the bladder, the vesicopelvic ligament represents the fusion of perivesical and

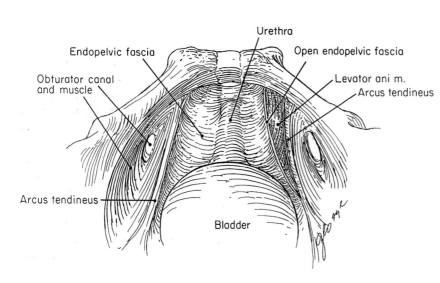

FIG. 43–2. Schematic diagram of the pelvic floor, specifically the levator ani musculature and its fascial condensations. The endopelvic fascia represents the abdominal side of the levator fascia. The arcus tendineus represents the insertion of the levator muscle into the obturator muscle of the lateral pelvic sidewall.

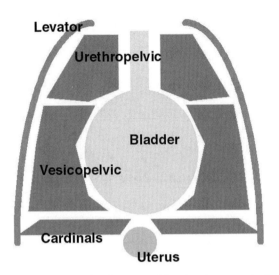

FIG. 43–3. Schematic diagram of the levator muscle fascia viewed from the vaginal side, with specifically named condensations that form supportive ligamentous structures for the urethra, bladder, and uterus.

endopelvic fascia attached to the tendinous arc. Such condensations of the endopelvic fascia create "ligamentous" structures that support the pelvic viscera, such as the pubourethral ligaments, urethropelvic ligaments, pubocervical fascia, and cardinal and uterosacral ligaments (Fig. 43–3). These represent discrete supportive structures that are part of a continuum of connective tissue surrounding the pelvic organs and serve as important surgical and physiological landmarks. An understanding of their individual contribution to pelvic visceral support is essential in reconstructive surgery. Therefore, these four fascial structures will be discussed in detail as a basis for understanding the pathophysiology of pelvic organ prolapse.

Pubourethral Ligaments

The pubourethral ligaments are a condensation of levator fascia connecting the inner surface of the inferior pubis to the midportion of the urethra. They provide support and stability to the urethra and its associated anterior vaginal wall. These ligaments divide the urethra into proximal and distal halves; the proximal or intraabdominal portion is responsible for passive or involuntary continence. The striated external urethral sphincter is located just distal to the pubourethral ligaments so that the midurethra is primarily responsible for active or voluntary continence. The distal one-third of urethra is simply a conduit and does not significantly change continence when damaged or resected. Weakening or detachment of the pubourethral ligament causes separation of the urethra from the inferior ramus of the pubic symphysis. This pathologic process has an unclear role in continence.

Urethropelvic Ligaments

The urethropelvic ligaments are comprised of a two-layer condensation of levator fascia that provides the most important anatomic support of the bladder neck and proximal urethra to the lateral pelvic wall (Fig. 43–4). The first layer is known as the periurethral fascia (vaginal side) and is located immediately beneath the vaginal epithelium, apparent as a glistening, white layer surrounding the urethra. The second layer of the urethropelvic ligament consists of the levator fascia covering the abdominal side of the urethra (endopelvic fascia), which fuses with the periurethral fascia. The two layers attach as a unit to the tendinous arc of the obturator fascia along the pelvic sidewall (Fig. 43–5). These lateral fusions of the levator and periurethral fascia provide important, elastic musculofascial support to the bladder outlet, thereby maintaining passive continence in women. Voluntary or reflex contractions of the levator or obturator musculature increase the tensile forces across these ligaments, increasing outlet resistance and continence. Thus, these ligamentous structures are critically important in the surgical correction of stress incontinence.

Pubocervical Fascia (Vesicopelvic Ligament)

The pubocervical fascia is a continuous sheet of connective tissue support from the pubic symphysis to the cervix, including the periurethral, perivesical, and endopelvic fascia that fuse to support the bladder to the lateral pelvic wall (Fig. 43–6). It is formed by the fusion

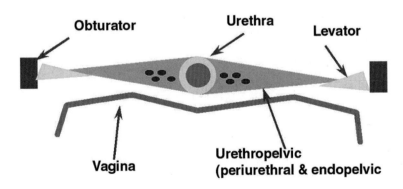

FIG. 43–4. Schematic diagram demonstrating the urethropelvic ligaments, a two-layer condensation of levator fascia that envelops the urethra and surrounding neurovascular structures and attaches to the lateral side wall.

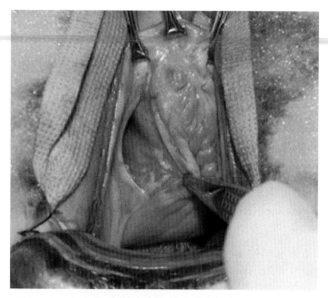

FIG. 43–5. Intraoperative photograph of the urethropelvic ligament as it attaches laterally to the tendinous arc.

of fascia from the bladder wall and anterior vaginal wall in the region of the bladder base. It is continuous distally with the periurethral fascia and proximally with the uterine cervix and cardinal ligament complex. This fascial condensation, sometimes referred to as the vesicopelvic ligament, fuses laterally with the endopelvic fascia, attaching to the pelvic sidewall at the tendinous arc and supporting the bladder base and anterior vaginal wall (Fig. 43–7). Attenuation of this lateral bladder support results in a lateral cystocele defect (paravaginal).

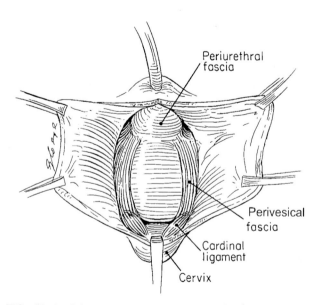

FIG. 43–6. Schematic diagram of the vaginal fascial condensations from the pubic symphysis to the cervix, including the periurethral fascia, perivesical fascia, and cardinal ligaments. This continuous sheet of fascial support is also known as the pubocervical fascia.

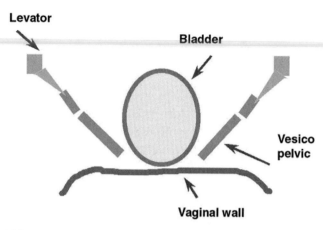

FIG. 43–7. Schematic diagram of the vesicopelvic ligament, the fascial condensation providing lateral support to the bladder base and anterior vaginal wall.

UTERINE AND VAGINAL VAULT SUPPORT

Cardinal–Sacrouterine Ligament Complex

The cardinal ligaments are thick, triangular condensations of pelvic fascia that originate from the region of the greater sciatic foramen. They insert into the lateral aspects of a fascial ring encircling the uterine cervix and isthmus as well as the adjacent vaginal wall, providing important uterine and apical vaginal support. In addition, the cardinal ligaments are an important mechanism of support for the bladder base and can be seen extending to the perivesical fascia. Often, it is difficult to differentiate the two structures surgically and sharp dissection is required. These ligaments contain numerous blood vessels branching from the hypogastrics that supply the uterus and upper vagina (4). The cardinal ligaments fuse posteriorly with the uterosacral ligaments (sacrouterine), which stabilize the uterus, cervix, and upper vagina posteriorly toward the sacrum. They originate from the second, third, and fourth sacral vertebrae and insert into the posterolateral aspect of the pericervical fascia and lateral vaginal fornices (3). The fascial unit is comprised of cardinal ligaments, uterosacral ligaments, and pubocervical fascia spread out posterolaterally on each side of the vaginal apex, uterus, and cervix to the pelvis (1).

The broad ligaments provide additional uterine support and are located more superiorly, covered by anterior and posterior sheets of peritoneum. They attach the lateral walls of the uterine body to the pelvic sidewall and contain the fallopian tubes, round and ovarian ligaments, and uterine and ovarian vessels.

POSTERIOR VAGINAL AND PERINEAL SUPPORT

Rectovaginal Septum

The rectovaginal septum represents a fascial extension of the peritoneal *cul-de-sac* between the vaginal apex and the anterior rectal wall. This septum is comprised of two distinct layers, the posterior vaginal fascia and the prerectal fascia, which fuse distally at their insertion into the perineal body. More proximally, these fascial layers fuse with the cardinal–uterosacral complex to provide support for the posterior vaginal apex. The proximal posterior vagina and intrapelvic rectum are supported by the pubococcygeus portion of the levator ani group, which inserts into the midline raphe between the vagina and rectum.

Perineum

The perineal body, a tendinous structure located between the anus and vagina in the midline, provides a central point of musculofascial insertion. This acts as an additional level of pelvic support that is elastic in nature, thereby allowing significant distortion and recoil during childbirth and intercourse (4). Two paired superficial transverse perineal muscles run on each side of the perineal body to the ischial tuberosities laterally, with a similar deeper pair of transverse perineal muscles found more superiorly. Voluntary contraction of these transverse perineal muscles effects lateral vaginal compression as well as stability of the perineum during acute increases in intraabdominal pressure.

The perineum can be conceptually divided into anterior and posterior triangular compartments by drawing a line between the two ischial tuberosities. The anterior, urogenital triangle in the female contains the clitoris, urethra, and vaginal vestibule in the midline. The ischiocavernosus muscles cover the clitoral crura at their attachments to the pubis. The bulbocavernosus muscles run on each side of the vaginal vestibule beneath the labia between the clitoris and the perineal body. The anal canal is found in the center of the posterior, anal triangle. The external anal sphincter is composed of two layers of fibers, the deeper layer completely encircling the anal canal and fusing with the pubococcygeus–puborectal muscles superiorly.

PATHOPHYSIOLOGY OF PELVIC FLOOR DYSFUNCTION

Mechanisms of Urethral Continence in Women

Bladder outlet resistance in women is attained by several factors working together to provide continence at rest and during stress maneuvers. Urethral anatomy, including functional length and elastic closure, is an important determinant of continence. In addition, activity of the muscular pelvic floor with its associated connective tissue elements helps maintain outlet resistance during times of increased intraabdominal pressure. The anatomic position of the urethra is another factor contributing to continence. Each of these entities will be discussed sepa-

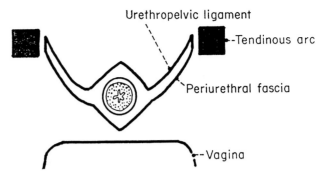

FIG. 43–8. Schematic diagram demonstrating weakness of the urethropelvic ligament, thereby allowing posterior and downward rotation of the urethra.

rately to provide a basis for understanding the pathophysiology of pelvic floor relaxation.

The urethra is made up of three functional anatomic components that result in an elastic, dynamic conduit with mucosal coaptation. The urethral mucosa is a transitional epithelium with numerous infoldings that allow distensibility and closure with excellent coaptation. Beneath the mucosa is a spongy tissue made up of vascular networks analogous to the corpus spongiosum in the male. Surrounding the spongy tissue is a thin musculofascial envelope, the periurethral fascia, which appears as a glistening, white membrane. These three components create a coaptive seal.

Both the bladder neck and urethra are normally maintained in a high retropubic position relative to the more dependent bladder base, creating a valvular effect. The bladder neck and urethra are supported by a musculofascial layer that suspends these structures from the pubic bone and pelvic sidewalls, thereby preventing their descent during increases in intraabdominal pressures (8). A limited degree of bladder base rotation against a well-supported urethra occurs with increased abdominal pressures, further creating a valvular effect between these two structures (5). Further, direct transmission of intraabdominal forces to a well-supported proximal urethra increases its resistance and promotes coaptation (9). Relaxation of the pelvic floor as well as weakening of the urethropelvic ligaments and midurethral complex produces significant posterior and downward rotation of the urethra and bladder neck (Fig. 43–8). This anatomic repositioning of the urethra and bladder neck to a more dependent pelvic position eliminates the valvular effect.

REFERENCES

1. Baden WF, Walker T. The anatomy of uterovaginal support. In: Baden WF, Walker T, eds. *Vaginal defects*. Philadelphia: Lippincott, 1992: 25–50.
2. DeLancey JO. Surgical anatomy of the female pelvis. In: Rock JA,

Thompson JD, eds. *Te Linde's operative gynecology*. Philadelphia: Lippincott–Raven, 1997:63–93.

3. DeLancey JOL, Richardson AC. Anatomy of genital support. In: Hurt WG, ed. *Urogynecologic surgery*. Gaithersburg, IL: Aspen Publishers, 1992:19–33.

4. Klutke CG, Siegel CL. Functional female pelvic anatomy. *Urol Clin North Am* 1995;22:487–498.

5. Raz S, Little NA, Juma S. Female urology. In: Walsh PC, Retik AB, Stamey TA, Vaughan ED, eds. *Campbell's urology*. Philadelphia: WB Saunders, 1992:2782–2829.

6. Redman JF. Surgical anatomy of the female genitourinary system. In: Buchsbaum HJ, Schmidt JD, eds. *Gynecologic and obstetric urology*. Philadelphia: WB Saunders, 1993:25–60.

7. Tanagho EA. Anatomy of the lower urinary tract. In: Walsh PC, Retik AB, Stamey TA, Vaughan ED, eds. *Campbell's urology*. Philadelphia: WB Saunders, 1992:40–69.

8. Blaivas JG, Romanzi LJ, Heritz DM. Urinary incontinence: Pathophysiology, evaluation, treatment overview, and nonsurgical management. In: Walsh PC, Retik AB, Vaughan ED, Wein AJ, eds. *Campbell's Urology*. Philadelphia: WB Saunders, 1998:1007–1043.

9. Enhorning G. Simultaneous recording of intravesical and intraurethral pressure. *Acta Chir Scand* 1961:276:3.

CHAPTER 44

Vaginal Hysterectomy

Karyn S. Eilber, Nirit Rosenblum, and Shlomo Raz

Uterine prolapse is a relatively common condition. From 1988 to 1990, 16.3% of hysterectomies performed in this country were for prolapse (8). Approximately 70% of the hysterectomies performed are done through the abdominal approach. Compared to the abdominal approach, the vaginal approach avoids the morbidity associated with an abdominal incision and is preferred when there is associated vaginal prolapse. By understanding the female pelvic anatomy and thus allowing control of the uterine vascular pedicles, a transvaginal hysterectomy can effectively be performed with minimal morbidity.

The uterus is supported mainly by the pelvic floor musculature and three sets of ligaments. The pelvic floor musculature involved in uterine support includes the levator ani muscle group (pubococcygeus, iliococcygeus, puborectalis) and the coccygeal muscles. The three sets of ligaments providing uterine support are the uterosacral, cardinal (Mackenrodt's), and broad ligaments. The body of the uterus is enclosed between the double-layered broad ligaments. The broad ligaments each contain a fallopian tube, the round and ovarian ligaments, and the uterine and ovarian vessels and extend from the lateral aspect of the body of the uterus to enter the internal inguinal ring. No significant uterine support is provided by the broad ligaments.

The uterosacral and cardinal ligaments extend from the cervix to the sacrum and arcus tendineus, respectively, and are fused posteriorly. These ligaments represent localized thickenings of the endopelvic fascia and provide the major uterine and apical vaginal (cervical) support. When performing a transvaginal hysterectomy, the fusion of the cardinal and uterosacral ligaments becomes clinically significant as will become apparent in the subsequent description of the technique.

De Lancey described the pathophysiology of uterine prolapse in terms of the interactions of the ligamentous support of the uterus and pelvic floor:

1. Level I—support of the upper vagina and cervix by the cardinal–uterosacral complex.
2. Level II—support of the midportion of the vagina to the arcus tendineus.
3. Level III—support involving the fusion of the anterior, lateral, and posterior vagina to the urethra, levator ani, and perineal body, respectively (5).

A defect in level-I support results in uterine prolapse. Attenuation of the cardinal–uterosacral ligament complex occurs either because of trauma (childbirth) or atrophy and the cervix is allowed to move anteriorly. The uterus then begins to shift posteriorly such that the intraabdominal pressure is directed on the anterior surface of the uterus. The uterus becomes progressively more retroverted until the axis of the uterus is essentially vertical. This position allows uterine prolapse to occur (4).

The exact etiology of pelvic prolapse is still unclear. Predisposing factors include increasing age, multiparity, maximal birth weight, postmenopausal status, chronic constipation, prior surgery for prolapse, and decreased pelvic floor muscle strength (5,11,13).

DIAGNOSIS

The clinical evaluation of the patient with uterine prolapse includes a complete history and physical examination and a limited number of ancillary tests. Considerations such as symptoms, prolapse of other organs, pelvic pathology, urinary incontinence, reproductive status, and sexual function all influence the management of the patient with uterine prolapse.

The classic presentation of a patient with uterine prolapse is a vaginal mass or bulge that is aggravated by standing and relieved in the supine position. Other complaints include perineal pressure, dyspareunia, or difficulty with ambulation. Urinary or bowel symptoms may be present if there is prolapse of other organs. Less commonly, a patient presents because uterine prolapse was incidentally found on routine physical examination.

An important piece of information in the patient's history is whether the patient has had a previous hysterectomy. Often, what is assumed to be uterine descent is only cervical descent resulting from a supracervical hysterectomy. It is also important to determine the presence of any known uterine disease. Endometriosis of unknown extent, large fibroids, and malignancy are contraindications for a vaginal hysterectomy.

Physical examination should be performed both in the supine and standing positions. The severity of prolapse may not be appreciated in the supine position. In both positions the patient needs to perform a Valsalva maneuver to fully elicit the prolapse.

Uterine examination includes determination of the level of descensus, uterine size, uterine mobility, and any abnormal gross pathology. The anterior, posterior, and apical vaginal walls are examined separately with the aid of a speculum to assess the presence of other prolapse such as cystocele, rectocele, or enterocele. The size of the introitus and evidence of vaginal stenosis should be noted as a size disproportion between the uterus and vagina may limit transvaginal delivery of the uterus.

The physical examination should be repeated at the time of surgery with the patient under anesthesia. Often, with anesthesia the degree of uterine descent and other prolapse become more pronounced.

A urinalysis and postvoid residual urine volume are obtained for all patients. Urodynamic evaluation is not routinely performed for patients with uterine prolapse and no history of stress or urge incontinence and normal residual urine. For patients with urinary symptoms or elevated residual urine, we recommend assessment of the lower urinary tract with a urodynamic evaluation and cystoscopy. Stress incontinence may be masked by the prolapse. As many patients with prolapse are elderly, detrusor instability secondary to obstruction versus hyperreflexia secondary to an occult neurological condition must be identified. Cystoscopy is useful to rule out any intrinsic urethral or bladder abnormalities that may be causing lower urinary tract symptoms.

Imaging of the upper urinary tracts is recommended as patients with uterine prolapse are more likely to have associated hydronephrosis compared to other vaginal prolapse and it may be severe enough to cause renal failure. Our preferred imaging modality to assess the presence of hydronephrosis as well as other pelvic pathology is dynamic magnetic resonance imaging (MRI). Dynamic MRI is a relatively simple, noninvasive test that takes only minutes to complete. No contrast is used as the bladder is distinct on T_2-weighted images. Sagittal images are taken of the pelvis with the patient at rest and then with a Valsalva maneuver. Uterine or other pelvic organ prolapse is readily identified with this imaging modality (Fig. 44–1).

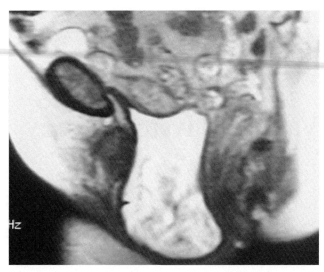

FIG. 44–1. Magnetic resonance imaging (MRI) of the pelvis. Dynamic MRI of the pelvis demonstrating uterine and bladder prolapse.

Another advantage is its ability to accurately determine uterine and ovarian pathology.

The Pelvic Organ Prolapse Quantification System (POP-Q) is a commonly used staging system for describing vaginal prolapse and is based on physical examination (2). We classify uterine prolapse based on the dynamic MRI. Prolapse is classified in reference to the puborectalis hiatus (sling). The puborectalis hiatus is formed by the puborectalis muscle (the most inferior part of levator ani) and includes the urethra, vagina, and rectum. The degree of prolapse is measured by 2-cm increments: Mild uterine prolapse is 0 to 2 cm distal to the hiatus, moderate prolapse is 2 to 4 cm, and severe prolapse is greater than 4 cm distal to the hiatus (1).

ALTERNATIVE THERAPY

Alternative therapy is either no treatment or pessary. Patients who are candidates for surgery are in general not well served with these alternatives.

SURGICAL TECHNIQUE

Hysterectomy alone is not sufficient to treat uterine prolapse as the defect is not with the uterus itself but with the pelvic support. Thus, every effort must be made to restore normal pelvic anatomy with adequate support and create a functional vaginal vault.

Prophylactic antibiotics are administered preoperatively. Following administration of anesthesia, the patient is placed in the high lithotomy position. If no contraindication exists, spinal anesthesia is preferred. An iodine-based solution is used to cleanse the skin from the suprapubic area to the posterior perineum. Sutures are used to

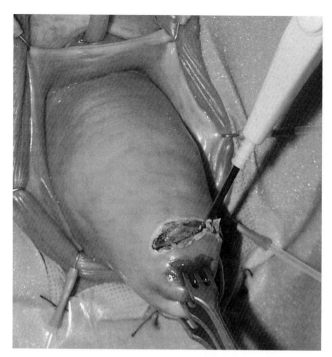

FIG. 44–2. Incision. A circumferential incision is made approximately 1 cm from the cervical os with electrocautery.

retract the labia laterally and a weighted speculum is inserted for vault exposure. If a sling or cystocele repair is planned, a Lowsley retractor is used to place a suprapubic catheter. The bladder is drained by the urethral and/or suprapubic catheter(s). A ring retractor with elastic stays is used for exposure. Two Lahey clamps are used to grasp the cervix. Electrocautery is used to make a circumferential incision approximately 1 cm from the cervical os (Fig. 44–2). The uterus is dissected free from the

bladder using sharp dissection, and the vesicoperitoneal space is developed (Figs. 44–3A and 44–3B). This dissection is facilitated by placing gentle downward traction on the Lahey clamps and retracting the bladder anteriorly with a Heaney retractor. Maneuvers to avoid an inadvertent cystotomy include dissection in the midline of the uterus, pointing the curve of the scissors toward the uterus, and remaining parallel to the glistening white surface of the uterus.

The posterior peritoneal fold is exposed in a similar fashion to the vesicoperitoneal fold and the posterior peritoneum is opened sharply. Adhesions are lysed and the cul-de-sac is inspected for any pathology. If difficulty is encountered when attempting to enter the peritoneum, the hysterectomy can be initiated in an extraperitoneal fashion by severing the uterosacral ligament and caudal portions of the cardinal ligament close to the cervix. This maneuver mobilizes the uterus to provide better visualization. Another Heaney retractor is placed in the posterior peritoneum.

Division of the uterosacral–cardinal ligaments is now performed. With the cervix under slight traction, a large right-angle clamp is introduced into the cul-de-sac parallel to the cervix. The right-angle clamp is used to expose the ligament, which is then grasped with a Phaneuf clamp and divided with electrocautery (Figs. 44–4A and 44–4B). The stumps are oversewn with figure-of-eight suture ligatures (0 Vicryl or Dexon). The ends of the sutures are left long and then placed in the grooves of the retractor ring. At this point the uterus can be manually everted and brought outside the introitus (Fig. 44–5). Safe entry into the anterior peritoneum can be made by placing a finger anteriorly over the uterine fundus to elevate the peritoneum. Electro-

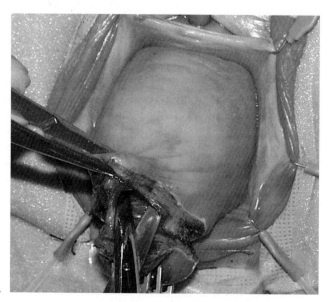

A

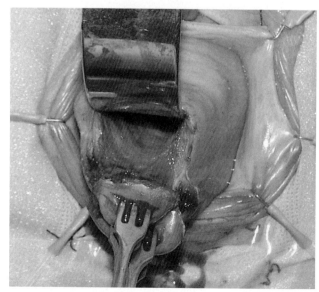

B

FIG. 44–3. Exposure of the anterior uterus. Sharp dissection is used to **(A)** expose the anterior uterus and **(B)** develop the vesicoperitoneal space.

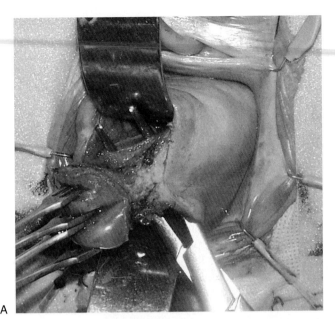 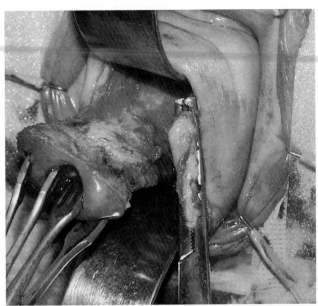

A   B

FIG. 44–4. Isolation of cardinal–uterosacral ligaments. Right-angle and Phaneuf clamps are used in succession to **(A)** better delineate the cardinal–uterosacral complex before **(B)** transection.

cautery can then be used to incise the peritoneum overlying the surgeon's finger. The broad ligaments are now ligated as above (Figs. 44–6A and 44–6B). If an oophorectomy is not planned, their attachments are also now divided. The uterus is finally removed. A circular

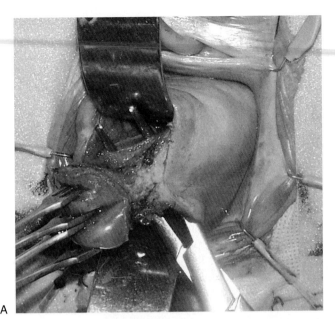

FIG. 44–5. Eversion of the uterus. After the bilateral cardinal–uterosacral ligaments have been ligated, the uterus is manually everted.

arrangement of the six ligated pedicles and their attached sutures remain (Fig. 44–7).

Two methods are employed to provide vault support and vaginal depth: (a) Perivesical and prerectal fascia are approximated to close the cul-de-sac and (b) a modified McCall culdoplasty is performed. The culdoplasty is performed first. Bilateral 0 Panacryl sutures are brought from outside the vaginal wall into the peritoneal cavity (in the area of the ligated cardinal–uterosacral complex). Figure-of-eight sutures incorporate the area lateral to the rectum and the uterosacral ligaments as they cross the iliococcygeus muscle in the posterolateral pelvic wall (Fig. 44–8). These sutures are approximately 8 to 10 cm from the vaginal cuff and are tagged at this time. They will not be tied until after the vaginal cuff is closed. It is usually necessary to pack the peritoneal cavity with moist laparotomy sponges for maximal exposure.

Two pursestring sutures of 0 Panacryl are now placed to close the vaginal cuff. These sutures incorporate the prerectal fascia, the cardinal–uterosacral ligament complex, the broad ligaments, and the perivesical fascia. It is important to stay in the midline when incorporating the perivesical fascia. Sutures placed too lateral may cause ureteral injury. The pursestring sutures are also tagged and not tied at this time. The sutures of the previously ligated pedicles of the broad ligaments and the cardinal–uterosacral ligament complex are identified on each side and tied in the midline. The pursestring sutures are now cinched and tied. If simultaneous repair of other prolapse is planned, it is now performed. The culdoplasty sutures are tied last. Vaginal depth is restored when the culdoplasty sutures are tied. Excess vaginal wall is excised before closure with an absorbable suture.

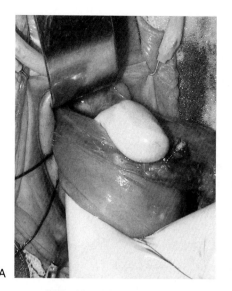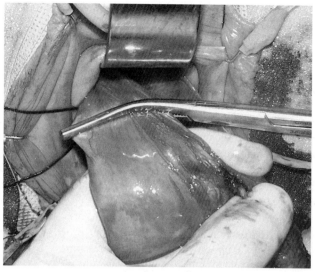

A

B

FIG. 44–6. Division of the broad ligament. The surgeon's index finger is **(A)** inserted into the peritoneal cavity and hooked around the broad ligament, which is **(B)** then ligated in the same fashion as the cardinal–uterosacral ligaments.

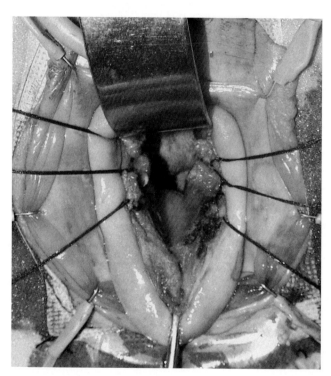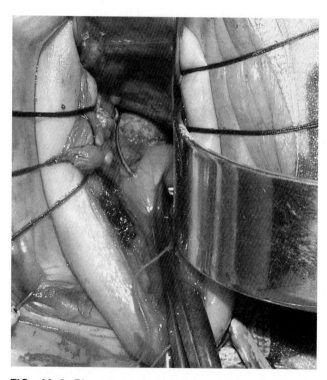

FIG. 44–7. Transected uterine pedicles. Arrangement of the transected pedicles of the cardinal, uterosacral, and broad ligaments before approximation.

FIG. 44–8. Placement of culdoplasty sutures. Inside the peritoneal cavity, a figure-of-eight culdoplasty suture approximates the area lateral to the rectum and the uterosacral ligaments as they cross the iliococcygeus muscle.

OUTCOMES

Complications

Short-term complications include hemorrhage, infection, and adjacent organ injury although these complications occur less frequently compared to the abdominal approach (6,7,12). Ileus may also occur but usually responds to conservative treatment. Interestingly, bladder and ureteral injury occurs less commonly with the vaginal approach. It has been proposed that traction applied to the cervix in combination with anterior retraction of the vesicouterine peritoneal fold provide sufficient displacement of the ureters such that injury is avoided (9).

Long-term complications include recurrence of prolapse and urinary fistula. The majority of recurrent prolapse involves only the upper vagina and is asymptomatic. Prolapse that develops following hysterectomy may be an enterocele that was missed at the time of surgery or, more commonly, that occurred because of insufficient closure and/or support of the cuff. An enterocele may also develop postoperatively if other pelvic floor relaxation is not repaired. Absence of the normal vaginal axis promotes prolapse of the cuff.

Ureterovaginal and vesicovaginal fistulas occur in 0.09% to 0.5% and 0.6%, respectively (4). Adequate anterior retraction of the bladder, ligation of the pedicles close to the cervix, and avoidance of lateral placement of the pursestring sutures in the perivesical fascia aid in the prevention of bladder and ureteral injury.

Results

In regard to overall postoperative genitourinary function, Vierhout concluded that there is minimal to no effect of nonradical hysterectomy on lower urinary tract function (14). Sexual function has always been a concern following hysterectomy. Recent data indicates that hysterectomy actually improves sexual functioning and overall quality of life. Rhodes and associates found that following hysterectomy the occurrence of sexual relations and orgasm increased while the rates of dyspareunia and low libido decreased (10). Similarly, researchers from the Maine Medical Assessment Foundation concluded that hysterectomy relieved pelvic pain, fatigue, depression, and sexual dysfunction and improved the overall quality of life 1 year after surgery (3).

Uterine prolapse is a condition that, depending on severity of prolapse and symptoms, may require surgical treatment. When there is no contraindication, vaginal hysterectomy avoids the morbidity associated with an abdominal hysterectomy and has lower rates of bladder and ureteral injury. Preoperative consideration must be given to uterine size, uterine and/or adnexal pathology, and bladder and bowel function.

REFERENCES

1. Barbaric ZL, Marumoto AK, Raz S. Magnetic resonance imaging of the perineum and pelvic floor. *Top Magn Reson Imag* 2001;12:83–92.
2. Bump RC, Mattiasson A, Bo K, Brubaker LP, et al. The standardization of terminology of female pelvic organ prolapse and pelvic floor dysfunction. *Am J Obstet Gynecol* 1996;175:10–17.
3. Carlson KJ, Miller BA, Fowler FJ Jr. The Maine Women's Health Study I: Outcomes of hysterectomy. *Obstet Gynecol* 1994;83:556–572.
4. Chopra A, Stothers L, Raz S. Uterine prolapse. In: Raz S, ed. *Female urology*, 2nd ed. Philadelphia: WB Saunders, 1996:457–464.
5. De Lancey JOL. Anatomic aspects of vaginal eversion after hysterectomy. *Am J Obstet Gynecol* 1992;166:1717–1724.
6. Dicker RC, Greenspan JR, Strauss LT, et al. Complications of abdominal and vaginal hysterectomy among women of reproductive age in the United States. The collaborative review of sterilization. *Am J Obstet Gynecol* 1982;144:841–848.
7. Gitsch G, Berger E, Tatra G. Trends in thirty years of vaginal hysterectomy. *Surg Gynecol Obstet* 1991;172:207–210.
8. Graves EJ, Kozak LJ. Detailed diagnoses and procedures, National Hospital Discharge Survey, 1996. *Vital Health Stat 13* 1998;138:1.
9. Hofmeister FJ, Wolfgram RL. Methods of demonstrating measurement relationships between vaginal hysterectomy ligatures and the ureters. *Am J Obstet Gynecol* 1962;83:938–948.
10. Rhodes JC, Kjerulff KH, Langenberg PW, et al. Hysterectomy and sexual functioning. *JAMA* 1999;282:1934–1941.
11. Samuelsson EC, Arne Victor FT, Tibblin G. Signs of genital prolapse in a Swedish population of women 20 to 59 years of age and possible related factors. *Am J Obstet Gynecol* 1999;180:299–305.
12. Scott JR, Sharp HT, Dodson MK, et al. Subtotal hysterectomy in modern gynecology; a decision analysis. *Am J Obstet Gynecol* 1997;176:1186–1191.
13. Swift SE. The distribution of pelvic organ support in a population of female subjects seen for routine gynecologic health care. *Am J Obstet Gynecol* 2000;183:277–285.
14. Vierhout ME. Influence of nonradical hysterectomy on the function of the lower urinary tract. *Obstet Gynecol Surv* 2001;56:381–386.

CHAPTER 45

Female Urethral Diverticulum

Jeffrey M. Carey and Gary E. Leach

The first case of a female urethral diverticulum was reported by Hey in 1805 (4). While the true incidence of urethral diverticula is unknown, the reported incidence varies from 1.4% to 5% depending on the population of women studied. Although diverticula are reported in all age groups, they most commonly present in the third through fifth decades. Historically, the incidence of diverticula was reported as higher in women of African descent, but modern series have not confirmed any racial predilection (3).

Female urethral diverticula arise from the wall of the urethra and consist of fibrous tissue lined with epithelium. Chronic inflammation may result in loss of the epithelial lining with subsequent adherence to the neighboring periurethral fascia and/or anterior vaginal wall.

The exact mechanism of diverticula formation is unknown. Rarely a diverticulum may be congenital in origin, but the most commonly accepted theories implicate the periurethral glands. Obstruction of the periurethral gland duct results in subsequent infection and abscess formation. Rupture of the abscess into the urethral lumen from trauma or tissue necrosis results in diverticula formation.

The complications of female urethral diverticula may include infection (either acute or chronic), stone formation, and malignancy. The incidence of malignancy is rare, as only 63 cases have been reported in the literature—accounting for less than 5% of all urethral carcinoma. The histopathology of female urethral diverticular carcinoma has been identified in 60 cases: adenocarcinoma 61% (37/60), transitional cell carcinoma 27% (16/60), and squamous cell carcinoma 12% (7/60) (8). The predominance of adenocarcinoma rather than squamous cell carcinoma is consistent with the pathophysiological hypothesis of an occluded periurethral gland.

DIAGNOSIS

The presenting symptoms of a urethral diverticulum vary considerably. (Table 45–1) (3). The classic symptoms of the three *D*s (*dysuria, postvoid dribbling,* and *dyspareunia*) are not the most common presenting symptom complex. Dysfunctional voiding, incontinence, infection, and pain symptoms predominate. The differential diagnosis of a urethral diverticulum is extensive and may include simple or chronic bacterial cystitis, interstitial cystitis, pelvic inflammatory disease, endometriosis, nonspecific or gonococcal urethritis, urothelial carcinoma *in situ*, detrusor instability, and bladder outlet obstruction. Two percent to 11% of urethral diverticula are asymptomatic and found incidentally on routine pelvic examination or radiographic imaging (3).

Physical examination should include a systematic pelvic examination, including palpation of the anterior vaginal wall and urethra. Compression of the anterior vaginal wall in patients with a diverticulum may reveal tenderness, mass, or drainage at the urethral meatus (purulent material, urine, or blood). Although the size of diverticula has not correlated well with symptoms, in the authors' experience, all urethral diverticula of significant size (greater than 1 cm) have been suspected by demonstrating periurethral tenderness or mass on pelvic exami-

TABLE 45–1. *Percentage of presenting symptoms in 627 women with urethral diverticula calculated from published reports*

Symptom	Range (%)	Mean (%)
Frequency	31–83	56
Dysuria	32–73	55
Recurrent Infection	33–46	40
Tender Mass	12–63	35
Stress Incontinence	12–70	32
Postvoid Dribbling	3–65	27
Urgency	8–40	25
Hematuria	7–26	17
Dyspareunia	12–24	16
Purulence per Urethra	2–31	12
Urinary Retention	3–7	4
Asymptomatic	2–11	6

nation. Induration or hardness in the area of a diverticulum suggests the possibility of malignancy or stone. Other causes of periurethral masses tend to fall into two primary categories: embryological and neoplastic. Embryological anomalies may include: Skene's gland abscess, Gartner's duct cyst, ectopic ureterocele, and vaginal wall inclusion cyst. Neoplastic periurethral masses may include urethral carcinoma, periurethral myoma, hemangioma, urethral varices, endometriosis, sarcoma botryoides, and vaginal wall metastasis.

Magnetic resonance imaging (MRI) is currently considered the best imaging modality for identifying and characterizing female urethral diverticula. MRI is considered superior to other imaging modalities given its outstanding soft-tissue resolution and anatomic detail, including its ability to identify loculated collections that do not communicate with the urethral lumen. In addition, MRI is less invasive than other studies as it does not require patient catheterization. Compared to surrounding tissues, urethral diverticula appear as high signal intensity periurethral masses on T_2-weighted images and low signal intensity masses on T_1-weighted images (Fig. 45–1). There has been controversy over the relative benefits of endoluminal versus surface coil MRI. In the authors' opinion, endoluminal MRI is neither widely available nor does it provide any distinct advantage over modern surface coil technology. In addition, endoluminal MRI is more expensive and may be more uncomfortable to the patient if diverticula are infected or inflamed.

Prior to the advent of MRI, a properly performed voiding cystourethrogram (VCUG) was considered by many to be the best radiographic test to confirm the presence, extent, and configuration of a urethral diverticulum (Fig.

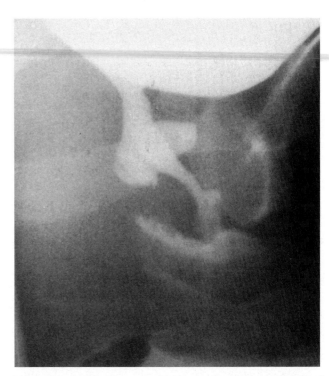

FIG. 45–2. Voiding cystourethrogram showing the details of a urethral diverticulum.

45–2) (10). VCUG is no longer considered the imaging study of choice as it is not as sensitive as MRI. The higher false negative rate of VCUG is attributed to incomplete distension of the diverticulum secondary to poor urinary flow rates, loculations, or narrow diverticular ostia.

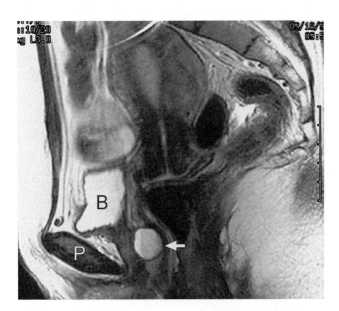

FIG. 45–1. T_2-weighted magnetic resonance image showing midurethral diverticlum identified by white arrow. B, bladder; P, pubic symphysis.

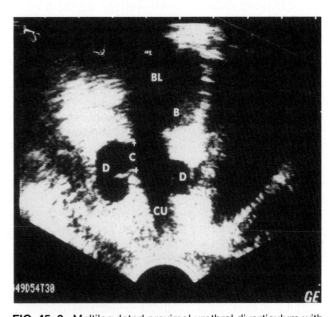

FIG. 45–3. Multiloculated proximal urethral diverticulum with its communication into the proximal urethra just below the bladder neck (between plus signs) as seen on transvaginal ultrasound. B, Foley catheter balloon; BL, bladder; C, diverticular communication; CU, Foley catheter in the urethra; D, multiloculated diverticulum.

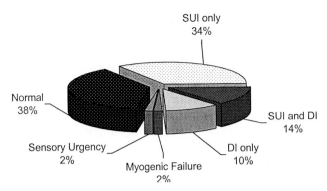

FIG. 45–4. Percentage urodynamic findings in 58 women with urethral diverticulum. DI, detrusor instability; SUI, stress urinary incontinence.

Other less beneficial imaging studies include intravenous urography (IVU), retrograde (double-balloon) positive-pressure urethrography, and ultrasonography. Despite the limitations of IVU, the authors frequently perform IVU prior to diverticulectomy as failure to recognize an ectopic ureter may result in excision and subsequent total urinary incontinence (1). Practically, retrograde positive-pressure urethrography is a difficult, time-consuming, and unsatisfactory procedure. Endoluminal ultrasound utilizes a 6.2 Fr or 9 Fr catheter-based transducer inserted per urethra (Fig. 45–3). This technique may aid surgical planning by identifying the diverticular orifice, contents, or multiloculation. In addition, endoluminal ultrasonography has been shown to identify diverticula that might otherwise have been missed at surgery (2).

Cystourethroscopy is recommended in addition to imaging studies. The use of a 20 Fr "short-beaked" female sheath is preferred because standard sheaths do not adequately expand the urethral wall, making diagnosis more difficult. Palpation of the suburethral mass with the cystoscope in place allows better appreciation of the location, size, and consistency of the diverticulum. Communication sites with the urethral lumen may be visualized during compression of the mass by extrusion of purulent material at the site(s) of communication.

Urodynamics should be considered preoperatively for patients with a history of stress, urge, or mixed urinary incontinence. Urodynamics were found to be abnormal in over one-half of patients with urethral diverticula (Fig. 45–4). The identification of preoperative detrusor insta-

bility (DI) is important as it may affect postoperative care and patient counseling. Video/fluorourodynamic studies should be used to differentiate "paradoxical" incontinence from true stress urinary incontinence (SUI). Paradoxical incontinence is identified by leakage of contrast from the diverticulum with stress maneuvers without the loss of contrast across the bladder neck.

Classification of urethral diverticula is usually according to the L/N/S/C³ classification system, which describes the diverticulum and allows the clinician to document all pretreatment factors before diverticulectomy (6). The acronym represents descriptive parameters as follows: L, location (distal, mid, proximal urethra with or without extension behind the bladder); N, number (single or multiple); S, size (centimeters, in two dimensions); C1, configuration (single, multiloculated, or saddle); C2, communication (proximal, mid, distal); and C3, continence. In our series of 63 patients, urethral diverticula were most commonly single in number (90%) and configuration (65%). The location of the diverticular swelling (57%) and ostia (55%) was most commonly midurethral (Table 45–2). The L/N/S/C³ classification system not only provides a means of documenting all pretreatment factors but also serves as a method of outcomes comparison within and between series.

INDICATIONS FOR SURGERY

The authors recommend urethral diverticulectomy if the patient is symptomatic and/or the diverticulum is of significant size. Patients who present with diverticular abscess and fail to respond to antibiotics may be managed with transvaginal aspiration prior to formal diverticulectomy. The authors preferred repair is transvaginal complete excision of the diverticula with a three-layer nonoverlapping vaginal flap technique.

A Martius labial fat pad graft is interposed between the urethra and vaginal wall after diverticulectomy in selected cases (7). The indications for the Martius graft include fibrotic and scarred tissues, history of radiation therapy, absent or tenuous periurethral fascia, and recurrent diverticula.

Anti-incontinence procedures are not performed at the time of diverticulectomy due to the high rate of recurrent SUI, and the risk of obstruction or erosion of the reconstructed urethra. Patients are counseled regarding the risk of postoperative stress incontinence based on preopera-

TABLE 45–2 *Preoperative classification of female urethral diverticulum (L/N/S/C3) in the authors' experience of 63 women*

Location (L)	Number (N)	Size (S)	Configuration (C1)	Communication (C2)	Continence (C3)
Beneath Bladder Neck (9)	Single (57)	0.2cm to 6.0cm	Multiloculated (22)	Proximal (16)	Dry (26)
Proximal Urethra (7)	Multiple (6)		Single (41)	Mid (35)	Stress (30)
Midurethra (36)			Saddle-shaped (14)	Distal (12)	Urge (3)
Distal urethra (11)					Mixed (4)

tive urodynamics and diverticular anatomy. The development of postoperative stress incontinence is then managed by transvaginal sling once healing is complete. Typically, a sling may be safely performed approximately 3 months after diverticulectomy.

ALTERNATIVE THERAPY

Lapides described transurethral "saucerization" by opening the diverticulum into the urethral lumen with a knife electrode (5). Modifications of this technique include using a 10 Fr pediatric resectoscope with a Collins knife or Pott scissors. Endoscopic procedures may be useful in primary or recurrent diverticula situated in the distal urethra. This creates a wide-mouthed diverticulum that drains freely. The use of endoscopic techniques in mid- or proximal urethral diverticula should be avoided as it greatly increases the risk of iatrogenic urinary incontinence.

Spence and Duckett described marsupialization by incising the urethral floor through the diverticulum to the level of the diverticular orifice (9). The vaginal and urethral epithelium is then coapted by a running absorbable suture and a Foley catheter is left in place for 2 to 3 days. This procedure should be considered for distal diverticula only, as use of this technique on mid- or proximal diverticula significantly increases the risk of subsequent incontinence. Other complications of this procedure include recurrent diverticula, vaginal voiding, and spraying of urine with micturition.

Other options described include: incision and packing of the diverticular cavity with oxidized cellulose (Oxycel or Gelfoam), partial ablation by transvaginally opening the diverticulum and using the sac as a second layer after closing the orifice, excision of the diverticulum and closure of the periurethral fascia in vest-over-pants fashion, and a two-layer vaginal flap technique.

SURGICAL TECHNIQUE

The night before and the morning of the operation, the patient performs Betadine vaginal douches. Because most diverticula are filled with purulent material, perioperative suppressive oral antibiotics are given the week prior to surgery and parenteral antibiotics are administered the day of surgery.

After induction of general or spinal anesthesia, the patient is placed in the modified dorsal lithotomy position after application of intermittent pneumatic calf compression. The vagina and lower abdomen are prepared and draped with isolation of the rectum from the operative field. The bladder is filled and an 18 Fr suprapubic Foley catheter is placed as a "safety valve" for bladder drainage using a modified Lowsley tractor or a Chiou percutaneous dilator technique. Simultaneous cystourethroscopy is performed to check the position of the suprapubic catheter and reconfirm the urethral communication site. A 14 Fr Foley catheter is inserted per urethra. Saline is infiltrated in the anterior vaginal wall and a U-shaped incision is then made with the apex distal to the diverticulum.

The authors prefer a three-layer closure with suture lines oriented in different directions to avoid overlapping and decrease the risk of urethrovaginal fistula formation. The anterior vaginal flap is reflected toward the bladder neck using scissors for sharp dissection in the correct plane on the shiny white surface of the vaginal wall (Fig. 45–5A). Dissection in the wrong tissue plane (usually too deeply) results in entry into either the periurethral fascia or the diverticulum itself. Premature entry into either structure makes the remainder of the dissection more difficult. Preservation of the periurethral fascia is important to provide a second layer of closure between the urethra and the vaginal wall.

The urethral diverticulum is usually readily apparent once the vaginal flap is reflected inferiorly. Next, the periurethral fascia is incised transversely to allow subsequent exposure of the diverticulum beneath this fascial layer (Fig. 45–5B). The plane between the periurethral fascia and the underlying diverticulum is defined using sharp dissection. Dissection is carried away from the midline with care taken not to dissect too deeply, avoiding premature entry into the diverticulum. Once this portion of the dissection is complete, the periurethral fascia can be opened like "leaves of a book" to completely expose the underlying diverticulum (Fig. 45–5C). The borders of the diverticulum are carefully defined by sharp dissection until the communication with the urethra is identified. Rarely, when there is difficulty identifying the diverticulum or its communication site, urethroscopy is performed. A probe or curved pediatric sound is then passed under visual control from the urethral lumen into the diverticulum for vaginal palpation. The diverticulum is then excised in its entirety including its communication with the urethra and the adjacent urethral wall (Fig. 45–5D). Thus, a large urethral defect is created. When the diverticulum is multiloculated, it should be opened and inspected to ensure that all intercommunicating pockets are identified and removed. It is important that all attenuated tissue at the urethral communication site be excised to reduce the risk of recurrent diverticula formation. On the other hand, excessive resection of urethral wall should be avoided.

The urethral defect is then closed vertically without tension using a running, locking 4-0 polyglactic acid (PGA) suture starting at the proximal margin. Care is taken to incorporate the full thickness of the urethral wall in the closure. A watertight closure is essential to reduce the risk of postoperative extravasation. The periurethral fascia is then closed transversely with a running 3-0 PGA suture. The sutures are placed to obliterate any "dead space" beneath the periurethral fascia. When indicated, a

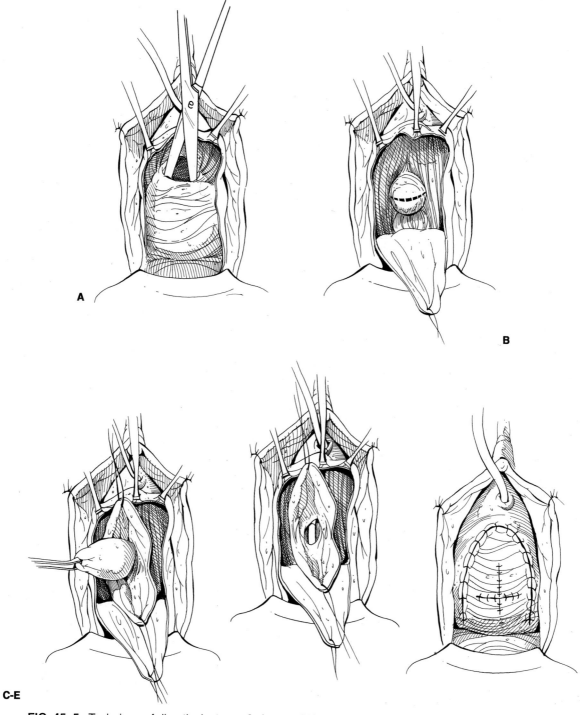

FIG. 45–5. Technique of diverticulectomy. **A:** Inverted-U incision and dissection of anterior vaginal wall flap. **B and C:** After transverse incision of the periurethral fascia, anterior and posterior flaps are mobilized to expose the underlying diverticulum. **D:** Excision of the diverticulum, creating a large urethral defect. **E:** Completed closure of the vaginal flap, with avoidance of overlapping suture lines.

Martius labial fat pad graft is harvested and placed between the periurethral fascia and the anterior vaginal wall closure (Fig. 45–6) (7). As mentioned previously, transvaginal bladder neck suspension is no longer performed given the high rate of recurrent stress inconti-

nence with these procedures. The anterior vaginal wall is closed with a running 2-0 PGA suture. Thus, the wound is closed in three layers: the urethral wall vertically, the periurethral fascia horizontally, and the overlying vaginal wall flap covering the underlying suture lines (Fig.

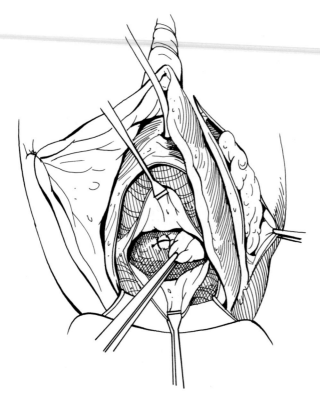

FIG. 45–6. Labial fat pad (Martius graft) after mobilization passed through the medial tunnel from the labial area to the fistula/diverticulectomy closure site and fixed in position with absorbable sutures.

45–5E). At the end of the procedure, an antibiotic-soaked vaginal pack is placed and both the suprapubic and urethral catheters are placed to gravity drainage.

Perioperative parenteral antibiotics are continued for 24 hours, followed by oral antibiotics until the catheters are removed. Belladonna and opium suppositories are given postoperatively until the patient can tolerate oral anticholinergics (oxybutynin or tolterodine and imipramine hydrochloride) to prevent bladder spasm. The vaginal packing is removed on postoperative day 1. Seven to 10 days postoperatively vaginal examination is performed to confirm an intact vaginal flap and suture lines. Anticholinergics are then discontinued 24 hours prior to performing a VCUG. During the VCUG the urethral catheter is removed and the bladder is filled with contrast through the suprapubic tube. The urethra is then carefully observed fluoroscopically during voiding. Should any extravasation occur (as noted in approximately 50% of patients), the patient is asked to stop voiding and the bladder is returned to drainage via the suprapubic catheter. The urethral catheter is not replaced and anticholinergics are resumed. The VCUG is then repeated 7 to 10 days later.

When there is no extravasation on the initial VCUG, the patient is allowed to empty her bladder; if the postvoid residual urine volume is less than 100 mL, the suprapubic catheter is removed. The suprapubic catheter is removed only after satisfactory bladder emptying is established. Intermittent self-catheterization is avoided for fear of disrupting the site of urethral reconstruction.

OUTCOMES

Complications

The urethral diverticulum may recur as a result of incomplete excision of the diverticulum and its urethral communication site. The likelihood of recurrence can be reduced by preoperatively identifying the presence of multiple diverticula and/or communication sites. Complete excision during the operation removes all pockets of a multiloculated diverticulum. Care should also be taken to completely close the urethral defect to prevent formation of a pseudodiverticulum between the layers of closure. The VCUG should be performed postoperatively to rule out extravasation from the urethral closure site before the patient resumes voiding.

Recurrence of a diverticulum is in general suggested by persistent or recurrent symptoms, periurethral mass, tenderness along the urethra, or recurrent urinary tract infection (UTI). Recurrent diverticula may be managed with a second excision procedure with Martius fat interposition. A small distal recurrent diverticulum may also be satisfactorily treated with transurethral saucerization or the Spence marsupialization procedure.

Urethrovaginal fistula is also a well-described complication of urethral diverticulectomy. In the authors' experience, fistula formation occurs with techniques involving vertical vaginal incisions and overlapping suture lines. Urethrovaginal fistula can be repaired transvaginally without excising the fistula using the three-layer anterior vaginal wall flap technique and interposition of Martius labial fat pad graft (7) (Fig. 45–6).

Bladder injury has also been described, in particular during dissection of a large proximal urethral diverticulum extending beneath the trigone. Such injuries result in an iatrogenic vesicovaginal fistula. Instillation of indigo carmine into the bladder and cystoscopy should be performed to rule out bladder injury prior to closure.

Urinary incontinence may occur postoperatively for the following reasons: persistent SUI, *de novo* SUI, recurrent diverticulum with paradoxical stress incontinence, urethrovaginal or vesicovaginal fistula, and/or detrusor instability. Postoperative incontinence is evaluated and appropriately treated depending on the etiology.

Postoperative irritative voiding symptoms may be caused by UTI or bladder dysfunction. Preoperative urodynamic evaluation is essential to identify candidates likely to develop postoperative detrusor instability. In our recently published series, 12 women had preoperative detrusor instability during urodynamic studies and it per-

TABLE 45–3. *Results and complications of diverticulectomy from published series compared to authors' series*

Complication	Published range (%)	Authors' series (%)
Recurrent Diverticulum	1–25	3.6
Urethrovaginal Fistula	0.9–8.3	1.8
Stress Incontinence	1.7–100	16.1
Recurrent Urinary Infection	7.1–31.3	0
Urethral Stricture	1.7–5.2	0

sisted in four women (33%) after diverticulectomy (3). Persistent detrusor instability is treated with anticholinergic medications, while *de novo* bladder dysfunction requires further evaluation to rule out obstruction.

Finally, postoperative narrowing of the urethra may occur by removing excess urethral wall during excision of the diverticular communication site. Sufficient urethral wall should be preserved to close over a 14 Fr Foley catheter. Urethral stricture after diverticulectomy may require additional urethral reconstruction.

Results

The results of urethral diverticulectomy from published series are summarized in Table 45–3. In our series, a urethral diverticulum was diagnosed in 63 women and urethral diverticulectomy was performed in 56 women (88.9%) (3). With a mean follow-up of 70 months (range, 6 to 136 months), 48 women (85.7%) had relief of their presenting symptoms. Two recurrent diverticula (noted at the distal urethral closure site) were documented by periurethral mass and/or tenderness on follow-up vaginal examination. Both recurrent diverticula were managed satisfactorily with transurethral saucerization. Early UTIs were identified and treated satisfactorily in six women, but none of these patients developed recurrent UTIs. Four women who had persistent detrusor instability after surgery noted significant urgency symptoms. No patient developed a postoperative wound infection or urethral stricture.

The overall continence status in the treatment group of 56 women with a mean follow-up of 70 months may be summarized as follows: Forty-five women (80.4%) were totally continent or minimally incontinent (dry or no pad for protection); ten women (17.9%) were moderately incontinent (1 or 2 minipads per day for protection); and one woman (1.8%) had severe incontinence (several pads per day for protection) because of detrusor hyperreflexia secondary to cerebellar degeneration.

REFERENCES

1. Blacklock AR, Shaw RE, Geddes JR. Late presentation of ectopic ureter. *Br J Urol* 1982;54:106–110.
2. Chancellor MB, et al. Intraoperative endo-luminal ultrasound evaluation of urethral diverticula. *J Urol* 1995;153:72–75.
3. Ganabathi K, et al. Experience with the management of urethral diverticulum in 63 women. *J Urol* 1994;152(5, Pt 1):1445–1452.
4. Hey W. *Practical observations in surgery*. Philadelphia: James Humphreys Publishers, 1805:303.
5. Lapides J. Transurethral treatment of urethral diverticula in women. *J Urol* 1979;121:736–738.
6. Leach GE. Urethrovaginal fistula repair with Martius labial fat pad graft. *Urol Clin North Am* 1991;18:409–413.
7. Leach GE, et al. L N S C3: a proposed classification system for female urethral diverticula. *Neurourol Urodynam* 1993;12:523–531.
8. Rajan N, et al. Carcinoma in female urethral diverticulum: case reports and review of management. *J Urol* 1993;150:1911–1914.
9. Spence HM, Duckett JW Jr. Diverticulum of the female urethra: clinical aspects and presentation of a simple operative technique for cure. *J Urol* 1970;104:432–437.
10. Zimmern P. The role of voiding cystourethrography in the evaluation of the female lower urinary tract. In: Paulson D, ed. *Problems in urology*. Philadelphia: JB Lippincott Co, 1991:23–41.

CHAPTER 46

Closure of Bladder Neck in the Male and Female

Robert W. Frederick and Philippe E. Zimmern

Bladder neck closure (BNC) is an uncommon procedure that has by tradition been reserved as a final alternative for the management of the female patient with neurogenically induced intractable incontinence arising from long-term Foley catheter drainage (4,9). It has also been used in the treatment of nonneuropathic conditions such as traumatic urethral destruction or recalcitrant fistula. BNC in the male is usually reserved for patients with neurogenic bladder or a history of incontinence secondary to trauma or urethrocutaneous fistula failing multiple prior attempts at surgical correction or artificial sphincter placement. In recent years, salvage prostatectomy and BNC in the management of recurrent prostate cancer after radiation therapy and in the management of severe complications after salvage cryotherapy has been reported (3,6).

With the many other options that exist for the treatment of these complex conditions, there is a limited but distinct role for BNC. Although initially fraught with a high failure rate, patient selection and technical refinements have allowed some authors to achieve a success rate of nearly 100% (9). This chapter will focus on the technique of both abdominal and vaginal bladder neck closure in the female and abdominal bladder neck closure in the male with emphasis on the principles necessary to achieve both successful and durable results.

DIAGNOSIS

Preoperative evaluation and patient selection is extremely important to the success of BNC. A careful history should include special attention to prior abdominal or pelvic surgeries including prior reconstructive flaps or grafts. During the physical exam it is important to carefully assess the presence of lower-extremity contractures that may limit access to the vagina, perineal skin integrity

or presence of decubiti, and the potential for intermittent catheterization to be carried out successfully. In the patient with adequate manual dexterity or a reliable caregiver, a catheterizable efferent limb from the bladder may be chosen for postoperative drainage. When intermittent catheterization is not feasible, options for postoperative bladder drainage primarily consist of suprapubic tube or incontinent ileovesicostomy.

Study of the upper urinary tract by either ultrasonography or intravenous pyelography is important to exclude hydronephrosis or ureteral obstruction as often the same processes responsible for the patient's incontinence may promote upper-tract deterioration. When upper-tract deterioration is noted, strong consideration must be given to supravesical diversion or preserving the bladder and lowering intravesical pressures by augmentation cystoplasty. A static or voiding cystogram assists in detecting bladder diverticula, vesicoureteral reflux, and calculi. In the case of urethral fistula or stricture, a retrograde urethrogram or fistulogram can document the nature and extent of the patient's underlying disease.

Cystoscopy with biopsy to exclude bladder malignancy is essential for the patient who has been managed for an extended period with an indwelling catheter. The extent of urodynamic evaluation is tailored to the choice of postoperative bladder management. In the patient who desires continent, catheterizable access to the bladder, preoperative urodynamic evaluation of bladder storage parameters such as compliance and detrusor overactivity must be documented to determine the need for concomitant augmentation cystoplasty. When the bladder outlet is patulous, occlusion of the outlet during urodynamic evaluation can be readily accomplished using gentle traction on an inflated Foley catheter.

A sterile urine culture should be documented preoperatively. When it is impossible to completely sterilize the urine, culture-specific preoperative parenteral antibiotics must be administered to ensure adequate tissue levels at the time of surgery.

INDICATIONS FOR SURGERY

The indications for bladder neck closure in the non-neurogenic patient are urethral destruction, severe intrinsic sphincteric deficiency that is not amenable to or has failed conventional treatment, and urethrovaginal fistula failing prior attempts at repair. Patients suffering from neurogenic incontinence often have intractable leakage from urethral destruction due to the long-term effects of an indwelling urethral catheter. A common indication is the patient with advanced multiple sclerosis and neurogenic detrusor overactivity resulting in catheter bypassing and extrusion. In such patients, if continence without a chronic Foley catheter can be achieved a significant improvement in quality of life has been demonstrated. Although control of incontinence has been achieved by some using a pubovaginal sling, many patients with urethral destruction and reduced urethral length are not suitable candidates for this procedure. Likewise, for the female patient who has failed attempts at urethrovaginal fistula closure BNC with a continent catheterizable efferent channel, incontinent vesicostomy, or suprapubic tube may represent a viable option for management.

The vaginal approach is favored in the patient without history of prior radiation who desires suprapubic tube drainage. An abdominal approach is desirable for the patient with a history of radiation in whom vaginal tissues may be poorly vascularized and in whom omental interposition between the bladder neck and vagina is desirable. It is also the approach of choice in the patient who elects for a continent efferent limb (bowel or appendix) or incontinent ileovesicostomy or who has failed a prior attempt at vaginal closure of the bladder neck (Table 46–1).

The role of BNC in the male with benign disease resides in the management of refractory urethrocutaneous or urethrorectal fistula and in cases of severe neurogenic or postoperative incontinence (with low outlet resistance) when the artificial sphincter is not an option. It may also be used in the treatment of recalcitrant urethral strictures when reconstruction is impossible or undesired.

BNC may be considered in conjunction with salvage prostatectomy for locally recurrent prostate adenocarcinoma after radiation therapy. Incontinence rates with a vesicourethral anastomosis in this patient population are reported as high as 65%, and the risk of artificial sphincter erosion is high (5). Complications encountered after salvage cryotherapy may be amenable to prostatectomy with BNC as well. These complications include osteitis pubis, recurrent gross hematuria, bladder outlet obstruction, urinary incontinence, puboprostatic fistula, urethral stricture disease, and intractable perineal pain. Most of these patients will have more than one of these complications and have undergone multiple previous less definitive surgeries to alleviate their symptoms with short-lived success (3).

ALTERNATIVE THERAPY

Options for local reconstruction in females with severe incontinence or fistula are limited. Although urethral reconstruction with vaginal wall or bowel is an available option, maintaining a urethral outlet that is both patent and continent can prove extremely challenging. Continence following these reconstructive procedures may be provided by autologous or synthetic sling materials, injectable bulking agents (collagen or Durasphere), artificial urinary sphincter, or bladder neck reconstruction (Young–Dees). In the male with refractory incontinence or fistula, when previously irradiated tissue is not present the artificial urinary sphincter and formal fistula closure are other viable alternatives.

Historically, supravesical diversion and ureterosigmoidostomy (nonneurogenic patients) have been advocated for treatment of patients with this severity of incontinence. However, it is our opinion that BNC should be considered before embarking on these more extensive surgical options. BNC not only preserves the bladder but also preserves the integrity of the ureterovesical junction, thereby protecting the upper tracts.

TABLE 46–1. *Comparison of approaches to bladder neck closure in the female patient*

Factor	Vaginal closure	Abdominal closure
Multiple prior abdominal procedures	Preferred Approach	Alternate Approach
Prior Radiation	No Prior Pelvic Radiation	History of Pelvic Radiation
Postoperative Drainage	Suprapubic Tube Drainage	Desires incontinent Vesicostomy or Catheterizable Bladder Drainage
Vascularized Interposition	Martius Flap	Omentum; Rectus Flap; Peritoneal Flap
Lower Extremity Flexibility	Adequate	Impaired
Perineal Skin Condition	Adequate	Decubiti or Infected

SURGICAL TECHNIQUE

The goals of the procedure are the same for both male and female patients regardless of the approach utilized. These goals include wide mobilization of the bladder neck to allow for tension-free closure, multilayer closure of the outlet without overlapping suture lines, thereby reducing the opportunity for fistula, interposition of vascularized tissue between the vesical outlet and urethral stump or vagina, and adequate postoperative bladder drainage with a large-bore catheter.

Vaginal Approach in the Female

The vaginal approach is preferred in the female who desires suprapubic tube drainage, has no history of prior radiation, and is not undergoing a concomitant abdominal procedure. Preoperative preparation includes antibiotics, vaginal douching, enema, and deep venous thrombosis prophylaxis. The patient is placed in the high lithotomy position with careful attention to padding of all pressure points and extremities. A Lonestar ring retractor (Houston, TX) is suggested along with a weighted vaginal speculum and headlight to provide maximal vaginal exposure. In the case of a small contracted bladder, the curved Lowsley retractor is employed to place a suprapubic tube. The patient is placed in the deep Trendelenburg position to displace bowel contents and the curved retractor is introduced through the urethra and directed to the anterior abdominal wall 1 to 2 cm above the symphysis pubis. A small suprapubic incision is made over the tip of

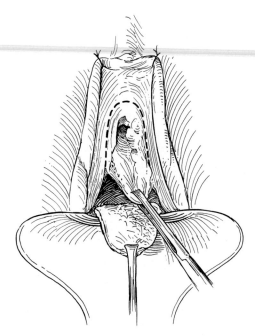

FIG. 46–2. Elevation of the vaginal flap.

the Lowsley, which can be palpated beneath the fascia. The tip of the retractor is then pushed out through the skin incision and a 20 Fr Foley catheter is grasped between the open jaws and delivered back into the bladder. Its intravesical position can be confirmed with cystoscopy or irrigation with normal saline.

A waterproof surgical ink pen marks the proposed inverted U-shaped vaginal wall incision. A dilute solution of vasopressin (60 U per 100 cm) (3) can be injected into the periurethral tissues and anterior vaginal wall to facil-

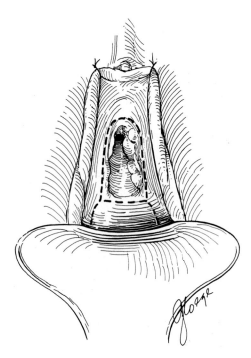

FIG. 46–1. Proposed incision for closure of the bladder neck.

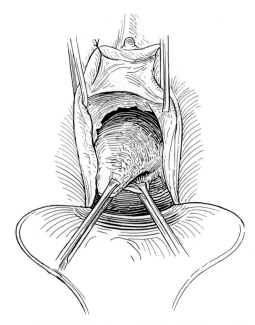

FIG. 46–3. Detachment of the bladder neck.

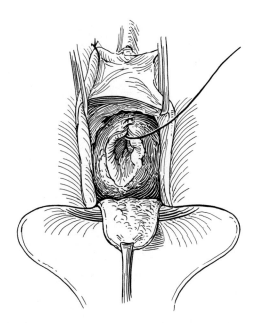

FIG. 46–4. Primary closure with tension-free anastomosis.

itate dissection of both the urethra and anterior vaginal flap and reduce local bleeding (Fig. 46–1).

After a circumscribing incision has been made around the urethral meatus, the broad-based vaginal flap is elevated using sharp scissors dissection (Fig. 46–2). This flap not only aids in the exposure of the remainder of the urethral dissection but serves as an advancement flap to close over the amputated vesical outlet and interposed labial fat pad. When dissecting in the proper plane, the vaginal wall exhibits a distinctly recognizable white glistening surface. Significant venous bleeding may be

encountered when the dissection is carried out too deep and into the venous sinuses of the bladder wall. Sharp dissection is then used to free the urethra from its lateral and anterior fascial attachments. To achieve a tension-free closure, the bladder neck must be completely detached from its surrounding (mostly anterior) attachments (Fig. 46–3). The pubourethral ligaments are sharply transected and the endopelvic fascia is perforated bilaterally using blunt or sharp dissection. After entering the retropubic space, blunt dissection is used to free the lateral and anterior aspects of the bladder neck. Indigo carmine is given intravenously to aid in visualizing the ureteral orifices and the urethral edges may be trimmed to expose fresh healthy tissues for formal closure.

The bladder neck is first closed in a vertical fashion with absorbable 3-0 polyglycolic acid (PGA) sutures (Fig. 46–4). The integrity of the closure is then checked by filling the bladder through the suprapubic tube. A second horizontal layer of interrupted 2-0 PGA serves to both imbricate the first layer and transfer the closed bladder outlet to a position high behind the symphysis pubis, thus rotating it into a nondependent position (Fig. 46–5). This technique not only avoids a dependent closure but also directs the force of bladder spasms away from the vagina, thereby reducing the likelihood of secondary vesicovaginal fistula.

The use of a Martius flap is recommended to reinforce the bladder neck closure and reduce the risk of fistula. The technique relies on a well-vascularized fibrofatty labial pad (from the labia majora) that is based posteriorly on a labial branch of the internal pudendal artery (8). The Martius flap is tunneled beneath the vaginal wall and fixed in place over the bladder neck closure with 3-0

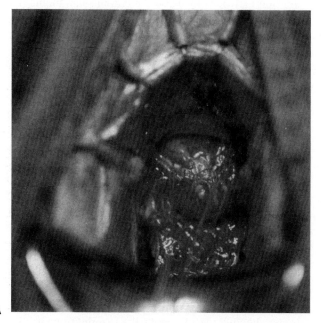

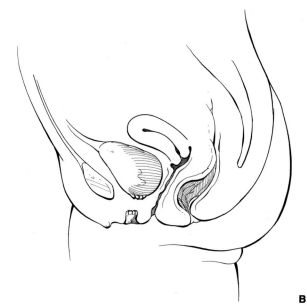

FIG. 46–5. A: Photograph of closure of the bladder neck. **B:** Lateral view of bladder neck closure.

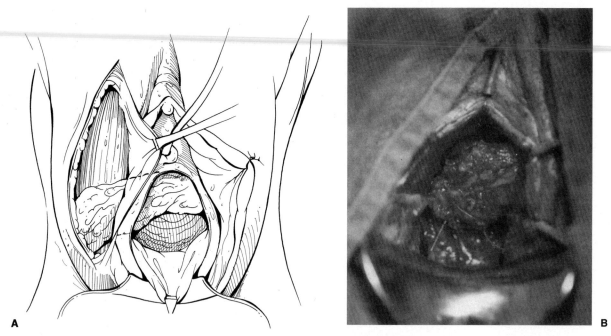

FIG. 46–6. A: Martius flap tunneled beneath the labia minora. **B:** Intraoperative photograph of Martius flap to close over the bladder neck.

PGA sutures (Fig. 46–6). The vertical labial incision can be closed with absorbable sutures over a small suction drain. The vaginal flap is trimmed and advanced to close the vaginal incision with a running 3-0 PGA suture (Fig. 46–7). The suprapubic tube is then irrigated to ensure patency and the vagina is packed for 24 hours with an antibiotic-soaked pack.

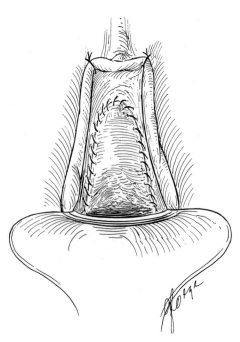

FIG. 46–7. Closure of the vaginal flap.

Abdominal Approach in the Female

The patient is placed in the low lithotomy position to provide continuous access to the vagina. Alternatively, if lower-extremity contractures prohibit the lithotomy position, the supine position may be appropriate. A urethral Foley catheter is placed and an infraumbilical midline incision made. This incision not only provides excellent exposure but also can be extended for omental harvest or use of bowel for an efferent catheterizable limb. A Pfannenstiel incision may be considered if a chronic suprapubic tube is chosen for postoperative bladder management. The rectus muscles are retracted laterally and the prevesical space (Retzius) is developed bluntly. The peritoneum is retracted superiorly, and a self-retaining retractor (Balfour or Bookwalter) provides exposure of the retropubic space.

With the aid of the Foley catheter and its balloon, the bladder neck and urethra are identified. A 2-0 PGA figure-of-8 suture is placed through the distal most aspect of the deep dorsal vein of the clitoris and the proximal urethra. Using electrocautery or sharp dissection, the anterior bladder neck is amputated from the pelvic inlet over the most distal aspect of the Foley catheter. The anterior bladder neck is grasped with traction sutures or Allis clamps and the Foley catheter is identified and delivered into the surgical field. After intravenous administration of indigo carmine, open-ended ureteral catheters may be placed to assist in a safe dissection of the posterior bladder neck (Fig. 46–8). A hand in the vagina can help identify and maintain the appropriate plane between the posterior bladder neck and the vaginal wall. Using electrocautery or sharp dissection, the posterior bladder

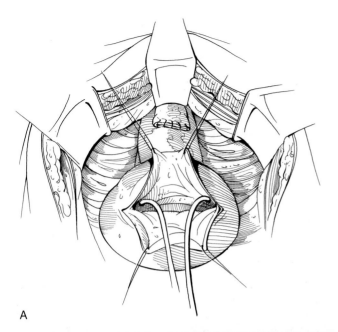

A

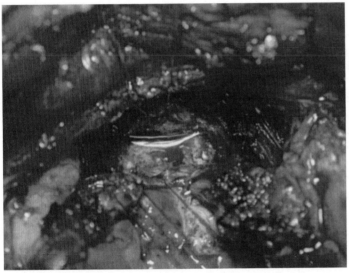

B

FIG. 46–8. **A:**Opened bladder with mobilization of the bladder neck. **B:**. Intraoperative photograph of divided urethral stump and mobilized open bladder neck.

neck is freed from the anterior vaginal wall. This division continues until the bladder neck is rolled up and out of a dependent position. The edges of the bladder neck are trimmed to allow approximation of healthy tissues and the ureteral stents are removed. When an incontinent vesicostomy or catheterizable efferent limb is selected for postoperative bladder drainage they may be fashioned at this time. Otherwise, a large-bore (24 Fr) Malecot or Foley catheter is placed through a stab wound in the bladder dome. The bladder neck is then closed in two layers as described for vaginal closure.

Approach in the Male

The technique of bladder neck closure in the male differs from the female in several distinct ways: (a) lack of

direct perineal access to the bladder neck; (b) options for vascularized tissue are more limited; and (c) the prostatic anatomy poses a challenge to both intraoperative closure and postoperative care.

The perineal approach to BNC, although conceptually and technically feasible, is not considered the procedure of choice in the male. Perineal access to the bladder neck necessitates either a concomitant prostatectomy with its own inherent morbidity or closure of the infraprostatic urethra, a procedure associated with a high rate of spontaneous fistulization. Infraprostatic closure of the urethra, although easily performed, is not desirable for the following reasons:

1. The surgical closure continues to remain in a dependent position.

2. With the exception of a gracilis or gluteal flap, there is little opportunity for interposition of a large healthy segment of vascularized tissue.

3. Prostate secretions can only drain in a retrograde fashion into the bladder or, in dyssynergic patients, remained trapped in the prostatic fossa, resulting in a high rate of fistulization.

4. Perineal closure does not preserve antegrade ejaculation and compromises future fertility.

The abdominal approach to bladder neck closure has two distinct advantages over perineal closure: (a) The bladder neck can be rotated anteriorly and out of a dependent position and (b) the choices for vascularized interposition are abundant (omentum, rectus flap, and peritoneal flap). Two techniques have historically been employed for abdominal closure of the bladder neck in men with benign disease: supraprostatic and infraprostatic closure. Supraprostatic bladder neck closure has been our choice as it offers several distinct advantages over infraprostatic closure. It is technically easier and does not involve deep pelvic dissection or transection of the dorsal venous complex. It allows for a better mobilization of the bladder neck, resulting in a tension-free closure. Last, it provides opportunity for future fertility as an antegrade flow of ejaculate is preserved.

When BNC is to be performed in conjunction with salvage prostatectomy, the extirpative portion of the procedure is performed first. Description of this portion of the procedure is beyond the scope of this chapter, but those who have published reports on the care of these patients (3,6) describe it as technically challenging. A distinct advantage of this operation, when compared to salvage prostatectomy with vesicourethral anastomosis, is that it allows for wider excision, in particular at the apex of the prostate.

After supine or low lithotomy positioning, the patient is prepped and a catheter is placed in a sterile fashion. An infraumbilical vertical midline incision is performed and the retropubic space is accessed as described earlier. The bladder neck is identified and absorbable suture is used to ligate the superficial dorsal venous complex at the prostatovesical junction. The prostate and vesical neck are grasped and electrocautery or sharp dissection is then used to amputate the anterior vesical neck from the prostate. Once the bladder neck mucosa is entered, the Foley balloon may be deflated and removed to permit visualization of the posterior vesical neck. Indigo carmine and ureteral catheters are used as previously described. The posterior bladder wall is transected and the plane between the bladder and the rectum identified. Mobilization of the posterior bladder neck from Denonvillier's fascia and rectum should continue until the vesical outlet has reached an anterior, nondependent position. Excessive mobilization should be avoided to prevent injury to the ureters or vascular pedicles of the bladder. A large-bore (22 to 24 Fr Malecot or Foley) suprapubic tube

is then placed through a separate stab incision. If an alternative bladder drainage method is desired (incontinent vesicostomy, catheterizable efferent limb), it may be constructed at this time.

Depending on its size, bladder neck closure can be performed by one of two methods. In the patient with a small bladder neck, a series of two absorbable pursestring sutures of 3-0 PGA may be used to invert the outlet similar to the inversion of an appendiceal stump. For a larger bladder neck, or where closure is more difficult, the outlet may be closed in two layers as described above. Placement of a well-vascularized flap of omentum, rectus muscle, or peritoneum in the fossa between the bladder neck closure and prostate is performed to not only facilitate healing but to help prevent fistulization (Fig. 46–9).

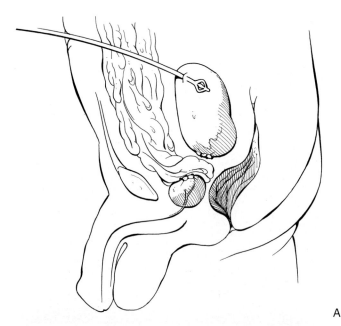

A

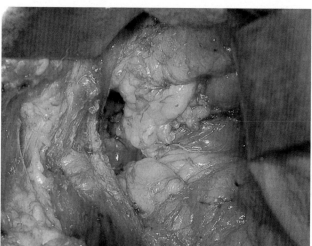

B

FIG. 46–9. A: Omental interposition in the male. **B:** Intraoperative photograph showing omental wrap over bladder neck closure to prevent secondary vesicourethral fistula.

Recently, a technique of BNC in combination with prostatectomy and intestinal interposition has been described (7). After removing the prostate, the bladder neck is incorporated into a transverse cystotomy that leaves the ureterovesical junction undisturbed. A segment of bowel is then mobilized and sutured in a single layer as an augmentation. Depending on the segment used, a continent catheterizable diversion was then fashioned. This technique may be desirable when a continent diversion is planned and an augmentation cystoplasty is necessary. It in addition has the advantage of incorporating nonirradiated tissue into the BNC of a previously irradiated pelvis, as in the case of salvage prostatectomy.

Concomitant prostatectomy may be indicated in the case of a strictured urethra or prostatorectal fistula that poses a problem to postoperative prostatic drainage. Some advocate performing prostatectomy in conjunction with BNC in those patients with preexisting complete erectile dysfunction as it facilitates the mobilization of the bladder neck away from urethral pathology (7). Because prostatectomy is not necessary to successfully accomplish BNC, its indication should be based on clear separate indications.

Following the BNC it is highly advisable to interpose vascularized tissue between the bladder neck and the pelvic outlet to reduce the risk of secondary fistula. Choices for interposition include omentum, a flap of adjacent peritoneum, or a rectus flap. We prefer omentum because of its size, reliable blood supply, and abundant lymphatic drainage. In patients with a generous omentum, a tongue may be easily mobilized with only limited dissection (8). If, however, the patient is extremely thin or has had radiation or prior intraabdominal surgery, a more extended incision may be needed and the omentum may be mobilized on a pedicle supplied by the right gastroepiploic artery. The right side is preferred due to its more dependent position in the abdomen and its more generous blood supply. The omentum is positioned between the BNC and the pelvic outlet and sutured in place with absorbable sutures. When a rectus flap is selected, it may be mobilized and based on an inferior epigastric vascular pedicle with careful attention to tie all lateral vascular collaterals. The mobilized rectus flap is then rotated downward and positioned as described above for omentum. Alternatively, a paravesical peritoneal flap may be interposed; however, its vascular supply may not be as reliable as omentum or rectus flap (8). A suction drain is left in the pelvis and brought out through a separate stab wound along with the suprapubic catheter.

POSTOPERATIVE CARE

Postoperative intravenous antibiotics are used for 3 to 5 days, after which patients are placed on daily oral antibiotic suppression. The suction drain is usually left for 1 to 2 days. In our experience a nasogastric tube is not usually necessary. The suprapubic tube is carefully secured to avoid kinking or dislodgement. Patients are kept on either oral or rectal anticholinergic medication (oxybutynin with or without imipramine or belladonna and opium suppositories) to prevent bladder spasms. A cystogram is obtained at 2 to 3 weeks to document the integrity of bladder neck closure. If there is no evidence of leak or fistula, the suprapubic tube may be changed or removed if a catheterizable stoma was chosen for bladder drainage.

OUTCOMES

Complications

The primary complication of bladder neck closure is postoperative fistula. Such a fistula may occur as early as 1 week postoperatively or as late as 1 year. Prevention of fistula formation is accomplished by careful debridement of the bladder neck edges, use of two nonoverlapping suture lines, nondependent positioning of the bladder neck, interposition of well-vascularized tissue over the closure, and avoidance of postoperative bladder spasms. When a fistula is suspected, the patient should undergo a cystogram with a mixture of 30% iodinated contrast and methylene blue dye. The site of leakage (vagina or perineum) should then be assessed both visually and radiographically. If a small fistula is encountered early in the postoperative period, bilateral percutaneous nephrostomies may be used to divert the urine away from the fistulous site. Reoperation is a more complex but reliable method of dealing with postoperative fistula. When the initial procedure was performed from a vaginal or perineal approach, reoperation should be performed suprapubically to allow extensive bladder mobilization and allow for interposition of a large, well-vascularized omental flap. Supravesical diversion is reserved for patients in whom all other attempts at repair have failed.

Loss of access to the bladder may also represent a source of postoperative morbidity. Loss of a suprapubic tube and closure of its tract is an underreported but not uncommon complication. Access may be reestablished by using a flexible cystoscope or ureteroscope and may require fluoroscopy to negotiate the tract and pass a flexible wire down to the bladder. If this procedure fails, the patient may be given a fluid bolus and the bladder may be percutaneously accessed under sonographic guidance. Once access has been established, the tract may be dilated and a council catheter passed over the wire. Inability to catheterize a continent efferent limb may be treated similarly and endoscopic negotiation of the conduit usually suffices to reestablish access.

Results

Although a number of authors have reported their results with BNC, most series have been small, retrospective, and with a great deal of variability in technique (2,4,9). Consequently, long-term outcomes and overall success rates are difficult to judge. In series where the bladder neck is anteriorly mobilized and appropriate vascularized interposition is utilized, long-term continence rates range from 86% to 100% with a 7% to 8% reoperation rate (4,9). In series where these principles have not been employed, fistula formation and reoperation rates range from 30% to 46% and 25% to 46%, respectively (1,2). In one series where female multiple sclerosis patients were treated with vaginal urethral closure and suprapubic cystostomy, approximately 80% of the patients who were continent (± an early revision) and available for reliable follow-up remained continent at an average follow-up of 6.5 years (range, 2 to 17 years) (2). Upper-tract deterioration has been noted in a single series (11%) and has been causally related to use of continent, catheterizable efferent channels in patients with persistent bladder dysfunction (1).

REFERENCES

1. Andrews HO, Shah PJR. Surgical management of urethral damage in neurogenically impaired female patients with chronic indwelling catheters. *Br J Urol* 1998;82:820.
2. Eckford SB, Kohler-Ockmore J, Feneley RCL. Long-term follow up of transvaginal urethral closure and suprapubic cystostomy for urinary incontinence in women with multiple sclerosis. *Br J Urol* 1994; 74:319.
3. Izawa JI, Ajam K, McGuire EJ, Scott S, Eschenbach AC, Skibber J, Pisters LL. Major surgery to manage definitively severe complications of salvage cryotherapy for prostate cancer. *J Urol* 2000;164:978.
4. Jayanthi VR, Churchill BM, McLorie GA, Koury AE. Concomitant bladder neck closure and Mitrofanoff diversion for the management of intractable urinary incontinence. *J Urol* 1995;154:886.
5. Martins FE, Boyd SD. Post-operative risk factors associated with artificial urinary sphincter infection-erosion. *Br J Urol* 1995;75:354.
6. Pisters LL, English SF, Scott SM, Westney OL, Dinney CPN, McGuire EJ. Salvage prostatectomy with continent catheterizable urinary reconstruction: a novel approach to recurrent prostate cancer after radiation therapy. *J Urol* 2000;163:1771.
7. Ullrich N, Wessells H. A technique of bladder neck closure combining prostatectomy and intestinal interposition for unsalvageable urethral disease. *J Urol* 2002;167:634–636.
8. Windle B, Kursh E. Use of interposition pedicle material for vesicovaginal fistula repair. In: McGuire EJ, ed. *Female urology*. Philadelphia: JB Lippincott Co, 1994:393–402.
9. Zimmern PE, Hadley HR, Leach GE, Raz S. Transvaginal closure of the bladder neck and placement of a suprapubic catheter for destroyed urethra after long term indwelling catheterization. *J Urol* 1985;134:554.

CHAPTER 47

Reconstruction of the Female Urethra

Jerry G. Blaivas and Adam J. Flisser

Reconstruction of the female urethra is a surgical undertaking that can range from deceptively simple to extraordinarily difficult. While it is usually possible to restore anatomy and function with a single procedure, failure to do so exposes the patient to the risks of multiple operations with decreasing chances of success. For this reason, it is incumbent upon the physician to be technically skilled in the correct procedures and to perform a comprehensive diagnostic examination to understand the patient's pathophysiology prior to performing the repair. The goal of surgery should be repair of the damaged urethra in such a way as to allow the patient voluntary, unobstructed, and painless micturition.

In the developing world, the most common cause of urethral damage (Table 47–1) requiring reconstruction is urethrovaginal fistula resulting from obstetric trauma. Prolonged obstructed labor with compression of the fetal head against the symphysis pubis causes pressure necrosis of the urethra with the subsequent development of complicated fistulae (4,7). Caesarean section performed to relieve this condition also carries a greater risk of sub-sequent fistula formation (1,4). Where modern obstetric care is available to prevent this type of injury, urethral damage is more commonly the result of reconstructive surgery for urethral diverticulum (6) although it is also a reported complication of bladder neck suspensions, anterior colporrhaphy, and, rarely, vaginal hysterectomy. Urethrovaginal fistulae are also caused by erosion of synthetic materials placed during pelvic reconstructive surgery or antiincontinence procedures. Local malignancy can cause fistula formation or fistula can develop as a long-term complication of radiotherapy. Unusual causes of urethral injury have been reported, including damage from sutures placed for Shirodkar cerclage for cervical incompetence in the gravid woman, complications from operative vaginal delivery, and pressure necrosis from tightly placed Kelly plication sutures over an indwelling catheter. The presence of an indwelling catheter itself can cause urethral necrosis, typically in the population of paralyzed or comatose patients. Finally, pelvic trauma can cause laceration of the urethra through separation or fracture of the symphysis pubis (10).

TABLE 47–1. *Causes of urethral damage in a case series of 98 women*

Transvaginal Bladder Neck Suspension	27
Urethral Diverticulectomy	26
Anterior Colporraphy	13
Synthetic Pubovaginal Sling	9
Urethral Diverticulum	9
Childbirth	5
Urogenital Cancers	5
Trauma	2
Cesarian Section	1
Vaginal Hysterectomy	1
Total	98

From Blaivas JG. Vaginal flap urethral reconstruction: and alternative to the bladder flap neourethra. *J Urol* 1996;141: 542–545, with permission, and subsequent unpublished data.

DIAGNOSIS

In keeping with the dictates of modern medical training, a thorough history and physical examination should form the basic approach to a patient suspected to have urethral injury. In our experience, pelvic examination will reveal the vast majority of urethral injuries. If concurrent sphincteric urinary incontinence complicates the diagnosis, the urethral meatus can be occluded by the examiner's finger while the patient strains or coughs. If the anterior vaginal wall is visualized with the assistance of a speculum blade placed into the posterior fornix, transurethral urinary leakage can usually be detected.

Cystoscopic examination is an essential part of the diagnostic investigation. Cystoscopy enables visualization of the extent of the pathology as well as the evaluation of both concurrent injuries or defects and the quality of the surrounding local tissue that is available for use in a reconstructive procedure. The addition of methylene blue to the cystoscopy fluid can be useful if a fistula is suspected but has not been observed. After the surgeon occludes the urethra with a Foley catheter, the vagina is examined for signs of urinary leakage.

It is important to recognize that urethral damage alone causes neither urinary incontinence nor detrusor instability. In patients who have coexisting urologic symptoms, the physician should be suspicious of injury to the proximal urethra and/or vesical neck. Videourodynamic examination will provide vital information about the presence of involuntary bladder contractions, bladder outlet obstruction, ureteral reflex, and bladder compliance and may also identify concurrent fistulae or diverticula. A low urinary flow rate can suggest posttraumatic stricture.

Radiological imaging is of great value in patients with urethral and urovaginal pathology. Intravenous pyelography will often reveal complicated fistulae that are associated with obvious urethral pathology. Retrograde pyelography should be performed when ureteral injury is suspected and may be valuable even in patients with normal intravenous pyelograms.

INDICATIONS FOR SURGERY

Surgical intervention is usually undertaken due to the presence of urethral obstruction, sphincteric urinary incontinence, or associated vesicovaginal fistula. We advocate the simultaneous correction of all of the coexisting anatomic and functional pathologies that led to the surgery. In patients with sphincteric incontinence, we recommend autologous fascial pubovaginal sling with supporting labial fat graft interposed between the vesical neck and the sling, with the vaginal mucosa closed directly over the fascial sling; however, others have alternatively proposed transvaginal bladder neck suspension in patients with favorable anatomy and incontinence due to urethral hypermobility (5).

The majority of patients we have seen suffering from urethral damage who also have impaired detrusor contractility, low bladder compliance, or detrusor instability improve after urethral reconstruction; however, patients with radiation cystitis do not belong to this group. The poor tissue quality in this subset of patients makes successful anatomic repair difficult and often results in functional problems. In this situation, supravesical diversion is often the more prudent and successful choice.

Past teaching suggested that 3 to 6 months of delay was necessary to allow the quality of the local tissue to improve as inflammation and edema subsided; however, recent studies show that, although pliable tissue must be available and free of infection and inflammation, lengthy delay is not necessary and under the right conditions successful repair can be accomplished within days or weeks of the injury (2).

ALTERNATIVE THERAPY

Alternatives to vaginal wall flaps include anterior and posterior bladder flap techniques. Creating a neourethra using these methods is possible with a comparable degree of success to the procedures outlined above; however, continence is not as easily achieved, with success rates of about 50% (5,8,11). Accordingly, we have chosen to emphasize vaginal reconstruction with antiincontinence surgery as the preferred management of urethral injury associated with incontinence rather than employing these alternatives and their associated complications. Nonetheless, when extensive vaginal scarring in conjunction with large fistulae precludes vaginal flap reconstruction a bladder flap procedure is the next reasonable alternative (Fig. 47–1).

After the edges of the fistula are dissected free from the pubic rami and the anterior and inferior aspect of the bladder is separated from its attachments, a rectangular flap of anterior bladder wall is raised and rolled into a tube over a 16 Fr catheter. The distal end of this tube is sutured either to the vaginal portion of the remaining urethra or at the site of the new urethral meatus. "Fixation sutures" are used to attach the neourethra/tubular bladder flap to the pubic periosteum and a Martius fat pad is placed beneath the suture lines (5).

SURGICAL TECHNIQUE

Regardless of the specific nature of the pathology and the precise procedure chosen to correct it, certain general principles should be followed: The operative site should be clearly exposed and closure should be accomplished in a tension-free, multiple-layer fashion, with local flaps or relaxing incisions used to mobilize the anterior vaginal wall. Appropriate bladder drainage is also essential and is accomplished through the placement of a large suprapubic catheter as well as a urethral catheter employed as a stent.

It is usually helpful to employ a well-supplied pedicle flap to promote healing and prevent fistula formation; potential sources of this flap include the labia majora (5), rectus abdominus muscle (3), gracilis myocutaneous (2), or perineal artery axial fasciocutaneous (Singapore) flaps (13). Regardless of the specific anatomic findings and the choice of vascular supply the basic procedure is described as follows.

With the patient in the dorsal lithotomy position, cystourethroscopy is performed and the urethral orifices are visualized. In an effort to prevent inadvertent surgical injury to the ureter during the repair, ureteral stents are placed if the urethral orifices are located close to the fistula; the stents are typically removed at the conclusion of the case. A 14 Fr percutaneous suprapubic cystotomy tube is placed under direct visualization unless concurrent abdominal incisions are planned (such as those used

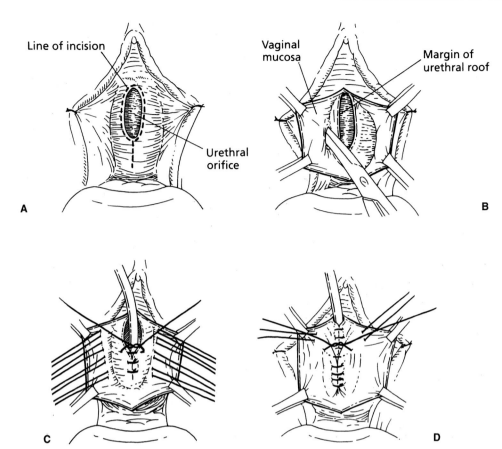

FIG. 47–1. Bladder flap reconstruction. Tanagho anterior bladder flap reconstruction can be used in lieu of vaginal flap reconstruction. (From Tanagho EA. Bladder neck reconstruction for total urinary incontinence: 10 years of experience. *J Urol* 1981;125: 321, with permission.)

in autologous fascial pubovaginal sling), in which case the placement of the tube is deferred until the end of the procedure. A 16 Fr urethral Foley catheter is placed and the balloon inflated to secure the catheter in place at the bladder neck.

There are several basic methods available for urethral repair, which are dependent on the anatomic defect and the availability of local tissue for flaps. Small urethral defects can be fixed with a tension-free *primary closure* (Fig. 47–2). The urethra is closed over a 16 Fr catheter with interrupted 3-0 or 4-0 chromic catgut sutures, which in our experience result in less dysuria and long-term urethral pain than do longer-acting synthetic absorbable sutures. If possible, a second layer of periurethral tissue is closed over the first. The vaginal mucosa is closed using lateral flaps elevated alongside the urethral repair or,

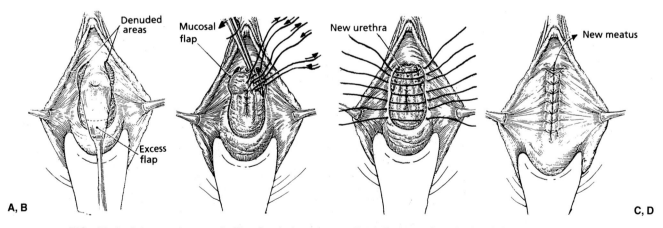

FIG. 47–2. Primary closure. **A:** The fistula is circumscribed. **B:** Lateral vaginal wall flaps are elevated and the lateral urethral walls are mobilized if possible. **C:** The urethra is closed primarily with interrupted sutures of 3-0 chromic catgut. The vaginal wall is closed either primarily or with a U-shaped flap depending on the availability of local tissue. (Modified from Mattingly RF, Thompson JD. In: *Telinde's operative gynecology*, 6th ed. Philadelphia: JB Lippincott Co, 1985:662, with permission.)

alternatively, using an inverted "U" incision of vaginal mucosa; chromic suture is also employed.

When insufficient urethral tissue exists for primary closure, rotation of a U-shaped *advancement flap* of anterior vaginal wall is a viable solution (Fig. 47–3). The cephalad aspect of the anterior vaginal wall is mobilized with a Metzenbaum scissor, advanced, and rotated to form the posterior and lateral walls of the neourethra, using the urethral catheter as a guide around which the tissue is suture. The harvested site in the vaginal wall can usually be repaired by closing the lateral and cephalad edges of the wound; however, pedicle flaps are sometimes necessary if the graft is large.

A larger vaginal wall flap can be employed as a *tube graft* (Fig. 47–4) in the case of extensive loss of urethral tissue. A rectangular incision is made with wide margins and the vaginal wall flap is rolled into a tube over the ure-thral catheter. It is best to provide a vascular pedicle flap for successful wound healing, and a pubovaginal sling is usually required if continence is to be achieved. As with vaginal advancement flaps, the vaginal wound is often too large for primary closure and a secondary rotational flap of vaginal wall or labia minora can be used to close the principal defect created by the initial tube graft incisions. In our experience, gracilis myocutaneous and rectus pedicle flaps have been necessary in only two of over 110 patients.

In cases of extensive vaginal scarring and urethral damage, there may be insufficient vaginal wall for use in the repair. A *labia minora pedicle graft* (Fig. 47–5) is a potential solution to this problem. The labia is cut as close as possible to the site of the urethral repair and in such a manner as to allow a rotational patch graft or tube graft of labial mucosa to be employed as a neourethra that is

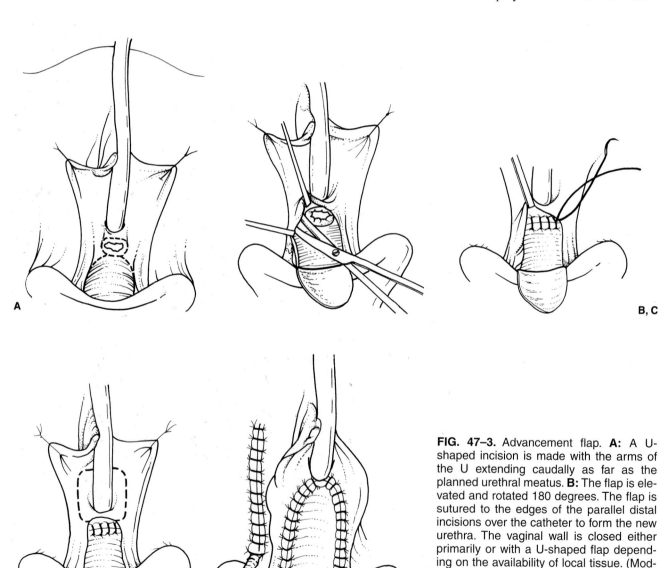

A

B, C

D,E

FIG. 47–3. Advancement flap. **A:** A U-shaped incision is made with the arms of the U extending caudally as far as the planned urethral meatus. **B:** The flap is elevated and rotated 180 degrees. The flap is sutured to the edges of the parallel distal incisions over the catheter to form the new urethra. The vaginal wall is closed either primarily or with a U-shaped flap depending on the availability of local tissue. (Modified from Mattingly RF, Thompson JD. In: *Telinde's operative gynecology*, 6th ed. Philadelphia: JB Lippincott Co, 1985: 660–661, with permission.)

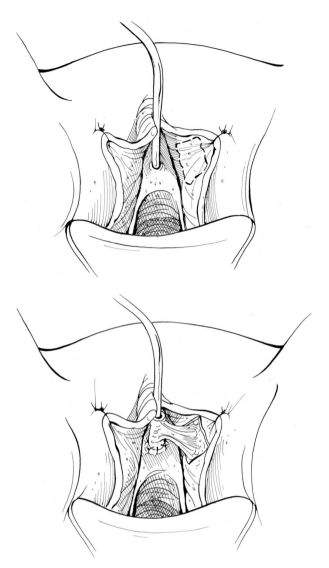

FIG. 47–4. Tube graft. **A:** An inverted U-shaped incision is made in the anterior vaginal wall with the apex of the U at the vesical neck just proximal to the urethral fistula. The fistula is circumscribed. **B:** A plane is created in the avascular plan just underneath the vaginal epithelium and the vaginal wall flap is reflected posteriorly. If a pubovaginal sling is to be performed, the dissection into the retropubic space is completed at this time. **C:** The urethrovaginal fistula is closed with interrupted sutures of 3-0 or 4-0 chromic catgut. **D:** Two parallel incisions are made alongside the Foley catheter and medially based flaps are elevated. **E:** The vaginal and labial wounds are closed. (From Blavais JG. Vaginal flap urethral reconstruction. An alternative to the bladder flap neurourethra. *J Urol* 1989;41:542–545, with permission.)

loosely approximated over the urethral catheter. The graft with underlying vascular supply is passed beneath the vaginal wall such that the mucosal surface forms the inner wall of the reconstructed urethra.

At the conclusion of the procedure, a Penrose drain is placed in the labial harvest sites if applicable, and is removed usually on postoperative day 1. The Foley

catheter should be fixed in a tension-free manner to the anterior abdominal wall to prevent trauma and pressure necrosis of the repair; this catheter is usually removed within postoperative days 2 to 5, before the patient is discharged from the hospital. A voiding cystourethrogram should be performed though the suprapubic catheter about 2 weeks after the procedure. If the patient successfully voids and there is no extravasation, the suprapubic catheter can be removed; if not, the voiding trial is repeated in another 2 weeks. None of our patients has required a catheter for longer than 4 weeks.

An autologous fascial pubovaginal sling can be prepared as part of the reconstructive procedure (Fig. 47–6) in cases associated with sphincteric incontinence or fistula where extensive dissection under the bladder neck puts the patient at risk for postoperative incontinence. Further, we recommend against the use of synthetic materials for concurrent incontinence surgery due to the risk of complications from erosion of the synthetic graft. It is crucial to note that if a pubovaginal sling is to be employed it is harvested but no vaginal dissection is performed until after the urethra is repaired; vaginal tissue should not be compromised by additional incisions until successful repair of the urethra is complete, leaving the widest variety of possible solutions to the patient's primary problem.

A Pfannenstiel incision is made approximately two finger breadths above the symphysis pubis. The surface of the rectus fascia is freed from adherent subcutaneous tissue and two parallel horizontal incisions are made in the midline, defining the 2- to 3-cm width of the rectus fascial strip that will become the sling. These incisions are extended laterally and superiorly until approximately 10 cm of fascia is marked by the parallel incisions. The fascial strip is then freed from the underlying muscle and scar using careful sharp dissection. Each end of the sling is then secured with long 2-0 nonabsorbable monofilament sutures and a running mattress suture directed across the width of the sling. The sling is then cut free and the security of the suspension sutures is checked by pulling each suture separately with moderate tension created by grasping each end of the fascia; it is then placed in a saline bath.

The lateral edges of the vaginal incisions are retracted laterally using Allis clamps and a closed Metzenbaum scissor is used to dissect bluntly into the retropubic space, keeping the scissor directed laterally by exerting pressure against the lateral aspect of the underside of the vaginal mucosa. There is usually a distinct and abrupt decrease in tissue resistance as the retropubic space is entered. The surgeon then places a fingertip into the dissected tract and further mobilizes the bladder neck and urethra through blunt dissection. With the surgeon's finger displacing the vesical neck medially, a long, curved clamp is fed abdominally under the inferior aspect of the free rectus fascia, against the pubic periosteum, and is then

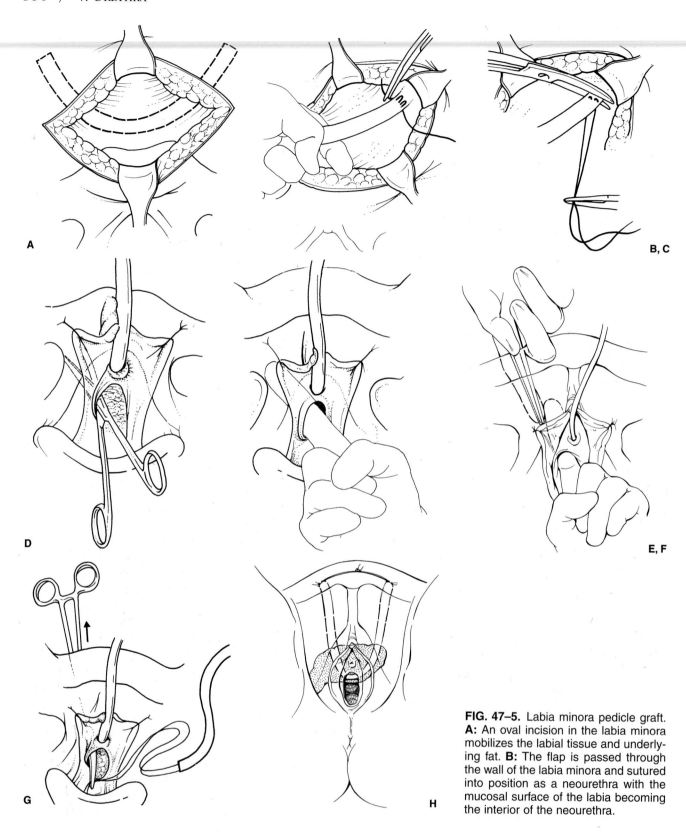

FIG. 47–5. Labia minora pedicle graft.
A: An oval incision in the labia minora mobilizes the labial tissue and underlying fat. **B:** The flap is passed through the wall of the labia minora and sutured into position as a neourethra with the mucosal surface of the labia becoming the interior of the neourethra.

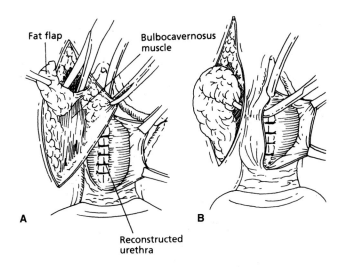

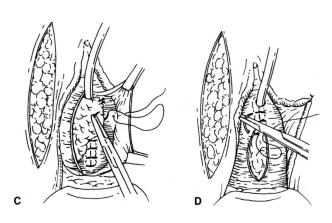

FIG. 47–6. Pubovaginal sling. **A:** A 2- to 3-cm wide graft is outlined with the incision kept parallel to the direction of the fascial fibers. The incision is extended laterally to the point where the fascia divides and passes to the internal and external oblique muscles. **B:** A 2-0 nonabsorbable running horizontal mattress suture is placed across the most lateral portion of the graft and the ends are left long. **C:** Each end of the fascial graft is transected approximately 1 cm lateral to the mattress suture. **D:** Dissection is begun with Metzenbaum scissors in the avascular plane just beneath the vaginal epithelium. The tips of the scissors are directed toward the patient's ipsilateral shoulder. **E:** The endopelvic fascia is perforated with the index finger and the retropubic space is entered. **F:** A long DeBakey clamp is passed from the abdominal to the vaginal wound lateral to the urethra. **G:** The fascial graft is passed around the urethra and brought to the abdominal wound on either side. **H:** The long ends of the sling are tied together in the midline with no tension. The labial fat pad is positioned between the sling and the vesical neck. (A–G from Blavais JG. Pubovaginal sling procedure. In: Whitehead ED, ed. *Current operative urology.* Philadelphia: JB Lippincott Co, 1990:93–101, with permission.)

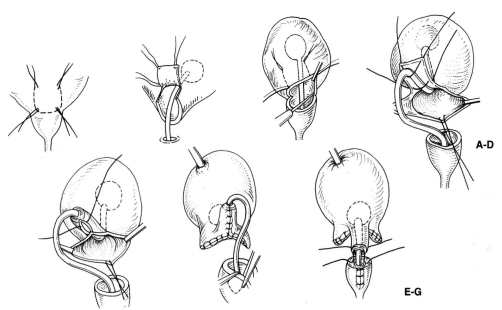

FIG. 47–7. Vascular pedicle graft. **A:** Incisions in the labia majora expose the underlying fat pad, which is suture ligated at its superior margin and mobilized posteriorly. **B:** The graft is drawn through a perforation in the vaginal wall. **C:** A 2-0 chromic catgut suture is used to fix the graft over the reconstruction. **D:** The vaginal wall is closed over the reconstruction. If a pubovaginal sling is performed it is placed beneath the vaginal wall prior to the closure. (Modified from Mattingly RF, Thompson JD. In: *Telinde's operative gynecology,* 6th ed. Philadelphia: JB Lippincott Co, 1985:663, with permission.)

TABLE 47–2 *Preoperative classification of female urethral diverticulum (L/N/S/C3) in the authors' experience of 63 women*

Reference	Number	Continence (%)	Cure/improved (%)	Anatomic repair (%)	Obstruction (%)
Bruce, 2000 (3)	6	83	100	100	0
Leng, 1998		4	75	75	100
Blaivac, 1996 (2)	49	90	92	96	2
Taneer, 1993 (12)	34	—	82	82	—
Elkins, 1990 (5)	20	50	55	90	10
Mundy, 1989 (9)	30	93	—	93	41
Patel, 1980	9	—	78	100	0
Morgan, 1978	9	56	89	100	11
Elkins, 1969	6	10	83	67	17
Hamlin, 1969	50	80	84	98	12
Gray, 1968	10	50	50	—	—
Symmonds, 1968	20	65	90	85	—

guided by the surgeon's abdominal hand onto the lateral aspect of the vaginal fingertip, thus protecting the bladder from injury.

The clamp is then fed through into the vagina, where it is used to grasp and pull through one of the nonabsorbable sling sutures into the abdominal wound. The procedure is repeated on the contralateral side, and the absorbable sutures are threaded through separate small stab incisions of the inferior leaf of the rectus fascia. Following this, the rectus fascia is closed using 0-PDS or Vicryl suture and the pubovaginal sling is positioned in the midline over the vaginal reconstruction. If a vascular pedicle graft is employed in the urethral reconstruction (Fig. 47–7), the graft is placed over the urethral repair and the sling is placed superficially over the graft. The vaginal mucosa is then closed and at the conclusion of the operation the long ends of the sling are tied together in the midline over the rectus fascia without any tension at all.

OUTCOMES

Complications

A review of published results reveals that successful anatomic reconstruction has been reported in 67% to 100% of cases, with emphasis on the need for vascular pedicle flaps to ensure viability of the repair (2,5,9,12). Continence varies from 55% to 93% of patients after a single operation and resulting urethral obstruction was varied from 2% to 41%; however, most studies did not specify the method of evaluating continence. It was clear that antiincontinence procedures were in general successful and dramatically improved the continence rates, with postoperative incontinence in 50% to 84% of patients who underwent anatomic reconstruction only.

We have performed 110 urethral reconstructive procedures in women [(2) and unpublished data]. All but one underwent primary or vaginal wall repairs, and the one Tanagho anterior bladder flap was unsuccessful. A Martius flap was used in all but four patients. We did not per-

form pubovaginal sling routinely until later in the series, and 50% of the early patients who underwent modified Pereyra procedures were incontinent; of these, all were subsequently cured by pubovaginal sling. For this reason we are strongly in favor of pubovaginal sling for concurrent antiincontinence surgery.

Three patients experienced necrosis of the flap, which in one case was associated with the development of sphincteric incontinence, and two other patients developed sphincteric incontinence. One patient had urinary obstruction from the pubovaginal sling and one patient had an unrecognized vesicovaginal fistula. All patients who suffered from incontinence were cured by successful reoperation and were dry at 1 year follow-up, except for one patient who declined surgery. No patients required intermittent catheterization.

Results

Urethral reconstruction in women can be highly complicated and requires considerable surgical expertise as well as a thorough diagnostic workup. In most women successful anatomic and functional repair can be achieved (Table 47–2) with a single surgical procedure employing vaginal flap reconstruction with grafted vascular supply and pubovaginal sling as an antiincontinence measure. Bladder flap techniques can also be used, especially in cases of extensive vaginal scarring.

REFERENCES

1. Bazeed M, Nabeeh A, El-Kenawy M, Ashamallah A. Urovaginal fistulae: 20 years' experience. *Eur Urol* 1995:27;34–38.
2. Blaivas JG. Vaginal flap urethral reconstruction: an alternative to the bladder flap neo-urethra. *J Urol* 1996;141:542–545.
3. Bruce RG, El-Galley RES, Galloway NTM. Use of rectus abdominis muscle flap for the treatment of complex and refractory urethrovaginal fistulas. *J Urol* 2000;163:1212.
4. Danso KA, Martey JOP, Wall LL, Elkins TE. The epidemiology of genitourinary fistulae in Kumasi, Ghana, 1977–1992. *Int Urogynecol J* 1996;7:117–120.
5. Elkins TE, Ghosh TS, Tagoe GA, Stocker R. Transvaginal mobilization and utilization of the anterior bladder wall to repair vesicovaginal fistulas involving the urethra. *Obstet Gynecol* 1993;79:455–460.

6. Guerriero WG. Operative injury to the urinary tract. *Urol Clin North Am* 1985;12:339–348.

7. Gray LA. Urethrovaginal fistulas. *Am J Obstet Gynecol* 1968;101:28.

8. Leadbetter GW Jr. Surgical correction of total urinary incontinence. *J Urol* 1964;91:261.

9. Mundy AR. Urethral substitution in women. *Br J Urol* 1989;63:80–83.

10. Perry MO, Husmann DA. Urethral injuries in female subjects following pelvic fractures. *J Urol* 1992;147:139–143.

11. Tanagho EA. Bladder neck reconstruction for total urinary incontinence: 10 years of experience. *J Urol* 1981;125:321.

12. Tancer ML. A report of thirty-four instances of urethrovaginal and bladder neck fistulas. *Surg Gynecol Obstet* 1993;177:77–80.

13. Zinman, L. Use of myocutaneous and muscle interposition flaps in management of radiation-induced vesicovaginal fistula. In: McDougal WS, ed. *Difficult problems in urologic surgery*. Chicago: Yearbook Medical Publishers, 1989:143–163.

CHAPTER 48

Urethral Stricture and Disruption

Brian J. Flynn and George D. Webster

Urethral stricture results from scarring induced by local tissue injury from trauma, inflammation, or ischemia. Trauma is the most common cause of local tissue injury and can occur from blunt perineal trauma such as straddle injury or pelvic fracture or may be due to penetrating knife or gunshot injury. More frequently, stricture may result from iatrogenic injury from urethral catheterization or endoscopic instrumentation. Inflammation due to gonococcal urethritis or lichen sclerosis can result in stricture formation. An uncommon cause of urethral stricture is malignancy, usually of urethral, penile, or lymphoid origin. The pathophysiology of urethral stricture involves progressive fibrosis of the epithelium with subsequent involvement of the underlying spongiosum. Narrowing of the urethral lumen results and may culminate in obliteration and—more rarely—fistula or abscess formation.

DIAGNOSIS

Urethral stricture most often presents with obstructive voiding symptoms although irritative symptoms, including frequency, urgency, and dysuria, may also occur. Hematuria, urethral bleeding, and pooling of urine in the dilated urethra proximal to the stricture leading to postvoid dribbling are not uncommon presentations. Recurrent urinary tract infection can accompany these symptoms. In cases of traumatic stricture, the history will include prior urethral instrumentation or an episode of external injury. Difficult catheter placement is sometimes the initial presentation of urethral stricture disease. Physical examination should include urethral palpation, which may help determine the severity of spongiofibrosis. Assessment of the character, color, and laxity of penile shaft skin and preputial skin when present is critical in determining flap and graft availability. Laboratory evaluation should include urine analysis and culture and assessment of renal function.

Conventional radiological studies provide the best means for evaluation of urethral strictures. Retrograde urethrography (RUG) should define the length, location, caliber, and multiplicity of the stricture (7). If the stricture is nearly obliterative, the urethra proximal to this point may not be adequately distended by RUG. In these instances, voiding cystourethrography (VCUG) may be utilized to evaluate the urethra proximal to the stricture. Simultaneous RUG–VCUG is indispensable in the evaluation of the obliterative urethral defect that follows pelvic fracture. In most office settings cystourethroscopy is more available then RUG and therefore more commonly utilized to evaluate the urethra. Although visual assessment of the urethra distal to the stricture permits evaluation of urethral vascularity is often not possible to visualize the urethra proximal to the point of narrowing, thereby limiting the evaluation. We therefore use urethroscopy primarily to rule out malignancy and complement the radiological findings. Transurethral ultrasound and magnetic resonance imaging have also been used in the evaluation of urethral disease but are not as widely available as RUG or endoscopy.

INDICATIONS FOR SURGERY

Urinary retention, recurrent urinary tract infection, and stone formation are accepted indications for the treatment of urethral stricture. Initial treatment is usually comprised of dilation or optical urethrotomy. Such intervention is rarely curative but usually temporizes the acute event for a variable duration (10). Urethroplasty is in general indicated if frequent urethral dilation is required or is complicated by false passage, diverticulum, fistula, bacteremia, or excessive pain and hemorrhage. In addition, strictures that occur in children or long, obliterative strictures justify earlier consideration for open repair. Numerous urethroplasty techniques have been described and it is true to say that no single technique is appropriate for all strictures. Techniques are broadly grouped into anastomotic and substitution repairs. In substitution repairs the urethral lumen is augmented with a flap or graft performed in single or multiple stages. Grafts, like flaps, have by tradition been obtained from genital skin; however, buccal mucosal grafts have emerged as the preferred urethral substitute in adults due to their favorable inherent qualities and consistent availability.

Procedure selection is determined primarily by the location, length, and etiology of the stricture. In addition, the presence of local adverse features such as fistulae, inflammation, or scarring may impact procedure selection. The goals of any surgical repair should be to achieve durable urethral patency without compromising sexual function or penile cosmesis.

ALTERNATIVE THERAPY

There are a number of nonsurgical alternatives for the treatment of urethral stricture. These include watchful waiting, self-calibration, dilation with filiform and followers or by balloon catheter, and optical urethrotomy using cold knife, electrocautery, or laser. More recently transurethral placement of metallic urethral stents has been utilized. In general, urethrotomy is contraindicated in the pendulous urethra due to the paucity of surrounding spongy tissue that is necessary for urethral reepithelialization. In addition, urethral stenting is discouraged in the pendulous urethra due to patient discomfort and potential compromise of erectile function. In the bulbar urethra all of the mentioned options are available. In terms of cure rates, optical urethrotomy has no advantage over urethral dilation (10). Further, if one urethrotomy or dilation fails to cure a patient then subsequent procedures are rarely if ever successful (5). Strictures that may be cured by dilation or urethrotomy are usually short (less than 1 cm) bulbar strictures, while longer strictures or those of the pendulous urethra are rarely cured by dilation or urethrotomy.

SURGICAL TECHNIQUE

General Surgical Principles

The urine culture should be negative prior to surgery and on-call parenteral antibiotics are given. If the patient has a suprapubic catheter, then broad-spectrum antibiotics are given for 24 hours prior to surgery. General endotracheal anesthesia is necessary for buccal mucosa harvest or for more extensive repairs, but for other repairs spinal anesthesia is acceptable. Most urethroplasties are performed in the lithotomy position, taking care to pad all pressure points. Exaggerated lithotomy is rarely necessary and carries a higher risk of neuronal injury and compartment syndrome. Methylene blue instilled per urethra

differentially stains the urethral scar from healthy urethra mucosa, thereby accentuating the stricture margins. "Table-fixed" ring retraction design (Bookwalter or Omni) is ideal for bulbar or posterior urethroplasty while nonfixed ring retraction design (Lonestar) is optimal for pendulous urethroplasty. Polyglycolic acid (PGA) suture material has ideal tensile strength, absorption rate, and tissue reactivity, and 5-0 is in general used. Wound drainage when necessary is accomplished with a 7 Fr closed-suction drain. Dressings should be supportive and noncompressive.

Urinary drainage is accomplished with a 12 Fr silicone urethral catheter, which causes the least mucosal irritation. In the bulbar or posterior urethra the catheter is fenestrated to promote drainage of the operative site, especially in cases where a graft or flap was utilized (Fig. 48–1). Suprapubic catheter drainage facilitates postoperative urethral stent management, allowing removal of the urethral catheter without requiring the patient to void. The duration of urethral catheterization is determined by the type of repair and is shortest for meatal or glanular repairs (5 to 7 days), intermediate for anastomotic repairs (10 to 14 days), and longest for one-stage graft repairs (21 days). Catheter removal and specifically voiding per urethra should be preceded by pericatheter RUG for all urethroplasties proximal to the glanular urethra. If there is no extravasation at the repair site, the catheter is removed and the patient resumes normal voiding. Continued review and RUG is then performed at 3 and 12 months following repair. Subsequently, symptomatic follow-up is indicated and some use periodic uroflow studies.

Strictures of the Glanular Urethra

Strictures in the glanular urethra are most commonly due to inflammatory conditions, instrumentation, or improper circumcision. Simple meatotomy, a glans-based Y–V advancement flap for very distal stenosis, or a ventral shaft skin onlay flap in the case of stricture involving the entire fossa navicularis may accomplish surgical repair. For Y–V advancement a V-shaped incision is made on the dorsal aspect of the glans with the apex terminating at the urethral meatus (Fig. 48–2). A dorsal midline extension of this incision is made into the urethra to widen the lumen to accept a 22 Fr sound. The glans flap can be elevated using skin hooks and sharp dissection to allow its mobilization into the most proximal limit of the dorsal urethral incision, where it is anchored with a 4-0 PGA suture. Care must be taken to leave this glans flap with a wide base to avoid vascular compromise.

More extensive strictures of the glanular and distal penile urethra may result from lichen sclerosis (LS). These are best repaired with nongenital skin as the penile skin is considered blighted and may eventually develop

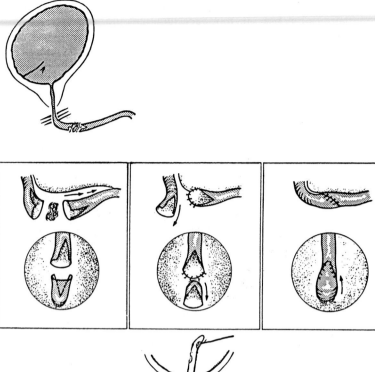

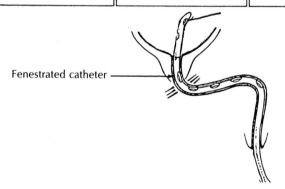

Fenestrated catheter

FIG. 48–1. The fenestrated urethral catheter is optimal following urethroplasty. Both a balloon or straight catheter may be used, and fenestrations are made in the catheter shaft in the region of repair. The fenestrations allow debris and exudate to be washed away from the site of repair. Bladder irrigation cannot be performed unless the catheter is inserted all the way into the bladder so that the most distal fenestration is intravesical.

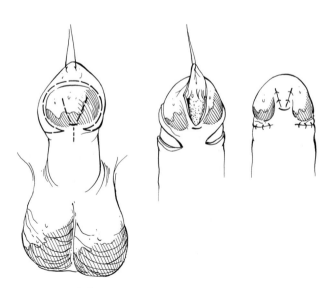

FIG. 48–2. Glans flap meatoplasty.

LS. In these cases, the diseased urethra is excised and buccal mucosa is inlayed and the urethra is left open. A second stage where the urethra is then tubularized occurs 6 to 12 months later after the graft matures and adjacent urethra is observed for further development of LS. If extensive stricture disease is unrelated to LS then a flap of skin obtained from the penile shaft allows repair in a single stage. The flap may be fashioned as an onlay or as a tube, depending on the extent of the disease (Fig. 48–3).

Strictures of the Pendulous Urethra

Pendulous urethral strictures are most often repaired using an onlay flap of penile skin. Although many variations of this technique have been described, the laterally based pedicled island flap originally described by Orandi gives excellent results and is technically forgiving. It is in general suitable for repairs measuring up to 8 cm (depending on penile length), although longer repairs can be performed by harvesting a penile "J" flap that has a

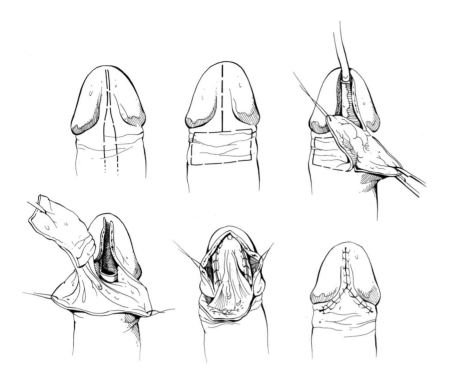

FIG. 48–3. Repair of meatal and distal penile urethral stricture using a pedicled island of distal penile skin. This procedure allows for reapproximation of glans tissue around the neourethra, giving an excellent cosmetic and functional result.

vertical and a distal circumferential component. A flap width up to 25 mm can be used without compromising penile skin closure. The patient is placed in either the lithotomy or a supine frog-legged position. An incision is made along the ventral penile raphe through Buck's fascia down to the strictured segment of urethra. Using skin hooks to elevate the flap and fine scissors for dissection, one skin margin is mobilized from the corpus cavernosum for 10 to 15 mm, staying deep to Buck's fascia (Fig. 48–4). With the urethra adequately exposed, a suitable catheter or filiform is placed in the urethral lumen as a guide and the urethra incised ventrally along the stricture. This incision is then extended to expose at least 1 cm of healthy urethra proximal and distal to the stricture. An onlay flap of suitable width to achieve a 24 Fr lumen (in general 18 to 25 mm) is then outlined on the mobilized lateral penile shaft skin. The flap length corresponds to the length of the urethrotomy and is tapered at the proximal and distal ends. Care must be taken not to incorporate a significant segment of hair-bearing shaft skin in the repair.

Once the flap has been outlined, the projected new skin edges are approximated in the midline to ensure that wound closure with minimal tension is possible. The lateral aspect of the flap is then incised through the subcutaneous connective tissue, leaving the underlying dartos and deeper Buck's fascia intact. With exposure of the correct tissue plane, the lateral penile shaft skin will retract with minimal additional dissection. The medial border of the island flap is then anchored to the lateral edge of the

incised urethra with 5-0 PGA stay sutures. The flap is sutured to the urethra beginning at the distal margin, using a running 5-0 PGA suture, incorporating the urethral epithelium in the closure. When the lateral suture line is complete, the free edge of the island flap can be rolled over and secured with 5-0 PGA stay sutures to the contralateral margin, recreating the urethral lumen. A similar running suture line is performed with 5-0 PGA to complete the onlay repair. Local wound drainage may be accomplished with a suction drain placed underneath the vascular pedicle along the length of the flap to obviate hematoma or urinoma formation, which could compromise the flap.

Wound closure is performed in two layers using 5-0 interrupted PGA sutures. Care must be taken when approximating the subdermal connective tissue of the skin margins to avoid injury to the flap pedicle. This first layer of closure serves to cover the exposed urethral suture line and minimize the risk of fistula formation. Final skin closure is performed with a running subcuticular 5-0 PGA suture. The wound is supported with adhesive strips and covered with a gauze and loosely applied Coband dressing to reduce edema formation. The urethral catheter is secured to the abdominal wall and remains in place for up to 3 weeks. If a suction drain is used it is removed within 24 hours and the supportive dressing taken down on postoperative day 2. The patient is allowed to ambulate on postoperative day 1 and the procedure is usually performed as an outpatient.

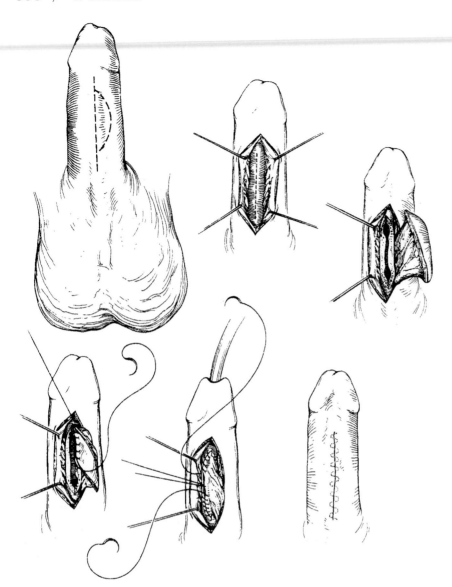

FIG. 48–4. Onlay urethroplasty of a pendulous urethral stricture (Orandi repair). The stricture is approached through a ventral penile incision. The outline of the skin island to be used for onlay is marked once the stricture has been opened and its length and caliber determined. The skin island is raised on a subcutaneous vascular pedicle and rotated inward and sutured as an onlay to augment urethral caliber. Skin closure is in at least two layers to avoid fistula formation.

Bulbar Urethral Stricture Repair

Anastomotic Urethroplasty

Strictures in the bulbar urethra are most often of traumatic origin from straddle injury, endoscopic instrumentation, or catheterization. When less than 1 cm in length, these are best managed by stricture excision and primary anastomosis. The patient is placed in the lithotomy position with the buttocks at the edge of the table. A midline perineal incision is made and bifurcated posteriorly 2 cm above the anus. Subcutaneous tissue is divided to expose the underlying bulbospongiosus muscle. The bulbospongiosus is divided in the midline and separated from the underlying bulbar urethra. Circumferential mobilization of the bulbar urethra is facilitated by sharply dividing the reflection of Buck's fascia lateral to the urethra, where it drapes over the corporal bodies just proximal to the crus. A space deep to Buck's fascia and between the separating

corporal bodies is entered on each side, and a right-angle clamp can then be passed over the roof of the urethra to commence the dorsal dissection. This dorsal dissection, separating the urethra from the corporal bodies, is then continued sharply until the entire strictured urethra has been circumferentially mobilized. Further mobility of the proximal bulbar urethra is obtained by dividing the ventral attachments to the perineal body.

A 20 Fr catheter is advanced to the strictured segment and the urethra is transected at this location. The diseased segment is excised proximally to expose healthy urethral tissue. It should be emphasized again that complete removal of fibrotic tissue with exposure of healthy proximal and distal urethra is essential for successful repair, but no more than 1 cm of urethra should be excised. If the urethral ends appose in a tension-free fashion they are spatulated sharply for 1 cm. Ideally, the proximal urethral segment is spatulated on its ventral aspect and the distal

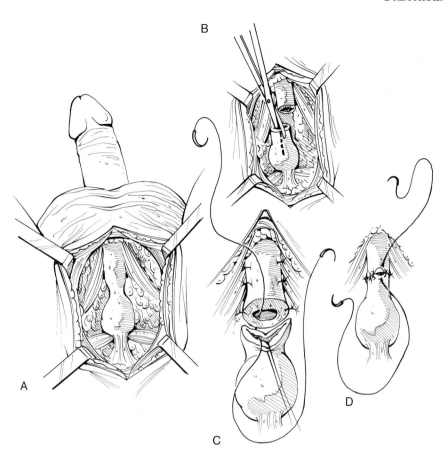

FIG. 48–5. Anastomotic repair of bulbar urethral stricture that may follow straddle injury. **A:** The urethra is exposed through a midline perineal incision and the stricture site identified and excised. **B:** Following stricture excision apposing spatulations of 1 cm are accomplished. **C:** The proximal urethral opening is spread-fixed to the underlying corporal body and spatulated anastomosis performed with interrupted sutures. **D:** The anastomosis is completed and additional tension-relieving sutures between urethral adventitia and adjacent corporal bodies are placed to avoid anastomotic tension during erection.

end on the dorsal aspect (Fig. 48–5). Using 5-0 interrupted PGA sutures the dorsal aspect of the proximal urethra is spread-fixed to the underside of the tunica albuginea of the corporal bodies to anchor and stabilize the anastomosis. Circumferential full-thickness anastomotic sutures complete the repair by approximating the distal spatulated urethra to the spread-fixed proximal segment. The bulbospongiosus and Colle's fascia are approximated in the midline with interrupted 4-0 PGA sutures. Final skin closure is made with interrupted 5-0 PGA sutures. The perineum is dressed and bolstered with fluff gauze and mesh underwear. The urethral catheter is secured to the abdominal wall to minimize traction and pressure on the urethra.

Augmented Anastomotic Urethroplasty

Excision of 1 cm of urethra and associated 1-cm spatulated repair results in a total of 2 cm of urethral shortening, an amount that can be easily accommodated by the elasticity of the mobilized bulbar urethra. If bulbar urethral strictures of greater than 1 cm in length are repaired by primary anastomosis there is a risk of causing penile chordee. If a 2-cm stricture is excised and a 1-cm spatulated anastomosis performed the total shortening would be 3 cm, and this may be excessive. We also prefer to not mobilize the urethra beyond the suspensory ligament of

the penis, as this also increases this risk of chordee. Hence, a variety of alternative procedures that avoid penile shortening and chordee may be used for strictures that are greater than 1 cm in length.

For strictures of up to 2 cm in length, stricture excision and augmented anastomotic repair is a good option. This procedure is similar to the above technique (anastomotic urethroplasty), the 2-cm segment being excised, but the urethra is then spatulated proximally and distally for 1 cm into healthy urethra on the same side. The anastomosis is then augmented with a graft (or a flap), the lumen increases avoiding the need for spatulation, which would result in an additional 1-cm loss. In the ventral onlay, spatulation is at the 6-o'clock position (floor) and the unspatulated dorsal (roof) strips are then reapproximated end-to-end after spread-fixation, thereby securing the anastomosed urethral roof strip to the overlying corporal body. The anastomosis is not completed circumferentially, resulting in a diamond-shaped ventral urethral defect into which is laid either a graft of penile skin or buccal mucosa or, alternatively, a diamond-shaped flap of penile skin mobilized on a pedicle through the scrotum. This repair is called an augmented roof strip anastomotic procedure, and it provides the advantages of an anastomosis while augmenting the repair to limit penile shortening to 2 cm, which is usually acceptable (Fig. 48–6). More recently (and our preference), this repair may be

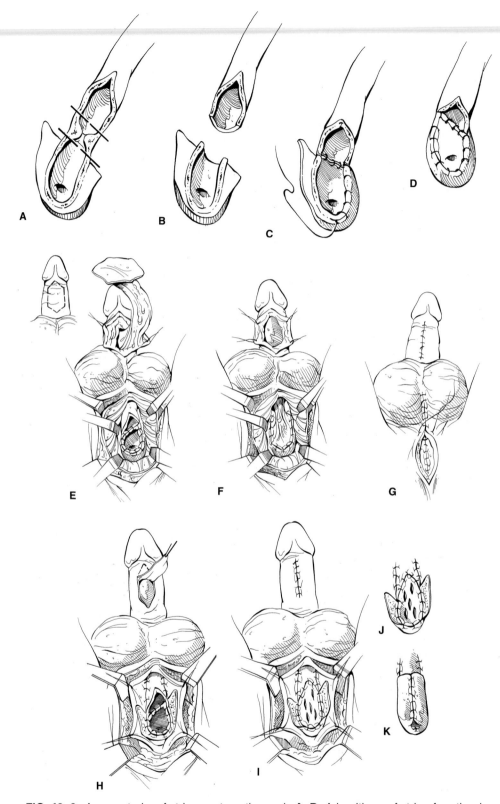

FIG. 48–6. Augmented roof strip anastomotic repair. **A–D:** A healthy roof strip of urethra is created by stricture excision and roof strip reanastomosis. **E–G:** An appropriately sized and shaped island of ventral penile skin is mobilized on its vascular pedicle, tucked through the scrotum, and sutured over the anastomosis augmenting its caliber (closure is in layers). **H–K:** This series illustrates the augmented roof strip anastomotic repair using a fenestrated full-thickness skin graft from the ventral penile shaft rather than a pedicled island of penile skin.

performed as a floor strip anastomosis, placing the augmenting graft on the dorsal aspect where it is spread-fixed to the overlying corporal body. This approach permits superior spread fixation of the graft and therefore reduces graft shrinkage and enhances graft take because of the reliable apposition to the corporal body and avoids graft or flap sacculation. Consequently, since 1996, analogous to Barbagli, we prefer the dorsal onlay in the bulbar urethra (1).

Onlay Bulbar Urethroplasty

More extensive bulbar strictures (over 2 cm in length) are usually inflammatory in etiology and it is rarely possible to complete any type of anastomotic repair without causing some penile chordee and tension on the anastomosis. In these situations we have found success using a buccal mucosal or skin graft onlay applied to the dorsal aspect of the strictured portion of the bulbar urethra (Fig. 48–7). The urethral bulb is exposed circumferentially as described earlier. A 20 Fr catheter is advanced to the site of narrowing and the urethra rotated 180 degrees to expose its dorsal aspect. Stay sutures of 4-0 silk are placed along the exposed dorsal aspect and the urethra is then incised along the strictured segment in the 12-o'clock (dorsal) position, extending the incision 1 cm into healthy urethra proximal and distal to the stricture.

Confirmation of proximal and distal patency is confirmed endoscopically and by calibration with a 24 or 26 Fr bougie à boule. A suitable skin donor site, selected on the ventral penile shaft or prepuce, or a buccal mucosa graft is harvested. The graft is spread-fixed on a paraffin block and defatted. It is then fenestrated with a scalpel and sized and shaped to fit the defect created by urethral incision. The graft is then anchored in a spread-fixed fashion to the corporal bodies opposing the dorsally incised strictured urethra. The urethra is then rotated back to its normal anatomic position and the margins of the urethral incision sutured to the fixed graft edge and corporal body using interrupted 5-0 PGA sutures. In this fashion, the dorsal graft becomes the new urethral roof, augmenting the urethral caliber at the stricture site. This dorsal approach mitigates blood loss from a ventral bulbar incision and provides excellent graft stabilization.

Panurethral Stricture or Failed Urethroplasty

The management of extensive stricture of the anterior urethra involving both the pendulous and bulbar portions can be extremely challenging. These are usually of inflammatory origin (often due to LS) and can be up to 20 cm in length. Urethral repair in these circumstances is undertaken either by combination repairs using grafts and flaps or, more conservatively, by multistaged repairs that may also use perineal inlays of full- or split-thickness skin graft.

One-Stage Combination Urethroplasty

One-stage combination procedures make use of both a flap repair for the pendulous portion of the urethra and a graft repair for the bulbar area with the two procedures being performed in continuity. The patient is placed in the lithotomy position for access to the perineum as well as the penile shaft. In the uncircumcised male the prepuce can be used as a skin graft donor site, leaving the remaining shaft skin for island pedicle flap construction. In the event there is insufficient penile skin, buccal mucosa may be used for the graft repair of the contiguous scrotal/bulbar urethra or buccal mucosa may be preferred even in cases where penile skin is sufficient.

A ventral incision is made over the pendulous urethra and this portion of the stricture is repaired using a ventral onlay repair in the fashion of Orandi, as described earlier. The more proximal scrotal portion of the stricture is then repaired in continuity by a dorsal or ventral onlay. This portion of the repair is approached through a separate incision in the perineum for exposure of the bulbar urethra. If a dorsal onlay is used, which is our preference, the bulbar urethra is circumferentially mobilized as far distally as the proximal limit of the penile flap repair and the urethra is then incised dorsally through the stricture, with the distal limit being the visible ventral onlay, and the dorsal onlay graft is then completed as described earlier. Hence, the long stricture is repaired by a ventral onlay flap for the pendulous portion and a dorsal onlay graft for the more proximal urethra, with the composite repair being completed nose to tail.

Staged Repair

Extensive anterior urethral stricture disease, in particular full-length strictures, strictures complicated by fistula or inflammation, long recurrent strictures following prior repair, and the absence of a reliable donor site for onlay, are best managed by a staged repair. Historically, such repairs were performed as scrotal inlay procedures with the resultant neourethra being constructed from hair-bearing scrotal skin, which experience has proven to be a suboptimal substitute. Variations on this theme now inlay fenestrated full-thickness preputial skin, split-thickness thigh skin, or buccal mucosa alongside the marsupialized urethra in the first stage. In the second stage, the neourethra is formed by tubularization of the graft. Full-thickness skin is superior for this purpose but is not often available in communities where circumcision is common. If split-thickness skin is to be used it is in general harvested from the thigh, which is easily accessed with a patient in the lithotomy position. The strictured anterior urethra is exposed through a ventral midline perineal incision that may bifurcate the scrotum and the urethra is then incised along the length of the stricture to healthy urethra proximally and distally. This again is confirmed

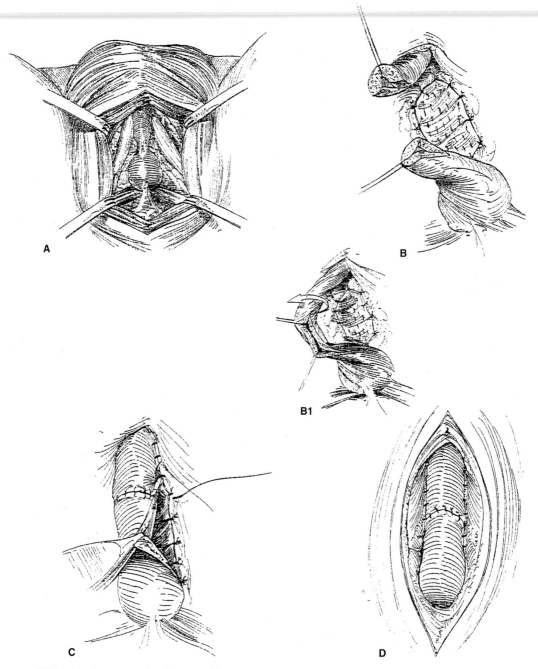

FIG. 48–7. The dorsal onlay graft bulbar urethroplasty. **A:** Exposure of the urethra. **B, B1:** Fenestrated graft sutured to the undersurface of the corporal body. Strictured portion of the urethra either excised or rotated. **C:** Suture of the opened urethra to dorsal onlay graft. **D:** Completed repair.

by calibrating the urethra with a 24 to 28 Fr bougie à boule, which should pass easily through each ostium. Using a dermatome set to 20 thousandths of an inch, a split-thickness graft is harvested from the thigh and meshed to a ratio of 1.5:1. A strip of meshed graft measuring 3 to 5 cm is then inlayed around the marsupialized strictured urethra (Fig. 48–8). Medially it is sutured to the incised urethral margin and laterally to the incised scrotal and perineal skin edges using 5-0 PGA. This width of graft accounts for the up to 50% shrinkage that may occur with split-thickness skin, resulting in suitable graft width for future neourethra. If buccal mucosa is inlayed (preferable but not always adequately available), a fenestrated graft of 2.5 to 3 cm in width is usually adequate because it undergoes less contraction. A suprapubic tube is placed for urinary diversion in the postoperative period and the graft is dressed with an Adaptic gauze and a tiedown dressing of sterile cotton fluffs soaked in Bunnell's solu-

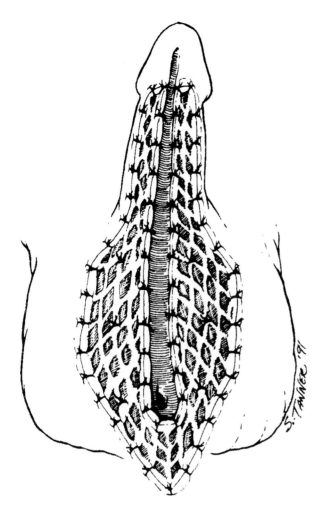

FIG. 48–8. Staged urethroplasty for full-length stricture disease using meshed split-thickness skin graft. The meshed graft is laid alongside the marsupialized urethra so that the neourethra will be tubularized from the graft rather than from hair-bearing scrotal skin. Tubularization of the neourethra is delayed for 3 to 6 months.

tion. The graft is keep moist by periodic application of Bunnell's solution until the dressing is removed after 5 days. Graft take is in the order of 95% or greater.

The second stage is performed a minimum of 3 months and in practice usually 6 to 12 months later to allow thorough vascularization of the graft and to allow adjacent stricture disease to declare itself. The proximal and distal urethral openings should again freely calibrate to 28 and 24 Fr, respectively, prior to second-stage closure. If the ostia have narrowed, revision rather than dilation should be undertaken, usually using a Y–V advancement technique. Second-stage repair is begun by incising the graft circumferentially to a width that will allow neourethral tubularization to approximately 28 Fr. The tubularization is performed by midline anastomosis with a running 5-0 PGA suture, interlocking every third pass, followed by a multilayer wound closure. Urethral stenting occurs for 14 to 20 days.

Posterior Urethroplasty

Posterior urethral stricture or defect most commonly occurs as a consequence of pelvic fracture and may occur in up to 10% of cases. Other less common causes include penetrating trauma, instrumentation, radiation, or infection. Optimal timing (immediate vs. delayed) and surgical approach (endoscopic vs. open) of pelvic fracture urethral distraction defect (PFUDD) remains controversial. Endoscopic approaches are primarily utilized in the acute setting when immediate realignment is indicated due to concomitant bladder neck injury, severe prostatomembranous dislocation, or rectal injury. Immediate or early endoscopic realignment may also decrease the length of subsequent strictures and place the disrupted ends in closer alignment, which may lessen the difficulty of delayed perineal repair. Delayed endoscopic "cut-to-the-light" procedures have also been performed utilizing a variety of techniques, usually for short, well-aligned defects.

In most instances delayed repair usually more than 3 months from the time of injury is appropriate and can be invariably accomplished through the perineum alone, resulting in stricture-free healing and minimal associated morbidity. In our experience substitution urethroplasty is reserved for the rare patient who has concomitant anterior urethral disease (i.e., stricture, hypospadias). The occasional indication for an abdominoperineal approach is the "complex posterior urethral defect." These include concomitant urethral or bladder base fistulae to the rectum, skin, or periurethral cavity requiring debridement and omentoplasty. In most cases we no longer consider an open bladder neck on preoperative VCUG an indication for concomitant bladder neck reconstruction at the time of posterior urethroplasty, which would necessitate an abdominoperineal approach.

One-Stage Perineal Anastomotic Repair

The patient is positioned in standard lithotomy and prepped and draped to give access to the perineum, genitalia, and suprapubic region. A midline perineal skin incision that is bifurcated posteriorly to improve perineal access is made. The midline dissection is deepened and the bulbospongiosus muscles are then divided and reflected from the bulbar urethra. The operative technique then progresses through four sequential maneuvers based on the intraoperative findings until a tension-free anastomosis is accomplished:

1. *Circumferential urethral mobilization.* The bulbar urethra is mobilized proximally to the point of obliteration (identified by the passage of a 20 Fr catheter) and distally as far as the suspensory ligament of the penis (Fig. 48–9). A descending 24 Fr van Buren sound is then passed through the suprapubic cystotomy tract and negotiated through the bladder neck into the prostatic urethra. Midline perineal scar inci-

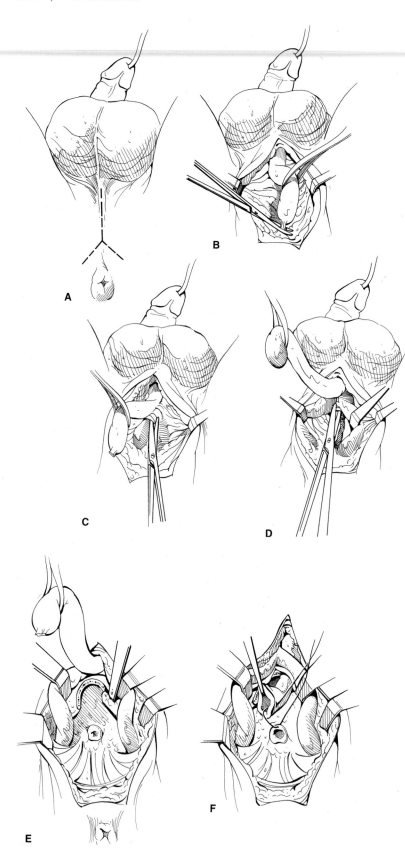

FIG. 48–9. Perineal repair of pelvic fracture urethral distraction defects. **A:** A midline perineal incision is bifurcated posteriorly. **B:** After dissecting the bulbospongiosus muscle from the bulbar urethra, it is circumferentially mobilized proximally to the obliterative defect. Incision of the posterior urethral attachments (scissors) facilitates mobilization. **C:** Once transected posteriorly the urethra is mobilized distally as far as the suspensory ligament of the penis, if necessary. **D:** Penile corporal bodies are separated, right from left, from the crus distally for 5 to 7 cm. The dorsal penile vessels dorsal to the corpora lie beneath the inferior rami of the pubis above. **E:** A channel is excised from the inferior ramus of the exposed pubis between the separated corporal bodies using bone osteotome and/or bone rongeur. **F:** The corporal body is circumferentially dissected and the mobilized urethra rerouted around it and through the resected bony defect. The mobilized bulbar urethra is spatulated dorsally for anastomosis to the posteriorly spatulated prostatomembranous urethra.

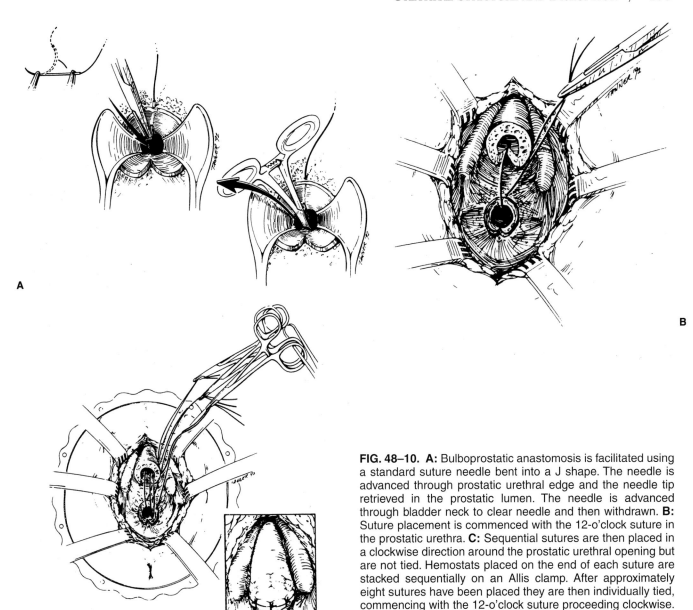

FIG. 48–10. A: Bulboprostatic anastomosis is facilitated using a standard suture needle bent into a J shape. The needle is advanced through prostatic urethral edge and the needle tip retrieved in the prostatic lumen. The needle is advanced through bladder neck to clear needle and then withdrawn. **B:** Suture placement is commenced with the 12-o'clock suture in the prostatic urethra. **C:** Sequential sutures are then placed in a clockwise direction around the prostatic urethral opening but are not tied. Hemostats placed on the end of each suture are stacked sequentially on an Allis clamp. After approximately eight sutures have been placed they are then individually tied, commencing with the 12-o'clock suture proceeding clockwise. A catheter is inserted following suture placement and tying.

sion is then performed until the tip of the sound is encountered. In cases where the defect is long, the tip of the descending van Buren sound is not palpable through the scar and one must boldly make a vertical incision in the perineal scar just behind the symphysis until the tip is encountered.

2. *Corporal body separation.* If a tension-free anastomosis cannot be achieved, the corporal bodies are separated, beginning at the level of the crus and progressing distally along a relatively avascular midline plane for approximately 4 to 5 cm. Further distal separation is usually not possible due to the more intimate connection between the corporal bodies. This separation allows the urethra to lie between the separated corporal bodies, thereby shortening the distance to the anastomosis.

3. *Inferior pubectomy.* If tension still exists, the dorsal penile vessels are displaced laterally or ligated and a wedge of bone is excised from the inferior aspect of the pubis using an osteotome and bone rongeurs, the wedge being large enough to allow the urethra be redirected cephalad to lie within the groove, resulting in an additional 1 to 2 cm of apparent urethral length. This maneuver also exposes the anteriorly displaced prostate, thereby facilitating the anastomosis.

4. *Supracrural rerouting.* The final maneuver is rerouting the urethra around the corporal body through a bony defect created by further pubectomy, shortening the distance to anastomosis by up to an additional 2 cm (Fig. 48–9). For this maneuver one corporal body is circumferentially mobilized at or just proximal to the suspensory ligament. The dissection is carried

out away from the surface of the corporal body to avoid injury to neurovascular structures. This maneuver does not cause significant penile torsion or chordee.

The urethra is then prepared by spatulation of the distal urethral stump at the 12-o'clock position and the proximal urethra at the 6-o'clock (posterior) position, allowing for identification of the healthy prostatic urethral mucosa and the verumontanum. The posterior incision in the scar is deepened until the hiatus is wide enough to easily accept the index finger (40 Fr), and the proximal limit of the incision approximates the verumontanum. Judicious pelvic floor scar excision, in particular anterolaterally, will prevent damage to the cavernous nerves. The anastomosis is then accomplished with interrupted 4-0 PGA sutures utilizing an advance-and-retrieve method through a long-bladed nasal speculum that is negotiated through the spatulated prostatic urethra. Suture placement is best performed by straightening a standard needle into a J shape (Fig. 48–10). The hub of the needle is then grasped "end on" with the needle driver and the needle tip pushed through the proximal urethral wall from the outside in. Once the needle tip appears inside the prostatic urethral lumen it is grasped with the needle driver and advanced until the needle hub clears the urethral wall and the needle is then withdrawn. The needle is then passed through the corresponding portion of the bulbar urethra. Sutures are placed clockwise and tagged independently with a hemostat and stacked in order. Once all sutures have been placed they are then tied in the order in which they were inserted. In general, 8 to 12 sutures are required to create a watertight anastomosis. A fenestrated 12 Fr urethral catheter is inserted and the suprapubic catheter is replaced. The patient is mobilized from the bed the same day of surgery and usually discharged the next day. The urethral catheter is removed 3 weeks following the repair if extravasation is absent on the pericatheter RUG. The suprapubic catheter is removed after a successful voiding trial, usually on the same day.

OUTCOMES

Complications

Hematoma or hemorrhage is in general rare if meticulous attention is paid to hemostasis during the repair. Wound infection is an uncommon complication that in general presents with erythema, induration, and fluctuance at the incision site.

Flap necrosis is uncommon in experienced hands and is most often due to technical errors in preparation of skin flaps or poor flap selection. Flap viability may also be adversely affected by prior surgery, infection, tissue ischemia, tobacco usage, and malnutrition. Contraction of 15%

to 25% is anticipated for full-thickness skin grafts and must be accounted for during preparation. Removal of subcutaneous fat and fascia must be achieved for adequate exposure of the subdermal vascular plexus but should not be so excessive as to convert the graft to a split-thickness variety. Fenestration of free grafts will promote drainage of the graft bed, and a well-vascularized graft bed must be assumed, sometimes requiring redeployment of spongy tissue. Split-thickness grafts are not advocated for one-stage urethroplasty because their shrinkage is unpredictable and may be excessive (up to 50%).

Fistula is in general uncommon in adult urethral surgery but is on occasion encountered in the setting of underlying infection or vascular compromise. It most commonly occurs following repair of pendulous urethral strictures. Suprapubic urinary diversion may allow for spontaneous healing of fistulas encountered within the first few weeks following urethroplasty. Fistulae that fail to close with proximal diversion in general need reoperation after a minimum of 6 months.

With use of an oversized or poorly supported ventral onlay flap or graft, in particular in the bulbar urethra, there is on occasion formation of a redundant urethral segment in which urine may pool, leading to poor urethral emptying and recurrent infection. Urethral stones can form as a result of urinary stasis in the diverticulum or as a result of retained hair on flaps and grafts. Proper measurement of flaps and grafts to provide a 26 to 28 Fr lumen, as well as adequate spread fixation of the onlay, may obviate sacculation. Preoperative epilation and proper selection of donor sites can prevent the hairy urethra.

Penile curvature may result because of inappropriate procedure selection in attempting anastomotic repair or long-graft onlay repair to the pendulous urethra distal to the suspensory ligament. It may also follow excessive urethral excision (greater than 2 cm) when performing anastomotic repair in the bulbar urethra. Although considerably longer defects are bridged in the anastomotic repair of PFUDD, the tension-relieving maneuvers and the elasticity of the healthy bulbar urethra in general prevent chordee.

In experienced hands erectile dysfunction as a result of anterior or posterior urethroplasty is rare. Temporary (3 months or less) impotence occurs in 53% in those who undergo anastomotic urethroplasty and 33% those who patch repair. However, permanent impotence was unusual, 5% and 0.9%, respectively (2). Further, Coursey et al. reported that erectile dysfunction after anterior urethroplasty is no more common than in men who undergo circumcision (2). In our recent series of posterior urethroplasty only 3% of patients had worsened erectile function following repair (3). These results can be attributed to judicious scar excision, minimal use of electrocautery, and dissection away from the dorsally based neurovascular structures.

Results

As understanding of urethral anatomy and tissue transfer techniques has grown, so too has the effectiveness of urethral reconstruction for stricture disease. Patency rates in excess of 90% are reported for anastomotic repairs in both posterior urethral distraction injury and bulbar strictures (3,9,11). With regard to substitution repairs, tube grafts fare less well than onlay procedures, both of which are best applied to the more proximal portion of the anterior urethra. A pessimistic constant annual attrition rate of 5% per year has been reported for substitution urethroplasty at follow-up of 10 years, although this is not these authors' experience (8). For repair of pendulous urethral strictures, flaps perform best in terms of patency and avoidance of penile curvature. Buccal mucosal grafts show promise and conceptually seem to be superior, but long-term data is necessary to define their emerging role in urethral reconstruction. Certainly the most common cause for stricture recurrence appears to be ongoing fibrosis in the adjacent unmanaged urethra, in particular that proximal to the repair.

From May 1991 to May 2001, Webster has performed a one-stage anastomotic perineal repair of PFUDD in 120 patients for an overall success rate of 97% (3). Anastomotic repair was accomplished utilizing our four-step progressive approach that required step 1 in 9%, step 2 in 37%, step 3 in 13%, and step 4 in 41% (3). Recurrent strictures were rare and usually occurred within the first 3 postoperative months. In most instances these strictures were short in length, located at the prior anastomosis, and responsive to either urethrotomy or secondary anastomotic perineal repair (3,11). The operation has not caused erectile dysfunction in those in whom potency has been preserved following their injury, and continence was not compromised for it resides at the bladder neck level.

REFERENCES

1. Barbagli G, Selli C, Tosto A, Palminteri E. Dorsal free graft urethroplasty. *J Urol* 1996;155:123–126.
2. Coursey JW, Morey AF, McAninch JW, et al. Erectile function after anterior urethroplasty. *J Urol* 2001;166:2273–2276.
3. Flynn BJ, Delvecchio FC, Webster GD. Perineal repair of pelvic fracture urethral distraction defects: experience in 120 patients over the past 10 years. *J Urol* 2003;170(5):1877–1880.
4. Guralnick ML, Webster GD. The augmented anastomotic urethroplasty: indications and outcome in 29 patients. *J Urol* 2001;165:1496–1501.
5. Heyns CF, Steenkamp JW, deDock MLS, Whitaker P. Treatment of male urethral strictures: is repeated dilation or internal urethrotomy useful? *J Urol* 1998;160:356–358.
6. Iselin CE, Webster GD. Dorsal onlay graft urethroplasty for repair of bulbar urethral stricture. *J Urol* 1999;161:815–818.
7. McCallum RW. The adult male urethra: normal anatomy, pathology and method of urethrography. *Radiol Clin North Am* 1979;17:227–244.
8. Mundy AR. The long-term results of skin inlay urethroplasty. *Br J Urol* 1995;75:59–61.
9. Santucci RA, Mario LA, McAninch JW. Anastomotic urethroplasty for bulbar urethral stricture: analysis of 168 patients. *J Urol* 2002;167:1715–1719.
10. Steenkamp JW, Heyns CF, deKock MLS. Internal urethrotomy versus dilation as treatment for male urethral strictures: a prospective, randomized comparison. *J Urol* 1997;157:98–101.
11. Webster GD, Ramon J. Repair of pelvic fracture posterior urethral defects using an elaborated perineal approach: experience with 74 cases. *J Urol* 1991;145:744–748.

CHAPTER 49

Surgery for Urethral Trauma

Michael J. Metro and Jack W. McAninch

Injury to the urethra can affect the anterior and posterior portions, and suspicion should be based on the nature of the trauma and findings on physical examination. Although the mechanism of injury can be either blunt or penetrating, blunt trauma accounts for more than 90% of urethral injuries. Early recognition and diagnosis and careful initial intervention are crucial to successful management and preventing long-term complications.

ANTERIOR URETHRAL INJURIES

The anterior urethra extends from the membranous urethra to the external meatus and is encompassed by the corpus spongiosum and Buck's fascia along its entire length. It is divided into two segments, the bulbar and pendulous urethra. The more proximal bulbar urethra lies under the bulbocavernosus muscle and roughly corresponds to the penoscrotal junction inferiorly and the suspensory ligaments superiorly. The pendulous or penile urethra extends distally to this. Just before the urethral meatus, the urethra widens to form the fossa navicularis (Fig. 49–1).

Blunt injury to the anterior urethra is often caused by motor vehicle accidents or direct blows to the perineum (e.g., "straddle" injuries), where force directed upon the relatively immobile bulbar urethra may crush it against the pubis. Penetrating injuries occur from gunshot or stab wounds and can affect the pendulous or bulbar urethra.

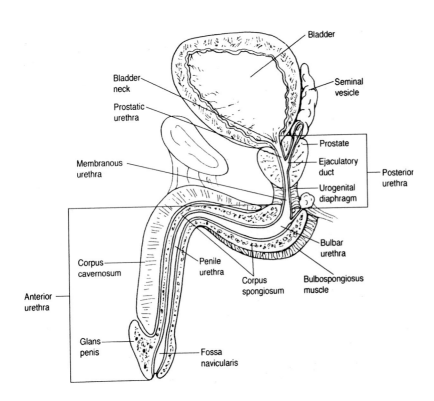

FIG. 49–1. Anatomy of the anterior and posterior urethra.

408

Anterior urethral injuries are rarely associated with pelvic fracture, but are seen in approximately 20% of penile fractures (9).

Diagnosis

A careful history will raise suspicion of acute urethral injury. Patients with penetrating trauma to the penis or perineum will likely be seen immediately after injury, but those with straddle injuries will often delay presentation (in 60%) until prompted by symptoms of voiding dysfunction.

Symptoms of acute injury include pain, blood at the meatus in 75%, inability to void, and hematuria. Urine or blood may extravasate and form characteristic hematomas, depending on which fascial covering contains the extravasation. When Buck's fascia remains intact, the hematoma extends only to the base of the penis. When Buck's fascia is violated, a characteristic "butterfly" hematoma is seen over the perineum contained by the dartos fascia and extending along the abdominal wall to Colles' and Scarpa's fascia.

All patients in whom a urethral injury is suspected should undergo dynamic retrograde urethrography (RUG) before any attempt at catheterization. The patient is positioned obliquely at a 45-degree angle with the bottom leg flexed at 90 degrees and the top leg kept straight (Fig. 49–2).

A scout film is taken to ensure proper positioning and exposure and to assess for the presence of foreign bodies. A 12 or 14 Fr Foley catheter is inserted into the fossa navicularis, and the balloon is filled with 2 to 3 mL of water to prevent dislodging during the study. Approximately 20

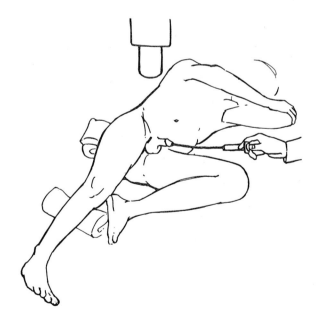

FIG. 49–2. Proper positioning for retrograde urethrography. The patient is placed obliquely at a 45-degree angle with the bottom leg flexed and the top leg straight. Slight traction on the penis during injection of contrast helps avoid telescoping of the urethra and allows more accurate characterization of the injury.

to 30 mL of undiluted water-soluble contrast agent is injected. A film is taken during injection with the penis held on slight stretch to prevent telescoping of the urethra. Films are taken again after injection and after emptying.

Extravasation of contrast is diagnostic of urethral injury. Complete transection must be considered when contrast fails to enter the bladder; partial disruption is present if some contrast enters the bladder. An error of technique should be suspected if contrast neither extravasates nor enters the bladder. If a catheter is in place at the time of urologic consultation it should not be removed, and its position within the bladder should be documented via irrigation. The urethra can be evaluated with a voiding cystourethrogram (VCUG) after a period of observation when a urethral injury is highly suspected.

Anterior urethral injuries are classified into three groups according to radiographic findings. *Contusions* appear as normal on RUG or as urethral elongation from compression from periurethral hematoma. *Incomplete disruptions* are demonstrated on RUG when extravasation is documented, but contrast still enters the bladder and urethral continuity is preserved. *Complete disruptions* are present when extravasation is seen without filling of the posterior urethra or bladder.

Indications for Surgery

Primary surgical repair of an acute anterior urethral injury should be avoided except in patients with concomitant penile fracture or penetrating injuries.

Alternative Therapy

Blunt injuries causing urethral transection are in general managed with suprapubic cystostomy diversion until the associated inflammatory response of the corpus spongiosum and soft tissue subsides. Percutaneously placed suprapubic cystostomy is preferred in patients with penetrating urethral trauma and hemodynamic instability, multiple associated injuries, or a known large urethral defect. Broad-spectrum antibiotics are indicated in the presence of extravasated blood or urine. Urinary diversion is maintained for 3 weeks, after which a VCUG is obtained.

In partial disruption, we believe the urologist may gently attempt passage of a 16 Fr Coudé urethral catheter without worsening the injury. If this is unsuccessful, realignment is not further attempted and a trocar suprapubic cystostomy (SPT) is done. Often, urethral reconstruction is not needed after SPT diversion. The preservation of any segment of urethral mucosa will often permit reepithelialization sufficient for adequate luminal recanalization. The reported stricture formation rate after partial urethral disruption is 45% to 67% (1,5), but the resulting scar is usually minimal and without functional significance, requiring no treatment.

Surgical Technique

When immediate repair is necessary, the patient is placed supine or in the low lithotomy position and is draped widely as penetrating injuries often require exploration for associated injuries to the penis, testes, perineum, and on occasion the rectum. Clean wounds need only minimal debridement followed by urethral closure with 6-0 Maxon sutures over a 16 Fr catheter. When the wound is contaminated, thorough irrigation and debridement of devitalized tissue are mandated.

When bulbar injuries are diagnosed, the patient is placed in the high lithotomy position and a vertical perineal incision is made. The urethra is exposed after division of the bulbocavernosus muscle and the corpus spongiosum is mobilized at the site of injury. Principles of repair are similar to those for elective urethroplasty for stricture: Bulbar defects less than 25 mm can be repaired with end-to-end anastomosis; longer defects should not be repaired acutely, as grafts or flaps will be required and contamination can compromise the repair. Necessary urethral length is gained via liberal dissection distally. The urethral ends are spatulated—the distal end dorsally and the proximal end ventrally (Fig. 49–3)—and the anastomosis is carried out with 5-0 and 6-0 Maxon sutures to create a tension-free, watertight closure. The dorsal surface is closed in one layer, with 5-0 Maxon sutures incorporating the urethral mucosa and spongiosal adventitia, and the ventral surface is closed in two layers with 6-0 Maxon (Fig. 49–4).

Pendulous injuries are exposed via a subcoronal circumferential incision. Penile urethral repairs carry a greater risk of chordee if the repair is under tension. Both repairs are completed over a 16 Fr silicone catheter that is removed after 2 to 3 weeks, when a VCUG is obtained.

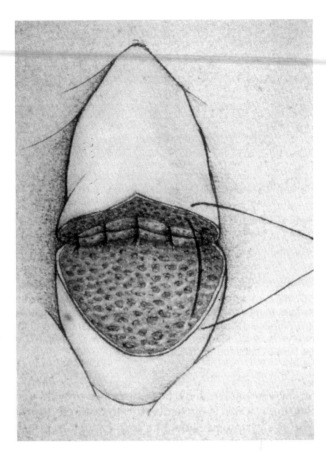

FIG. 49–4. Repair of bulbar urethral injuries. Anastomosis is carried out with a single-layer dorsal closure and a two-layer ventral closure using interrupted 5-0 or 6-0 Maxon sutures.

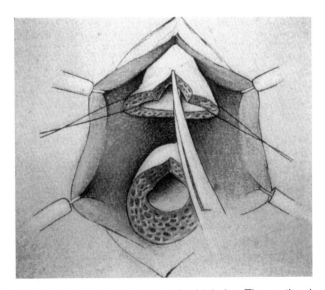

FIG. 49–3. Repair of bulbar urethral injuries. The urethra is mobilized and spatulated in preparation for tension-free end-to-end anastomosis.

Outcomes

Complications

The complications of anterior urethral injury include infection and stricture formation. As discussed, some strictures have minimal functional significance but others will require intervention with dilation, incisional urethrotomy, or formal urethral reconstruction. Extravasated blood or urine can lead to periurethral abscess formation, which can progress to necrotizing gangrene, urethrocutaneous fistulas, and periurethral diverticula (5). Incontinence and impotence, although common in posterior urethral injuries, are uncommon in anterior injuries.

Results

Anastomotic urethroplasty (end-to-end) can be done in a high percentage of patients who sustain a straddle injury requiring surgery. The procedure, as described above, has an overall success rate of more than 90%. Should a stricture develop after repair, internal urethrotomy provides an excellent solution.

POSTERIOR URETHRAL INJURIES

The posterior urethra includes the membranous and prostatic urethra. Injuries are often complex and frequently have multiple associated injuries. Indeed, in contrast to anterior urethral injuries, almost all membranous injuries from blunt trauma have associated pelvic fractures (although only about 5% to 10% of pelvic fractures have an associated urethral injury). Injury is not uncommon as the membranous urethra is positioned between two relatively fixed points. The prostatic apex is attached to the pubis via the puboprostatic ligaments, and the proximal bulbar urethra is fixed in the perineum just distal to the urogenital diaphragm. A shearing force can avulse the urethra here as it passes under the pubic arch. Disruption of the prostatomembranous urethra is therefore a potentially devastating injury, entailing great risk of urologic complications.

Diagnosis

The diagnosis of posterior urethral injury is not difficult as long as suspicion is high. Almost all patients will have blood at the external meatus and many have a palpably distended bladder (7). In patients with pelvic trauma, rectal exam may reveal the classic "high-riding" prostate owing to the accumulation of significant pelvic hematoma. However, in patients in whom bleeding is not severe the prostate will not be displaced, and in some younger men the prostate is indistinguishable from pelvic hematoma.

RUG should be performed in all patients with suspected posterior urethral injury before any attempt at urethral catheterization. If findings are normal, a Foley catheter should be gently advanced into the bladder and a formal cystogram should be obtained to assess for bladder perforation (occurring in 15%) (3).

Posterior urethral injury has been classified into three types based on the integrity of the urethra and urogenital diaphragm (2,10,11): type I, urethral stretching without disruption; type II, urethral rupture but intact urogenital diaphragm; and type III, disruption of both the urethra and urogenital diaphragm. A urethral catheter can be passed in type I injury, and cystography can then be performed. In patients with type II or III injury, urethral catheterization should be avoided (Fig. 49–5).

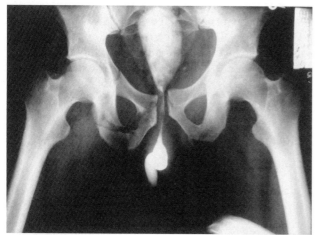

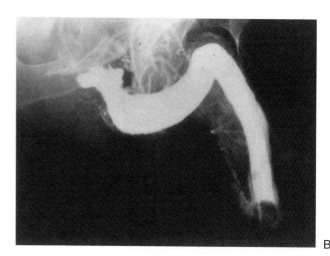

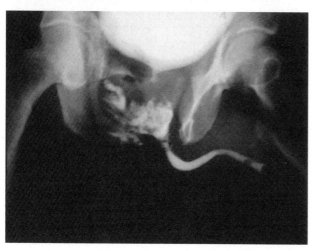

FIG. 49–5. Posterior urethral injuries. **A:** Type I— stretched urethra without rupture. Note the displaced and compressed bladder and fractures of the right symphysis and superior and inferior rami. **B:** Type II—complete rupture of the membranous urethra with intact urogenital diaphragm. Note the limited extravasation and venous filling. **C:** Type III—Note the pattern of extravasation when the urogenital diaphragm is disrupted, as compared with type II. (From Dixon CM. Diagnosis and acute management of posterior urethral disruptions. In: McAninch JW, ed. *Traumatic and reconstructive srology.* Philadelphia: WB Saunders, 1996:347–355, with permission.)

A

B

C

Indications for Surgery

Controversy still exists regarding whether primary realignment or suprapubic diversion is the optimal management for membranous urethral disruption. Those who perform primary realignment report a lower rate of subsequent stricture formation—69% versus 100% when suprapubic diversion alone is used. This potentially avoids a second surgery in almost one-third of patients (12). Subsequent repair may also be easier because of the alignment of the prostate and urethra.

Advocates for delayed reconstruction cite the benefits of the ease and speed of suprapubic catheter placement in the severely traumatized patient. Also, because periprostatic dissection is avoided, the risk of impotence is minimized. Webster et al. reported an 11% incidence of erectile dysfunction in patients treated with delayed reconstruction in comparison with 44% of those with primary realignment; incontinence was also lower (2% vs. 20%) (12). Finally, most injuries result in obliterative strictures that are short (less than 2 cm) and can be repaired with a greater than 90% success rate via a perineal approach 4 to 6 months later (8). For these reasons, we believe that suprapubic diversion with delayed repair is the optimal treatment.

Alternative Therapy

We believe open suprapubic cystotomy tube placement should be performed in all patients with posterior urethral disruptions because of the association with bladder rupture. If the patient is unable to undergo operative exploration and placement, the cystotomy tube can be placed percutaneously with ultrasound guidance if necessary. Immediate urethral repair or reapproximation is indicated if the patient requires exploration for associated rectal or vascular injury, if bladder neck laceration is suspected, or if the bladder is fixed high in the pelvis by its attachment to comminuted bone fragments. This condition, known as "pie-in-the-sky" bladder, leads to very long strictures that may be difficult to repair in a delayed fashion.

Surgical Technique

For open cystotomy tube placement, certain principles should be followed. The patient is placed in the supine position and the genitalia is prepped. A lower midline incision is made to gain access to the prevesical space anterior to the dome of the bladder. Dissection in the space of Retzius and in the lateral perivesical space should be minimized to avoid disturbing the pelvic hematoma. The bladder should be opened vertically with electrocautery and the cystotomy should be long enough to inspect the bladder and repair bladder neck injury if present. Bladder lacerations, if present, should be repaired in two layers with a 2-0 Dexon suture in the

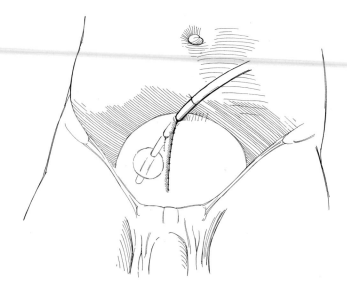

FIG. 49–6. A large-caliber Foley catheter is placed in the bladder dome after inspection for concomitant bladder laceration. With the catheter placed through the superior end of the midline incision, bladder neck identification is facilitated at the time of subsequent reconstruction.

detrusor and a 4-0 chromic suture in the mucosa. A silicone Foley catheter is placed in the dome and brought through the upper part of the midline incision (Fig. 49–6). This position facilitates bladder neck identification during subsequent reconstruction. A larger-caliber catheter should be used if hematuria is expected to be an issue postoperatively. No drains are used unless bowel injury is present.

Outcomes

Complications

Complications of treatment are directly related to the severity of injury. Initial complications include infection of the pelvic hematoma and blood loss at pelvic exploration (obviated by minimizing dissection and avoiding drains where possible); delayed complications include impotence or incontinence as well as stricture formation.

Results

At our institution delayed reconstruction is preferred in most patients with posterior urethral injury. However, we believe that incontinence and impotence are related more to the severity of injury than to the method of urethral management. Overall, impotence occurs in 50% to 80% of patients, but delayed return of potency is seen in up to 63% after definitive urethroplasty (4,6–8). Nearly all patients remain continent if their bladder neck continence mechanism is undamaged, regardless of treatment method. Endoscopic treatment, either initial or delayed, is safe and well tolerated, but multiple subsequent internal urethrotomies are required in up to 90% of patients.

REFERENCES

1. Cass AS, Godec CJ. Urethral injury due to external trauma. *Urology* 1978;11:607–611.
2. Colapinto V, McCallum RW. Injury to the male posterior urethra in fractured pelvis: A new classification. *J Urol* 1977;118:575–580.
3. Corriere JN Jr. Trauma to the lower urinary tract. In: Gillenwater JY, Grayhack JT, Howards SS, Duckett JW, eds. *Adult and pediatric urology*, 3rd ed. St. Louis, MO: Mosby–Year Book, 1996:563–585.
4. El-Abd SA. Endoscopic treatment of posttraumatic urethral obliteration: Experience in 396 patients. *J Urol* 1995;153:67–71.
5. Jackson DH, Williams JL. Urethral injury: a retrospective study. *Br J Urol* 1974;46:665–676.
6. Koratium MM. The lessons of 145 posttraumatic posterior urethral strictures treated in 17 years. *J Urol* 1995;153:63–66.
7. McAninch JW. Traumatic injuries to the urethra. *J Trauma* 1981;21:291–297.
8. Morey AF, McAninch JW. Reconstruction of posterior urethral injuries: Outcome analysis in 82 patients. *J Urol* 1997;157:506–510.
9. Nicolaisen GS, Melamud A, Williams RD, McAninch JW. Rupture of the corpus cavernosum: surgical management. *J Urol* 1983;130:917–919.
10. Sandler CM, Harris JH Jr, Corriere JN Jr, Toombs BD. Posterior urethral injuries after pelvic fracture. *AJR* 1981;137:1233–1237.
11. Sandler CM, Phillips JM, Harris JD, Toombs BD. Radiology of the bladder and urethra in blunt pelvic trauma. *Radiol Clin North Am* 1981;19:195–211.
12 Webster GD, Mathes GL, Selli C. Prostatomembranous urethral injuries: A review of the literature and a rational approach to their management. *J Urol* 1983;130:898–902.

CHAPTER 50

Artificial Urinary Sphincter for Incontinence

John J. Smith III and David M. Barrett

Among the critical functions of the bladder is the requirement to maintain continence in a low-pressure reservoir. Humans are socially continent creatures, yet estimates of 16 to 20 million Americans with some type of urinary leakage are reported. When we lose the ability to remain dry, whether from bladder dysfunction, neurological disease, or as a result of surgery, the social and psychological consequences can be overwhelming. Fortunately, for those patients with specific intrinsic urethral dysfunction the artificial urinary sphincter (AUS), an implantable prosthetic device, can restore urinary control.

While early attempts at a solution for incontinence after prostatectomy were frustrating and unsuccessful, Scott persisted and implanted the first series of reliable prosthetics in 1972 (19). Some 30 years later, evolution of the device has led to a versatile dependable implant. Among the advances was a design change to include a narrow-backed cuff in 1987 to decrease the potential for urethral erosion and reinforced color-coded kink-resistant tubing to assure proper assembly.

The entire system consists of three components: a reservoir, a cuff, and a pump mechanism. The pressure balloon reservoir has various preset pressure ranges whose selection is based on the location of the cuff. The cuff also is available in various sizes depending on the location of its use, be it at the urethral bulb, bladder neck, or for a continent reservoir. Last, the pump is a simple ingenious device with a deactivation button, manual pump and delayed refill resistor. Once activated, the cuff remains open for 2 to 4 minutes as fluid initially leaves the cuff, only to slowly return through the refill resistor in the control mechanism (pump), again restoring continence. The deactivation button prevents the transfer of fluid and therefore pressure back to the cuff (Figs. 50–1A and 50–1B).

DIAGNOSIS

The evaluation of patients with sphincteric incontinence begins with a good clinical history and a voiding diary. Physical examination (supine and erect), neurological exam, and upper and lower urinary tract function should be assessed. This assessment, although tailored to the individual, usually includes cystoscopy and a formal urodynamic study. When performed with fluoroscopy, vesicoureteral reflux can be ruled out or if discovered be treated at the time of implantation of the AUS. Urodynamic findings will also aid in surgical planning. For example, in a patient with a flaccid large bladder, requiring intermittent catheterization, it may be best to place the cuff at the bladder neck rather than urethral bulb and risk erosion. In a patient with low-volume, high-pressure hyperreflexia, an augmentation cystoplasty, autoaugmentation, or other therapy may be required in conjunction with an AUS.

Cystoscopy should be part of the initial workup to rule out bladder neck contracture, urethral stricture, urethral diverticulum, false passage, and even foreign body and stones. These complicating factors need to be definitively managed prior to implantation of the AUS.

INDICATIONS FOR SURGERY

The most common indication for implantation of the AUS is incontinence after prostatectomy. A minimum of 6 months should be allowed after prostatectomy before placement of an AUS as many patients can significantly improve their control. If there has been no significant change in the moderate to severely wet patient in this time frame, one is unlikely to see further improvement.

Other conditions associated with urinary incontinence due to poor urethral function include congenital conditions like exstrophy–epispadias complex, myelomeningocele, and sacral agenesis. In addition, indications could include patients with incontinence following a pelvic fracture, urethral reconstruction, specific spinal cord injury, and rarely following radiation therapy to the pelvis. These patients must have documented stable bladders or plans to control any intravesical pressure with

414

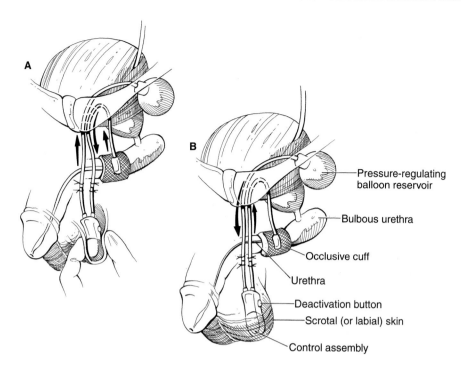

Pressure-regulating
balloon reservoir

Bulbous urethra

Occlusive cuff

Urethra

Deactivation button

Scrotal (or labial) skin

Control assembly

FIG. 50–1. Components and cycling of the AS 800 AGUS. **A:** Squeezing of the scrotal/labial pump transfers fluid out of the compression cuff and into the reservoir, initiating voiding. **B:** A delayed refill resistor slowly allows the cuff to refill automatically over 3 to 5 minutes.

anticholinergic medication or even augmentation cystoplasty.

The only absolute contraindications to an artificial sphincter are patients with poor bladder compliance, low-volume detrusor hyperreflexia, detrusor sphincter dyssynergia, and recurrent urethral stricture disease. It is also critically important that patients have both the physical dexterity and mental capabilities to work the prosthesis. Any active stone disease or recurrent bladder tumors represent relative contraindications.

Special mention of women with incontinence treated by AUS should be noted. Today, most women with intrinsic sphincter deficiency are treated by a suburethral sling. The AUS is usually an option of last resort in women or used only in the suitable neurogenic female at the level of the bladder neck. These patients must be instructed in clean intermittent catheterization prior to implantation. Last, while childbearing is possible deactivation of the AUS during the last trimester is suggested and delivery by cesarean section is strongly recommended (2).

ALTERNATIVE THERAPY

AUS is not the only option for patients with sphincteric urinary incontinence. Patients may remain without treatment if they so desire. Depending on the patient preference, protective pads, clamps, urethral inserts, and external devices can be used. The long-term track record of urethral bulking agents is poor. Other patients may wish to have a catheter or even a urinary diversion.

The male suburethral sling has also been recommended for some patients with stress incontinence. There

are little data to suggest which patients are ideally suited for this approach and even less data on long-term success, follow-up, and complications.

SURGICAL TECHNIQUE

Like any implantation of a mechanical device it is imperative to have proper antibiotics in a timely fashion, proper skin care, and sterile urine. A 12 Fr Foley catheter is placed in a male and a 16 Fr catheter in a female. The patient is placed in the dorsal lithotomy position for urethral cuff placement. If bladder neck placement is entertained, then abduction of the legs in a modified extended position is utilized. In the male a rectal tube is placed to aid in identification of the rectum; a vaginal pack or EEA sizer is placed in the female to outline the vagina. The patient is scrubbed for 10 minutes and during draping a special adhesive drape covers the rectal area to prevent fecal contamination.

The three components of the device should be kept separate from the surgical field until ready for implantation. Liberal use of antibiotic solution in the field is helpful. Limited use of sharp instruments avoids injury to the tubing. Use of predetermined isoosmotic contrast material is preferred. If device malfunction occurs postoperatively, function and component location can be documented by radiographs.

Male Cuff Placement

In the adult male, the vast majority of cuffs are placed in the bulbous urethra. A midline perineal incision is

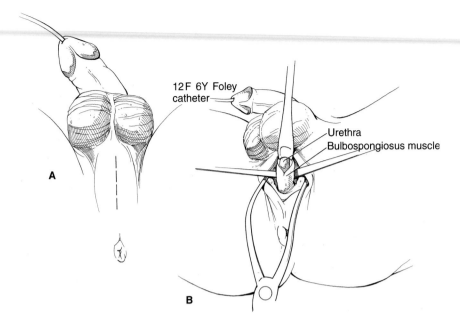

FIG. 50–2. **A:** Bulbous urethral perineal raphe incision for placement of bulbous urethral cuff. **B:** Sharp dissection and circumferential isolation of 2-cm length of bulbous urethra.

made to expose the underlying tissues until the bulbocavernous muscle can be identified (Figs. 50–2A and 50–2B). A self -retaining retractor is used to expose the urethra. Care is taken in dissecting the urethra laterally first and then circumferentially. Traction on the urethra itself, provided by grasping the urethra and Foley together, can greatly facilitate dissection. The most difficult dissection is anteriorly at the 12-o'clock position, where a septum between the two corporal bodies and the urethra can be found. A 2-cm wide plane must be developed to accommodate the cuff. The 4.5-cm cuff is the most common size in adult males. The cuff, which has a small amount of contrast in it, is carefully clamped with a rubber shod to prevent leakage of contrast fluid or air getting into the system.

Attention is now turned to the abdomen on the dominant hand of the patient. A small midline incision or small transverse incision is made. A small space is developed below the rectus in the paravesical space to place the reservoir. In general, a 61- to 70-cm water balloon is chosen. On occasion, a 51- to 60-cm reservoir is available for use in patients with a previous history of radiation or urethral surgery to decrease the risk of erosion. A counterincision is made in the rectus fascia to bring the tubing out (Fig. 50–3). This separates pocket and exit site, facilitating closure. Next, 22 cc of contrast solution is placed in the reservoir. Proper setting of the balloon reservoir in the space is confirmed before closure.

The pump mechanism is placed in the scrotum by developing a subcutaneous plane above Scarpa's fascia. The pocket can be developed bluntly and/or with Hegar's dilators. It is important to assure good positioning of the pump for the patient to grasp it without struggle. Once this space is ready, a path below Scarpa's fascia from the

same area to the perineal incision is made. The cuff tubing, doubly clamped, is carefully transferred to the abdominal incision site. Now that all components are in place, they can be trimmed to appropriate length and connected with quick connectors. The device is tested two to three times before deactivation to confirm its function. Care should be taken to leave enough fluid in the pump to allow activation from the deflated state. This is best assured by waiting approximately 30 seconds after activation before deactivating the system for a number of weeks. The AUS is deactivated for 6 weeks to permit healing. The incisions are closed in layers with absorbable suture material. The Foley catheter is left for 24 hours.

In some male patients, the bladder neck cuff placement is best. In this case, the retropubic space is entered

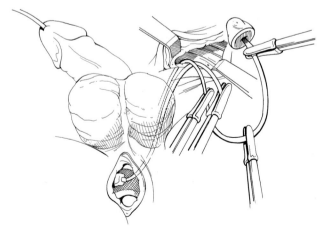

FIG. 50–3. A counterincision is made in the rectus fascia to bring the tubing out.

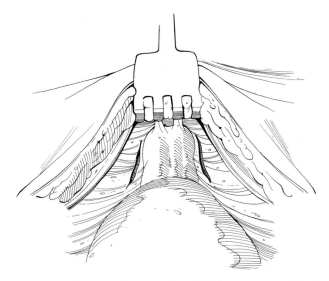

FIG. 50–4. A plane between the bladder neck posteriorly and the rectum is developed.

through a midline incision. The anterior rectus fascia is opened sharply. Staying extraperitoneal, the space of Retzius is developed through blunt and sharp dissection. The endopelvic fascia is identified, cleaned off, but not opened. A plane between the bladder neck posteriorly and the rectum is developed (Fig. 50–4). In an adult male, the plane is proximal to the prostate and distal to the ureterovesical junction. Careful, deliberate, sharp, and occasional blunt dissection, creating a 2-cm tunnel, in the region between the prostate and bladder neck is critical to avoid injury to the ureters, bladder, or rectum (Fig. 50–5). If the dissection is extremely difficult, consider opening

the bladder in the anterior midline. Do not carry the incision down to the bladder neck as this may jeopardize a future erosion. Open the anterior bladder enough to visualize and palpate where the dissection can safely continue. An 8- to 14-cm cuff is usually required in the adult male. Once the cuff tubing has been securely passed around the bladder neck, it is passed through the posterior segment of the rectus muscle and onto the anterior rectus fascia.

The balloon pressure reservoir is placed in the prevesical space. This should be easy as the space has already been developed. A 61- to 70-cm water pressure reservoir is routinely used although at times a larger cuff is used and requires a 71- to 80-cm water pressure balloon. Finally, the pump mechanism is put in the ipsilateral hemiscrotal pocket developed as described earlier. The quick connectors are used to connect the segments and the system is tested two to three times (Fig. 50–6).

It may be prudent during the early dissection of the bladder neck to periodically check the integrity of the bladder. This is done by filling the bladder with antibiotic solution mixed with methylene blue. Any bladder injury identified that is small can be repaired in two layers. If a rectal injury is suspected and testing from the rectal tube proves to be positive, the operation should be abandoned after the rectal wall is repaired.

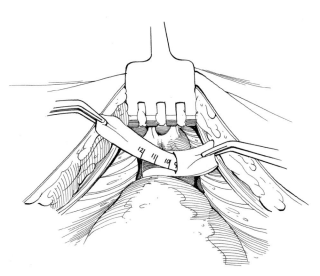

FIG. 50–5. Careful, deliberate, sharp, and occasional blunt dissection, creating a 2-cm tunnel, in the region between the prostate and bladder neck is critical to avoid injury to the ureters, bladder, or rectum

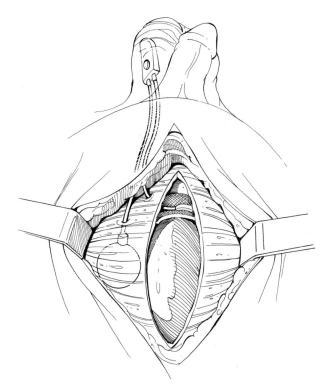

FIG. 50–6. The quick connectors are used to connect the segments and the system is tested two to three times.

Female Cuff Placement

The cuff for females is placed around the bladder neck, which can be approached from the abdomen or the vagina. The abdominal approach mirrors that of the male. The space of Retzius is entered after a midline or Pfannenstiel incision. A plane above the endopelvic fashion is developed. A Betadine-soaked sponge should be in the vagina during dissection. The proper plane is superior to the pelvic wall (endopelvic fascia) and caudad to the ureters as they enter the trigone (Fig. 50–7). A 2-cm circumferential width is required to pass the cuff behind the bladder neck safely with a right-angle clamp. Again, periodic testing of the bladder integrity is performed to rule out a small injury. Should a small tear in the bladder or vagina be noted, it should be closed and the procedure can continue.

Once the cuff is in place, its tubing is passed through the rectus about 4 to 5 cm above the pubis in preparation for connection to the pump tubing. Sizing of the cuff in women is crucial and most patients require a 6- to 8-cm cuff. Anything larger suggests too wide a dissection in the soft tissue near the bladder. Measurement needs to be accomplished with a 12 Fr Foley catheter in place.

The pump mechanism in the female is placed in the ipsilateral labia majora by creating a subcutaneous pocket with Hegar's dilators. The pocket created needs to be accessible and dependent for ease of manipulation. Once placed, the tubing is trimmed and connections made. The system is then tested and finally deactivated (Fig. 50–8).

In 1988 Appel reported a transvaginal technique for placement of the AUS cuff. He advocated an inverted "U" incision, with the apex at the midurethra. It is the authors' limited experience that a midline incision may have less chance of infection, vascular compromise, and erosion. Nonetheless, the retropubic space is entered as for performing a sling. The tips of blunt curved Mayo scissors

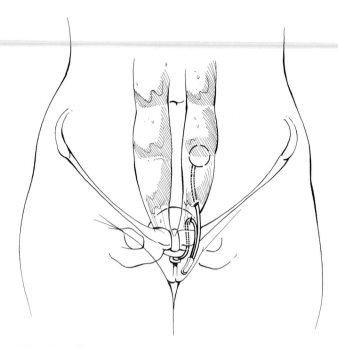

FIG. 50–8. Once placed, the tubing is trimmed and connections made. The system is then tested and finally deactivated.

pointing to the ipsilateral shoulder carefully enter the retropubic space. Once through, the scissors are slowly spread and blunt finger dissection behind the pubis usually results in excellent exposure. A small, moist vaginal tape can be placed into the retropubic space for more blunt dissection. Done in this fashion it is rare to need to make a counterincision above the urethra to complete a urethrolysis. The area above the urethra at the level of the bladder neck can be palpated from either side. A measuring tape can confirm the proper cuff size. The cuff is then passed behind the vesical neck and secured in place with the knob of the cuff perivesically and not against the vaginal epithelium (Figs. 50–9A and 50–9B). A small abdominal incision is made at this time to place a reservoir in the prevesical space. Once completed, the cuff tubing is transferred to the ipsilateral side into the retropubic space and through the rectus fascia. A subcutaneous pocket, as previously described, is created. The reservoir is filled with 22 mL of isoosmotic contrast and all components are connected. The vaginal and abdominal incisions are closed with absorbable sutures.

Placement of Cuff in Children

In selective children AUS is a consideration to establish continence (9,12) providing the child is old enough to perform self-catheterization. Most boys are able to be taught by about 6 to 7 years old, whereas girls are usually 8 to 9 years old. The more physically mature the child, in particular in females, the easier the placement of some of the components. The dissection, in particular in the

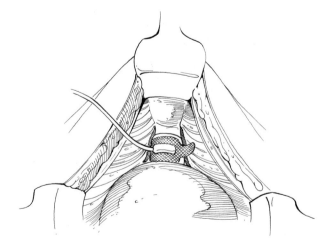

FIG. 50–7. The proper plane is superior to the pelvic wall (endopelvic fascia) and caudad to the ureters as they enter the trigone.

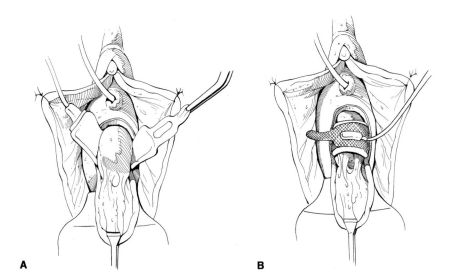

A   **B**

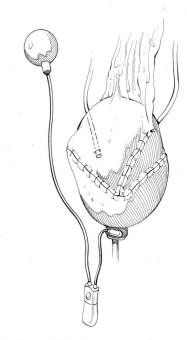

FIG. 50–9. The cuff is then passed behind the vesical neck and secured in place with the knob of the cuff perivesically and not against the vaginal epithelium.

female, must be precise because the urethral and vaginal tissues are soft and fragile. The older female has a more well-developed labia to discretely place the pump in. In both sexes, the only site for cuff placement is the bladder neck. The extraperitoneal approach is the same as in the adult from above. Again, purposeful cystotomy can facilitate dissection in some females. The usual cuff size is 6 to 8 cm. A low-pressure reservoir (61 to 70 cm) is used to avoid atrophy and cuff erosion. Despite these precautions, complications in children are higher. Bosco et al. (4) and Adams et al. (1) reviewed complications resulting in removal of devices in 13% to 25% of patients for erosion or infection. The only other revision child and parent need to be aware of is the lengthening of the pump tubing into the scrotum or labia commensurate with growth.

AUS and Intestinal Segments

The goal of reconstructive bladder surgery is a low-compliant, good capacity reservoir that is continent. While the AUS addresses the later issue, on occasion a reservoir needs to be constructed. The enterocystoplasty or augmentation cystoplasty can increase the bladder capacity, lower the bladder leak pressure, but in some instances requires an AUS to provide continence. Many authors have reported simultaneous augmentation and AUS placement, although in general the enterocystoplasty is performed first (7,13,15). The cuff is always placed around the bladder neck as previously described or through a mesenteric window (Fig. 50–10). In simultaneous procedures, a suprapubic tube is left for 3 weeks. The Foley catheter can be removed in 48 hours to minimize tissue ischemia in the area of the recently dissected bladder neck. Sterile technique is a must in bowel cases with AUS implantation. Voluminous amounts of antibiotic solution throughout the augmentation procedure should be routine. Any gross contamination should defer placement of the AUS to another time. Any drains used peri-

operatively should be removed as soon as feasible to avoid contamination. If the patient cannot void because of edema postoperatively, a small catheter can be used for clean intermittent catheterization for a short time until the incontinent state returns.

Penile Prosthesis and AUS

Similar controversy exists regarding same time or delayed placement of AUS and a penile prosthesis. In a two-staged approach either prosthetic can arguably be placed first. Regardless of the patient's preference, the second prosthesis should be preceded by a careful review of the original operation and multiple radiographs are

FIG. 50–10. The cuff is always placed around the bladder neck as previously described or through a mesenteric window.

recommended to ascertain the actual position of the device. In the case of simultaneous implantation, the sphincter should be placed first. This permits testing of the three components before insertion of the penile prosthesis. In addition, a semirigid rod or unicomponent device, which can be placed subcoronally, may avoid prolonged exposure of the perineum and facilitate successful two-prosthetic implantation. Parulkar and Barrett (17) reported a satisfactory continence rate of 95% and a functional penile prosthesis in 98% in combination patients. In the event of an infection, it is highly likely all components will be involved and need to be removed.

Radiation and AUS

Pelvic radiation is known to increase the likelihood of complications in implantation of an AUS. Most of these are infection–erosion problems requiring surgical revision in 25% to 57% of cases (14,21). The host response to a foreign body is different in irradiated tissue because radiation arteritis and other changes induce fibrosis and atrophy. This can represent a precursor condition to infection or erosion. Patients with a high risk of local pelvic recurrence of tumor may be better suited for a urinary diversion.

OUTCOMES

Complications

Postoperative urinary retention is common. In men this can be resolved by placing a small catheter in the bladder after the sphincter mechanism has been examined to confirm deactivation of the cuff. In women it is wise to preoperatively instruct them in clean intermittent catheterization. In both cases, postoperative edema, usually responsible for the retention, resolves in 48 to 72 hours. Another early problem can be a hematoma in the labia or scrotum. Only a large symptomatic hematoma should be evacuated. Antibiotic therapy and local care are usually sufficient. The device will not be manipulated or activated for 6 to 8 weeks, plenty of time for this to resolve.

The overall infection rate with the AUS is approximately 1% to 3% (3,6). Infection most commonly presents months later or even years following the implantation. Most often the first sign of infection is pain or tenderness with pump manipulation or pain in the scrotum. There may initially be no swelling. The most common organisms are *Staphylococcus epidermidis* and *Staphylococcus aureus* (20). Delayed and late infections usually are indolent, less virulent pathogens such as gram-negative bacteria. All patients with a prosthetic implantation should take antibiotics before any dental work or invasive surgical procedure. Further, we strongly urge patients to carry and wear identifying information to alert other healthcare providers of the presence of the implanted AUS. While some physicians have tried to salvage or drain locally, in most instances the entire prosthesis must be removed. After 3 to 6 months, one can consider reimplantation.

Cuff erosions can occur as a result of infection, an unrecognized urethral injury at surgery, too thin a dissection around the urethra, or from tissue atrophy over time. The presenting complaint may be referred pain to the tip of the penis, recurrent incontinence, bloody discharge, or pain or swelling in the perineum. Cystoscopy can confirm the erosion. Delayed erosions have become less frequent with the introduction of the narrow-backed cuff system. If a cuff must be removed, the tubing from the pump mechanism can be plugged with a stainless steel plug in preparation for a reimplant in 3 to 6 months. After successful reimplantation, in particular in irradiated patients, purposeful deactivation on a nightly basis can be taught to the patient in an attempt to reduce the chances of tissue atrophy or erosion.

Persistent or recurrent incontinence can be systematically evaluated. If there is no erosion by cystoscopy and the system seems to cycle further diagnostic tools are needed. A videourodynamic study may reveal poor urethral resistance, low leak point pressure, or possible bladder instability or lack of compliance. Instability can be treated medically with any number of anticholinergic drugs and fluid management. If a very low leak point is found, a tandem cuff is suggested (5,11). This can be performed by using a "Y" connector and adding 3 mL to the reservoir. The device does need to be deactivated for 6 to 8 weeks as though it were new. If, however, the leak pressure is higher, changing the balloon pressure reservoir is indicated, in particular in patients with a bladder neck cuff because the reservoir is much more accessible than the cuff. Last, a reduction in cuff size or relocation to a more proximal site can also be entertained as solutions. In the female patient persistent incontinence should prompt an evaluation to rule out a vesicovaginal fistula.

If leakage of the device is suspected, surgical exploration may be required. A fluoroscopic unit can be helpful if contrast is in the system. The cuff is first exposed through a perineal incision. If the cuff is fine, the tubing should be examined. Each element of the device can usually be tested from the inguinal or abdominal incision. The area of the connections, usually over the pubic bone, should be explored and each limb identified. The cuff is the most common source for leakage and the pump is the least likely source of leakage. Once the leakage is identified, the individual component is replaced. In the rare event that no fluid is in the system, the entire prosthesis should be replaced. As a last effort before complete removal, an ohmmeter if available can be used to identify the site or component that is failing (18).

Female patients who have become pregnant must be followed or observed closely. Many authors have recommended device deactivation in the third trimester and during labor. In addition, those female patients with an augmentation cystoplasty and AUS should strongly consider cesarean delivery (8,16). The patient should be sure her gynecologist is in touch with a urologist familiar with the workings of the AUS.

Results

Gundian et al. (10) in 1989 reviewed the Mayo Clinic experience in 117 patients receiving an AUS for incontinence following radical retropubic prostatectomy. Ninety percent of the patients were improved or cured of their incontinence. The infection rate was 2.5%. The most recent study by Elliott and Barrett in 1998 showed 90.4% of patients were alive with a functioning device. The reoperation rate was 12% and 186 of the 323 patients had undergone a radical prostatectomy. The experience with females has also been positive, with rates of continence between 86% and 93%.

REFERENCES

1. Adams MC, Mitchell ME, Rink RC. Artificial urinary sphincters in the pediatric population. Presented at Meeting of the American Urological Association, Dallas, TX, May 1989.
2. Barrett DM, Parulkar BG. The artificial sphincter (AS-800). Experience in children and young adults. *Urol Clin North AM* 1989;16: 119–132.
3. Blum MD. Infections of genitourinary prosthesis. *Infect Dis Clin North Am* 1989;3:259–274.
4. Bosco PJ, Bauer SB, Colodny AH, Mandell J, Retik AB. The long term results of artificial sphincters in children. *J Urol* 1991;146:396–399.
5. Brito CG, Mulcahy JJ, Mitchell ME, Adams MC. Use of a double cuff AMS800 urinary sphincter for severe stress incontinence. *J Urol* 1993;149:283–285.
6. Carson CC. Infections of genitourinary prosthesis. *Urol Clin North Am* 1989;16:139–147.
7. de Badiola FI, Castro-Diaz D, Hart-Austin C, Gonzalez R. Influence of preoperative bladder capacity and compliance on the outcome of artificial sphincter implantation in patients with neurogenic sphincter incompetence. *J Urol* 1992;148:1493–1495.
8. Fishman IJ, Scott FB. Pregnancy in patients with the artificial urinary sphincter. *J Urol* 1993;150:340–341.
9. Gonzalez R, Koleilat N, Austin C, Sidi AA. The artificial sphincter AS800 in congenital urinary incontinence. *J Urol* 1989;142 (2, Pt 2): 512–521.
10. Gundian JC, Barrett DM, Parulkar BG. Mayo Clinic experience with use of the AMS 800 artificial urinary sphincter for urinary incontinence following radical prostatectomy. *J Urol* 1989;142:1459–1461.
11. Kowalczyk JJ, Spicer DL, Mulcahy JJ. Long-term experience with the double-cuff AMS 800 artificial urinary sphincter. *Urology* 1996;47: 895–897.
12. Light JK, Hawila M, Scott FB. Treatment of urinary incontinence in children: the artificial sphincter versus other methods. *J Urol* 1983; 130:518–521.
13. Light JK, Lapin S, Vohra S. Combined use of bowel and the artificial urinary sphincter in reconstruction of the lower urinary tract: infectious complications. *J Urol* 1995;153:331–333.
14. Martins FE, Boyd SD. Artificial urinary sphincter in patients following major pelvic surgery and or radiotherapy: are they less favorable candidates? *J Urol* 1995;153:1188–1193.
15. Nurse DE, Mundy AR. One hundred artificial sphincters. *Br J Urol* 1988;61:318–325.
16. Parulkar BG, Barrett DM. Application of the AS-800 artificial sphincter for intractable urinary incontinence in females. *Surg Gynecol Obstet* 1990;171:131–138.
17. Parulkar BG, Barrett DM. Combined implantation of artificial sphincter and penile prosthesis. *J Urol* 1989;142:732–735.
18. Parulkar BG, Lamontagne DP, Vickers MA Jr. Detection of leakage in inflatable genitourinary devices. *Urology* 1996;47:97–101.
19. Scott FB, Bradley WE, Timm GW. Treatment of urinary incontinence by implantable prosthetic sphincter. *Urology* 1973;1:252–259.
20. Shandera KC, Thompson IM. Urologic prosthesis. *Emerg Med Clin North Am* 1994;12:729–748.
21. Walsh IK, Williams SG, Mahendra V, et al. Artificial urinary sphincter implantation in the irradiated patient: safety, efficacy and satisfaction. *Br J Urol* 2002;89:364–368.

CHAPTER 51

Urethral Cancer in Women

John A. Heaney

Primary urethral carcinoma is an extremely rare entity, accounting for less than 1% of all adult malignancies. It is one of the few urologic malignancies for which the incidence in women is greater than that in men, with a 4:1 female:male ratio. Most cases of female urethral carcinoma occur in patients who are postmenopausal. The mean age at diagnosis is 55 to 60 years (7).

The etiology of urethral cancer is unknown, and the risk factors for its occurrence are undefined in the majority of patients. Associations between urethral cancer and chronic irritation and infection have been made, including a correlation between the occurrence of cancer and a prior history of urethral caruncle and urethral diverticula.

The most common type of urethral cancer is squamous cell carcinoma (55%), followed by transitional cell carcinoma (17%) and adenocarcinoma (16%) (8,9). However, in cases of urethral cancer occurring in diverticula the most common histological type is adenocarcinoma (8). The least common types of urethral cancer include clear-cell carcinoma, undifferentiated carcinoma, and melanoma (8,9). The disease tends to spread first by local invasion into the muscularis of the urethra and then into the periurethral connective tissue, the anterior vaginal wall and vulva, the bladder neck, and the pubic arch. Lesions in the distal one-third of the urethra spread to the superficial and deep inguinal nodes, whereas proximal lesions spread via the deep pelvic lymphatics to the periaortic chain (9). Clinically evident adenopathy in patients with urethral cancer is likely to represent metastatic disease, with 80% to 90% of grossly enlarged lymph nodes harboring metastatic deposits (4). Although distant metastases are uncommon at presentation, distant disease can eventually occur via hematogenous spread to the liver, lung, bone, and brain. Patients tend to fail both locally and at distant sites, with prognosis more dependent on the clinical stage at presentation than on the histological type or grade of the primary tumor (1,9).

DIAGNOSIS

Because the symptoms of urethral cancer are subtle, the diagnosis is usually delayed and patients commonly present with locally advanced disease at the time of diagnosis. The most prevalent symptom at presentation is urethral bleeding, spotting, or hematuria. Other symptoms include dysuria, urgency, frequency, urethral discharge, or dyspareunia. A palpable anterior vaginal wall mass can be found on bimanual examination or an ulcerated lesion may be found on examination of the urethral meatus. Women with urethral carcinoma are often misdiagnosed with other entities such as urethral diverticuli, stenosis or prolapse, polyps, hemangiomas, fistulas, caruncles, or atrophic vaginitis on original evaluation but continue to have symptoms despite medical therapy. Thus, any patient with persistent symptoms that do not respond to standard therapies should be evaluated for carcinoma with urethroscopy and transurethral biopsy of any suspicious lesion.

The Grabstald staging system for urethral carcinoma is in most common use and is compared to the tumor–node–metastasis (TNM) staging system shown in Table 51–1. Careful examination of the external genitalia and bimanual examination under anesthesia at the time of tumor biopsy will help determine if the tumor is resectable. A helpful technique is to palpate the tumor while the cystoscope sheath is in the urethra to determine the local extent of the tumor. Evaluation of the bladder neck and proximal urethra via endoscopy and biopsy should also be performed if bladder preservation approaches are to be considered. The inguinal nodes should be carefully examined because palpable lymphadenopathy usually represents malignancy.

Chest radiograph and computed tomography (CT) scanning of the abdomen and pelvis are performed to look for distant metastases or significant adenopathy in the groin, pelvis, or abdomen. In the presence of enlarged

TABLE 51–1. *Staging of female urethral carcinoma*

Grabstald[a]	TNM[b]	
	Tx	Primary Tumor Cannot be Assessed
	T0	No Evidence of Primary Tumor
Stage 0	Tis	Carcinoma *In Situ* (CIS)
	Ta	Noninvasive Papillary, Polypoid, or Verrucous
Stage A	T1	Invades Lamina Propria
Stage B	T2	Invades Periurethral Muscularis
Stage C1	T3	Invades Anterior Vaginal Muscle or Bladder Neck
Stage C2		Invades Anterior Vaginal Mucosa
Stage C3	T4	Invades adjacent Structures Including Clitoris, Labia, or Pubis
Stage D1	N1	Regional Metastasis to Inguinal Lymph Nodes (TNM = Single Node <2 cm)
Stage D2	N2	Regional Metastasis to Pelvic Lymph Nodes (TNM = Single Node >2 cm but <5 cm or Multiple <5 cm)
Stage D3	N3	Metastasis to Lymph Nodes Above the Aortic Bifurcation (TNM = > cm Node)
Stage D4	M1	Distant Metastasis (With Any Primary Tumor)

[a]From Grabstald H. Tumors of the urethra in men and women. *Cancer* 1973;32:1236, with permission.
[b]Modified from Beahrs OH, et al, eds. *Manual for staging of cancer*, 3rd ed. Philadelphia: JB Lippincott Co, 1988:120, with permission.

lymph nodes, ultrasound- or CT-guided lymph node biopsy or laparoscopic node dissection can be performed; the presence of pelvic nodal metastasis portends a poor prognosis and is a contraindication to exenterative surgery unless complete response follows neoadjuvant chemotherapy.

INDICATIONS FOR SURGERY

Without treatment, most urethral cancers will progress with a mean survival of only 12 months (1). If the patient has clinically localized disease and has a reasonable life expectancy, then curative treatment is indicated. The presence of metastatic disease or pelvic lymph node involvement is a contraindication to performing radical surgery. For superficial, noninvasive urethral lesions, topical tumor ablative treatments can be used (1,9). For distal urethral lesions, a less invasive distal urethrectomy can be performed in selected cases (see below). However, the presence of a histologically confirmed invasive urethral carcinoma is an indication that radical excision of the tumor and the surrounding tissues is needed. In the absence of inguinal adenopathy, there is no need for inguinal node dissection because there is no clear benefit for prophylactic lymphadenectomy (6). Patients may be considered for bladder preservation surgery with continent cutaneous urinary diversion if they are compliant, have adequate hand–eye coordination to perform intermittent self-catheterization, and have a creatinine less than 2.0 to avoid electrolyte disorders. If the patient cannot manage the complexities of a continent diversion, then noncontinent forms of urinary diversion, such as a suprapubic tube, ileocutaneous vesicostomy, or ileal conduit, are preferable.

ALTERNATIVE THERAPY

For superficial lesions of the urethra, endoscopic fulguration of the lesion can be performed. However, because no pathologic material is obtained during fulguration of the lesion, adequate biopsies of the lesion must be obtained before tumor destruction to rule out the presence of any invasive disease. The neodynium:YAG or holmium:YAG laser can be used safely to destroy the lesion through an endoscope, with the advantage that the laser energy penetrates up to 3 mm (at a power setting of 60 W) into the urethral tissue and can provide for a therapeutic margin. Use of laser has the potential risk of postoperative urethral stricture from injury to the underlying spongiosum of the urethra. For treating urethral lesions, the noncontact laser beam is applied to the tumor site for 0.5 to 1 seconds up to a maximum power level of 25 to 30 W (9).

Radiation therapy (either interstitial or external beam) can also be used to cure low-stage urethral cancer. However, when it has been used for high-stage disease the response rates to radiation therapy were low and the complication rates high. Side effects such as incontinence, stricture, fistula, or radiation cystitis occurred in almost 50% of patients (2). There is evidence that external beam radiation therapy, especially when combined with brachytherapy, may confer a survival advantage when it is used as an adjuvant to surgery, either in cases where the tumor is locally excised or where a larger exenteration has to be performed because of the presence of high-stage disease (2,9).

SURGICAL TECHNIQUE

With the exception of transitional cell carcinoma, urethral cancers represent lesions that originate in the squamous and columnar epithelium of the urethra. As such, urethral cancer does not involve a "field defect" change in the entire urothelium, and the bladder transitional cell epithelium should be spared from involvement if the tumor has not grossly invaded the bladder by direct extension (5). In patients with either a squamous cell carcinoma or an adenocarcinoma of the urethra, a bladder-preserving procedure can decrease patient morbidity without compromising the outcome of the cancer surgery. If a transitional cell carcinoma is found in the urethra, then the entire lower urinary tract urothelium must be considered at risk and the patient treated accordingly.

Treatment of Distal Urethral Tumors

The technique of distal urethrectomy can be used for patients with urethral tumors that are clinically localized to the distal one-third of the urethra. Ideally, the lesion should be restricted to the meatus because resection of more than 1 cm of the urethra can result in incontinence.

The patient is placed in the lithotomy position on an operating table where the footrest can be either lowered or removed and the perineum rests at the edge of the table, allowing for the placement of a weighted vaginal speculum. Number 1 silk sutures are placed into the labia and tacked to the medial thigh to separate the labia and improve exposure to the vaginal introitus. A Scott ring retractor is also placed to provide vaginal exposure. A Foley catheter is placed to facilitate palpation of the urethra and the tumor during dissection.

A circumscribing incision is made around the urethral meatus as shown in Figure 51–1. After sharp dissection has been performed through the epithelium of the vagina, sharp dissection with Metzenbaum scissors and Bovie electrocautery are used to dissect along the urethra in a circumferential manner, using palpation of the Foley as a guide to the dissection. If the distal urethra is firmly adherent to the anterior vaginal wall, it is easier sometimes to resect the anterior vaginal wall with the urethra instead of trying to preserve the anterior vaginal wall that is attached to the urethra.

A figure-of-eight, 0 silk stay suture or Allis clamp is placed at the meatus, and gentle traction allows exposure of the urethral wall during dissection. A small right-angle clamp is used to facilitate dissection along the anterior and lateral aspects of the urethra, and bleeding sites along these planes are identified and fulgurated. Dissection is extended to a point 0.5 to 1 cm beyond the palpable tumor. An anterior incision is made in the urethra beyond the tumor to the level of the Foley, and 3-0 catgut stay sutures are placed in the urethra to prevent retraction of the urethra after the distal urethra is transected. The remaining circumference of the urethra is then divided and the specimen is removed. Frozen sections of the margins are sent to confirm that there is no residual tumor in the urethral stump. If local involvement of the anterior vaginal wall is suspected, a portion of the anterior vaginal wall can be excised in continuity with the specimen. This is done by incising the vaginal wall epithelium 0.5 to 1 cm around the periphery of the urethral mass.

Pinpoint electrocautery is used to achieve hemostasis. The urethral meatus is then reconstructed by suturing the edges of the urethral stump to the edges of the vaginal incision using 3-0 chromic catgut sutures. After the urethral meatus is reconstructed, the remaining defect in the vaginal wall is approximated with interrupted 3-0 polyglactic acid sutures or chromic sutures. A vaginal pack and urethral catheter are placed. The vaginal pack is removed on postoperative day 1 and the Foley catheter is removed 7 days after surgery.

Treatment of Larger Distal Lesions

For patients with squamous cell carcinoma or adenocarcinoma of the urethra not involving the bladder neck, a bladder-preserving approach can be used. The bladder neck is closed and a continent cutaneous bladder drainage is created with either an ileocecal segment for augmentation or the appendix using the Mitrofanoff principle. However, if the primary tumor is transitional cell carcinoma of the urethra the entire bladder urothelium is also at risk and cystourethrectomy should be performed.

The patient is placed in the low lithotomy position with the legs extended in Allen stirrups to allow for perineal access without interference of the abdominal exploration. A weighted vaginal speculum is placed, and no. 1 silk sutures are used to tack the labia laterally to improve exposure to the vaginal introitus. A Scott ring retractor is placed to provide further vaginal exposure. A Foley catheter is inserted to facilitate palpation of the urethra, bladder neck, and the tumor during dissection.

After examination under anesthesia and careful palpation of the inguinal nodes, a midline transperitoneal lower-abdominal incision is performed. The incision runs from the pubis at least to the umbilicus; it is extended superiorly as needed. Bilateral pelvic node dissections are completed and the specimens sent for frozen section. If the lymph nodes are positive, most surgeons will only do a palliative procedure. If there is no evidence of nodal involvement, the bladder neck is mobilized from the lateral attachments to the pelvis by incising the endopelvic fascia. The attachments of the urethra to the urogenital diaphragm are exposed and divided lateral to the urethra with electrocautery. The uterus and ovaries are preserved.

After the anterior urethra and bladder neck have been mobilized through the retropubic space, dissection is then initiated through a transvaginal approach to excise the urethra and distal bladder neck along with a margin of anterior vaginal wall. This is done by extending the circumscribing perimeatal incision into the anterior vaginal wall to a point that is 0.5 to 1 cm from the periphery of the palpable tumor. The pubourethral ligaments that con-

A

B

C

D

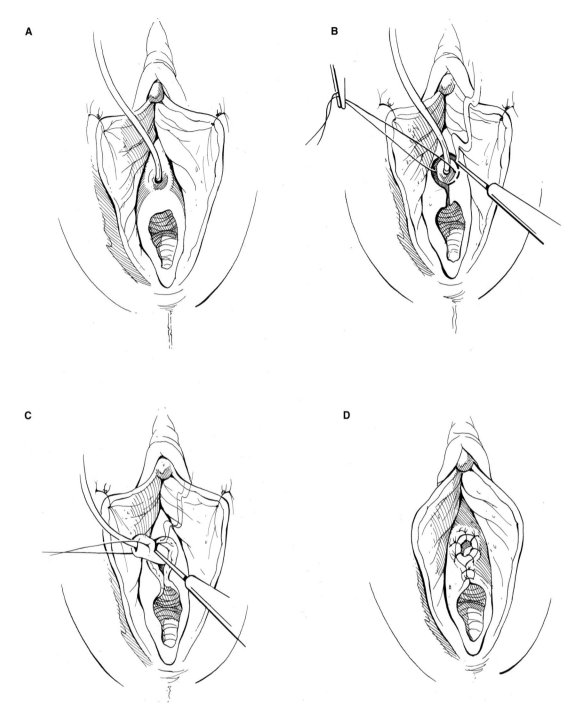

FIG. 51–1. Technique of distal urethrectomy.

nect the distal urethra to the inferior surface of the symphysis are identified using blunt dissection with a right-angle clamp; the ligaments are then divided with electrocautery. The dissection is extended under the pubic rami to the base of the bladder.

Through the abdominal incision, the bladder neck is then opened anteriorly with electrocautery. The ureteral orifices are then identified, and the ureters may be can-

nulated with 5 Fr whistle-tip catheters. The trigone is transected distal to the orifices with the incision extended through the vaginal wall to complete the resection (Fig. 51–2). Frozen sections of the margins are obtained to confirm that all disease has been excised. The bladder neck is closed in two layers with synthetic absorbable sutures (please see Chapter 49 for a more detailed description). Just before completion of bladder neck clo-

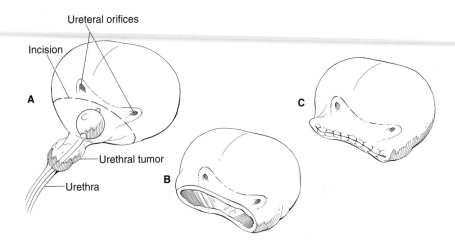

Ureteral orifices

Incision

A

Urethral tumor

Urethra

B

C

FIG. 51–2. Technique of urethrectomy and bladder preservation by excision of the tumor at the level of the bladder neck, with subsequent bladder neck closure.

sure, the ureteral catheters are removed. Ureteral stenting is not required if the ureters were not injured during the dissection.

If there is adequate vaginal tissue remaining, the vagina can be closed primarily with 2-0 polyglactin sutures. However, if there is inadequate vaginal tissue, or if the patient wants to preserve sexual function, then we reconstruct the vagina by mobilizing pedicled skin flaps from the gluteal region (Fig. 51–3). For creation of a gluteal flap, a U-shaped incision is created, running from

the defect into the vagina and toward the gluteus along the posterior–medial thigh. Sharp dissection is performed along the incisions, going deep into the subcutaneous tissue to create an advancement flap that has a thickness of 2 cm. Hemostasis is achieved with pinpoint cautery. This flap is then advanced and rotated to fill in the vaginal wall defect. The vaginal epithelium is anastomosed to the advancement flap with 3-0 synthetic absorbable sutures, and the external skin on the medial thigh is then approximated with a subcuticular closure.

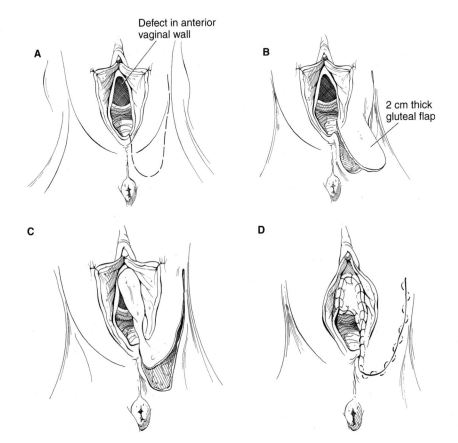

Defect in anterior vaginal wall

A

B

2 cm thick gluteal flap

C

D

FIG. 51–3. Creation of gluteal flap. An inverted-U incision is created on the posterior medial thigh. A 2-cm-thick flap is created and rotated into the defect in the anterior vaginal wall. A running closure is then used to secure the flap to the remaining vaginal epithelium, completing the reconstruction.

The continent cutaneous diversion is then performed, using an ileocolic segment for augmentation (see illustrations in Chapter 55); if the bladder capacity is adequate and the appendix present, a continent efferent limb may be created using the Mitrofanoff principle (Chapter 80). Postoperatively, the patient is managed with a 14 Fr catheter running through the stoma, a 22 Fr suprapubic tube, a vaginal pack, and a pelvic drain. Usually it is not necessary to use a nasogastric tube for intestinal decompression after performing an ileocolic anastomosis, although the patient is kept fasting until the full return of bowel activity. The vaginal pack is removed 24 to 48 hours after surgery. The enterocystoplasty is irrigated with normal saline beginning on postoperative day 1, and the patient is taught how to irrigate the pouch before discharge to home. The patient is maintained on antibiotic suppression until all of the drains and catheters are removed. Three weeks postoperatively, a cystogram is performed and all tubes are removed if no leak is detected. The patient is then managed with clean intermittent catheterization. Patients who have an ileocutaneous vesicostomy or Mitrofanoff continent limb will be taught stoma care prior to discharge.

Treatment of Proximal Urethral Tumors or More Locally Advanced Lesions

For patients who have large tumors or tumors involving the bladder base, bladder-preserving approaches are not feasible and anterior pelvic exenteration is indicated. A stoma site on the abdomen is selected preoperatively for urinary diversion, and the patient should meet with an enterostomal therapist preoperatively to help prepare for surgery. The patient undergoes a full mechanical bowel prep preoperatively.

Radical cystourethrectomy, pelvic lymph node dissection, and urinary diversion are then performed in the standard fashion (see Chapters 24, 77, and 78). For larger lesions, wide excision of the vulva, pelvic floor, and pubic rami may also be indicated. In such circumstances, closure of the perineal defect with a gracilis myocutaneous flap will be needed after removal of the tumor.

OUTCOMES

Complications

Treatment of urethral tumors in the distal one-third of the urethra by partial urethrectomy is well tolerated and relatively free of complications. Incontinence has not been reported as a complication of this procedure because the internal sphincter of the bladder is located at the proximal one-third of the urethra near the bladder neck. Meatal stenosis is another potential complication that is easily managed with intermittent dilation or meatoplasty.

Complications of continent cutaneous diversion include stomal stenosis, incontinence, electrolyte disorders, vitamin B_{12} deficiency, upper-tract deterioration, pyelonephritis, and pouch rupture. These patients require ongoing education to properly manage their cutaneous diversion to avoid complications. Further, careful long-term monitoring is required to detect and treat the complications described above.

Results

Long-term outcomes following treatment for advanced urethral cancer have been poor. Overall outcome data have been difficult to categorize because of the scarcity of cases, but prognosis depends more on the stage of the tumor at the time of presentation than on the histology of the primary tumor and the type of treatment utilized (1,9). In a large study of 72 women, the 5-year overall survival was 32%; it was 78% for low-stage and 22% for high-stage tumors (1). Patients with tumors of the anterior urethra were less likely to die of cancer than those who had tumors of the posterior or whole urethra. Only 30% to 40% of patients who undergo anterior exenteration for locally advanced tumors remained disease free after 5 years of follow-up (7,9). Of the recurrences that were seen, 57% were localized to the pelvis and 43% were associated with distant disease. After recurrence occurred, the mean survival overall was only 8 months, although sporadic cases have been cured with resection of the local recurrence alone.

In contrast, local recurrence of disease has not been a major problem in the patient who undergoes a partial or total urethrectomy for tumor treatment. This may reflect the better prognosis that is associated with smaller, distal urethral lesions as much as it represents the success of the surgical method. Five-year survival using local tumor excision in carefully selected patients to treat distal urethral carcinomas approaches 100% (7,9). Similar excellent results have been seen in patients selected for bladder-preservation approaches. In a recent series of five well-selected patients who underwent bladder-preservation surgery for urethral carcinoma, no patient had local recurrence with a mean follow-up of 39 months (5). One patient in that series died of a concurrent ovarian cancer, and the remaining four remained free of disease at last follow-up.

Narayan and Konety reported a 55% survival in patients with advanced urethral carcinoma treated with radiotherapy and surgery compared to 34% with radiation alone (9). Because there has been little improvement in survival rates of women with aggressive tumors over the last four decades, combined modality management with chemotherapy, surgery, intraoperative brachytherapy, and/or adjuvant external beam radiation has been proposed and initial experience has shown improved outcomes and good tolerance (2,3).

ACKNOWLEDGEMENT

This chapter is modified and updated from that of J. Naitoh, W. J. Aronson, and J. B. DeKernion in the 5th edition of this book.

REFERENCES

1. Dalbagni G, Zhang ZF, Lacombe L, Herr HW. Female urethral carcinoma: an analysis of treatment outcome and a plea for a standard management strategy. *Br J Urol* 1998;82:835.
2. Dalbagni G, Machele DS, Pascal E, et al. Results of high dose rate brachytherapy, anterior pelvic exenteration and external beam radiotherapy for carcinoma of the female urethra. *J Urol* 2001;166:175.
3. Gheiler EL, Tefilli MV, Tiguert R, et al. Management of primary urethral cancer. *Urology* 1998;52:487.
4. Grabstald H. Tumors of the urethra in men and women. *Cancer* 1973;32: 1236.
5. Hedden BJ, Husseinzadeh N, Bracken RB. Bladder sparing surgery for locally advanced female urethral cancer. *J Urol* 1993;150:1135.
6. Levine RL. Urethral cancer. *Cancer* 1980;45:1965.
7. Mayer R, Fowler JE, Clayton M. Localized urethral cancer in women. *Cancer* 1987;60:1548.
8. Mostofi FK, Davis CJ, Sesterhenn IA. Carcinoma of the male and female urethra. *Urol Clin North Am* 1992;19:347.
9. Narayan P, Konety B. Surgical treatment of female urethral carcinoma. *Urol Clin North Am* 1992;19:373.

CHAPTER 52

Carcinoma of the Male Urethra

John A. Heaney

Urethral carcinoma in men is rare, representing less than 1% of urinary tract tumors. The age incidence of urethral cancer in men ranges from 40 to 70 years, most urethral cancers being diagnosed at over age 50. Causal factors may include chronic irritation, in particular from urethritis and venereal disease, and urethral stricture disease. Two studies have suggested a causal role for human papilloma virus 16 (HPV-16) in squamous cell carcinoma of the urethra (1,6).

To best understand the pathophysiology, treatment, and prognosis of urethral cancer in men, we can divide the urethra into three anatomic units: (a) the penile urethra, (b) the bulbar and membranous urethra, and (c) the prostatic urethra. The most frequent cell type is squamous cell carcinoma, occurring in 78% of patients, followed by transitional cell carcinoma in 15% and adenocarcinoma

occurring in 6% (3,4). Other cell types including carcinoid and melanoma have been reported. Squamous cell carcinoma occurs most commonly in the penile and bulbomembranous urethra, and transitional cell carcinoma occurs most commonly in the prostatic urethra (Fig. 52–1).

Squamous cell carcinoma of the urethra usually spreads by direct extension to adjacent structures or to the superficial and deep inguinal nodes, which then drain to the external iliac nodes. Whereas squamous cell carcinoma of the urethra usually spreads by direct extension to adjacent structures and to regional lymph nodes, primary transitional cell carcinoma of the prostatic urethra has a propensity for hematogenous dissemination, and patients usually succumb to their disease from distant metastases.

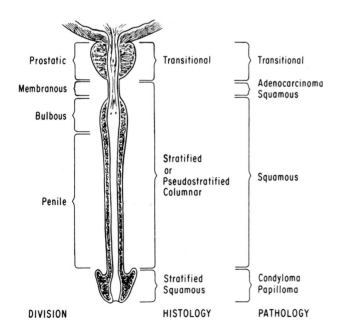

FIG. 52–1. Changes in the histology of the epithelial lining within the divisions of the male urethra tend to dictate the pathology of the tumor most likely to occur. (From Webster GD. The urethra. In: Paulsen DF, ed. *Genitourinary surgery*. New York: Churchill Livingstone, 1983:567, with permission.)

DIAGNOSIS

A diagnosis of urethral cancer should be suspected in men with recurring urethral stricture disease that is progressing and refractory to treatment. Retrograde urethrography should be performed in all patients with recurring or progressing urethral stricture disease to define the extent of any benign stricture and be combined with urethroscopy and biopsy to rule out urethral carcinoma. One should have an increased suspicion of urethral cancer when urethral stricture disease is associated with complicating factors such as a bloody urethral discharge, a urethral or penile mass, phlegmon, or urethrocutaneous fistula.

The diagnosis of urethral cancer is confirmed by percutaneous or transurethral biopsy of the lesion or mass. Biopsies may need to be repeated if initial biopsies are negative and the disease process persists. If local therapy or penile- or urethral-sparing surgery is being considered, then biopsies of the more proximal urethra should be performed to ensure a negative margin and exclude a "skip" lesion.

A careful physical exam should be performed to establish the degree of local invasion including the urethra, corpora cavernosa, and perineum, which should be palpated to evaluate for induration. A digital rectal exam and a bimanual exam may detect invasion into the membranous and prostatic urethra and rectum. The inguinal nodes should be carefully palpated because clinically suspicious nodes in men with urethral cancer usually represent metastases.

Magnetic resonance imaging (MRI) gives excellent resolution of the primary lesion and can identify tumor invasion into the tunica albuginea and the septum between the corpora cavernosa (5) and may also identify the presence of local invasion into the pubic bone, which will help to determine preoperatively if bone resection will be required. An MRI scan or a computed tomography (CT) scan should be performed to evaluate the inguinal, pelvic, and paraaortic nodes, and a chest x-ray should be obtained to evaluate the lungs. The most useful staging system for urethral carcinoma was proposed by Ray and associates (4) and is shown with the equivalent tumor–node–metastasis (TNM) stages in Table 52–1.

INDICATIONS FOR SURGERY

Urethral carcinoma is a highly aggressive and lethal disease. The median survival with no treatment or with only palliative treatment is 3 months, and the longest survival with no treatment is 15 months. If the metastatic workup demonstrates distant disease, then only palliative treatments should be performed.

For patients with biopsy-proven squamous cell carcinoma of the penile urethra, cure depends on adequate local control. Squamous cell carcinoma of the urethra tends to recur locally, and death in these patients usually results from complications related to local disease. For highly selected patients with localized stage-0 or stage-A tumors, local resection may suffice. This can be accomplished with transurethral resection or open resection of the involved urethra with an end-to-end anastomosis. These tumors may also be vaporized or fulgurated with laser using the neodynium:YAG, holmium:YAG, or CO_2 wavelengths.

For tumors involving the penile or distal bulbar urethra but confined to the corpus spongiosum and if negative margins of the corpus spongiosum and a 2-cm margin of tumor-free urethra can be obtained, penile-sparing surgery is an option. It is important in these cases to have a careful examination of frozen and permanent sections and close postoperative follow-up.

In general, patients with invasive carcinoma of the penile urethra should be treated with partial penectomy if a 2-cm tumor-free margin can be obtained and the patient is still able to direct his stream with the residual penile stump; otherwise, total penectomy is indicated. An alternative approach in some patients is subcutaneous penectomy with preservation of the glans and later phalloplasty. If a 2-cm tumor-free margin of urethra cannot be obtained, then more extensive surgery is indicated. If the initial surgery performed fails to obtain adequate tumor-free margins, then the surgeon should not hesitate to reoperate if adequate local resection is feasible.

Patients with carcinoma involving the bulbomembranous urethra have a worse prognosis and usually present in advanced stages with direct tumor extension into adjacent tissues or regional node involvement. If the pelvic lymph nodes are negative, then a variety of options exist

TABLE 52–1. *Staging of male urethral carcinoma*

Ray	TNM	
Stage 0	Tis	Confined to Mucosa Only (*In Situ*)
Stage A	Ta	Into But Not Beyond Lamina Propria
Stage B	T2	Into But Not Beyond Substance of Corpus Spongiosum or Into But Not Beyond Prostate
Stage C	T3, T4	Direct Extension Into Tissues Beyond Corpus Spongiosum (Corpora Cavernosa, Muscle, Fat, Fascia, Skin, Direct Skeletal Involvement), or Beyond Prostatic Capsule
Stage D1	N1, N2	Regional Metastasis Including Inguinal and/or Pelvic Lymph Nodes (With any Primary Tumor)
Stage D4	M1	Distant Metastasis (With Any Primary Tumor)

for resecting the primary tumor. Usually, those patients in whom the tumor abuts or invades the pubic bone require total penectomy, total urethrectomy, prostatectomy, and partial pubectomy. If biopsies of the bladder neck are negative and adequate tumor-free margins can be obtained, then one may perform bladder neck closure combined with a continent cutaneous bladder augmentation or an ileocutaneous vesicostomy. If negative margins cannot be obtained at the bladder neck, then one should proceed with radical cystectomy and urinary diversion. In general, total penectomy is required for these patients with subcutaneous penectomy remaining an option.

Primary transitional cell carcinoma of the prostatic urethra is best treated by radical cystoprostatectomy and *en-bloc* urethrectomy, and urinary diversion is indicated.

If the inguinal nodes are palpably negative in patients with invasive carcinoma of the penile or bulbomembranous urethra, then only serial exams of the inguinal nodes is indicated. In patients with suspicious inguinal nodes, first perform a bilateral pelvic lymph node dissection. If frozen section reveals the pelvic nodes to be negative, then one proceeds with resection of the superficial and deep inguinal nodes on the involved side and transposes the sartorius muscle over the exposed femoral vessels. On the contralateral side, if the inguinal nodes are not clinically suspicious for malignancy then perform a modified inguinal node dissection to include the superficial nodes, with the lateral border of the femoral artery being the lateral margin.

ALTERNATIVE THERAPY

Radiation therapy has had limited success in treating carcinoma of the anterior urethra. The complications are significant and include stricture and woody penile edema as well as local recurrence resulting in death (2). Chemotherapy has had limited success for treating urethral cancer and, like radiation therapy, is usually reserved for palliative treatment of advanced disease. Preoperative radiation therapy and chemotherapy has been proposed for bulky disease and in high-risk patients appears to result in better local control but does not improve survival.

SURGICAL TECHNIQUE

Carcinoma of the Penile Urethra

Preoperatively an enema is given the morning of surgery. Ampicillin and gentamicin (or a third-generation cephalosporin) are given 1 hour before surgery as prophylaxis. For invasive carcinoma of the penile urethra, either partial penectomy or total penectomy should be performed, and these procedures are described in Chapter 66 .

Penile-sparing surgery can be performed in patients with carcinoma of the penile urethra or carcinoma of the distal bulbar urethra if the disease is limited to the corpus spongiosum. Usually this is not the case, and patients require either partial or total penectomy. To perform penile-sparing urethrectomy, the patient is placed in the dorsal lithotomy position and an inverted-U incision is made medial to the ischial tuberosities and below the base of the scrotum (Fig. 52–2). The superficial fascia is incised vertically, and the bulbospongiosus muscle is identified, incised, and resected. The urethra is dissected off of the corpora cavernosa and surrounded with a vessel loop. While traction is placed on the urethra with the vessel loop, the remainder of the distal penile urethra is dissected off the corpora cavernosa using pinpoint electrocautery. Bleeding from the corpora cavernosa is oversewn with 3-0 polyglycolic acid (PGA) sutures. The urethral dissection proceeds distally to the fossa navicularis, resulting in inversion of the penis. The penis is everted, the urethral meatus and fossa navicularis are excised with the electrosurgical unit using cutting current, and the urethra is drawn into the incision in continuity. The meatus is oversewn with two interrupted 3-0 PGA sutures. The urethra proximal to the lesion is dissected and divided to ensure a 2-cm margin of normal urethra. A 0.25-in. Penrose drain is placed and brought out through a skin incision.

A small circle of skin is excised several centimeters ventral to the anus, and the urethra is spatulated 1 cm and sewn to the skin edges with interrupted 3-0 chromic sutures. Carefully inspect the urethra to make sure that it is not twisted or kinked and pass a catheter to rule out obstruction. The superficial perineal fascia is closed with a running 3-0 PGA suture and the skin is closed with a running 4-0 PGA subcuticular suture. The drain is removed 24 to 48 hours postoperatively and the catheter is removed 48 hours postoperatively.

Carcinoma of the Bulbomembranous Urethra

Rarely, radical surgery can be performed with sparing of the corpora cavernosa, and, in general, total penectomy combined with prostatectomy and urinary diversion is required for these patients. If a bladder-sparing procedure is being considered, obtain biopsies of the bladder neck before the procedure. If the primary tumor is large, a plastic surgeon may be needed to assist with creation of a muscle flap to fill the perineal defect resulting from the radical surgery.

For home bowel preparation, begin the patient on clear liquids 2 days before the procedure, and the morning before the procedure have the patient drink 4 L of GoLytely or 500 mL of Fleet's Phosphasoda to be completed by noon. Oral erythromycin and neomycin are begun the evening before surgery, and the patient is given a Fleet's enema the morning of the procedure. Ampicillin, gentamicin, and metronidazole are given intravenously 1 hour before the procedure.

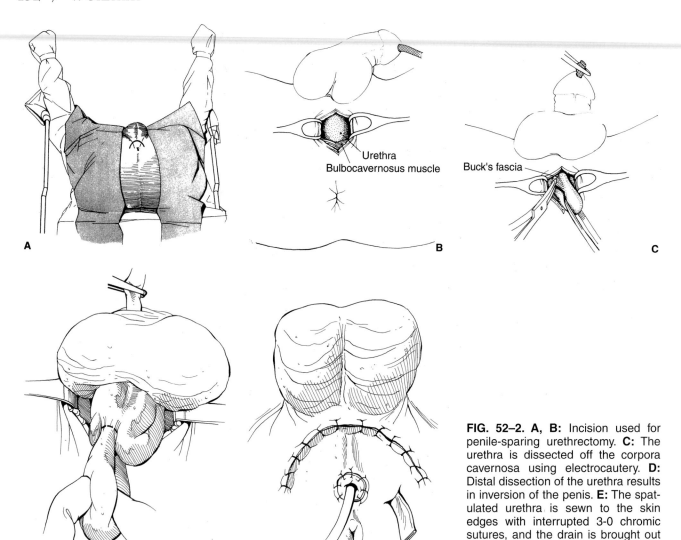

A

B Urethra
Bulbocavernosus muscle

C Buck's fascia

D

E

FIG. 52–2. **A, B:** Incision used for penile-sparing urethrectomy. **C:** The urethra is dissected off the corpora cavernosa using electrocautery. **D:** Distal dissection of the urethra results in inversion of the penis. **E:** The spatulated urethra is sewn to the skin edges with interrupted 3-0 chromic sutures, and the drain is brought out through a separate stab incision.

The patient is positioned in the low lithotomy position to allow simultaneous exposure to the abdomen and perineum with the table flexed above the iliac crests to allow better exposure to the pelvis and all pressure points are well padded. A midline incision is made from 3 cm above the umbilicus down to the pubis, the peritoneum is entered, and the abdomen is explored to rule out metastatic disease. A bilateral pelvic lymph node dissection is performed with the limits being the bifurcation of the common iliac artery proximally, the genitofemoral nerve laterally and superiorly, Cooper's ligament distally, and the obturator nerve inferiorly. The nodes are sent for frozen section examination; if they are positive, the radical procedure is terminated and palliative management is indicated. If the nodes are negative, the operation is continued through a perineal approach. A circumferential incision is made around the base of the penis extending down the median raphe of the scrotum, and the incision extended down the perineum (Fig. 52–3). The dartos fascia is divided in the midline with electrocautery without

entering the tunica vaginalis, as is the superficial perineal fascia. The suspensory ligament of the penis and the neurovascular bundle of the penis are divided between 0 silk ties. The corpora cavernosa are then divided between clamps at the ischial tuberosities, and the ends are oversewn with a running 2-0 PGA suture. Resect the bulbar urethral mass with great care to avoid leaving positive tumor margins. If the tumor invades the scrotum, then total scrotectomy with or without orchiectomy may be required. Part or all of the urogenital diaphragm may need to be resected. If the tumor is invading the superficial periosteum of the pubic arch, then resect the periosteum with electrocautery. If there appears to be more extensive invasion of the pubic arch, the pubic arch is scored with electrocautery with the cutting current to obtain a 1-cm negative margin and the inferior portion of the pubic arch is resected with an orthopedic hammer and chisel.

The surgeon then proceeds with resection of the tumor mass up to the apex of the prostate. Through the abdomi-

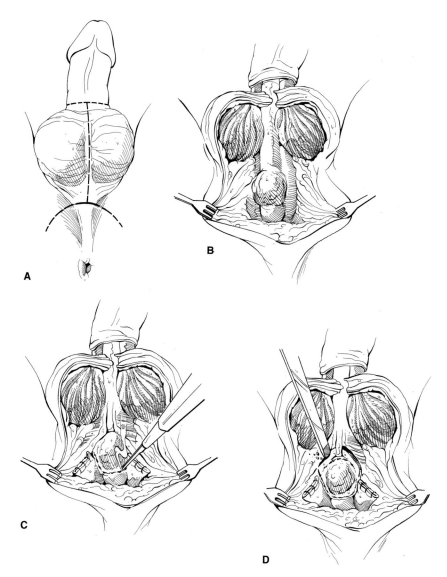

FIG. 52–3. A, B: Incision used to gain access to the perineum for total penectomy, total urethrectomy, radical prostatectomy, and continent cutaneous bladder augmentation. **C:** Electrocautery and suture ligatures are used to resect the urethral mass. **D:** If pubic bone invasion is present, the pubic arch is first scored with electrocautery; then, an orthopedic hammer and chisel are used to resect the inferior pubic arch to ensure a negative margin.

nal incision the prostatectomy is performed in an antegrade fashion by starting at the bladder neck and working distally. First, the endopelvic fascia is incised bilaterally and the prostate is dissected from the bladder neck with electrocautery along with the seminal vesicles and vas deferens. The lateral prostatic pedicles are divided between clips or ties. The puboprostatic ligaments are sharply divided, and the dorsal venous complex is identified and divided between 0 PGA ties. The entire surgical specimen is submitted *en bloc* for frozen sections to confirm that the tumor margins at the bladder neck and throughout the specimen are negative. If any margins are positive, then a deeper resection is indicated where possible.

If the bladder neck margins are negative, the bladder neck is closed after verifying patency of the ureters by intravenous administration of indigo carmine or the passage of pediatric feeding tubes. The bladder neck mucosa and inner muscle is opposed with interrupted 2-0 PGA sutures and the outer muscle with a running 0 PGA

suture. The perineal defect is packed with laparotomy pads and the urinary diversion is performed through the abdominal incision.

Urinary diversion may be achieved with either ileocutaneous vesicostomy or continent cutaneous bladder augmentation.

For continent cutaneous bladder augmentation, a 15-cm segment of cecum and a 10-cm segment of adjacent ileum are isolated on its vascular pedicle (Fig. 52–4). In cases where a long appendix is present, a cecal augmentation and continent cutaneous efferent limb may be fashioned using the Mitrofanoff principle (Chapter 80). After bowel continuity has been restored, the cecum is opened along the antimesenteric border and the appendix is removed if it is not to be used as the efferent limb. The ileum is tapered around a 14 Fr catheter using a GIA stapler. The serosa is incised along the anterior tinea of the cecum and the tapered ileal segment within this groove is secured with interrupted 3-0 PGA sutures. A cruciate

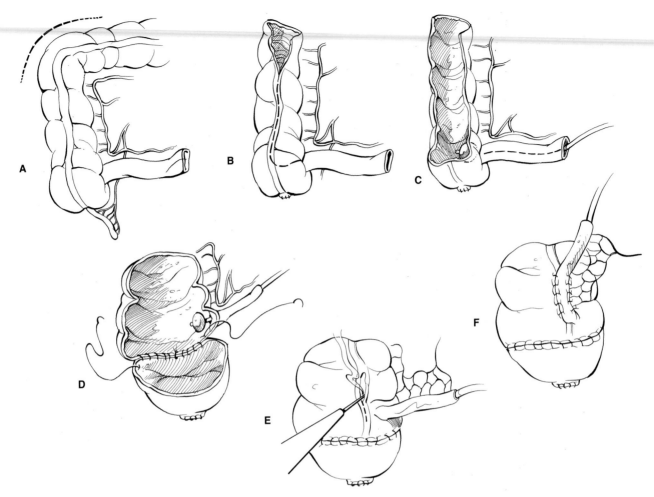

FIG. 52–4. A: Mobilize a 15-cm segment of cecum and adjacent 10 cm of ileum. **B:** Excise the staple lines and detubularize the cecum by incising along the tinea as shown. **C:** Taper the ileum over a 14 Fr catheter using a GIA stapler. **D:** Suture the detubularized cecum to the bladder. **E:** Create flaps of the posterior tinea. **F:** Secure the tinea flaps to the lateral wall of the ileal efferent limb.

incision is made in the bladder dome with electrocautery, and the cecal patch is attached to the bladder with running locking 2-0 PGA sutures and interrupted 2-0 PGA sutures. The distal ileum is brought out to the skin at a preselected stoma site, any redundant ileum is excised, and it is verified that the 14 Fr catheter passes easily through the ileal stoma into the bladder. Alternatively, instead of tunneling the efferent limb, continence can be obtained by reinforcing the ileocecal valve with interrupted 3-0 silk sutures. The pouch is drained with a 14 Fr catheter running through the efferent limb of ileum and a 24 Fr suprapubic tube.

The pelvic defect may be closed by sewing Marlex mesh to the urogenital diaphragm with interrupted 0 Proline sutures. Alternatively, a gracilis muscle flap or rectus abdominis muscle flap can be dissected by a plastic surgeon and used to close the pelvic defect. The superficial perineal fascia is closed with a running 3-0 PGA suture and the skin is closed with a running 4-0 chromic suture. If there is insufficient skin to bring the skin edges together, then a pedicled gluteal flap can be created to close the skin defect (see Chapter 54). A Jackson–Pratt drain is placed between the mesh and the superficial perineal fascia and is brought out through the perineum. Large Penrose drains are also placed through the abdominal wall into the pelvis before the abdominal wall fascia is closed. A cystogram is performed 3 weeks postoperatively, and if there are no leaks the drains are removed and the patient is taught self-catheterization. Antibiotics are continued until all drains are removed.

Subcutaneous Penectomy

To avoid the severe disfigurement of total penectomy in patients with early invasion through the corpus spongiosum, the penile skin and glans penis can be left intact. To accomplish this, the spongiosum and cavernosum are resected completely while the penile skin and the dorsal neurovascular bundle supplying the glans are meticulously dissected and preserved. This is a less mutilating procedure, and the glans penis and penile skin may be used for reconstruction at a later date, if desired.

OUTCOMES

Complications

Complications of transurethral resection or laser treatment of superficial urethral carcinoma include urethral stricture and urethrocutaneous fistula. These patients need to be followed closely postoperatively and, at the first sign of urethral stricture disease, treated with daily self-dilation. If this is unsuccessful, then more extensive urethroplasty procedures may be required.

The main complication resulting from partial and total penectomy is stenosis of the meatus or perineal urethrostomy. This can be managed either with self-dilation or meatoplasty. Local recurrence of tumor can cause outlet obstruction at the meatus or anywhere along the urethra, and suspicious lesions must be biopsied and treated accordingly.

The primary complications of radical resection of bulbar urethral tumors include pelvic abscess and perineal wound breakdown. This can subsequently lead to severe intraabdominal complications and sepsis. These are extremely morbid complications and can only be prevented by careful attention to all technical aspects of the original operation, including placement of large pelvic drains.

Postoperative management must include ongoing irrigation of mucus plugs from a continent cutaneous diversion and ongoing monitoring of the pelvic drains with careful attention to assure that the drains are not prematurely removed. Delayed postoperative fever requires appropriate imaging and prompt drainage of any fluid collections to prevent a large abscess from developing. Resection of the pubic bone may lead to osteitis pubis and may require orthopedic consultation and long-term antibiotics.

Results

In well-selected patients with superficial squamous cell carcinoma or transitional cell carcinoma of the urethra, transurethral resection, laser fulguration, or local excision offers excellent cure rates approaching 100% (7). Recurrence in these patients is not uncommon, and close follow-up is mandatory. In patients with squamous cell carcinoma of the penile urethra who undergo partial penectomy, in whom a 2-cm tumor-free margin is obtained, the results are also excellent and approach 100% (7). Results of radical penectomy for squamous cell carcinoma of the urethra are not as good, and the disease-free rate reported is roughly 40%. This probably reflects the fact that these patients initially present with more advanced disease. In patients with carcinoma of the bulbar urethra, serious consideration should be given to performing more radical surgery to obtain good tumor-free margins. The overall survival for patients presenting with squamous cell carcinoma of the proximal bulbar and membranous urethra is roughly 10% because of the advanced nature of this disease. Of patients with disease amenable to surgery who undergo radical excision including radical penectomy and prostatectomy with or without cystectomy, 38% are reported to be free of disease.

ACKNOWLEDGMENT

This chapter is modified and updated from that of W. J. Aronson, J. Naitoh, and J. B. DeKernion in the 5th edition of this book.

REFERENCES

1. Cupp MR, Reza MS, Goellner JR, Espy MJ, Smith TF. Detection of human papillomavirus DNA in primary squamous cell carcinoma of the male urethra. *Urology* 1996;48:551.
2. Dalbagni G, Zhang ZF, Lacombe L, et al. Male urethral carcinoma: analysis of treatment outcome. *Urology* 1999;53:1126–1132.
3. Krieg R, Hoffman R. Current management of unusual genitourinary cancers. Part 2: urethral cancer. *Oncology* 1999;13:1511–1520.
4. Ray B, Canto AR, Whitmore WF Jr. Experience with primary carcinoma of the male urethra. *J Urol* 1977;117:591.
5. Vapnek JM, Hricak H, Carroll PR. Recent advances in imaging studies for staging of penile and urethral carcinoma. *Urol Clin North Am* 1992; 19:257.
6. Wiener JS, Liu ET, Walther PJ. Oncogenic human papillomavirus type 16 is associated with squamous cell cancer of the male urethra. *Cancer Res* 1992;52:5018.
7. Zeidman EJ, Desmond P, Thompson IM. Surgical treatment of carcinoma of the male urethra. *Urol Clin North Am* 1992;19:359.

SECTION VI

Vas Deferens and Seminal Vesicle

Section Editor: Larry Lipshultz

CHAPTER 53

Seminal Vesicle and Ejaculatory Duct Surgery

Paul J. Turek

SEMINAL VESICLE SURGERY

The seminal vesicle is a uniquely male organ, derived from the mesonephric duct beginning at 13 fetal weeks. The normal adult seminal vesicle is 5 to 8 cm in length and 1.5 cm in width and has a volume of 10 mL. Histologically, the organ wall is composed mainly (80%) of smooth muscle and is lined by columnar epithelium. The blood supply is derived from the deferential artery or, on occasion, from branches of the inferior vesical artery. The seminal vesicles receive primary innervation from adrenergic fibers supplied from the hypogastric nerve.

Primary pathologic states of the organ are rare. Secondary lesions constitute the major reason for organ removal. Congenital lesions of the seminal vesicles include ureteral ectopy, seminal vesicle cysts, and aplasia. The vast majority of men with cystic fibrosis, and 1% of infertile men, present clinically with absence of the vas deferens and seminal vesicles. Infections of the seminal vesicles are uncommon, but tuberculosis and schistosomiasis are not infrequent causes of masses, abscesses, and calcifications in developing countries. Chronic bacterial seminal vesiculitis, a rare and difficult diagnosis, is presumably a consequence of bacterial prostatitis. Benign tumors of the seminal vesicles include papillary adenoma, cystadenoma, fibroma, and leiomyoma. Malignant neoplasms are extremely rare (100 reported cases) and include papillary adenocarcinoma and sarcoma (1,13). Radical excision of the organ is the accepted treatment for seminal vesicle malignancies. Far more common than primary malignancies is secondary involvement from carcinoma of the bladder, adenocarcinoma of the prostate or rectum, and lymphoma.

Diagnosis

The normal seminal vesicle is not palpable on digital rectal examination. The area superior to the prostate can be enlarged and compressible in the presence of seminal vesi-

cle dilation or firmly indurated if the organ contains tumor. These findings require further evaluation. Transrectal ultrasound (TRUS) is the diagnostic modality of choice to evaluate seminal vesicle size and pathology. In addition to high-resolution delineation of anatomy, TRUS facilitates needle aspiration for cytology or core biopsy for tissue diagnosis. Even greater anatomic detail can be obtained with computed tomography (CT) scan or magnetic resonance imaging (MRI), although their use should be limited to the staging of solid lesions within the pelvis and to confirm the hemorrhagic nature of suspicious masses. In infertile patients who present with azoospermia, or in patients with hematospermia or coital pain, TRUS is the initial imaging study. Contrast vasography accurately images the vas deferens and ampullary–seminal vesicle junction but is less reliable than TRUS for seminal vesicle pathology.

Indications for Surgery

Most procedures performed on the seminal vesicles are related to radical surgery for the treatment of urethral, prostate, bladder, or rectal cancer. Treatments specific to the seminal vesicle include transrectal aspiration of cysts or abcesses, transurethral unroofing of abscesses, obstructing cysts, or allowing stone passage, and open resection for refractory infections to excise an ectopic ureter or remove benign or malignant masses.

Cysts are treated in the presence of symptoms referable to a mass effect. Surgical drainage of abscesses usually follows the failure of antibiotic therapy. The excision of solid lesions of the seminal vesicles is warranted after aspiration or biopsy confirmation of pathology. This section discusses open and laparoscopic surgical approaches to the seminal vesicle.

Alternative Therapy

Few established alternatives to surgery exist for tumors of the seminal vesicles. Infections can often be treated with antibiotics. Many asymptomatic congenital anomalies can be observed.

Surgical Technique

Although a variety of open surgical approaches to the seminal vesicles have been described, the most useful are the transvesical, transperineal, paravesical and retrovesical, and transcoccygeal methods, as illustrated in Figure 53–1. In addition, a laparoscopic retrovesical approach to organ removal has gained popularity recently, with a total of eight published cases to date (2,8). The approach that is chosen depends on the nature of the lesion to be excised and, more importantly, surgeon experience. For most procedures, consideration should be given to having 1 U of autologous blood available for emergency use.

Transvesical Approach

The patient is positioned supine and an infraumbilical extraperitoneal incision is made (10). The incision can be midline or Pfannenstiel. The rectus muscles are separated and the space of Retzius entered. A Balfour retractor is used to expose the anterior bladder wall. The bladder wall is opened with a vertical (7 to 10 cm) incision that extends to no closer than 2 to 3 cm from the anterior bladder neck. Full-thickness bladder wall stay sutures of 2-0 Vicryl are placed at either end of the incision for traction and also to prevent tearing of the incision with retraction. The lateral blades of the Balfour retractor are repositioned within the bladder to expose the trigone and posterior wall. Several moist 4–8 sponges are packed in the bladder dome; a Deaver blade is placed superiorly to stretch the bladder interior and flatten the posterior wall.

One may intubate the ureters with no. 8 feeding tubes or ureteral stents to define the course of the intramural ureters. With a cutting Bovie stylet, a 5-cm vertical incision is made through the trigone (Fig. 53–2A). Beyond the thick muscle of the bladder wall near the bladder neck, the ampullae of the vas can be recognized (Fig. 53–2B). With sharp dissection, the seminal vesicles are identified lateral to the ampullae at the prostate base. In the absence of prior inflammation, the plane around the seminal vesicles is easily entered. They are dissected free, ligated at the prostate base with 2-0 chromic sutures, and then divided. A metal clip placed across the cut end of the seminal vesicle minimizes spillage of organ contents. The distal vascular pedicle should be identified and controlled with small metal clips or ties and the organ removed.

Prior inflammation can make the dissection difficult. In this situation, ureteral catheters are useful to help avoid ureteral injury. It is also important to avoid too deep a dissection and risk violating Denonvillier's fascia and entering the rectum.

The posterior bladder incision is closed in two layers: a running 2-0 absorbable suture for the muscle layer and a running 4-0 absorbable suture in the mucosal layer. After removal of the sponge packs and stents, a urethral catheter is placed and the anterior bladder wall is closed in a manner similar to the posterior wall. Suprapubic drainage of the bladder is optional. A suction drain is left for 2 to 3 days and removed if drainage is less than 60 mL per day. The urethral catheter is removed in 7 to 10 days. Early postoperative ambulation is the rule. Patients may

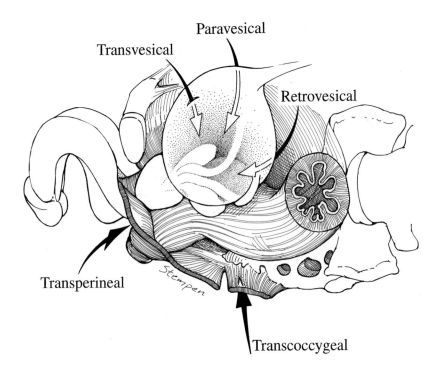

FIG. 53–1. The four different surgical approaches to seminal vesicle surgery.

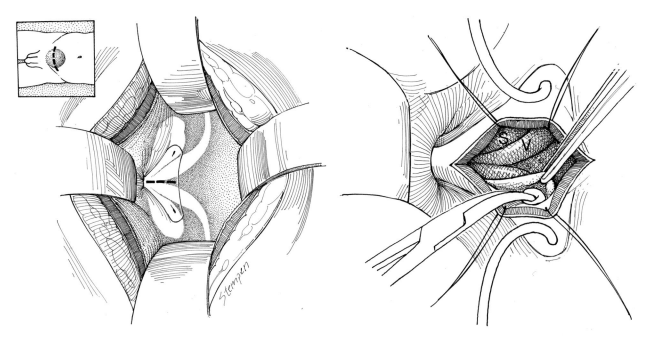

FIG. 53–2. The transvesical approach to the seminal vesicle. **A:** Vertical incision in the trigone to expose the retrovesical seminal vesicle. **B:** Dissection of the vas ampullae and seminal vesicles.

be discharged with or without the drain when pain is controllable with oral medication, in general within 2 to 3 days of surgery.

Transperineal Approach

The patient should undergo preoperative outpatient bowel preparation with citrate of magnesia or Go-Lytely and receive broad-spectrum antibiotics systemically before the procedure. Intermittent compression stockings are recommended to prevent thromboembolic events.

The transperineal approach to seminal vesiculectomy is virtually identical to radical perineal prostatectomy described elsewhere. An exaggerated dorsal lithotomy position is used to elevate the perineum so that it is parallel to the floor. An inverted-U incision is made in the perineum and the central tendon is divided (Fig. 53–3A). An anterior retractor stretches the rectal sphincter superiorly, allowing visualization of the glistening anterior rectal fascia fibers. The rectourethralis is divided near the prostatic apex and a weighted speculum is placed, dropping the tented rectum. To adequately expose the seminal vesicle, the rectum should be dissected off the posterior surface of the prostate to a point higher than that needed for perineal prostatectomy. Denonvillier's fascia is then incised transversely or in the midline (if nerve-sparing) on the prostate near the base of the seminal vesicles.

Seminal vesicle dissection is facilitated by posterior traction on the prostate provided by placement of a Lowsley retractor in the bladder. Medially, the ampullae and seminal vesicles are apparent after Denonvillier's fas-

cia is incised (Fig. 53–3B). The ampullae can be spared for the excision of a simple seminal vesicle cyst or small tumor but may need resection in the setting of cancer or infection. After dissection of the seminal vesicle at the prostatic base, an absorbable tie of 2-0 suture is used to ligate the gland (Fig. 53–3B). Before division of the seminal vesicle, a clip is placed on the cut end of the organ to minimize spillage. An Allis or Babcock clamp is then placed on the freed base of the seminal vesicle to ease the apical dissection. I have found that dividing the organ at the base of the prostate first and dissecting distally along the seminal vesicle is easier than tip dissection followed by base ligation. The vascular pedicle at the apex of the gland is usually observed within 1 cm of the tip and is ligated with small metal clips, allowing gland removal. The wound is closed in layers as outlined for perineal prostatectomy. A Penrose drain is left in the area of dissection for 24 hours or until no drainage is noted. This approach is well tolerated, and patients are usually discharged within 24 to 48 hours of surgery.

Paravesical and Retrovesical Approaches

The paravesical approach is suitable for large, unilateral seminal vesicle cysts and for the correction of congenital anomalies in children. A vertical infraumbilical midline or Pfannenstiel incision is used to expose the space of Retzius; the bladder is bluntly dissected away from the pelvic sidewall. The vas deferens is tracked medially toward the bladder base to help locate the seminal vesicle. The plane between the bladder and seminal

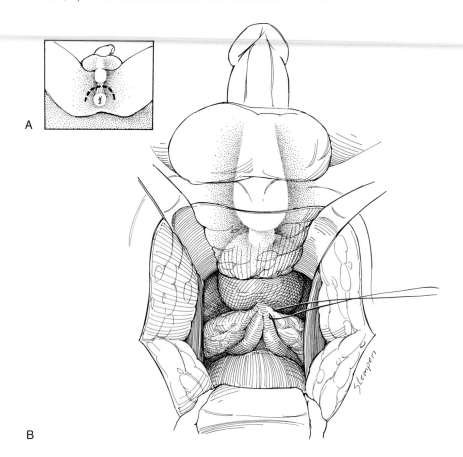

A

B

FIG. 53–3. The transperineal approach. **A:** U-shaped incision in the perineum with takedown of the central tendon. **B:** Exposure and ligation of the seminal vesicles after incising Denonvillier's fascia.

vesicle is developed from laterally to medially, a dissection facilitated by emptying the bladder with a Foley catheter. As the seminal vesicle is dissected, be aware that the vas deferens crosses over the ureter and that the ureter can easily be injured. As the plane between the bladder and seminal vesicle develops, roll the bladder medially for better exposure. At the level of the prostate, do not dissect lateral to the seminal vesicles as this may damage the neurovascular bundle. The neck of the seminal vesicle is defined at the prostate base and the organ ligated with 2-0 absorbable sutures. A drain may be left in place in the bed of the dissection and brought out through a separate stab incision. Usually the drain and Foley catheter can be removed 24 hours later. The recovery time is rapid, with discharge 48 hours after surgery.

The retrovesical approach is appropriate in cases of bilateral seminal vesicle excision for small cysts or tumors (3). In general, a midline, infraumbilical, intraperitoneal incision is made to gain access to the dome of the bladder and the *cul-de-sac* between bladder and rectum (Fig. 53–4A). With intraabdominal exposure, the small and large bowels are gently packed superiorly and the peritoneal reflection near the posterior bladder is incised transversely over the rectum (Fig. 53–4B). It is important not make the incision too deep and risk injury to the rectum. With careful sharp dissection, the bladder is peeled forward off of the rectum until the ampullae and the seminal vesicle apices are visualized (Fig. 53–4C). In

a manner similar to the paravesical approach, the seminal vesicles are dissected to the prostatic base, the neck of the gland encircled, and the organ ligated with 2.0 absorbable sutures. A suction drain can be left in the bed of dissection and secured as described above. Postoperative care is similar to the paravesical approach except that the return of bowel function may be delayed 24 hours with intraabdominal dissection.

The retrovesical approach can also be performed laparoscopically (8). After anesthesia is induced, with the patient in the supine, head-down position, a Foley catheter is placed. Transperitoneal access is obtained after Veress needle pneumoperitoneum through a 10-mm subumbilical trocar. Under visualization, three additional laparoscopic ports are accessed: the midline suprapubic area (5 mm) and the left (5 mm) and right (12 mm) lateral borders of the rectus muscle (Fig. 53–4D). After retracting the bladder, the retrovesical space is entered by incising the peritoneum just medial to where the vas deferens crosses the medial umbilical ligament, across the posterior *cul-de-sac* to the same point on the other side. This is a similar dissection to that performed in the open retrovesical approach (Figs. 53–4B and 53–4C). After dissecting the peritoneal reflection, the retrovesical space is developed and the apex of the seminal vesicles realized. Ideally, the dissection is performed to completely free the seminal vesicles down to their junction with the ampullary vas deferens. The organ is secured with clips

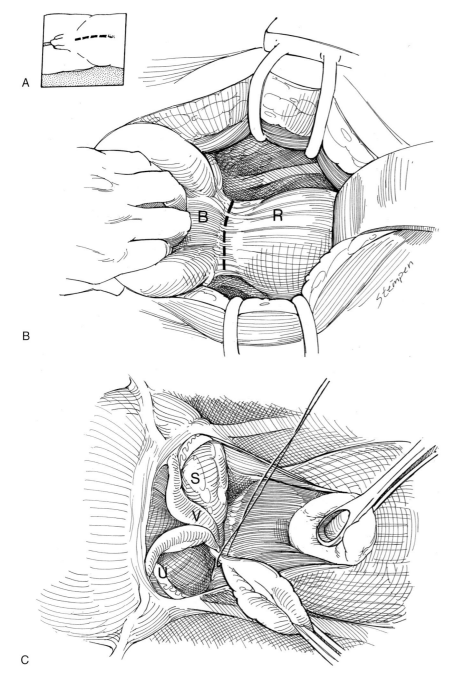

FIG. 53–4. The retrovesical approach. **A:** Midline infraumbilical incision. **B:** Incision of the posterior peritoneum over the rectum in the *cul-de-sac.* **C:** Exposure of the vas ampulla and seminal vesicle behind the bladder.

(Continued on next page)

proximally and distally and transected. Cysts are in general circumferentially dissected and lightly aspirated to allow for better visualization during more caudal dissection. The retrovesical peritoneum is reapproximated with intracorporeal 0 absorbable sutures and the larger port sites closed with Vicryl sutures. The skin is secured with adhesive strips.

Postoperatively, patients are discharged the next day and the Foley catheter removed within 18 hours postoperatively. Oral intake can in general be resumed within 6 hours. Regular activity is encouraged as early as 10 days after the procedure.

Transcoccygeal Approach

Urologists are in general not as familiar with transcoccygeal surgery as they are with other approaches (7). This dissection is appropriate for individuals in whom the perineum or lower abdomen is not accessible because of limitations in patient positioning or due to multiple prior surgeries in these anatomic regions. Because it is an uncommon surgical approach, it will be discussed only briefly.

The patient is placed in the prone, jackknife position. An incision is made along the coccyx and angled into a gluteal cleft (Fig. 53–5A). The coccyx is removed and the

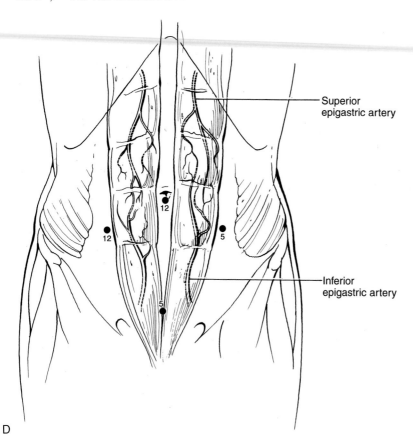

FIG. 53–4. (*Continued*) **D:** Optimal sites (black spots) of access for transabdominal laparoscopic seminal vesicle excision. Numbers represent trocar size in millimeters.

Superior epigastric artery

Inferior epigastric artery

D

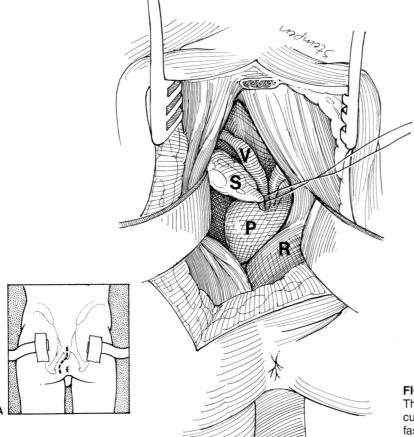

FIG. 53–5. The transcoccygeal approach. **A:** The incision is made over the coccyx and curved along the gluteal cleft. **B:** Denonvillier's fascia is incised deep to the rectum to expose the prostate and seminal vesicles.

A

B

TABLE 53–1. *Relative complication rates of the different surgical approaches to the seminal vesicle*

Approach	Rectal Injury	Impotence	Bladder or Ureteral Injury	Risk for Blood Transfusion	Other risks
Other	Moderate	High	Moderate	Moderate	Thromboembolic
Transvesical	Low	Low	High	Low	Fistula
Transperineal	High	High	Moderate	Moderate	Thromboembolic
Para/Retrovesical	Moderate	Low	Moderate	Low	
Transcoccygeal	High	High	Low	Low	Low
Laparoscopic	Low	Low	Unclear	Low	Air Embolism

gluteus maximus muscle layers retracted laterally to expose the rectosigmoid colon. After Denonvillier's fascia is incised medial and deep to the rectum, it is dissected off the prostate with exposure of the seminal vesicles (Fig. 53–5B). Injury to the neurovascular bundle is more likely with this approach because it is superficial to the prostate and therefore directly in the path of dissection. After the seminal vesicles are removed, the rectum is carefully inspected for injury. The wound is closed in anatomic layers and a drain is placed. Postoperative recovery is usually rapid.

Outcomes

Complications

Each approach to seminal vesicle surgery is associated with unique complications. The relative complication rates with these approaches are outlined in Table 53–1. Limited extraperitoneal rectal injuries can be handled with formal two-layer closure. Rectal injury with the retrovesical approach is intraabdominal, however, and may require the placement of omentum over the repair or even temporary colostomy. Most bladder injuries can be closed primarily. The most important point about ureteral injuries is their recognition. Most ureteral injuries can be treated adequately with stents for 7 to 10 days.

Results

Resection of the seminal vesicles for cystic and inflammatory diseases is in general successful, although large case series are rare. Seminal vesicle extirpation for cancer has also been successful, but the rarity of this indication prohibits an accurate assessment of survival and cure rates. Strict categorization of the 100 reported cases of primary seminal vesicle cancer reveals that fewer than 50% are truly primary to the seminal vesicle (1,13). In general, reconstructive surgery in children using these approaches has resulted in satisfactory outcomes.

EJACULATORY DUCT SURGERY

The ejaculatory ducts are paired, collagenous, tubular structures that commence at the junction of the vas defer-

ens and seminal vesicle, course through the prostate, and empty into the prostatic urethra at the verumontanum. As illustrated in Figure 53–6, there are three distinct anatomic regions to the ejaculatory duct: the proximal and largely extraprostatic portion, the middle intraprostatic segment, and a distal segment that is incorporated into the lateral aspect of the verumontanum in the prostatic urethra (5)

The duct consists of three histological layers: an outer muscular layer, a collagenous middle layer, and an inner mucosal layer (9). The muscular layer is absent in the distal segment.

Diagnosis

Ejaculatory duct obstruction causes infertility in 5% of azoospermia men. Duct obstruction can result from seminal vesicle calculi, of mullerian duct (utricular) or wolffian duct (diverticular) cysts, postsurgical or postinflammatory scar tissue, calcification near the verumontanum, or congenital atresia (11). Classically, this condition presents as hematospermia, painful ejaculation, or infertility with azoospermia. Associated risk factors include evidence of prior urinary tract infection or trauma and perineal pain or discomfort. It is important to discontinue medications that may impair ejaculation. An abbreviated list of these medications is found in Table 53–2. Ejaculatory duct obstruction is suggested by finding enlarged, palpable seminal vesicles on rectal examination. The diagnosis is confirmed by a combination of findings:

1. An ejaculate volume less than 2.0 mL and a pH less than 7.2 that contains no sperm or fructose.
2. A TRUS demonstration of dilated seminal vesicles (greater than 1.5 cm width) or dilated ejaculatory ducts (greater than 2.3 mm) in association with a cyst, calcification, or stones along the duct.

Recently, high-resolution TRUS has virtually replaced the more invasive vasography for this diagnosis. MRI with endorectal coil is recommended in suspicious cases without TRUS findings as it is excellent for the detection of small cysts. To complete the evaluation for infertility, it is important that the serum follicle-stimulating hormone (FSH) and testosterone be normal. Testicular vol-

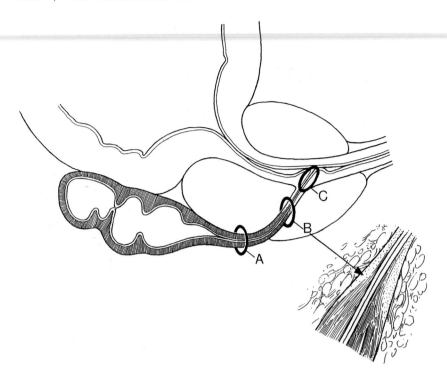

FIG. 53–6. Illustration of the three anatomic regions of the ejaculatory duct from the seminal vesicle to the prostatic urethra. **Inset:** How longitudinal muscle layer becomes attenuated in middle segment. (From Nguyen HT, Etzell J, Turek PJ. Normal human ejaculatory duct anatomy: a study of cadaveric and surgical specimens. *J Urol* 1996;155: 1639–1642, with permission.)

ume should also be normal. A testis biopsy confirming ongoing sperm production is also helpful.

TRUS-Assisted Diagnostic Techniques

Not all patients with ejaculatory duct obstruction have dilated seminal vesicles and not all patients with dilated seminal vesicles have ejaculatory duct obstruction. This has led to refinements in diagnostic techniques. Jarow described seminal vesicle sperm aspiration with TRUS to more accurately define affected patients (5). With a 30-cm, 21-gauge needle (Williams, Chiba, or oocyte retrieval needle), the seminal vesicles are aspirated transrectally or transperineally during TRUS (Fig. 53–7A). The aspirate is then examined under 400× phase microscopy for sperm. The finding of more than three sperm per high-power field is considered positive and suggestive of obstruction. Importantly, the duration of sexual abstinence prior to aspiration can influence the findings. Seminal vesicle aspiration should be performed with less than 24 hours of sexual abstinence. Despite the fact that aspiration does not anatomically localize the site of blockage or differentiate between physical blockage and functional obstruction, it

confirms that spermatogenesis is ongoing and that epididymal obstruction is unlikely.

Injection of nonionic contrast (50% Renografin) into the seminal vesicles after seminal vesicle aspiration followed by formal radiographic imaging can be a useful retrograde study of seminal vesicle and vasal anatomy in suspected obstruction (Fig. 53–7B). Also, a good quality pelvic and inguinal vasogram can be obtained in most patients (Fig. 53–7B). Fluoroscopy or a kidney-ureter-bladder (KUB) plain film is taken after the injection of 5, 10, and 20 mL of contrast to delineate excurrent duct anatomy. Helpful maneuvers include (a) having the patient in the 15- to 30-degree reverse Trendelenburg position for radiographs to "open up" the pelvic outlet and minimize overlying pelvic bone density and (b) placing a Foley catheter with 5 mL of water in the balloon on slight traction during contrast injection to reduce the spillage of contrast into the bladder that "clouds" the radiograph. As seminal vesiculography is more invasive than simple aspiration, it may require mild intravenous sedation and is best performed at the time of transurethral surgery.

Injection of diluted indigo carmine or methylene blue (1:5 dilution with saline) into the seminal vesicle with TRUS instead of contrast is termed *seminal vesicle chromotubation.* When performed with cystoscopy it can assess whether or not there is antegrade flow of dye from the seminal vesicle into the prostatic urethra (Fig. 53–7C). In fact, "patency," with chromotubation, defined by the presence of dye egressing from the ejaculatory duct orifices after seminal vesicle injection may be the most accurate way to diagnose complete ejaculatory duct obstruction, unilateral or bilateral (14).

TABLE 53–2. *Medications associated with impaired ejaculation*

Antihypertensive Agents
  α-Adrenergic Blockers (Prazosin, Phentolamine)
  Thiazides
Antipsychotic Agents

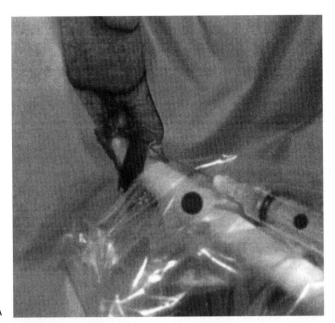

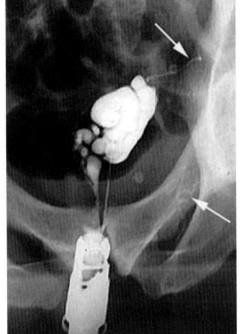

FIG. 53–7. A: Illustration of working setup for transrectal ultrasound (TRUS) aspiration of seminal vesicles. Large black dot points out the TRUS probe inserted into the rectum and small grey dot is placed on the syringe and needle used for aspiration. **B:** Illustration of a normal TRUS seminovesiculogram showing seminal vesicle and ejaculatory ducts with contrast. Arrows show the pelvic and inguinal vas deferens. **C:** Normal TRUS chromotubation. Cytoscopic view of methylene blue egressing from both ejaculatory duct orifices (white Xs) after injecting the seminal vesicles.

Indications for Surgery

Patients with ejaculatory duct obstruction sufficient to cause coital discomfort, recurrent hematospermia, or infertility should be considered candidates for transurethral treatment. Infertility with duct obstruction can present with low ejaculate volume and azoospermia or low ejaculate volume with decreased sperm density (less than 20×10^6 sperm per mL) or impaired sperm motility (less than 30% motility). Anatomic findings suggestive of obstruction and lesions located within approximately 1 to 1.5 cm of the verumontanum are usually amenable to transurethral management.

Alternative Therapy

Discontinuation of the medications listed in Table 53–2 may improve states of ejaculatory dysfunction. Anatomic lesions are most appropriately treated with surgery.

Surgical Technique

Transurethral resection of the ejaculatory ducts (TURED) is performed in the outpatient setting. Following the administration of light general or regional anesthesia and a single dose of a broad-spectrum antibiotic, the patient is placed in the dorsal lithotomy position with a rectal drape (O'Connor). Formal cystourethroscopy is

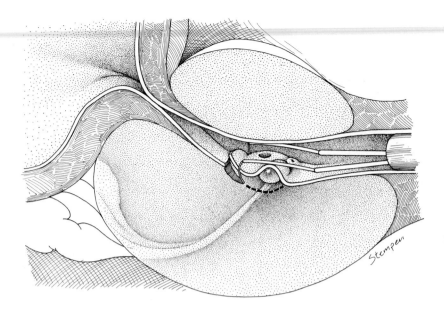

FIG. 53–8. Transurethral resection for ejaculatory duct obstruction. Midline resection of the verumontanum is shown. Lateral and deeper resection may be necessary depending on the site and reason for duct obstruction. (Conceptualized by Paul Stempen)

performed. Careful examination is made of the areas lateral to the verumontanum within the prostatic urethra to visualize either ejaculatory duct orifice. A small resectoscope (24 Fr) and electrocautery loop are inserted and the verumontanum resected in the midline (Fig. 53–8). The resection is performed with pure cutting current to minimize cauterization of the delicate ejaculatory ducts. Often several passes of the cutting loop are required to visualize the ejaculatory duct openings within the prostate. This can mean relatively deep dissection in a small prostate gland, a situation that can make even an experienced transurethral surgeon feel uneasy. At the correct level of resection, cloudy, milky fluid can usually be seen refluxing from the opened ducts. After resection, large bleeding blood vessels are lightly cauterized, with care taken to avoid fulguration of the duct openings. Because the area of resection is at the prostatic apex, near both the external urethral sphincter and the rectum, careful and constant positioning of the resectoscope is essential. A finger placed in the rectum can help avoid rectal injuries and assist in keeping the resectoscope tip proximal to the external sphincter. A small Foley catheter is placed for 24 to 48 hours and removed on an outpatient basis. Oral antibiotics are given while the catheter is in place. After such treatment for infertility, intercourse is resumed after 7 days, and a formal semen analysis is checked as early as 2 weeks and then at regular intervals thereafter, until semen quality stabilizes.

Several useful aids can ensure that the resection is performed safely and completely. With an endoscopic needle, the milky ejaculatory duct fluid can be sampled transurethrally during the procedure and inspected with microscopy for sperm. The use of simultaneous, real-time TRUS during the resection is a valuable addition to this procedure. The exact location of the lesion to be resected can be determined by TRUS and the depth of resection continuously assessed during the resection. Similarly, TRUS can be used to guide the instillation of indigo carmine or methylene blue into the seminal vesicles with a long, 20-gauge Chiba needle before the resection. The dye is subsequently visualized on relief of obstruction.

Outcomes

Complications

The expected complication rate from TURED surgery is approximately 20% (12). The most common complications are self-limited hematospermia, hematuria requiring recatheterization, and urinary tract infection. More concerning, but less frequent, are epididymitis and a "watery" ejaculate. High-volume watery ejaculate is presumed secondary to the reflux of urine retrograde through the ejaculatory ducts into the seminal vesicles or into opened cysts, as suggested by the finding of creatinine in the ejaculates of TURED patients. In addition to the social implications of this, the exposure of sperm to urine may impair fertility potential. Several potentially major but rarely reported complications include retrograde ejaculation, rectal perforation, urinary incontinence, and recurrent seminal vesicle infection.

Results

Long-term relief of postcoital and perineal pain after TURED can be expected in 60% of patients (4). Hematospermia has also been effectively treated with TURED, but the literature on this indication remains anecdotal. There is convincing evidence from several large series of patients treated for infertility that a 20% to 30%

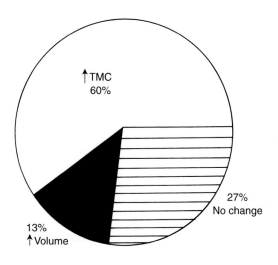

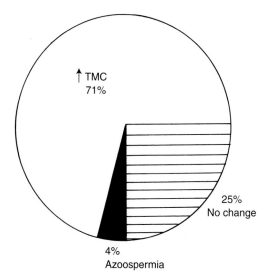

FIG. 53–9. Expected outcome of transurethral resection of the ejaculatory ducts for the indications of low-volume azoospermia and low-volume oligoasthenospermia (TMC, total motile count rise of greater than 50% after surgery). (Adapted from Turek PJ, Magana JO, Lipshultz LI. Semen parameters before and after transurethral surgery for ejaculatory duct obstruction. *J Urol* 1996;155:1291–1293, with permission.)

pregnancy rate can be expected from TURED (11,12). In one series, men treated for either low-volume azoospermia and low-volume oligoasthenospermia were equally likely (65% to 70%) to show improvements in semen quality after TURED (12) (Fig. 53–9). From a recent series, it appears that obstruction due to cysts responds better to TURED than that due to calcification (6).

Several caveats of TURED surgery should be emphasized to the patient preoperatively. Roughly 13% of men treated by TURED for low-volume azoospermia will convert to normal-volume azoospermia. Among these patients, we have found evidence of secondary obstruction at the level of the epididymis that requires epididymovasostomy. Epididymal obstruction may reflect the effects of time and blockage on other portions of the delicate male ductal system. Notably, 4% of patients treated for low-volume oligoasthenospermia may become azoospermic after TURED, presumably from scar tissue formation. We now recommend preoperative sperm cryopreservation if TURED is planned for this indication.

REFERENCES

1. Benson RC Jr, Clark WR, Farrow GM. Carcinoma of the seminal vesicle. *J Urol* 1984;132:483.
2. Cherullo EE, Meraney AM, Bernstein LH, Einstein DM, Thomas AJ, Gill IS. Laparoscopic management of congenital seminal vesicle cysts associated with ipsilateral renal agenesis. *J Urol* 2002;167:1263.
3. DeAsis JS. Seminal vesiculectomy. *J Urol* 1952;68:747.
4. Farley S, Barnes R. Stenosis of ejaculatory ducts treated by endoscopic resection. *J Urol* 1973;109:664.
5. Jarow JP. Seminal vesicle aspiration in the management of patients with ejaculatory duct obstruction. *J Urol* 1994;152:899.
6. Kadioglu A, Cayan S, Tefekli A, Orhan I, Engin G, Turek PJ. Does response to treatment of ejaculatory duct obstruction in infertile men vary with pathology? *Fertil Steril* 2001;76:138.
7. Kreager JA, Jordan WP. Transcoccygeal approach to the seminal vesicles. *Am Surg* 1965;31:126.
8. McDougall EM, Afane JS, Dunn MD, Shalhav AL, Clayman RV. Laparoscopic management of retrovesical cystic disease: Washington University experience and review of the literature. *J Endourol* 2001; 15:815.
9. Nguyen HT, Etzell J, Turek PJ. Normal human ejaculatory duct anatomy: a study of cadaveric and surgical specimens. *J Urol* 1996; 155:1639–1642.
10. Politano VA, Lankford RW, Susaeta R. A transvesical approach to total seminal vesiculectomy: a case report. *J Urol* 1975;113:385.
11. Pryor JP, Hendry WF. Ejaculatory duct obstruction in subfertile males: analysis of 87 patients. *Fertil Steril* 1991;56:725.
12. Turek PJ, Magana JO, Lipshultz LI. Semen parameters before and after transurethral surgery for ejaculatory duct obstruction. *J Urol* 1996;155: 1291–1293.
13. Williams RD. Surgery of the seminal vesicles. In: Walsh PC, Retik AB, Stamey TA, Vaughan ED, eds. *Campbell's urology*, 6th ed. Philadelphia: WB Saunders, 1992;2942–2955.
14. Wu DS, Shinohara K, Turek PJ. Ejaculatory duct chromotubation as a functional diagnostic test in ejaculatory duct obstruction. *J Urol* 1999; 161:1357A.

CHAPTER 54

Vasectomy

Jon L. Pryor

Elective vasectomy is a popular method of permanent sterilization for men. Approximately 500,000 men undergo this procedure in the United States each year. Despite being considered a minor office procedure, vasectomy has been noted to be the most common procedure involved in malpractice claims against urologists. The urologist needs to be thoroughly versed in the management of men seeking surgical sterilization. This chapter reviews the preoperative evaluation, surgical techniques, complications, and failure rates of vasectomy.

DIAGNOSIS

A brief physical examination, in a warm room, of the genitalia is critical to make sure both vasa are palpable. Large varicoceles, hydroceles, or a vas that is difficult to palpate because of a contracted (tight) scrotum may warrant doing the procedure in an operating room.

INDICATIONS FOR SURGERY

No strict criteria exist for determining which patient should be offered vasectomy. Patients who are unmarried, have no children, or have no clear indication for the procedure should be thoroughly counseled as vasectomy may not be appropriate for these men. Involvement of the spouse in the decision making and in witnessing the consent, although not required in most states, is recommended.

ALTERNATIVE THERAPY

Vasectomy is the only form of male birth control that is currently available. All other forms of birth control are directed at the female partner, including oral contraceptives, tubal ligation, and other forms of contraception.

SURGICAL TECHNIQUE

The introduction of the no-scalpel vasectomy (NSV) in the United States by Li in 1986 has played a major role in refining the procedure. In our opinion, major contributions of this variation of vasectomy have been threefold: the use of a single midline approach at the median raphe of the scrotum, the use of the external spermatic sheath injection for anesthetizing the vas, and the three-finger method for fixation of the vas. We describe our vasectomy technique, which relies on some aspects of the NSV but employs the scalpel to incise the skin.

Shaving of the scrotum, although not mandatory, is preferred. The vas deferens is held using the three-finger technique (Fig. 54–1). The middle finger of the nondominant hand is used to manipulate the right vas deferens to the skin at the median raphe of the scrotum. The vas is then tensed over the middle finger, with the thumb and index finger used to stretch the skin over the vas while positioning the vas as superficial to the skin as possible. A 25- or 27-gauge 1.5-in. needle is used for injection. One percent to 2% plain lidocaine (i.e., without epinephrine) is injected in a transverse fashion across the median raphe between the thumb and index finger to raise a superficial skin wheal 1 to 1.5 cm in diameter. Apply pressure on the skin wheal using a gauze sponge for a few seconds to enhance palpation of the vas deferens. Once the superficial wheal is made, the needle is advanced its full length immediately adjacent and parallel to the vas (Fig. 54–2), following a path that is in the general direction of the external inguinal ring. Two to 5 mL of lidocaine is injected within the external spermatic sheath as the needle is withdrawn. After injection, the right vas deferens is released and the left vas is manipulated to the median raphe. The left vas is anesthetized using the same technique as on the right vas. If this is done properly, the referred abdominal discomfort that occurs with manipu-

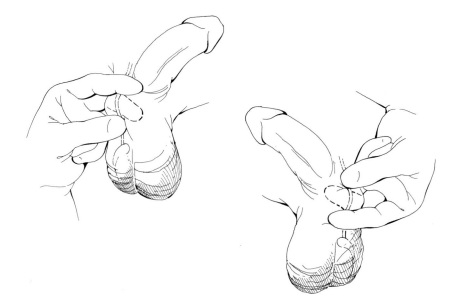

FIG. 54–1. The three-finger technique for isolating the **(A)** right and **(B)** left vas deferens.

lation of the vas during vasectomy is usually eliminated using this anesthetic technique.

After local anesthesia has been accomplished, the right vas is again fixed under the skin wheal with the nondominant hand. The vas should be held as superficial to the skin as possible. The scalpel is used to make a 1.0-cm transverse incision over the vas deferens (Fig. 54–3A). The incision is carried down until the vas is identified. Grab the vas or its sheath with a towel clip to ensure that the vas does not slip away. The vas sheath is then incised vertically until the bare vas wall is clearly seen. An Allis clamp or Adison tissue forceps is used to grasp only the vas, with care taken to avoid including the vasal sheath in the clamp or forceps (Fig. 54–3B). The vas should be eas-

ily pulled out of its sheath; if not, the surgeon most likely did not completely incise the sheath. At this point the vas should be covered only on the posterior aspect by the vas sheath. A mosquito clamp is passed along the undersurface of the vas and gently spread to strip the sheath and vasal vessels away from the vas (Fig. 54–4A). This maneuver should result in a 1.5- to 2.0-cm bare segment of vas.

The testicular end of the isolated vas segment is ligated with a 2-0 Vicryl or silk suture, leaving a long free end of suture to hold the vas with a mosquito clamp. The vas is then transected 1 cm from the ligature with Iris scissors or a scalpel, exposing the lumen of the vas (Fig. 54–4B). (Note: At this point some surgeons irrigate the abdominal

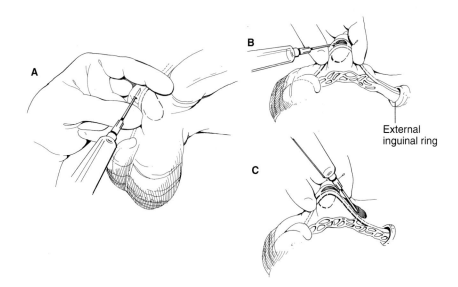

External inguinal ring

FIG. 54–2. The right vas deferens is manipulated to the midline raphe and anesthetized.

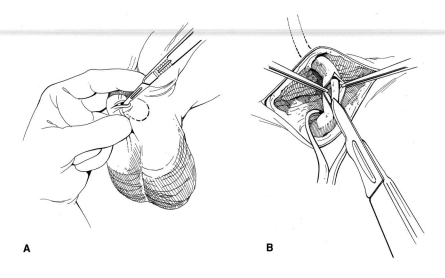

A   **B**

FIG. 54–3. A: A 1-cm transverse incision is made over the vas deferens. **B:** The vasal sheath is incised vertically and the vas deferens is grasped.

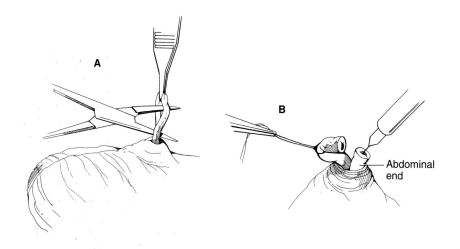

A

B

Abdominal end

FIG. 54–4. A: The vasal sheath and vessels are stripped away from the vas deferens. **B:** Transection of the vas deferens and cauterization of the lumen of the abdominal end.

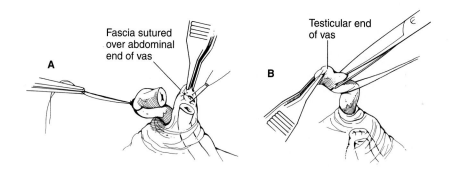

Fascia sutured over abdominal end of vas

A

Testicular end of vas

B

FIG. 54–5. The vasal sheath is closed over the vas deferens stump and a segment of vas is transected.

end of the vas to accelerate clearance of sperm; however, there is no evidence that irrigation accelerates the clearance of sperm and therefore irrigation is not recommended.) A battery-operated hot wire is passed 0.5 cm into the lumen of the abdominal end of the vas. The needle is slowly withdrawn as current is applied to the lumen. The surgeon should avoid a full-thickness burn of the lumen as this can cause necrosis of the vas and increases the risk of recanalization. The idea is to create enough injury to cause fibrosis of the vasal lumen, which results in permanent occlusion of the vas. The vas is then released, allowing the abdominal end to retract. The vasal sheath is then grasped with forceps and pulled over the abdominal end of the vas. A single interrupted 3-0 chromic suture is used to close the fascial edges of the sheath over the abdominal end of the vas (Fig. 54–5). This maneuver isolates the abdominal vas from the testicular end of the vas, which decreases the risk of recanalization. The testicular end of the vas is then transected next to the suture so as to allow a 1-cm segment of vas to be removed. This segment of vas can be sent to pathology for formal confirmation of vasectomy or saved for future pathologic analysis, if necessary. The free end of suture is cut and the testicular end of the vas is allowed to retract into the scrotum.

The left vas deferens is then manipulated to the same incision using the same three-finger technique and the procedure is repeated as described for the right vas. Once the left side has been completed, the incision is observed for bleeding. Hemostasis is meticulously obtained with electrocautery as any bleeding can cause a large scrotal hematoma. A single interrupted 3-0 chromic suture can be used to approximate the skin edges, but this is sometimes not required as the incision usually contracts and approximates itself. Antibiotic ointment is applied to the wound. Gauze is applied and held in place with a scrotal support. A jockstrap is recommended, but brief underwear can also be used.

OUTCOMES

Complications

Scrotal hematoma is the most worrisome complication of vasectomy and occurs in up to 3% of patients. Not surprisingly, one study found that the rate of scrotal hematoma was higher for physicians who performed fewer than 50 vasectomies a year (5): The hematoma rate was 4.6% for physicians with fewer than 10 vasectomies per year versus 1.6% for those who performed more than 50 per year. Most scrotal hematomas are small and do not require drainage. Warm compresses, nonsteroidal antiinflammatory medications, and restricted activity result in resolution of the majority of these hematomas. On occasion, the hematoma expands underneath the pliable skin of the scrotum and becomes large. These hematomas require surgical drainage, which results in relief of discomfort and a quicker recovery.

Incisional infections occur in 1% to 3% of patients. Most infections are superficial and resolve with a course of oral antibiotics. Rarely does an abscess form, which would then require surgical incision and debridement.

Chronic scrotal pain after vasectomy is not uncommon and has been reported to occur in up to 33% of patients. Of the patients with chronic scrotal pain, one-half stated that the pain was troublesome; however, only 9 of 172 (5%) sought medical attention for the symptoms. The general belief is that the scrotal pain after vasectomy is secondary to congestion of the epididymal tubule and is sometimes associated with epididymal blowout causing an epididymal granuloma. The symptoms, which can be exacerbated by sexual activity and ejaculation, are in general self-limiting. Nonsteroidal antiinflammatory medications are recommended to treat the inflammatory process, which usually leads to resolution of the symptoms. Patients with persistent pain despite conservative therapy can be treated with epididymectomy. Vasovasostomy has also been recommended but has the drawback of fertility.

Sperm granuloma at the vasectomy site occurs in 1% to 10% of patients. These granulomas form as a result of blowout of the testicular end of the vasal occlusion. Most granulomas are asymptomatic. The majority of patients only need reassurance that the lump in the scrotum is not cancer or something bad. Patients who experience discomfort from the granuloma should be treated initially with nonsteroidal antiinflammatory medications. If the symptoms do not resolve, excision of the granuloma is recommended.

There have been numerous methods described for closure of the vasal ends matched only by the number of techniques described for isolating the vas. Multiple authors have reported no recanalization with the use of luminal fulguration of both vasal ends and interposition of the fascial sheath over the abdominal end, as described previously. The luminal burn causes a fibrotic reaction that seals the vasal lumen, and the interposed fascial sheath enhances the closure. This method is easy to master, leaves minimal foreign material in the scrotum, and does not jeopardize the chances of future vasectomy reversal. The authors recommend this technique as the method for closing the vasal ends; however, we do feel that a single ligature on the testicular stump prevents leakage of sperm long enough to allow fibrosis of the abdominal end to occur. Recanalization rates or failure rates of less than 1% can be expected with this technique.

Results

The patient should be instructed to lie supine as much as possible during the first 12 to 24 hours following the procedure. Most vasectomies are done in the afternoon so that by the next morning the patient can ambulate. Intermittent application of an ice pack to the scrotum during the first 8 hours is highly recommended. The cooler temperature causes contraction of the scrotum and compression of any bleeding sites, decreasing the risk of hematoma formation.

Patients may return to work the next day, but strenuous activity should be avoided for at least 1 week. Patients should abstain from sexual activity for 1 week to allow fibrosis of the vas to occur. Patients need to be instructed on the importance of using contraception until they have two azoospermic semen analyses.

Studies have shown that the time to azoospermia is more dependent on the number of ejaculations than the time interval after vasectomy. In one study, 66% of patients were azoospermic after 12 ejaculations, whereas 98% were azoospermic after 24 ejaculations (6). When the time interval following vasectomy was the dependent variable, 67% to 98% were azoospermic at 3 months. We recommend that the patient should return in approximately 3 months for the first semen analysis and have ejaculated at least 24 times during that period. Most recanalizations occur early so a second semen analysis is obtained 4 months postvasectomy to assure sterility. If the patient has two azoospermic semen analyses, he can discontinue contraception.

Approximately 2.5% of patients will have persistently low counts (less than 10,000 per mL) of nonmotile sperm on semen analysis up to 7 months after vasectomy. Proper handling of these patients has been reviewed extensively in the literature (2,3,9). There have been no reported pregnancies in this group. These authors conclude that patients with less than 10,000 nonmotile sperm per mL can be given special clearance to have unprotected intercourse provided that the patient is aware of the extremely low risk of pregnancy. This "special clearance" appears to be accepted in the British literature but has rarely been discussed in the US literature. Patients with motile sperm in the semen analysis at 3 months should be advised to undergo repeat vasectomy.

Early recanalization or failure rates is in general defined as significant numbers of sperm or any motile sperm that persists beyond 4 months from vasectomy. This definition excludes patients with less than 10,000 nonmotile sperm per mL (i.e., the special clearance patients). It is estimated that 1 in 200 patients will have recanalization or vasectomy failure. These patients will need a repeat vasectomy. Late recanalization, which is the detection of sperm after two azoospermic samples, has been shown to occur in 15 of 2250 (0.67%) of patients at 1 year following vasectomy (4). These patients typically have very low sperm concentrations and subsequent semen analyses are usually azoospermic. Because most patients do not return for a semen analysis after being cleared for unprotected intercourse, patients with late recanalization are unlikely to be picked up in clinical practice. Evidence that these patients are usually not fertile is that the pregnancy rate after the initial semen analyses are azoospermic is around 1 in 3000 patients, much less than the 1 in 150 patients with late recanalization (1,4). Again, the 1 in 3000 patients who report a pregnancy after the initial semen analyses show azoospermia reminds us (and our patients) that a vasectomy is not perfect and future conception cannot be guaranteed.

Vasectomy is a safe and relatively easy procedure to perform and should continue to be offered to men who desire a permanent form of contraception. The no-scalpel technique has introduced modifications that have improved the efficiency of the procedure. Surgeons performing this procedure should attempt to do at least 50 vasectomies per year, as proficiency in this technique has been shown to decrease complication rates. The evidence to date indicates that vasectomy is not associated with any long-term adverse sequelae.

REFERENCES

1. Alderman PM. The lurking sperm: a review of failures in 8879 vasectomies performed by one physician. *JAMA* 1988;259:3142.
2. Benger JR, Swami SK, Gingell JC. Persistent spermatazoa after vasectomy: a survey of British urologists. *Br J Urol* 1995;76:376.
3. Davies AH, Sharp RJ, Cranston D, Mitchell RG. The long-term outcome following "special clearance" after vasectomy. *Br J Urol* 1990;66:211.
4. Haldar N, Cranston D, Turner E, MacKenzie I, Guillebaud J. How reliable is a vasectomy? Long-term follow-up of vasectomised men. *Lancet* 2000;356:43.
5. Kendrick JS, Gonzales B, Huber DH, Grubb GS, Rubin GL. Complications of vasectomy in the United States. *J Fam Pract* 1987;25:245.
6. Marshall S, Lyon RP. Variability of sperm disappearance from the ejaculate after vasectomy. *J Urol* 1972;107:815.
7. McCormack M, LaPointe S. Physiologic consequences and complications of vasectomy. *Can Med Assoc J* 1988;138:223.
8. McMahon AJ, Buckley J, Taylor A, Lloyd SN, Deane RF, Kirk D. Chronic testicular pain following vasectomy. *Br J Urol* 1992;69:188.
9. Philp T, Guillebaud J, Budd D. Complications of vasectomy: review of 16,000 patients. *Br J Urol* 1984;56:745.
10. Schmidt SS. Vasectomy by section, luminal fulguration and fascial interposition: results of 6248 cases. *Br J Urol* 1995;76:373.

CHAPTER 55

Vasoepididymostomy

Richard S. Lee and Richard E. Berger

Azoospermia may be caused by obstruction of the vas deferens, ejaculatory duct, or epididymis. Epididymal obstruction may be caused by congenital abnormalities, infection, vasectomy, trauma, or iatrogenic causes. The most common cause of epididymal obstruction is epididymal tubule breakage after vasectomy. To bypass the epididymal obstruction, a vasoepididymostomy must be performed.

Vasoepididymostomy can be a much more technically demanding procedure than vasovasostomy. Vasoepididymostomy involves suturing a relatively large muscular organ, the vas deferens, to a smaller, very fragile organ, the epididymis. Success of the procedure depends on the skill of the surgeon and the location of the obstruction, and use of the operating microscope is mandatory. The surgeon performing vasoepididymostomy needs to be technically prepared and skilled in microsurgery because vasoepididymostomy is probably the most difficult microsurgical urologic procedure.

DIAGNOSIS

Men with epididymal obstruction are typically azoospermic with a normal semen volume, alkaline pH, and fructose positive. Physical examination should find normal vasa deferentia, indicating the patient does not have congenital absence of the vas deferens (CAVD). The epididymis may be easily palpable or congested. If obstruction is high in the epididymis, it may be only swollen near the head. Testicles should be relatively normal in size and testicular biopsy should reveal spermatogenesis with 20 to 30 mature spermatids per round tubule. Laboratory evaluation should reveal a normal serum follicle-stimulating hormone, luteinizing hormone, and testosterone level, which is associated with normal spermatogenesis.

INDICATIONS FOR SURGERY

The indications for performing a surgery to correct obstruction are a healthy male who desires natural conception and is a suitable surgical candidate. The partner's ovulatory and tubal status should be determined prior to surgery. Finding an abnormal fertility status of the partner could influence the decision on weather to perform vasoepididymostomy or *in vitro* fertilization (IVF).

ALTERNATIVE THERAPY

Indications for alternative therapy would be testicular failure, extensive trauma to the lower genitourinary system requiring major reconstruction, significant erectile or ejaculatory dysfunction, or female problems requiring IVF (11). In most cases, vasoepididymostomy is more cost effective than IVF/ intracytoplasmic sperm injection (ICSI) after sperm retrieval from the testicle or epididymis (4,12).

SURGICAL TECHNIQUE

The patient is positioned in the supine position with the arms either at the side or on the chest. Because of the length of the procedure (2 to 5 hours), the patient should be appropriately padded at all pressure points. Epidural agents have the benefit of eliminating lower-body movement. Regional or local anesthetic combined with sedation is usually adequate if the surgeon is experienced and the surgery is limited to the scrotal region. However, local anesthetic may not be adequate if the procedure becomes very extensive, the patient cannot remain still, or if abdominal or inguinal vas deferens or ejaculatory duct obstruction is found. If obstruction is found in the abdominal or inguinal vas deferens or ejaculatory duct, an epidural or general anesthesia may be required.

Equipment and surgical instruments used for this procedure include a microsurgical needle holder, microsurgical forceps and scissors, and bipolar cautery. Sutures utilized include 5-0 Prolene, 9-0 nylon suture on a cutting needle, and a 10-0 nylon suture on double-armed 70-μm tapered needles. Other supplies include Penrose drains, normal saline or Ringer's lactate irrigation, and isotonic glycine solution. We perform the surgery under a 20× surgical microscope.

455

Vasoepididymostomy Not Associated with Previous Vasectomy

One task for the surgeon is to determine definitively that obstruction is in the epididymis. This determination is made at the time of surgery after the patient has been informed of all surgical possibilities, risks, and outcomes. The vas deferens is isolated at the junction of the straight and convoluted portions so as to preserve as much vas deferens as possible. Using an operative microscope, the vasal vessels are spared while the vasal sheath is vertically incised. A clean segment of bare vas is delivered and transected with a no. 2 or 3 nerve cutter. The proximal vasal fluid is examined for sperm under a phase contrast microscope at 400×. Absence of sperm or sperm fragments is consistent with epididymal obstruction; however, obstruction at a testicular or vas deferens level is still possible.

The seminal vesical end of the vas is cannulated with a 24-gauge angiocatheter and injected with normal saline or Ringer's lactate to confirm patency. Glycine should not be used because it can potentially precipitate and obstruct the vas deferens. If the fluid passes easily, a formal vasogram is not necessary. If any doubt exists, indigo carmine dye may be injected and the bladder catheterized. Presence of blue or green dye in the urine confirms patency. Use of methylene blue should be avoided because of its possible inflammatory effects on the vas deferens (9). Indigo carmine when diluted four times or more had minimal effect on sperm motility (9). If patency is not confirmed, formal vasography should be performed with water-soluble radiographic contrast medium (Renografin) (10) to locate the obstruction.

Vasoepididymostomy Associated with Previous Vasectomy

Determine that the vas deferens is patent in a similar manner as someone without previous vasectomy, except open the vas just proximal to the vasectomy site (3). Vasoepididymostomy is performed when epididymal obstruction exists. Absence of a sperm granuloma at the vasectomy site and absence of sperm in the proximal vasal fluid may indicate epididymal obstruction. On inspection of the epididymis, the epididymal tubules will often be dilated at the head and then become small or nonvisible as you proceed toward the tail. On occasion, a sperm granuloma will be found within the epididymis. The more time that has elapsed since a vasectomy increases the likelihood that an epididymal blowout will lead to obstruction (1).

Surgical Incision

An appropriate sized scrotal incision should be made to allow for retrieval of the vas deferens and isolation of the epididymis. Two scrotal incisions may be required for bilateral vasoepididymostomies if the patient has had a previous high vasectomy. If a patient is known to have bilateral obstruction from a previous vasectomy repair and a bilateral vasoepididymostomy is to be performed, a midline scrotal incision can be made. The advantage of a midline incision is easy access to both the left and right epididymis and vas deferens with a minimal incision. If abdominal or inguinal vasa obstruction is found, it may be impossible to get enough vas deferens length to perform a vasoepididymostomy (5).

The surgeon should be prepared to perform fluoroscopy or a static abdominal pelvic film in the case that the patency of the vas deferens cannot be confirmed with irrigation of saline or indigo carmine through the vas deferens. If the ejaculatory ducts are obstructed, a transurethral resection of the ejaculatory ducts can be performed in conjunction with the vasoepididymostomy. The patient should be made aware of this possibility prior to beginning the procedure. Because the vas deferens has been mobilized and opened at this point, we prefer to complete the vasoepididymostomy and the ejaculatory duct resection at the same setting if the patient has consented and appropriate anesthesia is available. Alternatively, it is possible to perform the transurethral ejaculatory duct resection at another time (5).

Once it is determined that spermatogenesis exists, the vasa are patent, and a vasoepididymostomy is to be performed, an appropriate segment and length of the vas deferens and epididymis must be mobilized and prepared for anastomosis. Prior to exploring the epididymis, the vas deferens and its blood supply are dissected free from surrounding tissue and brought to the lateral side of the epididymis. Care must be taken not to dissect the blood supply away from the cut end of the vas. Appropriate length of the vas deferens must be mobilized to create a tension-free anastomosis. If appropriate length is not available, the scrotal incision can be extended cephalad for further mobilization of the vas deferens. If an appropriate length of vas cannot be mobilized, such as when the patient has had a higher vasectomy, the tale and midportion of the epididymis can be mobilized to help bridge the gap in some cases (5).

The operating microscope is brought into the operative field. Using this scope, the epididymis is examined and the initial sight of anastomosis is determined. Identify the most distal dilated epididymal tubule with the fewest overlying blood vessels. Frequently, the epididymal tubules will be dilated to a certain point and then become small and nonvisible. The point of the dilated epididymal tubule furthest from the head should be chosen. The epididymal tubule is exposed by creating a 2-mm × 2-mm window in the epididymal tunic with microscissors. The tubule is further exposed by carefully dissecting the adventitial tissue over the tubule.

Single Tubule End-to-Side Anastomosis

To perform the single tubule end-to-side anastomosis (Figs. 55–1A to 55–1F), the dilated epididymal tubule is

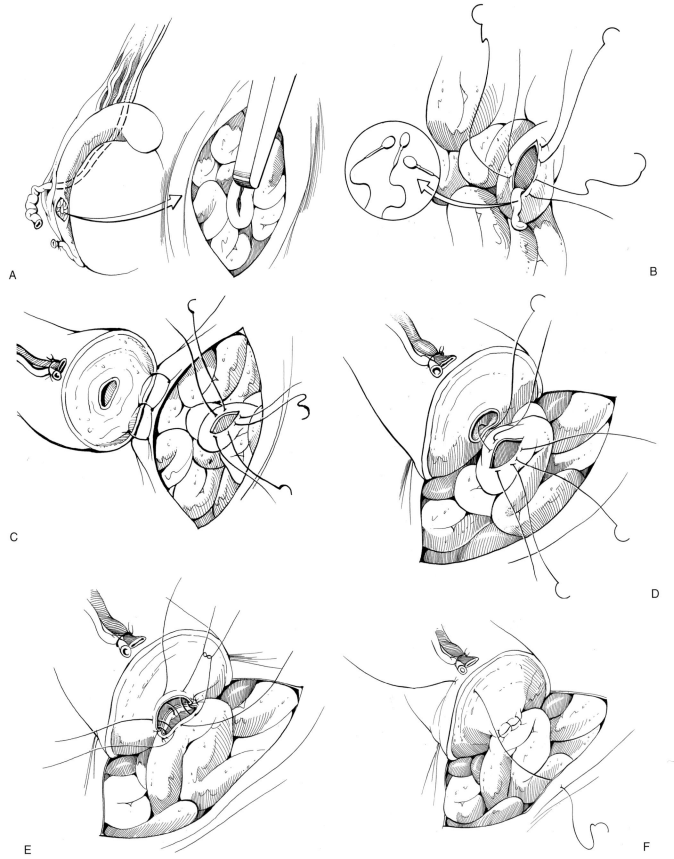

FIG. 55–1. A: Longitudinal incision into the epididymal tubule. **B:** Placement of 10-0 nylon identification sutures 120 degrees apart. **C:** The vas deferens is secured to the epididymal tunic with 9-0 nylon. **D:** Placement of identification suture in the vas deferens. **E:** The sutures are tied. **F:** Second stabilization suture of 9-0 nylon from the vas adventitia to the epididymal tunic.

localized and incised in the longitudinal axis with a microknife or opened using a microscissors. Unobstructed segments will efflux fluid that should be touch prepped for sperm. If sperm are observed and fluid continues to emit from the tubule, this tubule site may be used for the anastomosis. If sperm are not seen and fluid continues to flow, another touch prep should be performed and examined after a few minutes. If still no sperm are seen, another site of the proximal epididymis should be prepped and examined in the same fashion.

Once sperm are found, the tubule is prepared for anastomosis. The cut end of the mobilized vas deferens is freshened with a razor blade and then brought into the field through a window in the mesentery of the testicle so that the cut face of the vas should be juxtaposed to the window created in the tunic of the epididymis. This is achieved by placing two interrupted 5-0 Prolene sutures in the tunic of the cord to the adventitia of the vas deferens.

Two to four sutures of 9-0 nylon are then placed to suture the posterior muscular layer of the vas deferens to the epididymal tunic. The epididymal tubule anastomosis to the vasal lumen is performed by placing six to eight 10-0 nylon double-armed sutures with 70-μm taper-point needles into the epididymal tubule inside to out of the epididymal lumen and outside to in on the vas deferens in a symmetrical fashion. All the sutures are passed inside to out in the cut end of the vas deferens prior to tying. Alternatively, sutures with needles on each end may be passed inside out on both sides. After completing the inner mucosal layer anastomosis, the remaining muscularis and adventitia are secured to the tunic of the epididymis with interrupted 9-0 double-armed nylon sutures. The testis is then returned to the tunica vaginalis and closed in a running fashion.

Triangulation End-to-Side Anastomosis

After determining that vasoepididymostomy is to be performed, the vas deferens and epididymis are mobilized and prepared in the same fashion as previously mentioned. Unlike the end-to-side anastomosis, the triangulation technique (Figs. 55–2A to 55–2H) secures the vas deferens to the tunic of the epididymis prior to opening the epididymal tubule.

Three posteriorly placed 9-0 nylon tension-free sutures are placed in the muscular layer of the vas deferens to the opening of the epididymal tunic. At this time, the epididymal tubule is reidentified and the surgeon places one arm of a double-armed 70-μm tapered 10-0 nylon suture in the epididymal tubule parallel to the open face of the vas deferens. This suture is placed superficially into and out of the epididymal tubule so that it incorporates most of the surface of the epididymal tubule facing the surgeon. Care is taken to not place the needle deeply and into the back wall of the epididymis.

Placement of the first suture often results in leakage of a small amount of fluid that can be checked for sperm using a touch prep. If sperm are found, the surgeon can then proceed with the rest of the anastomosis. If no sperm are seen, the suture can be pulled free and used in a different anastomosis; the procedure takes little more time than initially making a window in the epididymal tubule and looking at the fluid prior to placing single sutures, as in the technique of a single tubule end-to-side anastomosis described in the previous section.

If the touch prep confirms sperm, two other sutures are then placed so that a roughly equilateral triangle is formed by the loops of sutures in the epididymal wall with an apex of the triangle pointing toward the vasal lumen. Great care is taken to not incorporate the back wall of the epididymis in these sutures.

A small opening in the epididymal tubule is then made in the center of the triangle using the cutting edge of a microneedle. Alternatively, the center of the triangle can be punctured and lifted with the tip of the 70-μm needle and a window cut in the tubule beneath the needle using a microscissors. Care must be taken not to cut the sutures. There are three double-armed sutures triangulated in the opened epididymal tubule. The needles of the sutures forming the right apex of the triangle are then placed in the right side of the vas deferens lumen. These are placed at the 5- and 3-o'clock positions into the vas lumen, at one-half to three-fourths of the distance from the lumen to the adventitial of the vas. The left-sided sutures are then placed at the 7- and 9-o'clock positions. Finally, the first suture placed is put in at the 11- and 1-o'clock positions in an inside-out fashion in the lumen of the vas deferens. Each suture is then tied, starting with the lateral sutures and finishing with the dorsal suture. Tying the sutures invaginates the epididymal tubule into the lumen of the vas deferens.

The anastomosis is then inspected for any leakage. Sutures are then cut. The attachment of the outside layer of the muscular layer of the vas deferens to the epididymal tunic is then completed using interrupted 9-0 nylon sutures. The testicle and epididymis are then placed back into the scrotum and the operation completed.

In the authors' opinion, the triangulation vasoepididymostomy is much easier and takes less time than traditional end-to-side vasoepididymostomy. Currently, the average time for bilateral vasoepididymostomy is no different than for bilateral vasovasostomy: Both take about 2.5 hours. Placing the three double-armed sutures prior to opening the epididymal tubule greatly simplifies the procedure. During placement of the sutures, the epididymal tubule is full, not collapsed as in the traditional procedure. Also, there is decreased leakage of the epididymal fluid from the epididymal tubule during suture placement and therefore it is easier to see the tubule. Because the sutures are placed in the epididymal tubule parallel to the face of the vas and not perpendicular to it, more tissue

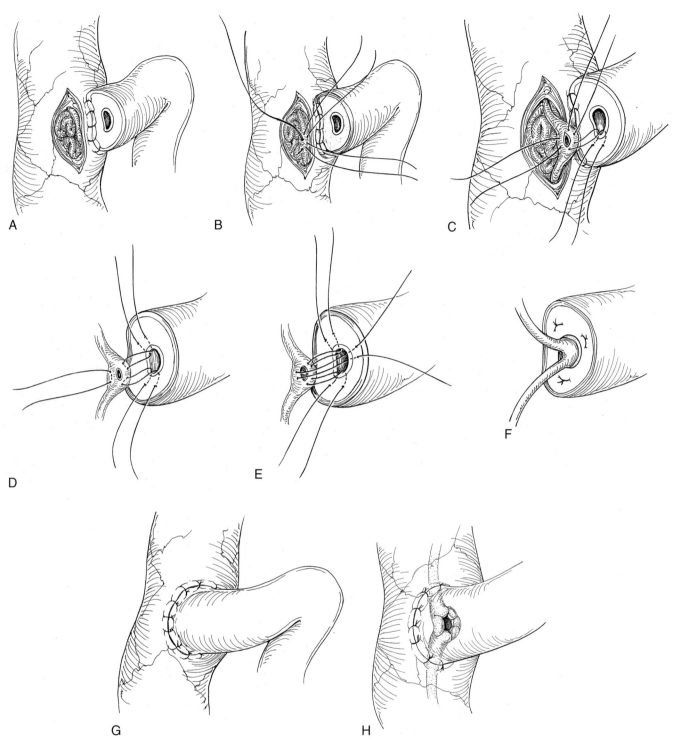

FIG. 55–2. A: An opening has been made in the epididymal tunic and the adventitia cleared from the epididymal tubule. The vas deferens has been sewn through the opening in the epididymal tubule using interrupted 9-0 nylon sutures. **B:** 10-0 double-armed sutures on a tapered needle have been placed in a triangulated fashion into the anterior wall of the unopened epididymal tubule. **C:** All sutures have been placed in the epididymal tubule and an opening made in the center of the resulting triangle using the cutting edge of a microneedle. The sutures on the right-hand side have been brought out approximately one-half of the way into the muscular layer. **D:** The sutures on the other side have been brought into the epididymal tubule in a similar fashion. **E:** Finally, the third sutures are brought into the epididymal lumen and out the muscular layer. **F:** The sutures are then tied successively, beginning with the lateral sutures and finishing with the dorsal suture. **G:** The outside layer is then completed, anastomosing the muscular layer of the vas deferens to the adventitial of the epididymal tubule. **H:** A cutaway view of the sutures tied showing imbrication of the epididymal tubule into the vas deferens.

from the epididymal tubule is incorporated into sutures to support the tension as it is tied. Although it is possible to place the sutures and then find that there are no sperm in the epididymal tubule, the fluid leaking around the first suture is checked after placement. This method may actually take less time than it takes to open the epididymal tubule carefully. The invagination of the epididymal tubule into the vas deferens should potentially decrease sperm leakage from the anastomosis. The sutures are brought inside out into the vasal lumen and then halfway out the muscular layer. The muscle therefore keeps the two ends of the suture apart. This technique is essentially the equivalent of using six individual sutures between the vas deferens and the epididymal tubule. However, placing only three sutures shortens the operative time and makes the procedure easier. A comparative randomized trial is needed among the various methods of vasoepididymostomy to determine the procedure with the best patency and ultimately the best pregnancy rate.

Meticulous hemostasis is absolutely necessary as expandability of the scrotum and lack of pressure can allow small amounts of bleeding to become large hematomas. Reexploration of a delicate microsurgical anastomosis can be deleterious to the surgical outcome. Scrotal Penrose drains are placed bilaterally and removed in 3 to 4 hours.

An alternative to placing three double-armed sutures into the epididymis is to use only two sutures. Prior to securing the vas to the epididymal tunic, two 10-0 nylon sutures are aligned parallel to each other in a Styrofoam block to allow a microblade tip between them. The needles are then grasped with a microneedle holder, and the tips of the needles are passed through a distended epididymal tubule so that the needles remain parallel. A jeweler's forceps is used to advance the remainder of the needle through the tubule. A microblade is then used to make the tubulotomy between the two sutures. A touch prep of the fluid is then checked for sperm (6).

Three 9-0 nylon sutures are used to secure the freshened vas deferens to the tunic of the epididymis. Each 10-0 nylon suture is then placed 1 mm into the vas lumen and out the muscularis at the 8- and 10-o'clock positions on the left side and 2- and 4-o'clock positions on the right. The tubule is invaginated into the vas deferens by placing lateral retraction on the sutures. Prior to tying the last intraluminal suture, a 9-0 nylon suture is placed in the anterior vas to the epididymal tunic to stabilize the vas and reduce tension. The final intraluminal suture is tied and three to four sutures are placed from the vas deferens to the epididymal tunic to complete the anastomosis (6).

POSTOPERATIVE CARE

Postoperatively, patients are provided with oral analgesics. Ice is placed on the scrotum or suprapubic area. Patients are requested to stay flat in recovery for 3 to 4 hours; drains are also removed at this time. Patients are provided with scrotal support, and it is recommended to use this support for the first 2 postoperative weeks. Strenuous lifting and activity is restricted for the first month. Sexual activity is also discouraged for 3 weeks. Patients are asked to provide a semen analysis every 3 months until pregnancy occurs. If no sperm are present in the semen after 1 year, a reoperation, testicular aspiration, and ICSI are presented to the patient as alternatives.

OUTCOMES

Complications

Complications from vasoepididymostomy are rare. The most serious complication is testicular atrophy resulting from inadvertent injury to the arterial blood supply to the testicle. This complication can be minimized and avoided by meticulous dissection when dissecting out the vas deferens from the cord structures and limiting dissection where the blood supply enters the testicle. Scrotal hematoma is another complication but can be avoided with meticulous hemostasis. Infection, including epididymitis and scrotal infections, can be limited by careful preoperative evaluation, the use of preoperative antibiotics, and attentive perioperative care.

Results

Success of this surgery can be measured by patency of the repair or by conception, and different success rates have been reported for each technique. The patency of bilateral microsurgical vasoepididymostomy is reported to be from 52% to 92% (12). It has also been reported that repeat vasoepididymostomy can be successful in 66% of patients who have a previously failed vasoepididymostomy (8).

We have reported that 92% of patients treated with triangulation end-to-side vasoepididymostomy achieved patency (2). We feel that the triangulation end-to-side technique is an easier procedure than the traditional end-to-side anastomosis and may lead to better results. Motile sperm often return to the ejaculate in 6 weeks to 3 months.

A variation of the triangulation end-to-side technique, in which only two double-armed sutures are simultaneously placed into a full epididymis, was reported to have a 77.7% patency rate in bilateral procedures and a 85.7% patency rate in unilateral procedures (6).

Goldstein compared the triangulation intussusception technique versus the end-to-side technique in male Wistar rats and found that the triangulation technique was superior to the conventional end-to-side technique. The triangulation technique had a 91.7% patency rate and fewer sperm granulomas (20.8%) as compared to the conventional end-to-side technique (54.1% and 58.4%) (7).

ACKNOWLEDGMENTS

Special thanks are extended to Noelani Chamberlain for copyediting and manuscript support.

REFERENCES

1. Belker AM, Konnak JW, Sharlip ID, et al. Intraoperative observations during vasovasostomy in 334 patients. *J Urol* 1983;129:524–527.
2. Berger RE. Triangulation end-to-side vasoepididymostomy. *J Urol* 1998;159:1951–1953.
3. Berger RE. Vasoepididymostomy triangulation pull-through technique. In: Goldstein M, guest ed. *Atlas of the Urologic Clinics of North America, surgery for male infertility*, vol. 7, no. 1. Philadelphia: WB Saunders, 1999:91–96.
4. Deck AJ, Berger RE. Should vasectomy reversal be performed in men with older female partners? *J Urol* 2000;163:105–106.
5. Goldstein M. Surgical management of male infertility and other scrotal disorders. In: Walsh, Retick, Vaughn, Wein, eds. *Campbell's urology*. Philadelphia: WB Saunders, 1998:1331–1377.
6. Marmar JL. Modified vasoepididymostomy with simultaneous double needle placement, tubulotomy and tubular invagination. *J Urol* 2000;163:483–486.
7. McCallum S, Li PS, Sheynkin Y, et al. Comparison of intussusception pull-through end-to-side and conventional end-to-side microsurgical vasoepididymostomy: prospective randomized controlled study in male Wistar rats. *J Urol* 2002;167:2284–2288.
8. Pasqualotto FF, Agarwal A, Srivastava M, et al. Fertility outcome after repeat vasoepididymostomy. *J Urol* 1999;162:1626–1628.
9. Sheynkin YR, Starr C, Li PS, et al. Effect of methylene blue, indigo carmine, and Renografin on human sperm motility. *Urology* 1999;53:214–217.
10. Thomas AJ, Nagler HM. Testicular biopsy and vasography for evaluation of male infertility. *Urol Clin North Am* 1987;14:167–176.
11. Thomas AJ. Vasoepididymostomy. In: Graham SD Jr, ed. *Glenn's urologic surgery*, 5th ed. Philadelphia: Lippincott–Raven, 1998:493–499.
12. Thomas AJ Jr. Vasoepididymostomy. In: Goldstein M, guest ed. *Atlas of the Urologic Clinics of North America, surgery for male infertility*, vol. 7, no. 1. Philadelphia: WB Saunders, 1999:65–90.

CHAPTER 56

Vasovasostomy

Arnold M. Belker

Vasovasostomy is performed most commonly to reverse an elective bilateral vasectomy. There now is virtually universal agreement among urologists that microsurgical anastomotic methods of vasovasostomy achieve better results than formerly were achieved with macrosurgical methods. Accordingly, only microsurgical techniques will be considered in this chapter. Although fibrin glue and laser welding anastomotic methods have been described, they have not been utilized by most urologic surgeons and therefore will not be discussed.

DIAGNOSIS

There are no standard or specific diagnostic studies performed prior to vasovasostomy. The preoperative scrotal examination may help predict the possibility for success after vasovasostomy. Epididymal induration suggests that an epididymal sperm granuloma has occurred as a result of increased epididymal tubular pressure after the vasectomy and that vasoepididymostomy will be required (13).

Approximately two-thirds of men develop serum antisperm antibodies after undergoing vasectomy (9). However, experts do not agree about whether or not such antibodies are likely to impair a man's fertility after a vasectomy reversal procedure. Urologic surgeons do not commonly obtain serum antisperm antibody tests to advise a man about his fertility potential if he undergoes a vasectomy reversal.

INDICATIONS FOR SURGERY

The request for a vasectomy reversal usually results from the male partner's divorce and subsequent remarriage. Much less frequent reasons for a vasectomy reversal are the loss of a child and azoospermia caused by unintended surgical injury to both vasa deferentia. The latter most often results from bilateral inguinal herniorrhaphy during infancy.

ALTERNATIVE THERAPY

Alternatives to vasovasostomy include adoption, various forms of sperm aspiration and *in vitro* fertilization (IVF), and vasoepididymostomy. Some couples inquire about the possibility of epididymal or testicular sperm retrieval for IVF with intracytoplasmic sperm injection (ICSI) instead of a vasectomy reversal. An analysis of the cost–effectiveness of microsurgical vasovasostomy compared to sperm retrieval for IVF with ICSI was performed by Pavlovich and Schlegel (11). They concluded that microsurgical vasovasostomy not only was a considerably more cost-effective approach but also that it had a better chance of resulting in the delivery of a child after a single intervention. In a similar study, Kolettis and Thomas found microsurgical vasoepididymostomy to be more cost-effective than sperm retrieval for IVF with ICSI (8).

Following vasectomy hydrostatic pressure in the epididymal tubule increases significantly, which may result in rupture of the epididymal tubule and the formation of an epididymal sperm granuloma (10). Silber emphasized that an epididymal sperm granuloma causes obstruction to the passage of sperm below the location of the sperm granuloma in the epididymis (13). When an epididymal sperm granuloma has caused epididymal obstruction after a vasectomy, vasoepididymostomy, rather than vasovasostomy, is required to reverse the vasectomy successfully.

SURGICAL TECHNIQUE

Vasovasostomy may be performed using spermatic cord block, epidural, spinal, or general anesthesia. When any method of anesthesia other than general anesthesia is chosen, it is useful to employ intravenous sedation, which helps avoid undesirable patient movement during microsurgical anastomotic suturing. Vasovasostomy is performed as an outpatient procedure regardless of the method of anesthesia.

Vasovasostomy commonly is performed using vertical scrotal incisions at the level of the vasectomy on each side. When either an unusually long segment of the vas deferens was resected at the time of the vasectomy or when the vasectomy was performed at an extremely high level, an infrapubic incision is useful to mobilize a maximum length of the abdominal end of the vas deferens (2). In such situations, modified infrapubic incisions are placed lateral to each side of the base of the penis (Fig. 56–1) (3).

A folding approximating clamp facilitates performance of anastomotic suturing. This clamp always is applied to the vasal ends from the assistant's side, which makes it necessary for the assistant rather than the surgeon to manipulate instruments around the hinge post of the folded clamp. Securing a suture that approximates spermatic fascia at the base of the isolated ends of the vas to the surgical drapes on the surgeon's side and a double wrap of umbilical tape around the hinge post of the folding approximating clamp to the surgical drapes on the assistant's side (Fig. 56–2) stabilizes the anastomosis bilaterally (4).

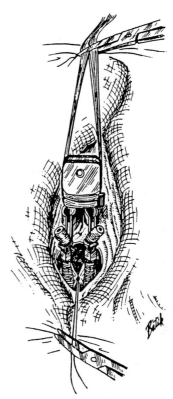

FIG. 56–2. The suture used to approximate spermatic fascia is tagged to the drapes on the surgeon's side. The folding approximating clamp is applied to position the hinge post on the assistant's side. After the approximating clamp is applied and folded, a double wrap of umbilical tape is placed around the hinge post of the clamp and tagged to the drapes on the assistant's side. The vasal ends thus are stabilized during anastomotic suturing. (From Belker AM. Microsurgical repair of obstructive causes of male infertility. In: *Seminars in Urology*, vol. 2. Philadelphia: WB Saunders, 1984:93, with permission.)

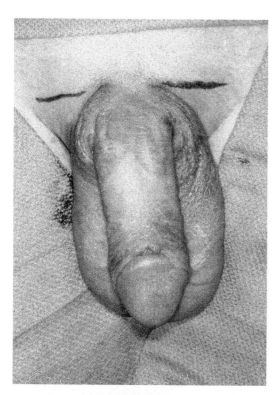

FIG. 56–1. The planned location of separate infrapubic incisions just lateral to each side of the base of the penis is indicated by lines drawn on the skin of the patient. This type of incision is useful when the vasectomy was performed very high in the scrotum or when an unusually long length of the vas was resected during the vasectomy. (From Belker AM. Microsurgical vasovasostomy: two-layer technique. In: Goldstein M, ed. *Surgery of male infertility.* Philadelphia: WB Saunders, 1995:63, with permission.)

Modified one-layer microsurgical vasovasostomy is performed by placing six to eight interrupted sutures of 9-0 nylon through the full thickness (adventitia, muscularis, and mucosa) of the vas. After these sutures are tied, more superficial outer muscular-layer sutures of 9-0 nylon are placed between adjacent full-thickness sutures. To obtain the best approximation of mucosal edges with this anastomotic method, it is advisable to place the full-thickness sutures in a "triangular" manner rather than in a "square" manner, as shown in Figure 56–3 (5).

The microsurgical method of two-layer vasovasostomy using a folding vas approximating clamp is shown in Figures 56–4 and 56–5, in which the mucosa has been stained with a dye to make it more apparent. Seven to ten interrupted sutures of 10-0 nylon (depending upon the amount of dilation of the testicular end lumen) are placed to approximate the mucosal edges and eight to ten interrupted sutures of 9-0 nylon to approximate the outer muscular-layer edges.

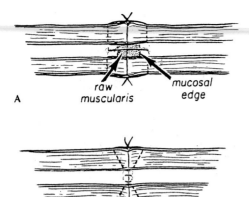

A

raw
muscularis

mucosal
edge

B

FIG. 56–3. A: Full-thickness "square" suture does not enter lumen near mucosal edges, leaving retracted mucosal edges and possibility for scar formation and resulting stenosis. **B:**. Full-thickness "triangular" suture is placed so that suture enters lumen near mucosal edges, assuring good approximation of mucosal edges. (From Belker AM. Vasovasostomy. In: Resnick MI, ed. *Current trends in urology*, vol. I. Baltimore: Williams & Wilkins, 1981:30, with permission.)

When intact spermatozoa are present in the intraoperative vasal fluid, vasovasostomy is performed. When only sperm heads (without tails) are found in the intraoperative vasal fluid, there is not universal agreement concerning whether vasovasostomy or vasoepididymostomy is indicated. The Vasovasostomy Study Group found that when only sperm heads were present in the intraoperative vasal fluid bilaterally sperm were seen in follow-up semen analyses in 75% (55/73) of patients after bilateral microsurgical vasovasostomy (6). Thus, many surgeons feel that vasovasostomy should be performed even when only sperm heads are present in the intraoperative vasal fluid, although other surgeons consider performing vasoepididymostomy when only sperm heads are present.

When no sperm or sperm parts are identified in the intraoperative vasal fluid, the surgeon should sample several more specimens of vasal fluid. If no sperm are found in any intraoperative specimen, Ringer's solution should be instilled through a 24-gauge blunt-tip needle into the testicular end of the vas without occlusion of the vas around the needle. Avoiding occlusion of the vas around the needle prevents rupture of the epididymal tubule that otherwise could be caused by the pressure of the instilled fluid. After Ringer's solution has been instilled, sperm

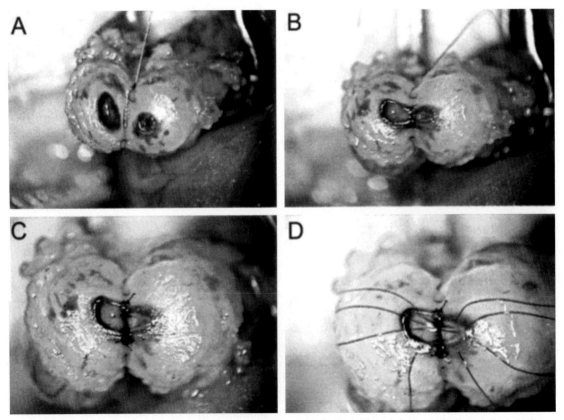

FIG. 56–4. The vasal ends have been placed in a folding approximating clamp and the clamp has been folded. Mucosa has been stained with a dye to make it more apparent. **A:** Completed posterior muscular layer suturing. **B–D:** Progression of mucosal layer suturing. (From Urology Surgical Associates, P.S.C., Louisville, KY, 2002, with permission.)

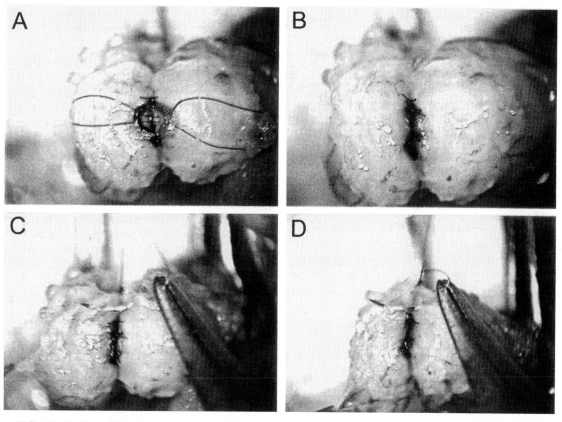

FIG. 56–5. A and B: Progressive tying of mucosal sutures. **C and D:** Placement of muscular layer sutures. (From Urology Surgical Associates, P.S.C., Louisville, KY, 2002, with permission.)

may be identified in the fluid that subsequently effluxes from the testicular end of the vas. If sperm are present in the effluxing fluid, vasovasostomy is performed.

When sperm or sperm parts are not present in the intraoperative vasal fluid, the choice of vasovasostomy or vasoepididymostomy depends upon several factors. Inspection of the epididymis may reveal a clear level of demarcation above which the epididymal tubule appears dilated and below which it appears collapsed, in which case vasoepididymostomy must be performed above the obvious level of obstruction. If there is no apparent point of epididymal obstruction, then the surgeon may be influenced by the gross appearance of the vasal fluid. When sperm were absent bilaterally from the intraoperative vasal fluid and the fluid was watery (clear, colorless, and transparent), the Vasovasostomy Study Group reported that sperm were seen in follow-up semen analyses after bilateral vasovasostomy in 80% of patients. When sperm were absent bilaterally from the intraoperative vasal fluid and the fluid appeared cloudy, sperm returned to the semen in 75% of men after bilateral vasovasostomy (6). However, when sperm were absent bilaterally from the intraoperative vasal fluid and the fluid appeared creamy only 26% of men had positive semen analyses. Thus, when sperm are absent from the intraoperative vasal fluid

vasoepididymostomy seems to be indicated when the vasal fluid is thick and creamy. The surgeon also may be influenced by the duration of the obstructive interval (time from vasectomy until its reversal), as subsequently discussed.

Patients are instructed to remain at home for 1 week postoperatively, avoid heavy physical activity and use a scrotal support for 1 month, and avoid sexual intercourse for 2 weeks after vasovasostomy. Prior experience showed that earlier return to daily activity resulted in separation of the anastomosed ends of the vas in several patients during repeat vasectomy reversal procedures. The 2-week postoperative prohibition of intercourse is based upon Schmidt's observation that histological sections of canine vasal anastomoses demonstrated virtually complete regeneration of the approximated tissue edges by 2 weeks postoperatively.

OUTCOMES

Complications

Perioperative complications of microsurgical reconstruction of the vas deferens include scrotal bleeding and swelling as well as possible disruption of the vasal anastomosis. Long-term potential complications are vasal obstruction and sperm granulomas.

Results

Results from microvascular vasal reconstruction can be expressed as either spermatozoa in follow-up semen analyses or subsequent pregnancy. The results of modified one-layer microsurgical vasovasostomy and two-layer microsurgical vasovasostomy are comparable (6).

The most important intraoperative factors influencing results are the presence or absence of sperm or sperm parts in the vasal fluid and the gross appearance of the vasal fluid when sperm are absent. The significance of these factors was discussed earlier in this chapter.

An important factor concerning the chance for success of vasovasostomy is the duration of the obstructive interval, which is the time from the vasectomy until its reversal. The Vasovasostomy Study Group reported rates of return of sperm to the semen and of pregnancy, respectively, of 97% and 76% when the obstructive interval was less than 3 years, 88% and 53%, respectively, when the interval was 3 to 8 years, 79% and 44%, respectively, for 9 to 14 years, and 71% and 30%, respectively, for 15 years or longer (6). Patients who have brief obstructive intervals thus are the most favorable candidates for vasovasostomy. A comparable correlation of more favorable pregnancy rates with briefer obstructive intervals was found by Abdelmassih et al., who reported results of epididymal sperm retrieval for IVF with ICSI according to the duration of the obstructive interval after vasectomy and according to the female partner's age (1). They concluded that pregnancy and embryo implantation rates after IVF with ICSI using epididymal sperm from vasectomized men both are more favorable the shorter the time interval is from vasectomy. This correlation could not be explained purely by male or female aging.

Length of the proximal vasal end correlates with intraoperative recovery of spermatozoa and postoperative success of vasovasostomy (14). If the length of the testicular vasal end is longer than 2.7 cm, intact spermatozoa are found in the intraoperative vasal fluid in 94% (30/32) of vasa, whereas if the testicular end vasal remnant is shorter than 2.7 cm intact spermatozoa are found in the intraoperative vasal fluid in only 15% (3/20) vasa.

The presence of a nodule at the transected testicular end of the vas suggests that a sperm granuloma may have formed at this location. Although a sperm granuloma at this site is associated with better intraoperative vasal fluid sperm quality, rates of return of sperm to the semen and of pregnancy after vasovasostomy do not seem to be influenced by the presence or absence of a sperm granuloma at the transected testicular end of the vas (6).

The influence of preoperative antisperm antibodies upon the results of vasovasostomy remains unclear, as previously discussed. My unreported experience has been that the fertility of men after vasovasostomy is influenced infrequently by the presence of such antibodies.

The age and fertility status of the female partner is extremely important in evaluating subsequent pregnancy rates. If the female partner has a history of irregular menses, pelvic inflammatory disease, or previous difficulty achieving a conception, she should have a reproductive gynecologic evaluation to determine the advisability for the male to undergo vasovasostomy. A woman's fertility potential decreases slightly between the ages of 31 and 35 and significantly declines at 36 to 40, while the chance for a pregnancy to occur in a woman older than 40 is extremely low (12). Fuchs and Burt stressed the importance of the female partner's age when microsurgical vasectomy reversal was performed 15 years or longer after the vasectomy. Sixty-two percent of their patients underwent either bilateral vasoepididymostomy or unilateral vasoepididymostomy with contralateral vasovasostomy (7). The overall pregnancy rate was 43% when the obstructive interval was 15 years or longer, and the most important predictor of postoperative pregnancy was the age of the female partner, with a progressive decline in the pregnancy rate as the age of the female partner increased.

REFERENCES

1. Abdelmassih V, Balmaceda JP, Tesarik J, et al. Relationship between time period after vasectomy and the reproductive capacity of sperm obtained by epididymal aspiration. *Hum Reprod* 2002;17:736–740.
2. Belker AM. Infrapubic incision for specific vasectomy reversal situations. *Urology* 1988;32:413–415.
3. Belker AM. Microsurgical vasovasostomy: two-layer technique. In: Goldstein M, ed. *Surgery of male infertility*. Philadelphia: WB Saunders, 1995:61–66.
4. Belker AM. Microsurgical repair of obstructive causes of male infertility. *Sem Urol* 1984;2:91–98.
5. Belker AM. Vasovasostomy. In: Resnick, MI, ed. *Current trends in urology*, vol. 1. Baltimore: Williams & Wilkins, 1981:20–41.
6. Belker AM, Thomas AJ Jr, Fuchs EF, et al. Results of 1,469 microsurgical vasectomy reversals by the Vasovasostomy Study Group. *J Urol* 1991;145:505–511.
7. Fuchs EF, Burt RA. Vasectomy reversal performed 15 years or more after vasectomy: correlation of pregnancy outcome with partner age and with pregnancy results of in vitro fertilization with intracytoplasmic sperm injection. *Fertil Steril* 2002;77:516–519.
8. Kolettis PN, Thomas AJ Jr. Vasoepididymostomy for vasectomy reversal: a critical assessment in the era of intracytoplasmic sperm injection. *J Urol* 1997;158:467–470.
9. Linnet L. Clinical immunology of vasectomy and vasovasostomy . *Urology* 1983;22:101.
10. Lyons RC, Petre JH, Lee CN. Spermatic granuloma of the epididymis. *J Urol* 1967;97:320–323.
11. Pavlovich CP, Schlegel PN. Fertility options after vasectomy: a cost-effectiveness analysis. *Fertil Steril* 1997;67:133–141.
12. Schwartz D, Mayaux BA. Female fecundity as a function of age: results of artificial insemination in 2139 nulliparous women with azoospermic husbands. Federation Cecos. *N Engl J Med* 1996;306:404–406.
13. Silber SJ. Sperm granuloma and reversibility of vasectomy. *Lancet* 1977;2:588–589.
14. Witt MA, Heron S, Lipshultz LI. The post-vasectomy length of the testicular vasal remnant: a predictor of surgical outcome in microscopic vasectomy reversal. *J Urol* 1994;151:892–894.

CHAPTER 57

Microsurgical Varicocelectomy

Shafquat Meraj and Harris M. Nagler

The prevalence of varicoceles in the general population is estimated to be 15%, whereas the prevalence within the infertile population is approximately 40% (9). Despite extensive study, the precise mechanism by which the varicocele leads to male infertility remains unknown. Several theories have been postulated in an attempt to explain the relationship between the varicocele and impaired spermatogenesis. Proposed pathophysiological mechanisms include:

1. Venous stasis leading to hypoxia.
2. Abnormal testicular temperature regulation.
3. Reflux of toxins of either renal or adrenal origin.
4. Changes in the testicular endocrine milieu.

The cofactor hypothesis has also been proposed in an attempt to explain the variable effect of the varicocele on spermatogenesis. This hypothesis states that the deleterious effects of varicoceles may become manifest when varicoceles exist in conjunction with other unidentified gonadotoxins (8). Although the pathophysiology of the varicocele has yet to be elucidated, it continues to be thought of as the most common correctable cause of male infertility. Infertility is the most common indication for varicocelectomy

DIAGNOSIS

The diagnosis of a varicocele is made during an office examination. The most common presentation is an adult male seeking evaluation for infertility. On occasion, the patient may provide a history of dull scrotal ache or heaviness upon prolonged standing. Patients or their partner may be aware of or complain of a scrotal mass. The physical examination should be performed in a warm, well-lit examination room with the patient in a supine and then an upright position. The grading system proposed by Dubin and Amelar (2) is widely employed. Grade 3 varicoceles are visible during physical examination while grade 2

varicoceles are palpable but not grossly visible. Grade 1 varicoceles are detected with the Valsalva maneuver only. A portable Doppler stethoscope may be used during the physical examination to confirm the physical examination findings and differentiate a thickening of spermatic cord associated with the cremasteric reflex from reflux. It is also important to measure the testicular size using an orchidometer to document any disparity in testicular size. This is critical in the examination of an adolescent male in whom the only manifestation of a varicocele might be differential growth of the testicle.

Semen analysis remains the cornerstone in the evaluation of any male with infertility. Abnormalities may be observed in sperm density, morphology, and motility. Improvement in semen parameters after the correction of the varicocele can also be assessed by postoperative semen analysis, which is monitored beginning 4 months after surgery and then every 2 months until it normalizes, a pregnancy ensues, or alternative therapies are employed.

The evaluation of the patient with a varicocele is tailored to the presentation. The infertile male requires a minimum of two baseline semen analyses and routine hormonal evaluation (testosterone, follicle-stimulating hormone, and luteinizing hormone). These studies may or may not be warranted in the evaluation of the symptomatic male with a varicocele. Certainly, the potential impact of a varicocele should be discussed and diagnostic options reviewed. Because varicoceles are in general asymptomatic, the symptomatic patient warrants scrotal ultrasonography to rule out any intrinsic testicular pathology that may be the cause of the patient's symptoms.

INDICATIONS FOR SURGERY

The mere presence of a varicocele in an otherwise asymptomatic male is not an indication for its correction. Some of the common indications for correcting a varicocele include:

1. Abnormal semen parameters or abnormal sperm function tests in an infertile male when the partner is thought to be fertile.
2. Impaired testicular growth in an adolescent.
3. Testicular pain associated with varicoceles in the absence of other pathology.
4. Cosmetic reasons.
5. Psychological concerns regarding future fertility.

Although some investigators still question the relationship between varicoceles and male infertility, the majority of studies support the surgical correction of varicoceles in infertile males with varicoceles and impaired semen parameters. A review of the literature supporting or refuting the role of varicocelectomy in the treatment of the infertile male is beyond the scope of this chapter. Suffice it to say that of the infertile males who undergo varicocelectomy approximately two-thirds demonstrate improved semen parameters and ultimately 30% to 50% of these couples are able to achieve pregnancy (10).

ALTERNATIVE THERAPY

Several different surgical approaches have been described for the ligation of the dilated spermatic veins. The most common approaches employed include inguinal, subinguinal, retroperitoneal, and laparoscopic. In the European community an antegrade scrotal sclerotherapy approach is also employed. While the efficacy in terms of improving semen parameters when the varicocelectomy is technically successful is in general comparable among these different approaches, the complication rates do vary significantly (1).

We employ the subinguinal approach and perform the dissection of the spermatic veins, artery, and lymphatic vessels with the assistance of a surgical microscope and Doppler sonography. The enhanced magnification along with the Doppler sonogram is essential to the meticulous dissection and proper identification of all vessels and lymphatic channels. This meticulous dissection minimizes the chances of recurrence and the formation of hydroceles—the two most common complications of nonmicrosurgical varicocelectomy. Although excellent exposure to the spermatic cord can be obtained using either the inguinal or subinguinal incisions, the subinguinal incision obviates the need for incision of the aponeurosis of the external oblique muscle. This decreases operative time and minimizes the chance of ilioinguinal nerve injury. In addition, this approach leads to less postoperative pain and faster recovery. This approach will be described in detail in this chapter.

SURGICAL TECHNIQUE

As discussed above, several surgical techniques have been described for the correction of varicoceles. We pre-

fer the subinguinal approach as described by Marmar et al. (5). The inguinal area is prepped and draped in the standard sterile fashion. We do not recommend the use of routine prophylactic antibiotics.

A small transverse incision is made just inferior to the level of the external ring result (Fig. 57–1). In the case of bilateral varicocelectomies the incision should be symmetrical, thereby resulting in a more cosmetically acceptable result. These incisions should be marked prior to prepping and draping the patient to assure appropriate placement and symmetry of the incisions (for bilateral incisions).

The Campers and Scarpa's fascia is divided using electrocautery. Roux retractors or a self-retaining retractor provides access to the spermatic cord as it traverses the pubic tubercle. The spermatic cord is then bluntly mobilized. The retractors are removed and the surgeon's index finger is passed beneath the spermatic cord (Fig. 57–2). This maneuver is facilitated by rolling the spermatic cord over the operating surgeon's index finger with a Mixter or peanut sponge. Once the cord has been adequately mobilized a Penrose drain is passed beneath the spermatic cord. Gentle traction on the Penrose elevates the spermatic cord to the level of the incision. Care should be taken to avoid overzealous retraction as this may result in occlusion of the spermatic artery. The ilioinguinal nerve is identified and gently retracted away from the field of dissection, ideally placing it outside of the field behind the Penrose drain.

The external spermatic fascia is then opened in the direction of the fibers using bipolar electrocautery. The use of bipolar electrocautery minimizes the potential for thermal injury to adjacent structures. The vas deferens is then identified and a white vessel loop is placed around it (Fig. 57–3).

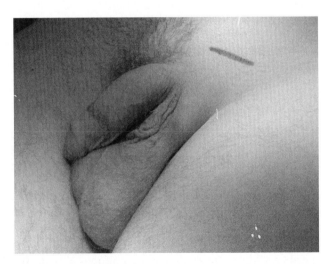

FIG. 57–1. Location of the subinguinal incision. The incision measures approximately 3 cm and is located just inferior to the level of the external ring.

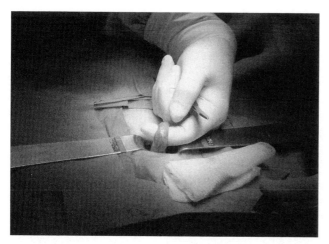

FIG. 57–2. The inguinal cord is lifted to the level of the incision and a Penrose drain is placed around it.

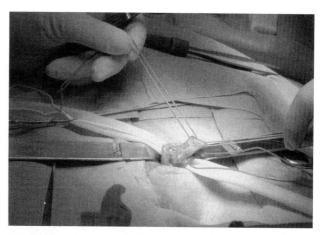

FIG. 57–4. The vas deferens is encircled with a white vessel loop. The bundle of vessels containing the testicular artery is tagged with a red vessel loop. A blue vessel loop is used to identify the veins.

The vascular packet within the spermatic cord is immediately visualized. The internal spermatic artery and the surrounding veins are usually easily identified at this point. We employ multiple vessel loops of different colors to aid in the dissection and identification of the veins, artery, vas, and lymphatics (Fig. 57–4). The location of the internal spermatic artery is then confirmed with a handheld intraoperative Doppler device. The remainder of the venous channels are then encircled with a blue vessel loop.

If the artery is clearly identified, the larger veins can be clipped or ligated and then divided. A representative segment of a vein is submitted for pathologic confirmation. The dissection to this point can be safely performed under the magnification of surgical loupes. However, the more delicate dissection and skeletonization of the testicular artery are performed with the assistance of the surgical microscope.

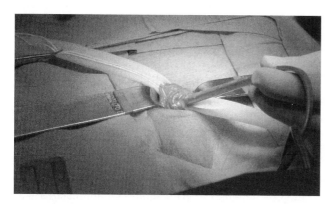

FIG. 57–3. The external cremasteric fascia is opened. A white vessel loop encircles the vas deferens, which is gently retracted. A handheld Doppler device is used to make a preliminary assessment of the testicular artery.

A successful varicocelectomy requires that the artery be skeletonized and that all other blood vessels are divided. This approach prevents the complications of recurrence, testicular injury, and hydrocele formation. These goals are accomplished by continuing the dissection under the operating microscope. Small-caliber arteries can often vasoconstrict during the manipulation. A small amount of papaverine can relieve the vasoconstriction and aid in the proper identification and isolation of the artery visually and with Doppler sonography. It is not unusual to encounter minor bleeding during the dissection of the blood vessels. Local pressure with a peanut sponge or gauze is usually sufficient to control this bleeding. For the more recalcitrant bleeders, a small amount of Avatine is adequate. When necessary a bipolar cautery may be employed. This is rarely necessary.

The use of a surgical clip applier significantly reduces operating time, especially when multiple veins are encountered. All venous channels should be either clipped or ligated and then divided. The spermatic, cremasteric, and deferential arteries are preserved, as are the lymphatics. The lymphatics are easily identified under the operation microscope and should be preserved to prevent the formation of a hydrocele (Fig. 57–5).

Once all the venous channels are ligated, the area external to the spermatic cord is examined for the presence of external cremasteric vessels. Upward traction on the Penrose drain will expose these vessels, which are seen perforating the floor of the canal and entering the cord distally. External cremasteric veins are clipped and divided while the arteries are preserved.

The incision site is then irrigated with normal saline and the cord structures are returned to their normal anatomic position. Gentle traction of the ipsilateral testicle allows the testicle and the cord to return to their nor-

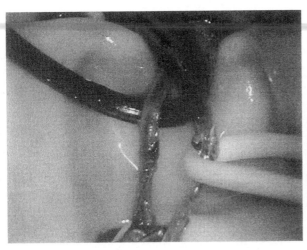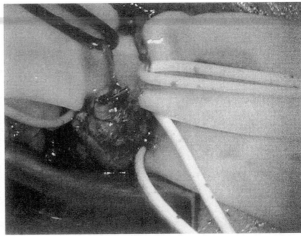

FIG. 57–5. As seen under the magnification of a surgical microscope, the testicular artery and the lymphatics are identified and spared. The darker (red) vessel loop is around the testicular artery

mal anatomic position. Pieces of Surgicel applied around the spermatic cord may help in achieving further hemostasis.

The Scarpa's fascia is closed using 3-0 plain stitches and the skin is approximated using 4-0 Monocryl sutures in a subcuticular fashion. A sterile dressing consisting of steristrips and Tegaderm is applied over the incision sites.

OUTCOMES

Complications

The complications following surgical correction of varicoceles may be divided into immediate and long-term complications. Immediate or perioperative complications are common to any type of surgery and include infection, bleeding, and/or hematoma formation. The infection rate associated with varicocele repair is extremely low and routine use of antibiotics is not encouraged. Testicular ischemia due to inadvertent injury to the testicular artery can manifest itself as severe testicular pain. The incidence of testicular ischemia following varicocele ligation is very low secondary to the presence of multiple arteries that supply the testes. In addition to the testicular artery, the vasal and cremasteric arteries contribute to the blood supply of the testicle.

The formation of hydrocele can be a common complication following varicocelectomy. Hydrocele formation occurs due to lymphatic obstruction during a varicocele repair when the lymphatic vessels are not properly identified and ligated with the spermatic and cremasteric veins. Greater magnification of the surgical microscope allows identification and preservation of the lymphatic vessels, thereby significantly decreasing the risk of hydrocele formation to less than 1% (8).

The incidence of varicocele recurrence is dependent upon the technique employed during the surgical repair. The highest rates have been associated with the retroperitoneal approach, which is commonly used for the repair of pediatric varicoceles (7). Even the smaller collateral veins that are left undivided can enlarge over time and lead to varicocele recurrence. In addition, this approach does not provide access to the external cremasteric vessels, which have been reported to be present in approximately 10% of patients (4). The microsurgical approach again allows the proper identification and ligation of even the smallest of veins. The incidence of varicocele recurrence with the microsurgical approach is well below 1% (6).

Results

Sixty percent to 80% of men will have improvement in their semen parameters following varicocelectomy. Of these, 20% to 60% are able to achieve pregnancy with their partners (10). Madgar et al. (3) showed a pregnancy rate of 44% at 1 year in a group of men who were surgically treated for varicoceles, while a control group who decided to forgo surgery had a pregnancy rate of only 10%.

Although controversial, studies have also shown that the size of the varicocele relates to the improvement that is seen in semen parameters following surgery. Steckel et al. (11) reported that men with grade 3 varicoceles had lower sperm counts compared to grade 2 and 1 varicoceles and showed a significantly better improvement in sperm count following microsurgical varicocelectomy than the men with smaller varicoceles.

Surgery for relief of pain should be approached with caution. However, Yaman et al. (12) showed complete resolution of pain in 88% of 119 patients who underwent subinguinal microsurgical varicocelectomy for painful varicoceles.

In conclusion, microsurgical varicocelectomy is a safe and effective procedure for the treatment of male infertility associated with varicoceles. It can be performed on an outpatient basis with minimal morbidity and excellent long-term outcome.

REFERENCES

1. Barbalias GA, Liatsikos EN, Nikiforidis G, et al. Treatment of varicocele for male infertility: a comparative study evaluating currently used approaches. *Eur Urol* 1998;34:393–398.
2. Dubin L, Amelar RD. Varicocele. *Urol Clin North Am* 1978;5:563–572.
3. Madgar I, Weissenberg R, Lunenfeld B, et al. Controlled trial of high spermatic vein ligation for varicocele in infertile men. *Fertil Steril* 1995;63:120–124.
4. Mali W, Oei H, Arndt J, et al. Hemodynamics of the varicocele. Part I & II. Correlation among the clinical, phlebographic and scintigraphic findings. *J Urol* 1986;135:483–493.
5. Marmar JL, DeBenedictis TJ, Praiss D, et al. The management of varicoceles by microdissection of the spermatic cord at the external inguinal ring. *Fertil Steril* 1985;43:583–588.
6. Marmar JL, Kim Y. Subinguinal microsurgical varicocelectomy: a technical critique and statistical analysis of semen and pregnancy data. *J Urol* 1994;152:1127–1132.
7. Misseri R, Gershbein AB, Horowitz M, et al. The adolescent varicocele II: the incidence of hydrocele and delayed recurrence after varicocelectomy in the long-term follow up. *Br J Urol* 2001;87:494–498.
8. Peng BC, Tomashefsky P, Nagler HM. The cofactor effect: varicocele and infertility. *Fertil Steril* 1990;54:143–148.
9. Pryor JL, Howards SS. Varicocele. *Urol Clin North Am* 1987;14:499–513.
10. Schlesinger MH, Wilets IF, Nagler HM. Treatment outcome after varicocelectomy. A critical analysis. *Urol Clin North Am* 1994;21:517–529.
11. Steckel J, Dicker AP, Goldstein M. Relationship between varicocele size and response to varicocelectomy. *J Urol* 1993;149:769–771.
12. Yaman O, Ozdiler E, Anafarta K, et al. Effect of microsurgical subinguinal varicocele ligation to treat pain. *Urology* 2000;55:107–108.

CHAPTER 58

Testis Biopsy and Testicular Sperm Extraction (TESE): Microscopic and Macroscopic Techniques

Carin V. Hopps and Peter N. Schlegel

The field of male infertility has progressed rapidly with modifications not only in the technique of testicular biopsy but also in the indications for biopsy. Testicular biopsy may be done percutaneously or with an open approach. It may be done to diagnose various abnormalities of spermatogenesis or intratubular germ cell neoplasia. Biopsy can also be utilized as a therapeutic testicular sperm extraction (TESE) technique to retrieve spermatozoa for use in *in vitro* fertilization (IVF) with intracytoplasmic sperm injection (ICSI), wherein a single spermatozoon is injected directly into an oocyte. The observation that seminiferous tubules containing sperm can be differentiated from those tubules with impaired or absent spermatogenesis based upon appearance under the microscope led to the introduction of microdissection TESE. This technique provides optimal sperm retrieval rates despite removal of a limited volume of tissue in patients with limited sperm production (5).

DIAGNOSIS

Of men who present for fertility evaluation, those with azoospermia may require a testis biopsy to determine the etiology of azoospermia so that options for treatment can be delineated. The diagnosis of azoospermia is made when centrifugation of the semen specimen at 3000 g for 15 minutes and thorough examination of the pellet reveals no sperm on two semen analyses obtained at least 4 weeks apart. Thorough reproductive history, medical history, physical examination, and hormone evaluation contribute significantly to determination of the etiology of azoospermia. Elevated follicle-stimulating hormone (FSH) and soft testes measuring less than 10 cc in volume associated with a flat epididymis are typical findings in nonobstructive azoospermia secondary to primary testic-

ular failure. Low testosterone, low FSH, and low luteinizing hormone (LH) are diagnostic of hypogonadotropic hypogonadism (secondary testicular failure), which should be treated medically before consideration of biopsy. Normal FSH and normal testicular volume are associated with obstructive azoospermia. Although the etiology of azoospermia can be determined based upon clinical evaluation for most patients, rarely diagnostic testis biopsy may be necessary to distinguish between obstructive and nonobstructive azoospermia.

INDICATIONS FOR SURGERY

Testis Biopsy

The most common indication for open testis biopsy is differentiation of obstructive from nonobstructive azoospermia in cases where the diagnosis is not clinically obvious. Men in whom the diagnosis is unclear usually have normal semen volume, normal testis size and consistency, palpable vasa deferentia, and a normal hormone profile. Biopsy is performed bilaterally regardless of testicular size or size discrepancy. Evidence of congenital bilateral absence of the vas deferens on physical examination (with normal FSH and testicular volume) precludes the need for biopsy, as these patients reliably have normal sperm production.

Diagnostic biopsy that reveals nonobstructive azoospermia can provide predictive value for sperm retrieval rates with microdissection TESE. The most advanced pattern, but not the predominant pattern, of spermatogenesis found on biopsy can predict the chances of successful sperm retrieval. When hypospermatogenesis, maturation arrest, or Sertoli cell only are found as the most advanced pattern of spermatogenesis on the biopsy, sperm retrieval rates are 79%, 47%, and 24%, respectively (8). Although parameters such as testicular volume and serum FSH have not been found to correlate with the chance of finding sperm by TESE (6), complete deletions of the AZFa or AZFb region of the Y chromosome portends a very poor prognosis for sperm retrieval (1). In summary, diagnostic biopsy should be done if the etiology of azoospermia is unclear, intratubular germ cell neoplasia is suspected, or results of the biopsy will affect the couple's decision to undergo TESE–ICSI. A couple that will proceed with ICSI only if the chance for sperm retrieval is above 24% (as seen with Sertoli-cell-only histology) should have a biopsy done to avoid unnecessary ovarian hyperstimulation.

Diagnostic testis biopsies should be quantitatively analyzed to evaluate the level of sperm production within the testis. Seminiferous tubules cut in perfect cross-section are identified and the number of condensed, oval spermatids per tubule are counted. Men with normal spermatogenesis will have an average of greater than 10 to 15 oval, condensed spermatids per tubule identified. Men with less than 5 spermatids per tubule on average may have inadequate sperm production for sperm to reach the ejaculate, even if an obstruction is identified and corrected. Patients with a limited number of tubules (as may be seen after percutaneous biopsy) or an indeterminate number of spermatids per tubule (5 to 10) may not be unequivocally diagnosed with obstructive or nonobstructive azoospermia.

Testicular Sperm \Extraction

Men with obstructive azoospermia who have obstruction of the excurrent ductal tract not amenable to surgical reconstruction, men who elect to forego surgical reconstruction, and couples for whom ICSI is indicated secondary to female factor infertility, such as advanced female age, may benefit from sperm retrieval techniques. Microepididymal sperm aspiration (MESA) yields the largest number of high-quality spermatozoa in men with obstructive azoospermia and normal spermatogenesis and is indicated for those couples who wish to have sufficient aliquots of sperm for multiple ICSI cycles, precluding the need for multiple percutaneous procedures. MESA is an open procedure that requires the experience of a surgeon trained in microsurgical technique. However, if a patient wishes to avoid an open procedure, a microsurgeon is not available, or the couple plans to proceed with only one ICSI cycle then a percutaneous sperm retrieval technique is appropriate in the patient with obstructive azoospermia. Percutaneous procedures include testicular fine-needle aspiration (TFNA), percutaneous epididymal sperm aspiration (PESA), and percutaneous testicular biopsy (PercBiopsy). Of the percutaneous procedures, PercBiopsy, performed with a 14-gauge biopsy needle, yields the greatest number of sperm with superior motility (7) and therefore is the authors' preference over other percutaneous techniques. Percutaneous procedures overall are associated with a slightly higher incidence of complications when compared with open procedures.

Because spermatogenesis in men with nonobstructive azoospermia is focal, the efficacy of random testicular biopsy is limited. Only 28% of men will have sperm found on the first random biopsy compared with 58% who will have sperm found with an average of 8.9 biopsy attempts overall (6.4 biopsies for those in whom sperm were retrieved) (4). Sperm may not be found until the fourteenth random biopsy. A controlled comparison of microdissection TESE versus random biopsies demonstrated that approximately one-third of men with sperm present in the testes will have unsuccessful treatment with random biopsies alone (5). In addition, greater yield of sperm was achieved with less tissue removed when microdissection TESE was applied. Removal of minimal Leydig cell volume is important to preserve testosterone production in these men with diminished testis volume. Spermatozoa have not been found within the testes of men with complete deletion of the AZFa or AZFb region of the Y chromosome in our experience and, as such, these microdeletions represent a significantly adverse prognostic finding for treatment of these men (1). Thus, microdissection TESE is the sperm retrieval technique indicated for men with nonobstructive azoospermia with the exception of those with microdeletion of the AZFa or AZFb region of the Y chromosome.

ALTERNATIVE THERAPY

There are no alternatives to these techniques that will yield comparable information.

SURGICAL TECHNIQUE

Open Testis Biopsy

Testis biopsy performed for the purpose of histological diagnosis or sperm retrieval may be done under local, regional, or general anesthesia. When local anesthesia is employed, a cord block is necessary. The cord is stabilized between the thumb and index finger and 5.0 cc of 1% lidocaine or 0.25% bupivacaine is instilled with a 25-gauge needle, taking care not to inject into a vascular structure. The skin and dartos muscle are also infiltrated with lidocaine or bupivacaine at the site of planned incision.

The testis is held firmly with the skin drawn tightly over the testis and a 1.5-cm transverse skin incision is made between blood vessels coursing transversely (Fig. 58–1). If bilateral testis biopsy is planned, two symmetrical scrotal incisions or one median raphe incision can be made to access both testes through one incision. The incision is deepened through the dartos muscle until tunica vaginalis is exposed. The tunica vaginalis is incised and each edge grasped with a hemostat to prevent retraction and facilitate later closure (Fig. 58–2). A stay suture is passed through the tunica albuginea to prevent retraction of the testis.

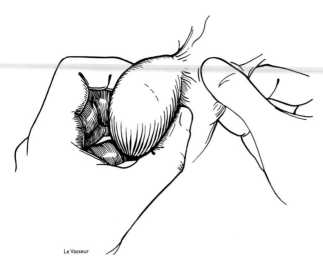

Le Vasseur

FIG. 58–1. Open testis biopsy. The skin is held tightly against the testis and a 1.5-cm skin incision is made transversely between cutaneous blood vessels (blood vessels not pictured). For bilateral biopsy, two symmetrical incisions can be made or one incision along the median raphe, through which both testes can be accessed.

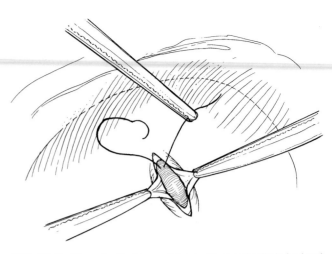

FIG. 58–2. Open testis biopsy. The tunica vaginalis is incised and the edges secured with hemostats. A stay suture is placed through the tunica albuginea.

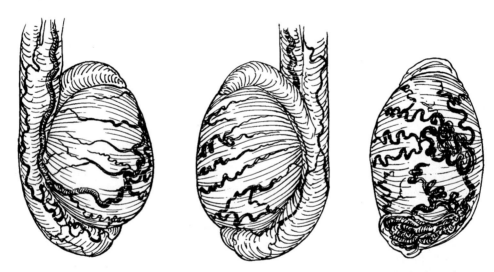

FIG. 58–3. Blood supply enters the testicular parenchyma near the efferent ducts, but also courses transversely in a series of end arteries subjacent to the tunica albuginea before delving into the parenchyma. (From Schlegel PN. Microsurgical techniques of epididymal and testicular sperm retrieval. *Atlas Urol Clin North Am* 1999;7:109–129, with permission.)

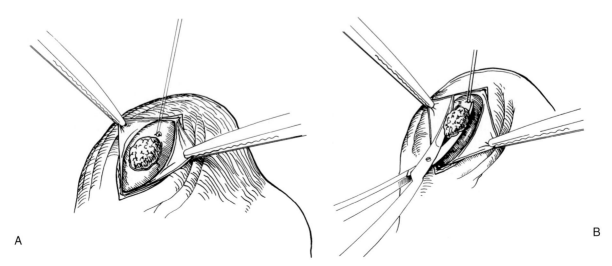

A

B

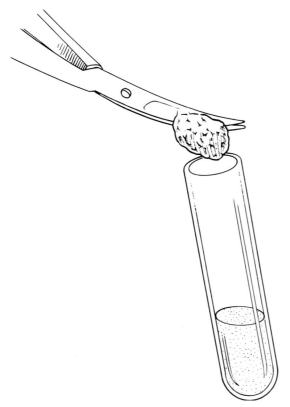

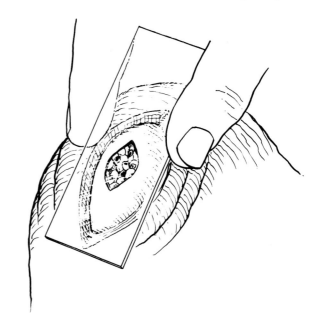

FIG. 58–6. Touch-prep cytological examination. A slide is touched to the cut surface of epididymal tubules. This fluid is examined under a bench microscope for the presence of sperm.

FIG. 58–5. The testis biopsy is placed into Bouin's solution for histological diagnosis or into human tubule fluid medium for cryopreservation. Formalin should never be used.

Blood supply to the testis enters the parenchyma near the efferent ducts and also courses subjacent to the tunica albuginea in a series of end arteries that enter the parenchyma at different levels (Fig. 58–3). Multiple incisions made within the tunica albuginea with numerous blind biopsies may disrupt the blood supply to the parenchyma, resulting in devascularization and atrophy. Testis biopsy performed with the operating microscope, providing 6 to 25× magnification, has been shown to result in significantly fewer complications such as hematoma formation and testicular atrophy when compared with a nonmicroscopic approach (2). Therefore, optical magnification is recommended for making an incision in the tunica albuginea for testis biopsy.

A relatively avascular area of the tunica albuginea is selected for the 0.5- 1.0-cm incision, which is made with a microknife, taking care to avoid vessels subjacent to the tunica albuginea. Bleeding from the transsection of small vessels may be controlled with bipolar electrocautery. With gentle pressure on the testis, the parenchyma exudes from the incision (Fig. 58–4A), and with a razor-sharp

curved Iris scissor a wedge of tissue can be easily excised (Fig. 58–4B). A biopsy done for histological diagnosis should immediately be placed in Bouin's solution, and a specimen for sperm retrieval is placed in human tubule fluid medium (Fig. 58–5). *Testicular tissue should never be placed in formalin as it severely distorts testicular cytoarchitecture.*

Following the biopsy, touch-prep cytological evaluation may be done to assess the biopsied region for the presence of spermatozoa (Fig. 58–6). A glass slide is simply touched to the cut surface of the testis, a coverslip is placed on top of the fluid, and the slide is examined under a separate bench light microscope under 400× magnification for the presence of sperm. An alternative to the touch prep is squash-prep cytological examination. A small piece of testicular parenchyma is removed through the same tunical incision and is placed onto a glass slide (Fig. 58–7). The tissue is teased apart with two 25-gauge needles, a coverslip is placed over the minced tissue, and the slide is examined under the microscope for the presence of sperm.

The incision in the tunica albuginea is closed with interrupted or running 5-0 polypropylene sutures. Permanent sutures are used to mark the biopsy site in the case that future sperm retrieval is necessary. The tunica vaginalis is reapproximated with running 5-0 Vicryl, the dar-

FIG. 58–4. Open testis biopsy. **A:** An incision is made in the tunica albuginea and parenchyma projects through the incision. **B:** A segment of parenchyma is removed with a sharp, curved Iris scissor.

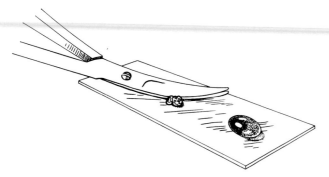

FIG. 58–7. Squash-prep cytological examination. A small piece of testicular tissue is placed onto a glass slide and is vigorously teased apart with two 25-gauge needles before placing a coverslip onto the tissue and examination under the microscope.

tos muscle with running 4-0 Biosyn, and the skin with 5-0 Monocryl in a subcuticular manner. Bacitracin is placed on the skin incision and a scrotal supporter is placed on the patient.

Percutaneous Testis Biopsy

Percutaneous biopsy may be done for sperm retrieval in men with obstructive azoospermia or as a diagnostic procedure. Its value is limited by the small volume of tissue and by the small number of sperm and tubules sampled. This procedure is readily performed in an office setting under local anesthesia with a cord block (see previous section for cord block technique). Once adequate anesthesia is achieved, the scrotal skin is held tightly against the testis. The testis is held between the

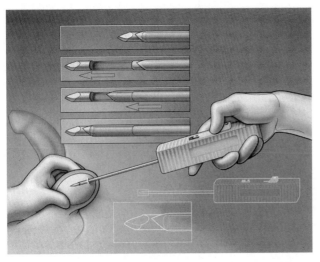

FIG. 58–8. Percutaneous testis biopsy. A 14-gauge biopsy gun is used to obtain a core of parenchyma for sperm retrieval in obstructive azoospermia. (From Sheynkin YR, Schlegel PN. Sperm retrieval for assisted reproductive technologies. *Contemp Urol* 1997;9:21–36, with permission.)

thumb and index finger and a 2-mm incision is made in the scrotal skin with a no. 11 scalpel blade or 16- to 18-gauge needle. The tip of a 14-gauge biopsy gun with 1-cm excursion is passed into the skin incision, advanced through the dartos muscle to the level of the tunica albuginea, and fired in an oblique direction along the longitudinal axis of the testis from the inferior pole toward the rete testis (Fig. 58–8). The biopsy needle is withdrawn and the core of tissue placed into human tubule fluid medium for processing by the IVF laboratory. Multiple biopsies may be done through the same entry site. Pressure is held at the biopsy site for 5 minutes and Bacitracin applied to the skin defect. A scrotal supporter is placed and ice applied to the scrotum after the procedure.

Microdissection Testicular Sperm Extraction

Several factors must be considered prior to sperm retrieval with microdissection TESE. Thorough evaluation of the female partner must be done prior to consideration of TESE to establish suitability of ICSI. Because up to 20% of men with inadequate sperm on preoperative semen analysis will actually have sperm usable for ICSI on the day of oocyte retrieval, a repeat semen analysis should always be performed on the day of planned sperm retrieval, which may allow cancellation of the procedure and use of ejaculated sperm for ICSI. Optimal results may be achieved with the use of fresh sperm, and TESE should ideally be scheduled on the same day as oocyte retrieval or on the day before with incubation of testicular tissue in medium overnight (3). Because sperm production is marginal in nonobstructive azoospermia, TESE should be delayed for at least 6 months following diagnostic testis biopsy, inguinal or scrotal surgery, or previous TESE to allow restoration of spermatogenesis. Finally, microdissection TESE is ideally performed with an embryologist present in the operating room to thoroughly evaluate samples of tissue for the presence of spermatozoa.

Scrotal exploration is performed through a median raphe incision under local, regional, or general anesthesia. If local anesthesia is utilized, cord block (as described for open testis biopsy) with subcutaneous block is provided. To accurately examine the testis and avoid injury to the epididymis, the testis is delivered through the incision. Eight to 15× optical magnification is utilized to visualize the blood vessels subjacent to the tunica albuginea. With a microknife, an incision is made within an avascular region at the midportion of the anterior, lateral, and medial surface of the testis, carefully avoiding capsular vessels as seen under the operating microscope (Figs. 58–9A and 58–9B). The incision should be large enough to directly visualize a wide area of testicular parenchyma (Figs. 58–9C and 58–9D).

The microdissection technique involves removal of very small, 2 to 3 mm, 1 to 5 mg, pieces of testicular tis-

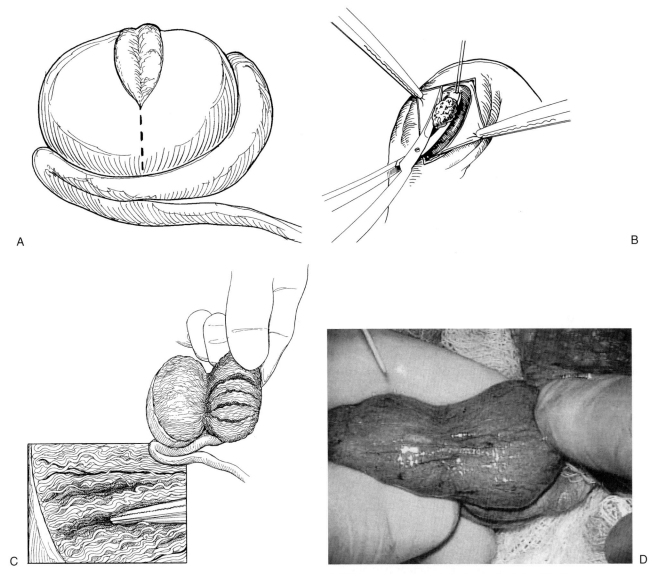

FIG. 58–9. Microdissection TESE. **(A)** Diagram and **(B)** intraoperative photograph depicting the transverse incision made within the tunica albuginea with use of the operating microscope to avoid subtunical vessels. **C, D:** With such an incision, a large surface area of seminiferous tubules may be easily visualized and the septae can be separated for further identification of normal-appearing tubules. (A and C from Hopps CV, Goldstein M, Schlegel PN. The diagnosis and treatment of the azoospermic patient in the age of intracytoplasmic sperm injection (ICSI). *Urol Clin North Am* 2002;29:895–911, with permission.)

sue. Tubules that contain sperm can be identified with an operating microscope at 15 to 25× magnification (Fig. 58–10). The tubules appear larger and more opaque when compared with tubules that do not contain sperm, which appear thin and thread-like. Individual normal tubules can be teased away from the adjacent parenchyma with microsurgical forceps.

The tissue is placed into human tubule fluid culture medium supplemented with 6% Plasmanate. The volume of tissue removed is small, limiting the difficulty of finding sperm within the suspension of tissue in the operating room. To release spermatozoa from within the tubules,

the specimen is cut with Iris scissors and the suspension passed through a 24-gauge angiocatheter to disrupt the tubules. The sample is then examined in the operating room under phase contrast at 200× power to determine if sperm are present in the removed tissue.

The dissection is terminated when it has been reliably determined that enough sperm have been found for use in ICSI. The finding of one sperm in a representative sample of excised tissue by the embryologist may be sufficient to conclude that an adequate number of sperm are present in the remainder of the sample to inject all available oocytes. If no sperm are retrieved, then additional samples of tissue

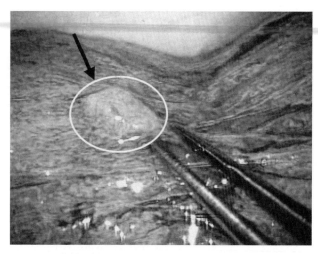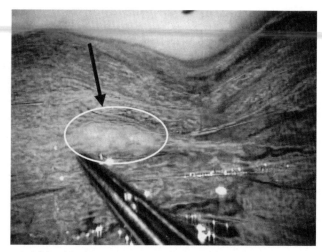

FIG. 58–10. Microdissection TESE. Dilated, opaque tubules (circle) with active spermatogenesis can be differentiated from the surrounding thin, stringy tubules with absent spermatogenesis under 15 to 25× magnification. Individual tubules can be teased away from the surrounding parenchyma with microsurgical forceps and are then prepared to determine the presence of sperm.

are obtained microscopically through the same tunical incision. If sperm are still not found, then a continued search is necessary in the contralateral testis. Extended efforts to remove large numbers of sperm from the testis are of limited value because the sperm may not survive cryopreservation. After ICSI has been performed, excess aliquots of tissue are processed for cryopreservation.

OUTCOMES

Complications

Testis biopsy is rarely associated with complications (2). The most common complications are hematoma formation and testicular atrophy. A hematoma may become large enough to require drainage. Intratesticular bleeding from disruption of subtunical vessels may result in high intratesticular pressures with subsequent ischemia and atrophy. In addition, multiple, poorly placed incisions within the tunica albuginea may disrupt a significant number of end arteries supplying the parenchyma, potentially resulting in testicular atrophy. For this reason, multiple incisions in the tunica albuginea should be avoided whether open testis biopsy or microdissection TESE are employed for sperm retrieval. Both use of the operating microscope to avoid subtunical vessels and bipolar electrocautery for precise hemostasis reduce the incidence of complications. Great care must be taken at time of biopsy to avoid the epididymis, as inadvertent injury to this structure may result in epididymal obstruction. Wound infection is exceedingly rare.

The percutaneous approach to testis biopsy, a blind procedure, may result in injury to the epididymis and the testicular artery. Percutaneous procedures are associated with slightly greater risk of hematoma formation when compared with open procedures.

Results

The sperm retrieval rate with open testis biopsy in men with nonobstructive azoospermia is 45% and increases to 63% with microdissection TESE (5). Microdissection TESE yields a greater number of sperm with less parenchyma removed due to the microsurgical removal of individual tubules rather than removal of a wedge of tissue, as is done with open biopsy. Sperm have also been found by microdissection TESE within the testes of men who have had open biopsies done previously without the finding of sperm.

The type of azoospermia (obstructive vs. nonobstructive) determines the manner in which a couple's infertility is approached as well as the sperm retrieval technique. Open testis biopsy, percutaneous testis biopsy, and microdissection TESE may be very successful sperm retrieval techniques in appropriately selected patients.

REFERENCES

1. Hopps CU, Mielnik A, Goldstein M, et al. Detection of sperm in men with Y chromosome microdeletions of the AZFa, AZFb and AZFc regions. *Hum Reprod* 2003;18:1660–1665.
2. Dardashti K, Williams RH, Goldstein M. Microsurgical testis biopsy: a novel technique for retrieval of testicular tissue. *J Urol* 2000;163: 1206–1207.
3. Levran D, Ginath S, Farhi J, et al. Timing of testicular sperm retrieval procedures and in vitro fertilization–intracytoplasmic sperm injection outcome. *Fertil Steril* 2001;76:380–383.
4. Ostad M, Liotta D, Ye Z, et al. Testicular sperm extraction (TESE) for non-obstructive azoospermia: results of a multi-biopsy approach with optimized tissue dispersion. *Urology* 1998;52:692–697.
5. Schlegel PN. Testicular sperm extraction: Microdissection improves sperm yield with minimal tissue excision. *Hum Reprod* 1999;14:131–135.
6. Seo JT, Ko WJ. Predictive factors of successful testicular sperm recovery in non-obstructive azoospermia patients. *Int J Androl* 2001;24:306–310.
7. Sheynkin YR, Ye Z, Menendez S, et al. Controlled comparison of percutaneous and microsurgical sperm retrieval in men with obstructive azoospermia. *Hum Reprod* 1998; 13:3086–3089.
8. Su LM, Palermo GD, Goldstein M, et al. Testicular sperm extraction with intracytoplasmic sperm injection for nonobstructive azoospermia: testicular histology can predict success of sperm retrieval. *J Urol* 1999;161:112–116.

CHAPTER 59A

Epididymal Sperm Procurement Techniques (Microscopic Epididymal Sperm Aspiration and Percutaneous Epididymal Sperm Aspiration)

David M. Nudell and Larry I. Lipshultz

With the advent of *in vitro* fertilization (IVF) and intracytoplasmic sperm injection (ICSI), the epididymis has become the preferred organ for the surgical procurement of sperm. Highly motile sperm can usually be found that can be used either immediately for an IVF cycle or reliably cryopreserved for future use.

DIAGNOSIS

In patients with either epididymal blockage or congenital absence of the vas deferens (CBAVD), it is critical that genetic testing and counseling be done for cystic fibrosis gene mutations prior to sperm harvesting as these mutations occur in a high number of patients with such anatomic abnormalities. If testis volume on physical exam and serum follicle-stimulating hormone concentrations are normal, a testis biopsy to assess spermatogenesis is usually unnecessary prior to epididymal sperm aspiration (8).

INDICATIONS FOR SURGERY

Epididymal sperm aspiration is usually done in patients following failed vasectomy reversal, patients with blockages of the epididymis, or those with congenital absence of the vas deferens. The goals of epididymal sperm aspiration are to (a) obtain a high number of motile sperm for use in a current IVF cycle, (b) obtain additional sperm to allow cryopreservation for any future cycles, and (c) inflict minimal damage to the epididymal tubules.

ALTERNATIVE THERAPY

There are two methods for the surgical removal of epididymal sperm: Microscopic epididymal sperm aspiration (MESA) and percutaneous epididymal sperm aspiration (PESA). MESA is done through a small, open incision and requires the use of an operating microscope. PESA is done transcutaneously using a butterfly-type needle (Table 59A–1). MESA has the advantage of a more anatomic approach to the epididymal tubule, resulting usually in higher yields of motile sperm. This is especially useful if sperm cryopreservation is desired. Damage to the epididymis is minimized by this direct approach. Disadvantages include the need for an operating microscope and basic microsurgical skills, cost, and patient recovery time. PESA can be done in an office set-

TABLE 59–1. *Comparison of advantages and disadvantages of MESA and PESA procedures*

Procedure	Advantages	Disadvantages
MESA	Anatomic approach to the epididymis Less epididymal damage Higher yield of sperm Cryopreservation possible	Operating eoom and microscope required Cost Longer recovery time
PESA	Office procedure Local anesthesia Cost Shorter recovery time	Blind procedure Multiple excursions of needle often needed Less sperm harvested May not be able to cryopreserve sperm

ting under local anesthesia with or without intravenous sedation but usually results in less sperm harvested, leading to less sperm being available for cryopreservation (1,7). It is important when doing PESA to have a "backup" plan should inadequate quality or numbers of sperm be aspirated by this technique. This usually involves either MESA or aspiration of testicular sperm.

SURGICAL TECHNIQUE

If the procedure is done on the same day as egg retrieval, it is important to coordinate timing between the urologist and reproductive endocrinologist. Optimally, the embryologist who will be performing the IVF procedure should be present to evaluate sperm characteristics in the procedure room. This helps the urologist know when enough high-quality sperm has been aspirated. Alternatively, if the procedure is being done electively prior to the initiation of IVF it is important to evaluate the sperm quality at the time of the procedure to know when adequate numbers of sperm have been obtained. Typically, it is practical to cryopreserve approximately 1 million motile sperm per tube. If multiple tubes are frozen, this allows only one tube to be thawed at the time of each IVF cycle.

In the nonobstructed epididymis, better quality, more mature sperm are usually found in the more distal aspects of the gland (cauda epididymis). In the obstructed epididymis, however, better quality sperm are found much more commonly in the body or even head of the epididymis. Seminal fluid from the distal epididymis in this case is usually devoid of motile sperm and contains a large number of white blood cells. In patients with CBAVD, there is usually only a small epididymal head remnant present, possibly making PESA more difficult to perform than MESA.

MESA

MESA is a microscopic approach to the epididymal tubule followed by controlled aspiration of sperm. Optical magnification using an operating microscope is necessary. Ideally, a microscope with an opposing head at 180 degrees should be used to allow for an assistant to sit across from the surgeon to aid in aspiration. General anesthesia allows for less patient movement, but regional or even local anesthesia can also be used. The procedure is begun on the side with the largest testicular volume or the one in which less surgical procedures have been performed. Adequate numbers of sperm can usually be obtained from one-sided aspiration, but patients should be aware that bilateral aspiration may be necessary. A transverse scrotal incision just large enough to deliver the testis is made down through the tunica vaginalis to deliver the testis and epididymis into the field. It is not necessary to dissect the plane between the tunica vaginalis and the overlying dartos muscle as this will lead to increased postoperative swelling. Techniques in which the epididymis can be directly accessed without complete delivery of the testis have also been described (5). The testis and epididymis are inspected under low-power optical magnification and the epididymis is grasped between the thumb and index finger of the nondominant hand. Under high power, the tunica vaginalis covering the epididymal tubule is incised using a fine microdissecting scissors. This is usually begun in the midcauda epididymis or in obvious areas of epididymal tubule dilation. If areas of dark yellow or green fluid inside the epididymal tubule are seen, these are usually devoid of sperm. It is important to coagulate bleeding vessels from the cut edge of this tunica prior to incising an epididymal tubule to minimize red blood cell contamination of the specimen. This is best accomplished with a microtipped, bipolar forceps.

Prior to incising any tubules, two or three tuberculin (1-mL) syringes are prepared. This is done by placing a small amount (1 to 2 mL) of suitable tissue culture fluid [HTF-HEPES (Irvine Scientific) with soluble-specific substance (Irvine Scientific)] into the bottom of a 5-mL tissue culture tube (Falcon). This "reservoir" of media will act to store sperm during the aspiration and should be kept close to

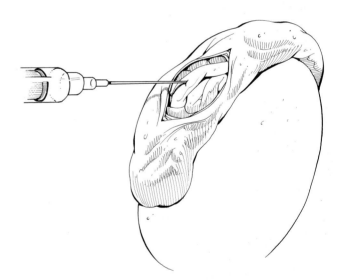

FIG. 59A–1. Microscopic epididymal sperm aspiration (MESA). After the epididymis has been isolated by delivery of the testis, the tunica overlying the epididymal tubule is incised with a curved microscissors under the operating microscope. Small bleeding vessels from the cut edge of the tunica should be coagulated with a fine-tipped bipolar cautery forceps to prevent red blood cell contamination of the specimen. A suitable dilated tubule in the corpus region is chosen and incised with an ophthalmic blade. Expelled contents are aspirated into a tuberculin syringe attached to a 24-guage Angiocath (needle removed). If motile sperm are seen, aspiration is continued in this area. It may be necessary to incise nearby tubules if the output from the initial tubule declines before adequate numbers of sperm are harvested. If no sperm are seen, it is usually necessary to move more proximal in the epididymis until adequate sperm motility is found.

37°C. The tuberculin syringes are capped with 24-gauge Angiocath catheters with the needles removed. Each one is "charged" by drawing up 0.1 mL of media. If this is not done, it will be difficult to expel the aspirated fluid into the reservoir and sperm will be lost in the catheter tip. During the aspiration, the seminal fluid is aspirated into the syringe until the plunger reaches the top. Care must be taken at this point not to disrupt the tip of the Angiocath as most of the sperm will be stored within it and not within the syringe itself. The syringe is inverted over the reservoir and the Angiocath tip advanced down into the reservoir media and the contents are expelled. The syringe is then "recharged" with media form the reservoir itself, thereby preventing the continued dilution of the reservoir fluid that would occur if fresh media were used to charge the catheters each time.

A suitably dilated epididymal tubule is incised using a fine, ophthalmic microblade and the expelled contents immediately examined on a slide under 40× power on a separate microscope. If highly motile sperm are encountered, aspiration can take place in this location (Fig. 59A–1). If no sperm or nonmotile sperm are found in this location, it is necessary to move more proximal in the epididymis until motile sperm are found. Once aspiration begins, gentle pressure is applied to the epididymis proximal to the open tubule with the back end of a jeweler's forceps. It may be necessary to make several separate incisions in one area for the maximum yield of sperm. Periodically, a small drop of fluid from the reservoir is examined to assess sperm quality. Aspiration is continued until the embryologist is satisfied with the yield or until enough motile sperm is present to allow for cryopreservation of several tubes containing approximately 1 million motile sperm each.

If enough sperm have been harvested from one side, the open epididymal tubules are cauterized to prevent continued leakage of sperm. If time permits, the epididymal tunic can be approximated over the tubules with a 9-0 nylon running suture. The testis and epididymis are replaced back into the tunica vaginalis in anatomic manner and the tunica is closed with a running, locking 3-0 absorbable suture. The dartos and skin are then closed with running or interrupted absorbable sutures.

PESA

For PESA, sperm within the epididymal tubule are accessed percutaneously, usually under local anesthesia. As with the MESA procedure, it is important to work closely with the reproductive endocrinologists who should be available at the procedure to assess sperm quality and quantity. This is especially true for PESA when compared to MESA due to the lower overall sperm recovery rates.

PESA is best done with a combination of intravenous sedation and a cord block. After adequate anesthesia, the inferior portion of the testis is stabilized by an assistant and the epididymis is held between the surgeon's thumb and forefinger (Fig. 59A–2). The skin overlying the epididymis is pulled taut. A 21-gauge butterfly needle attached to a 20-mL syringe is inserted into the caput epididymis and withdrawn gently while applying steady backpressure on the plunger until fluid can be seen entering the tubing of the aspiration setup. Once the plunger has reached 20 mL, the tubing is clamped and the needle removed. The syringe is replaced with a 5-mL syringe containing a small amount of tissue culture media (same as used above for MESA) and the contents of the needle and tubing are "backflushed" into a suitable tissue culture tube. A small amount of this fluid is then examined under a microscope (40×) to assess sperm presence and quality. The procedure is repeated until adequate amounts of epididymal fluid are retrieved.

The most significant drawback of PESA is the "blind" nature of the procedure, often requiring multiple, poten-

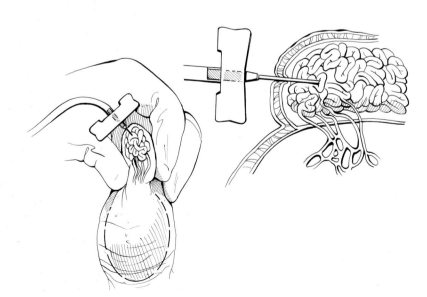

FIG. 59A–2. Percutaneous epididymal sperm aspiration (PESA). After immobilization of the epididymal caput region between the thumb and index finger of the nondominant hand, a 23-guage butterfly needle is inserted into the epididymis, directing the tip from caput to corpus. The needle is gently withdrawn while applying steady backpressure on the syringe plunger until fluid is aspirated. To prevent accidental discharge of the fluid when the plunger is released, the tubing is clamped and a second syringe containing tissue culture media is attached to the tubing. The clamp is removed and the contents of the tubing are expelled by forcing a small amount of media back through the tubing. Often, several passes of the needle will be necessary to obtain adequate numbers of sperm.

tially damaging needle insertions into the epididymis. The delicate, coiled anatomy of the epididymal tubules are easily damaged with such maneuvers. In patients with CBAVD, it may be difficult to access the epididymal head remnant if it is small using percutaneous approaches. However, despite this potential drawback, success rates up to 89% have been reported (3). While PESA may be successful for an initial IVF cycle, future cycles will usually require repeated procedures due to the lower chance of sperm cryopreservation using this technique. Another potential problem with PESA is the contamination of sperm with both white and red blood cells. This can usually be avoided during a MESA procedure and may require additional steps on the part of the reproductive endocrinology team to purify the sperm for successful IVF.

OUTCOMES

Complications

Complications of MESA and PESA are rare and are similar to those encountered after any epididymal procedure. These include skin infection, epididymo-orchitis, and hematoma formation. Injury to the spermatic cord blood vessels is rare, but this would lead to testis atrophy and further impairment to fertility. Both MESA and especially PESA can lead to progressive scarring of the epididymis. This may impair future IVF attempts should they be necessary. This is usually not as critical for patients following MESA as they usually have had large numbers of motile sperm cryopreserved. For PESA patients, this may be only a theoretical risk as multiple aspirations on the same ipsilateral epididymis have been reported to yield good results.

Results

In general, high success rates have been reported for both MESA and PESA with similar fertilization and pregnancy rates per IVF cycle. Success rates for MESA are in the range of 85% to 100% for sperm retrieval for concurrent IVF cycles and 80% to 90% for the ability to cryopreserve excess motile sperm (2,5). For PESA, sperm retrieval rates are slightly lower, ranging from 62% to 95% (1,2). Sperm cryopreservation rates for PESA are not reported in many studies, although in one large study only 54% of patients were able to have sperm cryopreserved (1). The need may arise for repeat PESA in those men who do not undergo sperm cryopreservation if the concurrently performed IVF cycle fails. In these cases, repeat PESA, at least for the first two repeated cycles, appears equally successful as the initial PESA attempt in some studies (3,4,6). Whether continued, repeated percutaneous access to the epididymis results in decreased sperm retrieval rates is not known.

The epididymis has become the preferred organ for sperm harvesting for IVF. This is due to the highly motile and abundant sperm that can be found even in cases of CBAVD, where most of the epididymis is also absent. MESA offers a controlled, microscopic approach that usually results in high enough numbers of sperm for concurrent use in an IVF cycle and cryopreservation of excess sperm. Other advantages include limited damage to the epididymal tubules and less specimen contamination with red blood cells. Disadvantages include patient cost, convenience, and recovery times. PESA is a percutaneous approach to epididymal aspiration that can be done using local anesthesia. Advantages include decreased cost, more rapid recovery, and a lack of need for microscopic skills and equipment. Disadvantages include the common need for multiple, blind needle passes through the epididymis and a less likely chance for sperm cryopreservation. With either approach, it is critical to coordinate the procedure closely with the reproductive endocrinologist so that adequate numbers and quality of sperm are obtained.

REFERENCES

1. Levine LA, Lisek EW. Successful sperm retrieval by percutaneous epididymal and testicular sperm aspiration. *J Urol* 1998;159:437–440.
2. Lin YM, Hsu CC, Kuo TC, et al. Percutaneous epididymal sperm aspiration versus microsurgical epididymal sperm aspiration for irreparable obstructive azoospermia—experience with 100 cases. *J Formos Med Assoc* 2000;99:459–465.
3. Meniru GI, Gorgy A, Podsiadly BT, et al. Results of percutaneous epididymal sperm aspiration and intracytoplasmic sperm injection in two major groups of patients with obstructive azoospermia. *Hum Reprod* 1997;12:2443–2446.
4. Meniru GI, Gorgy A, Batha S, et al. Studies of percutaneous epididymal sperm aspiration (PESA) and intracytoplasmic sperm injection. *Hum Reprod Update* 1998;4:57–71.
5. Nudell DM, Conaghan J, Pedersen RA, et al. The mini-micro-epididymal sperm aspiration for sperm retrieval: a study of urological outcomes. *Hum Reprod* 1998;13:1260–1265.
6. Rosenlund B, Westlander G, Wood M, et al. Sperm retrieval and fertilization in repeated percutaneous epididymal sperm aspiration. *Hum Reprod* 1998;13:2805–2807.
7. Tournaye H. Surgical sperm recovery for intracytoplasmic sperm injection: which method is to be preferred? *Hum Reprod* 1999;14[Suppl 1]:71–81.
8. Tournaye H, Camus M, Vandervorst M, et al. Surgical sperm retrieval for intracytoplasmic sperm injection. *Int J Androl* 1997;20[Suppl 3]:69–73.

Epididymectomy

David M. Nudell and Larry I. Lipshultz

The epididymis is a complex tubular network that connects the testicular efferent ducts to the vas deferens. In total, the single epididymal tubule measures 3 or 4 m. In its coiled form, the epididymal tubule is contained within the tunica vaginalis of the epididymis, creating a cres-cent-shaped organ intimately attached to the posterolateral aspect of the testis. The epididymis is anatomically divided into caput, corpus, and cauda regions (head, body, and tail, respectively) (Fig. 59B–1). While there are histological differences in the delicate epididymal tubule between these regions, there are no gross and discreet dividing lines between the regions. The blood supply to the caput and body of the epididymis arises from a division of the testicular artery. The cauda epididymis is usually supplied by a branch of the vasal artery, but rich anastomotic connections usually exist. The epididymis functions primarily in sperm transport and maturation.

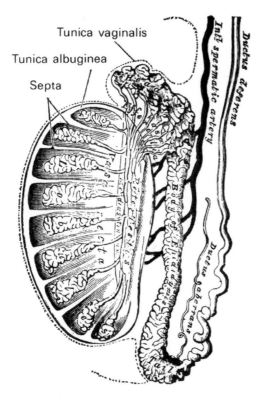

FIG. 59B–1. Sagittal section of the testis and epididymis. The epididymis is seen attached to the posterolateral aspect of the testis. The efferent ducts (vasa efferentia) of the testis consist of 10 to 20 channels draining individual lobes of the testis into the globus major of the epididymis. The epididymal tubule gradually gains more smooth muscle components as it progresses toward the vas deferens, which is seen exiting the inferior, most distal aspects of the epididymis.

DIAGNOSIS

This procedure is performed rarely and the diagnostic steps are individualized to each patient.

INDICATIONS FOR SURGERY

Currently, epididymectomy is done more commonly for complex epididymal cystic disease, chronic scrotal pain, or postvasectomy pain syndromes. Other indications are for abscess or chronic infections of the epididymis.

ALTERNATIVE THERAPY

Surgical removal of all or part of the epididymis is done uncommonly, especially with the availability of broad-spectrum antibiotics. In the past, most cases were performed for abscess, chronic infection, or tuberculosis of the epididymis. In cases of scrotal abscess, the epididymis may be removed in an attempt to save the testis from overwhelming orchitis (1). If tuberculosis is suspected, it is critical to obtain appropriate cultures at the time of surgery.

SURGICAL TECHNIQUE

After administration of appropriate antibiotics if necessary, either general or local anesthesia is induced. If local anesthesia is used, a generous cord block and infiltration of the skin overlying the incision will be adequate. A transverse scrotal incision is made that is just large enough to deliver the testis, epididymis, and distal vas deferens. The initial incision may be carried down through the tunica vaginalis without extensive dissection of the plane between the tunica vaginalis and dartos muscle layer. This will allow delivery of the intravaginal contents. Often, the distal vas deferens can be accessed in this way as well. If extensive scarring or infection has occurred, it may be necessary to dissect the tunica vaginalis free of the dartos muscle layer due to dense adhesions. In these cases, sharp dissection of the testis and epididymis from the undersurface of the tunica vaginalis will usually be necessary as well. In cases performed for postvasectomy pain, it is important to remove the epididymis and vas all the way up to and including the vasectomy site or sperm granuloma (2). If performed for other reasons, the vas may be divided and ligated at the junction of the convoluted and straight vas with an absorbable suture. In patients with complex cystic disease, it is critical to ascertain the patient's desire for future fertility. If fertility is still desired, epididymectomy should be avoided. If surgery is necessary in this situation, the larger cysts should be removed from the epididymis individually with the use of an operating microscope to avoid epididymal tubular obstruction.

After the vas is divided, it is dissected back to the vasoepididymal junction and dissection begun in the plane between the epididymis and the testis (Fig. 59B–2). Optical loupe magnification can be helpful in maintaining the correct plane and avoiding injury to the testis or spermatic cord vessels. The dissection is done sharply with fine Iris-type scissors and Bovie cauterization. The epididymis is grasped between the thumb and index finger of the nondominant hand and elevated off the testis as the dissection progresses from inferior to superior. The epididymal artery may be encountered midway up the dissection of the epididymis, but its exact location may be variable. If encountered, the artery should be ligated. The main spermatic cord blood supply containing the testicular artery will usually be found medial and posterior to the dissection in the region of the head or proximal body of the epididymis (Fig. 59B–2). In cases where the normal anatomy is distorted, it is important to avoid dissection into the spermatic cord as this will lead to testicular infarction and subsequent atrophy. The most superior attachment of the epididymis to the testis consists of the testicular efferent ducts. These can be ligated with a single absorbable suture or cauterized. At this point, the specimen can usually be removed intact.

After irrigating the area, the epididymal bed is inspected closely for bleeding. Vessels can be cauterized or ligated with small, absorbable sutures. The edges of

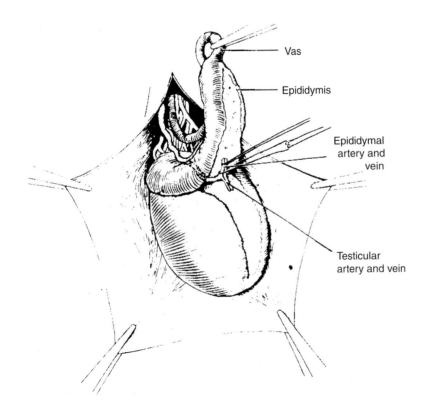

Vas

Epididymis

Epididymal artery and vein

Testicular artery and vein

FIG. 59B–2. Drawing demonstrating the correct plane of dissection during epididymectomy. The main spermatic cord structures are seen posterior and medial as they enter the testis. Injury to these structures can be avoided by dissecting only the plane between the epididymis and testis, which will usually contain only epididymal blood supply. The vascular pedicle to the epididymis may be encountered in the dissection plane between the testis and epididymis. The exact location of this blood supply can be variable.

the tunica along the bed of the epididymis should be approximated with several absorbable sutures for further hemostasis and to prevent leakage of testicular sperm from the efferent ducts. If extensive dissection has been performed or purulent material was encountered, a drain should be left in place that exits in a dependent fashion. Otherwise, the tunica vaginalis is closed with a running absorbable suture followed by closing the dartos layer and skin with interrupted or running absorbable sutures.

OUTCOMES

Complications

Complications of epididymectomy include hematoma formation, orchitis, skin infection, chronic pain, and infertility. Inadvertent injury to the spermatic cord during a difficult dissection may lead to testis atrophy.

Results

The results of epididymectomy vary with the indications for surgery. In patients with complex, symptomatic cystic disease, patient satisfaction is usually high following surgical removal (3). In patients with chronic orchalgia, epididymectomy has produced poor results, with around 50% improvement rates in several series (3–5). This may not be surprising given the high incidence of perineural fibrosis found in the pathology specimens from patients undergoing epididymectomy for pain syndromes (2). However, in well-selected patients satisfaction as high as 90% has been obtained (5). Poor predictors of success include pain extending into the groin region, failure to alleviate pain following a well-placed spermatic cord block, and normal appearance of the epididymis on preoperative ultrasound (5). Selective denervation of the spermatic cord may be another alternative to epididymectomy for chronic pain syndromes (6). This technique involves skeletonizing the spermatic cord surgically, leaving only the vas deferens, a few lymphatic channels, and the testicular artery intact. This procedure is best accomplished through a subinguinal incision with the use of an operating microscope. Long-term results of this relatively new approach remain to be determined.

For patients with postvasectomy pain syndromes, epididymectomy results have been mixed. In general, about 50% of patients report long-term satisfaction and prevention of ongoing pain following epididymectomy (2). As mentioned, it is important in these cases to include the vas deferens up to and including the vasectomy site in the surgical specimen.

Epididymectomy is performed most commonly for complex cystic disease, chronic pain syndromes, postvasectomy pain syndromes, and nonhealing infections. There are slight but important differences in the technique used for each of these indications. For example, during epididymectomy performed for postvasectomy pain syndromes, excision of the proximal vas up to and including the vasectomy site is necessary. This is not necessary in patients with cystic disease or with idiopathic orchalgia. In patients with cystic disease who desire fertility, epididymectomy should be avoided and the larger cysts, if necessary, should be removed microsurgically. In patients with infection, it is important to obtain appropriate intraoperative cultures and insert a dependently directed drain.

REFERENCES

1. Chen TF, Ball RY. Epididymectomy for post-vasectomy pain: histological review. *Br J Urol* 1991;6:407–413.
2. Heidenreich A, Olbert P, Engelmann UH. Management of chronic testalgia by microsurgical testicular denervation. *Eur Urol* 2002;41:392–397.
3. Padmore DE, Norman RW, Millard OH. Analyses of indications for and outcomes of epididymectomy. *J Urol* 1996;156:95–96.
4. Sweeney P, Tan J, Butler MR, et al. Epididymectomy in the management of intrascrotal disease: a critical reappraisal. *Br J Urol* 1998;81:753–755.
5. West AF, Leung HY, Powell PH. Epididymectomy is an effective treatment for scrotal pain after vasectomy. *BJU Int* 2000;85:1097–1099.
6. Witherington R, Harper WM IV. The surgical management of acute bacterial epididymitis with emphasis on epididymotomy. *J Urol* 1982;128:722–725.

Testis

SECTION EDITOR: David A. Sulanson

Anatomy

Sam D. Graham, Jr.

The testes are paired organs suspended in the scrotum by their respective cords. Embryologically, the testes develop at the urgenital ridge and descend into the scrotum via the inguinal canal at birth.

The scrotum is a cutaneous pouch which contains the testes and parts of the spermatic cords. It is divided into two lateral portions by a septum which corresponds the the median raphe on the skin surface. The scrotum is comprised of two layers, the skin which is heavily rugated and dartos tunic. Dartos tunic is a thin layer of muscle continuous with Scarpa's and Camper's fascia (Figure SVII-1).

The cord has several layers of fascia and muscle, the outer layer being the external spermatic fascia which is a continuation of the intracrural fascia from the inguinal ring. Below the external spermatic fascia are the cremasteric muscle fibers which are a continuation of the internal oblique muscle of the abdomen. The transversalis fascia is continued along the cord as the internal spermatic fascia. The tunica vaginalis lines the scrotal compartment with a parietal layer as well as a layer (visceral) overlying the testis. The tunica is a continuation of the peritoneum, but is obliterated through the majority of the cord.

The spermatic cord is a combination of the internal and external spermatic arteries as well as the artery to the vas deferens (Figure SVII-1). The internal spermatic artery is a branch of the abdominal aorta. Though the internal spermatic artery is the main supply to the substance of the testes, it branches to supply the epididymis and vas deferens as well as freely anastamoses with the artery of the vas deferens. The external spermatic artery is a branch of the inferior epigastric artery and supplies the coverings of the cord as well as anastamoses with the internal spermatic artery. The artery of the vas deferens is a branch of the superior vesical artery.

The venous structures of the cord include the spermatic veins which emerge from the back of the testis and coalesce with tributaries from the epididymis. As they progress up the cord, they form a convoluted plexus (pampiniform plexus). The plexus unites below the inguinal ring to form three or four veins and continue to combine to one or two veins within the abdomen. On the right, the spermatic vein enters the vena cava at an acute angle, while the left spermatic vein joins the left renal vein.

The testes are suspended in the scrotum by the cords, the left usually being lower than the right. The average testicle is 4 cm to 5 cm in length, approximately 2.5 cm in width and 3 cm deep. The epididymis is attached to the posterior testicle and consists of three portions–the head, the body, and the tail which is continuous with the vas deferens (Figure SVII-2). The head of the epididymis is attached to the convoluted tubules of the testes at the mediastinum testes (Figure SVII-3).

There are three coverings of the testes–the tunica vaginalis, the tunica albuginea, and the tunica vasculosa. The tunica vaginalis is the serous covering of the testis that is the continuation of the peritoneum. The tunica albuginea is the fibrous covering of the testis and is a dense membrane. Excepting where the epididymis attaches to the testicle at its posterior border, the entire tunica albuginea is covered by the tunica vaginalis. Internally thetestis has numerous septae that segment the convoluted tubules.

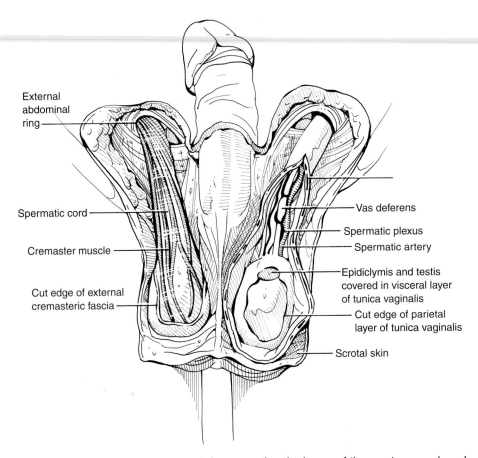

External
abdominal
ring

Spermatic cord

Cremaster muscle

Cut edge of external
cremasteric fascia

Vas deferens

Spermatic plexus

Spermatic artery

Epidiclymis and testis
covered in visceral layer
of tunica vaginalis

Cut edge of parietal
layer of tunica vaginalis

Scrotal skin

FIG. SVII–1. Anatomy of the testis and cord demonstrating the layers of the scrotum, cord, and scrotal compartments.

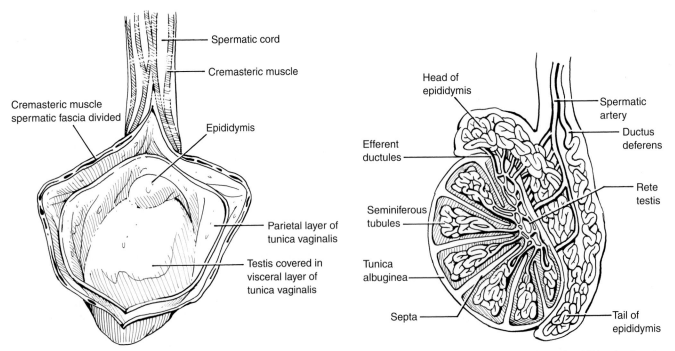

Spermatic cord

Cremasteric muscle

Cremasteric muscle
spermatic fascia divided

Epididymis

Parietal layer of
tunica vaginalis

Testis covered in
visceral layer of
tunica vaginalis

Head of
epididymis

Spermatic
artery

Ductus
deferens

Efferent
ductules

Seminiferous
tubules

Rete
testis

Tunica
albuginea

Septa

Tail of
epididymis

FIG. SVII–2. The scrotal compartment with the layers as well as the appendages of the testis and epididymis.

FIG. SVII–3. Dissection of the testis and epididymis showing the relationships of the vessels and the connection of the epididymis to the convoluted tubules at the rete testes.

CHAPTER 60

Simple Orchiectomy

Sherri M. Donat

Simple orchiectomy involves the removal of one or both testes at the distal cord, usually through an anterior transscrotal approach although it has also been described through a transpubic approach (8). It is used in the treatment of benign intrascrotal processes and as a method of hormonal ablative therapy in patients with advanced prostate cancer.

Among men in the United States, prostate cancer is the most commonly diagnosed malignancy, with 189,000 new cases identified in 1996 and approximately 30,200 deaths attributed to it (1). Since Huggins and Hodges first demonstrated the therapeutic benefit of hormonal ablation in the treatment of advanced prostate cancer, bilateral scrotal orchiectomy has been commonly utilized as a means of removing the testosterone-producing tissue, thereby bringing serum levels to castrate levels (6). Although it has been by tradition used only for treatment in patients with advanced or metastatic disease, it is currently being evaluated for patients with presumed localized disease in both neoadjuvant and adjuvant settings to determine if it has any benefit in decreasing the chance of local or systemic recurrence and improving survival when used in combination with the traditional monotherapies of surgery or radiation (3).

DIAGNOSIS

The initial diagnosis of prostate cancer is usually made through a combination of digital rectal exam, prostate-specific antigen level, patient symptoms, and transrectal ultrasound-directed biopsy, although it is on occasion found incidentally on transurethral resection for obstructive benign disease. Advanced disease may involve lymph nodes, bone, or, less commonly, visceral or soft-tissue lesions and may be documented by physical exam, elevated prostatic acid phosphatase levels, abnormal bone scan, computed tomography scan, magnetic resonance imaging, plain film bone survey, or chest x-ray. Lymph node involvement may be determined by biopsy of enlarged nodes seen on imaging studies or unexpectedly during the pelvic lymph node dissection for a radical prostatectomy.

Benign intrascrotal processes such as epididymal orchitis or devitalization of testicular tissue by trauma or torsion are diagnosed by physical exam, patient symptoms, nuclear testicular exams, color Doppler ultrasonic exam, and/or surgical exploration. In general, inflammatory processes show increased flow on both nuclear scans and Doppler flow studies and processes causing devascularization show decreased or no flow on nuclear and Doppler flow studies. However, if there is any question as to whether an acute scrotum represents a testicular torsion versus an epididymal orchitis it should be surgically explored immediately to answer the question and render the appropriate treatment.

INDICATIONS FOR SURGERY

The primary indication for bilateral scrotal orchiectomy is advanced prostate cancer requiring hormonal ablation as treatment. Other indications for simple orchiectomy include benign intrascrotal disorders such as a traumatic injury to the testis requiring partial or complete removal of the devitalized tissue, testicular necrosis following prolonged torsion, and severe epididymal orchitis that is refractory to antimicrobial therapy.

Removal of testicular neoplasms through a transscrotal approach is contraindicated because of the increased risk of local recurrence; therefore, if there is any question of a testicular mass it should be approached through an inguinal incision.

ALTERNATIVE THERAPY

There are now several agonist analogs of gonadotropin-releasing hormone that inhibit the pituitary gonadal axis, resulting in the downregulation of luteinizing hormone-releasing hormone receptors and subsequent decrease in gonadotropin secretion. These are equally effective in achieving hormonal ablation and provide an alternative to orchiectomy in patients for whom the psychological implications of the surgery are too great (3). The cost effectiveness of surgery is certainly superior to chemical castration. Alternatives to the total removal of the testis and epididymis have been explored and include subcapsular orchiectomy and subepididymal orchiectomy (2,5,7,11). These give the cosmetic effect of a testis being present but also achieve the therapeutic goal of androgen ablation. There has been some controversy (9) over the efficacy of subcapsular orchiectomy since it was first described in 1942 by Riba (11); however, multiple modern studies have demonstrated its efficacy and suggest that any residual testosterone production is most likely a result of incomplete removal of the intratesticular contents (2). Testicular prostheses are also available for use in patients who desire a better cosmetic result, and may be placed in either the tunica vaginalis or within the tunica albuginea (12). Kihara and Oshima (7) have also described an epididymal-sparing orchiectomy with insertion of a pedicled fibrofatty tissue graft to preserve scrotal cosmesis after bilateral orchiectomy. This type of procedure may be complicated by epididymitis, which can be minimized by performing a vasectomy at the same time of the procedure (5). Advantages of a fibrofatty tissue graft over implants/prosthesis are that there are no risks of developing autoimmune disorders and rupture or migration complications.

SURGICAL TECHNIQUE

Simple Orchiectomy

This procedure may be performed with local, regional, or general anesthesia. Local anesthetic sensory blockade is obtained by infiltrating the spermatic cord in the region of the vas deferens in the high scrotum just below the pubic tubercle with a 0.5% bupivacaine solution. Care must be taken to ensure that the block is not injected intravascularly by drawing back on the syringe prior to injecting the medication. The same solution is then injected subcutaneously at the site of the anterior scrotal incision. Sensory blockade should then be tested by pinprick before the beginning of the procedure.

Scrotal Approach

The anterior scrotal wall is shaved to remove existing hair and the scrotum and genitalia are prepped in a sterile manner. A 2.5- to 3-cm midline incision is made just through the skin along the median raphe in the anterior scrotal wall using a no.15 blade scalpel while the assistant pushes a testicle toward the incision between his thumb and index finger so that the testicle lies directly under the incision (Fig. 60–1). By electrocautery, the incision is then

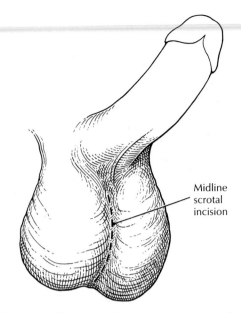

FIG. 60–1. A midline scrotal incision over the median raphe allows access to both testes.

carried down through the dartos and cremasteric layers until the parietal portion of the tunica vaginalis is incised directly over the testis. This is usually notable for a gush of fluid from the peritesticular space. The incision in the tunica vaginalis is lengthened in both directions far enough to allow exposure of the entire testicle through the wound. The surrounding tunics are freed from the spermatic cord by a combination of blunt and sharp dissection. Meticulous hemostasis may be obtained in each layer as it is entered with electrocautery. Once the spermatic cord is isolated, the vas deferens is separated, doubly clamped, divided, and ligated with 2-0 Vicryl ties (Fig. 60–2). The remainder of

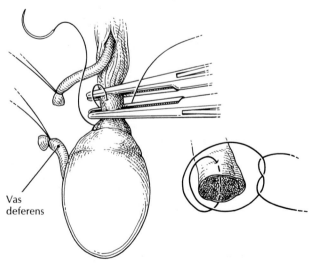

FIG. 60–2. The vas deferens is ligated separately from the vascular structures of the cord. The vascular structures are double ligated with both a free tie proximally and a suture ligature distally using 0 Vicryl.

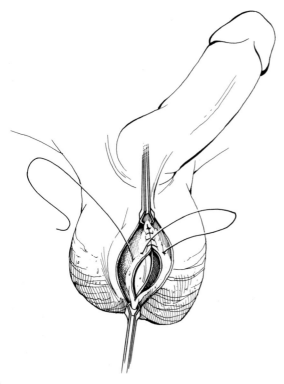

FIG. 60–3. Closure of the deep layers of the scrotum including the dartos musculature and testicular tunics laterally and the midline septum in one running layer.

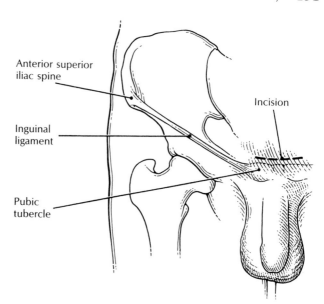

FIG. 60–4. A midline suprapubic incision 2 to 3 cm above the pubis allows access to both testes at a level just below the external ring.

the cord structures may be divided into one or more bundles and are doubly clamped on the proximal side and singly clamped on the distal side. Once divided, the proximal portion of the cord is ligated with a 0 Vicryl free tie behind the most proximal clamp, which is then removed, and an 0 Vicryl suture ligature is placed just distal to the free tie (Fig. 60–2). Before the cord is released to retract proximally, the tunics, dartos, and subcutaneous areas are again inspected for hemostasis. Once this is felt adequate, the cord is allowed to retract and attention is turned to the opposite testicle. It is then removed through the same midline incision in the same manner. This leaves two openings in the tunica vaginalis and dartos layers, which are separated by a median septum. These deep layers are then closed in one layer using a 3-0 Vicryl running suture. Allis clamps are placed at either end of the median septum to facilitate the exposure (Fig. 60–3). The skin is then closed with interrupted 3-0 chromic sutures and a gauze dressing is applied. Drains are not required but can be considered if there is doubt about hemostasis. Compression or turban dressings may also be used if there is concern over postoperative hemostasis or edema.

Suprapubic Approach

This approach is advantageous in patients in whom you want to avoid a scrotal incision and/or place testicular prostheses at the time of the orchiectomy. The patient

again is placed in the supine position and the suprapubic area is shaved. A 4- to 5-cm transverse incision is made in the midline approximately 2 to 3 cm above the pubic symphysis (Fig. 60–4). This is extended down through the subcutaneous tissues to the level of the rectus fascia using electrocautery. The subcutaneous tissue is then swept bluntly toward the external inguinal ring, exposing the distal spermatic cord, which is then isolated just distal to the ring in the upper scrotum (Fig. 60–5). Right-angle retractors are helpful to obtain exposure during this dissection by moving the incision toward the side being worked on. The spermatic cord is looped with a Penrose

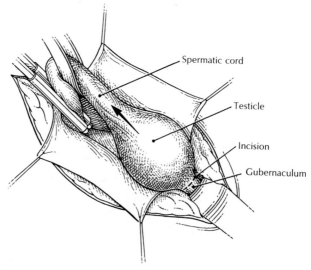

FIG. 60–5. Isolation of the cord with a Penrose drain. Division of the gubernaculum allows complete mobilization of the testis from the scrotum.

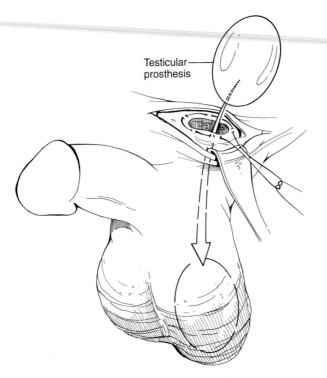

FIG. 60–6. If a prosthesis is desired, it is placed into the empty hemiscrotum. To prevent migration, a pursestring suture is used to close the neck of the hemiscrotum, eliminating the need for an anchoring suture.

drain and the testicle is delivered into the wound by placing upward pressure on the scrotum and testicle, with simultaneous upward traction on the cord with the Penrose drain. The gubernaculum is then divided, which mobilizes the testicle (Fig. 60–5). The vas deferens and spermatic cord are then divided as previously described. If testicular prostheses are desired, they are then placed into the empty scrotum after adequate hemostasis is ensured, and a pursestring suture of 3-0 silk is used to close the neck of each hemiscrotum (Fig. 60–6). Scarpa's fascia is closed with 3-0 Vicryl suture and the skin is closed with a 4-0 Vicryl subcuticular suture reinforced with benzoin and steristrips.

Subcapsular Orchiectomy

This approach is used in patients who desire the cosmetic effect of testicles being present without the use of testicular prosthesis. The operation is approached through the anterior scrotum as previously described (Fig. 60–1). Once the testicle is delivered to the wound, the tunica albuginea is opened in midline in a cephalad-to-caudad fashion. Hemostats are placed on the edges of the capsule to provide traction and an index finger is placed behind the capsule to invert it (Fig. 60–7). This maneuver facilitates the removal of the parenchymal contents, which are swept to the midline using a gauze sponge. The midline

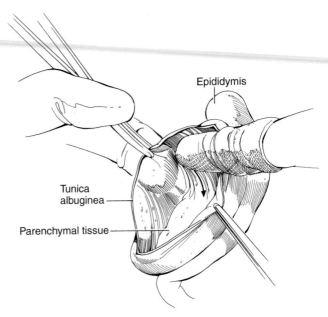

FIG. 60–7. The tunica albuginea is opened in midline opposite the epididymis and the contents are swept bluntly to the midline attachment.

attachment of the parenchyma is divided using electrocautery and the remainder of the interior capsule is cauterized to ensure hemostasis and complete destruction of all testicular parenchyma (Fig. 60–8). This technique has also been described using a CO_2 laser (13). The tunica albuginea is then closed using a running 3-0 Vicryl suture (Fig. 60–9) and the residual testicular tunics, adnexa, and cord are returned to the scrotum. The deep layers of the scrotum are closed in one layer as previously described, as is the skin (Fig. 60–3).

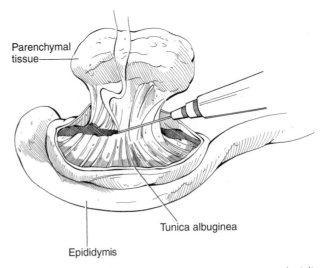

FIG. 60–8. The parenchymal tissue is then removed at its midline attachment with electrocautery and the internal surface of the capsule is cauterized.

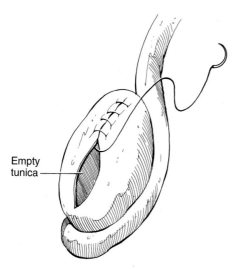

FIG. 60–9. The tunica albuginea is reapproximated with a running 3–0 Vicryl suture.

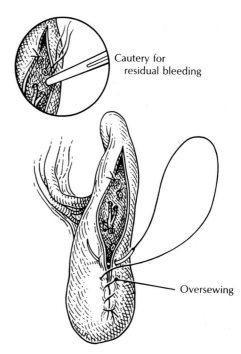

Cautery for residual bleeding

Oversewing

FIG. 60–11. After removal of the testis and further hemostasis with electrocautery, the tunica of the epididymis is closed over the raw surface using a running suture.

Subepididymal Orchiectomy

This is another procedure offered as an alternative to simple scrotal orchiectomy for a more acceptable cosmetic result. Again, the initial exposure to the testicles is the same as previously described for the anterior scrotal approach (Fig. 60–1). Once the testicle is delivered to the wound, a vasectomy is performed including double ligation and division to minimize the possibility of postoperative epididymitis (5). A line of dissection between the cleavage plane of the testis and the epididymis is utilized (Fig. 60–10). Dissection is started at the head of the epididymis, and the epididymal tissue is clamped for hemostasis. Care must be taken to secure the spermatic artery entering the testis at a point between the midportion and the tail of the epididymis. The clamped epididymal tissue

is ligated using a 3-0 Vicryl suture. Meticulous hemostasis is then obtained using electrocautery, and a running 3-0 Vicryl suture on a tapered needle is used to approximate the edges of the tunica albuginea over the raw surface of the epididymis (Fig. 60–11). The remaining spermatic cord and epididymis are replaced into the scrotum, which is closed as previously described.

OUTCOMES

Complications

Complications can include infection, hematoma, edema, and the inadvertent removal of a testicular neoplasm through the scrotal approach. Of these, hematoma can be a significant problem because of the distensible nature of the scrotum, which prevents any tamponade effect. Reexploration with evacuation of the hematoma and placement of a drain may be required but can be ineffective when the bleeding dissects subcutaneously in the dartos layer. This has led to the development of several preventative measures to achieve adequate compression of the area postoperatively, including turban-type dressings or compression of the scrotal wall over a gauze bolster as described by Oesterling (10). These techniques should not be substituted for being meticulous in obtaining hemostasis at the time of the procedure.

Infection, depending on the degree of severity, is managed by incision and drainage of any abscess pockets. This is followed by local wound care, which may include

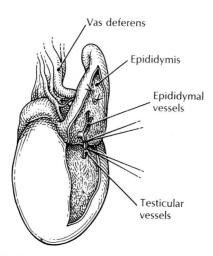

Vas deferens

Epididymis

Epididymal vessels

Testicular vessels

FIG. 60–10. Dissection of the testis from the epididymis, ligating the epididymal side over clamps with Vicryl suture.

wet-to-dry dressing changes, sitz baths, and whirlpool with debridement of any devitalized tissue. Antibiotics can be used in cases where there is induration only and no abscess to drain or in combination with the incision and drainage procedure if needed. If antibiotics are used, they should be directed by the results of wound cultures.

If a testicular neoplasm has been inadvertently removed through a scrotal approach, the remaining inguinal spermatic cord should be removed, as well as a wide excision of the scrotal scar. The hemiscrotum should also be removed if there was any known tumor spillage during the transscrotal procedure. This usually results in cure rates similar to those for conventional initial radical inguinal orchiectomy (4).

Results

The effectiveness of scrotal orchiectomy in terms of achieving adequate hormonal ablation in patients with prostate cancer can be easily determined by measuring serum testosterone levels postcastration, which are reduced by approximately 90%. Castrate levels of testosterone have reportedly been achieved by 2 and 15 hours after surgery (2,3). Prostate-specific antigen levels, patient symptoms, and patient survival may be followed to determine the procedure's effectiveness in terms of disease control. Side effects may include loss of libido, impotence, and hot flashes.

For benign intrascrotal processes such as epididymal orchitis unresponsive to antibiotics, or devitalized tissues secondary to torsion or trauma, simple orchiectomy is curative.

REFERENCES

1. Ahmedin J, Thomas A, Murray T, Thun M. Cancer Statistics, 2002. *CA Cancer J Clin* 2002;52:23.
2. Arcadi JA. Rapid drop in serum testosterone after bilateral subcapsular orchiectomy. *J Surg Oncol* 1992;49:35.
3. Cassady JR, Hutter JJ, Whitesell LJ. Prostate cancer. In: Vogelzang NJ, Scardino PT, Shipley WU, Coffey DS, eds. *Comprehensive textbook of genitourinary oncology*. Baltimore: Williams & Wilkins, 1996:557–828.
4. Giguere JK, Stablein DM, Spaulding JT, et al. The clinical significance of unconventional orchiectomy approaches in testicular cancer. A report from the Testicular Cancer Intergroup Study. *J Urol* 1988;139:1225.
5. Glenn JF. Subepididymal orchidectomy: the acceptable alternative. *J Urol* 1990;144:942.
6. Huggins C, Hodges CV. Studies on prostatic cancer: the effect of castration, of estrogen, and of androgen injection on serum phosphatases in metastatic carcinoma of the prostate. *Cancer Res* 1941;1:293.
7. Kihara K, Oshima H. Cosmetic orchiectomy using pedicled fibrofatty tissue graft for prostate cancer: a new approach. *Eur Urol* 1998;34:210.
8. Klein EA, Herr HW. Suprapubic approach for bilateral orchiectomy and placement of testicular prosthesis. *J Urol* 1990;143:765.
9. O'Conor VJ, Chaing SP, Grayhack JT. Is subcapsular orchiectomy a definitive procedure? *J Urol* 1963;89:236.
10. Oesterling JE. Scrotal surgery: a reliable method for the prevention of postoperative hematoma and edema. *J Urol* 1990;143:1201.
11. Riba LW. Subcapsular castration for carcinoma of the prostate. *J Urol* 1942;48:384.
12. Solomon AA. Testicular prosthesis: a new insertion operation. *J Urol* 1972;108:436.
13. Wishnow KI, Johnson DE. Subcapsular orchiectomy using the CO_2 laser: a new technique. *Lasers Surg Med* 1988;8:604.

CHAPTER 61

Inguinal Orchiectomy

David A. Swanson

Testicular tumors are relatively rare (only two to three cases per 100,000 men; an estimated 7,500 new cases in the United States in 2002) (5). When they occur, 94% are germ cell tumors and the rest are tumors of the gonadal stroma and secondary tumors of the testis. In black men throughout the world, germ cell tumors occur infrequently, but because they do occur this diagnosis cannot be excluded on the basis of race alone. Although the etiology of testicular tumors is not known, there is a relatively high association (reported in up to 12% of tumors) with a history of cryptorchidism; in 20% of such cases, the tumor is in the normally descended testis. Orchidopexy does not prevent the subsequent development of tumor; it simply makes the diagnosis easier to establish. Carcinoma *in situ* (CIS) is also known to be associated with cryptorchidism, and data support the hypothesis that at least some, if not all, germ cell tumors originate as CIS (8).

DIAGNOSIS

Most testicular tumors present as a palpable nodule or painless swelling of the testis, often discovered incidentally by the patient or his sex partner. The differential diagnosis of a testicular mass includes tumor, epididymitis and epididymoorchitis (the two most common diagnoses other than cancer), torsion (the diagnosis of which also requires surgery), and, less commonly, hernia, hydrocele, spermatocele, varicocele, hematoma, and hematocele. The patient with cancer may complain of a dull ache or sense of heaviness. Acute onset of pain is relatively rare and usually indicates bleeding within the tumor or associated epididymitis. Signs and symptoms may be secondary to metastatic spread.

When careful bimanual examination of the testis reveals an intratesticular mass, with or without an associated epididymal mass or tenderness, testicular tumor must be suspected. A transscrotal ultrasound is a widely available, rapid, sensitive, noninvasive, and inexpensive

way to determine whether there is a solid mass within the tunica albuginea (10). Color Doppler ultrasound might on occasion help differentiate testicular torsion. Magnetic resonance imaging can also demonstrate the presence of an intratesticular mass but has no established advantage over a careful physical examination plus ultrasound exam. With rare exceptions, all solid masses within the testis should be considered malignant until proven otherwise, and all require surgical intervention.

Patients with testicular tumors commonly have elevated tumor markers, in particular β-human chorionic gonadotropin and α-fetoprotein. However, the presence of normal marker levels does not exclude malignancy, and there is in general no advantage to waiting for the marker results before operating, although blood should always be drawn for these tests before orchiectomy (10).

INDICATIONS FOR SURGERY

The presence of an intrascrotal mass that cannot be clearly localized to outside the tunica albuginea is sufficient indication for surgical exploration through an inguinal approach. Although a sense of urgency is appropriate, it is not necessary to consider inguinal orchiectomy an emergency procedure; it can be scheduled during regular operating hours.

ALTERNATIVE THERAPY

For the patient who has equivocal findings on physical examination and ultrasound that make the diagnosis of epididymitis tenable, a short course of antibiotics may be tried. If there is no prompt improvement (less than 10 to 14 days), or if the serum tumor markers are elevated, inguinal exploration should be performed. Although radical (inguinal) orchiectomy is standard therapy for a solid lesion within the tunica albuginea, partial orchiectomy might be appropriate in the patient with a solitary testis or bilateral testicular masses or in the patient whose preoperative evaluation makes the diagnosis of an epidermoid cyst of the testis highly likely (2–4,9). The selection criteria, technique, and results will be presented in Chapter 60.

SURGICAL TECHNIQUE

Although regional anesthesia is acceptable, general anesthesia is preferred because of the short duration of the surgery and the possible reflex response to traction on the testicle and cord. With the patient in the supine position, and after adequate anesthesia, the lower abdominal wall, penis, and scrotum are cleaned with a surgical scrub and draped in a sterile fashion so that the palpable testicular mass and ipsilateral hemiscrotum are accessible in the surgical field. By tradition, an oblique skin incision is made approximately 2 cm superior to the inguinal ligament, extending parallel to that ligament from just above the pubic tubercle laterally approximately 8 to 10 cm to a point overlying the internal inguinal ring. I prefer a more horizontal incision, extending approximately 5 to 8 cm from one finger breadth above the superior aspect of the external inguinal ring laterally toward the internal inguinal ring, which might be slightly more cosmetic (Fig. 61–1).

Deepen the incision with the knife or electrocautery through the subcutaneous tissue until the external oblique aponeurosis is reached. There are usually one or two significant veins that traverse this incision. They should be isolated and secured with hemoclips or 3-0 plain or chromic catgut sutures before being cut. When the external oblique aponeurosis is cleaned sufficiently to be well

visualized, it is helpful to place one or two small self-retaining Gelpi (or similar) retractors in the wound to improve exposure. Next, use the scalpel to make a small incision in the external oblique aponeurosis midway between the internal and external inguinal rings, in the direction of its fibers. Insert Metzenbaum scissors through this opening and push the closed scissors with slight upward pressure underneath the aponeurosis to the external inguinal ring and then laterally toward the internal ring (Fig. 61–2A). This helps ensure that the ilioinguinal nerve will not be cut during the next step, which is to push the partially opened Metzenbaum scissors from the point of incision into the external inguinal ring and then laterally toward the internal ring as required, thus splitting the aponeurosis and opening the roof of the inguinal canal (Fig. 61–2B). Careful inspection will usually reveal the ilioinguinal nerve, which should be freed up carefully by blunt and sharp dissection for the length of the incision. It can then be retracted out of the surgical field by passing two small hemostats underneath the nerve, grasping the superior edge of the aponeurosis, and retracting it in a cephalad direction. It may also help to grasp the inferior edge of the aponeurosis and retract it as well to fully expose the inguinal canal.

This will expose the spermatic cord, although it may not appear distinct because of the cremasteric muscle fibers surrounding the cord, which merge into the internal oblique muscle. Using a gauze sponge wrapped around the fingertip (Fig. 61–3A or a peanut (Küttner) sponge (Fig. 61–3B), bluntly develop the plane between the spermatic cord and floor of the inguinal canal until it can be encircled with a thumb and forefinger. It is usually easiest to both initiate the dissection and completely encircle the cord at the level of the pubic tubercle. Once you have ascertained that all components of the cord are included, pass a 0.5-in. Penrose drain around the cord (Fig. 61–3C), elevate it with gentle traction, and free up the cord laterally to the internal ring using predominantly blunt dissection, although some sharp dissection may be required. Be careful as you approach the internal ring that the inferior epigastric vessels are not injured, and inspect the spermatic cord carefully to ensure that an indirect inguinal hernia, which could contain bowel or bladder, is not present. At this point, occlude the spermatic cord firmly with either a soft rubber-shod clamp or, as I prefer, a 0.5-in. Penrose drain encircled twice around the cord, tightened in a tourniquet fashion, and secured with a Kelly or right-angle clamp (Fig. 61–4). Be sure to leave enough spermatic cord distal to the internal ring to permit it to be double-clamped later without first removing the tourniquet.

It is now possible to mobilize the testis from the scrotum and through the opened external inguinal ring into the inguinal canal and surgical field. Upward pressure on the external skin of the hemiscrotum and testis, coupled with gentle traction on the spermatic cord, will in general

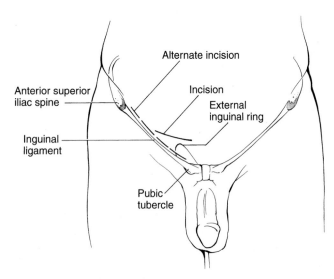

FIG. 61–1. An almost horizontal incision from just cephalad to the external inguinal ring laterally almost to the internal ring provides adequate exposure and an excellent cosmetic result. Alternatively, the incision may be made parallel to the inguinal ligament.

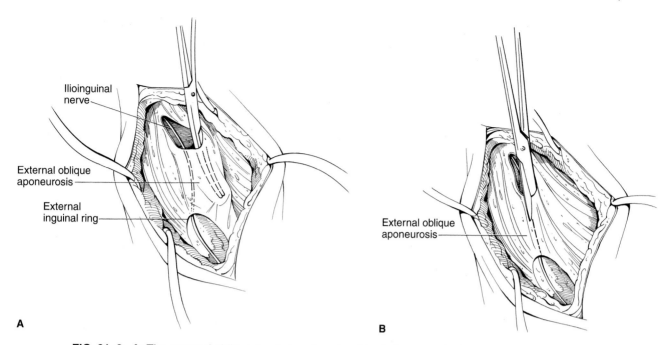

FIG. 61–2. A: The external oblique fascia is entered and tented up over the length of the inguinal canal before cutting to help ensure that the ilioinguinal nerve is not injured. **B:** The external oblique fascia is incised over the spermatic cord and the incision is extended into the external ring.

define the circumferential fibromuscular attachments that need to be cut or, better, electrocoagulated to completely free up the testis (Fig. 61–4). At the most inferior aspect of the testis, there may be a well-defined gubernaculum that needs to be clamped and cut, with care taken to exclude scrotal skin, and tied with 2-0 or 3-0 chromic catgut.

At this point, isolate the testis and spermatic cord, now free to the level of the internal ring, with sterile towels and carefully inspect the testis. If the diagnosis is still in doubt, you may open the tunica vaginalis and expose the tunica albuginea of the testis. If doubt still persists, which should happen only rarely, a small incision may be made in the tunica albuginea to permit insertion of a finger for palpation of the testicular parenchyma. If all of these maneuvers fail to exclude tumor, the surgeon should proceed with radical orchiectomy rather than risk returning a testis with tumor to the scrotum. I want to emphasize that it is only rarely necessary to open even the tunica vaginalis and far more rare to open the tunica albuginea or perform a biopsy.

To complete the orchiectomy, double-clamp the spermatic cord at the level of the internal ring and proximal to the Penrose tourniquet with two Kelly or heavy right-angle clamps; add a third clamp to occlude the cord just distal to the Penrose tourniquet (Fig. 61–5). Transect the cord and remove the testicle, with attached spermatic cord, from the surgical field. The cord is tied behind the most proximal clamp with a 0 silk tie, and a suture ligature of 0 silk is placed behind the most distal clamp. Leave one of the two sutures long for later identification

of the stump of the cord if a retroperitoneal lymph node dissection is performed. Some surgeons prefer to tie the cord in two portions, separating the spermatic vessels and the vas deferens, and double-tying both portions of the cord. In either case, after the cord is securely tied allow it to retract through the internal ring into the retroperitoneum.

Next, carefully inspect the entire floor of the inguinal canal as well as the scrotal compartment by everting the scrotal wall into the surgical field with upward external pressure on the most dependent portion of the hemiscrotum. Control all sites of bleeding, even tiny ones, with electrocautery and then irrigate with sterile water. It is prudent to perform a final inspection for complete hemostasis at this point before closure. Begin the closure by careful inspection of the inguinal floor. If it seems weak, it can be reinforced with several interrupted sutures in a standard hernia repair. If not, release the ilioinguinal nerve and close the external oblique aponeurosis with interrupted 2-0 silk or 2-0 Prolene sutures, placing the sutures at varying distances from the aponeurotic edge to prevent a linear tear and taking care to exclude the ilioinguinal nerve (Fig. 61–6). The closure should begin at the level of the internal ring and extend medially as close to the pubic tubercle as possible because there is no longer any reason to have an external inguinal ring. A drain is not necessary or advisable. Irrigate the wound once again and close the skin incision with clips or with a running subcuticular suture of 4-0 Vicryl. Cover the wound with a dry sterile dressing and gently compress the scrotum with either fluffed gauze sponges held in place with an athletic

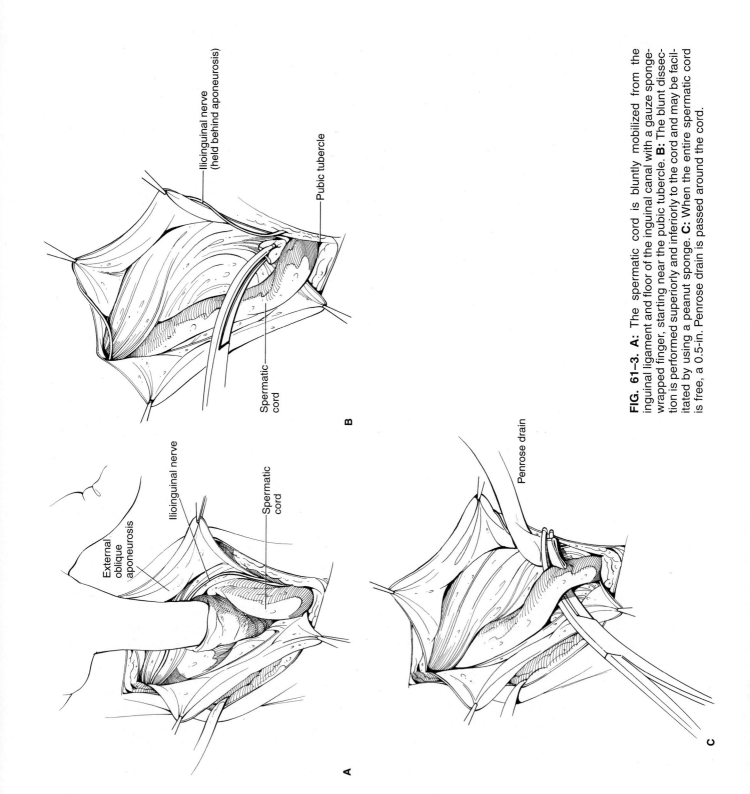

FIG. 61–3. A: The spermatic cord is bluntly mobilized from the inguinal ligament and floor of the inguinal canal with a gauze sponge-wrapped finger, starting near the pubic tubercle. **B:** The blunt dissection is performed superiorly and inferiorly to the cord and may be facilitated by using a peanut sponge. **C:** When the entire spermatic cord is free, a 0.5-in. Penrose drain is passed around the cord.

Ilioinguinal nerve
(held behind aponeurosis)

Pubic tubercle

Spermatic
cord

B

External
oblique
aponeurosis

Ilioinguinal nerve

Spermatic
cord

A

Penrose drain

C

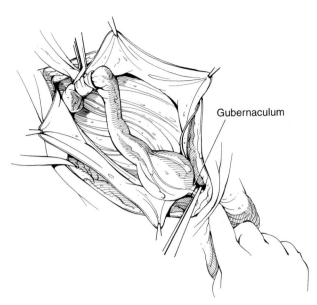

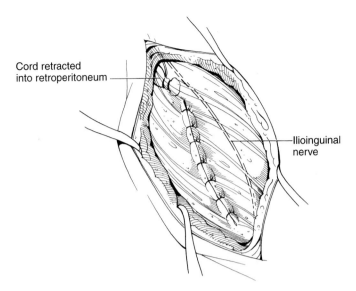

FIG. 61–4. The Penrose drain is encircled twice around the cord just distal to the internal ring and clamped to act as a tourniquet. A finger outside the scrotum helps push the testis into the surgical field. The gubernaculum is clamped and cut and the scrotal side of the gubernaculum is tied.

FIG. 61–6. The stump of the cord retracts back through the internal ring into the retroperitoneum; one suture is left long. The external oblique fascia is closed with interrupted sutures placed at varying distances from the cut edge and completely closing the external ring.

supporter or by gently wrapping the scrotum with a loosely applied turban dressing of Kling, Kerlix, or Coban. Avoid using an ice pack because it has little impact on swelling and is a source of considerable discomfort.

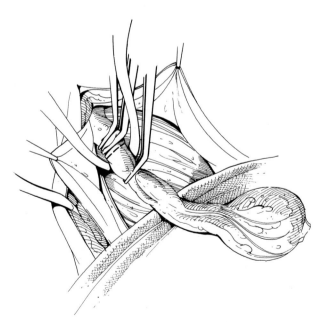

FIG. 61–5. The spermatic cord is triple-clamped just distal to the internal ring (two clamps proximal and one distal to the Penrose tourniquet) and cut after careful inspection of the testis, which has been isolated from the surgical field on a sterile towel.

Patients may resume a regular diet and ambulation when completely awake and may be discharged. Most patients require oral narcotic analgesics for pain control for several days.

OUTCOMES

Complications

Many would consider the most serious complication to be scrotal violation, which in the past required hemiscrotectomy and now requires irradiation to the scrotum (for seminoma). In truth, no data demonstrate reduced survival following scrotal contamination (6). Nonetheless, there is virtually no reason why the testis should be approached transscrotally if the diagnosis of possible testicular tumor has been even considered. At the least, a transscrotal approach prevents early control of venous outflow in the cord before manipulation of the tumor, leaves spermatic cord behind, potentially alters lymphatic drainage of the testis, risks tumor contamination of the scrotum, and may preclude consideration of surveillance as a treatment option, although even this has been challenged (1,7).

The most common actual complication is probably an intrascrotal hematoma. Because the scrotum is such an expansile organ with loose areolar tissue beneath the dermis, bleeding may continue because of a lack of tamponade, and the resulting hematoma may grow quite large. These scrotal hematomas usually become organized and quite firm and may even raise the question of residual or recurrent tumor. Nonetheless, if the hematoma does not become infected (which would require surgical drainage) it can almost always be followed expectantly and will eventually regress. Ideally, this complication should be prevented. The depths of the inguinal canal and entire inner surface of the scrotal wall should be thoroughly and compulsively inspected and electrocoagulated to ensure hemostasis. The surgeon can facilitate this, as described earlier, by everting the scrotal wall with a finger positioned on the most dependent portion of the external scrotal wall. After hemostasis appears adequate, irrigate with sterile water and inspect again. Although the turban dressing used in bilateral orchiectomy, which completely collapses the scrotum, is not possible, it is possible to use a modified turban dressing that is wrapped firmly enough to collapse the hemiscrotum ipsilateral to the orchiectomy but not so tight as to cause pain because of pressure on the remaining testis.

It is also possible to get a retroperitoneal hematoma if the ligature(s) on the spermatic cord pull off or if there is an injury to one of the inferior epigastric vessels. The first cause can be prevented by a properly tied ligature with adequate length of spermatic cord distal to it so it cannot slip off. A suture ligature on the spermatic cord offers a measure of security. Injury to the epigastric vessels can be avoided by careful dissection of the proximal spermatic cord at the level of the internal inguinal ring. This complication is usually discovered incidentally at the time of further staging evaluation with a computed tomography scan, although an unexplained and occult blood loss may prompt investigation. If bleeding has stopped when the problem is discovered, it virtually never requires specific treatment; the hematoma should ultimately be reabsorbed.

Results

Properly performed inguinal orchiectomy with the spermatic cord taken at the level of the inguinal ring is potentially curative if the tumor is still confined to the testis. Except for treatment of a complication, reoperation is virtually never required, although additional surgical procedures may be performed later to remove regional lymph nodes.

REFERENCES

1. Aki FT, Bilen CY, Tekin MI, Ozen H. Is scrotal violation per se a risk factor for local relapse and metastases in stage I nonseminomatous testicular cancer? *Urology* 2000;56:459–462.
2. Berger Y, Srinivas V, Hajdu SI, Herr HW. Epidermoid cysts of the testis: role of conservative surgery. *J Urol* 1985;134:962–963.
3. Heidenreich A, Engelmann UH, Vietsch HV, Derschum W. Organ preserving surgery in testicular epidermoid cysts. *J Urol* 1995;153:1147–1150.
4. Heidenreich A, Weissbach L, Höltl W, Albers P, Kliesch S, Köhrmann KU, Dieckmann KP, for the German Testicular Cancer Study Group. Organ sparing surgery for malignant germ cell tumor of the testis. *J Urol* 2001;166:2161–2165.
5. Jemal A, Thomas A, Murray T, Thun M. Cancer statistics, 2002. *CA Cancer J Clin* 2002;52:23–47.
6. Leibovitch I, Baniel J, Foster RS, Donohue JP. The clinical implications of procedural deviations during orchiectomy for nonseminomatous testis cancer. *J Urol* 1995;154:935–939.
7. Pizzocaro G. Editorial comment. *J Urol* 1995;154:939.
8. Rajpert-De Meyts E, Giwercman A, Skakkebaek NE. Carcinoma *in situ* of the testis–a precursor of testicular germ cell cancer: biological and clinical aspects. In: Vogelzang NJ, Shipley WU, Scardino PT, Coffey DS, eds. *Comprehensive textbook of genitourinary oncology*, 2nd ed. Baltimore: Lippincott Williams & Wilkins, 2000:897–908.
9. Sloan JC, Beck SDW, Bihrle R, Foster RS. Bilateral testicular epidermoid cysts managed by partial orchiectomy. *J Urol* 2002;167:255–256.
10. Steele GS, Kantoff PW, Richie JP. Staging and imaging of testis cancer. In: Vogelzang NJ, Shipley WU, Scardino PT, Coffey DS, eds. *Comprehensive textbook of genitourinary oncology*, 2nd ed. Baltimore: Lippincott Williams & Wilkins, 2000:939–949.

CHAPTER 62

Organ-Preserving Surgery in Testicular Tumors

Axel Heidenreich

Testicular germ cell tumors (TGCTs) are the most common neoplasms in young men, with bilateral simultaneous and sequential tumors arising in 2% to 3% of the patients. Bilateral orchiectomy is still recommended as the gold standard treatment resulting in infertility, lifelong dependency on androgen substitution, and psychological distress due to castration at a young age. Because most testicular cancer patients are going to be long-time survivors with modern therapeutic approaches, long-term morbidity should be omitted whenever possible; cure of cancer might only be achieved if quality of life following therapy can be restored to pretreatment levels. Considering these quality of life issues, organ-sparing surgical approaches have been developed in patients with bilateral testicular cancer or in selected patients with a germ cell tumor arising in a solitary testicle.

DIAGNOSIS

The diagnosis of testicular cancer is usually made by the appearance of a mass in the testicle that on ultrasonography appears solid or to have some cystic components (2). Serum markers including β-human chorionic gonadotropin and α-fetoprotein are routinely drawn prior to surgery.

INDICATIONS FOR SURGERY

Patients in whom preservation surgery is contemplated should have enough testicular parenchyma for maintaining physiological testosterone synthesis, which requires that the diameter of the tumor should not exceed 2 cm (3,7). Preoperative serum testosterone and serum luteinizing hormone (LH) levels should be in the normal range. Elevated LH levels in the presence of normal testosterone levels indicate compensated Leydig cell insufficiency. These patients bear a high risk to develop hypogonadism with the need for androgen substitution following surgery. In addition, a semen analysis should

be obtained to assess fertility and discuss the option of cryopreservation (3,5). Also, testicular ultrasonography must be performed preoperatively because this usually represents the imaging modality of choice to assess intratesticular location and diameter of the tumor. Scrotal magnetic resonance imaging appears only to be necessary if there is more than tumor suspected or if there is a very high suspicion for a benign testicular lesion (6).

ALTERNATIVE THERAPY

The alternative to testicular-sparing surgery is bilateral orchiectomy, which will require lifelong hormonal replacement. Other problems associated with bilateral orchiectomy include infertility and the psychological impact of the procedure on the patient, who is usually a young male.

SURGICAL TECHNIQUE

An inguinal approach is chosen with the skin incision being made about two finger breadths above and parallel to the inguinal ligament (Fig. 62–1). The incision extends from the external inguinal ring cephalad for about 5 cm and it is carried down to the external oblique fascia (Fig. 62–2). Care is taken not to injure the ilioinguinal nerve, which runs laterally just underneath the fascia.

The spermatic cord is identified and isolated at the level of the pubic tubercle (Fig. 62–3), secured with a half-inch Penrose drain, mobilized back to the internal inguinal ring (Fig. 62–4). As in the case of radical orchiectomy, the spermatic cord might be cross-clamped with a rubber-shod clamp prior to delivering the testicle in the operating field. In this scenario, all following manipulations should be performed under cold ischemia by placing the testicle in crushed ice.

On the other hand, it is also possible to deliver the testicle into the operating field without cross-clamping the

501

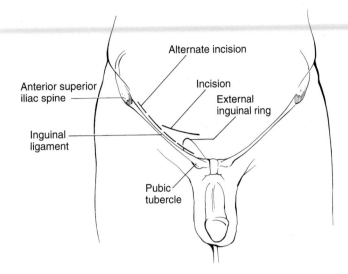

FIG. 62–1. Inguinal incision for exploration of the testicle in relation to anatomic landmarks of the groin.

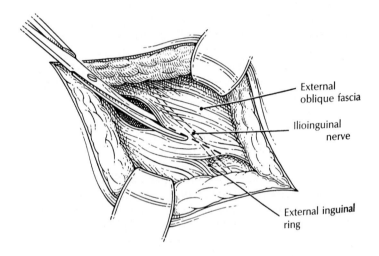

FIG. 62–2. Incision of the external oblique fascia and its close relationship to the ilioinguinal nerve.

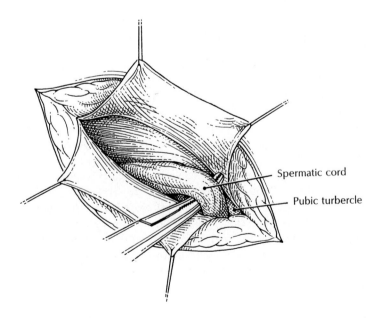

FIG. 62–3. Delivery of the spermatic cord after the external oblique fascia has been opened.

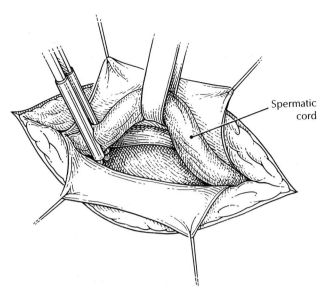

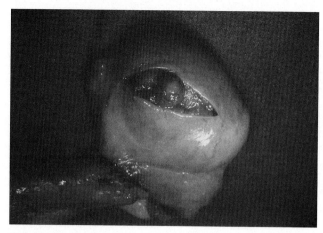

FIG. 62–6. Incision of the tunica albuginea just above the testicular tumor.

FIG. 62–4. Mobilization of the spermatic cord up to the internal inguinal ring; the cord may be cross-clamped if desired.

spermatic cord; we know that simple tumor cell shedding will not result in an increased frequency of distant metastases unless the tumor cells harbor molecular characteristics enabling them to adhere to the vascular endothelium, invade adjacent organs, and induce neovascularization. The testicle is delivered by slight traction on the spermatic cord and inversion of the scrotum; the gubernaculum is divided between two clamps and suture ligated with 3-0 silk ties (Fig. 62–5).

The operating field is draped with laparotomy pads and the tunica vaginalis is opened anteriorly; depending on the size and the intratesticular location of the tumor, it might be located underneath the tunica albuginea by sim-

ple palpation. In the presence of small testicular lesions, intraoperative ultrasonography with a 7.5-MHz scanner might be used for visualization and detection (1).

The tunica albuginea is incised just above the tumor (Fig. 62–6); because small testicular lesions usually present with a pseudocapsule, the surrounding testicular parenchyma can be scraped away with the blade of a scalpel (Fig. 62–7). Following the enucleation procedure, four additional biopsies are taken from the tumor bed to exclude tumor infiltration (Fig. 62–8) and all specimens are sent for frozen section examination (FSE). At least in our hands, FSE has turned out to represent a reliable technique to differentiate between tumors of benign or malignant dignity. Another biopsy is taken from the peripheral testicular parenchyma, fixed in Bouin's or Stieve's solution, and sent for pathohistological analysis to exclude associated testicular intraepithelial neoplasia. After careful bipolar coagulation of small intratesticular blood ves-

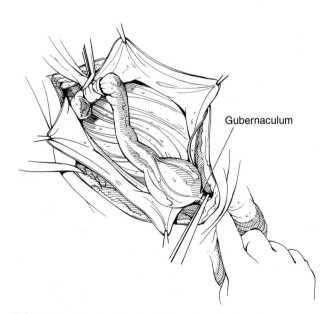

FIG. 62–5. The testicle is delivered and the gubernaculum may be divided and suture ligated.

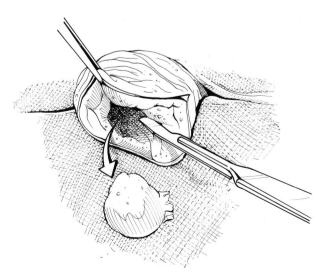

FIG. 62–7. The tumor is surrounded by a firm pseudocapsule.

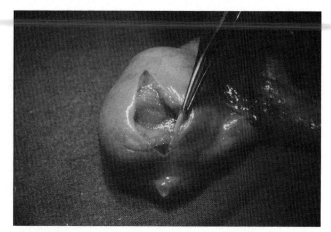

FIG. 62–8. Additional quadrant biopsies following the enucleation procedure.

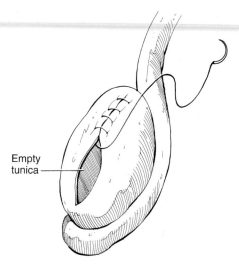

Empty
tunica

FIG. 62–9. Running suture of the tunica albuginea.

sels, the tunica albuginea is closed with a 4-0 Vicryl running suture (Fig. 62–9), the tunica vaginalis is closed with a Vicryl 3-0 running suture, and the testicle is replaced in the scrotum, taking care not to twist the spermatic cord. A formal orchidopexy for the testicle is not necessary. The skin is closed with an absorbable, intracutaneous running suture; usually, no drains are placed. Postoperatively, the patient should receive potent analgesics and antiphlogistics to reduce uncomfortable testicular pain.

OUTCOMES

Complications

Potential complications include hemorrhage and loss of the testicle. Eight-five percent to 92% of patients have maintained adequate androgen levels (5).

Results

The initial study showed a 5-year survival rate of 92% and the maintenance of physiological testosterone serum levels in 92% without the need for androgen substitution in a limited number of patients (5). These results resulted in the German Testicular Cancer Study Group-defined criteria for proper patient selection, surgical technique, and follow-up based on the review of a large patient cohort with a median follow-up of more than 8 years. The disease-free survival rate was 99%, local recurrences developed in 5.5%, and normal testosterone serum levels were maintained in 85% of the patients.

The use of testicular-sparing surgery in testicular cancer requires that there be close follow-up for possible recurrence. The best modality for local follow-up is transscrotal ultrasonography. We recommend the first ultrasound to be done 4 to 6 weeks postoperatively, a time when scar tissue has replaced the intraparenchymatous traumatic edema; thereafter, scrotal imaging should be performed at 2-months intervals for the first year to ade-

quately document the developing scar tissue for further follow-up studies (5). In patients having undergone local radiation therapy postoperatively, periodic ultrasonography can be safely omitted and the patient should be educated to self-palpate the testicle. In patients not having undergone adjuvant local radiation periodic ultrasonography should be performed twice annually due to the high risk of local recurrence. In patients developing a local recurrence secondary orchiectomy has to be performed and androgen substitution has to be initiated (3–5).

In summary, organ-preserving surgery in patients with testicular germ cell tumors is feasible in patients with bilateral testis cancer or germ cell tumor in a solitary testicle. The procedure should be performed in conjunction with biopsies of the tumor bed and the resection rim and frozen section analysis as well as a biopsy of the peripheral parenchyma. Follow-up in these patients should be either postoperative radiation of the remaining testicle with 18 Gy or very close follow-up. As this is still a controversial procedure, it may be best performed in a center experienced in the management of testicular cancer.

REFERENCES

1. Buckspan MB, Klotz PG, Goldfinger M, et al. Intraoperative ultrasound in the conservative resection of testicular neoplasms. *J Urol* 1989;141: 326–327.
2. Fuse H, Shimazaki J, Katayama T. Ultrasonography of testicular tumors. *Eur Urol* 1990;17:273–275.
3. Heidenreich A, Bonfi R, Derschum W, et al. A conservative approach to bilateral testicular germ cell tumors. *J Urol* 1995;153:10–13.
4. Heidenreich A, Höltl W, Albrecht W, et al. Testis-preserving surgery in bilateral testicular germ cell tumors. *Br J Urol* 1997;79:253–257.
5. Heidenreich A, Weissbach L, Höltl W, et al., for the German Testicular Cancer Study Group. Organ sparing surgery in malignant germ cell tumors of the testis. *J Urol* 2001;166:2161–2165.
6. Menzner A, Kujat C, König J, et al. MRI in testicular diagnosis: differentiation of seminoma, teratoma and inflammation using a statistical score. *Rofo Fortschr Geb Rontgenstr Neuen Bilgeb Verfahr* 1997;166:514.
7. Weissbach L. Organ preserving surgery of malignant germ cell tumors. *J Urol* 1995;153:90–93.

CHAPTER 63

Retroperitoneal Lymphadenectomy

Michael A.S. Jewett and Rishikesh R. Pandya

Carcinoma of the testis arises from the germinal epithelium and is the most frequent malignancy in young men aged 20 to 35. Most patients are curable with appropriate management. There are two principal histological subtypes: seminoma and nonseminoma (the latter include embryonal carcinoma, teratocarcinoma, teratoma, yolk sac tumor, and choriocarcinoma). After radical inguinal orchiectomy, seminomas are usually treated by radiation and/or chemotherapy. Retroperitoneal lymphadenectomy (RPL) or lymph node dissection (RPLND) is indicated in patients with nonseminoma for staging and treatment of early stage disease and after chemotherapy for residual masses. It is rarely employed for seminoma unless there is a persistent residual retroperitoneal mass.

DIAGNOSIS

Characteristically, patients present with a painless mass in one testis. Ultrasound of the scrotum is usually employed to confirm the presence of the mass within the testicular parenchyma. Less commonly, the tumor will have an inflammatory component that produces pain and tenderness that can be mistaken for epididymitis. Up to 5% of tumors are bilateral, but they are usually asynchronous in presentation. Nonseminomas have a high propensity for metastases. The majority of metastases are lymphatic, although up to 10% appear to be hematogenous. The regional nodes that are involved are in the retroperitoneum, where the testis formed embryologically and draws its blood supply. Primary landing zones for lymphatic nodal metastases differ between sides (2).

Right-side tumors first metastasize to the interaortocaval nodes with less frequent involvement of the high preaortic and paracaval nodes. Left-side tumors metastasize to the left paraaortic region and the interaortocaval nodes. They rarely cross to the right side unless there is extensive metastatic disease. Extension via the thoracic duct to the supraclavicular node and systemic circulation

occurs in approximately 40% of patients at presentation, who will characteristically have lung metastases.

Clinical staging terminology is changing but groupings are defined as follows: stage I (formerly stage A, now pT1-4N0M0S0), tumor confined to the testis; stage II (formerly stage B, now pT1-4N1-3M0S0-1), metastatic disease confined to the retroperitoneal lymph nodes; and stage III (formerly stage C, now pT1-4N1-3M0-1S0-3), those with systemic metastases, usually to the lung (6).

The retroperitoneum is assessed by a computed tomography (CT) scan that includes the pelvic area with special attention to the renal hilar area down to the inferior mesenteric artery, which is the level at which most metastases will occur. Lung metastases are identified by chest x-ray and/or CT scan. The tumor markers a-fetoprotein (AFP) and b-human chorionic gonadotropin (HCG) are elevated in 70% to 80% of patients before orchiectomy and will usually remain elevated if there is metastatic disease. The half-lives are up to 5 days and up to 24 hours, respectively, for the two markers so that repeated determinations should be taken to discriminate between naturally decaying markers and ongoing secretion after orchiectomy. The overall accuracy for staging in stage I is 70%, i.e., all tests are negative but occult metastasis has occurred, usually to the retroperitoneum. For stage II, accuracy has been reported to be 70% to 80% with approximately equal false positive and false negative rates of 20% to 30%, respectively, but better imaging techniques have probably improved accuracy. Patients with pure embryonal carcinoma are more likely to have metastatic disease, in particular if vascular invasion is seen in the primary tumor. Choriocarcinoma rarely occurs in its pure form and usually metastasizes hematogenously.

INDICATIONS FOR SURGERY

The principal treatment alternatives after orchiectomy are surveillance, retroperitoneal lymphadenectomy, or primary chemotherapy. Patients with nonseminomatous stage I tumors can be stratified by risk of metastases using the primary tumor characteristics (5). Low-risk patients could be followed closely with a less than 20% risk of progression. Those with pure embryonal carcinoma plus vascular/lymphatic invasion have more than a 50% chance of metastases, and RPL or chemotherapy should be considered. Patients with persistent elevation of markers as the only evidence of disease are considered as a distinct stage group (stage IS) and are in general treated with primary chemotherapy because of the high rate of systemic metastases, although RPL is an option.

In patients with stage-II nonseminomatous tumors, RPL is the standard but if the nodal disease is less than 5 cm in diameter (stage N1-2), or if there are multiple small nodes, primary chemotherapy should be considered because of the high rate of concurrent systemic metastases. Some centers use initial chemotherapy for disease greater than 2 cm in diameter (stage N2).

Patients with stage-III disease are managed with initial chemotherapy, but all residual disease should be excised after the induction phase of therapy. Large retroperitoneal masses rarely completely disappear. The possibilities of residual carcinoma or teratoma that can expand are the indications for surgery if a persistent mass is seen on CT of the retroperitoneum after three or four cycles of chemotherapy. The histology is useful to determine future treatment as residual carcinoma may be an indication for further chemotherapy (11).

In patients with seminoma, occasional persistent retroperitoneal disease occurs after radiation or chemotherapy, often because there are nonseminomatous elements despite the fact that the primary was pure seminoma. These patients should be considered for RPL. It must be remembered that retroperitoneal masses in seminoma disappear slowly, over as long as a 1 year after radiation therapy, so the vast majority will not need surgery or further therapy.

ALTERNATIVE THERAPY

Patients with tumors confined to the testis (stage T1) who do not have vascular or lymphatic invasion and have elements of teratoma are less likely to have occult metastases and can be considered for surveillance (10). Up to 90% of patients will require no further therapy, but follow-up must be close, in particular during the first 2 years. Surveillance protocols should include at least two monthly visits for the first 2 years with a CT scan of the abdomen every 4 months. Each visit should include a history, physical examination, markers, and a chest x-ray. The mean time to progression is 6.5 months.

For stage II, primary chemotherapy when retroperitoneal metastatic disease is identified risks overtreatment, as up to 30% of these patients have false positive CT scans. There is clearly a tumor volume cut point beyond which occult systemic metastases are so likely

that primary chemotherapy is indicated. Our practice is to use primary chemotherapy for patients with a greater than 5 cm in any dimension CT mass and/or marker levels that are greater than 100. Radiation rarely has a role in nonseminoma management.

Infertility may occur as a result of RPL because of damage to the sympathetic postganglionic nerves in the retroperitoneum with loss of antegrade ejaculation. Therefore, patients should be advised to consider sperm banking. Infertility may also be preexistent in approximately 25% of patients (9). Even poor-quality semen should be stored, as new reproductive technologies can use the DNA or immotile sperm. Laparoscopic RPL is an advanced laparoscopic procedure and is now being done in some centers (7).

SURGICAL TECHNIQUE

Primary Procedure (No Previous Treatment)

We use a midline abdominal incision for the surgical approach, but the thoracoabdominal approach is an alternative, in particular with early stage left-sided tumors, when the dissection may be limited to the left paraaortic and interaortocaval nodal areas. An anterior transabdominal midline approach is more commonly practiced and is made from the tip of the xiphoid to the midlower abdomen around the left side of the umbilicus to avoid the falciform ligament (Fig. 63–1A). Laparotomy is then carefully performed to assess the extent of retroperitoneal disease and rule out other pathology. The small bowel and right colon are mobilized so that they can be rotated out of the abdomen and placed on the chest. The hepatic flexure can be taken down although this may not be necessary in all cases, followed by incision of the posterior peritoneum along the right colic gutter to the cecum (Fig. 63–1B). Care must be taken to identify the right ureter during mobilization of the right colon, and the rest of the small-bowel mesentery is incised cephalad to Trietz's ligament (Fig. 63–1C). Lymphatics can be coagulated or preferably ligated when divided.

The inferior mesenteric vein is routinely divided. Division of the vein allows rotation of the pancreas superiorly to allow better access to the retroperitoneum. Using blunt and sharp dissection, a plane is developed between the bowel including the pancreas and the anterior surface of the perinephric fascia. The small bowel and the right colon are then placed into a bowel bag and rotated out of the abdomen onto the chest.

With the retroperitoneum now fully exposed, the limits of dissection can be defined. There is some controversy regarding the extent of dissection required, but the following recommendations are based on the observed pattern of metastases:

1. For the grossly normal retroperitoneum, it seems reasonable to remove a template of nodes that for right-

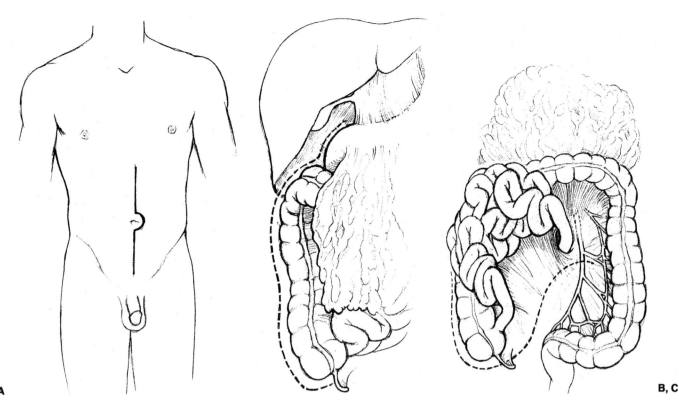

FIG. 63–1. A: Midline incision from xyphoid to symphysis. **B:** Incision of the line of Toldt to allow reflection of the right colon and exposure of the retroperitoneum. **C:** Continuation of line of peritoneal incision around the root of the bowel mesentery.

sided tumors would include left paraaortic nodes lateral to the ureter from the upper border of the renal vein to the level of the inferior mesenteric artery below, all the interaortocaval nodes, and the precaval and paracaval nodes; also, the nodes along the right common iliac should be removed to its bifurcation with the right ureter as the right lateral limit (Fig. 63–2A) (3). The sympathetic nerves can be identified and preserved within the template.

For left-sided tumors, dissection would include the same left paraaortic nodes from the renal vein to the bifurcation of the common iliac lateral to the left ureter and nodes on the front of the aorta and in the interaortocaval region inferior to the renal vein to the inferior mesenteric artery (Fig. 63–2B). These limits will include the primary landing sites for nodal metastases but microscopic metastases can occur in the interaortocaval nodes so these may be removed as well. Postganglionic sympathetic nerves important for emission may be injured in this area so dissection should be done by surgeons familiar with nerve identification and preservation. Any suspicious nodes outside these boundaries should be biopsied and, if positive, a bilateral dissection performed.

2. In the presence of multiple gross nodes but fewer than five and none greater than 2 cm, use the same limits, recognizing that with right-side tumors there

may be left paraaortic nodal involvement in up to 17% and left iliac in up to 7% that will be missed with the template (4). Two percent of patients might have a suprahilar node in the interaortocaval region, but that might well be grossly recognized and removed. It would seem reasonable, therefore, to omit this region for this stage of disease. If one of the grossly enlarged nodes is greater than 2 cm in diameter but smaller than 5 cm, or if there are more than five nodes, a full bilateral RPL should be done (Fig. 63–2C). There will be no significant additional patient morbidity if more dissection is performed unless the additional dissection involves dividing further lumbar arteries, which may contribute to some back pain postoperatively.

For bilateral dissection, the limits are the ureters laterally, superiorly the inferior border of the superior mesenteric artery extended bilaterally at a level 1 to 2 cm above the renal arteries, and inferiorly to at least the midpoint of the ipsilateral external iliac artery and to the bifurcation of the contralateral common iliac artery including the aortic bifurcation (Fig. 63–2C) the anterior spinal ligament and psoas muscles are cleared (8). Full bilateral dissection is begun by incising the retroperitoneal tissue in the midline anterior to the inferior vena cava (IVC). The left side of the cava is exposed from the left renal vein to its

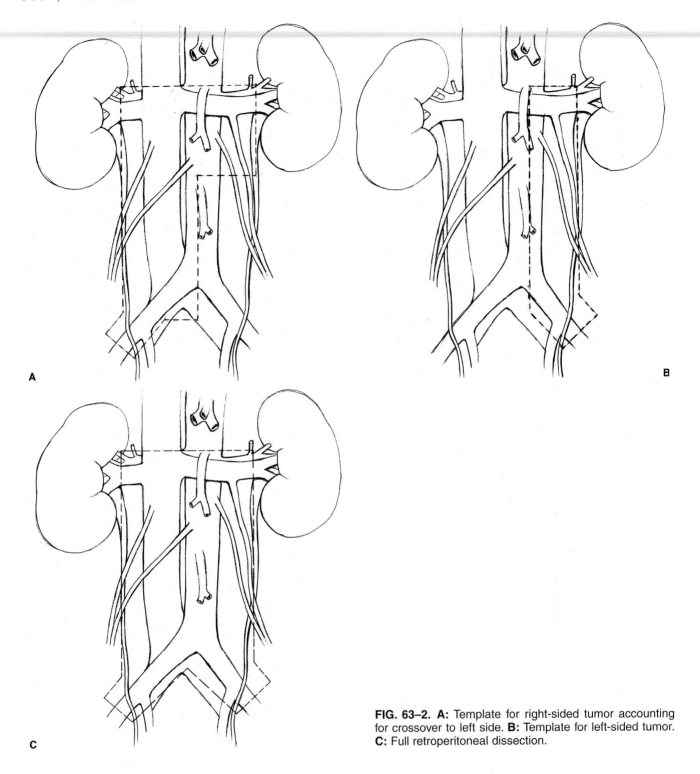

A

B

C

FIG. 63–2. A: Template for right-sided tumor accounting for crossover to left side. **B:** Template for left-sided tumor. **C:** Full retroperitoneal dissection.

origin at the left common iliac vein by peeling the adipose and lymphatic tissue medially, taking care to cauterize or ligate small vessels (Fig. 63–3A). The IVC is carefully rolled laterally with ligation and division of the left lumbar veins as required (Fig. 63–3B). The right sympathetic chain lies posterior to the midline of the cava (Fig. 63–4). A review of the anatomy of the retroperitoneal sympathetics is

important because nerve-sparing techniques specifically identify and preserve these nerves while still performing a thorough lymphadenectomy.

Seminal emission results from sympathetic stimulation of the seminal vesicles and vas deferens with deposition of semen in the posterior urethra. The sympathetic fibers arise from the sympathetic trunk as postganglionic nerves

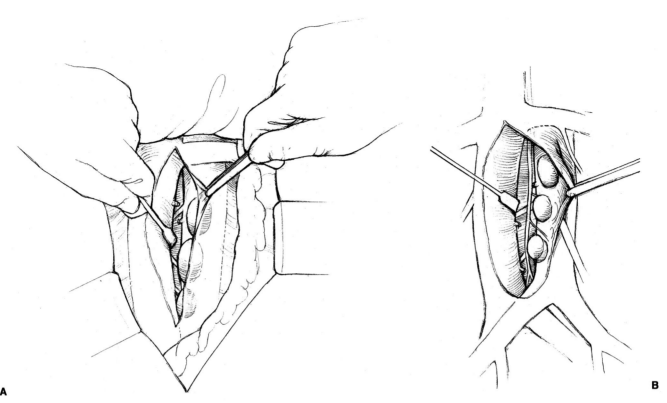

A **B**

FIG. 63–3. **A:** Dissection between the vena cava and aorta. **B:** Retraction of the great vessels allows exposure of the lumbar vessels, which should be ligated.

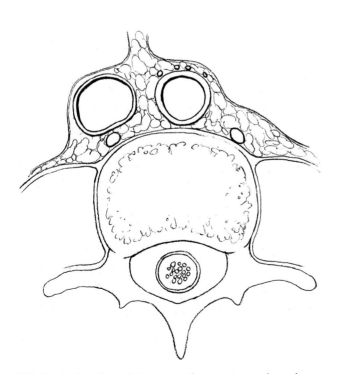

FIG. 63–4. Relationship between the great vessels and sympathetic trunks.

(specifically T12–L3). The paired sympathetic trunks run along the medial margin of the psoas, lateral to the lumbar vertebrae. The ganglia that comprise the sympathetic chain in this area usually number four or five (range, two to six) and are rounded or fusiform in shape with diameter 1 to 10 mm. Variation of number with fusion of adjacent ganglia is common. The overlying aorta partly conceals the left trunk, with the right trunk being partly covered anteriorly by the IVC (Fig. 63–4).

The lumbar sympathetic nerves arise from the ganglia opposite the first, second, and third lumbar vertebral bodies (Fig. 63–5). These nerves course in a variable fashion anteromedially to form a network of fibers lying on the anterior surface of the aorta. In addition, one often sees small groups of ganglion cells. Condensation of these nerve fibers and ganglia occurs with the formation of several nerve plexuses: superior mesenteric plexus, inferior mesenteric plexus, and hypogastric plexus. There is a high degree of variability in location of these plexuses, with their nomenclature approximating adjacent aortic branches (intermesenteric nerves, which have no constant pattern, connect the plexuses). The lowermost plexus, the hypogastric plexus, can usually be found anterior to the bifurcation of the aorta and in the interiliac angle. From this plexus, the right and left inferior hypogastric nerves run inferiorly to form the pelvic nerves that will eventu-

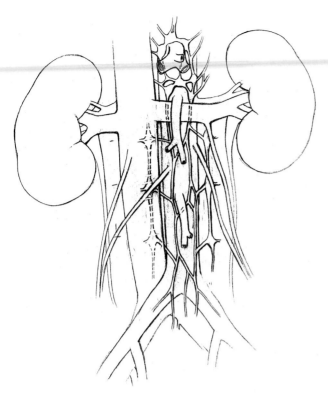

FIG. 63–5. Anatomy of the lumbar sympathetic nerves.

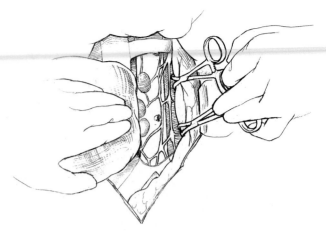

FIG. 63–6. Reflection of the left ureter and adipose tissue

ally supply sympathetic fibers to the bladder, prostate, urethra, periurethral glands, vas deferens, and seminal vesicles. The right lumbar veins can be followed posteriorly behind the cava as a guide to identify it. Although these lumbar veins normally run medial to the sympathetic chain, on occasion they can be lateral and even branch around the sympathetic chain. From the fusiform ganglia, fine postganglionic nerve fibers can be seen coursing anteromedially and inferiorly to the right side of the aorta. These fibers are the lumbar splanchnic nerves and can be individually skeletonized from the underlying interaortocaval lymphatic tissue, which is ultimately mobilized posteriorly from the anterior spinal ligament and withdrawn inferiorly, leaving the web of sympathetic nerves.

Before the surgeon proceeds further, the left ureter is visualized by creating a plane across the midline anterior to the retroperitoneal lymphatic tissue but behind the inferior mesenteric artery in the sigmoid mesocolon. This dissection may rarely require division of the inferior mesenteric artery, but it should be several centimeters distal to its origin. The left ureter can be exposed to the perinephric tissue, which is reflected laterally to visualize the left psoas muscle, leaving the left paraaortic retroperitoneal adipose tissue containing the lymph nodes intact (Fig. 63–6). This bulk of tissue is carefully reflected medially to expose the left sympathetic chain. The lumbar vessels on the left are also identified with this dissec-

tion as they course directly medially past the sympathetic chain and can be sacrificed as needed. The lumbar splanchnic nerves are identified originating from the sympathetic ganglia coursing medially and anteriorly. Superiorly, there may be a branch anterior to the renal artery coming from a higher ganglia, but this may be difficult to preserve.

At this point, the surgeon has a sense of the individual patient's sympathetic anatomy, which is variable. The aorta can now be exposed in the midline by mobilizing the left renal vein and splitting the soft tissue over it. Dissection is carried close to the aorta. The individual sympathetic nerve branches, having been identified on both right and left sides from preceding dissection, are seen on the anterior and lateral surfaces of the aorta. They are skeletonized, with care taken to preserve those branches that form variable plexuses on the anterior aorta. This allows withdrawal of the interaortocaval lymphatic tissue and the left paraaortic tissue from between the anterior spinal ligament posteriorly and the nerves anteriorly. The plexus at and below the level of the inferior mesenteric artery condenses to form the two hypogastric nerves that pass over the aorta and proceed inferiorly into the pelvis. Identification and preservation of these two nerves allow all lymphatic tissue over the aortic bifurcation and common iliac veins down to the sacral promontory to be removed without sacrificing ejaculation. Inferiorly, it is our practice to limit the dissection to a point approximately midway along the ipsilateral external iliac artery and to the bifurcation of the contralateral common iliac artery. The remnant of the spermatic cord is removed ipsilaterally with as much of the vas deferens as is easily removable along with the spermatic vessels to their attachments in the retroperitoneum.

Frequently, nodal metastases or tumor masses are immediately adjacent to or involve nerves. It is not necessary to preserve all postganglionic nerves to ensure ejaculation. Therefore, the surgeon should not hesitate to sacrifice nerves unilaterally or even in a limited manner bilaterally to ensure complete removal of disease.

The retroperitoneum defined by the selected surgical margins should now be clear of all lymphatic and fatty tissue surrounding the great vessels, with the postganglionic sympathetic nerves remaining beside and on the aorta. The contents of the bowel bag are placed back into the abdomen, and the large- and small-bowel peritoneal reflections are closed in their normal relationships using a running suture of no. 1 absorbable suture. The abdominal incision is closed using a running no. 1 polyglycolic suture with interrupted figure-of-eight sutures. Drains are not used.

Postchemotherapy Procedure

Patients with residual retroperitoneal disease pose particular problems. A full bilateral dissection remains the procedure of choice, although many patients appear to have a localized mass. Some centers advocate "lumpectomy" rather than a more extensive dissection, but this controversy is not resolved. Microscopic disease may occur in nodes adjacent to the gross disease. The potentially extensive nature of the tumor may on occasion require nephrectomy *en bloc,* resection of part or all of the aorta, and even resection of the IVC. Vascular surgical skill may therefore be necessary. Small lacerations or punctures of the great vessels may occur and require suture with fine no. 5-0 monofilament.

The approach and limits of dissection are similar. Nerve sparing may be possible in up to 50% of these patients if the mass is confined. The areas of greatest challenge are at the points at which the masses adhere to the great vessels. A combination of sharp and blunt dissection is required with good proximal and distal control where the vessels are normal. The actual plane of dissection may appear to be under the adventitia. The locations of small neovascularization vessels are difficult to predict but manageable. Comfort with normal anatomy is mandatory, and this surgery is not for the inexperienced. Distortion of normal anatomy and the frequent anomalies of retroperitoneal vessels can be challenging. Sudden blood loss may occur, so patients need close monitoring intraoperatively by an experienced anesthetist. Finally, intraoperative biopsy can be misleading and is not recommended for treatment decisions.

OUTCOMES

Complications

Intraoperative complications are unusual and are mainly confined to vascular damage of the renal or great vessels (1). Topical papaverine to reduce vessel spasm is used throughout the procedure. It is now rare to experience vascular injury without significant volume of disease. In removing a bulky mass from the aorta, care is taken to define the appropriate plane of dissection. It is easy to dissect in a subadventitial plane on the aorta, leaving a weakened vessel for potential aneurysmal dilation. If an appropriate plane of dissection cannot be developed, it may be safer to resect part of the vessel wall with primary closure or placement of a synthetic graft. In addition, vein or Gore-Tex patches have been used to close caval defects.

The meticulous obliteration of lymphatics by ligature or cautery will decrease the incidence of lymphocele and ascites postoperatively. On occasion, a lymphocele can become symptomatic because of a local mass effect resulting in vague abdominal or flank discomfort. Rarely, obstruction of the small bowel or ureter can occur secondary to the lymphocele mass. Management usually is by the percutaneous drainage if symptomatic, with ultrasound or CT scan used for guidance. Most resolve spontaneously, however.

Early postoperative complications with RPL are similar to those for any major abdominal procedure. Aggressive chest physiotherapy should be commenced immediately postoperatively in all patients to minimize the risk of atelectasis and pneumonia, which occurs in approximately 1% of patients. A potential pulmonary complication seen in testis cancer patients is related to pulmonary fibrosis secondary to previous bleomycin chemotherapy. Intraoperatively, the patient is maintained on a lower inspired oxygen concentration and a slight negative fluid balance is maintained. Following the recognition of this association with chemotherapy, only the rare patient will have a serious complication from his chest.

Finally, late bowel obstruction, which occurs in about 1% of patients, can be minimized with careful reapproximation of the retroperitoneum during closure or by employing the thoracoabdominal approach.

Results

It is anticipated that 70% of patients with clinical stage-I disease do not need further treatment. The majority of the remaining 30% have retroperitoneal metastases that can be resected. Patients selected with low-volume stage II disease who have complete resections now fail in approximately 30% of cases without adjuvant chemotherapy. Therapy may therefore be reserved for those patients when they progress. Alternatively, all positive-node patients may have adjuvant treatment. Stage I and II patients should have cure rates of virtually 100%. Patients with very bulky retroperitoneal disease or systemic disease have a lower survival rate and, with multidisciplinary management and use of initial chemotherapy followed by salvage surgery, approximately 70% should be curable.

REFERENCES

1. Baniel J, Foster RS, Rowland RG, et al. Complications of postchemotherapy retroperitoneal lymph node dissection. *J Urol* 1995;153: 976–980.

2. Donohue JP, Maynard B, Zachary M. The distribution of nodal metastases in the retroperitoneum from nonseminomatous testis cancer. *J Urol* 1982;128:315–320.

3. Donohue JP. Nerve-sparing retroperitoneal lymphadenectomy for testis cancer. Evolution of surgical templates for low-stage disease. *Eur Urol* 1993;23:44–46.

4. Donohue JP, Thornhill JA, Foster RS, et al. The role of retroperitoneal lymphadenectomy in clinical stage B testis cancer: the Indiana University experience (1965 to 1989). *J Urol* 1995;153:85–89.

5. Freedman LS, Jones WG, Peckham MJ. Histopathology in the prediction of relapse of patients with stage I testicular teratoma treated by orchidectomy alone. *Lancet* 1987;2:294–298.

6. Greene F, Page D, Fleming I, et al. *AJCC Cancer Staging Manual*, 6th ed. New York: Springer, 2002:35–41.

7. Janetschek G, Peschel R, Hobisch A, Bartsch G. Laparoscopic retroperitoneal lymph node dissection. *J Endourol* 2001;15:449–453; discussion 453–445.

8. Jewett MA, Kong YS, Goldberg SD, et al. Retroperitoneal lymphadenectomy for testis tumor with nerve sparing for ejaculation. *J Urol* 1988;139:1220–1224.

9. Lange PH, Chang WY, Fraley EE. Fertility issues in the therapy of nonseminomatous testicular tumors. *Urol Clin North Am* 1987;14:731.

10. Read G, Stenning SP, Cullen MH, et al. Medical Research Council prospective study of surveillance for stage I testicular teratoma. *J Clin Oncol* 1992;10:1762–1768.

11. Steyerberg EW, Gerl A, Fossa SD, et al. Validity of predictions of residual retroperitoneal mass histology in nonseminomatous testicular cancer. *J Clin Oncol* 1998;16:269–274.

CHAPTER 64

Torsion of the Testicle

Paul G. Espy and Harry P. Koo

Testicular torsion is a surgical emergency that demands prompt recognition and treatment to preserve testicular function. This condition occurs when the spermatic cord twists upon itself, leading to vascular compromise and testicular loss with prolonged ischemia. The need for timely assessment and intervention is heightened by the fact that hours often elapse between the onset of symptoms and the urologist's evaluation. Despite the continuing advancements in radiological imaging of the acute scrotum, a history and physical examination consistent with acute testicular torsion are often sufficient to warrant immediate surgical exploration.

Torsion of the spermatic cord has been recognized in all age groups, although the majority of patients present during adolescence. The peak incidence has uniformly been seen in the 12- to 18-year-old age range, with a second, much smaller peak in the perinatal period (13). Although the incidence decreases with age after adolescence, all age groups are susceptible. The annual incidence of testicular torsion in men under the age of 25 is estimated to be 1 in 4,000 (13). One large study found that 6.8% of cases involved an undescended testicle and it was speculated that testicular torsion was 10 times more common in patients with undescended testes (13). Curiously, a number of investigations have demonstrated unequal laterality, with the left testicle being affected more frequently. Bilateral torsion is said to account for fewer than 5% of all cases (13).

Testicular torsion can be classified as extravaginal or intravaginal based on whether the twisting is above or below the reflection of the tunica vaginalis onto the spermatic cord (Fig. 64–1). *Extravaginal* torsion occurs when the tunica vaginalis is not securely attached to the scrotum, allowing the testicle and the tunica vaginalis to rotate as a unit along the longitudinal axis. This variant is virtually always limited to the perinatal population and may take place antenally or postnatally—a distinction that has important prognostic and therapeutic implica-

tions. A review by Das and Singer found that 72% of perinatal torsions happen *in utero* (4). With *intravaginal* torsion, twisting of the spermatic cord occurs entirely within, but does not involve, the tunica vaginalis. This type of torsion affects patients outside of the perinatal age group, although it has been reported on rare occasion in newborns. Several anatomic factors contribute to intravaginal torsion. In the "bell-clapper" deformity, the tunica vaginalis inserts at an abnormally high location on the spermatic cord, thus preventing scrotal contact with the testicle. In addition, the mesorchium may have a narrow attachment onto the testicle, allowing the testis to assume a more horizontal position within the scrotum. These factors contribute to increased testicular motility within the tunica vaginalis and facilitate rotation of the testis about the spermatic cord.

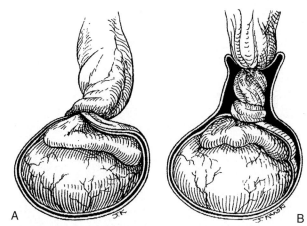

FIG. 64–1. (A) Extravaginal torsion, typical of a neonatal testicular torsion. The tunica vaginalis is involved with the twist of the spermatic cord. **(B)** Intravaginal torsion, usually seen after the neonatal period, involves the spermatic cord below the reflection of the tunica vaginalis onto the spermatic cord.

DIAGNOSIS

Perinatal Torsion

In the newborn, local and systemic symptoms of torsion may be scarce, delaying presentation and diagnosis. The patient with antenatal torsion may present with a large, firm, painless scrotal mass. Parents may report a swollen scrotum with discolored skin. In postnatal torsion, similar symptoms develop in a newborn with a previously normal scrotal examination. However, torsion that occurs after birth is more likely to cause systemic symptoms such as irritability or lack of appetite. Parents may also note an acute onset of redness and swelling of the scrotum.

In newborns, the physical exam may be the only indicator of testicular torsion. The neonate is usually in no acute distress, although a postnatal onset is more likely to cause general discomfort. An abdominal or inguinal mass may be found in the case of an undescended testis. More often a firm, large, nontender mass that fails to transilluminate is present in the scrotum (Fig. 64–2). The scrotal skin may be discolored, ranging from erythematous to blue–black depending on the degree and duration of torsion. Chronic changes are more frequently seen with antenatal torsion.

Torsion in Children, Adolescents, and Adults

Torsion outside of the perinatal population is usually associated with a more acute symptomatology. The classic presentation is described as a sudden onset of severe, unilateral testicular pain, with swelling of the testicle. With time, the patient may complain of swelling and redness of

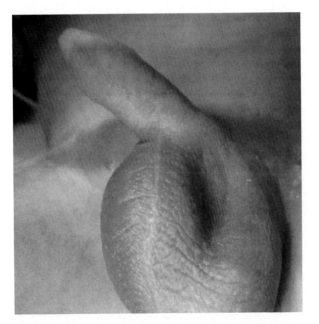

FIG. 64–2. Physical exam of an infant with extravaginal torsion reveals a firm, enlarged mass of the right scrotum.

the scrotum. Pain in the groin or abdomen, with associated nausea and vomiting, is not uncommon. One-third of patients may report previous episodes of testicular pain and swelling (13). Urinary symptoms and fever are infrequent.

Older patients typically have more acute findings on physical exam. Almost invariably, the testicle will be swollen and exquisitely tender. Scrotal edema and erythema are usually present. In many cases the affected testicle assumes a retracted, horizontal lie. Loss of the cremasteric reflex is suggestive of testicular torsion, and in several series was universally absent. These characteristic findings all point toward an etiology of testicular torsion, but it must be remembered that no single finding is pathognomonic.

Torsion of Testicular Appendages

Four testicular appendages have been identified: the appendix testis (hydatid of Morgagni), the appendix epididymis, the paradidymis (organ of Giraldés), and the vas aberrans of Haller. Each of these is susceptible to torsion, but the overwhelming majority of twisted appendages involve the appendix testis. Torsion of a testicular appendage is often characterized by a gradual onset and few systemic symptoms. Early in the course of torsion of the appendix testis, physical examination may reveal a tender mass located at the upper pole of the testicle, sometimes adherent to the overlying skin. In our experience, it has been rare to see a small area of ecchymotic skin at the upper pole ("blue dot sign"), which is pathognomonic for torsion of the appendix testis. In almost all cases the testicle has a normal orientation and the cremasteric reflex is intact (12). With time, torsion of the testicle and torsion of an appendage can become clinically indistinguishable. Imaging with Doppler ultrasound may show a hyperechoic mass at the upper pole of a normal-appearing testicle. If the clinician is completely confident in the diagnosis of appendage torsion, the condition can be treated symptomatically. Therapy consists of bedrest, scrotal elevation, and nonsteroidal antiinflammatory agents as needed. Symptoms should begin to resolve within 1 to 2 weeks as the infarcted appendage is gradually resorbed. If testicular torsion cannot be ruled out with certainty, urgent surgical exploration is needed.

DIAGNOSTIC STUDIES

Testicular torsion is a clinical diagnosis and is proven at the time of surgery. Radiological studies may support the diagnosis, but negative imaging should not preclude exploration when clinical suspicion is high. Nonetheless, diagnostic examinations should be performed when testicular torsion is considered unlikely and the clinician has concluded that the patient has a nonsurgical condition.

Color Doppler ultrasound is widely utilized in the evaluation of scrotal abnormalities and has been studied in

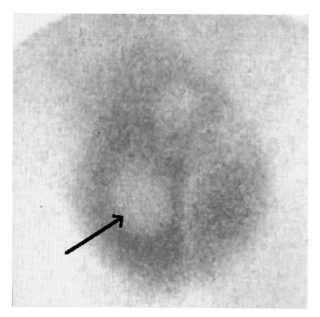

FIG. 64–3. Nuclear scintigraphy shows the characteristic "cold spot" in the right testicle (*arrow*).

patients with testicular torsion. The capacity to view both blood flow and anatomic detail is particularly useful in assessing the scrotal contents and can provide valuable information about other pathologic conditions. A recent study found that color Doppler has a sensitivity of 89% in diagnosing testicular torsion (1). It has also been used to diagnose testicular torsion *in utero*. Lack of intratesticular blood flow and testicular enlargement are characteristic findings. However, arterial blood flow ceases only after venous obstruction and edema develop, which can lead to a false negative result early in the torsion. Intermittent torsion may also go undiagnosed. As with many radiographic technologies, interpretation is highly dependent on the experience of the technician or radiologist.

Nuclear blood flow scan with technetium-99m pertechnetate is well known for its diagnostic accuracy, with a sensitivity of 80% to 100% (8). The positive scan will show a "cold spot," which represents decreased perfusion in the affected testis, with a surrounding area of increased uptake (Fig. 64–3). One drawback of nuclear scintigraphy is the inability to evaluate testicular and scrotal anatomy. Further, results in pediatric patients can be challenging to interpret due to small blood vessels size and decreased rate of blood flow. Nuclear scans are in general more time consuming and expensive than color Doppler studies.

INDICATIONS FOR SURGERY

Management of the newborn with testicular torsion is an area of controversy. To understand treatment in this age group it is important to define the condition as prenatal or postnatal. Torsion that presents acutely after birth requires emergent surgical exploration. The nonviable testicle should undergo orchiectomy while evidence of viability should prompt detorsion with orchidopexy. We recommend fixation of the contralateral testis regardless of the condition of the affected testicle. In the case of bilateral torsion (both prenatal and postnatal), the threshold for performing bilateral orchidopexy should be lower in an effort to preserve testicular function. The most common scenario in the perinatal period is the case of prenatal torsion, in which the baby is found to have chronic changes and a nonviable testicle. These neonates should undergo elective orchiectomy with contralateral testis fixation once anesthesia risk assessment has been stabilized (within 1 to 2 days of diagnosis). Operative risk is a concern, but in a recent series of 27 patients with perinatal torsion who underwent exploration 2 hours to 2 months after birth there were no surgery- or anesthesia-related complications (9). Regular follow-up is needed to assess testicular size and pubertal development, and the services of an endocrinologist should be considered when hormonal dysfunction is expected (e.g., bilateral torsion). The option for testicular prosthesis placement in childhood should be discussed with the parents of orchiectomy patients.

The principles of management for patients beyond infancy are similar to those for newborns, although the more acute presentation in the older group provides greater opportunity for testicular salvage. To reiterate, a history and physical exam consistent with testicular torsion demands immediate surgical exploration. Orchiectomy is needed for the nonviable testicle, while a viable testis should be untwisted and fixed to the scrotum. Orchidopexy should be performed to protect the contralateral testicle. Testicular prostheses are available for adults and can be placed during the initial operation or at a later date. Evidence of testicular atrophy should be noted during follow-up visits. Further, it is important to discuss with patients the increased risk of subfertility.

ALTERNATIVE THERAPY

Some clinicians recommend that manual detorsion should be attempted. Studies evaluating the success rate for manual detorsion have produced conflicting evidence. Clinicians who adopt this strategy must do so on the premise that it does not substitute for or delay surgery. Because the majority of testes twist inward (right testicle clockwise and left counterclockwise as viewed from the foot of the bed), manual detorsion should occur in the opposite direction. Nerve block of the spermatic cord can facilitate this maneuver, but it may also conceal the relief of detorsion or the pain of manipulation in the wrong direction. Successful manual detorsion should be followed by immediate surgical exploration.

While currently limited to animal models, medical adjuncts may one day be implemented, along with surgical management, to minimize the sequelae associated with testicular torsion. Pentoxyfylline, a methyl xanthine derivative that decreases blood viscosity and platelet aggregation, appears to improve blood flow to both testes after unilateral torsion (11). Nitric oxide has been shown to have a protective effect against histopathologic changes in the contralateral testicle, presumably through the regulation of blood flow (5).

SURGICAL TECHNIQUE

Aside from the choice of incision, the surgical treatment for perinatal and childhood/adult (intravaginal) testicular torsion is essentially the same. For perinatal torsion, we use an inguinal approach on the affected side. The reason for doing so is that with extravaginal torsion (Fig. 64–4), there is a rare chance that another problem may exist, such as hernia or tumor, that is best treated superior to the scrotum.

For intravaginal torsion, a vertical midline scrotal incision is our preferred approach to explore both testes. Two separate hemiscrotal incisions may also be used with excellent cosmetic results. Following incision to the level of the dartos muscles, the affected testis is moved under the midline incision. The layers of tunicae can be gently separated using a hemostat to minimize bleeding. The final few layers of tunicae are opened in a vertical fashion to expose

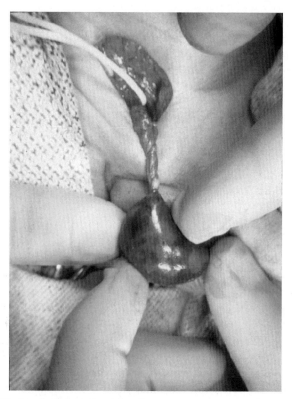

FIG. 64–4. Exposure of the right spermatic cord and testicle through an inguinal incision reveals a case of extravaginal torsion. *Note*: This is the same patient whose physical exam is seen in Figure 64–2.

the testis. A torsed testis usually appears dark blue or black. Following manual detorsion, the testis is inspected for viability. If the viability of the testis is in question, the detorsed testis is wrapped in a warm moist sponge to recover while the contralateral testis is being pexed. If there still remains concern about the viability, a small nick can be made in the tunica albuginea to expose the seminiferous tubules, which should appear dusky rose to pink.

A nonviable testis should be removed to avoid continued symptoms or possible infection and reduce the possibility of contralateral testicular damage from antisperm antibodies. We do not routinely place a testicular prosthesis at the time of orchiectomy. For individuals who request a testicular prosthesis, we have performed delayed placement of solid silicone prostheses through a low inguinal incision.

The techniques for fixation of the viable, detorsed testis and the contralateral testis still remain debated. Some of the controversy includes fixation with or without eversion of the tunica vaginalis, the use of absorbable or nonabsorbable sutures, and fixation at two or three sites on the testis (3,7,10). We believe that the most important step in the fixation is the eversion of the tunica vaginalis (Figs. 64–5A and 64–5B). This step produces two effects: (a) The testis is in an extravaginal position and thus would not be at risk for intravaginal torsion; (b) everting the tunica vaginalis allows for contact between tunica albuginea and the dartos. As an additional step, we perform two-point fixation of superior and inferior peritesticular tissue using absorbable (Vicryl) or nonabsorbable (Prolene) sutures.

OUTCOMES

Complications

The most significant complication of testicular torsion is infarction of the gonad. This event depends on the duration and degree of torsion and is managed by orchiectomy. A testicle that is viable at the time of surgery may later become atrophic despite orchidopexy, and must be monitored closely by physical exam. Abnormal semen analysis and contralateral testicular apoptosis are also recognized sequelae following testicular torsion (2,6). As such, the risk of subfertility should be discussed with the patient. Although rare, torsion of a previously pexed testicle may occur.

Results

The primary determinants of testicular viability are the degree to which the spermatic cord twists and the duration of torsion. The literature reports dismal salvage rates in newborns (as low as 5%); however, these accounts do not always distinguish between prenatal and postnatal torsion. Few cases of testicular salvage have been reported with an antenatal event. An aggressive approach

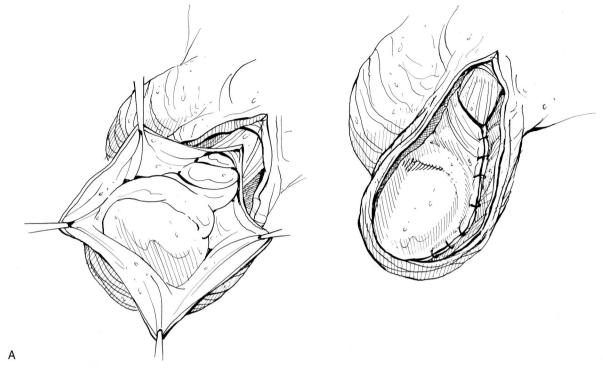

FIG. 64–5. A: Scrotal incision with open tunica vaginalis reveals an intravaginal torsion. **B:** Tunica vaginalis is everted following detorsion of the testicle.

to postnatal torsion is likely to improve the rate of testicular salvage for this subset of patients, which was 20% in a recent study (9). Long-term assessment of fertility in patients with perinatal torsion is lacking.

Determining the duration of symptoms is easier in patients outside of the newborn age group for obvious reasons. Workman and Kogan found that patients who underwent surgery within 6 hours of onset have testicular salvage rates of 83% to 97% (14). This figure dropped to 55% to 85% between 6 to 12 hours of onset, and after 24 hours the salvage rate fell to less than 10% (14). These statistics are consistent throughout the literature. Notably, testicular salvage does not necessarily imply normal testicular function. A number of studies have demonstrated that men with testicular torsion are prone to subfertility and abnormalities of the contralateral testicle.

In summary, testicular torsion is a urologic emergency that is diagnosed clinically and treated by immediate surgical exploration. The decision to perform orchiectomy versus orchidopexy of the affected testicle is based on the viability of the testis at the time of exploration. In either case, contralateral orchidopexy should be performed. The anatomic abnormalities that predispose the patient to testicular torsion are well established; however, the mechanisms responsible for long-term testicular dysfunction and contralateral testicular damage are under investigation. Rates of testicular salvage have improved dramatically since the first recorded case of testicular torsion in 1840. With heightened awareness of the signs and symptoms on the part of patients and physicians, along with a

better understanding of the pathophysiological mechanisms, immediate and long-term outcomes of testicular torsion will continue to improve.

REFERENCES

1. Baker LA, et al. An analysis of clinical outcomes using color Doppler testicular ultrasound for testicular torsion. *Pediatrics* 2000;105(3): 604–607.
2. Bartsch G, et al. Testicular torison: Late results with special regard to fertility and endocrine function. *J Urol* 1980;124:375–378.
3. Bellinger MF, et al. Orchiopexy: an experimental study of the effect of surgical technique on testicular histology. *J Urol* 1989;142:553–555.
4. Das S, Singer A. Controversies of perinatal torsion of the spermatic cord: a review, survey and recommendations. *J Urol* 1990;143: 231–233.
5. Dokucu AI, et al. The protective effects of nitric oxide on the contralateral testis in prepubertal rats with unilateral testicular torsion. *BJU Int* 2000;85:767–771.
6. Hadziselimovic F, et al. Increased apoptosis in the contralateral testes of patients with testicular torsion as a factor for infertility. *J Urol* 1998;160:1158–1160.
7. Lent V, Stephani A. Eversion of the tunica vaginalis for prophylaxis of testicular torsion recurrences. *J Urol* 1993;150:1419–1421.
8. Melloul M, et al. The value of radionuclide scrotal imaging in the diagnosis of acute testicular torsion. *Br J Urol* 1995;76:628–631.
9. Pinto KJ, et al. Management of neonatal testicular torsion. *J Urol* 1997; 158:1196–1197.
10. Rodriguez LE, Kaplan GW. An experimental study of methods to produce intrascrotal testicular fixation. *J Urol* 1988;139:565–567.
11. Savas C, et al. Pentoxifylline improves blood flow to both testes in testicular torsion. *Int Urol Neph* 2002;33:81–85.
12. Van Glabeke E, et al. Acute scrotal pain in children: results of 543 surgical explorations. *Ped Surg Int* 1999;15:353–357.
13. Williamson RCN. Torsion of the testis and allied conditions. *Br J Surg* 1976;63:465–476.
14. Workman SJ, Kogan BA. Old and new aspects of testicular torsion. *Sem Urol* 1988;VI:146–157.

CHAPTER 65

Scrotal Trauma and Reconstruction

Gerald H. Jordan

The anatomy of the male genitalia is quite complex, in particular in the scrotum, where there are multiple fascial layers (Fig. 65–1). From the standpoint of trauma, however, most of the fascial layers are relatively unimportant. Buck's fascia is related to the deep penile structures and is important in the containment of periurethral processes or the occasional hematoma associated with injury to the corpora cavernosa. In the scrotum, the analogous fascia to Buck's fascia—the external spermatic fascia—is usually uninvolved with scrotal trauma. The dartos fascia of the penis becomes the tunica dartos in the scrotum and then reflects onto the perineum as Colles' fascia. Those

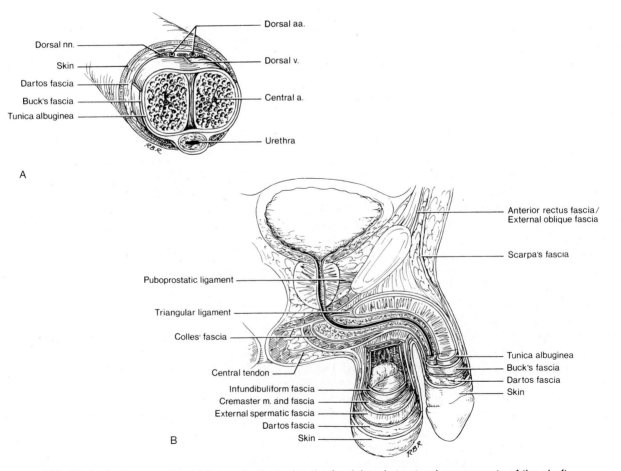

FIG. 65–1. A: Cross section of the penis illustrating the fascial and structural components of the shaft of the penis. **B:** Sagittal section of the pelvis demonstrating the fascial layers and structural component.

fascial layers are in continuity with Scarpa's fascia over the abdomen and reflect over the thighs to become contiguous with the fascia lata (Fig. 65–2) (1,3).

The deep internal pudendal arteries depart Alcock's canal. They give off prominent superficial branches, the perineal artery and the posterior scrotal artery. They then continue as the common penile artery with its many branches (Fig. 65–3). The blood supply to the testicles is based on the spermatic artery and the paravasal arteries. These two blood supplies join via connections close to the testicle and also within the hilum of the testicle. The posterior scrotal branches arborize to become the fascial plexuses of the tunica dartos of the scrotum. Large skin islands can be carried on this blood supply (Fig. 65–4). There often also are vessels within the scrotal raphe that further add to the dependability of these scrotal fascial flaps. Further blood supply to the scrotum is via the perineal artery, which arborizes to become the fascial blood supply and is the basic blood supply to the skin lateral to the scrotum, the basis for the "perineal axial fasciocutaneous flap" (Singapore flap). The superficial external pudendal vessels, the vessels of the medial circumflex artery, and the deep external pudendal arteries likewise send branches onto the scrotum to arborize there and become a portion of the fascial blood supply (Fig. 65–4).

The venous anatomy of the deep structures of the penis is essentially in reverse of the arterial supply, with the subcoronal plexus becoming the deep dorsal vein and, in about 60% of cases, the superficial dorsal vein of the penis. The deep dorsal vein drains to the median periprostatic plexus, and the superficial veins drain laterally into the iliofemoral system. The crural and cavernosal veins, those that are oriented medially, drain medially, to Santorini's plexus, and those departing laterally drain to the iliofemoral system (Fig. 65–5).

Culp has classified injuries to the external male genitalia into five categories: nonpenetrating, penetrating, avulsion, burns, and radiation injuries (both direct and indirect) (3). Nonpenetrating injuries result from either a crushing or sudden deforming force to the scrotum. These forces can cause severe damage to the internal structures without disrupting the skin. With any nonpenetrating trauma to the scrotum or perineum, one must suspect and rule out injury to the corpus spongiosum and urethra.

Penetrating injuries to the genitalia can involve the urethra. Most of the injuries require exploration, irrigation, and removal of foreign-body material, if any, with anatomic repair and drainage. If there is any suspicion of urethral injury, retrograde urethrogram should be performed, and cystoscopy performed if further clarification of the injury is required. Saline should be used for irrigation in these cases. Because of the position of the urethra beneath the scrotum and perineum, significant penetrating injuries to the scrotum can also often miss the urethra.

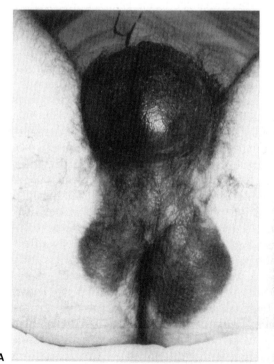

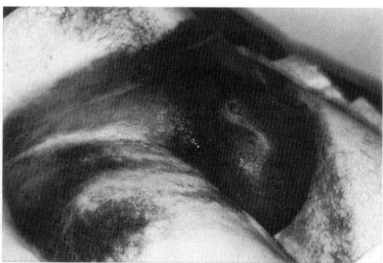

A

B

FIG. 65–2. A: Perineal view of a trauma patient illustrating a hematoma contained by Colles' fascia (classic butterfly hematoma). **B:** Same trauma patient illustrating the containment of the hematoma by the extended Colles' layer, i.e., the fascia lata of the thigh and extending onto the abdomen beneath Scarpa's fascia.

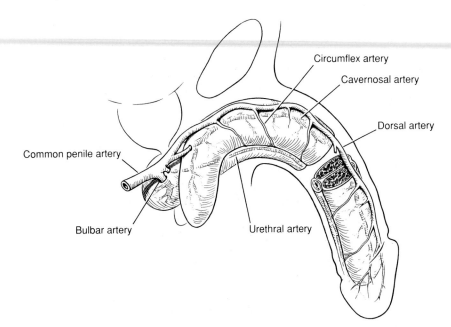

FIG. 65–3. Illustration of the distribution of the common penile artery.

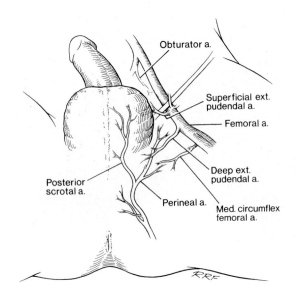

FIG. 65–4. Illustration of the blood vessels felt to contribute to the fascial blood supply of the scrotum.

Avulsion injuries of the genital skin most frequently involve the scrotal skin and occur when the patient's clothing becomes entangled in machinery. The loose scrotal tissues entangle, and as the clothing is ripped off so is the loose genital skin. These avulsion injuries vary from minimal injuries, which are essentially nothing more than lacerations, to emasculating injuries, which take not only the skin but also the deep structures. It is not unusual for a testicle to be avulsed along with the skin. The deep penile structures, however, are usually not avulsed. Avulsion, fortunately, usually takes only the skin and the tunica dartos, leaving the underlying Buck's fascia of the penis and the fascial layers surrounding the tes-

ticle intact. In most of these cases bleeding is not a problem, as the skin and fascia are avulsed in a plane between the fascial structures related to the deep structures and the superficial fascia.

Burns to the genitalia are usually not isolated injuries but reflective of a wider area of body burn. Chemical burns are in general only superficial and involve the skin. Thermal injuries can be deep, but often, even with extensive deep burns proximate to the genitalia, the multiple clothing layers (i.e., underwear and other clothing) can protect the genitalia. Electrical burns disseminate via the deep vascular and neurological structures, and what may appear to be a minimal burn to the skin and scrotum may have significant deep injury associated with it, and this can be devastating. However, usually the deepest burns associated with electrical contact occur at the site of the current inflow and the ground site. These sites are usually not the genitalia. However, it is not uncommon to have thermal burns in concert with the electrical burns, as frequently the clothing is ignited by the electrical spark. Thus, with electrical burns, fortunately, if the genitalia are involved it is usually a more superficial process.

Radiation injuries to the genitalia can occur either from direct exposure to the genitalia or from the effects of radiation on the venous and lymphatic drainage. Now, by and large, we do not see complications of direct radiation to the genitalia because radiation for penile lesions is rarely undertaken. The secondary effects of radiation, as seen in the scrotum, are usually manifested by chronic lymphedema, chronic lymphangiectasia, and, in some cases, chronic recurring cellulitis.

To this list must be added the patient who has required significant debridement because of rapidly progressive, multiorganism fasciitis (Fournier's gangrene). Fournier's gangrene is often seen with processes of the rectum, such

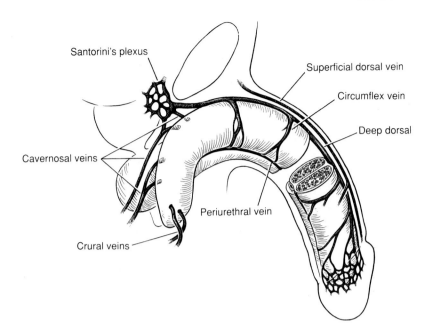

FIG. 65–5. The venous drainage of the deep structures of the penis.

as missed perianal abscess, or with processes involving the urethra, such as periurethral abscess, many times associated with other comorbidities such as diabetes mellitus. Many of these patients present late, and excision, while lifesaving, usually leaves a significant defect. If the fasciitis is associated with pathophysiology of the urethra and/or anus, then these situations must be managed and resolved before reconstruction (5).

Also, in recent years we have seen several patients who have attempted to enhance the size and bulk of their genitalia with the injection of lipid-containing substances such as paraffin or petroleum jelly or inert substances such as silicone. In these cases, one is confronted, often, with a fulminant cellulitis that must be treated with broad-spectrum antibiotics. Later, the process is that of a sclerosing granuloma process. In some cases, the skin must be excised along with the deeper involved structures, but it is not unusual to be able to excise the deep process and leave the skin that survives on its random dermal blood supply.

DIAGNOSIS

A contusion of the scrotum, i.e., scrotal hematoma, can be confused with a fracture of the testicle. The latter injury implies disruption of the tunica albuginea of the testicle. With a scrotal contusion the hematoma usually is noted to be posterior and lateral to the testicle (Fig. 65–6), whereas with fracture of the testicle the parenchyma of the testis is not normal and is often associated with a hematocele (Fig. 65–7). In the presence of

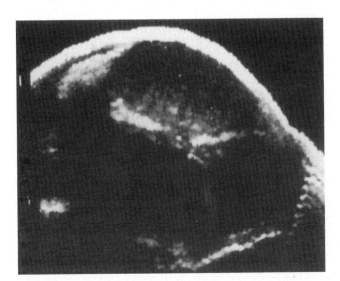

FIG. 65–6. B-scan ultrasound demonstrating the classic distribution of a scrotal contusion (scrotal wall hematoma). Note the testis displaced anteriorly, with the hematoma contained in the multiple fascial layers of the scrotum.

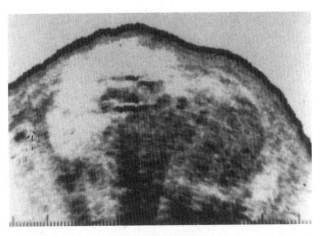

FIG. 65–7. B-scan ultrasound of a patient with a fracture of the testicle. Note the disrupted parenchymal pattern of the testicle, the hematocele, and the demonstration of extruded seminiferous tubules within the hematocele.

penetrating trauma to the genitalia, a retrograde urethrogram is always indicated because of the close proximity to the urethra. In all cases of genital avulsion, other than a simple scrotal avulsion, a complete evaluation of the urethra must be done, along with a rectal examination and possibly flexible sigmoidoscopy.

INDICATIONS FOR SURGERY

Exploration of the scrotum would be indicated if there are indications of injury to the testicle (blunt or penetrating). Scrotal reconstruction would be required following complex lacerations or penetrating injury to the scrotum, avulsion injuries, excisions for chronic cellulitis, lymphangiectasia and lymphedema, following significant burns to the scrotal skin, and for the other processes, just enumerated above.

ALTERNATIVE THERAPY

Contusions of the scrotum are usually treated with bedrest, analgesia, and scrotal elevation. Scrotal elevation can be accomplished very efficiently with a Bellevue-style bridge or with scrotal support.

SURGICAL TECHNIQUE

Scrotal Hematomas and Blunt Testicular Injury

There is little to be accomplished in exploring the scrotal hematoma secondary to external blunt trauma, as the hematoma is usually disseminated throughout the highly elastic layers of the scrotum and does not form a drainable hematoma per se. On the other hand, if there is a testicular injury, exploration and repair of the testicle is indicated (Fig. 65–8). Exploration consists of exposure of the testicle.

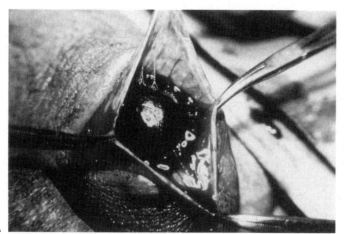

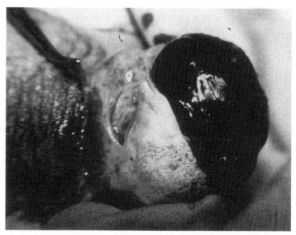

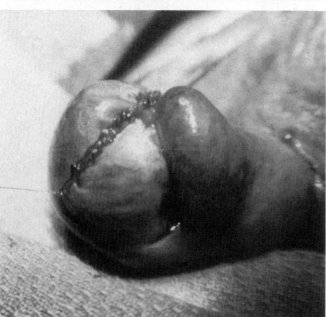

FIG. 65–8. A: Patient with fractured testicle; the skin has been opened, as has been the vaginal space. Note the draining hematocele fluid with clots affixed to the seminiferous tubules. **B:** The testicle has been delivered. Note the clot attached to the extruded tubules. **C:** Appearance of the testicle following repair.

The space of the tunica vaginalis is opened, the hematocele is drained, seminiferous tubules are debrided, and the tunica albuginea is closed. In the past polyglycolic (PGA) suture was used; however, now we use polydioxanone suture, although Monocryl is also an option. The parietal tunica vaginalis is left open and is reflected as would have been done for a hydrocele. The scrotum is drained and closed with 3-0 PGA suture, chromic suture, or Monocryl.

Penetrating Injuries to the Genitalia

Penetrating injuries have been subclassified as either simple or complicated. By and large, complicated injuries imply urethral involvement, amputation, or near-total amputation and, with regard to the scrotum, imply amputation or injury of the testicle, with or without amputation of the overlying scrotal skin (Fig. 65–9). Simple lacera-

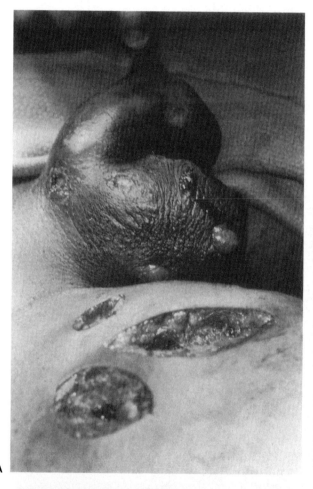

A

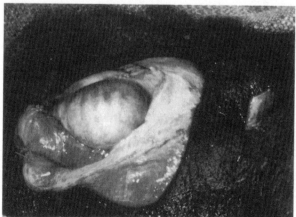

C

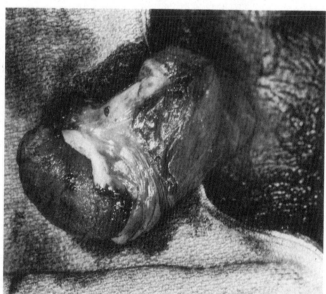

B

FIG. 65–9. **A:** Young patient with complex penetrating trauma to the thigh and genitalia. Retrograde urethrogram, rectal examination, and flexible sigmoidoscopy were normal. The patient's scrotum was explored. **B:** The patient's right testicle is delivered; note the intact seminiferous tubule pattern with virtual complete disruption of the tunica albuginea. **C:** Appearance of the same testicle (B) following reconstruction of the tunica albuginea with primary closure. **D:** Appearance of the genitalia with the gunshot wounds debrided and the right hemiscrotum drained. Coburn has assembled a series of patients with similar injuries to that illustrated. In those cases, the testicle was closed with a parietal tunica vaginalis patch. He reports good results with this technique.

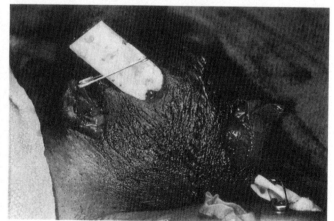

D

tions are managed with primary closure and drainage if indicated. In the case of amputation of the testicles, testicular microreplantation has been performed including vasovasostomy, along with reapproximation of the vasculature of the spermatic cord (Fig. 65–10). The testicle is placed, as quickly as possible, in a sterile bag in saline-soaked gauze, and that bag is placed in a second bag filled with saline slush for cold preservation. Unlike amputation of the penis, where successful replantation has been done as long as 18 hours from the injury, the testicle must be replanted by 6 to 8 hours because of the very high metabolic rate of testicular tissue.

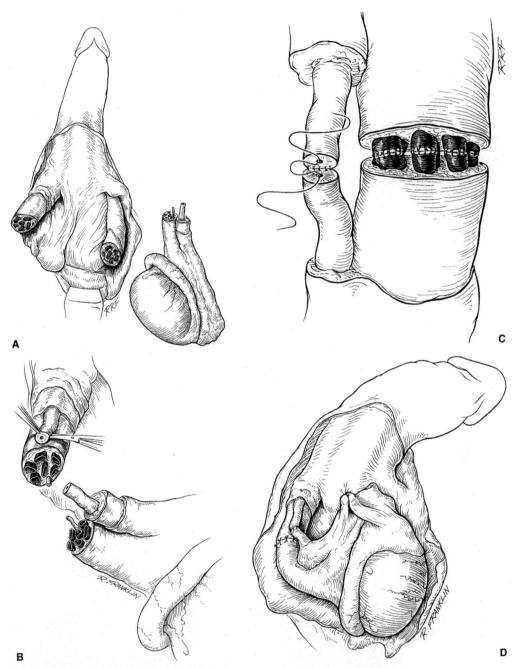

FIG. 65–10. A: Appearance of a patient following bilateral testicular amputation and scrotal amputation. The patient presented with only his right testicle. The left testicle could not be found at the trauma scene. **B:** The right testicle is reanastomosed to the left (longer) spermatic cord. **C:** Note the appearance of the debrided spermatic cord and the debrided distal spermatic cord going to the testicle. Vasovasostomy was performed with a two-layer microscopic technique. Microscopic coaptation of the spermatic artery and multiple spermatic veins was performed. **D:** Appearance of the replanted testicle before closure of the scrotum.

There can be some difficulty in identifying the vessels in the spermatic cord, although they are somewhat compartmentalized. Identifying the artery proximally is not difficult, and identification of the distal artery in the severed organ can be aided by examining the relationship of the compartments to the vas deferens. Coaptation of the artery and a number of veins is optimal using 9-0 or 10-0 Prolene, depending on the size of the respective vessels. Vasovasostomy can be done using 9-0 or 10-0 Prolene or nylon sutures either with a classic microscopic two-layer technique or a single-layer "tricorner" technique depending on the surgeon's preference.

If possible, the testicle should not be covered with a graft but either placed in a thigh pouch and later liberated or, if there is some remaining redundancy of the scrotum, covered primarily with reapproximation of the remaining scrotal tissues.

Obviously, if the patient arrives without his amputated testicle then hemostasis must be assured. Usually the vessels are in spasm, but they clearly can come out of spasm later. The wound should be irrigated and, if contaminated, packed to be closed by secondary intention. If the wound is clean, then primary closure or primary grafting can be performed.

Avulsion Injuries

Small scrotal avulsions are managed as simple lacerations with either primary or delayed closure and drainage, as would be indicated for any laceration (Fig. 65–11). For larger injuries, the emergency management consists of allowing the injury to completely declare (Fig. 65–12).

The area of the avulsed scrotum should be managed with cold saline packs and observed over 12 to 24 hours. Clear demarcation will occur and allow the surgeon to debride only the tissue that is nonviable. Debridement with closure is then performed.

If a primary closure cannot be accomplished with the remaining scrotal tissue, then the surgeon has several options. One option is to place the testicles in thigh pouches to be later liberated and replaced to the area of the scrotum. The preferable option is to perform a primary reconstruction of the scrotum using a mesh split-thickness skin graft. The graft should be harvested 0.016 to 0.018 in. thick and then meshed on a 1.5 to-1 meshing template. The testicles must be fixed in position using permanent suture or absorbable suture that is slowly absorbed so that they do not migrate beneath the graft. The meshing of the graft allows for escape of serum and blood products from beneath the graft but also allows the graft to configure to the complex contours of the underlying testicles. The vaginal space is left open, and the parietal tunica vaginalis is reflected to fix the testicle in place. The graft is then applied immediately to the testicles, suturing it to the surrounding skin. It is the opinion of some authors that grafting directly on the visceral tunica vaginalis or tunica albuginea can lead to a situation where there is chronic testicular pain. This has not been the author's experience. Unless the wound is markedly contaminated, cases so managed have yielded very successful results.

The grafts should be bolstered using Xeroform gauze or one of the other commercially available fine meshed gauzes applied directly to the graft with Dacron batting

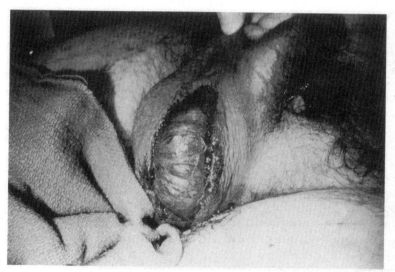
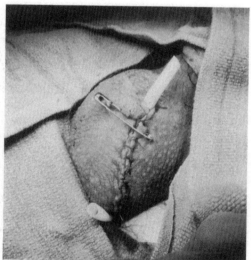

FIG. 65–11. A: Appearance of a left scrotal avulsion injury. Patient was injured in a motorcycle accident in which his trousers were ripped off as he departed the motorcycle. **B:** Appearance after closure. Primary closure is performed with drainage.

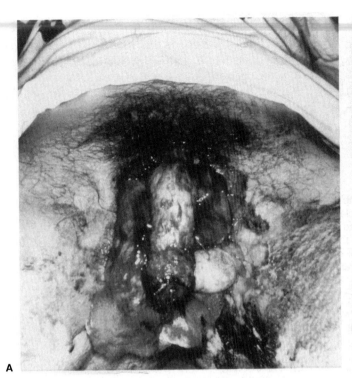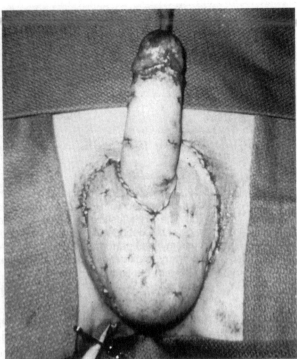

A   B

FIG. 65–12. A: Large avulsion injury of the genitalia. Patient was injured when his clothing was ensnared in the power takeoff mechanism of a tractor. Note the exposed shaft of the penis and the exposed testicles bilaterally. **B:** The appearance after reconstruction with a split-thickness skin graft. The patient was observed for 24 hours, allowing the wounds to demarcate. In this case, both the shaft of the penis and the scrotum were reconstructed with a sheet split-thickness skin graft.

soaked in saline and mineral oil placed over the fine meshed gauze. Lately we have favored the use of the N-Terface product. The bolster is held in place with 2-0 chromic sutures. Unless associated with a urethral injury, the patient can be "diverted" with a soft Foley catheter. In patients in whom the avulsion injury extends near to the anus, colostomy may be required. It must be emphasized that local skin flaps are not recommended for primary closure in these cases.

Should the testicles be avulsed, replantation is not an option. During the avulsion injury, the vasculature is stretched before giving way to the force, and the endothelial damage can be significant and unpredictable.

In patients in whom the avulsion injury is tantamount to emasculation, these injuries are often associated with significant injuries to the adjacent tissue. Reconstruction assumes a very secondary position as these patients require lifesaving steps. The vast majority of these patients will require colostomy, suprapubic cystostomy, and multiple dressing changes over the post-trauma course, and often present with significant bleeding.

Genital Burns

The emergency therapy of genital burns is similar to that for any burn. The scrotum can be dressed open with topical antibiotic ointments such as Silvadene, or a closed antibiotic dressing regimen can be used. The integrity of the urethra must be determined when the patient presents. A Foley catheter can be placed in the patient who has burns to his genitalia. If there were evidence of urethral burn, then most would suggest diversion with suprapubic cystostomy. If the burns to the genital and perineal area are extensive, then an occasional patient will require colostomy. If the subscrotal urethra is involved in the burn, no attempt at initial reconstruction should be made.

The genital tissues are remarkably vascular; debridement of the genitalia, in general, should be accomplished carefully. Aggressive debridement should be avoided as many of the tissues will recover and are nonreproducible. Whirlpools and tank soaks are useful for gentle debridement and cleansing and may be done early on, two to three times per day.

Chemical burns rarely involve the structures deep to the skin and are managed with copious irrigation and

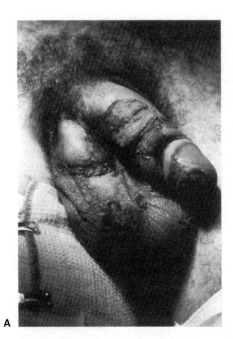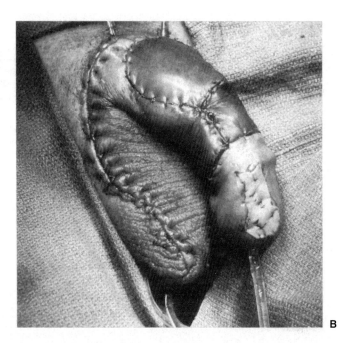

FIG. 65–13. A: The appearance of the genitalia in a patient who was burned in a steam-line accident. Note the burns to the glans, the dorsum of the shaft of the penis, and the right hemiscrotum. **B:** In this particular case, reconstruction of the glans was accomplished with a small split-thickness skin graft. Reconstruction of the shaft of the penis was accomplished with a penile skin island flap; the patient was uncircumcised, and the ventral skin was mobilized to the dorsum. The scrotal burn was completely excised, and primary reconstruction of the right hemiscrotum was accomplished. This particular patient demonstrates all of the possibilities for reconstruction following burn debridement.

then as with a thermal burn. If a patient has evidence of an electrical burn to the area of the genitalia, the patient must be observed for 12 to 24 hours and then explored. In electrical burns, the initial management is aimed at debridement, and reconstruction can be offered later as the situation dictates (Fig. 65–13).

Radiation Injuries

Just as there can be lymphedema of the scrotum in men, there can be lymphedema in the vulva of women. Although it is not the topic of this chapter, some mention should be made in that the management of lymphedema of the vulva and secondary reconstruction is different from the management of lymphedema of the scrotum with reconstruction. In women, the most common cause of lymphedema is idiopathic. The treatment for lymphedema of the labia is vulvectomy. If the vulvectomy involves excision of the vaginal tissues, then the lateral hair-bearing tissue should not be sutured into the vagina. Instead, reconstruction of the labia can be accomplished using either the rectus abdominis flap, gracilis flaps, or posterior thigh flaps. One should select the flap so that the flap drainage is away from the lymphatic distribution affected by the radiation.

In the case of the man with scrotal lymphedema and recurrent cellulitis, all layers of the scrotum should be excised, down to the level of the external spermatic fascia (Fig. 65–14). It is not uncommon for the patient also to have large hydroceles (2).

The vaginal space should be opened and the parietal tunica vaginalis then reflected and incorporated in the orchidopexy. Reconstruction can be accomplished, using split-thickness skin grafts, as already discussed, and on the scrotum these grafts can be meshed as discussed earlier. The meshing allows for the graft to better comply to the contours of the testicle and to allow the rather significant serous drainage noted in these patients to escape from beneath the graft. In addition, the meshing seems to improve the cosmetic result by giving a pseudorugated appearance to the tissue. Neither full-thickness skin grafts nor local skin flaps should be used. The cosmetic results achieved in these patients, so reconstructed, are excellent.

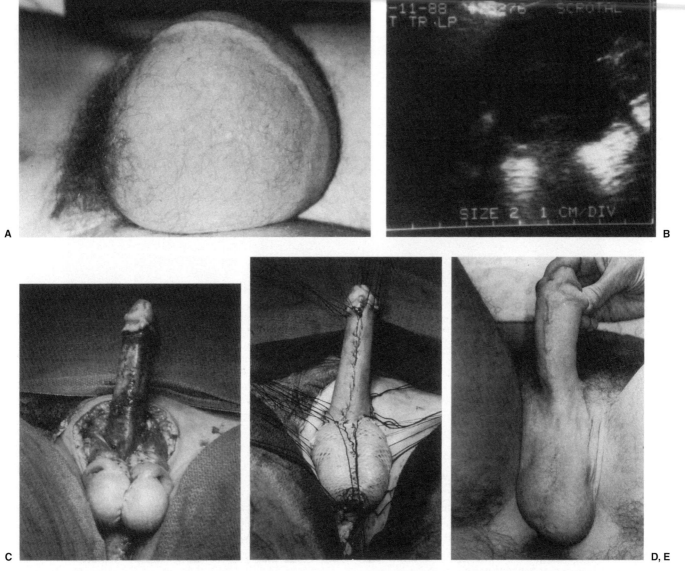

FIG. 65–14. Appearance of a young man with chronic genital lymphedema following irradiation therapy for Hodgkin's lymphoma. **A:** Appearance of the massively lymphedematous scrotum. **B:** B-scan ultrasound demonstrating the large hydrocele. Note the normal testis posteriorly. **C:** Appearance of the genitalia after debridement of the lymphedematous tissue. Note orchidopexy has been performed. **D:** Immediate appearance following reconstruction of the shaft of the penis with a split-thickness skin graft and reconstruction of the scrotum with a meshed split-thickness skin graft. **E:** Appearance of that same patient 6 months postoperatively. Note the small amount of residual lymphedema of the preputial cuff. Further note the redundant appearance of the scrotal graft.

Fournier's Gangrene

If the primary process has resulted in extensive debridement of the scrotum, the testicles can be placed in thigh pouches with the intention of later replacing the testicles in their normal anatomic area and for scrotal recon-

struction (Fig. 65–15). The lateral defects on the thigh can often be closed *per primam* or can be grafted.

For most patients, however, the scrotal excisions do not necessitate placing the testicles in thigh pouches, but instead they can be dressed in the wound. These patients often require multiple dressing changes and wet-to-dry

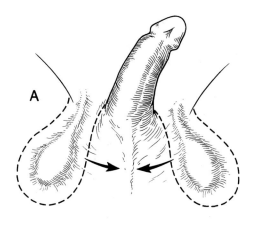

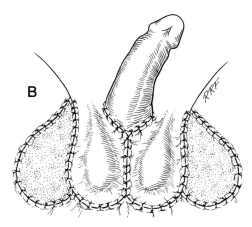

FIG. 65–15. Technique after McDougal for liberation of testicles that have been placed in thigh pouches. Note that the testicles are mobilized with random thigh skin flaps and transposed to the midline to reconstruct the scrotum. The lateral defects can be closed *per primam* or can be grafted.

debridements. When reconstruction is undertaken, the testicles must be fixed in their normal anatomic position. It is my custom to open the parietal tunica vaginalis and reflect it, and, as already described, graft techniques can be utilized to restore the scrotum. Although local flaps can be used, the cosmetic results achieved with local flaps are usually less than optimal when compared to reconstruction techniques utilizing split-thickness skin grafts. Interestingly, these mesh split-thickness skin grafts not only remain supple but, in many cases (as has been shown), will actually become redundant.

OUTCOMES

Complications

Complications of scrotal trauma and reconstruction are primarily related to inadequate appreciation of the degree of injury with subsequent necrosis of additional skin. It is important for the surgeon to adequately debride the devitalized skin, which may require more than one trip to the operating room. The failure of a skin graft to take is usually a result of technical errors such as accumulation of fluid under the graft, inadequately prepared graft bed, or continual slippage of the graft over the bed, which does not allow capillary ingrowth.

Results

In general, the scrotal skin is highly distensible and even a small fragment can be expanded to cover a large defect with a good anatomic result. There has been concern regarding the effect of implantation of the testes in thigh pockets on spermatogenesis, although there is little clinical data to support this concern.

REFERENCES

1. Arneri V. Reconstruction of the male genitalia. In: Converse J, ed. *Reconstructive plastic surgery*, 2nd ed. Philadelphia: WB Saunders, 1977:3902–3921.
2. Charles RH. The surgical technique and operative treatment of elephantiasis of the generative organs based on a series of 140 consecutive successful cases. *Ind Med Gaz* 1901;36:84.
3. Jordan GH, Gilbert DA. Male genital trauma. *Clin Plast Surg* 1988;15:431.
4. Jordan GH, Gilbert DA. Management of amputation injuries of the male genitalia. *Urol Clin North Am* 1989;16:359–367.
5. Jordan GH, Schlossberg SM, Devine CJ. Surgery of the penis and urethra. In: Walsh PC, et al., eds. *Campbell's urology*, 7th ed., vol. 3. Philadelphia: WB Saunders, 1997:3316–3394.

Penis/Scrotum

Section Editor: Gerald H. Jordan

Anatomy

Sam D. Graham, Jr.

The penis is composed of three columnar bodies, a pair of which are larger, dorsally located, and extend the length of the penis (Figure SVIII-1). These two columnar bodies contain cavernosal vascular tissue and are called the corpora cavernosa. Proximally the corpora cavernosa taper to form the crus and are attached to the pubic arch. Each corpora is closely applied to the other, separated only by a septum, for most of the distal penis. The corpora cavernosus is supported at its base by the ischiocavernosus muscles which arise from the inner surface of the ischial tuberosity and are innervated by the perineal nerves.

The third columnar body, the corpora spongiosa, contains the urethra and the distal end is bulbous forming the glans penis. The corpora spongiosa is attached proximally to the perineal membrane and at the most proximal portion is larger forming the bulb.

Each of the corporal bodies is encased in its own tunica albugnea and the 3 corporal bodies are surrounded by Buck's fascia which is a continuation of Colle's fascia. (Figure SVIII-2). Buck's fascia is attached posteriorly to the urogenital diaphragm and anteriorly forms the suspensory ligament. There is little vascular communication between the corpora cavernosa and the corpora spongiosa. There is, however, vascular communication between the two corpora cavernosa via pectiniform septa in the distal corpora.

VASCULAR ANATOMY

The superficial penile artery lie between the superficial and Buck's fascia and originates from the external pudendal artery which in turn is a branch of the femoral

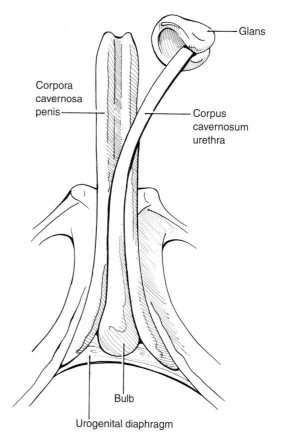

FIG. SVIII–1. Anatomy of the three corporal bodies comprising the penis.

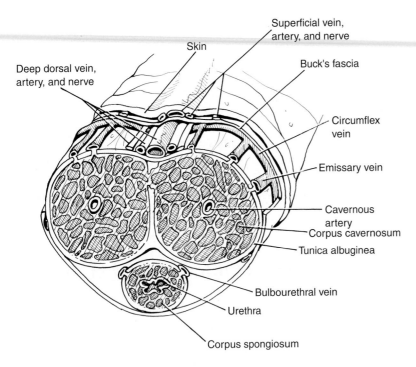

FIG. SVIII–2. Cross-section of the penis demonstrating fascial layers as well as vascular and neuroanatomy

artery. This artery, along with a corresponding vein supplies the penile skin and is located between the superficial penile fascia and Buck's fascia. The deep arterial supply arises from the internal iliac artery which initially branches into the internal pudendal artery and then into the penile artery. As the penile artery exits the urogenital diaphragm it branches into the bulbourethral, cavernosus, and urethral artery. The cavernosus artery is the direct supply of the corpora cavernosa. The penile artery continues along the corpora cavernosa as the dorsal artery.

The corpora spongiosa is supplied by the bulbourethral artery proximally, circumflex arteries from the dorsal artery along its shaft. The glans is supplied by the dorsal artery. The dorsal artery, deep dorsal vein, and the dorsal nerve are enclosed within Buck's fascia.

The superficial penile vein drains into the external pudendal vein. The circumflex and deep dorsal vein drain into the Plexus of Santorini as do the crural and cavernosal veins (Figure SVIII-3).

LYMPHATIC ANATOMY

The lymphatics of the penile skin drain into the superficial inguinal and subinguinal lymph nodes. The lymphatics of the glans penis empty into the subinguinal and external iliac nodes. The deep lymphatics drain into the hypogastric and common iliac nodes.

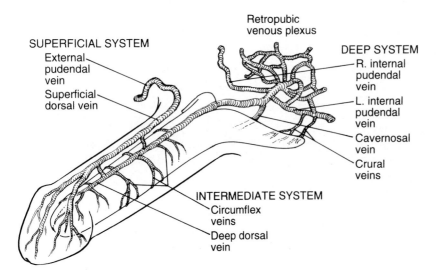

FIG. SVIII–3. Venous drainage of the penis.

CHAPTER 66

Partial and Total Penectomy in the Management of Invasive Squamous Cell Carcinoma of the Penis

Antonio Puras Baez

Penile carcinoma is usually an epidermoid tumor arising in the glans or mucosal lining of the prepuce. Its incidence follows a distinct geographic and racial distribution. It has been reported to constitute up to 16.7% of all cancers in some regions of India (9) and 12.2% of all cancers in Uganda (4). In Brazil it represents 2.1% of all malignancies, although in some regions of the country it constitutes up to 17% of all neoplasms (2). In Puerto Rico the age-adjusted incidence is around 5 per 100,000 males (6), whereas in the United States and Europe it accounts for only 0.4% to 0.6% of all malignancies in males (7).

The tumor is age related, showing an age-specific rate of increase with each decade, having its peak incidence at the fifth and sixth decades. An earlier age of onset and a high proportion of younger patients have been reported in areas of high incidence.

The precise etiology of penile carcinoma remains undetermined. Numerous factors have been associated with the risk of developing squamous cell carcinoma of the penis, such as chronic irritation, poor genital hygiene, the presence of an intact foreskin, phimosis, smegma, and viruses. This tumor is rarely seen in populations performing ritual neonatal circumcisions and is extremely rare among Jews, who practice circumcision at birth. Although this neoplasm can occur in men who were circumcised at birth, such reported cases involve patients who had incomplete circumcision or occurrence of scars in traumatic procedures. In a series of 1,581 patients with penile carcinoma, 90% of these patients were not circumcised, and of those who had been circumcised only 5 had the procedure early in life (8). It appears, therefore, that newborn circumcision may prevent carcinoma of the penis but does not confer the same protection later in life.

There is increasing evidence for a sexually transmitted viral etiology in penile cancer. Human papilloma viruses (HPV), especially types 16 and 18, have been detected in around 50% of penile carcinomas. It appears that an enclosed prepucial environment associated with a poor genital hygiene of the foreskin, chronic irritation, and exposure to certain etiologic agents such as viruses, smegma, hydrocarbons, and sterols may also play a causative role in the development of the tumor.

DIAGNOSIS

Patients with penile carcinoma may present with lesions that may vary from a subtle induration or erythema of the glans or foreskin, papule, a warty growth, or a large exophytic lesion with purulent discharge and cellulitis. Uncircumcised patients may present with edema of the foreskin and purulent discharge. These lesions are usually nonpainful and there is a delay in patient presentation due to self-denial, ignorance, fear, and personal neglect.

Sufrin and Huben (11) reviewed reports of more than 3,500 patients with penile cancer and found that the presenting symptoms consisted of a penile mass, lump, or nodule in 47% of patients, a penile ulcer or sore in 35%, and inflammatory lesion or bleeding from the external surface of the penis in 17%. Less than 1% of patients were found incidentally during the course of an adult circumcision. The most frequent location of the primary lesion is on the glans, the coronal sulcus, and the prepuce (8). This anatomic variation may be due to constant exposure of the glans, coronal sulcus, and inner prepuce to active carcinogenic irritants contained within the prepucial sac.

533

Penile cancers usually begin as a small lesion on an uncircumcised male with evidence of chronic irritation and/or poor genital hygiene. If left unattended, the lesion will gradually grow to involve the entire glans and/or prepuce. Buck's fascia, which is rich in elastic fibers, acts as a temporary natural barrier, protecting the corporeal bodies and urethra from tumor invasion. As the malignant tumor progresses, there will be infiltration of Buck's fascia and the tunica albuginea with invasion of cavernous erectile tissue and potential vascular and lymphatic infiltration. Untreated tumors continue to grow, producing progressive erosion and destruction of the penis. Most lesions will develop secondary infection resulting in a foul-smelling discharge with or without cellulitis of the surrounding tissue. Ulcerative tumors are usually less differentiated and have a tendency for earlier nodal metastasis.

Penile lesions such as erythroplasia of Queyrat, leukoplakia, cutaneous horn, balanitis xerotica obliterans, condyloma acuminatum, and giant condyloma may resemble squamous cell carcinoma of the penis and must be considered in the differential diagnosis.

Penile lesions should be examined thoroughly and assessed in regard to location, tumor growth, size, and infiltration of the corpora bodies or urethra. Careful examination of the inguinal area and pelvis is of extreme importance. The lesion should be cultured and the patient started on appropriate antibiotic therapy. Any suspicious growth or ulceration should be biopsied and the depth

and type of invasion, the presence of microvascular permeation, and the histological grade of the tumor assessed prior to initiation of any therapeutic modality.

The definitive diagnosis is secured by biopsy of the lesion (Fig. 66–1) following appropriate antibiotic therapy. Adequate anesthesia is obtained with 1% local lidocaine and a 1.5-cm elliptical wedge of tumor tissue is removed. The biopsy should include tumor growth and adjacent neighboring normal tissue to be examined for tumor infiltration. The incision is closed with interrupted 3-0 chromic catgut. I prefer to perform a biopsy as a separate procedure and discuss with the pathologist the tumor grading, type of growth, and presence of microvascular permeation prior to initiation of any therapeutic modalities. Patients with tight phimosis who have a purulent discharge and a mass or induration concealed underneath the foreskin are managed with a dorsal slit incision, long enough to retract the prepuce and adequately examine and biopsy any suspicious lesion or growth.

INDICATIONS FOR SURGERY

Survival of carcinoma of the penis depends primarily on the tumor grade, depth of invasion, and the status of the regional nodes. The primary therapeutic goal in the management of penile carcinoma should be complete tumor excision, regional lymphatic control, and a functional, cosmetic penis. Surgical excision plays a prominent role in the management and control of the primary lesion. If adequately performed, it will assess the histological grade, depth, and type of tumor invasion and in many instances can be curative.

ALTERNATIVE THERAPY

Various other therapeutic modalities, including radiation therapy, chemotherapy, and combinations of these, have been used in the treatment of the primary lesion. Penile-sparing procedures such as micrographic excision (Mohs microsurgery) and laser procedures have been utilized in other cutaneous malignancies and have been investigated in penile cancer.

Mohs microsurgery is a technique of excision of the lesion in thin horizontal layers using microscopic examination of the entire undersurface of each layer and systematic use of frozen sections. Two techniques by which microscopic control of the tumor is achieved have been described. The first technique is a fixed tissue technique in which the tissues are subjected to *in situ* chemical fixation with zinc chloride paste before excision of successive layers. In the fresh tissue technique, a local anesthetic is injected and the tissues excised in fresh, unfixed state and examined by frozen section. The fresh tissue technique is recommended for small tumors, whereas for larger infiltrative lesions the fixed tissue technique will

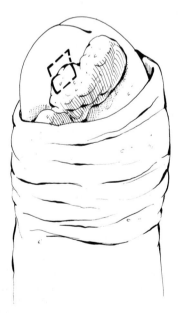

FIG. 66–1. Wedge biopsy of the penile lesion. (Redrawn from Das S, Crawford ED. Carcinoma of the penis: Management of the primary. In: Crawford ED, Das S, eds. *Current genitourinary cancer surgery.* Philadelphia: Lea and Febiger, 1990, with permission.) Biopsy should include tumor growth and adjacent neighboring normal tissue to be examined for tumor infiltration.

provide control of bleeding from the relatively noncontractile vessels of the erectile tissues of the glans and corpora cavernosa. Cure rates for low-stage lesions that are less than 1 cm in diameter are close to 100%, while cure rates for lesions over 3 cm dropped to around 50%. It appears that microscopically controlled tumor excision provides an effective treatment alternative to manage some types of penile cancer with excellent cosmetic and functional results. Complications related to most micrographic techniques are meatal stenosis and disfigurement of the glans.

The mayor advantages of laser therapy for carcinoma of the penis are destruction of the tumor with penile preservation and function; it also gives the advantage of tissue destruction, sealing of small vessels and nerve endings, and reducing the incidence of postoperative bleeding and pain. The main disadvantage of laser surgery is difficulty obtaining histological documentation and determining the depth of penetration by the tumor; it appears that the sight and depth of penetration of the primary lesion correlates with its curability. Malloy and associates were able to cure five of five patients with Tis lesions but only six of nine patients with T1 tumors (5). Bandieramonte and associates (1) were able to resect T1 tumors at the glans penis by using a very short pulse and a high peak power at the base of the lesion and at the meatus, providing precise excision of the specimen for histological examination; however, a 15% recurrence rate was reported (1).

SURGICAL TECHNIQUE

Circumcision and Tumor Excision

Patients with small lesions involving the prepuce may be adequately managed by wide circumcision with a 1.5-cm margin. Microscopic examination by frozen section should be performed to obtain a tumor-free margin due to the high risk of recurrence. The histopathologic slides should be reviewed with the pathologist with special attention to the patterns of tumor growth, grading, depth of invasion, and microvessel infiltration. Suspicious lesions at the glans or coronal sulcus should be biopsied and proved to be free of tumor. Selected patients with superficial tumors of the shaft can be managed with a wide excision excising around 2 cm of normal skin. The skin defect can be covered by a full-thickness skin graft.

Partial Penectomy

Invasive tumors involving the glans and coronal sulcus can be adequately managed by partial penile amputation excising around 1.5 to 2 cm of normal tissue proximal to the margin of tumor infiltration (Fig. 66–2). In most instances, this should leave a functional penis of over 4

cm in length, which allows standing micturition and enough rigidity and length for vaginal penetration. Frozen sections of the proximal margins are necessary to confirm tumor-free resection and a recurrent rate of 10% or less.

The procedure is performed under local, regional, or general anesthesia; the patient is placed in the supine position. The penis is prepped with povidone/iodine solution and the tumor isolated using a sterile condom glove that is sutured in place. The lesion and urine should be cultured preoperatively and appropriate parenteral antibiotics started prior to the surgical procedure. A 0.25-in. Penrose or 14 Fr Red Robinson catheter is applied as a tourniquet at the base of the penis. A circumferential incision is marked on the skin 1.5 to 2 cm proximal to the lesion. The skin is incised circumferentially and the superficial and deep dorsal veins are divided and ligated using 3-0 silk. Buck's fascia is incised onto the tunica albuginea of the corpora. The corpora cavernosa are sharply divided down to the urethra and the central cavernosal arteries ligated on each side.

The urethra is dissected free from the corpus spongiosum in such a manner that an approximately 1-cm stump projects distally to the transected corpora cavernosa. The urethral stump is then divided and the specimen removed. The urethral stump and transected corpora are then washed with gentamicin solution. The corporal ends are closed with horizontal mattress sutures of 2-0 Vicryl incorporating Buck's fascia, tunica albuginea, and intercavernous septum. The tourniquet is then released and all minor vessels are fulgurated until adequate hemostasis is obtained. The urethra is spatulated and sutured to the skin using 4-0 Vicryl. The remaining skin is closed using 3-0 Vicryl sutures. A 16 Fr Foley catheter is left indwelling to closed straight drainage for 48 hours and the wound is dressed.

Variations to this closure is to leave a flap of dorsal skin and make a crescentic button-hole incision in the dorsal skin flap; this flap is then rotated ventrally toward the urethra, which has been spatulated dorsally, and the urethra anastomosed to the button-hole opening with 4-0 Vicryl interrupted sutures. The skin flaps are then reapproximated with 3-0 Vicryl.

The other option is to leave a 1.5- to 2-cm urethral stump, spatulate the urethra ventrally, and the dorsal urethral flap will be rotated dorsally and anastomosed to the tunica albuginea of the corpora cavernosa and skin.

Total Penectomy

Patients with large, extensive, and infiltrating lesions involving the glans and midshaft of the penis in which the location precludes adequate excision with a functional residual remnant are managed by total penectomy (Fig. 66–3). The patient is placed in the lithotomy position and

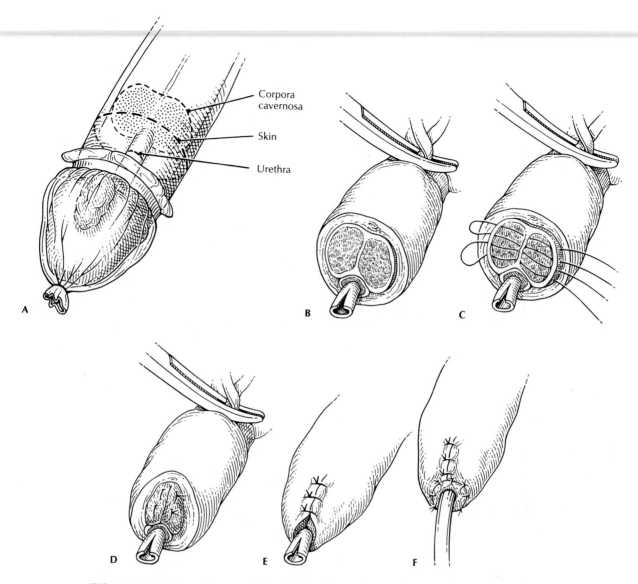

FIG. 66–2. Partial penile amputation. **A:** Condom catheter is placed over the tumor and a circumferential incision is marked on the skin 2 cm proximal to the lesion. **B:** A 14 Fr catheter or 0.25-in Penrose is placed as a tourniquet at the base of the penis. The skin and Buck's fascia are incised onto the tunica albuginea. Corpora cavernosa is sharply divided down to the urethra. The urethra is dissected free from the corpora spongiosum and a 1-cm stump projects distally to a transected corpora cavernosa. **C:** Spatulate the urethra on its dorsal surface and close the corporal ends with horizontal mattress sutures incorporating Buck's fascia, tunica albuginea, and intercavernous septum. **D:** Release the tourniquet and obtain adequate hemostasis. **E:** The dorsal skin is closed longitudinally. **F:** Start ventral approximation of the penile skin to the urethra and continue dorsally. The remaining dorsal skin is closed longitudinally.

the lesion is prepped with povidone/iodine solution; appropriate antibiotic therapy should be started before the procedure. A condom catheter or rubber glove is secured to the base of the penis with interrupted 3-0 silk sutures; an elliptical incision is made around the base of the penis and extended through the subcutaneous tissues until the surface of pubis is reached. All vessels and lymphatics are either fulgurated or ligated. The suspensory ligaments of the penis are isolated with a right-angle clamp and divided. The dor-

sal vein and penile arteries are identified, clamped, ligated, and divided. The penis is then reflected cephalad, Buck's fascia is opened ventrally, and the urethra is dissected free from the corpora cavernosa with sharp and blunt dissection. At the distal bulbar region the urethra is divided, leaving enough length to reach the perineum. The corpora cavernosa are dissected to the ischiopubic rami, sutured, and ligated with 2-0 Dexon and transected. The specimen should be removed with a 2-cm tumor-free margin.

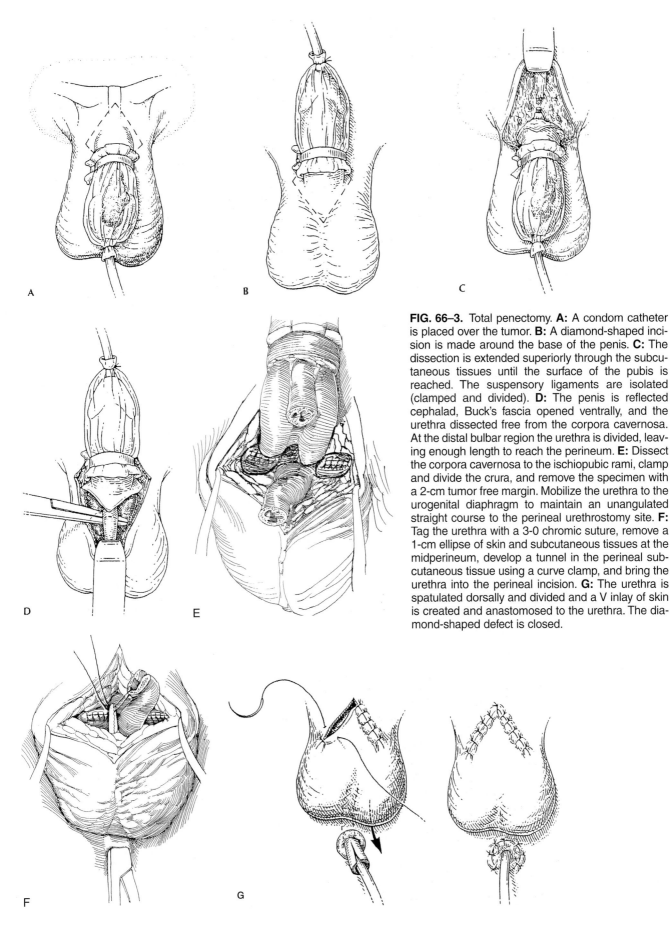

FIG. 66–3. Total penectomy. **A:** A condom catheter is placed over the tumor. **B:** A diamond-shaped incision is made around the base of the penis. **C:** The dissection is extended superiorly through the subcutaneous tissues until the surface of the pubis is reached. The suspensory ligaments are isolated (clamped and divided). **D:** The penis is reflected cephalad, Buck's fascia opened ventrally, and the urethra dissected free from the corpora cavernosa. At the distal bulbar region the urethra is divided, leaving enough length to reach the perineum. **E:** Dissect the corpora cavernosa to the ischiopubic rami, clamp and divide the crura, and remove the specimen with a 2-cm tumor free margin. Mobilize the urethra to the urogenital diaphragm to maintain an unangulated straight course to the perineal urethrostomy site. **F:** Tag the urethra with a 3-0 chromic suture, remove a 1-cm ellipse of skin and subcutaneous tissues at the midperineum, develop a tunnel in the perineal subcutaneous tissue using a curve clamp, and bring the urethra into the perineal incision. **G:** The urethra is spatulated dorsally and divided and a V inlay of skin is created and anastomosed to the urethra. The diamond-shaped defect is closed.

The urethra is then dissected to the area of the urogenital diaphragm to obtain an unangulated straight course to the perineal urethrostomy site. The urethra is tagged with 3-0 chromic catgut sutures. A 1-cm ellipse of skin and subcutaneous tissues are removed at the midperineum just midway between the rectum and scrotum. A tunnel is developed in the perineal subcutaneous tissue using a curve clamp so that the urethra will not be angulated and the urethra is drawn into the perineal incision. The urethra is spatulated dorsally; a V inlay of skin can be created and anastomosed to the urethra using 3 or 4 Vicryl. A watertight technique should be used to prevent urinary leakage under the flap. An 18 Fr Foley catheter is inserted and 0.25-in. Penrose drains are left to drain each side of the scrotum. The scrotal incision is closed transversally to allow elevation of the scrotum away from the perineal urethrostomy. Triple antibiotic is placed over the wound incision and around the perineal urethrostomy. A pressure dressing and scrotal support are applied for 24 hours. The Penrose drains are usually removed in 48 hours and the Foley catheter should be removed when the urethrostomy is well healed.

Lesions involving the perineum and anterior abdominal wall may need adjuvant preoperative chemotherapy in an attempt to downsize the tumor. If no adequate response is observed, the patient will need complete removal of the neoplasm with total emasculation. In some instances cystoprostatectomy with urinary diversion will be necessary.

OUTCOMES

Complications

The most common complication of partial and total penectomy is meatal stenosis. The V inlay technique has been used to decrease the stenosis at the urethral opening. Patients should be aware of this complication and instructed to start self-dilatation as soon as they notice a decrease in the urine stream.

Patients with partial or total penectomy suffer serious psychological and physical trauma with major changes in their quality of life. They should undergo psychiatric evaluation and counseling and receive emotional support in which the family and a team of social workers, psychologists, and physicians should take an active role. New techniques for penile reconstruction have been described and include the radial forearm flap and the use of innervated forearm osteocutaneous flap combined with big toe pulp for reconstruction of the glans.

Results

Surgery plays a prominent role in the treatment and control of the primary lesion. The presence and extent of metastasis to the inguinal nodes are the most important prognostic factors for survival in patients with penile cancer. Patients who are at risk or have persistent adenopathy following treatment to the primary should undergo early regional inguinal lymphadenectomy.

Several investigators have noted the correlation between tumor grade, survival, and regional metastasis. Well-differentiated tumors seldom demonstrate nodal involvement and have a high disease-specific survival. Penile tumors are classified according to the histological pattern of tumor growth (3). Tumors that exhibit a compact, vertical growth are usually high-grade neoplasms, associated with regional nodal metastasis. Most recently, Slaton et al. (10), in a series of 48 patients with invasive squamous cell carcinoma of the penis, examined the prognostic factors for lymph node metastasis using univariate and multivariate analysis. They concluded that the pathologic stage of the penile tumor, vascular invasion, and greater than 50% poorly differentiated cancer were independent prognostic factors for inguinal lymph node metastasis. This data clearly establishes the significance of histological grade, patterns of tumor growth, depth of invasion, and vascular permeation in predicting regional spread and survival.

Five-year survival for patients with negative groins or minimal nodal disease (two or less nodes involved) following curative regional lymphadenectomy should be over 80%. Survival drops significantly in the presence of multiple nodal involvement, pelvic metastasis, and extranodal extension of cancer. The therapeutic goals and objective in the management of a patient with penile cancer should be complete tumor excision of the primary lesion, leaving a cosmetic functional penis, and early regional lymphatic control.

REFERENCES

1. Banderiamonte G, Santoro O, Boracchi P, et al. Total resection of glans penis surface by CO_2: laser microsurgery. *Acta Oncol* 1988;27:575.
2. Brumini R. In: *Cancer in Brazil: Histopathological data, 1976–1980.* Rio de Janeiro: Ministry of Health, 1982.
3. Cubilla AL, Barreto J, Caballero C, et al. Pathologic features of epidermoid carcinoma of the penis: a prospective study of 66 cases. *Am J Surg Pathol* 1993;17:753–763.
4. Dodge OG, Linsell CA. Carcinoma of the penis in Uganda and Kenya, Africa. *Cancer* 1963;16:1255–1263.
5. Malloy TR, Wein AJ, Carpiniello VL. Carcinoma of the penis treated with neodymium:YAG laser. *Urology* 1988;31:26–29.
6. Marcial V, Puras A, Marcial VA. Neoplasms of the penis. In: Holland JF, Frei E, Bast R Jr, et al., eds. *Cancer medicine,* 4th ed. Baltimore: Williams & Wilkins, 1996:2165–2175.
7. Muir C, Waterhouse J, Mack T, Powel J, Whelan S, eds. *Cancer incidence in five continents.* Lyon, France: International Agency for Research on Cancer; 1987; Publication 88.
8. Puras A, Rivera J. Invasive carcinoma of the penis: Management and prognosis. In: Oesterling JE, Richie JP, eds. *Urologic oncology* 1st ed. Philadelphia: WB Saunders, 1997:604–617.
9. Reddy CRRM, Raghavaiah NV, Mouli KC. Prevalence of carcinoma of the penis with special reference to India. *Int Surg* 1975;60:470–476.
10. Slaton JW, Morgenstern N, Levy DA, et al. Tumor stage, vascular invasion and percentage of poorly differentiated cancer: Dependent prognosticators for inguinal lymph node metastasis in penile squamous cancer. *J Urol,* Vol. 165 2001;165:1138–1142.
11. Sufrin G, Huben R. Benign and malignant lesions of the penis. In: Gillenwater JY, Grayhack JT, Howards SS, et al., eds. *Adult and pediatric urology,* 2nd ed. St. Louis, MO: Mosby–Year Book, 1991:1643–1678.

CHAPTER 67

Lymphadenectomy for Penile Carcinoma

Shahin Tabatabaei and W. Scott McDougal

Squamous cell carcinoma of the penis tends to spread locally to regional lymph nodes long before distant metastasis occurs. Approximately 50% of patients have lymph node involvement at presentation. Metastatic spread to the locoregional lymph nodes occurs in a stepwise fashion along the normal route of penile lymphatic drainage. The disease first spreads to the superficial and deep inguinal nodes, followed by the pelvic nodes (i.e., external iliac and obturator lymph nodes). Although tumor metastasis to the contralateral inguinal nodes is common, pelvic cross-drainage has not been reported.

The most important prognostic factors for survival in men with invasive squamous cell carcinoma of the penis are the presence and extent of inguinal lymph node metastasis (8). Although penile carcinoma metastatic to the lymph nodes portends a poorer prognosis, aggressive surgical excision of the involved nodes is associated with increased long-term survival (3,8) with a possible cure in 30% to 60% of patients with inguinal lymph node metastasis. This is not true if the tumor has spread to the pelvic lymph nodes, however, in which case there is a less than a 10% survival rate. There is currently no effective chemotherapy for patients with disease beyond the inguinal nodes. Without treatment, patients with metastatic disease die within 2 years.

Until recently, inguinal lymphadenectomy had been associated with significant morbidity (30% to 90%) and up to 3% mortality. Further, previous studies reported up to a 50% false positive rate in patients with clinically enlarged lymph nodes. These reports have generated considerable controversy regarding the indications for a lymphadenectomy in patients with penile carcinoma.

DIAGNOSIS

The diagnosis is secured at the time of biopsy and definitive treatment of the primary lesion (Chapter 66). A computed tomography scan of the abdomen and pelvis is important for staging the pelvic nodes.

INDICATIONS FOR SURGERY

In the last two decades, improvements in surgical and perioperative techniques have decreased the complication rates of inguinal lymphadenectomy. In addition, accurate prognostic factors to predict lymph node involvement have been better defined. Therefore, a more proactive approach to treating penile cancer may be taken. Tumor grade and depth of invasion help predict the lymph node involvement (3,7,8). In patients with grade I squamous cell carcinoma (SCC) of the penis, 24% to 37% may have inguinal lymph node involvement, while almost 82% of patients with grade III tumors have positive inguinal lymph nodes (4,7). Patients with carcinoma *in situ* and verrucous carcinoma of the penis are considered low risk as there is no evidence that these lesions metastasize. Patients with tumor stage T2 or greater (invasion into the corpora) have a 30% to 66% incidence of positive nodes. When stage and grade are combined, those with grade III and/or those with stage T2 or greater have an 80% incidence of positive nodes (7).

We advocate early lymphadenectomy in high-risk patients with nonpalpable groin adenopathy. Figure 67–1 summarizes our current approach to managing inguinal lymph nodes in these patients. As shown in the algorithm, all patients with penile cancer undergo 4 to 6 weeks of antibiotic therapy before the inguinal lymphadenectomy. It has been shown that most patients with ulcerative, penile SCC have infectious lymphangitis. Inguinal lymphadenectomy in the absence of appropriate antibiotic treatment may significantly increase the complication rates of the surgery.

Controversies regarding unilateral versus bilateral groin dissection have been resolved by recent data and

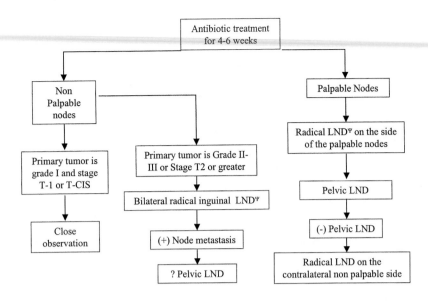

FIG. 67–1. Management of inguinal lymph nodes following primary surgery for carcinoma of the penis. LND, lymph node dissection.

studies indicating that lymphatic cross-drainage to the contralateral side does occur. Therefore, we strongly recommend bilateral inguinal lymphadenectomy.

The role of pelvic lymphadenectomy and whether the lymphadenectomy should start in the groin or pelvis is also controversial. Many studies indicate that involvement of pelvic lymph nodes is an ominous sign and almost all of these patients succumb to the disease in less than 2 years. Indeed, the knowledge of pelvic lymph node status has prognostic significance and may change the surgical approach. If the pelvic lymph nodes are positive, the surgical intention will be focused on palliation. In these situations, we still perform inguinal lymphadenectomy, but only on clinically palpable inguinal nodes, to prevent lesions from penetrating through the skin and/or invading into the femoral vessels, which may result in fatal femoral artery bleeding. In these cases, we do not proceed to contralateral inguinal lymphadenectomy for nonpalpable contralateral nodes.

In patients with negative palpable inguinal lymph nodes, who are at high risk for inguinal node involvement, several approaches have been proposed to minimize morbidity. These include: (a) modified inguinal lymphadenectomy, (b) sentinel lymph node biopsy (SLNB), and (c) intraoperative lymph node mapping (IOLM).

Some investigators suggest a modified inguinal lymphadenectomy for the side with nonpalpable inguinal lymph nodes and then radical lymphadenectomy only if the superficial lymph nodes are positive for cancer on the frozen section. This approach differs from radical dissection in four respects: (a) The skin incision is smaller, (b) the lymph nodes lateral to the femoral artery or dorsal to the fossa ovalis are spared, (c) the saphenous vein is preserved, and (d) the sartorius muscle is not transposed. Proponents of this approach point to evidence that there

is decreased morbidity without any increase in mortality (1). The main argument against this approach is that it relies heavily on intraoperative frozen section diagnosis of lymph node involvement, which may be inaccurate (6).

Another approach is sentinel node biopsy. Lymphangiograms performed via the dorsal penile lymphatics demonstrate drainage into a specific lymph node center, which is most often located between the superficial epigastric and the superficial external pudendal vein. Studies have suggested that the sentinel lymph node is the first site of metastasis and is often the only lymph node involved. Although the concept is intriguing, the location of the sentinel node varies and therefore clinicians have not found it in particular useful (9).

Based on the experience with breast and melanoma cancers, IOLM of the inguinal nodes has been proposed to address the shortcomings of SLNB. The technique involves injecting a vital blue dye and/or technetium-labeled colloid adjacent to the primary lesion and following its drainage to a specific node in the inguinal region. This node is designated the sentinel node. The goal is to eliminate the anatomic variability of the sentinel node location. Although preliminary results with IOLM are promising, lack of long-term follow-up, as well as the associated learning curve and technical difficulties of the procedure, limit its current use. We do not recommend IOLM as a standard approach at this time.

ALTERNATIVE THERAPY

The value of radiation therapy and chemotherapy is still uncertain. These treatments are currently considered palliative. In patients with positive inguinal lymph nodes the survival rate is significantly less when treated by radiation therapy than when treated with surgery. Based on the encouraging results of adjuvant radiation therapy in squamous cell carcinoma of the head and neck, some investigators advocate the use of preoperative radiation therapy in patients with large, fixed regional nodes (greater than 4 cm in size and/or extracapsular extension). We are not in favor of this approach as flap viability may be compromised and there is no proven survival benefit in penile cancer.

Experience with chemotherapy in penile carcinoma is hampered by a limited number of cases and lack of prospective trials. Cisplatin, bleomycin, vincristine, and methotrexate have all been shown to provide a partial response in selected cases (5). The use of chemotherapy as adjuvant or neoadjuvant therapy may be beneficial, although the optimum chemotherapy regimen remains to be determined.

SURGICAL TECHNIQUE

The lymphatics of the skin of the penis, scrotum, and perineum drain into the superficial and deep inguinal nodes. Extensive work by Daseler et al. on inguinal lymph node dissection suggests five node groups exist in the superficial inguinal area (2):

1. Central nodes at saphenofemoral junction.
2. Superolateral nodes around the superficial circumflex vein.
3. Inferolateral nodes around the lateral (femoral) cutaneous and superficial circumflex veins.
4. Superomedial nodes around the superficial external pudendal and superficial epigastric veins.
5. Inferomedial nodes around the greater saphenous vein.

Overall, 4 to 25 lymph nodes are present in the superficial groups (Fig. 67–2A). All of these nodes are situated below the globular fat of the superficial fascia called Camper's fascia.

The superficial fascia of the thigh (fascia lata) separates the superficial inguinal nodes from the deep nodes (Fig. 67–2B). The deep inguinal nodes are located medial to the femoral vein in the femoral canal. The most cephalad deep inguinal node, know as the node of Cloquet, is located between the femoral vein and the lacunar ligament.

Blood supply to the inguinal skin derives from superficial branches of the femoral artery (i.e., superficial external pudendal, superficial circumflex iliac, and superficial epigastric arteries). Corresponding veins parallel the arteries that join into the greater saphenous vein as it joins the femoral vein at the fossa ovalis. These arteries are ligated in the inguinal lymphadenectomy. Skin flap viability depends on anastomosing vessels within the superficial globular fat of Camper's fascia, which track from lateral to medial along the skin lines, parallel to the inguinal ligament. In theory, the transverse skin incision least compromises this blood supply.

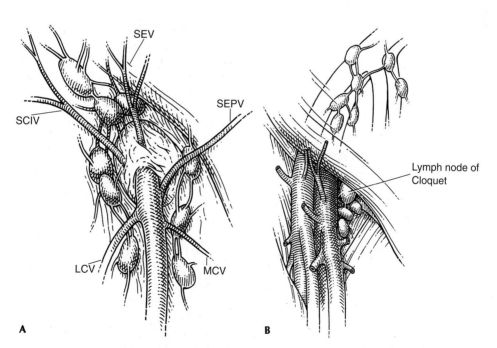

FIG. 67–2. A: Superficial lymph nodes and the five tributaries of the saphenous vein: medial (MCV) and lateral (LCV) cutaneous, superficial external pudendal (EPV), superficial circumflex iliac (SCIV), and superficial epigastric (SEV). These veins should be ligated and the surrounding package removed with preservation of the saphenous vein. **B:** Deep inguinal lymph nodes, which in general number two to four. The most cephalad lymph node is the node of Cloquet.

Radical Inguinal Lymphadenectomy

The patient is placed in the supine position with the ipsilateral hip abducted and the ipsilateral knee flexed (Fig. 67–3). The dissection margins for radical inguinal lymphadenectomy cover the area outlined superiorly by a line drawn from the superior margin of the external inguinal ring to the anterosuperior iliac spine (ASIS), medially by a line drawn from the pubic tubercle 15 cm down the medial thigh, and laterally by a line drawn from the ASIS extending 20 cm inferiorly (Figs. 67–3 and 67–4). A line drawn between the inferior end of the lateral and medial margins marks the inferior limit of the dissection. An incision is made 3 to 4 cm inferior and parallel to the inguinal crease over the medial thigh from the lateral to medial limits of the dissection. The femoral vessels should be palpable in the medial aspect of the incision.

Skin flaps are developed superiorly and inferiorly as the first step of the dissection. Elevation of the skin edges with skin hooks allows dissection within the superficial fatty fascia of the thigh. At the junction of the superficial globular fat and the deeper membranous fat, the tissues are separated. The skin and globular fat are elevated off of the deep membranous fascia and Scarpa's fascia cephalad to a point 4 cm above the inguinal ligament. The skin flaps are protected by gentle elevation with Deaver

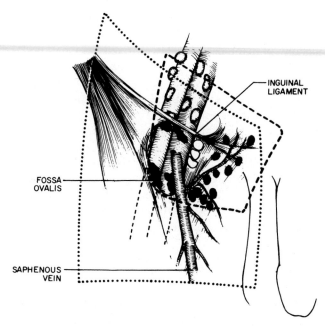

FIG. 67–4. Comparison of limits of dissection of modified inguinal lymphadenectomy (broken line) with classic groin dissection (dotted line). Note that with the modified groin dissection the dissection is medial to the midpoint of the femoral artery. Black, superficial inguinal nodes; white, deep inguinal nodes; gray, external iliac nodes. (From Catalona WJ. Modified inguinal lymphadenectomy for carcinoma of the penis with preservation of saphenous veins: technique and preliminary results. *J Urol* 1988;140:306–310, with permission.)

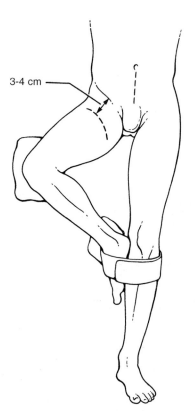

FIG. 67–3. The patient is positioned with the hip abducted and knee flexed. The skin incision is demarcated by the line drawn 2 finger breadths below the inguinal crease.

retractors placed over moist sponges. Inferior traction on the lymphatic package with a small sponge under the left hand provides countertraction to facilitate dissection in the proper plane.

Dissection is carried down through Scarpa's fascia onto the external oblique aponeurosis. The external inguinal ring and emerging spermatic cord are identified medially and retracted as dissection extends to the pubic tubercle. The fat and lymphatics are separated from the spermatic cord and base of the penis medially. Vascular and lymphatic channels are meticulously ligated to prevent fluid accumulation under the skin flaps. The fatty lymph packet is elevated off of the external oblique fascia to the inferior border of the inguinal ligament (Poupart's ligament), where the femoral vessels are identified within the femoral sheath (Fig. 67–5A).

The medial (adductor longus muscle) and lateral (sartorius muscle) borders of the dissection are identified next, and the fascia lata is incised over the muscles. The muscles are traced to their confluence at the apex of the femoral triangle, representing the inferior limit of dissection. The resulting triangular packet of lymphatics and fat needs only to be elevated off its deep margin to complete the dissection. Care must be taken not to retract the adductor longus medially or the sartorius muscle laterally

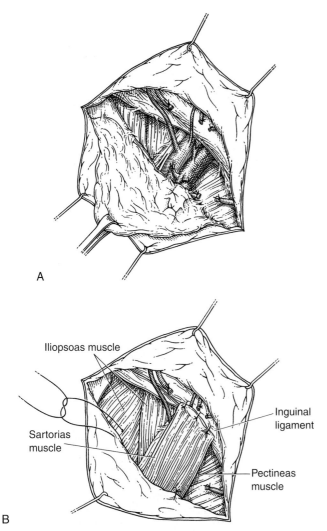

A

B

Iliopsoas muscle

Sartorias muscle

Inguinal ligament

Pectineas muscle

FIG. 67–5. A: Raised groin flaps and the completed groin dissection. **B:** The sartorius muscle is detached at the anterior superior iliac spine and moved medially, thus providing for coverage of the vessels. The transferred sartorius muscle is sutured to the inguinal ligament.

as the dissection will extend too far caudally (i.e., confluence of the two muscles will be displaced caudally).

The saphenous vein is identified medially and preserved if possible. Although this vessel is by tradition sacrificed during radical lymphadenectomy, this achieves no therapeutic benefit and may increase morbidity. If massive lymphadenopathy exists, the saphenous vein should be removed. The femoral sheath is incised over the femoral artery and vein. Medial dissection isolates the lymph node of Cloquet between Cooper's and Poupart's ligaments, lateral to the lacunar ligament. The femoral sheath is stripped inferiorly to the apex of the femoral triangle, as the fascia overlying the sartorius and adductor longus is stripped distally. The deep lymph nodes are removed from their location between the femoral artery and vein. The superficial cutaneous perforating arteries and veins are ligated as they are encountered on the sur-

face of the femoral artery and saphenous vein, leaving the intact saphenous to join the femoral vein, in the area of now absent fossa ovalis. It is important to limit the lateral aspect of dissection along the femoral sheath to the anterior surface of the femoral artery. Dissection laterally on the femoral sheath can injure the femoral nerve beneath the iliacus fascia (deep to the fascia lata), and posterolateral dissection can injure the profunda femoris artery.

When this dissection is complete, the superficial and deep lymphatics are removed together *en bloc*. The wound is irrigated liberally. The exposed femoral vessels are covered by mobilizing the sartorius from its insertion on the anterior superior iliac spine, transposing it over the vessels, and securing its cephalad margin to the inguinal ligament with 2-0 silk suture (Fig. 67–5B). Blood supply to the sartorius arises from its medial and inferior aspects, and care must be taken to protect these vessels during mobilization. The medial edge of the muscle can be tacked to the adductor longus to assure coverage of the femoral vein. If pelvic lymphadenectomy has been performed simultaneously, this dissection should join with the distal limit of the pelvic dissection and allow free communication with the pelvis. To prevent herniation, Cooper's ligament should be secured to the shelving edge of Poupart's ligament with permanent suture (2-0 Proline) without compromising the lumen of the femoral vein.

At this point the wound edges will be inspected for nonviable tissue. Any suspicious area with doubtful vascularization should be excised. Some have suggested giving an ampule of fluorescein intravenously and inspecting the skin edges with a Wood's lamp for viability. We have not found this technique to be particularly useful.

A Jackson–Pratt drain is placed beneath the subcutaneous tissue and brought out inferiorly. The skin flaps are tacked to the surface of the exposed muscles with 3-0 silk and the wound closed with nylon sutures or staples. A light-pressure dressing is applied for the first 12 hours. Care is taken not to apply excessive pressure, which might further compromise blood supply in the skin flaps.

Parenteral antibiotics are continued for 48 hours and then converted to oral agents. The patient is maintained on bedrest for 1 day. Deep vein thrombosis (DVT) prophylaxis, i.e., thromboembolic stockings pneumoboots, is crucial. The drain is removed when the patient is ambulatory and drainage is less than 30 cc per day. Patients are instructed to use thromboembolic stockings for at least 6 months after the surgery. Hospital stockings are converted to fitted compression stockings 1 month postoperatively.

Modified Inguinal Lymphadenectomy

The skin is incised transversely 2 cm below the groin crease for a distance of 10 cm. Skin flaps are raised in the same manner as described above for a distance of approximately 8 cm cephalad and 6 cm caudally. Cephalad dissection onto the external oblique is performed as in radical lymphadenectomy, and the medial extent of dissection is identical. The lateral dissection is more limited, however. After opening the femoral sheath, dissection lateral to the femoral artery is not performed. The sartorius is not exposed, and dissection inferiorly on the fascia lata and femoral sheath extends only to the caudal edge of the fossa ovalis (Fig. 67–4). The saphenous vein is preserved in the superficial nodal package, and the deep lymphatics below the fascia lata between the femoral vessels and medial to the femoral vein along the adductor longus fascia up to Cooper's ligament are removed. Postoperative management is similar to that for radical lymphadenectomy. We do not advocate this approach.

Inguinal Reconstruction After Inguinal Lymphadenectomy

Large groin defects may be created after inguinal lymphadenectomy for bulky metastatic penile cancer. Many types of flaps have been described and advocated to cover large defects in the groin, when extensive dissections are required. The goal is to provide muscle bulk to protect the femoral vessels and full-thickness skin for wound coverage. This will allow for the least morbidity postoperatively and the least likelihood of femoral vessel rupture should adjuvant radiotherapy be required. Flaps described to accomplish this purpose have included a tensor fascia lata myocu-

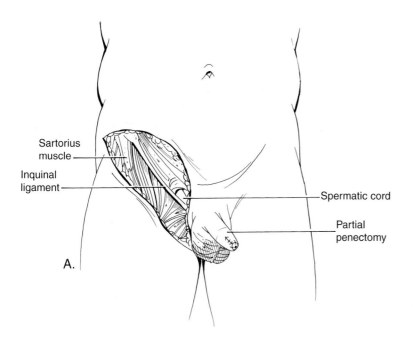

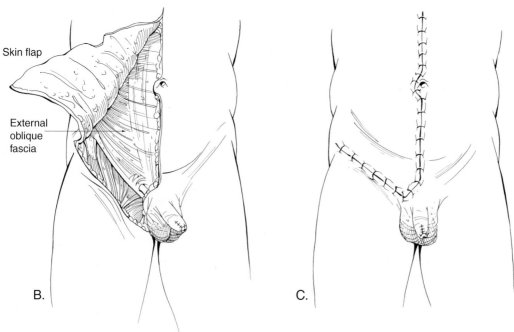

FIG. 67–6. A: On occasion overlying skin must be removed with the lymph nodes, thus creating a large groin defect that does not allow primary skin closure. An advancement flap is a convenient method of covering the defect. The lines of incision for raising the flap are indicated. **B:** The flap is raised superficial to the abdominal wall fascia. **C:** The flap is advanced and sutured over the defect, thus providing full-thickness skin coverage to the extensive groin defect.

taneous flap, a gracilis myocutaneous flap, an abdominal rotation flap, a rectus abdominis myocutaneous flap, a deep inferior epigastric artery myocutaneous flap, a thigh rotational skin flap, and a scrotal advancement flap. Most of these reconstructive procedures are performed in collaboration with a plastic/reconstructive surgeon.

Recently, we proposed the use of an abdominal cutaneous advancement flap as an alternative for primary skin closure of large groin defects (10). The procedure involves sartorius muscle transfer for vascular coverage followed by elevation of the ipsilateral abdominal wall, immediately anterior to the underlying rectus and external oblique fascia, cephalad to the level of the umbilicus. This provides enough mobility for closing a gap of up to 12 cm or less (Figs. 67–6A and 67–6B). For patients with larger (up to 20 cm) gaps, a midline incision is made to the xiphoid process and the entire overlying skin and subcutaneous tissue immediately superficial to the rectus abdominus and external oblique muscle is raised on the ipsilateral side of the defect. The flap is then moved caudad to cover the defect (Fig. 67–6C). Jackson–Pratt drains are employed beneath the flap. Postoperative management is similar to the standard inguinal lymphadenectomy described above. The simplicity, lower morbidity, and excellent cosmetic results are the main advantages of this procedure. The technique may be utilized for bilateral groin defects as well. The presence of abdominal scars (paramedian, appendectomy, Gibson or flank incision) may compromise the blood supply to the flap and are considered relative contraindications to this approach.

OUTCOMES

Complications

Skin necrosis, wound infection, vascular injuries, lower-extremity lymphedema, DVT, and death are some of the potential complications. Skin necrosis and wound infection are probably the most feared complications. Older series report up to 30% flap necrosis. Improved understanding of the cutaneous blood supply, avoidance of the vertical skin incision, improved surgical technique, and appropriate use of perioperative antibiotics have resulted in significant reduction in mortality, skin necrosis, and wound infection—to negligible levels—in several recent reports.

Results

Currently, surgical intervention is the most effective approach to treat SCC of the penis. Early inguinal lymphadenectomy can improve survival in the high-risk patient. Expectant follow-up may be offered to low-risk patients, with clinically negative groin nodes, who comply with comprehensive, close observation.

REFERENCES

1. Catalona WJ. Modified inguinal lymphadenectomy for carcinoma of the penis with preservation of saphenous veins: technique and preliminary results. *J Urol* 1988;140:306–310.
2. Daseler E, Hanson, BJ, Reimann AF. Radical excision of the inguinal and iliac lymph glands. *Surg Gynecol Obstet* 1948;87:679–694.
3. Horenblas S, van Tinteren H. Squamous cell carcinoma of the penis. IV. Prognostic factors of survival: analysis of tumor, nodes and metastasis classification system. *J Urol* 1994;151:1239–1243.
4. Horenblas S, van Tinteren H, Delemarre JF, et al. Squamous cell carcinoma of the penis. III. Treatment of regional lymph nodes. *J Urol* 1993;149:492–497.
5. Hussein AM, Benedetto P, Sridhar KS. Chemotherapy with cisplatin and 5-fluorouracil for penile and urethral squamous cell carcinomas. *Cancer* 1990;65:433–438.
6. Lopes A, Rossi BM, Fonseca FP, et al. Unreliability of modified inguinal lymphadenectomy for clinical staging of penile carcinoma. *Cancer* 1996;77:2099–2102.
7. McDougal WS. Carcinoma of the penis: improved survival by early regional lymphadenectomy based on the histological grade and depth of invasion of the primary lesion. *J Urol* 1995;154:1364–1366.
8. McDougal WS, Kirchner FK Jr, Edwards RH, et al. Treatment of carcinoma of the penis: the case for primary lymphadenectomy. *J Urol* 1986;136:38–41.
9. Pettaway CA, Pisters LL, Dinney CP, et al. Sentinel lymph node dissection for penile carcinoma: the M. D. Anderson Cancer Center experience. *J Urol* 1995;154:1999–2003.
10. Tabatabaei S, McDougal WS. Primary skin closure of large groin defects after inguinal lymphadenectomy for penile cancer using an abdominal cutaneous advancement flap. *J Urol* 2003;169:118–120.

CHAPTER 68

Surgical Treatment of Peyronie's Disease

Keith F. Rourke and Gerald H. Jordan

Peyronie's disease is characterized by the formation of a fibrous lesion within the tunica albuginea of the corpora cavernosa. This lesion or "plaque" is believed to be caused by repetitive microvascular trauma (2). It is proposed that trauma, either acute or chronic, is sustained during intercourse, with subsequent scar formation in susceptible individuals. The plaque's inelasticity results in a functional shortening of the corporal body on the most affected side, resulting in deformity during erection. The incidence of Peyronie's disease has recently been estimated at up to 3% of the general male population (7).

Patients most commonly present with dorsal curvature. It is the authors' opinion that the plaques, in true Peyronie's disease, are always associated with the insertion of the septal fibers. Extensive plaque formation may result in an hourglass deformity, significant penile shortening, or a "hinge" effect distal to the plaque. Fortunately, only a small proportion of patients with Peyronie's disease have deformity requiring surgical intervention. Surgical intervention should be regarded as palliation of the deformity only and not as cure.

The surgical management of Peyronie's disease requires a thorough understanding of the penile anatomy (Fig. 68–1). The penis is composed of three erectile bodies enveloped by fascial layers containing both sensory nerves and blood vessels. The corpus spongiosum lies in the ventral penile midline and expands distally to form the erectile tissue of the glans. The two corpora cavernosa make up the bulk of the penis. Proximally, the corpora cavernosa are fixed to the underside of the pubis and distally fuse to form a single blood space contained within a sheath of connective tissue called the tunica albuginea.

The tunica albuginea consists of two layers, an outer longitudinal layer and an inner circular layer. The outer layer attenuates in the ventral midline and the tunica albuginea becomes unilaminar. Buck's fascia is the next enveloping layer. Within Buck's fascia is the deep dorsal vein located in a dorsal midline groove. Flanking the deep dorsal vein within Buck's fascia are the coiled dorsal arteries and numerous tributaries of the dorsal nerve. The dartos fascia and skin compose the outermost layers of the penile shaft.

DIAGNOSIS

The diagnosis of Peyronie's disease can usually be made with a focused history and physical examination. On history, it is imperative to elicit the duration of symp-

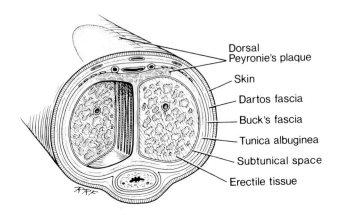

Dorsal
Peyronie's plaque

Skin

Dartos fascia

Buck's fascia

Tunica albuginea

Subtunical space

Erectile tissue

FIG. 68–1. Cross-sectional penile anatomy with dorsal Peyronie's plaque.

toms, progression of the penile deformity, and degree of sexual dysfunction. Erectile dysfunction, to some degree, is felt by many surgeons to be uniformly present. This may represent the psychological impact incurred from living with a genital deformity but may also be due to several other organic causes. Physical examination should be focused on delineating plaque location, size, and opposing plaque formation (if present). An attempt to elicit known disease associations such as Dupuytren's contracture or other elastic tissue fibromatosis should be made. Objective evaluation of penile curvature with a photograph of the erect penis is extremely helpful. Plain radiographs are effective in demonstrating plaque calcification, believed to be a sign of plaque maturity.

It is important to evaluate and define the surgical candidate's preoperative erectile function. Prospective surgical patients at our center are evaluated with color duplex Doppler ultrasound (CDDU) in the presence of pharmacologically induced erection. Abnormalities in the resistive index or end-diastolic velocity prompt further testing with dynamic infusion cavernosometry/cavernosography (DICC). In addition, one must determine if acceptable intercourse can be accomplished by enhancement of erectile rigidity alone. In this scenario, patients are best served with a pharmacological erection program as an alternative to surgery.

A frank discussion of treatment goals with the Peyronie's couple is imperative. The patient should be assured that the process is not malignant or life threatening. The goal of surgery is to straighten the penis and maintain erectile function such that satisfactory intercourse is achieved. Couples must be aware that preexisting penile shortening and erectile dysfunction will not be improved by straightening procedures. Evaluation with a sex therapist can help patients and partners adjust to these new sexual expectations.

INDICATIONS FOR SURGERY

Although medical treatments targeting resolution of scar tissue have largely been unsuccessful, an attempt at treating Peyronie's disease medically should be made in most patients prior to surgical intervention. A surgical candidate must meet certain criteria. First, the disease process must be stable and the plaque mature/quiescent. In review, the signs of disease quiescence include unchanged penile deformity for a minimum of 6 months, with the resolution of pain associated with erection. Moreover, before surgical intervention most investigators recommend a minimum 12-month waiting period from disease onset. The experienced examiner may recognize the clinical findings of a mature or calcified plaque and could elect to intervene earlier than this arbitrary time period. Once disease stability exists, indications for surgical intervention are penile deformity and/or erectile dysfunction that preclude intercourse.

Three general techniques exist for the surgical management of Peyronie's disease: (a) corporal plication procedures, (b) plaque incision/excision with grafting, and (c) penile prosthesis insertion with plaque modeling or incision. Many protocols have been published describing the treatment of Peyronie's disease, but the best outcome depends on an individualized approach. Plication procedures involve shortening the corpora cavernosum on the side opposite the plaque, but carry the advantages of being less technically demanding with a more rapid convalescence and probably a smaller risk of postoperative erectile dysfunction. Incision or excision of the Peyronie's plaque with grafting of the corporotomy defect is a more technically complex procedure and may incur a risk of graft-induced venoocclusive dysfunction. Patients with severe curvature, hourglass deformity, or inadequate penile length are more amenable to incision/excision with grafting over plication techniques that can further shorten or deform the erect penis. Plication procedures may be the preferred option for ventral curvatures as historically this subset of patients has demonstrated poor outcomes with grafting. Straightening techniques are appropriate for patients with adequate erectile function, in whom penile straightening alone will achieve satisfactory intercourse. At our institution we prefer the technique of plaque incision with grafting except for severely calcified plaques, which may require excision.

Last, insertion of penile prostheses for Peyronie's disease was once considered a panacea but is now reserved for patients with severe erectile dysfunction. In patients with severe curvature, prosthetic implantation can be done in conjunction with an incision and grafting procedure. Remodeling the plaque intraoperatively after prosthesis placement is remarkably successful and often avoids the need for incision (8). The technique of penile prosthesis insertion is covered in Chapter 70.

ALTERNATIVE THERAPY

Medical management includes oral agents, topical agents with or without ultrasound, and intralesional injection protocols. As mentioned, surgical management of Peyronie's disease should be viewed as a palliation of the mechanical effects of the disease rather than a cure.

SURGICAL TECHNIQUE

Plaque Incision

The initial skin incision is dependent on plaque location. As previously mentioned, plication procedures address the aspect of corpus cavernosum opposite the plaque while plaque incision/excision techniques approach the plaque directly. The dorsum of the corpora cavernosum is best exposed by a circumferential degloving incision. If the patient has been previously circum-

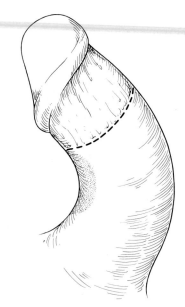

FIG. 68–2. Dorsal penile curvature with incision marked at the circumcision scar.

cised then the incision should be performed at the original surgical site (Fig. 68–2). Approaching the penis through the previous circumcision site has not been problematic, even when the scar is displaced proximally. Ventral exposure can also be achieved through a midline incision on the ventral aspect of the penis.

The penile shaft is degloved to its base by sharply dissecting the dartos fascia from the underlying Buck's fascia. This maneuver gives good exposure for midshaft and distal lesions. For proximal plaques or patients with a redundant prepuce, a second incision may be created on the scrotum or lateral to the base of the penis. Then, after degloving the shaft of the penis it is delivered into the counterincision, laying the shaft skin aside and covering it with a warm gauze dressing. This protects the penile skin from trauma until the end of the procedure, when it is returned to the shaft.

Plication Procedures

Several techniques have been described to "plicate" the curvature associated with Peyronie's disease. Procedures are performed via a degloving incision with the patient in the supine position. An artificial erection is created to accurately define the point of maximal curvature using a pressure infuser with 0.9% saline. The use of a tourniquet for control of bleeding or induction of an artificial erection is not favored as proximal curvatures can be concealed. Buck's fascia opposite the site of maximal curvature is sharply incised and elevated off of the underlying tunica albuginea. Correction of dorsal curvature requires identification of the corpus spongiosum ventrally. For ventral curvature, care must be taken to avoid injury to

the dorsal neurovascular structures. Once the tunica albuginea is exposed, plication of corpora can be performed in several ways. Creation of an ellipse corporotomy defect with reapproximation of the corporal edges using 3-0 PDS sutures effectively counteracts the opposing lesion (6). Tissue may be excised or more conveniently and safely placed underneath the corporotomy closure. Correction of curvature can also be achieved by plicating the corpora cavernosa using a series of "loosely tied" parallel nonabsorbable sutures without incising the tunica albuginea (3). Once acceptable straightening is achieved, the penis is closed anatomically in layers and a small-caliber closed-suction drain is placed superficial to Buck's fascia.

Plaque Incision and Grafting

After incision and degloving, exposure for dorsal plaque incision requires elevation of the dorsal neurovascular bundle concurrently with Buck's fascia. This can be approached by several techniques. One technique involves making bilateral incisions lateral to the corpus spongiosum, then dissecting Buck's fascia and the dorsal neurovascular bundle off the lateral and dorsal aspects of the corpora cavernosa. Alternately, a dorsal plaque can be approached through the bed of the deep dorsal vein with a modified vein dissection. This is done by sharply opening Buck's fascia over the path of the deep dorsal vein to the level of the penopubic ligaments (Fig. 68–3). The dorsal vein is elevated and ligated as proximally as possible without detaching the penopubic attachments and then distally to the vein "trifurcation" (Fig. 68–4). The circumferential veins are ligated at their junction with the deep dorsal vein. The lateral neurovascular structures are reflected off the tunica albuginea in concert with the inner lamina of Buck's fascia. Buck's fascia is widely mobilized from the base of the penis out to the coronal margin and to the lateral aspect of the penis (Fig. 68–5). Approaching the dorsal plaque through the bed of the dorsal vein appears to be a technically superior approach.

Once appropriately exposed, the extent of the plaque can be determined by palpating the surface of the tunica albuginea. After creation of an artificial erection, an H-

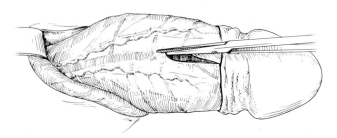

FIG. 68–3. Incision of Buck's fascia overlying the dorsal vein after penile degloving.

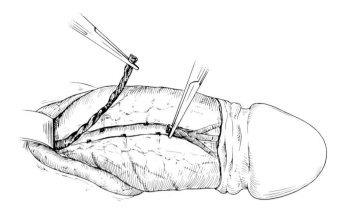

FIG. 68–4. Deep dorsal vein dissection and ligation.

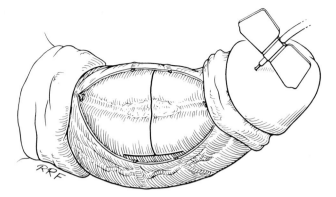

FIG. 68–6. An H-shaped incision marked at the point of maximal deformity.

shaped incision is marked at the point of maximal curvature (Fig. 68–6). Once the incision is created, the "flaps" of the H are elevated and allowed to "slide" (Fig.68–7). During this maneuver the septal fibers are divided. It is not necessary to remove thickened septal fibers and it is unnecessary and potentially harmful to remove any spongy erectile tissue. A square defect is then created by suturing the flap corners into place with interrupted 4-0 PDS sutures. If an indentation exists after corporotomy, darting incisions are made to allow for expansion of the scar (Fig. 68–8).

After the incision is completed, we measure the defect area with the penis at stretched length to ensure accurate graft coverage. The ideal graft material is not known. We have preferentially used dermis at our institution (1). Alternatively, corporotomy defects can be patched with saphenous vein (5). Temporalis fascia, tunica vaginalis, nonautologous pericardial grafts, and small intestinal submucosa (SIS) grafts have also been described. Tunica vaginalis lacks tensile strength and is best applied to small defects. Prosthetic (e.g., Gore-Tex, silastic) and nonautologous grafts, historically, have tended to fibrose and contract. The authors feel caution should be used when applying these "grafts" in the absence of concurrent prosthetic implantation.

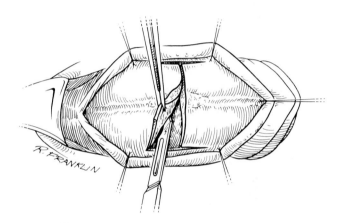

FIG. 68–7. Incision of the tunica albuginea.

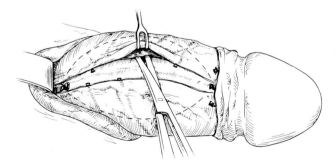

FIG. 68–5. Elevation of Buck's fascia concurrently with the dorsal neurovascular structures.

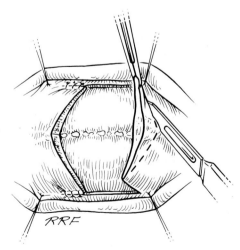

FIG. 68–8. Creation of a square defect in the tunica albuginea. Darting incisions are performed if indentation persists.

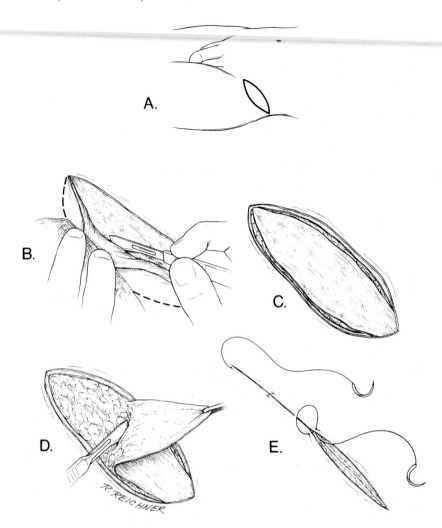

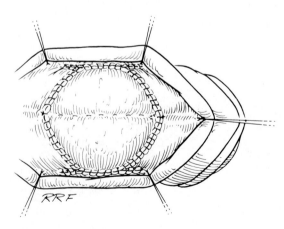

FIG. 68–9. Dermal harvest from the non-hirsute skin above the iliac crest.

The dermal graft is obtained from the nonhirsute area of abdominal skin located superior and lateral to the iliac crest (Fig. 68–9). The graft is deepithelialized freehand, using a scalpel and loupe magnification. After deepithelialization, a superficial incision is made through the epidermis and extended into the subcuticular adipose tissue. The dermis is harvested and is meticulously defatted. The donor site is closed primarily with absorbable monofilament sutures. The graft is marked 30% larger than the corporotomy defect in all dimensions, as the graft will "contract" when released from the inherent tissue tension at the donor site.

Once tailored, the dermal graft is sewn into the corporotomy defect using interrupted 4-0 PDS sutures followed by a running locked 4-0 PDS suture (Fig. 68–10). Artificial erection is performed after graft placement to ensure a watertight suture line and an acceptably straight penis. Any leaks, if present, are oversewn.

We have found that curvature can be corrected with incision and grafting alone in about 70% of instances. The remaining 30% will require an additional "touch-up" plication or in the rare case a second incision into the plaque. Incision as opposed to excision limits the size of the applied graft and may be more reliable in preserving erectile function. The penis is closed as described previously for surgical plication.

FIG. 68–10. Watertight closure of the corporotomy after dermal graft.

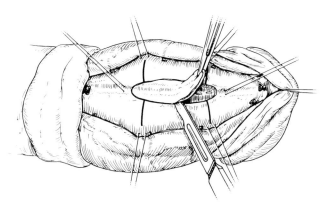

FIG. 68–11. Excision of Peyronie's plaque.

Plaque Excision and Grafting

Plaque excision (vs. incision) may be required in the patient with a severely calcified plaque. In this scenario the plaque is exposed as previously discussed. Prolene stay sutures are used to mark the plaque at the proximal and distal aspects. An incision outlining the plaque is made and the plaque is excised (Fig. 68–11). The corporotomy defect left by plaque incision is converted from ovoid to stellate by creating lateral incisions into the tunica albuginea (Fig. 68–12). Grafting and closure is then accomplished in the same manner as the technique of plaque incision.

POSTOPERATIVE CARE

A loosely applied Bioclusive dressing is used to dress the penis. A mildly compressing Kling gauze dressing is wrapped around the Bioclusive to reduce edema and keep the surgical spaces collapsed around the suction drains. The Kling dressing is removed in 4 hours and the glans is checked every 30 minutes during this interval. A 14 Fr Foley is placed intraoperatively and left for 24 hours. The

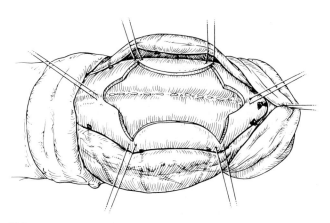

FIG. 68–12. Creation of stellate defect after plaque excision.

drains are in general removed on postoperative day 1 and the patient is discharged the same day. Erections are suppressed with diazepam and amyl nitrite for 2 weeks postoperatively.

After 2 weeks, patients are encouraged to have erections but refrain from intercourse. Erections during this time are beneficial as they may help prevent skin adherence to the deeper layers of the penis and with grafting techniques erections will stretch the graft, aiding in its maturation. At about 6 to 8 weeks postoperatively, patients may resume sexual intercourse.

OUTCOMES

Complications

Early postoperative complications include hematoma formation, wound infection, and persistent penile edema. Meticulous hemostasis with bipolar cautery, the use of small closed-suction drains, and careful tissue handling can minimize the risk of these complications. Patients should be informed of the risk of experiencing a change in glanular sensation. This applies predominantly to those patients requiring dissection of Buck's fascia dorsally. The vast majority of patients recover adequate glanular sensation and it is unusual for persistent neuropathies of the glans to occur. Other potential complications involve the risk of a bothersome granuloma ("lump") formation after the use of permanent sutures during a plication procedure.

Recurrent disabling curvature is uncommon but may occur. Patients requiring grafting with dermis should be counseled that during the late phase of maturation the graft tends to contract and may be inelastic enough to recreate some of the curvature. Patients can be ensured that this is transient and straightening will occur when the graft softens.

The most frequently encountered "complication" is that of diminished penile rigidity postoperatively. With plication procedures this occurs in approximately 5% to 6% of patients and with grafting procedures in approximately 10% to 12% of cases. Erectile dysfunction can occur as a consequence of surgery but may also represent the natural history of Peyronie's disease. Many of these patients benefit from the addition of pharmacological therapy to enhance their erectile function.

Results

A successful reconstructive procedure for Peyronie's disease results in a satisfactory straightening of the penis such that any residual deformity does not interfere with sexual intercourse. Second, adequate erectile function is required for this to occur. Surgical success correlates linearly with preoperative erectile function (4). Patients with good erectile function and accumulated intracorporal pressures have a surgical success rate in excess of 88% to 90%. Poor erectile function preoperatively correlates strongly with a poor surgical outcome and these patients may be best managed with prostheses placement. Those patients falling in between with fair erectile function demonstrate acceptable success rates in the 70% to 80% range.

Surgical intervention for Peyronie's disease is indicated when a stable plaque causes disabling penile deformity and/or erectile dysfunction. The goal of surgery is to resume satisfactory sexual intercourse by correcting penile curvature without further diminishing erectile function. Incision/excision with grafting should be considered over plication in patients with severe curvature, shortening, or deformity. With proper patient selection, surgical correction for Peyronie's disease yields excellent results.

REFERENCES

1. Devine CJ Jr., Horton CE. Surgical treatment of Peyronie's disease with a dermal graft. *J Urol* 1974;111:44.
2. Devine CJ Jr, Somers KD, Jordan GH, Schlossberg SM. Proposal: Trauma as the cause of the Peyronie's lesion. *J Urol* 1997;157:285.
3. Gholami SS, Lue TF. Correction of penile curvature using the 16-dot plication technique: A review of 132 patients. *J Urol* 2002;167:2066.
4. Jordan GH, Angermeier KW. Preoperative evaluation of erectile function with dynamic infusion cavernosometry/cavernosography in patients undergoing surgery for Peyronie's disease: Correlation with postoperative results. *J Urol* 1993;150:1138.
5. Lue TF, El-Sakka AI. Venous patch graft for Peyronie's disease. Part I: Technique. *J Urol* 1998;160:2047.
6. Pryor JP, Fitzpatrick JM. A new approach to the correction of the penile deformity in Peyronie's disease. *J Urol* 1979;122:622.
7. Schwarzer U, Sommer F, Klotz T, Braun M, Reifenrath B, Engelmann U. The prevalence of Peyronie's disease: Results of a large survey. *Br J Urol* 2001;88:727.
8. Wilson SK, Delk JR II. A new treatment for Peyronie's disease: Modeling the penis over an inflatable penile prosthesis. *J Urol* 1994;152:1121.

CHAPTER 69

Priapism

Derek J. Bochinski and Tom F. Lue

Priapism is a pathologic condition of a penile erection that persists beyond or is unrelated to sexual stimulation. Priapism may be classified as ischemic (venous, low flow) and nonischemic (arterial or high flow). The term low flow is misleading because there is no flow into or out of the corpus cavernosum in the ischemic priapism and therefore the term should not be used. Nonischemic priapism is often caused by a ruptured helicine artery pumping well-oxygenated blood into the corpora cavernosa; this may not need urgent surgical attention. Ischemic priapism is a "compartment syndrome" caused by a trapping of poorly oxygenated blood in the corpus cavernosum with associated ischemic damage; these patients must be treated as soon as possible. Untreated cases will lead to ischemia, necrosis, and severe scarring of the erectile tissue. After 24 hours there is evidence of irreversible smooth muscle necrosis, destruction of epithelium, and exposure of the basement membrane with thrombocytes adherent to it (5).

DIAGNOSIS

On initial evaluation, patients should have a detailed history and physical, with emphasis on possible causative factors. Historical features should include the length of the priapism episode and the occurrence of any previous episodes. Physical examination should assess for subtle neurological defects, pelvic masses, and perineal abnormalities as well as the characteristics of the penis. Patients with significant pain and with a rigid penis and soft glans are more likely to have ischemic priapism. Patients with nonischemic priapism usually have a semierect penis without pain. Laboratory tests should include complete blood count, urinalysis, reticulocyte count, and sickle cell anemia screen as well as urine toxicology screen for metabolites of cocaine (when appropriate).

Diagnosis of the type of priapism and the management of the ischemic type should commence as soon as possible (Fig. 69–1). Aspiration of penile blood may be diagnostic; acidotic, hypoxic blood (PO_2 less than 40, PCO_2 greaterh than 60, and pH less than 7.25) is suggestive of ischemic priapism. Color duplex ultrasound has proven to be another useful tool in discriminating between the different types of priapism. No cavernosal arterial flow is seen with ischemic priapism, while a ruptured artery with unregulated blood pooling in the area of injury can often be seen in trauma-induced nonischemic priapism. Before any invasive therapy, informed consent should be obtained. Patients should understand that there is a 50% chance of erectile dysfunction regardless of duration of priapism or method of management.

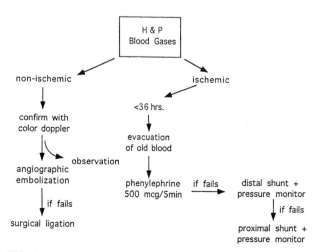

FIG. 69–1. Algorithm for the diagnosis and management of priapism.

INDICATIONS FOR SURGERY

If medical management is unsuccessful in allowing detumescence of the penis, surgical management should be considered for ischemic priapism. The immediate goal is to allow blood to flow readily in and out of the penis to prevent ischemic damage and relieve pain.

ALTERNATIVE THERAPY

For ischemic priapism, evacuation of the old blood followed by intracavernous injection of a diluted alpha-adrenergic agonist is successful. A variety of alpha-adrenergic agonists have been used; we have had the most success with aspiration plus diluted phenylephrine, 250 to 500 µg every 3 to 5 minutes until detumescence. This therapy is not recommended for high-flow priapism; it is ineffective and may cause systemic side effects.

SURGICAL TECHNIQUE

Surgical correction involves connecting the engorged cavernosal tissue with the glans, corpus spongiosum, or dorsal or saphenous vein. This surgically created fistula will allow blood to drain from the corpora cavernosa until the pathologic process has resolved. Ideally, the surgically created fistula will spontaneously close after the priapism-causing factors have resolved. On the basis of these principles, many techniques have been used for the urgent treatment of priapism.

Of the shunting procedures, we recommend distal cavernosum–glans shunt as the first choice because it is easier to perform and has fewer complications. The shunting procedure can be performed with a large biopsy needle (7) or a scalpel (2) inserted percutaneously through the glans. It can also be performed by excising a piece of the tunica albuginea at the tip of the corpus cavernosum through an incision on the glans (9). Of the three procedures, excision of both tips of the corpora cavernosa is the most effective and can be performed even if the two others fail. However, nonclosure of the shunt may contribute to postoperative erectile dysfunction.

In general, the distal shunting procedure is quite successful in reestablishing penile circulation in most cases except those with severe distal penile edema or tissue damage. In these cases, a proximal shunt such as between the corpus cavernosum and the saphenous vein (8) or dorsal vein (1) is performed. Alternatively, a shunt can also be created between the corpus cavernosum and the bulb of the corpus spongiosum (4). These procedures are time consuming and technically challenging. Pulmonary embolism associated with Grayhack's procedure and urethral fistula as well as purulent cavernositis associated with Quackels' procedure have been reported.

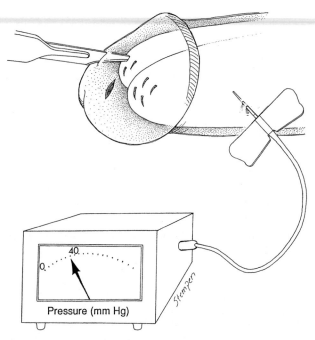

FIG. 69–2. After multiple glans–cavernosal shunts, monitoring intracavernosal pressure for 10 minutes after closure to ensure a pressure of greater than 140 mm Hg is essential for a successful repair.

The efficacy of the shunt can be tested intraoperatively to assess its success. This is best done by monitoring the intracavernosal pressure for 10 to 15 minutes after completion of the shunt (Fig. 69–2). A pressure of less than 40 mm Hg for longer than 10 minutes is necessary for a successful shunt. If this is not achieved, a larger shunt or a more invasive procedure will be needed.

Glans–Cavernosal Shunt

This is the least invasive technique for priapism management. Under local or general anesthesia, a pointed no. 11 knife blade is inserted through the glans to penetrate the tip of the corpus cavernosum. The knife is then twisted 90 degrees and pulled back to incise the tunica albuginea close to the tip of the cavernous body (2). After this shunt has been made, the skin on the glans is closed with fine chromic catgut. Good results are suggested by swelling of the glans and detumescence.

Al-Ghorab Procedure

Under local anesthesia, an incision is made on the dorsum of the glans penis 1 cm distal to the coronal ridge (6). The distal end of the glans is then hinged forward to expose the ends of the bulging corporal bodies. Using sharp dissection, a 5-mm segment of tunica at the tip of the corporal bodies is excised, including a portion of the septum. Dark blood should be draining from the corporal bodies. When detumescence has occurred, the skin is repositioned with chromic sutures in a way so as not to obliterate the spongy vascular space of the glans.

Quackles' Cavernosum–Spongiosum Shunt

Under regional or general anesthesia, an 18 Fr Foley catheter is placed into the bladder to aid in identifying the urethra. The patient is placed in the lithotomy position. A vertical incision is made in the perineal skin just posterior to the scrotum and overlying the bulbous urethra (Fig. 69–3). The bulbocavernous muscle is reflected off of the urethra and preserved. Identify the junction between the spongiosal and cavernosal bodies; the spongiosum should be easily compressible and flaccid. Corresponding 1-cm longitudinal incisions are made through the tunica of the spongiosal and cavernosal bodies close enough to each other so that they may be sewn together. Excising an elliptical segment of tunica rather than just incising may provide a better fistula. After one cavernosal body is opened, the old blood should be evacuated with manual milking until bright red blood is expressed. The shunt is completed by suturing the posterior wall followed by the anterior wall in a watertight fashion with 5-0 polydioxanone suture (PDS). If the intracavernosal pressures stay below 40 mm Hg after 10 to 15 minutes, then the skin may be closed. If the pressure is more than 40 mm Hg, then shunting on the other side should be done (4).

Cavernosal–Venous Shunts

In 1964, a venous bypass using saphenous vein was described for the treatment of priapism. Under general anesthesia, the patient is placed in the supine position with his legs slightly frog-legged. The first incision is made over the saphenofemoral junction 3 to 4 cm below the inguinal ligament; this incision may be extended distally along the course of the saphenous vein (Fig. 69–4). Extending distally from the fossa ovalis, the saphenous vein is mobilized for 8 to 10 cm, enough to be tunneled subcutaneously to the root of the penis without tension. At the distal extent of vein mobilization, it is ligated with 2-0 silk and sharply divided.

The second incision is a 1-in. vertical one over the lateral aspect of the penile shaft near the root of the penis and extending through all layers to the tunica albuginea. Blunt dissection is used to tunnel between the two incisions, after which the cut length of vein is passed to the medial incision without tension, twisting, or excessive angulation. With the ipsilateral corporal body identified, excise a small ellipse of tunica. Manually express and irrigate the old blood; then, spatulate the vein in preparation for anastomosis. The vein is sewn to the aperture in the tunica with 5-0 PDS in a running, watertight fashion (3).

Cavernosum–Dorsal Vein Shunt

This shunt (6) is based on the principle that the dorsal vein is not involved in priapism. A 4-cm skin incision is made at the base of the penis, extending through Buck's fascia. The superficial or deep dorsal vein is mobilized sufficiently that it will reach the desired site of tunical ellipse incision. After the cavernosal body has been opened and the vein is spatulated on its ventral surface, the anastomosis may be done using 5-0 PDS.

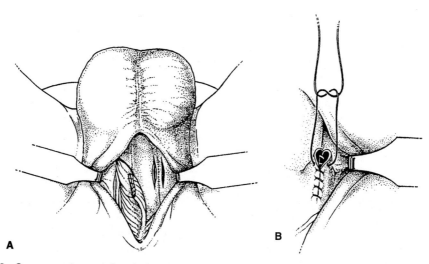

FIG. 69–3. Cavernosal–spongiosal shunt. **A:** Incisions on the tunica of the spongiosum and cavernosum. **B:** Anastomosis of the openings.

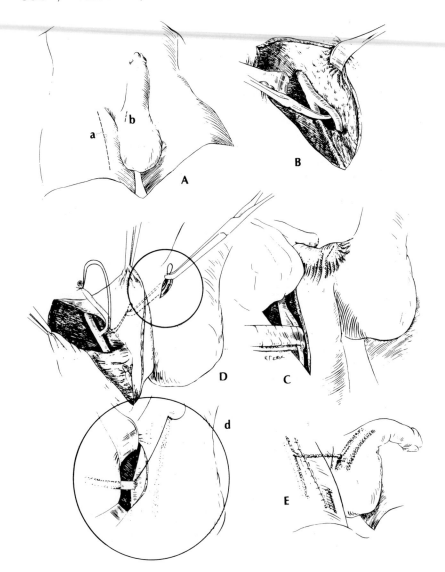

FIG. 69–4. Cavernosal–saphenous vein shunt.

POSTOPERATIVE CARE

After surgery, if detumescence is complete the patient can be discharged home. If not, the patient is admitted for intravenous antibiotics and supportive care. These shunting procedures will allow drainage through the dorsal or saphenous veins, glans, or corpus spongiosum. Circular compressive dressings should be avoided because they may decrease venous drainage and perpetuate the process. Intermittent manual squeezing and milking of tissue will help keep the shunt open and prevent a recurrence of priapism. The penis will likely appear partially erect even with an effective shunt because of postischemic hyperemia. If there are any questions, intracavernous blood gasses or color duplex ultrasound can be used to differentiate ischemic versus nonischemic situations. Recurrent (stuttering) priapism can be treated with self-injected diluted phenylephrine as described above. The most successful preventive measure is the adminis-

tration of antiandrogen or gonadotropin-releasing hormone agonist for 4 to 6 months.

NONISCHEMIC PRIAPISM

A history of perineal trauma with a nonpainful, intermittent erection is suggestive of nonischemic priapism. Cavernous blood gases will reflect nonischemic blood levels. Color duplex ultrasonography is the best diagnostic tool; it can identify the high-flow state and site of the ruptured artery.

After the diagnosis has been made, these patients may be observed for as long as several months to allow the fistula to spontaneously close. If this does not occur, then angiographic embolization of the ruptured artery should be performed. If the fistula persists, then suture ligation of the ruptured artery via a perineal approach can be done under ultrasound guidance.

OUTCOMES

Complications

Early complications include recurrence, bleeding, infection, skin necrosis, abscess, cellulitis, gangrene, urethral damage, urethrocutaneous fistula, and urethral stricture. Late complications include fibrosis of erectile tissue and failure of venous shunt to close spontaneously, leading to venogenic impotence. Careful handling of tissue, close immediate postoperative management, and judicious use of antibiotics will best minimize the risk of these complications.

Pulmonary embolism has been reported to occur following cavernosa–saphenous shunt. This serious complication should be considered in any patient with suggestive symptoms.

Results

The most common complication of priapism is loss of potency, which may be a function of the disease as well as a result of the procedure. Postmanagement potency rates range from 54% to 57%, and the impotence is in general considered to be a result of fibrosis of the corpora from the inflammatory response. The most critical factor in maintaining potency in patients with priapism is the duration of the priapism episode. Patients treated within 24 to 36 hours will more likely have a favorable response than those who delay treatment. Patients with prolonged or recurrent episodes are more likely to suffer impotence as a result of fibrosis. Other risk factors are older patients with cardiovascular disease and those with repeated episodes from sickle cell anemia. Traumatic priapism appears to have the best prognosis in preservation of erectile function.

REFERENCES

1. Barry JM. Priapism: treatment with corpus cavernosum to dorsal vein penis shunts. *J Urol* 1976;116:754.
2. Ebbehoj J. A new operation for priapism. *Scand J Plast Reconstruct Surg* 1975;8:241.
3. Odelowo EO. A new cavernospongiosum shunt with saphenous vein patch for established priapism. *Int Surg* 1988;73:130.
4. Quackles R. Cure of patient suffering from priapism by cavernospongiosal anastomosis. *Acta Urol Belgica* 1964; 32:5.
5. Spycher MA, Hauri D. The ultrastructure of erectile tissue in priapism. *J Urol* 1986;135:142.
6. Wendell EF, Grayhack JT. Corpora cavernosa–glans penis shunt for priapism. *Surg Gynecol Obstet* 1981;153:586.
7. Winter CC. Priapism cured by creation of fistulas between glans, penis, and corpora cavernosa. *J Urol* 1978;119:227–228.
8. Grayhack JT, McCullough W, O'Connor VJ, Trippel O. Venous bypass to control priapism. *Invest Urol* 1964;58:509–513.
9. Ercolo CJ, Pontes JE, Pioro JM Jr. Changing surgical concepts in the treatment for priapism. *J Urol* 1981;125:210–211.

CHAPTER 70

Penile Prosthesis Implantation

Culley C. Carson

While erectile dysfunction has been described since ancient times, adequate treatment has only been available for the last three decades. The era of implantable devices began with the development of silicone-based prosthetic materials in the late 1960s as a result of the space program (4). Modern penile prosthetic devices were first developed in the early 1970s when Small et al. (6) along with Scott et al. (5) reported the implantation of penile prosthetic devices into the corpora cavernosa to fill the corpora cavernosa and provide a physiologically functional erection with good cosmetic results. These devices have undergone multiple revisions and redesigns between the early prosthetic devices and the currently implanted inflatable penile prostheses. Mechanical malfunction rates in these early devices, however, were reported in excess of 60% of cases. Current inflatable prosthetic devices, however, have a far improved mechanical reliability. These current devices can be divided into semirigid, mechanical, and multiple-component inflatable penile prostheses of which there are two- and three-piece models available.

Semirigid rod and mechanical prostheses available today are the successors of the devices designed in the 1970s (Table 70–1). These devices, while easier to implant, have few advantages over the newer inflatable devices because infection and mechanical malfunction rates are similar. The semirigid devices consist of a central metal core and a silicone elastomer rod while the mechanical Duraphase implant is a series of disks held in

position by a central cable. The latter design facilitates positioning of the implant between uses.

The three-piece inflatable penile prostheses vary in construction from three-layer silicon/Dacron/Lycra to a single layer of silicon or Bioflex (Fig. 70–1). Options include girth expansion and/or length elongation. Aneurismal dilatation is rare with both of these cylinder designs but has been reported. Similarly, other design changes—including replacement of stainless steel connectors with plastic connectors, addition of nonkinked tubing, single design construction, Teflon cylinder input sleeves, and multiple-layer cylinders—have improved the longevity of these devices. These modifications have decreased mechanical malfunction rates from greater than 30% to less than 5%.

The three-piece inflatable penile prostheses continue to be the most satisfactory prostheses once they are implanted and while they remain functional. These prosthetic devices produce the most natural appearing erection in girth, length, and with satisfactory rigidity and

TABLE 70-1. *Penile prostheses*

Semirigid rods	Inflatable
AMS 600 (AMS)	700 CX (AMS)
Malleable (Mentor)	700 Ultrex (AMS)
Dura II (AMS)	Alpha 1 (Mentor)
	GFS (Mentor)
	Ambicor (AMS)

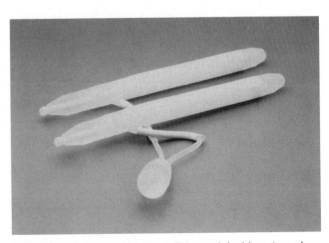

FIG. 70–1. American Medical Systems' Ambicor two-piece inflatable penile prosthesis.

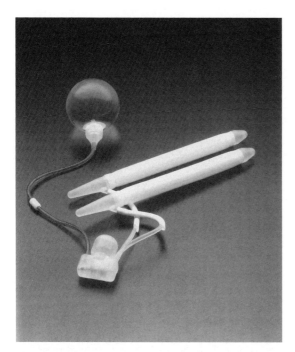

FIG. 70–2. American Medical Systems' AMS 700CX three-piece inflatable penile prosthesis.

excellent flaccidity for optimal concealment. They also have advantages for many patients with complex penile implantations because the flaccid position removes pressure from the corporal cavernosa and decreases the possibility of erosion in these highly difficult implantations.

To improve ease of surgical implantation and remove a portion of the prosthesis placed within the abdominal region, two-piece prostheses were designed (Fig. 70–2). Because these two-piece inflatable prostheses remove the separate reservoir, additional fluid is available either by a larger scrotal pump or a combination of proximal cylinder and pump reservoir. Although these devices provide adequate erection in many patients, the limited reservoir capacity decreases flaccidity and may, in some patients, diminish rigidity. These prostheses are especially difficult to deflate in patients with small penises and frequently provide inadequate rigidity of patients with longer penises. While less optimal than three-piece devices, these two-piece implants may be ideal for patients in whom reservoir placement is difficult or contraindicated. Such patients as renal transplant recipients and patients who have undergone significant radical pelvic exenteration procedures may benefit from two-piece devices.

DIAGNOSIS

The diagnosis of erectile dysfunction can be obtained by history. The clinician should determine whether the erectile dysfunction is situational or constant, whether the degree of dysfunction is partial or total, and also include the details of the relationship with the partner. Any coexisting conditions such as diabetes, vascular disease, smoking, medications (especially steroids, hormones, antihypertensives, or antidepressants), and use of alcohol or drugs should be identified. Physical examination should include the genitalia including the testes, hair distribution, femoral and distal lower-extremity pulses, and the penis for Peyronie's plaques or other abnormalities. Nocturnal tumescence studies, cavernosometry, cavernosography, or penile Doppler is useful in some patients in securing the diagnosis.

INDICATIONS FOR SURGERY

Although there are a variety of penile prosthesis designs currently available for implantation, not all patients with erectile dysfunction are candidates for penile prosthesis implantation. Careful counseling of patients before penile implant procedures will limit many of the problems with postoperative dissatisfaction. Once the discussion and demonstration of penile implant varieties has been carried out, patients can be counseled about the most appropriate penile prosthesis for their individual use. Patients may choose a specific prosthetic type based on their needs and preferences (1). Younger patients with normal manual dexterity and patients who wear stylish, form-fitting, athletic clothing or who shower in public at a health club or other athletic facility often choose a three-piece inflatable penile prosthesis because appearance in the flaccid position is better than other designs. For these patients, implantation of a semirigid rod penile prosthesis requires a significant lifestyle change and they are better served with an inflatable-type prosthesis. Similarly, patients with Peyronie's disease, secondary implantation, or significant peripheral neuropathy such as occurs in severe diabetes are best served with an inflatable penile prosthesis because interior tissue pressures are diminished between uses and the possibility of extrusion is diminished.

For patients in whom the convenience of inflation and deflation are not important, the risks and mechanical malfunctions may outweigh the disadvantage of a malleable penile prosthesis (Fig. 70–3). Such patients as paraplegics who require external urinary collection device, those with inadequate manual dexterity, or those with significant obesity may be better served with a malleable penile prosthesis.

ALTERNATIVE THERAPY

Alternative therapy includes sexual counseling, vacuum erection devices, intracavernosal injection therapy, intraurethral medication, or oral medications. Less commonly used therapies include penile vascular (arterial or venous) surgery.

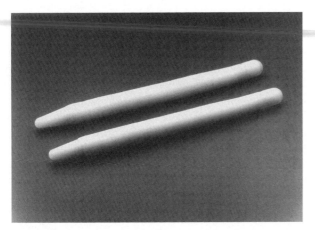

FIG. 70–3. American Medical Systems' AMS 600 malleable penile prosthesis.

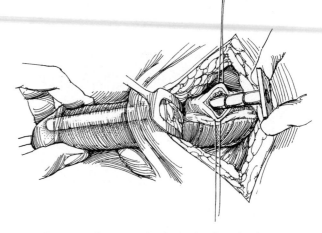

FIG. 70–4. Corporal dilation using Brooks dilators.

SURGICAL TECHNIQUE

Surgical implantation of penile prostheses can be carried out using a variety of surgical approaches and incisions. Semirigid and malleable prostheses can be implanted through a distal penile approach. Multiple-piece prostheses, however, can be implanted by the infrapubic or penoscrotal approach. While individual surgeons have a variety of rationales for each of these approaches, there does not appear to be any clear advantage in patient satisfaction or outcome of the two approaches. Patient anatomy may dictate appropriate choice. Patients with previous abdominal surgical procedures where reservoir placement is difficult may be better served with an infrapubic approach while patients with massive obesity may be better approached through a penoscrotal incision. Two-piece devices, because there is no separate reservoir, are best implanted through a penoscrotal incision.

Distal Penile Approach

A distal penile approach is usually the best approach for insertion of a semirigid or mechanical penile prosthe-

sis. This incision heals well, allows complete corporeal dilation, and facilitates rod placement. After placement of a Foley urethral catheter, a circumcoronal incision is carried out over 180 degrees of the subcoronal region of the penis. Dissection is carried down to the layer of Buck's fascia, taking care to avoid the dorsal penile nerves, which course within Buck's fascia. After the Buck's fascia is identified, stay sutures are applied to the two corpora through the tunica albuginea lateral to the penile nerves. These longitudinal incisions can be extended as much as is necessary for dilation and cylinder insertion. The corporal dilation is begun with Metzenbaum scissors to establish a track in the corporal tissue. Dilation then follows with Hagar, Brooks, or Dilamezinsert dilators to 9 to 11 cm depending upon required cylinder girth (Fig. 70–4). Once the corpora are sized using a Furlow or other dilator, the cylinders can be placed (Figs. 70–5 and 70–6). A small vein retractor can be used to facilitate placement of the distal end of the cylinder. The corporotomy is closed with 2-0 absorbable, synthetic sutures. With noninflatable cylinders, a penile block can be performed and a noncompression dressing is applied.

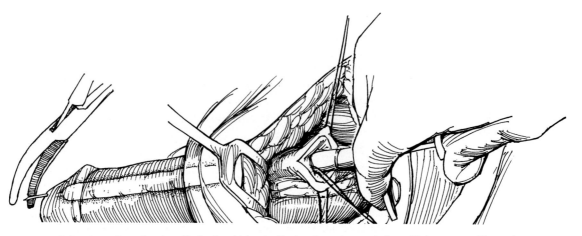

FIG. 70–5. Prosthesis cylinder loaded onto Furlow inserter and placed into corporal tunnel.

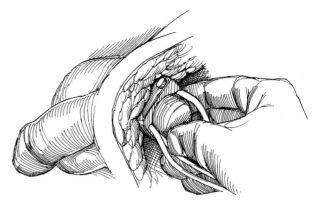

FIG. 70–8. Blunt dissection establishes a location for the pump device.

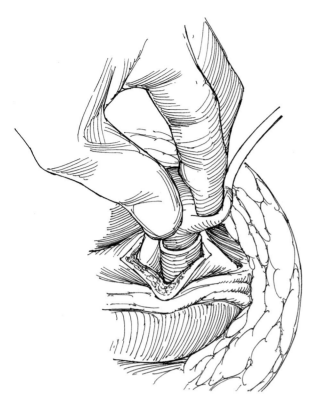

FIG. 70–6. Placement of proximal cylinder base.

Infrapubic Approach

The infrapubic approach allows better visualization of the reservoir placement than the penoscrotal approach. However, because of the proximity of the dorsal neurovascular bundle in the infrapubic approach, injury is possible, resulting in decreased distal penile sensation in some patients. The infrapubic approach is usually carried out with a horizontal incision approximately one finger breadth below the symphysis pubis, allowing implantation with an easily concealed incision once the pubic hair regrows (Fig. 70–7). In patients with significant obesity or a previous midline incision, however, a midline incision carried out just to the base of the penis facilitates

exposure of the corpus cavernosum and improves ability for corpus cavernosum dilation. After incision of the subcutaneous tissue, the dissection is continued to the rectus fascia. The rectus fascia is incised horizontally and dissected cephalad for approximately 2 to 3 cm. A midline separation of the rectus muscles is carried out using sharp and blunt dissection. A pouch is created bluntly beneath the rectus muscles to comfortably insert the inflatable reservoir without compression (Fig. 70–8).

Dissection is then carried out over the corpora cavernosa. Sharp and blunt dissection is begun on either side of the fundiform ligament identifying the dorsal neurovascular bundle. Note that the dorsal nerves of the penis lie approximately 2 to 3 mm lateral to the deep dorsal vain. Once Buck's fascia has been dissected free from the tunica albuginea, the shiny white tunica albuginea is fixed with traction sutures. A corporotomy incision is then carried out between the traction sutures and the corpora cavernosa entered (Fig. 70–9). The corporotomy

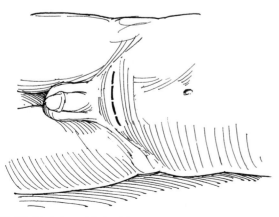

FIG. 70–7. Infrapubic incision for prosthesis implantation.

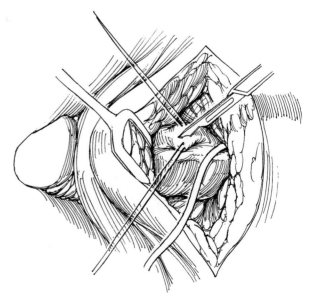

FIG. 70–9. Corporotomy incision between two stay sutures, avoiding the dorsal neurovascular bundles.

incision can be carried out with scalpel or electrocautery. Metzenbaum scissors are then used to carefully initiate the tunneling of the corpora cavernosa, gently spreading the cavernosal tissue both proximally until the ischial tuberosities and crura of the corpora are encountered and distally palpating the glans penis to identify the distal-most aspect of dilation. Hagar dilators from size 9 to 12 or Brooks, Pratt, or Dilamezinsert dilators can be used. If corporeal fibrosis is encountered, Rosillio cavernatomes can be used to dilate to size 12. Once dilation has been adequately carried out bilaterally, the Furlow introducer or Dilamezinsert is used to measure the corpora cavernosal length using a traction suture as a central point of reference. The proximal and distal measurements are added to identify total corporal length and obtain appropriately sized inflatable cylinders. A length slightly less than measurement is usually obtained to permit comfortable positioning of the cylinders. Rear tip extenders of size 0.5, 1, 2, or 3 cm or combinations thereof are placed on the proximal cylinder end to adjust length. Once measurement has been obtained, interrupted sutures can be placed for later corporotomy closure. The advantage to this technique is the elimination of suture needles close to the area of the inflatable cylinder, diminishing the possibility of cylinder damage during corporotomy closure. Other methods of corporotomy closure include running sutures with or without a locking technique. Once the corporotomy sutures are placed, cylinders are positioned in the dilated corpora cavernosa using the inserting tool with distal needle to pull the cylinders into position. Once positioned, it is essential to visualize the cylinder in the corpus cavernosum to ensure that there is no kinking and complete proximal and distal seating has taken place (Fig. 70–10). The corporal incision should be placed proximal enough to allow easy exit of the input tube and minimize cylinder/input tube contact. Closure of the corpora cavernosum is carried out with traction on the cylinder placement suture to maintain it in a flat, nonkinking position and ensure adequate seating. Following placement of cylinders and closure of the corporotomy inci-

sion, cylinder inflation can be tested by placing fluid in each of the cylinders through the input tubes, gently inflating the prosthesis to identify any abnormalities in position, curvature, or other problems.

A finger is then placed in the most dependent portion of the scrotum lateral to the testicle on the right or left side. The finger is then pushed to the area of the external inguinal ring and any adipose tissue in this area is dissected free to expose the Dartos fascia. Dartos' fascia is thoroughly cleaned to allow pump placement. Following development of this subcutaneous pouch for the pump, the pump is positioned in the most dependent portion of the scrotum and temporarily fixed into position using a Babcock clamp. The inflatable reservoir is then placed in the previously constructed subrectus pocket and filled with an appropriate volume of normal saline or water/radiographic contrast media. Before connection, it is important to release pressure on the filling syringe and determine if any backfilling is seen. This backfilling or backpressure may predict autoinflation in the postoperative period. Tubing connection is then carried out using quick connectors or suture tie plastic connectors. The snap-on connectors are used for Mentor prosthesis. In redo prosthesis in which a residual tubing segment is connected to a new device piece, suture tie plastic connectors must be used. The tubing is tailored to eliminate excessive length but to allow for adequate pump positioning is carried out prior to connection. Shodded clamps are used to compress the tubing and the ends of the tubing, once tailored, are flushed with inflation fluid to eliminate small particles and blood clots. After the tubing is connected, the adequacy of the connection is tested by gently pulling on the connectors. All shodded clamps are removed and the device is inflated and deflated on multiple occasions to ensure adequate location, placement, and erection.

Following testing, thorough irrigation with antibiotic solution is carried out and the rectus fascia closed with interrupted sutures. The wound is then closed in the standard fashion with two layers of subcutaneous tissue and a subcuticular skin suture. A dry sterile dressing is applied, a Foley catheter placed if necessary, and an ice pack applied. Suction drains could be used at the surgeon's discretion.

Postoperatively patients are instructed to maintain their penis in a Sutherland position for 4 to 6 weeks. Tight underwear and athletic supporters are not used in an effort to maintain the pump in its most dependent position.

Penoscrotal Approach

Three-piece inflatable penile prostheses as well as semirigid and two-piece prostheses can be implanted by a transverse or vertical penoscrotal incision. This approach has distinct advantages in obese patients and is widely used for routine penile prosthesis implantation. Because

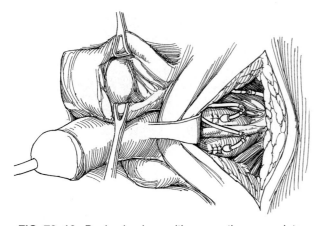

FIG. 70–10. Device in place with connections complete.

the penoscrotal approach requires differentiation from the corpus spongiosum during resection, initial placement of a Foley catheter is necessary for this approach. The incision is placed in the upper portion of the scrotum. The Scott/Lone Star retractor facilitates exposure with this incision. Once the skin incision has been carried out, dissection is continued lateral to the corpus spongiosum and urethra to expose corpora cavernosa. Incision and closure of the corpora cavernosa are similar to that described previously for the infrapubic incision, but synthetic absorbable sutures must be used with this approach because the suture line may be palpable postoperatively (Fig. 70–11). Pump placement is likewise in the most dependent portion of the scrotum just above Dartos fascia with positioning using a Babcock clamp.

Dissection for reservoir placements can be carried out with a second separate infrapubic incision but is more commonly performed through the penoscrotal incision (Fig. 70–12). The scrotal skin incision is retracted to the area of the external inguinal ring and dissection is carried out medial to the spermatic cord. The transversalis fascia is identified and incised sharply using Metzenbaum scissors placed firmly against the pubic tubercle. Dissection is carried out using a combination of sharp and blunt dissection. A reservoir insertion tool can be passed through the inguinal canal to allow reservoir placement. More often, however, dilation is carried out with the index finger after incision of the transversalis fascia and with gen-

tle blunt dissection using a large Kelly clamp. The reservoir balloon is then positioned over the index finger and placed in the perivesical space. Inflation of the reservoir is carried out with care that no backpressure is observed. If refilling of the syringe occurs, the reservoir is removed and reservoir pocket enlargement must be carried out. Once the reservoir is placed, inflated, and tubing connected as previously described, the device is tested in inflation and deflation (Fig. 70–13). Closure is carried out with a subcuticular suture in the standard fashion.

Perioperative antibiotic treatment is critical in diminishing incidence of perioperative infection and prosthetic removal. An initial perioperative dosage of an agent effective against the most common infectious pathogens should be administered 1 to 2 hours prior to surgery and continued for 48 hours postoperatively. Choice of an aminoglycoside with a first-generation cephalosporin, a cephalosporin alone, vancomycin, or a fluoroquinolone is appropriate for prophylaxis of the most common infections from *Staphylococcus epidermidis*. Patients are discharged for 7 days of continued antibiotic therapy. The use of antibiotic-coated penile implants, while reducing the incidence of postoperative infection, does not preclude the need for systemic, perioperative antibiotics. The penile prosthesis remains deflated for 4 weeks while healing occurs. Prior to activation, the patient is advised to retract the pump into his scrotum on a daily basis and tight underwear and athletic supports are avoided to

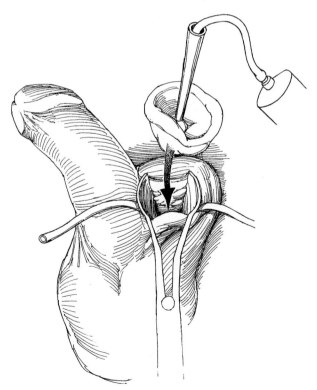

FIG. 70–11. Penoscrotal incision with exposure of corpora cavernosa.

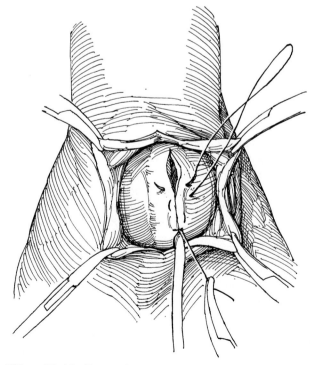

FIG. 70–12. Reservoir placement with penoscrotal approach.

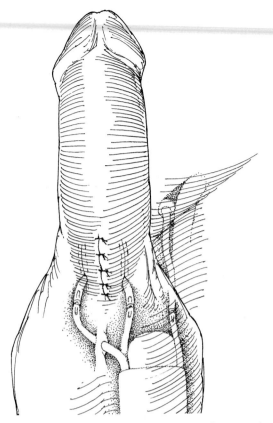

FIG. 70–13. Pump placed for penoscrotal approach.

maintain pump position. A return office visit for activation of the device is carried out once discomfort has resolved. Patients are advised to inflate and deflate the device on a daily basis for 4 weeks to allow tissue expansion around the prosthesis. Most patients can then begin use of their device 4 to 6 weeks after implantation.

OUTCOMES

Complications

Despite careful counseling, many patients enter penile prosthesis procedures with expectations that cannot be met by penile prosthesis surgery. Complaints about decreased penile length compared with preimplant state, decreased penile sensation, "coolness" of the penis and glans penis, and chronic pain, as well as partner dissatisfaction, are among the complaints patients may voice despite adequate surgical implantation and satisfactory mechanical functioning. Fortunately, these complaints are unusual and more than 90% of patients report satisfaction with their prostheses. Many patients who are dissatisfied with their penile prostheses will benefit from sexual counseling or continued counseling assistance from the implanting surgeon to be sure that they are able to operate the device satisfactorily and understand its use.

Most patient's dissatisfaction results from difficulty with operation of the device and unrealistic expectations. Preoperative discussions with patients should include the concept that penile prostheses do not create normal erections but only support the penis for sexual activity. Penile prosthesis surgery brings about the ability to resume sexual functioning and vaginal penetration but decreased penile sensation, length, and engorgement may result. Patients should also be advised that a penile prosthesis will not improve libido or ejaculation. Patients frequently report delayed or difficult ejaculation initially following penile prosthesis surgery. This delay is primarily a result of inadequate preparation, stimulation, and psychological adjustment to the prosthesis. Most patients require 3 to 6 months of prosthesis use with careful attention to presexual stimulation before ejaculation routinely returns to preoperative levels. Because the prosthesis neither improves nor detracts from preoperative ejaculatory ability, patients must be counseled regarding their preoperative ejaculatory ability before prosthesis placement.

The most worrisome postoperative complication is infection, which occurs in fewer than 10% of all patients. Perioperative prosthetic infections can, however, occur at any time in the postoperative period in patients with penile or other prosthetic devices. Patients continue to be at risk for hematogenously seeded infections from gastrointestinal, dental, or urologic manipulations as well as remote infections. Patients must be counseled to request antibiotic coverage if remote infections occur. Most periprosthetic infections are caused by Gram-positive organisms such as *S. epidermidis*, but fungi or Gram-negative organisms such as *Escherichia coli* and *Pseudomonas* are also common culprits. Severe gangrenous infections with a combination of Gram-negative and anaerobic organisms have also been identified and frequently result in significant disability and tissue loss. Patients at increased risk for perioperative infections include diabetics, patients undergoing penile straightening procedures or circumcision with prosthetic implantation, patients with urinary tract bacterial colonization, and immunocompromised patients, such as posttransplant patients. Spinal cord injury patients have also been reported to have a specially increased risk of infections, with rates reported as high as 15%.

Appropriate treatment of periprosthetic infections requires early and immediate identification with institution of parenteral antibiotic therapy and early prosthesis removal (2). Conservative treatment would dictate a healing period of 3 to 6 months followed by repeat prosthesis implantation. Satisfactory results with prosthesis removal, a 5 to 7 day course of antibiotic irrigation, followed by additional replacement has been reported for selected patients. Better long-term results with no additional morbidity can be achieved with the prosthesis salvage technique reported by Mulcahy. This technique—which requires removal of the infected implant and vigorous irrigation using solutions of antibiotics, provadone iodine, hydrogen peroxide, and a repeat of these solutions—is successful in more than 75% of infected prostheses (2).

The most common complication of penile prosthesis function is mechanical malfunction. Mechanical malfunction has declined from rates as high as 61% to levels below 5% since the 1970s (3,7). Aneurismal dilation of inflatable cylinders, both American Medical Systems and Mentor, tubing kinking, reservoir leakage, and pump malfunction have been limited by device modifications. Fluid leak, however, continues to be a problem for many inflatable penile prostheses. These mechanical malfunctions require replacement of the leaking portion of the inflatable portion of the prosthesis. If a nonfunctioning prosthesis has been in place more than 4 years, however, it is usual practice to replace the entire device to reduce further mechanical malfunction (1).

Semirigid rod penile prostheses are associated with fewer mechanical problems; the most common complication associated with these prostheses is cylinder erosion through skin or urethra. Prosthesis fracture or breakage has been reported and patients may return 6 to 8 years postimplantation with complaints of decreased rigidity of their semirigid rod, indicating fracture of central prosthetic cylinder wires. These wire fractures cannot usually be appreciated radiographically unless the prosthesis is put on stretch once it has been explanted. Replacement of these devices is indicated when patients note decreased rigidity. Prosthesis extrusion or erosion is most common in diabetics and spinal cord injury patients, especially those requiring urinary management with catheter placement or of condom catheter collection devices.

Extrusion can also occur beneath the penile skin distally from vigorous dilation or remotely from trauma or repeated use. These extrusions are characterized by distal penile pain with use. Correction can be carried out with the use of a patch graft, but a better approach is rerouting with no grafting material. Rerouting is associated with less infection and pain and a reduced recurrence rate.

Results

Long term function and use have been confirmed in studies of patients with implants as long as 10 years (3). While partner satisfaction notes are few, patients have a greater than 90% satisfaction and those with functioning devices for more than 5 years used them 27 times monthly (3). Other studies have confirmed that patient satisfaction is greater than any other ED treatment modality (1).

REFERENCES

1. Carson CC. Reconstructive surgery using urological prostheses. *Curr Opin Urol* 1999;9:233–239.
2. Carson CC. Penile prosthesis implantation and infection for Sexual Medicine Society of North America. *Int J Impotence Res* 2001;13(Suppl 5):S35–S38.
3. Carson CC, Mulcahy JJ, Govier FE. Efficacy, safety and patient satisfaction outcomes of the AMS 700CX inflatable penile prosthesis: results of a long-term multicenter study. AMS 700CX Study Group. *J Urol* 2000;164:376–380.
4. Mulcahy JJ. Long-term experience with salvage of infected penile implants. *J Urol* 2000;163:481–482.
5. Scott FB, Bradley WE, Timm GW. Management of erectile impotence. Use of implantable inflatable prosthesis. *Urology* 1973;2:80–82.
6. Small MP, Carrion HM, Gordon JA. Small-Carrion penile prosthesis. New implant for management of impotence. *Urology* 1975;5:479–486.
7. Wilson SK, Cleves MA, Delk JR, Jr.. Comparison of mechanical reliability of original and enhanced Mentor Alpha I penile prosthesis. *J Urol* 1999;162(3, Pt 1):715–718.

CHAPTER 71

Penile Venous Surgery

Mark R. Licht and Ronald W. Lewis

Although the exact incidence of vasculogenic impotence is not known, arterial insufficiency and/or venous leakage of varying etiology probably account for the majority of cases. Sustaining a rigid erection depends on both adequate perfusion pressure of the erectile bodies via arterial inflow and maintenance of intracavernosal pressure by increased venous outflow resistance. The trapping of blood within the expanding corporal bodies during erection by direct compression of subtunical venules as they exit through the tunica albuginea is known as the corporal venoocclusion mechanism. Venous leak impotence refers to the inability of an individual to maintain a rigid erection because of abnormal venous outflow from the corpora cavernosa secondary to failure of the corporal venoocclusive mechanism. In this chapter, we discuss the diagnosis of venogenic impotence and detail the surgical correction of this form of erectile dysfunction by penile venous dissection and ligation.

DIAGNOSIS

A history and a physical examination help identify patients who may have venous leak impotence. Patients present with either complete loss of erection, decreased penile rigidity, or rapid loss of erection during intercourse. Medication effect, significant cardiovascular disease, psychological disorders, and tobacco use should be excluded as contributing causes of impotence. Penile trauma, surgery for priapism, Peyronie's disease, and previous endoscopic incision of urethral strictures can all lead to focal defects in the corporal venoocclusive mechanism (7).

The first diagnostic test that we employ in the diagnosis of venogenic impotence is penile duplex Doppler ultrasonography. This test allows for the evaluation of both penile arterial inflow and venoocclusion as well as the erectile response to the intracavernosal injection of a vasodilating agent. Patients with measured end-diastolic

velocities over 3 cm per second for up to 15 to 20 minutes after the administration of the vasodilating agent despite normal arterial inflow, measured as peak systolic velocities greater than 30 cm per second, may have venogenic impotence (3). Patients who obtain a full rigid erection within 10 minutes of injection that lasts for 30 minutes probably have no clinically significant vascular disease. Patients who achieve tumescence only or who rapidly obtain a rigid erection that dissipates within 15 to 20 minutes are suspected of having a venous leak.

Infusion pharmacocavernosometry and cavernosography are the definitive tests for diagnosing venous leak impotence and visualizing the sites of leakage. Knowledge of the anatomy of the venous drainage of the penis is critical in interpreting this study (Fig. 71–1). The technique we employ has been described in detail elsewhere (6). After injection of a vasodilating agent, the need for a flow rate of less than 150 mL per minute of saline to maintain a rigid erection at an intracorporeal pressure of at least 90 mm Hg is indicative of corporal venoocclusive dysfunction. A maintenance flow rate between 30 and 50 mL per minute is considered borderline for venous leakage. Others have used lower flows to maintain as diagnostic cutoffs (6). Contrast material is infused into the corpora at the defined maintenance flow rate, and then AP and oblique radiographs of the penis are taken. The most common sites of venous leakage seen in patients with venoocclusive dysfunction are the deep dorsal vein, the cavernosal veins, and the circumflex veins at the base of the penis. A large amount of drainage into all of these systems is a contraindication to surgery because these patients do not do well.

INDICATIONS FOR SURGERY

Patients must meet strict criteria to be selected for venous surgery. Candidates must first have a history that is consistent with venous leak impotence, corroborated

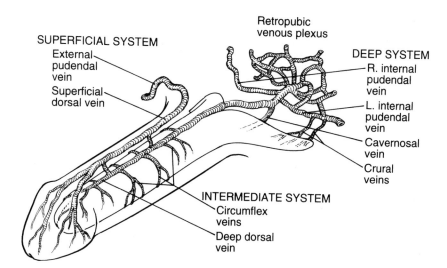

SUPERFICIAL SYSTEM
External pudendal vein
Superficial dorsal vein

Retropubic venous plexus

DEEP SYSTEM
R. internal pudendal vein
L. internal pudendal vein
Cavernosal vein
Crural veins

INTERMEDIATE SYSTEM
Circumflex veins
Deep dorsal vein

FIG. 71–1. Penile venous anatomy.

by duplex Doppler sonography and intracavernosal test injection findings. Other causes of impotence should be ruled out. Normal penile arterial inflow must also be documented in response to an intracavernosal injection agent because patients with concomitant arterial disease often have a poor outcome after venous surgery. Cavernosometry and cavernosography must confirm venoocclusive dysfunction and outline the sites of leakage. Patients should have no medical contraindications to surgery. There is no strict age limit, but we prefer to perform venous surgery on patients less than 65 years old.

Patients need to eliminate all tobacco use at least 6 months before surgery. Finally, patients must select venous surgery after presentation of alternative forms of therapy and discussion of expected success rates. We also perform venous surgery in conjunction with penile arterial revascularization in select patients with both focal arterial disease and venoocclusive dysfunction (8).

ALTERNATIVE THERAPY

Patients with venous leak impotence have some effective surgical and nonsurgical options to consider along with penile venous dissection and ligation. Patients with mild to moderate venoocclusive disorders will respond to oral sildenafil therapy for erectile dysfunction. Vacuum erection devices create an adequate erection by drawing blood into the penis with negative pressure in the vacuum tube. A constriction band placed at the base of the penis prevents outflow of blood and substitutes for a faulty venoocclusive mechanism. Self-injection of intracavernosal vasodilating agents at high doses can often produce a functional erection in patients with mild to moderate venous leak. Patients with severe leakage, however, will most often not respond to injection therapy. Combining self-injection with a constriction band is also helpful in maintaining an erection in some patients. Implantation of

a penile prosthesis effectively replaces the natural venoocclusive mechanism with a mechanical device capable of producing a sufficiently rigid erection. A goal-directed approach is used to help the patient select an appropriate form of therapy.

SURGICAL TECHNIQUE

Patients receive a dose of an intravenous cephalosporin 1 hour before surgery. Surgery is performed under either general intubated or spinal anesthesia. The patient is positioned supine with the legs abducted to allow easy access to the perineum. If crural ligation and banding are planned as part of the operative procedure, then a dorsal lithotomy position is preferred. A lighted suction device can facilitate illumination of the deep infrapubic dissection. An intraoperative Doppler probe can be helpful in localizing small arteries in this region. We do not routinely use optical magnification for the dissection. The operative field is prepped and draped in a sterile fashion from the umbilicus to the perineum, and an 18 Fr Foley catheter is placed for the purpose of bladder drainage and improved urethral identification.

An infrapubic curvilinear anterior peripenile scrotal incision is made with a no. 15 blade (Fig. 71–2). The superior extent of the incision is the inferior border of the pubis and the inferior extent is the median raphe of the scrotum below the penile shaft. Superficial tissue is dissected free of the corporal bodies with sharp and blunt dissection. Communicating veins joining the deep and superficial drainage systems are isolated, ligated with 3-0 plain gut sutures, and divided. The penile skin is then stripped away from the shaft and the penis is inverted into the wound to gain exposure to the superficial and deep venous systems (Fig. 71–3). Any other venous trunks of the superficial system that receive tributaries from the corpora are ligated with absorbable suture material and divided at this time (Fig. 71–4).

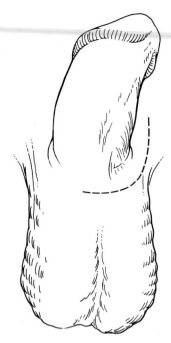

FIG. 71–2. Peripenile scrotal incision for penile venous surgery.

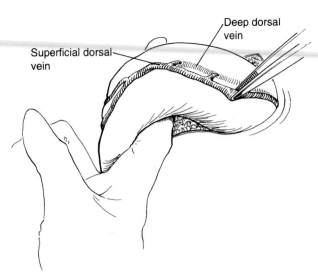

FIG. 71–4. Ligation of superficial veins with connections to the corpora.

A 19-gauge butterfly needle is placed into the base of the corpus cavernosum and fixed in place to the tunica albuginea with a 3-0 chromic suture (Fig. 71–5). The cavernosal tissue receives an injection of 30 mg of papaverine, followed 10 minutes later by indigo–carmine colored saline (12 mL in 250 mL of saline) to help visualize abnormally effluxing veins. The butterfly needle tubing is clamped for the duration of the procedure and is used again after the dissection to perform intraoperative cavernosometry. A 3/8-in. Penrose drain is looped around the

penile shaft between the corpora. The penile skin near the glans is clamped to the Mayo stand to retract the penile skin, elongate and stabilize the penile shaft, and afford exposure for the proximal dissection.

The superficial fundiform ligament is identified at the base of the penis and divided to expose the suspensory ligament. The suspensory ligament is then sharply divided close to the underside of the pubic symphysis (Fig. 71–6). The suspensory ligament must be completely taken down to expose the deep infrapubic region. Care is taken to identify and divide small veins emanating from the underside of the pubis and joining the superficial drainage system as well as veins perforating Buck's fascia to connect the deep and superficial systems at this level. Failure to ligate these vessels can lead to significant bleeding, which can be difficult to control and obscure exposure for the proximal portion of the venous dissection.

Deep in the infrapubic region, Buck's fascia is opened in the midline over the deep dorsal vein. The vein usually

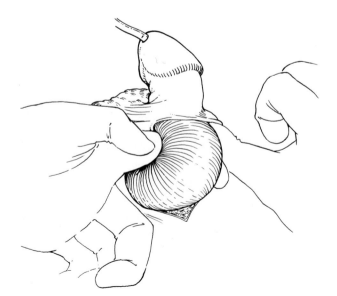

FIG. 71–3. Inversion of the penile shaft into the wound.

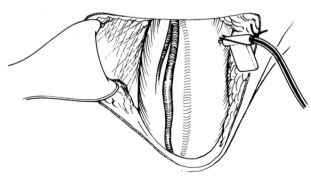

FIG. 71–5. Placement of a butterfly needle for intraoperative cavernosometry.

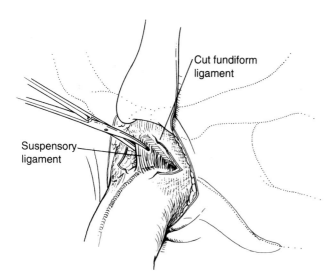

FIG. 71–6. The suspensory ligament is divided to expose the base of the penis.

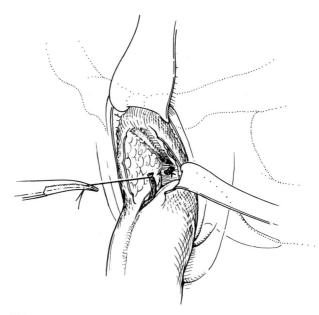

FIG. 71–7. Division of the deep dorsal vein in the infrapubic region.

has a single large main trunk at this level. The deep dorsal vein is dissected free of the tunica albuginea, ligated with 0 silk ties, and divided (Fig. 71–7). Inferior to the deep dorsal vein, the cavernosal veins can be identified in the penile hilum at this time. They may be divided if they are a major source of leakage. Great care is taken to preserve the cavernosal arteries and nerve trunks that lie lateral to these veins.

If the deep dorsal vein is a significant source of abnormal penile drainage, then it is dissected from the infrapubic region along the penile dorsal midline under Buck's fascia distally toward the glans. It is important to stay in the midline during the dissection to avoid the laterally

located dorsal arteries and nerves. Circumflex and emissary veins encountered on either side of the deep dorsal vein are ligated with 3-0 plain gut sutures and divided (Fig. 71–8). Bipolar electrocoagulation on a low setting can be used to cauterize some small vessels along the shaft.

Sometimes the deep dorsal vein is composed of two trunks along the penile shaft, and each must be dissected separately. Dissection continues until several fanning tributaries constitute the deep dorsal vein approximately 1 cm from the glans. Rarely, a large vein arises from the

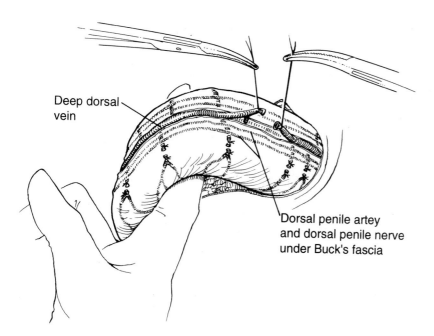

Deep dorsal vein

Dorsal penile artey and dorsal penile nerve under Buck's fascia

FIG. 71–8. Division of circumflex and emissary veins on both sides of the deep dorsal vein.

tunica albuginea and penetrates Buck's fascia to join the deep dorsal vein. Ligation of this vein creates a sinusoidal defect in the tunica, which must be closed with a 3-0 chromic figure-of-eight suture ligature. The junction between the corpora cavernosa and the spongiosum is carefully inspected as well, and circumflex veins connecting the two structures are ligated and divided.

After vein dissection and ligation are completed, 30 mg of papaverine is injected into the corpora via the butterfly needle and cavernosometry is performed 10 minutes later. If the abnormal draining veins have been eliminated, then a rigid erection is easily maintained at a flow of saline considerably less than 5 mL per minute (Fig. 71–9). Following this, the suspensory ligament is reapproximated with a 0 silk suture ligature between the infrapubic periosteum and the penile shaft. A no. 10 Jackson–Pratt fenestrated bulb suction drain is then placed in the wound with the tubing exiting via a separate stab incision lateral to the surgical incision. The subcuticular tissue is closed with a running 3-0 chromic suture, with care taken to approximate equal tissue planes to minimize the chance of scar formation resulting in fixation of the base of the penis. The skin edges are then reapproximated with a running subcuticular 3-0 Monocryl suture. The wound is covered with a standard sterile dressing and the penis is snugly wrapped with a self-adherent Coban wrap. Care is taken to avoid glanular edema from a dressing that is too tight. The Foley catheter and the dressing are removed the day after surgery. The drain is removed as soon as drainage is negligible, usually in 24 to 48 hours. Patients are discharged from the hospital on postoperative day 2 or 3. They are advised against engaging in intercourse for 6 weeks.

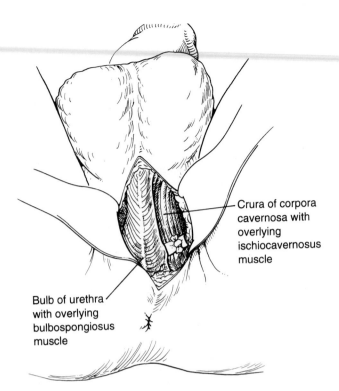

FIG. 71–10. Crural banding to correct venous leakage from crural veins.

Labels: Crura of corpora cavernosa with overlying ischiocavernosus muscle; Bulb of urethra with overlying bulbospongiosus muscle

Crural Banding and Other Procedures

If the crural veins are found to be the only source of major venous leakage by cavernosography, we perform a crural banding procedure. The crura are exposed near the bulb of the urethra via a perineal incision, and a 1/4-in. Mersilene ribbon (Ethicon, Inc.) is used to band the crura (Fig. 71–10). Veins draining from the edge of the crura are ligated as well. Crural banding is not routinely performed at the time of deep dorsal vein ligation and is usually a secondary procedure. Another secondary procedure that is rarely employed is spongiolysis. Via a penile scrotal incision, the corpus spongiosum is exposed and stripped away from the ventral surface of the corpora cavernosa. All communications between the two structures are ligated or coagulated.

OUTCOMES

Complications

Table 71–1 lists the complications that have been encountered after penile venous surgery (9). Complications can be divided into immediate and long-term. Most patients experience some superficial bruising of the shaft and scrotum. Penile edema is usually moderate and resolves within 2 to 3 weeks. The incidence of penile edema has decreased since our use of a compression dressing and a closed wound drainage system. Painful

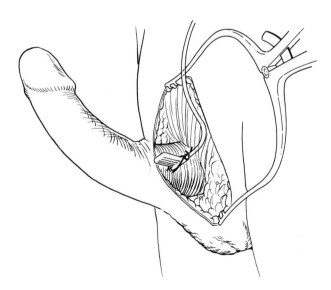

FIG. 71–9. Cavernosometry after completion of the dissection confirms correction of the venous leak.

TABLE 71–1. *Complications of penile venous surgery*

Immediate
    Common
        Penile and Scrotal Bruising
        Penile Edema
        Painful Nocturnal Erections
    Rare
        Wound Infection
        Hematoma
Long-Term
    Common
        Penile Shortening
        Decreased Penile Sensation
        Decreased Ability for Orgasm
    Rare
        Wound Scar Contractures/Penile Tethering

nocturnal erections often occur for the first 24 to 48 hours after surgery. Infrequently, they may last for longer than 1 week. Wound infection and true hematoma rarely occur. Care taken during the infrapubic portion of the dissection can eliminate the risk of postoperative hematoma.

Despite careful reapproximation of the suspensory ligament after the vein dissection is complete, approximately 20% of patients complain of penile shortening. The amount of perceived loss of length, however, is rarely clinically or functionally significant. Hypoesthesia or numbness of the glans or shaft of the penis is a common occurrence after surgery. Patients who report a loss of sensation often experience a diminished ability to achieve orgasm as well. In most cases, though, penile sensation returns completely within 7 to 9 months. Infrequently, wound scar contractures occur that lead to true penile tethering. In these cases, revision surgery is necessary, consisting of release of scar tissue and skin Z-plasty.

Results

Although individual reports of successful vein ligation procedures date back to the early 1900s, the modern era of penile venous surgery did not begin until the development of accurate and appropriate diagnostic and surgical techniques. A number of surgeons have since reported on the initial and long-term success rates for this procedure. Donatucci and Lue reported on 100 patients operated on between 1986 and 1988 (2). Forty-four patients (44%) had an excellent result, defined as a complete return of spontaneous erections rigid enough for penetration, and 24 patients (24%) noted some improvement in rigidity. All patients were followed for longer than 1 year after surgery.

Knoll et al. reported a 46% excellent response to surgery in 41 patients followed for an average of 28 months (4). Claes and Baert similarly reported a return of normal erectile function in 30 of 72 patients (42%) and a partial response in 23 others (32%) (1). Patients were all followed for more than 1 year.

Lewis recently reported on 60 patients, of whom 16 (27%) initially had return of normal erections (8). Seventeen other patients (28%) experienced improved rigidity and were able to have intercourse with the aid of intracavernosal pharmacological injections for a combined success rate of 55%. All patients were followed for at least 2 years. Over time, 13 of the 33 patients (39%) who initially experienced a successful result later reported failure of the procedure. Kropman et al. also reported a 40% late failure rate at a mean follow-up of 28 months in 10 of 20 patients who initially experienced a successful result from surgery (5).

The best long-term results were recently reported by Sasso et al. (10). Seventeen of 23 patients (74%) had normal erections within 1 year of venous ligation surgery and 12 of 17 maintained normal spontaneous erectile function long-term. The authors describe strict operative selection criteria, including the need to determine a crucial percent of smooth muscle in the corporeal tissue found on preoperative biopsy.

Several different factors can account for the approximately 40% failure rate of penile venous surgery. Inability to accurately diagnose concomitant arterial disease and less extensive venous dissection probably account for many of the early patient failures in the series reported above. With the use of stricter diagnostic inclusion criteria and a more aggressive surgical approach, many of these early failures could have been avoided.

Collateralization has limited the long-term success rates of other types of venous surgery as well. A final reason for failure is that the ligation of penile veins may not address the true underlying pathologic disorder in many patients. Sinus smooth muscle disease that prohibits the expansion of the tunica albuginea and the subsequent compression of subtunical venules have been postulated as a major cause of venoocclusive dysfunction (11). To date, though, no practical test is available to accurately diagnose this entity. Penile venous surgery remains a reasonable surgical option for highly selected patients with venous leak impotence.

REFERENCES

1. Claes H, Baert L. Cavernosometry and penile vein resection in corporeal incompetence: An evaluation of short-term and long-term results. *Int J Impotence Res* 1991;3:129.
2. Donatucci CF, Lue TF. Venous surgery: Are we kidding ourselves? In: Lue TF, ed. *World book of impotence*. London: Smith-Gorthdon and Co, 1992:221–227.
3. King BF, Lewis RW, McKusick MA. Radiologic evaluation of impotence. In: Bennett AH, ed. *Impotence. Diagnosis and management of erectile dysfunction*. Philadelphia: WB Saunders, 1994:52–91.
4. Knoll LD, Furlow WL, Benson RC. Penile venous ligation surgery for the management of cavernosal venous leakage. *Urol Int* 1992;49:33.
5. Kropman RF, Nijeholt AABL, Giespers AGM, Swarten J. Results of deep penile vein resection in impotence caused by venous leakage. *Int J Impotence Res* 1990;2:29.
6. Lewis RW. Diagnosis and management of corporal veno-occlusive dysfunction. *Sem Urol* 1990;8:113.

7. Lewis RW. Venogenic impotence. Diagnosis, management, and results. *Probl Urol* 1991;5:567.

8. Lewis RW. Venous surgery in the patient with erectile dysfunction. *Atlas Urol Clin North Am* 1993;1:21.

9. Petrou S, Lewis RW. Management of corporal veno-occlusive dysfunction. *Urol Int* 1992;49:48.

10. Sasso F, Gulino G, Weir J, Viggiano AM, Alcini E. Patient section criteria in the surgical treatment of veno-occlusive dysfunction. *J Urol* 1999;161:1145.

11. Wespes E, Moreira De Goes P, Sattar AA, Schulman C. Objective criteria in the long-term evaluation of penile venous surgery. *J Urol* 1994; 152:888.

CHAPTER 72

Penile Arterial Reconstruction

Ricardo Munarriz, John Mulhall, and Irwin Goldstein

Erectile dysfunction is defined as the consistent inability to obtain or maintain a penile erection satisfactory for sexual relations. Community epidemiological studies have revealed that 52% of men age 40 to 70 years have self-reported (17%), moderate (25%), and complete (10%) forms of impotence. While there are a large variety of surgical and nonsurgical options available for these patients, penile revascularization is currently the only modality of therapy that has the potential to permanently cure patients, i.e., allow return of spontaneously developing erections without the necessity for any internal or external devices.

The overall goal of penile revascularization surgery is to bypass obstructive arterial lesions in the hypogastric–cavernous arterial bed. The specific objective of the surgery is to increase the cavernosal arterial perfusion pressure and blood inflow in patients with vasculogenic erectile dysfunction secondary to pure arterial insufficiency. Young men, without other vascular risk factors, who have erectile dysfunction of a pure arteriogenic nature represent the ideal patient population for this procedure.

DIAGNOSIS

The diagnostic algorithm is aimed at ensuring that this operation is performed on the ideal candidate, i.e., one in whom there is erectile dysfunction purely on the basis of arterial insufficiency. All young patients with a history suggestive of trauma-associated impotence (pelvic fractures and perineal trauma) undergo a comprehensive history and physical examination. They have a routine endocrinologic evaluation to ensure adequate circulating levels of testosterone. These patients undergo a nocturnal penile tumescence test in an attempt to rule out neurogenic and psychogenic erectile dysfunction. Duplex Doppler ultrasonography provides diagnostic hemodynamic data (cavernosal peak systolic and end-diastolic

velocities) and preoperative information such as: (a) presence of communicating branches from the dorsal to the cavernosal artery (Fig 72–1A), (b) direction of flow through septal communicators (Fig 72–1B), and (c) dorsal artery diameters and peak systolic velocities (Figs. 72–1C and 72–1D), which are critical in the selection of the best recipient dorsal artery. Finally, vascular assessment by dynamic infusion cavernosometry/cavernosography (DICC) is required to demonstrate arterial pressure gradients between the brachial artery and the cavernosal arteries and to further evaluate the venoocclusive function. The criteria for the definition of pure arteriogenic erectile dysfunction are beyond the scope of this chapter and have been outlined elsewhere (2). The purpose of the testing is to rule out corporovenous occlusive dysfunction. Following hemodynamic diagnosis, if the patient has pure arterial insufficiency a selective internal pudendal arteriogram is performed to confirm the location of the obstructive lesion, which is in general in the common penile or cavernosal artery(ies), and select the best inferior epigastric artery. Only following this complete evaluation do we perform a penile revascularization procedure.

INDICATIONS FOR SURGERY

The success of this operation is based on the selection of the correct candidate and the microsurgical capabilities of the surgeon. To this end, we have developed a list of criteria that the patient and surgeon must meet to ensure optimum results. The criteria are as follows:

1. The patient's history is characterized by (a) strong libido, (b) a consistent reduction in erectile rigidity during sexual activity, (c) increased erection rigidity during morning erections, (d) variable sustaining capability with the best maintenance of the rigidity during early morning erections, and (e)

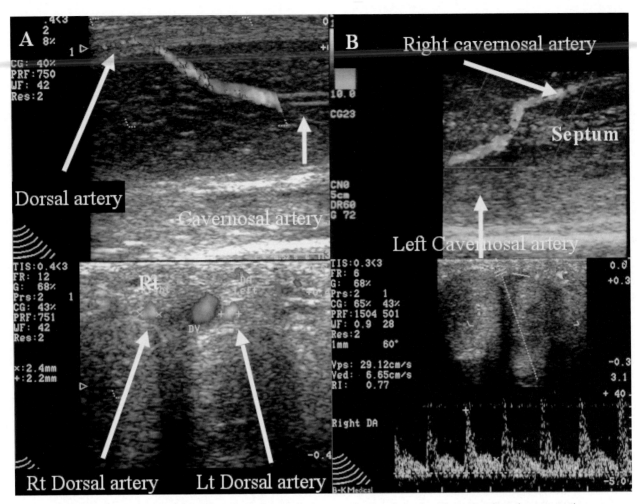

FIG. 72–1. Penile duplex Doppler ultrasound. **A:** Communicating branches from the dorsal artery to the cavernosal artery. **B:** Septal perforator from the right cavernosal artery to the left cavernosal artery. **C:** Dorsal artery diameters. **D:** Dorsal artery peak systolic velocities.

poor spontaneity of erections, taking much effort and excessive time to achieve the poorly rigid erectile response.

2. Normal hormonal and neurological evaluation.

3. Increased arterial gradients during cavernosal artery occlusion pressure determination at the time of DICC (Fig. 72–2A), indicative of arterial insufficiency.

4. Normal venoocclusive parameters (flow-to-maintain values, pressure decay values) during DICC (Fig. 72–2B).

5. The presence of an occlusive lesion in one or both hypogastric–cavernous arterial beds (Figs. 72–3A and 72–3B) located in the common penile artery or cavernosal artery that is amenable to distal bypass.

6. The presence of an inferior epigastric artery of sufficient length to allow anastomosis to the dorsal artery (Fig. 72–3C) without common trunks with the obturator arteries, which theoretically may diminish inferior epigastric arterial perfusion pressures (steal syndrome; Fig. 72–3D).

7. The presence of a communication branch(es) between the dorsal artery and the cavernosal artery distal to the occlusion that will allow the inflow of new blood flow and the development of increased intracorporal pressure.

8. Avoidance of any penile trauma, such as may occur during masturbation or a sexual encounter, for a period of 6 weeks postoperatively to avoid disruption of the anastomosis.

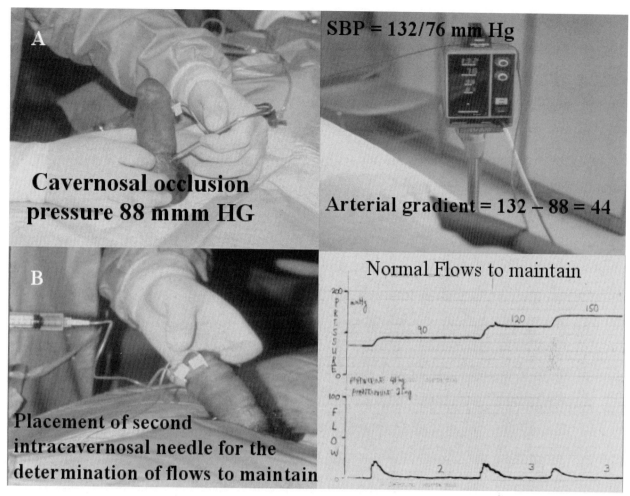

FIG. 72–2. Dynamic infusion cavernosometry and cavernosography. **A:** Arterial gradients between the brachial and the cavernosal arteries. **B:** Normal flows-to-maintain

ALTERNATIVE THERAPY

Nonsurgical treatment options for impotence include psychotherapeutic, hormonal, pharmacological, and external device interventions (4). Surgical treatment options consist primarily of penile prosthesis insertion (1).

SURGICAL TECHNIQUE

The patient is placed supine on the operating table and his arms secured next to his body to minimize upper-extremity nerve injuries. As this operation may last in excess of 5 hours, great care must be taken in the positioning and padding of the limbs, in particular the neurovascular points on the upper limbs. With the arms secured next to the patient's body and by alternating the position of the blood pressure cuff periodically throughout the procedure, we have not had any transient nerve palsies. General endotracheal anesthesia with complete muscle relaxation facilitates harvesting the donor vessel. The patient's abdomen and genitalia are carefully shaved, prepped, and draped, following which a 16 Fr Foley catheter is placed using sterile technique. The patient is given one dose of preoperative antibiotics (cefazolin or vancomycin if penicillin allergic).

From a technical standpoint, the operation can be divided into three stages: dorsal artery dissection, inferior epigastric artery harvesting, and microsurgical anastomosis (5,6).

Dorsal Artery Dissection

A curvilinear incision is made, in general on the side opposite to the planned abdominal incision for inferior epigastric artery harvesting (Fig. 72–4A). The incision is made 2 finger breadths from the base of the penis, from a point opposite the ventral root of the penis, to the scrotal median raphe. This incision is carried down through

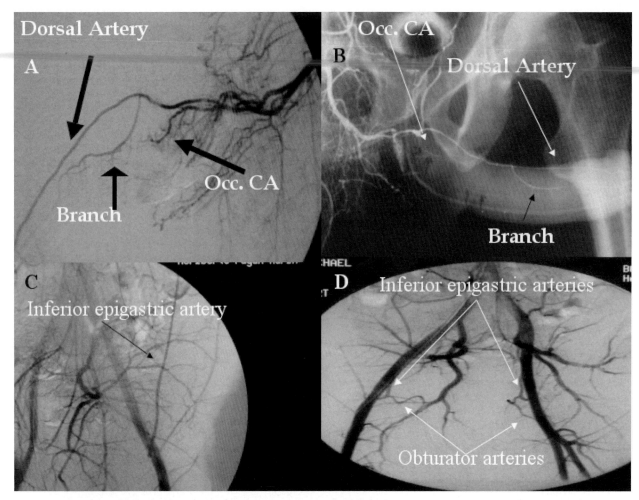

FIG. 72–3. Selective internal pudendal arteriogram. **A and B:** Obstruction of the cavernosal artery. **C:** Inferior epigastric artery with good length and no branches. **D:** Inferior epigastric arteries with bilateral common trunks with the obturator arteries.

the dartos layer using cautery. The advantages of this incision are that it offers (a) excellent proximal and distal exposure of the penile neurovascular bundle, (b) the ability to preserve the fundiform and suspensory ligaments preventing penile shortening, and (c) the absence of unsightly postoperative scars on the penile shaft or at the base of the penis. Use of a ring retractor with its elastic hooks maximizes operative exposure of the penis with a minimum of assistance.

The ipsilateral tunica albuginea is subsequently identified at the midpenile shaft. With the penis stretched, blunt finger dissection along the tunica albuginea is performed in a distal direction deep and inferior to the spermatic cord structures along the lateral aspect of the penile shaft, avoiding injury to the fundiform ligament. The penis is then inverted through the skin incision, with care taken to push the glans in fully (Fig. 72–4B). The penis must not be tumesced during this maneuver. If a partial erection is

present, intracavernosal α-adrenergic agonist (100 μg phenylephrine) should be administered. Blunt finger dissection around the distal penile shaft enables a plane to be established between Buck's fascia and Colles' fascia, and a Penrose drain is secured in this plane.

Exposure of the neurovascular bundle and, in particular, the right and left dorsal penile arteries is now performed. The arteries are usually obvious, located on either side of the deep dorsal vein and surrounded by the dorsal nerves. Isolation of the dorsal penile arteries for such arterial bypass surgery requires limited dissection at this time in the procedure; thus, ischemic, mechanical, and thermal trauma to the dorsal penile arteries may be minimized. To avoid injurious vasospasm, topical papaverine hydrochloride irrigation is applied frequently. In this way, preservation of endothelial and smooth muscle cell morphology during dorsal artery preparation is ensured. This is very critical as the room temperature of

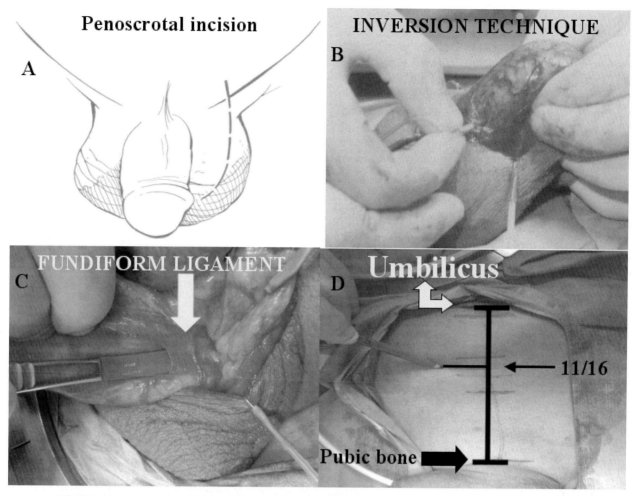

FIG. 72–4. Surgical technique. **A:** Inguinoscrotal incision. **B:** Penile inversion. **C:** Fenestration of the fundiform ligament. **D:** Abdominal incision for harvesting the epigastric artery.

the operating room, the use of room temperature irrigating solution, and even the skin incision can induce vasoconstriction, spasm, and possible endothelial cell damage. For intraluminal irrigation, we utilize a dilute papaverine, heparin, and electrolytic solution believed to be capable of inhibiting the early development of myointimal proliferative lesions during surgical preparation.

The right and left dorsal penile arteries are identified first in the midpenile shaft. Their course is followed proximally underneath the fundiform ligament, with care being taken to leave the fundiform ligament intact. A fenestration is fashioned in the fundiform ligament proximally, usually near the junction of the fundiform and suspensory ligaments at a location where the pendulous penile shaft becomes fixed proximally (Fig. 72–4C). Blunt dissection is performed under the proximal aspect of the fundiform ligament above the pubic bone toward the external ring. This dissection enables the inferior epi-

gastric artery to pass from its abdominal location to the appropriate location in the penis while simultaneously preserving the fundiform ligament. The penis is placed back on its normal anatomic position and the inguinoscrotal incision is temperately closed with staples.

Harvesting of the Inferior Epigastric Artery

A transverse semilunar abdominal incision following Langer's lines is the preferred incision, although a paramedian incision can be used especially if the desired inferior epigastric artery is short, has several branches, or the patient habitus precludes a standard transverse incision (Fig. 72–4D). The transverse incision provides excellent operative exposure of the inferior epigastric artery and heals with a more cosmetic scar compared to those observed with paramedian skin incisions. The starting point of the transverse incision is approximately 11/16 of the total distance from the pubic bone to the umbilicus in the midline. It extends laterally along the skin lines for approximately 5 cm. The rectus fascia is incised vertically. The junction between the rectus muscle and underlying preperitoneal fat is identified and the preperitoneal space is entered. The rectus muscle is reflected medially.

The inferior epigastric artery and its two accompanying veins are located beneath the rectus muscle in the preperitoneal plane. The ring retractor is again utilized to optimize operative exposure. It is critical to harvest an inferior epigastric artery of sufficient length to prevent tension on the microvascular anastomosis. Application of topical papaverine is utilized on the inferior epigastric artery throughout the dissection. Thermal injury is avoided using low-current microbipolar cautery set at the minimum level necessary for adequate coagulation and the vasa vasora are preserved by dissecting the artery *en bloc* with its surrounding veins and fat. Dissection of the

inferior epigastric is required from its origin at the level of the external iliac artery to a point at the level of the umbilicus (Figs. 72–5A and 72–5B). It is at this point that the artery bifurcates. In the past, we made every effort to use the bifurcation where possible to allow anastomoses to both dorsal arteries, but we have not seen a significant improvement in erectile function in patients who underwent anastomosis of the inferior epigastric artery to both dorsal arteries when compared to patients who had a single anastomosis. Thus, we are currently performing a single anastomosis, minimizing surgical time and preserving a dorsal artery in case a second penile revascularization is desired.

The transfer route of the neoarterial inflow source is prepared from the abdominal perspective prior to transecting the vessel distally (the penile transfer route has previously been dissected; Fig. 72–5C). The temporary scrotal staples are removed and the penis is reinverted.

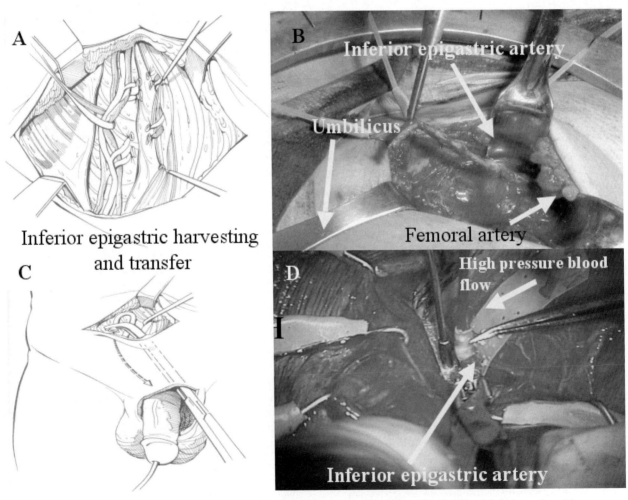

FIG. 72–5. Surgical technique. **A:** Inferior epigastric artery dissection. **B:** Mobilized inferior epigastric artery. **C:** Inferior epigastric artery transfer. **D:** Release of inferior epigastric artery clamp, documenting excellent arterial inflow.

The internal ring on the side of the harvested artery is identified lateral to the origin of the inferior epigastric artery. Using blunt finger dissection through the inguinal canal, a long fine vascular clamp is passed through the fenestration in the fundiform ligament, the external and internal inguinal rings, and a Penrose drain is placed to protect this transfer route.

The donor vascular bundle is transected at the level of the umbilicus between two ligaclips and carefully inspected for any proximal bleeding points. The long fine vascular clamp is brought through the internal inguinal ring again, this time to grasp the end of the transected inferior epigastric artery. The inferior epigastric vascular bundle is transferred to the base of the penis. It should be briskly pulsating and of adequate length. The origin of the inferior epigastric artery should be inspected for kinking or twisting. Following the achievement of complete hemostasis, closure of the abdominal wound is performed in two layers. The rectus fascia is closed utilizing a running 0 polyglycolic acid suture, one suture started at either end of the incision. The skin edges are apposed using skin staples.

Microvascular Anastomosis

A ring retractor and the associated elastic hooks are utilized once again on the inguinoscrotal incision and the fenestration of the fundiform ligament to gain exposure of the proximal dorsal neurovascular bundle. The pulsating inferior epigastric artery is placed against the recipient dorsal penile arteries and a convenient location is selected for the vascular anastomosis. The anastomosis (or anastomoses) is (are) created based on the arteriographic and duplex Doppler ultrasound findings. An end-to-end anastomosis is best under conditions whereby dorsal penile artery communications exist to the cavernous artery. In addition, an end-to-end anastomosis transfers perfusion pressure more effectively than an end-to-side anastomosis with less turbulence. It has been our experience that ligation of both dorsal penile arteries to perform bilateral proximal end-to-end anastomoses has never caused ischemic injury to the glans penis.

The appropriate dorsal penile artery segment is freed from its attachments to the tunica albuginea, with care being taken to avoid injury to any communicating branches to the cavernosal artery. Vascular hemostasis of this segment of the dorsal penile artery may be achieved with either gold-plated (low-pressure) aneurysm vascular clamps or vessel loops under minimal tension for the minimal of operating time. The only location where the adventitia must be carefully removed is at the site of the vascular anastomosis, i.e., the distal end of the inferior epigastric artery and the free end of the dorsal artery, to avoid causing subsequent thrombosis. If segments of adventitia enter the anastomosis, patency of the anastomosis is in jeopardy as adventitia activates clotting factors from the extrinsic clotting system. The remaining adventitia should be preserved in the vessels as the vasa vasorum provide a nutritional role to the vessel wall. The preservation of the adventitia is in addition important in terms of vessel innervation.

We use a plastic colored background material to aid in vessel visualization under the microscope. An end-to-end anastomosis is performed between the inferior epigastric artery and the dorsal artery using interrupted 10-0 nylon sutures (single-armed, 100-μm, 149-degree curved needle) under 10× magnification (Figs. 72–6A and 72–6B). Following release of the temporary occluding vascular clamps (or vessel loops) on the dorsal penile artery, the anastomosed segment should reveal arterial pulsations along its length and retrograde into the inferior epigastric artery. Such an observation implies a patent anastomosis. At this time, the inferior epigastric artery gold-plated aneurysm clamp may be removed (Fig. 72–5D). The intensity of the arterial pulsations in the anastomosis usually increases. On occasion, the application of a small amount of hemostatic material may be needed to aid in promoting hemostasis from suture needle holes in the vessel walls. After complete hemostasis has been achieved and correct instrument and sponge counts are assured, closure of the inguinoscrotal incision may begin. The dartos layer is reapproximated using a 3-0 polyglycolic acid sutures in a running fashion. The skin edges are closed with skin staples. The Foley catheter is left to closed-system gravity drainage overnight.

Modifications of the above-described procedure may be utilized. The most common alternative arterial anastomosis is an end-to-side anastomosis between the inferior epigastric artery and dorsal penile artery. A 10-0 suture is placed along the longitudinal axis of the dorsal penile artery in a 1-mm segment in the region of the intended anastomosis. After placing tension on the suture, an oval section of the artery wall is excised with a curved microscissors, resulting in a 1.2-to 1.5-mm horizontal arteriotomy (Fig. 72–6C). A temporary 2 Fr silastic stent is placed within the arteriotomy for clearer definition of the vessel lumen. The sutures are placed initially at each apex of the anastomosis and then subsequently three to five interrupted sutures are placed into each side wall. All sutures used to complete the anastomosis are inserted equidistant from each other to avoid an uneven anastomosis. One side of the anastomosis is completed prior to commencing the other side. If a temporary vascular stent is used, it is removed following placement of all sutures (Fig. 72–6D). The use of a temporary vascular stent enables careful inspection of the vessel back wall.

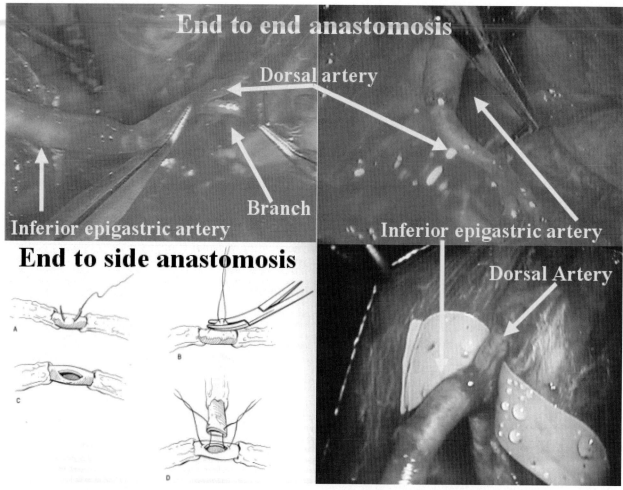

FIG. 72–6. Microsurgical anastomosis. **A and B:** End-to-end anastomosis. **C:** Microsurgical anastomosis technique. **D:** End-to-side anastomosis.

OUTCOMES

Complications

Mechanical disruption of the microvascular anastomosis and subsequent uncontrolled arterial hemorrhage may occur from blunt trauma in the first few postoperative weeks following coitus, masturbation, or from accidents. We recommend abstention from sexual activities involving the erect penis until 6 weeks postoperatively.

Other complications include penile pain and diminished penile sensation from injury to the nearby dorsal nerve (7). Loss of compliance of the suspensory and fundiform ligaments postoperatively may lead to diminished penile length. Preserving the two ligaments has markedly minimized those complications in our series. Glans hyperemia, once a complication seen when inferior epigastric artery to deep dorsal vein anastomoses (dorsal vein arterialization) were performed, is no longer seen because we no longer perform this form of anastomosis (3).

Results

We have reported on the objective postoperative hemodynamic status including steady-state equilibrium intra-cavernosal pressures and venoocclusive and arterial function testing parameters in patients who experienced successful as well as unsuccessful clinical results following microvascular arterial bypass surgery for impotence (Figs. 72–7A to 72–7D).

Of the 226 patients who underwent penile microvascular arterial bypass surgery from 1985 to 1992, 68 (30%) (mean age, 34 ± 10 years) underwent both preoperative and postoperative pharmacocavernosometry/graphy. The mean duration between the bypass procedure and follow-up postoperative testing was 8 ± 6 months. Surgical bypasses in these 68 patients included 65 inferior epigastric artery to dorsal penile artery including 30 with dual dorsal arterial anastomoses. There were, in addition, nine artery-to-deep-dorsal-vein anastomoses including six performed in conjunction with an arterial anastomosis.

Twelve patients (21%) with pure arteriogenic impotence had a postoperative mean increase in steady-state equilibrium intracavernosal pressure of 25 ± 12.3 mm Hg (range, 13 to 45 mm Hg). Of the remaining 56 patients, 49 had concomitant venous surgery. In this latter group, there was no significant change in mean steady-state equilibrium intracavernosal pressure,

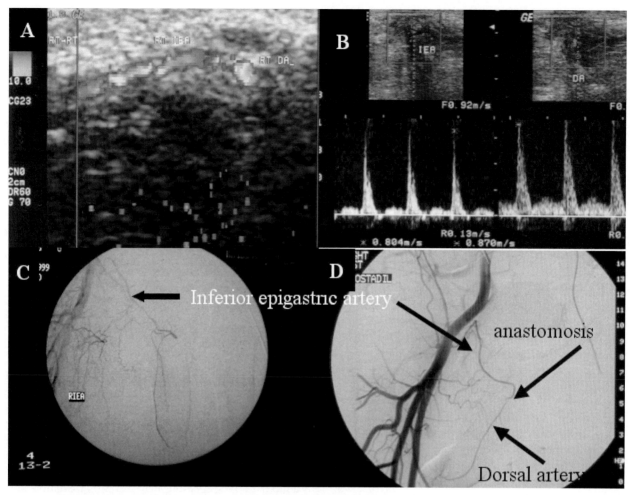

FIG. 72–7. Postoperative imaging. **A:** Color duplex ultrasound documenting anastomotic patency. **B:** Normal cavernosal artery peak systolic velocities. **C and D:** Postoperative arteriograms documenting an intact anastomosis between the inferior epigastric artery and the dorsal artery.

mean pressure decay in 30 seconds, or mean flow-to-maintain values. The remaining seven, who did not have venous surgery, had normal venoocclusive function pre- and postoperatively; however, the postoperative intracavernosal pressure did not increase (3).

REFERENCES

1. Goldstein I. Arterial revascularization procedures. *Sem Urol* 1986;4: 252–258.
2. Goldstein I. Vascular diseases of the penis. In: Pollack HM, ed. *Clinical urography*, 3rd ed. Philadelphia: WB Saunders, 1990:2231–2252.
3. Hatzichristou DG, Goldstein I. Arterial bypass surgery for impotence. *Curr Opin Urol* 1992;1:114.
4. Krane RJ, Goldstein I, Saenz de Tejada I. Impotence. *N Engl J Med* 1989;321:1648–1659.
5. Michal V, Kramer R, Popischal J, Hejhal L. Direct arterial anastomosis on corporal cavernosa penis in therapy of erectile dysfunction. *Rozhl Chir* 1973;52:587–590.
6. Michal V, Kramer R, Popischal J. Femoropudendal bypass, internal iliac thromboendarterectomy and direct arterial anastomosis to the cavernous body in the treatment of erectile impotence. *Bull Soc Int Chir* 1974;33: 341–345.
7. Zorgniotti AW, Lizza EF. Complications of penile revascularization. In: Zorgniotti AW, Lizza EF, eds. *Diagnosis and management of impotence.* Philadelphia: BC Decker, 1991.

CHAPTER 73

Penile Trauma

Daniel I. Rosenstein, Allen F. Morey, and Jack W. McAninch

Trauma to the penis is an uncommon event. Because of the relatively protected position of the penis between the thighs and pubic bone, it is usually able to avoid direct injury from external forces. Nonetheless, penile trauma may arise from both blunt and penetrating injuries. Such injuries present unique and difficult management problems to the urologic surgeon, in particular regarding long-term cosmesis, voiding function, and future potency. Major blunt penile injuries include penile rupture and skin loss from strangulation or degloving injuries. Penetrating penile trauma is usually secondary to stab or gunshot wounds and thus seldom occurs in the absence of associated genital, urethral, or major organ injury, except in the event of bites and self-inflicted wounds. Due to the wide disparity in the causes, diagnosis, and treatment, this chapter is divided into three parts: penile rupture, penile skin loss, and penetrating penile trauma.

PENILE RUPTURE

The most common blunt injury involving the penis is rupture of the corpora cavernosa, or penile fracture. This almost invariably occurs when the erect penis is forced to bend in an irregular fashion, such as when it accidentally impinges on the pubis or perineum after slipping out of the vagina during sexual intercourse (11). The remainder of cases are caused by falls out of bed with an erect penis, masturbation, or manipulation of the erect penis. The patient often reports a cracking or popping noise at the time of injury, leading to immediate detumescence and rapid onset of discoloration and swelling over the site of injury. There is frequently a delay in presentation to the hospital—presumably secondary to patient embarrassment.

The opinions expressed herein are those of the authors and are not to be construed as reflecting the views of the US Armed Forces or the Department of Defense.

Diagnosis

The diagnosis of penile rupture is easily made by physical examination along with the appropriate history. Swelling and discoloration may or may not be limited to the penis, depending on the integrity of Buck's fascia. If Buck's fascia is intact, the hematoma will be contained and will not usually spread below the base of the penis, resulting in the typical "eggplant" deformity (Fig. 73–1). However, if the laceration in the tunica albuginea involves Buck's fascia extravasation will be contained by Colles' fascia and ecchymosis will extend in a "butterfly" distribution over the perineum, scrotum, and lower abdomen. Examination may reveal angulation of the penis away from the side of rupture because of the mass effect of the hematoma. In addition, focal tenderness and a palpable defect in the tunica albuginea may help localize the fracture site. There is often a clot lying over or near the fracture site that corresponds to the site of cavernosal rupture.

Penile rupture can occur anywhere along the shaft including the base of the penis, where the corpora are fixed by the penile suspensory ligament. The fracture is typically located at the base of the penis, just proximal to the penoscrotal junction. In general only one corporal body is injured, although both corpora and the corpus spongiosum can be affected depending on the severity of the injury. Most patients are able to urinate normally, but the urologist must maintain a high index of suspicion for urethral injury. Failure to void spontaneously may signify compression of the urethra by hematoma but should lead to evaluation of urethral injury by retrograde urethrography (RUG). Urethral injury occurs in up to one-third of cases and usually consists of partial disruption, although complete transection can result (10). Retrograde urethrography is mandatory in all patients with blood at the urethral meatus, hematuria of any extent, or inability to void (11). However, because RUG is easy to perform and provides reliable results we perform it routinely in all

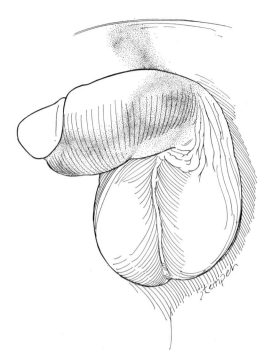

FIG. 73–1. Fractured penis displaying the pathognomonic "eggplant deformity" with swelling and discoloration extending to the base of the shaft. The penis usually bends away from the side of injury because of the hematoma.

cases of suspected penile rupture. Adjunctive imaging studies in penile fracture (including ultrasound, magnetic resonance imaging, and cavernosography) are usually unnecessary as the clinical picture is frequently adequate to initiate therapy.

Indications for Surgery

Although penile fractures can be managed nonoperatively, the literature shows a clear advantage to early operative repair (10,11). This approach results in faster recovery, shorter hospital stay, less morbidity, and less long-term penile curvature. The goals of acute exploration are evacuation of hematoma and primary repair of the laceration.

Alternative Therapy

Conservative treatment consists of cool compression dressings, antiinflammatory agents, and sedatives to reduce erections. This results in eventual resorption of the hematoma and scar formation at the site of the tunical rupture.

Surgical Technique

The patient is placed in a supine position and a Foley catheter is placed to facilitate identification of the urethra and urinary drainage. Exposure is usually obtained

through a subcoronal circumferential incision, and the penile skin is degloved down to the base. The distal circumferential incision is favored because it allows both exposure of the ruptured corpus and adequate assessment of the contralateral corpus and corpus spongiosum. Alternatively, an incision may be made on the shaft directly over the fracture site. This approach is only useful if the fracture is palpable preoperatively as the corporal bodies may not be easily explored through this incision. Further, the corpus spongiosum cannot be directly inspected via this approach.

Following the circumcising incision, the corpus spongiosum is carefully inspected to evaluate for potential urethral injury. Inspection of the fracture site usually reveals a transverse laceration, between 0.5 and 2.0 cm long, in the tunica albuginea of the proximal penile shaft (4). After evacuation of the hematoma and irrigation, minimal debridement of nonviable wound edges may be necessary before closure with interrupted 4-0 Maxon sutures (Fig. 73–2). The surgeon should not probe the exposed cavernous tissue unnecessarily as this may elicit troublesome bleeding. A tourniquet may be used intraoperatively to control hemorrhage. Lacerations may run directly under the dorsal neurovascular bundle located on the dorsal surface of the corpora at approximately the 10- and 2-o'clock positions (Fig. 73–3). This necessitates careful dissection of these structures off the corpora to allow a safe, watertight closure. Division of the deep dor-

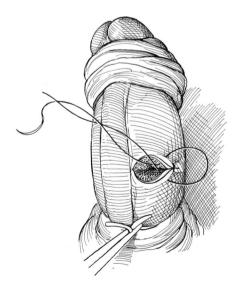

FIG. 73–2. Identification and repair of penile fracture. A distal circumferential subcoronal incision is made and skin and soft tissue are mobilized off the underlying corporal bodies down to the base of the penis. This maneuver exposes the transverse laceration in the tunica albuginea. The laceration is repaired using interrupted 4-0 Maxon with the knots buried. Exposed corporal erectile tissue should not be probed or explored as this may cause troublesome bleeding.

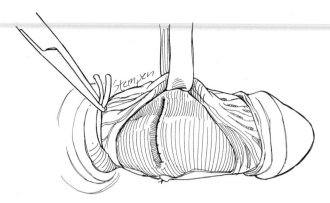

FIG. 73–3. Penile fracture extending beneath dorsal neurovascular bundles. Elevation of the ipsilateral dorsal neurovascular bundle facilitates repair of lacerations and protects these structures from inadvertent injury. Division of the deep dorsal vein in the midline provides access to the correct surgical plane beneath the ipsilateral neurovascular bundle.

sal vein facilitates unilateral dissection of the neurovascular bundle off the underlying corpus cavernosum. The penile skin is then replaced and the subcoronal incision is closed with interrupted 4-0 chromic sutures. If the patient is uncircumcised, the prepuce must be closely monitored for development of subcoronal edema. Postoperatively, a loose compression dressing (Coban) is gently placed, and the urethral catheter may be removed on postoperative day 1. Systemic antibiotics, antiinflammatory agents, and fibrinolytics are unnecessary. Most patients can be discharged home within 1 to 2 days of surgery. Sexual activity can be resumed at about 4 to 6 weeks. Painful erections may be present in the early postoperative period. Suppression of erections with benzodiazepines or amyl nitrate may provide symptomatic relief.

When urethral transection occurs in the context of penile rupture, we advocate primary repair with interrupted 5-0 or 6-0 Maxon sutures over a 16 Fr silicone catheter. In cases of complete urethral transection, additional urinary diversion through a percutaneous suprapubic cystostomy tube may be prudent (11). A voiding cystourethrogram (VCUG) should be carried out at approximately 14 days postrepair to document adequate healing before catheter removal.

Outcomes

Complications

Many patients treated conservatively or with delayed repair have some form of sexual dysfunction such as painful erection, disabling curvature, or erectile dysfunction secondary to cavernous–venous occlusive disease (1,14). Patients with a missed urethral injury associated with penile fracture are also at risk of periurethral abscess, stricture, and fistula formation.

Results

Patients who have operative repair within 48 hours of the injury have excellent functional results. In two relatively large studies, none of the patients with early operative repair experienced impotence, penile curvature on erection, or painful intercourse (4,11).

PENILE SKIN LOSS

Diagnosis

Penile skin loss can occur from necrotizing infection, burns, constrictive bands, or degloving injuries from blunt or penetrating trauma. Dog and human bites may also result in considerable penile skin loss. When the skin loss is secondary to infection (e.g., Fournier's gangrene), repeated debridement with antibiotics and moist dressing changes must be instituted to prepare the underlying tissue for delayed reconstruction. If the wounds are grossly contaminated, the testes may be placed in subcutaneous thigh pouches with a view toward delayed scrotal reconstruction. Avulsions are most often caused by power tool injuries or motor vehicle accidents, although this injury may rarely be self-inflicted secondary to insertion of the penis into vacuum cleaners and other suction devices (1). Because of the laxity of penile skin, the avulsion usually occurs just deep to the subcutaneous dartos layer, leaving the corporal bodies uninvolved. Immediate repair is frequently possible in cases of traumatic skin loss. If immediate closure is to be attempted, the wound edges must be clean and viable and hemostasis must be excellent to avoid delayed skin necrosis and sloughing.

Indications for Surgery

Partial penile skin loss, especially in the distal shaft, is best managed by rotational mobilization of a local skin flap. Primary closure may be appropriate if the defect is short and there is abundant remaining shaft skin. Extensive skin loss, whether from the injury itself or surgical debridement, usually requires tissue transfer for repair. In impotent patients, the penis can be buried under a scrotal flap with the glans left exposed to allow micturition (Fig. 73–4) (5). The penis may be liberated at a later date using the scrotal skin as a graft to cover the previously denuded area. In sexually active patients, a thick (0.016 to 0.018 in.), nonmeshed split-thickness skin graft is used. Thick split-thickness grafts are preferred because they are non–hair-bearing, have minimal contraction, and offer excellent cosmesis and viability. If sexual function is not a concern, a thinner skin graft may be harvested and meshed. The avulsed skin that is still attached on a viable pedicle can be gently washed and reapplied with the knowledge that it may need to be debrided at a later time. Completely avulsed penile skin will usually not survive as a free graft if reapplied to the denuded penile shaft.

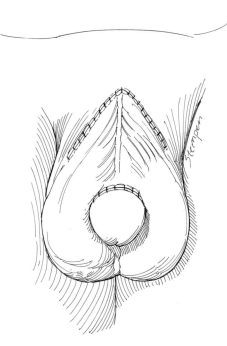

FIG. 73–4. Scrotal tunnel maneuver for penile skin coverage. The penis shaft may be buried beneath a flap of scrotal skin to provide skin coverage, leaving the glans exposed. This is a viable option in older patients who either were impotent before their injury or who have sustained severe associated injuries.

Alternative Therapy

There are no alternatives to surgery.

Surgical Technique

The patient is placed supine and both the genitals and a carefully chosen donor site are prepped into the field. The anterolateral thigh provides thickness, texture, and color resembling penile skin and is therefore the preferred donor site. Alternatively, the medial or posterior thigh or buttock may be used as a skin donor site. A Foley catheter is placed to prevent postoperative urinary contamination. The shaved donor site is coated with sterile mineral oil, and a Brown or Padgett dermatome (10-cm wide strip) is used to harvest the graft in at approximately 0.018-in. thickness. The graft is then tailored to fit the defect on the shaft. The donor site may be dressed with fine mesh gauze under slight pressure to ensure adequate hemostasis. Placement of a semipermeable plastic or silicone membrane (e.g., Biobrane) directly against the donor site helps reduce contamination. After about 24 hours, the Biobrane is adherent to the donor site and the redundant edges may be trimmed. This dressing usually falls off spontaneously after 2 weeks.

To prepare the penile shaft for grafting, it must be sharply debrided of all devitalized tissue and any chronic granulation tissue. It is imperative to prepare the recipient site so that the graft will have adequate blood supply. Debridement of the glans should be avoided, but all nonviable skin including the distal prepuce should be excised up to the coronal sulcus. Native penile skin distal to the graft will become edematous because of disruption of native lymphatic and venous drainage along the shaft. Hemostasis in the graft bed is essential to prevent hematoma formation under the graft.

Once prepared, the penis is stretched and the graft applied circumferentially around the shaft. The graft seam is placed at the ventral aspect to simulate the appearance of the median raphe (Fig. 73–5). The graft is sutured in place using interrupted 5-0 chromic sutures. Chordee formation has in general not been a problem because the graft will have minimal longitudinal contraction. The graft is secured to itself and along the shaft with interrupted 5-0 chromic sutures. Several 4-0 Vicryl sutures are placed at the proximal and distal graft edges and left long to use as bolster tieover sutures. A Xeroform dressing is placed directly on the graft. A bolster dressing is then fashioned using mineral oil-soaked cotton and fluffs. The whole dressing is secured in place using the bolster sutures, leaving the glans visible for inspection. To keep the penis in a vertical position, a padded plastic splint is placed around the bolster dressing. This housing may be fashioned out of a 500-cc sterile water container.

Postoperatively, the patient is kept at strict bedrest until the dressing is removed, usually after 5 days, when the Foley catheter is also removed. Immobilization of the

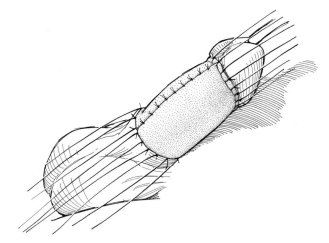

FIG. 73–5. Penile split-thickness skin graft. A thick (0.016 to 0.018 in.) split-thickness skin graft is applied to the denuded penile shaft. The distal skin is discarded to just beneath the corona when a circumferential graft is indicated. The graft is placed with the seam in the midline ventrally and secured with 5-0 chromic sutures to itself and along the shaft, while 4-0 silk sutures placed proximally and distally are left long to secure a bolster dressing.

penis in the extended position maintained by the bolster is critical for graft survival. Broad-spectrum antibiotics and administration of subcutaneous heparin for deep venous thrombosis prophylaxis are useful adjuncts. We do not routinely administer medications to reduce frequency of erections unless they are painful for the patient. Erections may provide natural tissue expansion and the grafts usually slide easily along the loose areolar tissue superficial to Buck's fascia. Once the penile dressing is removed, twice-daily sitz baths can be started to enhance epithelialization and reduce bacterial contamination.

Outcomes

Complications

The common causes of early failure of penile skin grafting are infection, shearing forces causing graft separation, and underlying hematoma. It is imperative that the graft bed be free of infected granulation tissue and any necrotic tissue. Shearing forces disrupt the blood supply to the new graft and are prevented by the penile splint and bolster dressing, provided the patient is cooperative with strict bedrest for 5 days. It is critical that the penis be maintained in the extended position within the bolster dressing as this will prevent folding or telescoping of the fresh graft on the penile surface. Hematoma causes failure by creating poor contact between the graft and the recipient bed. It is prevented by ensuring meticulous hemostasis of the graft bed prior to laying the graft in place. Meshed grafts allow better dissipation of hematoma fluid but are discouraged in potent patients because of their increased degree of contraction.

Results

Long-term results of reconstruction have been excellent, with successful graft take exceeding 90%. Sensation remains absent in the grafted skin but is retained in the glans and in deeper structures. Potency is unaffected by this type of reconstruction. Most patients have satisfactory intercourse after reconstruction. Cosmetic and functional results of nonmeshed, thick split-thickness penile grafts are superior to either meshed grafts or scrotal flaps.

PENETRATING PENILE TRAUMA

Penetrating trauma to the penis is most often caused by firearms but can also result from stab wounds, industrial accidents, self-mutilation attempts, and bites. In all cases, general principles of management include judicious debridement and hemostasis within the wound as well as careful exploration and repair of corporal and urethral injuries. Most civilian penile gunshot wounds are caused by low-velocity missiles, which cause damage only in the path of the bullet. Penetrating penile injuries are a more common genitourinary injury during wartime, possibly because of inadequate genital coverage by protective body armor (12). Associated wounds of the thigh and pelvis are common and may require urgent exploration and repair. Successful treatment of penetrating penile injuries must address and preserve normal voiding, potency, and penile cosmesis.

Diagnosis

Genital injury is determined by careful physical examination, with special attention paid to the trajectory of the bullet and initial hemostasis. The finding of a palpable corporeal defect in combination with an expanding penile hematoma or significant bleeding from the entry/exit wound is highly predictive of corporeal injury and should prompt expedient exploration (7). The exam should include a vascular (glanular capillary refill) and penile sensory assessment (9). Urethral injury, which occurs in 25% to 40% of penetrating injuries to the penis, should be excluded with RUG in all cases (6). The triad of no blood at the meatus, absence of hematuria, and normal voiding suggests that there is no urethral injury; however, penetrating trauma can cause urethral injury without clinical signs of damage. Cystography, intravenous pyelography, and scrotal ultrasonography may be necessary to evaluate associated urologic injuries. Cavernosography is rarely indicated in this setting (9).

Indications for Surgery

Penetrating injury to the penis most often requires surgical exploration. In addition, patients with unstable major organ injury will be unable to undergo immediate exploration. In these cases, initial treatment consists of hemostasis and packing of major wounds. Penetrating injury causing major skin loss will require tissue transfer for satisfactory coverage, but associated corporal and urethral injuries must be repaired before the skin grafting. Immediate primary closure or reconstruction should take place only with a clean wound that is in general less than 8 hours old.

Alternative Therapy

Single pellet wounds with small entrance sites and superficial stab wounds in which there is no active bleeding or hematoma may not require surgical exploration (3).

Surgical Technique

Operation consists of judicious debridement of devitalized tissue and hemostasis. The wound must be copiously irrigated to remove all foreign bodies, including powder from shotgun pellets and pieces of clothing. Bleeding almost always occurs from a lacerated corporal body but may also be from disrupted superficial veins. The primary objective of surgical exploration is control of corporal bleeding and repair of corporal defects. The corpora are well vascularized, and extensive debridement is usually unnecessary and will hinder future potency. We thus do not recommend extensive exploration of erectile or glanular tissue. Hemostasis is obtained by gentle compression and watertight closure of the tunica albuginea alone, usually with interrupted 4-0 Maxon sutures. Urethral injuries are repaired with 5-0 Vicryl sutures over a silicone catheter. Devitalized urethra must be carefully debrided, and primary repair with a tension-free anastomosis can usually be accomplished. Associated scrotal and spermatic cord injuries are treated with debridement and, if necessary, orchiectomy or ligation of the vas deferens. The skin can be closed primarily unless viable skin edges cannot be approximated. In contaminated wounds or those encountered after 8 hours, immediate skin closure or grafting is not recommended and the wound is packed instead. Once the wound is clean, delayed primary closure, staged reconstruction, or healing by secondary intention may be selected. An important contraindication to debridement and primary closure is the case of massive tissue destruction often associated with close-range shotgun blasts. These should be debrided and allowed to declare themselves in terms of the extent of injury. They may then be repaired in a staged fashion. It appears that longer-range injuries due to shotgun blasts may create multiple low-velocity wounds with less significant blast effect. Carefully selected longer-range shotgun injuries have been successfully managed with immediate debridement and primary repair (13).

Penile bites deserve special mention as they can rapidly progress to severe infection. Wounds should be copiously irrigated and all devitalized tissue debrided. All wounds should be left open and prophylactic antibiotics administered. Antibiotic treatment should cover gram-positive and gram-negative organisms as well as anaerobic gram-negative rods. The most common colonizing organisms in the mouth of a dog include *Pasteurella*, *Streptococcus*, and *Staphylococcus* species (2). Hospitalization with frequent wound inspection and intravenous antibiotics is necessary in those with delayed presentation or with increased risk factors such as steroid use, diabetes, or immunodeficiency syndromes. Close follow-up is mandatory in all outpatients.

Outcomes

Complications

Early complications of penetrating penile trauma include rebleeding and infection. Because the corpora are heavily vascularized, breakdown of repair in the tunica albuginea is rare. A small minority will report superficial sensory loss, pain with erection, and rapid detumescence. Complications attributable to the urethral injury include urethral stricture, periurethral abscess, and urethrocutaneous fistula.

Results

Excellent functional results can be expected except in those cases of high-velocity injuries where massive tissue destruction has occurred. Most patients report retained potency without penile curvature and with satisfactory cosmetic results (5,8). Patients who develop late penile curvature in the absence of palpable corporeal defects or plaques may have scarring and contraction of the underlying cavernosal tissues and the intercavernous septum (7).

REFERENCES

1. Armenakas NA, McAninch JW. Use of skin grafts in external genital reconstruction. In: McAninch JW, ed. *New techniques in reconstructive urology.* New York: Igaku-Shoin, 1996:127–141.
2. Cummings JM, Boullier JA. Scrotal dog bites. *J Urology* 2000;164:57.
3. Goldman HB, Dmochowski RR, Cox CE. Penetrating trauma to the penis: functional results. *J Urol* 1996;155:551.
4. Gomez RG. Genital injuries: presentation and management. In: McAninch JW, ed. *Problems in urology.* Philadelphia: JB Lippincott Co, 1994:279–289.
5. Gomez RG. Genital skin loss: reconstructive techniques. In: McAninch JW, ed. *Problems in urology.* Philadelphia: JB Lippincott Co, 1994: 290–301.
6. Gomez RG, Castanheira AC, McAninch JW. Gunshot wounds to the male external genitalia. *J Urol* 1993;150:1147.
7. Hall SJ, Wagner JR, Edelstein RA, Carpinito GA. Management of gunshot injuries to the penis and anterior urethra. *J Trauma* 1995;38:439.
8. McAninch JW. Management of genital skin loss. *Urol Clin North Am* 1989;16:387.
9. Miller KS, McAninch JW. Penile fracture and soft tissue injury. In: McAninch JW, ed. *Traumatic and reconstructive urology.* Philadelphia: WB Saunders, 1996:693–698.
10. Nicolaisen GS, Melamud A, Williams RD, McAninch JW. Rupture of the corpus cavernosum: surgical management. *J Urol* 1983;130:917.
11. Orvis BR, McAninch JW. Penile rupture. *Urol Clin North Am* 1989;16: 369.
12. Salvatierra O, Rigdon WO, Norris DM et al. Vietnam experience with 252 urological war injuries. *J Urol* 1969;101:615.
13. Tigert R, Harb JJ, Hurley PM, et al. Management of shotgun injuries to the pelvis and lower genitourinary system. *Urology* 2000;55:193.
14. Volz LR, Broderick GA. Conservative management of penile fracture may cause cavernous–venous occlusive disease and permanent erectile dysfunction. *J Urol* 1994;151:358A.

CHAPTER 74

Penile Replantation

Daniel I. Rosenstein and Gerald H. Jordan

Penile amputation is a rare injury in the Western world, arising largely from attempts at self-emasculation or as the result of violent assault. It may also arise secondary to industrial work accidents or as a war injury. Injuries amounting to penile amputation have also been reported as a rare complication of circumcision (7). The largest single series of penile amputation injuries stems from Thailand, where in the 1970s an epidemic of approximately 100 cases was reported (1). In these cases, adulterous husbands had their penises amputated by their humiliated wives while they slept. Unfortunately, only 18 of 100 cases in this series were successfully replanted because the amputated penis was often rapidly disposed of by the wife. Thus, experience with penile replantation is largely based upon case reports and smaller series. Despite the rarity of this injury, good functional and cosmetic results are routinely attainable using the microsurgical approach to penile replantation.

Psychotic patients who carry out self-emasculation may be broadly divided into two categories. The more common subgroup includes schizophrenic patients in a decompensated (actively psychotic) state. One study found that 87% of self-emasculating patients were psychotic at the time of injury (4). These patients are usually victims of command hallucinations that coerce the patient to mutilate his genitals. Because these patients respond well to psychiatric rehabilitation, they are unlikely to repeat an attempt at self-mutilation (8). They should therefore be replanted in a timely manner following penile amputation, with psychiatric support throughout the patient's admission and probably lifetime. Nonpsychotic patients who self-emasculate are often diagnosed with severe personality disorders. These patients are more difficult to rehabilitate (12).

While early attempts at penile replantation were frequently fraught with complications including skin and glans slough, the majority of these attempts were successful at salvaging the penis with corporal reapproxima-

tion alone. This field was revolutionized in 1976, when two independent groups described the first successful penile replantation using microvascular techniques (3,13). Since that time, microneurovascular repair has been considered the standard of care in penile replantation and has provided superior results with regard to postoperative sensation, erectile function, and overall graft viability (2).

The remarkable ability of an amputated penile tip to survive even in the absence of penile arterial and venous reanastomosis attests to the unique vascular supply of the penis. It seems that the sinusoidal blood within the corporal bodies closely approximates arterialized parameters, thus nourishing the distal bodies and skin early on without having to depend upon collateral vessel development. Microvascular reanastomosis has further decreased skin and glans slough because the skin may be perfused directly rather than via corporal perforators.

DIAGNOSIS

The physical diagnosis is obvious with complete loss of the distal penis. Patients who have self-inflicted wounds will have either a command psychosis or nonpsychosis with emasculation. The surgery staff should work closely with a psychiatrist in these patients because the emasculation is only a symptom of the underlying disease. Traumatic amputations either from an assault or industrial equipment will likely have postsurgical need for psychiatric evaluation. All patients should be aware of the potential for loss of the penis as well as the potential for impotence

INDICATIONS FOR SURGERY

Because penile tissue has a remarkable resistance to prolonged ischemia (11), all attempts to replant the available member should be carried out unless the penis has

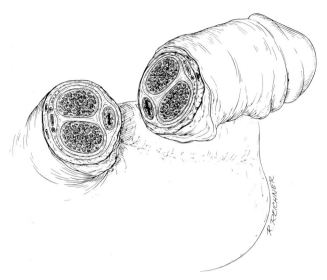

FIG. 74–1. The typical appearance of a penile amputation injury. (From Jordan GH, Gilbert DA. Management of amputation injuries of the male genitalia. *Urol Clin North Am* 1989; 16:359–367, with permission.)

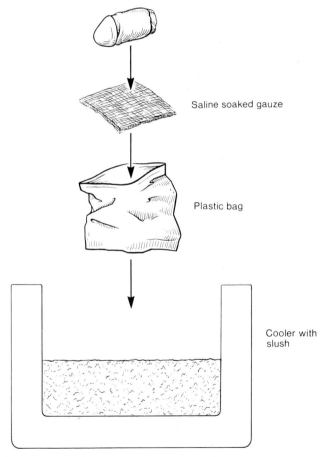

Saline soaked gauze

Plastic bag

Cooler with slush

FIG. 74–2. Illustration of the bag-within-a-bag technique of organ emergent cold storage. The amputated part of the penis is placed on a saline-soaked gauze sponge, within a sterile (if possible) plastic bag. The plastic bag is then immersed in a second container of iced slush. (From Jordan GH. Initial management and reconstruction of male genital amputation injuries. *Traumat Reconstr Urol* 1996;57:673–681, with permission.)

been extremely mutilated. Replantation has been successful despite hypothermic ischemic times of 24 hours or longer. Most patients have sharply lacerated their penises, with clear anatomic structures and vessels often visible both in the stump and the distal portion (Fig. 74–1). The penis should be preserved with the "bag-within-a-bag" technique (Fig. 74–2). This serves to increase ischemic tolerance. The amputated penis is wrapped in saline-soaked gauze in a sterile plastic bag. This bag is then immersed in ice slush. The patient should be kept warm and peripherally vasodilated throughout the procedure as well as in the postoperative period.

ALTERNATIVE THERAPY

Alternatives are limited and are basically to not reconstruct the penis and perform a urethrostomy.

SURGICAL TECHNIQUE

Microsurgical replantation should be carried out under optical microscopy (6), with systematic exploration and debridement of the corporal bodies and dorsal neurovascular structures as necessary (Fig. 74–3). The urethra should be spatulated and reanastomosed first as this provides stability to the remainder of the repair. A two-layer repair using 6-0 polydioxanone suture (PDS) or 6-0 Vicryl for the mucosa followed by 5-0 PDS for the spongy erectile tissue is appropriate. Coaptation of the cavernosal arteries does not seem to offer any advantage.

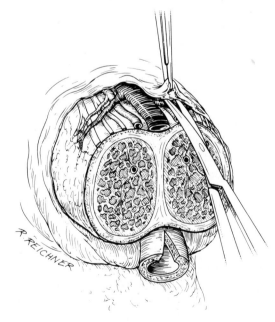

FIG. 74–3. The urethra, corpora cavernosa, and dorsal neurovascular structures are exposed and minimally debrided. (From Jordan GH, Gilbert DA. Management of amputation injuries of the male genitalia. *Urol Clin North Am* 1989; 16:359–367, with permission.)

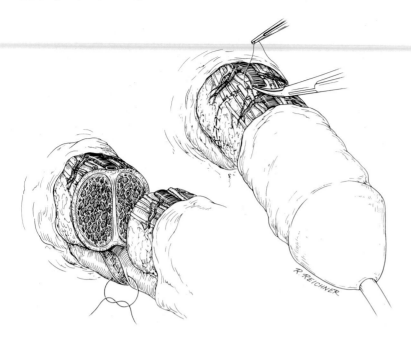

FIG. 74–4. A two-layer spatulated urethral anastomosis is completed. Microvascular coaptation of the dorsal vein, deep dorsal artery, and dorsal nerves is accomplished. (From Jordan GH, Gilbert DA. Management of amputation injuries of the male genitalia. *Urol Clin North Am* 1989;16:359–367, with permission.)

The tunica albuginea and the corpora cavernosa should then be meticulously closed with interrupted 4-0 or 5-0 PDS sutures.

The dorsal neurovascular structures are repaired next. Both dorsal penile arteries should be reapproximated using 11-0 nylon or Prolene, and the deep dorsal vein is then repaired with 10-0 nylon or Prolene. Following completion of the vascular anastomosis, the dorsal nerve bundles should be reapproximated with 10-0 nylon. The epineurium of each side should be placed in apposition so that fascicular regrowth is facilitated (Fig. 74–4). These nerves are branches of the pudendal nerve and are responsible for sensation within the glans. The autonomic cavernous nerves branch proximally within the corporal bodies and are not directly repaired (15).

Following completion of the microsurgical anastomoses, the dartos fascia should be reapproximated using 5-0 Vicryl sutures and the skin is loosely reapproximated using 6-0 Vicryl. Shaft skin should be preserved if at all possible as initially questionable skin may appear more viable in the postoperative period (Fig. 74–5). A diverting suprapubic cystotomy catheter should be placed and the urethra stented with a small soft silicone catheter. The penis should be immobilized and elevated to facilitate venous and lymphatic drainage. A subcutaneous suprapubic tunnel technique has been described for protection of the replanted penis in the early postoperative period (5).

If the microvascular approach to replantation is technically or otherwise not feasible, the penis should be replanted via corporal and urethral reapproximation. The denuded replanted penis may be buried in the scrotum followed by delayed liberation with scrotal skin cover, as described by McRoberts et al. (10). Although penile salvage is usually successful via this technique, it obviously requires a second procedure that leaves thick hair-bearing scrotal skin on the shaft of the penis or requires grafting.

If the amputated penis is absent or too mutilated for replantation, hemostasis should be achieved, followed by spatulation of the neomeatus. The proximal shaft may be buried in the surrounding skin or the residual corporal stumps may be covered by a split-thickness skin graft. In the unusual circumstance that perineal contamination precludes immediate replantation, temporary ectopic implantation (to the forearm) followed by delayed anatomic replantation has been employed successfully (9).

The patient should be kept on bedrest for a minimum of 1 week, with urinary diversion continuing for at least 3 weeks. During this period, the replanted penis should be closely monitored with frequent Doppler ultrasonography and signs of skin slough or decreased glans

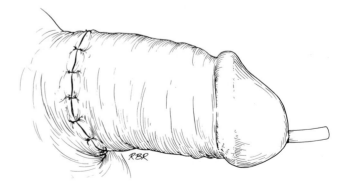

FIG. 74–5. Postoperative result. (From Jordan GH, Gilbert DA. Management of amputation injuries of the male genitalia. *Urol Clin North Am* 1989; 16:359–367, with permission.)

viability should be documented. The stenting catheter may be removed at the 3-week postoperative period, with a voiding urethrogram carried out to document the absence of urinary extravasation at the repair site. The use of daily aspirin in the postoperative period is recommended. More aggressive anticoagulation is usually not warranted but should be addressed on a case-by-case basis.

OUTCOMES

Complications

The frequency of skin necrosis, glans slough, and urethral complications have all been reduced with the microvascular approach to replantation. Several reports document the return of partial or complete erectile function in the months following the replantation (6,12,14). Patients who fail to achieve adequate return of erections may still respond to a pharmacological erection protocol.

Results

Given the uniformly good results of microvascular penile replantation from both a cosmetic and functional point of view, this approach should be performed if at all possible. If microsurgery is not feasible, macroscopic replantation should still be offered.

REFERENCES

1. Bhanaganada K, Chayavatana T, Pongnumkul C, et al. Surgical management of an epidemic of penile amputations in Siam. *Am J Surg* 1983;146:376.
2. Carroll PR, Lue TF, Schmidt RA, Trengrove-Jones G, McAninch JW. Penile replantation: current concepts. *J Urol* 1985;133:281–285.
3. Cohen BE, May JW, Daly JS, et al. Successful clinical replantation of an amputated penis by microneurovascular repair. *Plast Reconstr Surg* 1977;59:276.
4. Greilheimer H, Groves JE. Male genital self-mutilation. *Arch Gen Psychiatry* 1979;36:441.
5. Harris DD, Beaghler MA, Stewart SC, Freed JR, Hendricks DL. Use of a subcutaneous tunnel following replantation of an amputated penis. *Urology* 1996;48:628–630.
6. Jiminez-Cruz JF, Garcia-Reboll L, Alonso M, Broseta E, Sanz S. Microsurgical penis replantation after self-mutilation. *Eur Urol* 1995;27:246–248.
7. Jong KP, Jun KM, Hyung JK, Reimplantation of an amputated penis in prepubertal boys. *J Urol* 2001;165:586–587.
8. Jordan GH, Gilbert DA. Management of amputation injuries of the male genitalia. *Urol Clin North Am* 1989;16:359–367.
9. Matloub HS, Yousif NJ, Sanger JR. Temporary ectopic implantation of an amputated penis. *Plast Reconstr Surg* 1994;93:408–412.
10. McRoberts JW, Chapman WH, Ansell JS. Primary anastomosis of the traumatically amputated penis: case report and summary of the literature. *J Urol* 1968;100:751.
11. Mosahebi A, Butterworth M, Knight R, Berger L, Kaisary A, Butler P. Delayed penile replantation after prolonged warm ischemia. *Microsurgery* 2001;21:52–54.
12. Sanger JR, Matloub HS, Yousif NJ, Begun FP. Penile replantation after self-inflicted amputation. *Ann Plast Surg* 1992;29:579–584.
13. Tamai S, Nakamura Y, Motomiya Y. Microsurgical replantation of a completely amputated penis and scrotum. *Plast Reconr Surg* 1977;60:287.
14. Wells MD, Boyd JB, Bulbul MA. Penile replantation. *Ann Plast Surg* 1991;26:577–581.
15. Zenn MR., Carson CC, Patel MP. Replantation of the penis: a patient report. *Ann Plast Surg* 2000;44:214–220.

CHAPTER 75

Varicocele: General Considerations

Carin V. Hopps and Marc Goldstein

A varicocele is an abnormal dilation of the veins draining the testis, the internal spermatic veins, that can be palpated through the scrotal skin. While varicoceles are present in 15% of the male population overall, they are present in 35% of men with primary infertility and 81% of men with secondary infertility (3) Varicocele is the most common etiology of male factor infertility, and varicocelectomy (ligation of the internal spermatic veins) is the most commonly performed surgical procedure for men with infertility. Varicocele is associated with decreased testicular volume, impaired sperm quality, and a decline in Leydig cell function (13). Surgical repair of clinical varicocele has been shown to avert further damage to testicular function, improve spermatogenesis, and improve Leydig cell function. Large varicoceles are associated with greater testicular dysfunction than are small varicoceles, and repair of large varicoceles results in greater improvement in semen parameters when compared with repair of small varicoceles (10).

Varicoceles most commonly occur on the left. Whereas the right internal spermatic vein drains into the vena cava, the left internal spermatic vein drains into the left renal vein and therefore is significantly longer than the right vein, resulting in greater transmission of pressure to the pampiniform plexus. Contributing to increased venous pressure is the position of the left renal vein, which crosses anterior to the aorta and posterior to the superior mesentery artery, potentially causing compression of the renal vein, known as the "nutcracker effect." Retrograde flow of blood into the pampiniform plexus due to incompetent valves within the internal spermatic vein may also contribute to dilation of this venous system.

The pathophysiology by which varicocele impairs testicular function is poorly understood. Of several proposed mechanisms of injury, thermal testicular injury is the hypothesis most supported by animal and human studies. Animal models have demonstrated a clear adverse effect of heat on testicular function. Varicocele is thought to affect thermoregulation of the testis by interfering with the countercurrent heat exchange mechanism within the pampiniform plexus. Although the scrotal location of the testes appears to underscore the importance of temperature regulation, the mechanism by which varicocele causes injury to the testis is likely multifactorial.

DIAGNOSIS

Varicocele is diagnosed by thorough examination of the scrotal contents with the patient in both the supine and standing positions. Relaxation of the dartos muscle, facilitated by a warm scrotum (we favor a simple heating pad on the scrotum), is essential for proper examination of scrotal contents. Grade I varicocele is palpable with Valsalva maneuver only, grade II is palpable in the standing position, and grade III is visually apparent through the scrotal skin as a "bag of worms." Transscrotal ultrasound is not necessary to diagnose varicocele but may be utilized if physical examination cannot be adequately accomplished or findings on physical examination are equivocal. Internal spermatic vein diameter greater than 3 mm and demonstration of retrograde flow through the vein with Valsalva maneuver on ultrasound are consistent with the diagnosis of clinical varicocele. Varicoceles that do not meet these criteria are defined as subclinical.

INDICATIONS FOR SURGERY

Most varicoceles are not associated with infertility, decreased testicular volume, or pain and therefore do not require surgical correction. A clinical varicocele in a patient with abnormal semen parameters should be surgically corrected to reverse the process of progressive and duration-dependent decline in testicular function. Repair of subclinical varicocele has not been shown to confer a benefit to the patient with male factor infertility and is not recommended

(4). Varicocele associated with ipsilateral testicular atrophy or with ipsilateral testicular pain that worsens progressively throughout the day, but subsides in the recumbent position, should be repaired as well. Varicocele ligation in adolescents with ipsilateral testicular atrophy has been shown to result in a significant increase in testis volume (5), and therefore surgical correction is recommended in this group. Adolescents with small- to moderate-grade varicoceles in the absence of atrophy are followed with yearly examination to assess testicular growth; the occurrence of diminished growth on the side of the varicocele warrants varicocelectomy. A sound argument could be made for repair of all grade III varicoceles in adolescents to conserve testicular function. Approximately 3% of adolescent males have grade III varicoceles.

ALTERNATIVE THERAPY

For men with infertility, abnormal semen parameters, and clinical varicocele, few alternatives to varicocelectomy are available. Currently utilized nonsurgical techniques include percutaneous radiographic occlusion and sclerotherapy. The retrograde percutaneous approach employs cannulation of the femoral vein and placement of a balloon or coil within the internal spermatic vein. Although this technique is associated with preservation of the testicular artery and lymphatics, it has a high unperformable rate due to difficulty in accessing the internal spermatic vein, and these men ultimately require surgical intervention. Radiographic occlusion is also associated with complications such as migration of embolization material into the renal vein resulting in kidney loss or pulmonary embolization, thrombophlebitis, arterial injury, and allergic reaction to contrast materials. This technique may have a role in the management of varicoceles that persist or recur following open surgical repair to avoid reoperation through scar tissue. Antegrade varicocele occlusion performed by percutaneous cannulation of a scrotal pampiniform vein and injection of a sclerosing agent has been described. This technique is associated with higher performability rates but similar recurrence rates when compared with the retrograde approach, in addition to presenting risk of injury to the testicular artery.

SURGICAL TECHNIQUE

Ligation of the internal spermatic veins can be approached in several ways. The earliest described technique involved placing an external clamp on the veins through the scrotal skin. Surgical varicocele ligation techniques include retroperitoneal, inguinal or subinguinal ligation, laparoscopic, and microsurgical varicocelectomy.

Retroperitoneal (Polomo) Approach

The retroperitoneal (Polomo) approach (Fig. 75–1) has the advantage of isolating the internal spermatic veins proximally, near the point of drainage into the left renal

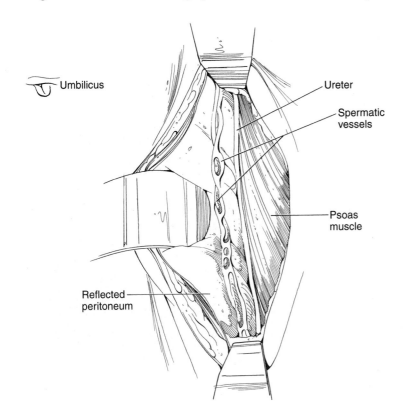

FIG. 75–1. Modified Palomo retroperitoneal approach for varicocelectomy. The internal spermatic vein is found on the posterior aspect of the peritoneum. It is isolated and divided between ligatures.

vein. At this level, only one or two large veins are present. In addition, the testicular artery has not yet branched and is often separate from the internal spermatic veins. A disadvantage to this approach is difficulty in preserving lymphatics, due to the poorly accessible retroperitoneal location of the vessels, leading to a higher incidence of postoperative hydrocele. In addition, a high recurrence rate is observed when the testicular artery is preserved due to preservation of the periarterial plexus of fine veins (venae comitantes), which may dilate with time and present as the source of recurrence. Parallel inguinal or retroperitoneal collaterals originating at the testis and joining the internal spermatic vein cephalad to the level of ligation in addition to cremasteric veins that are not ligated may contribute to recurrence. Intentional ligation of the testicular artery has been suggested in children to minimize recurrence, but in adults who present with infertility ligation of the testicular artery cannot be recommended as this is unlikely to enhance testicular function.

The patient is placed in the dorsal supine position on an operating table. A horizontal iliac incision equidistant from the umbilicus and anterior superior iliac spine is made (7 to 10 cm depending on the patient's body habitus). The external oblique aponeurosis is incised obliquely. The internal oblique is split 1 cm off the lateral edge of the rectus abdominis and the transversus abdominis is incised. The peritoneum is dissected free from the abdominal wall and retracted. The spermatic vessels appear adherent to the peritoneum, making it important to remain close to the peritoneum. Continued dissection along the abdominal wall would lead posteriorly to the psoas muscle. Retraction of the peritoneum allows easy identification of the spermatic veins, and in less than 10% of cases the spermatic artery is clearly visible, isolated from the rest of the spermatic structures, identified, and preserved.

The remainder of the operation depends on the intraoperative findings. In the case of a single vein and no collateral, the artery is identified and will only be preserved when it is not accompanied by a plexus of small veins indissociable from the artery. In the case of multiple veins, the collaterals are identified and all vessels from the ureter to the abdominal wall are ligated. Spermatic vessels are in general inspected over a distance of 7 or 8 cm and ligated by braided, permanent suture material.

After verification of hemostasis, the internal oblique, transversus abdominis, and the external oblique aponeurosis are reapproximated with absorbable suture. Scarpa's fascia is closed by a resorbable running suture. The skin is closed in subcuticular manner with absorbable suture.

Inguinal (Ivanissevich) Approach

The incision is made 2 cm above the symphysis pubis (Fig. 75–2). The external oblique aponeurosis is carefully divided to avoid injuring the underlying ilioinguinal nerve. The cord is mobilized and a Penrose drain is inserted beneath the cord and retracted to gain exposure of the cord. The spermatic fascia is then incised and the vessels are identified. Each vein is isolated, doubly ligated with nonabsorbable suture, and transsected. Intraoperative Doppler may be utilized to identify the testicular artery. After all collaterals are identified, the external oblique aponeurosis is closed with running absorbable suture and the skin is closed in subcuticular manner.

Laparoscopic Varicocele Repair

Laparoscopic varicocele repair is a modification of the retroperitoneal technique with similar advantages and disadvantages. The optical magnification afforded

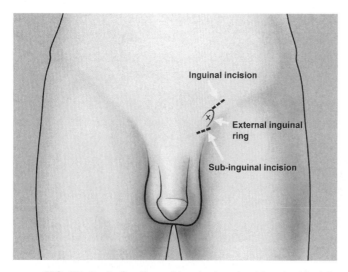

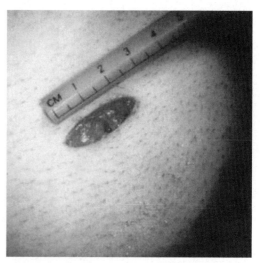

FIG. 75–2. A: Position of inguinal and subinguinal incisions. The external inguinal ring can be located by invaginating the scrotal skin with an index finger in a cephalad direction over the pubic tubercle. The location of the ring is marked on the skin. **B:** A subinguinal incision measuring only 2.5 cm in length.

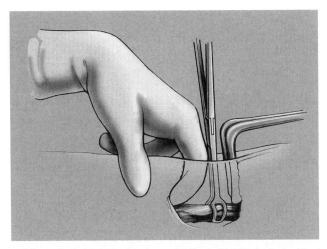

FIG. 75–3. Subinguinal approach. An index finger is hooked into the external inguinal ring retracting cephalad, while a small Richardson retractor retracts the soft tissues caudad toward the scrotum. The assistant grasps the spermatic cord with a Babcock clamp for elevation of the cord into the wound.

through the laparoscope provides the ability to preserve the lymphatics and the testicular artery while ligating the few internal spermatic veins present at this level and the venae comitantes adherent to the testicular artery. Laparoscopic technique introduces a unique set of complications including injury to bowel, intraabdominal vessels, and viscera in addition to air embolism and peritonitis, all of which are much more serious than those associated with open varicocelectomy.

Microsurgical Varicocelectomy

Microsurgical subinguinal or inguinal varicocelectomy is our preferred approach to varicocele ligation. The spermatic cord is elevated into the incision (Fig. 75-3), providing excellent exposure, and with use of the microscope providing 6 to 25× magnification the small periarterial and cremasteric veins can be readily ligated as can extraspermatic and gubernacular veins when the testis is delivered into the wound (Fig. 75–4). The external and internal spermatic fasciae are carefully opened to expose the vessels (Fig. 75-5). The testicular artery can be readily identified under the microscope and preserva-

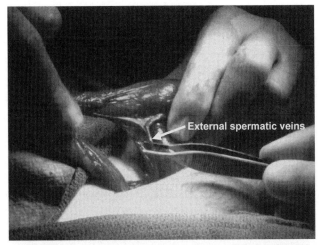

A

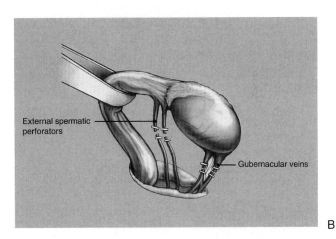

B

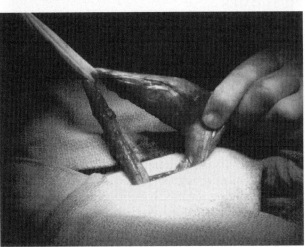

C

FIG. 75–4. A: Following delivery of the testis, the cord and gubernaculum are inspected for extraspermatic collateral veins. **B:** All external spermatic and gubernacular veins are doubly clipped and transected. **C:** The testis and cord following division of these veins. All remaining venous drainage is contained within the cord itself.

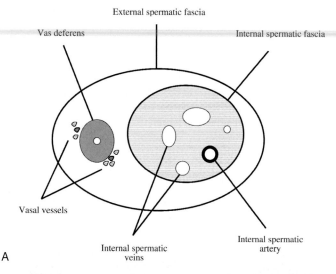

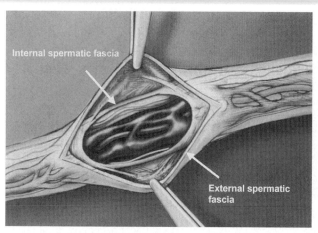

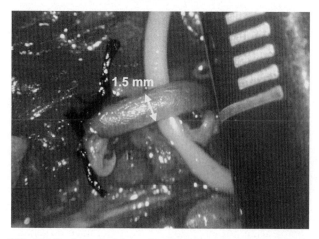

FIG. 75–5. A: Diagram of a cross-section of the spermatic cord, illustrating the anatomic relationship between the external and internal spermatic fascias. A **(B)** diagram and **(C)** intraoperative photo of the spermatic cord with opened external and internal spermatic fascias.

tion of the artery is more likely with enhanced visualization (Fig. 75-6). Lymphatics are also identified and preserved (Fig. 75-7), resulting in a lower incidence of hydrocele postoperatively.

OUTCOMES

Complications

The most common complication following varicocelectomy is hydrocele formation. The incidence of postoperative hydrocele following the nonmicrosurgical technique ranges from 3% to 33% with an average of 7%. Examination of the hydrocele fluid has shown that the fluid characteristics are consistent with obstruction of lymphatics (12). The effect of a hydrocele on sperm function and fertility is uncertain. Nearly half of postoperative hydroceles require surgical correction due to size. Use of magnification to identify lymphatics and preserve them has nearly eliminated the incidence of hydrocele formation (2,8).

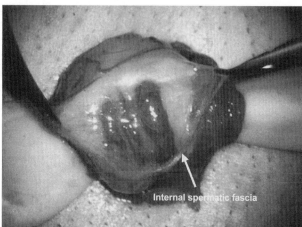

FIG. 75–6. A vessel loop is placed around the testicular artery for identification throughout the procedure. The artery has been dissected free of all adjacent veins and lymphatics.

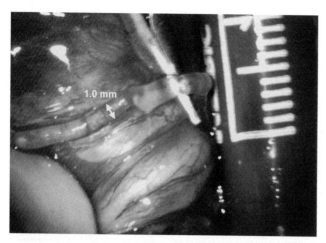

FIG. 75–7. A lymphatic measuring 1 mm in diameter is visualized under the microscope and preserved.

Testicular artery injury is a complication of varicocelectomy. Although the testis also receives blood supply from the cremasteric and deferential arteries, ligation of the testicular artery may result in atrophy and/or impaired spermatogenesis. Microscopic technique facilitates identification and preservation of the testicular artery, minimizing the risk of testicular injury (2).

Varicocele recurrence occurs in periarterial, parallel inguinal, midretroperitoneal, or transscrotal collaterals (6). Parallel inguinal collaterals are missed with retroperitoneal repair. Routine inguinal techniques without optical magnification miss scrotal collaterals and small veins adherent to the testicular artery. The microsurgical approach with delivery of the testis is associated with a varicocele recurrence rate less than 1% when compared with 9% for nonmagnified inguinal techniques (2,8).

Results

Varicocelectomy has been found to improve sperm concentration, motility, and morphology with a corresponding increase in pregnancy rate. A randomized controlled trial of surgery compared with no surgery (control group) showed that 60% of men who underwent varicocelectomy initiated a pregnancy within 1 year, whereas pregnancy was achieved in only 10% of those couples in which the varicocele went unrepaired (7). The control group then underwent varicocelectomy, and during the second year of the study 44% initiated a pregnancy. A series of 1,500 men who underwent microsurgical varicocelectomy resulted in 43% pregnancy at 1 year and 69% at 2 years when female factors were excluded (2). Varicocelectomy improves semen parameters sufficiently such that for most couples assisted reproductive techniques (ARTs) are either rendered unnecessary or the type of ART necessary to bypass the male factor is downstaged (1). In addition, up to 50% of men with nonobstructive azoospermia will respond to varicocelectomy with return of sperm to the ejaculate (9). In adolescents, a moderate to large varicocele can be responsible for testicular growth retardation and early ligation of the varicocele may reverse this process (5). Finally, varicocelectomy can increase serum testosterone levels for infertile men with varicoceles (11).

REFERENCES

1. Çayan S, Erdemir F, Özbey İ, et al. Can varicocelectomy significantly change the way couples use assisted reproductive technologies? *J Urol* 2002; 167:1749–1752.
2. Goldstein M, Gilbert BR, Dicker AP, Dwosh J, Gnecco C. Microsurgical inguinal varicocelectomy with delivery of the testis: An artery and lymphatic sparing technique. *J Urol* 1992;148:1808–1811.
3. Gorelick JI, Goldstein M. Loss of fertility in men with varicocele. *Fertil Steril* 1993;59:613.
4. Jarow JP, Ogle SR, Eskew LA. Seminal improvement following repair of ultrasound detected subclinical varicoceles. *J Urol* 1996;155:1287–1290.
5. Kass EJ, Belman AB. Reversal of testicular growth failure by varicocele ligation. *J Urol* 1987;137:475–476.
6. Kaufman SL, Kadir S, Barth KH, Smyth JW, Walsh PC, White RI. Mechanisms of recurrent varicocele after balloon occlusion or surgical ligation of the internal spermatic vein. *Radiology* 1983;147:435–440.
7. Madgar I, Weissenberg R, Lunenfeld B, et al. Controlled trial of high spermatic vein ligation for varicocele in infertile men. *Fertil Steril* 1995;63:120.
8. Marmar JL, Kim Y. Subinguinal microsurgical varicocelectomy: a technical critique and statistical analysis of semen and pregnancy data. *J Urol* 1994;152:1127–1132.
9. Matthews GJ, Matthews ED, Goldstein M. Induction of spermatogenesis and achievement of pregnancy after microsurgical varicocelectomy in men with azoospermia and severe oligoasthenospermia. *Fertil Steril* 1998;70:71.
10. Steckel J, Dicker AP, Goldstein M. Influence of varicocele size on response to microsurgical ligation of the spermatic veins. *J Urol* 1993; 149:769–771.
11. Su LM, Goldstein M, Schlegel PN. The effect of varicocelectomy on serum testosterone levels in infertile men with varicoceles. *J Urol* 1995;154:1752–1755.
12. Szabo R, Kessler R. Hydrocele following internal spermatic vein ligation: A retrospective study and review of the literature. *J Urol* 1984; 132:924–925.
13. World Health Organization. The influence of varicocele on parameters of fertility in a large group of men presenting to infertility clinics. *Fertil Steril* 1992;57:1289.

CHAPTER 76

Hydrocele and Spermatocele

John A. Nesbitt

Hydrocele and spermatocele both refer to common but abnormal collections of fluid within the scrotal sac. While the etiology of each is different, both may require surgical intervention for cure. These structures must be included in the differential diagnosis of scrotal masses.

HYDROCELE

A hydrocele (from the Greek *hydros* for water and *kele* for mass), literally a watery rupture or water in the scrotum, is an abnormal collection of fluid in the tunica vaginalis that may surround the testicle. The fluid is usually amber and is considered to be an exudate. A small amount of fluid, several cubic centimeters, is normally present around the testicle. This fluid is present between layers of the tunica vaginalis and is continuously secreted and reabsorbed by this mesothelial layer. Several types of hydroceles exist that may be associated with other pathologic findings. Many hydroceles occur congenitally. Most of these resolve spontaneously before age 1. Acquired hydroceles are found later in life. If due to local inflammation, these may resolve as well. Intervention is usually only required for size or discomfort.

During month 3 of gestation, the gubernaculum traverses the inguinal canal from the internal ring, through the external inguinal ring, and out into the scrotum, pulling with it the parietal peritoneal lining of the abdominal cavity (processus vaginalis). Late in the third trimester, the testis leaves its intraabdominal location, descending along the same route as the gubernaculum, through the inguinal canal and exiting the external ring posterolateral to the processus vaginalis. Normally, the segment of the processus vaginalis lying in the inguinal canal obliterates by the time of birth. A portion of the processus is left within the scrotum closely applied to the testicle. This structure is then termed the tunica vaginalis. Persistence of the inguinal portion of the processus may lead to a patent processus vaginalis, a hernia (indirect), or

a localized pocket of fluid lying within the inguinal canal known as a hydrocele of the cord.

Most acquired hydroceles are idiopathic; however, the clinician must be careful to consider other causes such as trauma, infection, or testicular tumor when evaluating a patient. Lymphatic obstruction due to ipsilateral inguinal or pelvic surgery may result in a secondary hydrocele. A common surgical cause for hydrocele is renal transplantation. In this scenario, the spermatic vessels and vas deferens are divided on the ipsilateral side, leading to hydrocele development. Epididymitis or orchitis may cause an acute hydrocele that usually resolves with resolution of the inflammation. Tropical infections such as filariasis may produce hydroceles where the tunica thickens due to lymphatic obstruction by the parasites. In these cases, the fluid is usually turbid due to the chylous drainage secondary to the lymphatic obstruction.

Diagnosis

In the pediatric population, hydroceles may present at birth or within the first year of life and are found in about 6% of full-term males. In general, a painless swelling is noticed in the scrotum. The swelling will transilluminate and may extend cephalad into the inguinal canal. The scrotal enlargement may increase or decrease in size if the processus is patent, allowing peritoneal fluid or bowel to enter the scrotum. If the processus is small, only fluid will enter. This persistence of the patent processus allowing the connection from the peritoneum to the scrotum is known as a communicating hydrocele. The change in size may not be apparent to the clinician but will be noticed by the parents.

In acquired hydroceles, the swelling may be accompanied by pain, especially if caused by an inflammatory process. The patient may report an enlargement within the scrotum, a tense sac, or some discomfort within the scrotum that may radiate inguinally or into the ipsilateral flank. The swelling is smooth, confined to the scrotum, and will usually transilluminate if the wall is not too thickened. With somewhat large and tense hydroceles, the testicle is not palpable. Because testicular neoplasms may also cause hydroceles, transscrotal ultrasonography is a useful preoperative diagnostic tool for imaging an otherwise inevaluable testicle in this case.

Indications for Surgery

Surgical intervention is indicated when the hydrocele is symptomatic either due to discomfort or the size impairing daily activity. Hydrocelectomy is inappropriate in the face of a testicular neoplasm.

Alternative Therapy

In congenital hydroceles, the treatment is usually observation initially unless the patient has an accompanying hernia. This is an important distinction to make because the later should be repaired surgically. When the diagnosis in uncertain, some have advocated repair. A period of observation would be appropriate in the absence of other symptoms. Many of these hydroceles will resolve in the first year of life if left untreated.

In acquired hydroceles requiring treatment, the approach is in general considered to be surgical. Various surgical techniques have been described, all of which yield satisfactory results (4). The surgical approach is in general preferred due to the high success and low recurrence rates. In symptomatic patients who are poor surgical risks alternative therapies may be considered. Hydroceles may be aspirated with some expected pain relief. In addition, a sclerosing agent such as tetracycline may be placed within the empty space in an effort to keep the fluid from reaccumulating. This treatment has met with mixed results and may be very painful. Other sclerosants have been used including ethanolamine oleate, polidocanol, sodium tetradecyl sulfate, and phenol. Sclerosing therapy typically requires up to three treatment sessions and, although high success rates have been reported (5), many still reserve this treatment for poor surgical candidates. The recurrence and complication rates associated with sclerotherapy are higher than the surgical approach and some side effects can include infection and testicular loss (7). Due to these risks some authors feel that sclerotherapy is not appropriate for young healthy patients (3).

Surgical Technique

There are several successful surgical techniques utilized to treat hydroceles. The scrotum is in general shaved and, along with the penis, the entire area is cleaned with antiseptic prep. The approach is usually midline scrotal or transverse between transversely running blood vessels

unless the diagnosis is in question. These cases should be approached inguinally. The incision should be carried down to the tunica vaginalis, where the blue hue of the hydrocele is seen. The hydrocele and testicle may be delivered through the incision. Blunt dissection and use of a surgical sponge will free any surrounding tissue from the hydrocele sac. Once this parietal layer of tunica vaginalis is exposed, one may select the type of procedure to perform. In general, the Lord procedure is suitable for more thin-walled hydroceles whereas the other described techniques are used with thicker sacs.

Andrews Procedure

This technique is commonly referred to as the "bottle operation." A 2- to 3-cm incision is made in the hydrocele sac near the superior portion (Fig. 76–1). The testicle is then delivered through the opening in the tunica vaginalis, everting the hydrocele sac around the testicle. The procedure may be completed by tacking the cut edges around the cord structures or leaving the everted sac open. A two-layer wound closure is then accomplished, reapproximating skin over the dartos layer.

Jaboulay or Winkleman Procedure

After delivering the testicle through an incision in the tunica, the majority of the sac is then resected, leaving a small cuff along the borders of the testicle. After everting the remnant, bleeding may then be controlled rapidly by a running suture closing the free edges around the cord structures (Fig. 76–2). Reapproximation of the edges is done loosely around the cord so as not to compromise the blood supply to the testicle. In another variation of this technique the parietal tunica vaginalis is resected nearly flush with the testis and epididymis. Electrocautery may be used around the edge to aid in hemostasis or bleeders

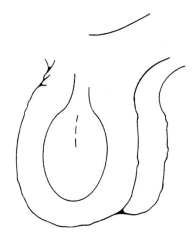

FIG. 76–1. The Andrews operation. A small incision is made high in the sac prior to eversion of the sac about the cord.

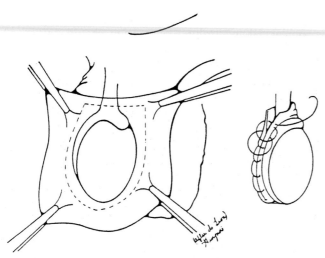

FIG. 76–2. The Jaboulay or Winkleman technique. The redundant sac is excised, leaving enough to be loosely closed about the cord. A running suture may be used to close the sac and rapidly control bleeding from the free edges.

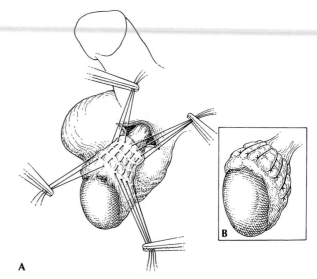

A

FIG. 76–4. The Lord operation. The testis is extruded through a small incision placed in the middle of the sac and interrupted plicating sutures are placed in a circumferential fashion.

may be ligated (Fig. 76–3). The standard two-layer closure is used to close the scrotum.

Lord Procedure

In utilizing this technique for hydrocelectomy, a small scrotal incision is made just large enough to deliver the testis into the field. The parietal layer of the tunica vaginalis is opened, without dissection from the dartos layer. Placing Allis forceps on the cut edges allows the testicle to be brought into the wound. Next, the edges are plicated circumferentially with interrupted 2-0 or 3-0 chromic catgut sutures, placing them about 1 cm apart. The bites should be approximately 1 cm as well (Fig. 76–4). As these sutures are tied the sac will accordion, forming a

collar around the testis and epididymis (Fig. 76–5). Wound closure is accomplished as discussed for the other procedures.

In general, any of these procedures may be performed without surgical drainage. When hemostasis is difficult to obtain, a small Penrose drain placed through a separate stab incision in the inferior aspect of the scrotum and left overnight is useful. This maneuver will also help prevent serous fluid from accumulating in the scrotum postoperatively. Because the scrotum is difficult to dress, fluff dressings held in place by a standard athletic supporter do well in this situation. An ice pack is kept in place for at least 24 hours to help diminish postoperative pain and swelling. Oral analgesics are utilized for several days. Antibiotics are usually not required.

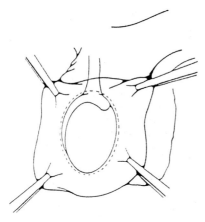

FIG. 76–3. Alternate technique. The sac is excised nearly flush with the testicle and epididymis and bleeders are ligated or fulgurated individually.

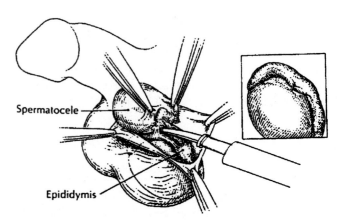

Spermatocele

Epididymis

FIG. 76–5. The sutures are tied and the sac will "accordion" into a collar superior to the testicle.

SPERMATOCELE

A spermatocele (from the Greek *spermatos* for sperm and *kele* for cyst or mass) is a cystic structure arising out of the epididymis, rete testis, or ductuli efferentes. These structures are filled with spermatozoa containing fluid that may be milky. These cysts are usually outside the tunica vaginalis and, as with hydroceles, transilluminate easily. They are frequently seen on scrotal ultrasound as an incidental finding and may be present in as many as 30% of males.

The etiology of most spermatoceles is idiopathic although trauma, infection, or an inflammatory process within the epididymis or scrotum may precede the development of a spermatocele. It is hypothesized that the epididymal ducts become obstructed, causing proximal dilation. The cause of the obstruction is thought to be the seminiferous epithelium continually shedding immature germ cells that are deposited in the efferent ducts, causing a blockage (1).

Diagnosis

Because most spermatoceles are asymptomatic, incidental discovery on self-examination or on physical exam by a physician are the most common ways a spermatocele is detected. The typical location within the scrotum is cephalad and sometimes posterior to the testicle; however, they may arise from any location on the epididymis.

These cystic structures are not usually painful, are round, and have distinct borders. The mass is easily separable from the testis.

Indications for Surgery

Most spermatoceles do not require intervention. Painful or large and embarrassing spermatoceles may require some intervention. Surgery should be entertained when there is a question of diagnosis of a potential tumor.

Alternative Therapy

In those requiring treatment, the options are aspiration with the use of sclerosing agents and surgery. Results are similar to those of hydrocele.

Surgical Technique

The spermatocele is approached through the same incision as for the hydrocele. The tunica vaginalis is incised and the testicle along with the spermatocele delivered into the incision. Utilizing sharp dissection, the cystic structure may be excised or "shelled out" from the epididymis without excessive mobilization of the epididymis or testis (Fig. 76–6). On occasion, an attachment to the epididymis can be identified and ligated. Hemostasis is accomplished with a needle-tip cautery or chromic

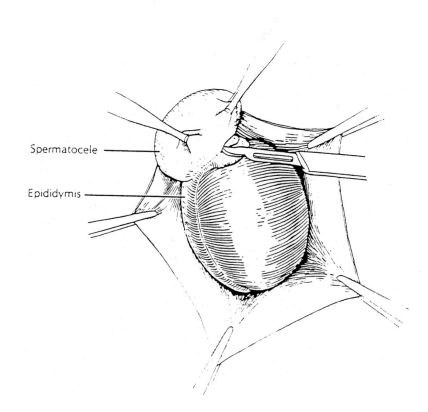

Spermatocele

Epididymis

FIG. 76–6. Spermatocelectomy. The spermatocele is separated from the globus major of the epididymis by sharp dissection and excised.

ligatures. The edges of the epididymis are reapproximated or a portion of adjacent fascia or tunica may be used to close the epididymal defect. It may be necessary to resect a portion of the tunica vaginalis in some cases or to perform a hydrocelectomy in conjunction with this procedure. Wound closure and postoperative management is similar to that for hydrocelectomy.

OUTCOMES

Complications

The usual surgical complications are seen with these procedures. The most common seen is hematoma, usually within the scrotum. Wound infection, scrotal abscess, and recurrent hydrocele or spermatocele complete the list but are much less common. There is some evidence that the Lord procedure for hydrocelectomy has fewer of these complications (2,6).

Results

Most patients have a successful outcome with a minimal incidence of recurrence.

REFERENCES

1. Itoh M, Li XQ, Miyamoto K, Takeuchi Y. Degeneration of the seminiferous epithelium with ageing is a cause of spermatocele? *Int J Androl* 1999;22(2):91.
2. Kaye K, Clayman RV, Lange PH. Outpatient hydrocele and spermatocele repair under local anesthesia. *J Urol* 1983;130:269.
3. Ku JH, Kim ME, Lee NK, Park YH. The excisional, plication and internal drainage techniques: a comparison of the results for idiopathic hydrocele. *Br J Urol Int* 2001;87:82.
4. Landes RR, Leonhardt KO. The history of hydrocele. *Urol Surv* 1967;17:135.
5. Nash JR. Sclerotherapy for hydrocele and epididymal cysts: a five year study. *Br Med J Clin Res* 1984;288(6431):1652.
6. Rodriguez WC, Rodriguez DD, Fortunado RF. The operative treatment of hydrocele: a comparison of four basic techniques. *J Urol* 1981;125:804.
7. Thompson H, Odell M. Sclerosant treatment for hydroceles and epididymal cysts. *Br Med J* 1979;2:704.

CHAPTER 77

Congenital Curvature

Kurt A. McCammon

Normal erectile function is not only dependent on normal vascular and neurological function but also requires elasticity and compliance of all tissue layers of the penis. During tumescence the penis begins to fill with blood and the corporal bodies and tunica albuginea reach their limits of compliance, causing rigidity. Patients with straight erections have normal and symmetrical expansion of the tunica albuginea. Those with curvature have an asymmetrical expansion of one aspect of their penis. This could be due to decreased compliance of one aspect of the tunica or foreshortening of one erectile body.

Patients usually present in their late teens to early 30s. Most men cannot remember their penis being straight and have always assumed their curvature was normal. After puberty and onset of sexual activity, they realize that the curvature impedes normal sexual relations. Some patients also notice that their curvature worsens with puberty. On occasion, a patient will present after the age of 30 either having been sexually active but found it difficult functionally or psychologically or, less commonly, sexually inactive due to the curvature and the embarrassment he feels.

Penile curvature is described as either congenital or acquired. There is some confusion with the terms "congenital curvature" and "chordee without hypospadias." Some use these terms interchangeably; however, we do not think they are synonymous. This curvature is associated with abnormalities of the ventral tissue planes or the corpus spongiosum.

Devine and Horton proposed a classification system for congenital penile curvature identifying five separate types of curvature (2). Types I to III can be collectively termed chordee without hypospadias (Fig. 77–1). This refers to an abnormal development of ventral penile tissue with the patient having a normally placed meatus. For patients with type I, none of the surrounding layers are normal and there is malfusion of the corpus spongiosum. Patients with type II curvature have a dysgenic band of

fibrous tissue lateral and dorsal to the urethra, which is believed to have formed from the mesenchyme that would have become Buck's and dartos fasciae. In type III congenital curvature, the patient's urethra, corpus spongiosum, and Buck's fascia are all developed normally.

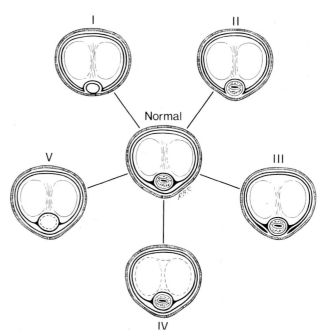

FIG. 77–1. Cross section of the penis displaying the forms of congenital curvatures of the penis. The normal penis is in the center. *Class I:* Epithelial urethra beneath the skin. Dysgenic tissue beneath it represents undeveloped corpus spongiosum, Buck's fascia, and dartos fascia. *Class II:* Normal urethra and spongiosum but abnormal Buck's and dartos fasciae. *Class III:* Abnormal dartos fascia only. *Class IV:* Normal urethra and fascial layers with abnormal corpocavernosal development. *Class V:* Congenital short urethra (rare). (From Devine CJ Jr, Horton CE. Bent penis. *Sem Urol* 1987;5:252, with permission.)

603

The abnormality in these patients is in the dartos fascia, which has an elastic band that causes the penis to bend sharply. Not infrequently these patients have a large and prominent mons pubis.

Type IV curvature is commonly referred to as congenital curvature of the penis by the authors. In type IV penile curvature development of the urethra, fascial layers, and corpus spongiosum is normal but there is also a relative shortness or inelastic area of the tunica albuginea. Experience with these patients has shown that they have a penis of normal length when flaccid but when erect the penis may be larger than expected, thought to be due to hypercompliance of the tunica albuginea. Many of these patients will note curvature prior to puberty but this becomes more accentuated after pubescence and the penile growth spurt that occurs during adolescence.

Type V curvature is the rarest of all types and some even question whether it exists. This type is known as the congenitally short urethra. The short urethra is not elastic enough or of adequate length, leading to ventral curvature during erections.

DIAGNOSIS

All patients should undergo a complete history, including an extensive sexual history and physical examination. Complete examination is done to rule out evidence of subclinical fracture or Peyronie's disease, which is obviously rare in the younger patient population. Patients are required to supply photographs of their erect penis for documentation of the curvature. The photographs are beneficial in distinguishing between congenital curvature and chordee without hypospadias. Psychological aspects of the disease also need to be addressed. On occasion, patients are evaluated preoperatively by a certified sex therapist and treated as needed.

Patients with chordee without hypospadias usually present with a ventral or ventral lateral curvature and are noted to have a penis that is normal or shorter than normal in length. As mentioned earlier these patients also have noted penile curvature throughout their whole life and may note some progression of the curvature during puberty. Many of these patients have abnormalities of the ventral penile skin. This may be a hooded preputial skin or a high insertion of the penoscrotal skin. The deep ventral tissues of the penis seem to be inelastic to examination and stretch. The inelastic tissue that is palpable is the dysgenic tissue that has replaced Buck's and dartos fasciae.

Some of these patients, because of their curvature and smaller than average length, have poor self-images. When identified, these are the patients who benefit from psychological counseling preoperatively.

INDICATIONS FOR SURGERY

Patients who have significant enough curvature to impair their sexual function are candidates for surgery. Surgery for chordee without hypospadias is successful in this patient population, with most curvatures repaired in a single procedure. Many times the curvature is corrected with excision of the dysgenic tissue on the ventrum of the penis and mobilizing the corpus spongiosum.

ALTERNATIVE THERAPY

There are no alternatives to surgery.

SURGICAL TECHNIQUE

There are a wide variety of surgical procedures to repair congenital curvature including incision and plication, incision with grafting, or penile disassembly. Most patients with congenital curvature are straightened completely with incision and plication.

Incision and Plication

If the patient has been previously circumcised an incision is made through the circumcision scar. Due to the previous circumcision there are new patterns of lymph and venous drainage and an incision proximal or distal to the old scar could lead to marked penile edema. The incision is made down to the superficial layer of Buck's fascia and the penis is degloved in this plane. Once completely degloved, an artificial erection is created using intravenous normal saline and a high-pressure pump. Perineal pressure may be needed initially, but prolonged pressure is not needed as these patients have normal erectile function. A tourniquet placed at the base of the penis is not recommended as this can mask the proximal extent of curvature.

The artificial erection demonstrates the degree and location of maximal curvature. In patients with ventral curvature a layer of dysgenic tissue may be noted that includes Buck's and dartos fasciae. This tissue is completely mobilized and excised. Care is taken not to injure the corpus spongiosum, which will need to be detached from the glans to the penoscrotal junction. If injured the urethra is closed primarily. Patients who suffer from a differential elasticity between dorsal and ventral aspects of the corporal bodies may receive some benefit from the excision of the inelastic dysgenic tissue but are rarely straight and often require further maneuvers to straighten the penis. An artificial erection is repeated after this and if straight the skin is closed (Fig. 77–2).

The options to straighten the penis are to either lengthen the short side with incisions and grafts or shorten the long side with excisions and/or incisions and plication. In the set of patients where penile length is not a major issue we usu-

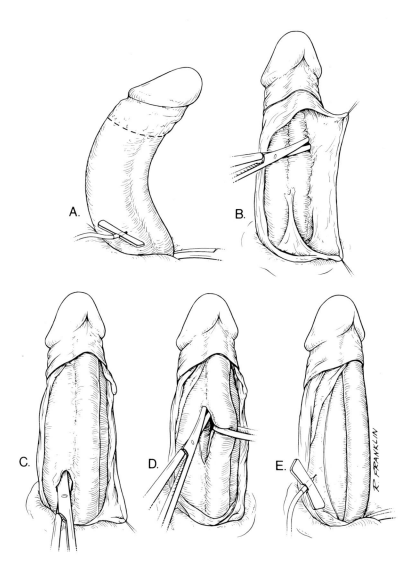

FIG. 77–2. Surgery for chordee without hypospadias. **A:** Ventral curvature demonstrated with artificial erection. **B:** Dysgenic dartos fascia is elevated and will be excised. **C:** The dysgenic layer of Buck's fascia is undermined by spreading the scissors. **D:** The inelastic fascia is excised as the corpus spongiosum and urethra are mobilized. **E:** Artificial erection demonstrates correction of the curvature.

ally choose to excise and perform plications. The patients recover from this more quickly and graft take is not an issue. Although rare, there is a possibility to induce venoocclusive dysfunction with dermal grafts (Fig. 77–3).

Once it has been determined to proceed with excision of tunica and dorsal plication, Buck's fascia is elevated incorporating the neurovascular structures via one of two techniques. One approach is to start lateral to the corpus spongiosum and carry the incision medially. The alternative approach is to excise the deep dorsal vein and approach the tunica from the dorsal midline. If done through this approach, after the dorsal vein is excised the inner layer of Buck's fascia is elevated off the tunica including the dorsal neurovascular structures; this dissection is carried laterally to the corpus spongiosum.

An artificial erection is again performed and the point of maximal curvature identified. The areas of ellipses are identified and marked. Edges of the planned ellipses are

opposed with a 3-0 polypropylene (Prolene) suture and a repeat artificial erection is performed. If this demonstrates adequate straightening the edges are marked, the suture is removed, and the ellipse of tunica is excised using a sharp scalpel. The underlying erectile tissue is left undisturbed by staying in the space of Smith. Watertight closure is performed with interrupted 4-0 PDS and a running 5-0 PDS. An artificial erection is performed after each ellipse is excised to determine results. If it is not straight further ellipses are excised to straighten the penis.

Once straight, Buck's fascia is closed. Two small suction drains are placed superficial to Buck's fascia. The skin is reapproximated with a 4-0 Vicryl suture and a small Foley is placed overnight. A bioocclusive dressing is placed. The Foley catheter is removed on postoperative day 1. One drain is removed in the morning as well and if output is low the other is removed that afternoon and the patient is discharged from the hospital.

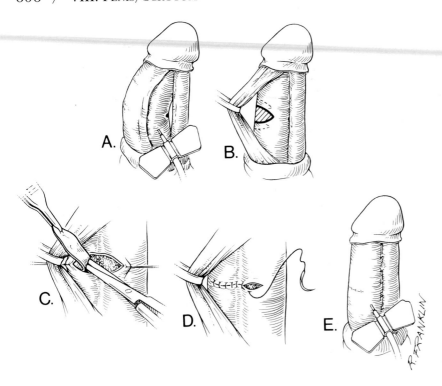

FIG. 77–3. Surgery for chordee without hypospadias. **A:** A circumcision incision has been made and the urethra has been mobilized by resecting the dartos and Buck's fasciae. The needle is in place for an artificial erection. The erection shows continuing chordee. The elastic urethra is not the cause of this curvature. The point of maximum concavity has been marked. **B:** An ellipse of tissue is outlined opposite the point of maximum concavity. As an alternative, two smaller ellipses are shown. **C:** Excision of the ellipse of tunica. Note the tips of the septal strands in the midline. **D:** Closure of the edges of the incision. **E:** Artificial erection revealing a straight penis. When the bend is more complex, ellipses must be excised in other locations. (From Devine CJ Jr, Horton CE. Bent penis. *Sem Urol* 1987;5:4, with permission.)

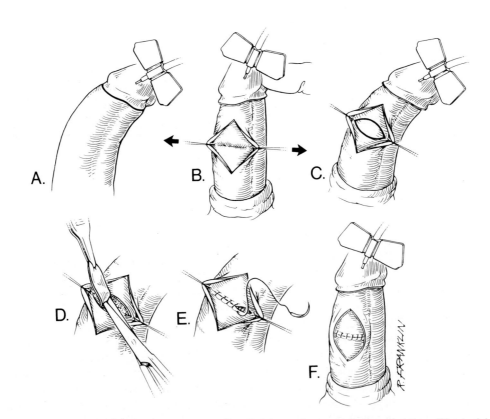

FIG. 77–4. Congenital lateral curvature. **A:** An artificial erection reveals the curvature. The incision to gain access to the potential ellipse of tissue is marked. **B:** The tunica albuginea has been exposed by mobilizing Buck's fascia, and Prolene sutures have been placed at the dorsal and ventral tips of the potential ellipse. While maintaining the artificial erection, tension is established on the two sutures as the penile shaft is straightened. The fold produced in the tunica is marked. **C:** When the penis is relaxed, this mark defines the ellipse of tunica to be removed. **D:** The tunica is excised. **E:** The edges are approximated. **F:** The penis is straight. Buck's fascia and the skin are closed.

Patients with lateral curvature may have associated ventral curvature or rarely dorsal curvature. On occasion, patients with lateral curvature may only have lateral curvature. In patients with only lateral curvature this can be approached through a small incision at the maximal point of curvature. After an artificial erection is obtained the point of maximal curvature is identified and a small incision is made on the contralateral side at the site of maximal convexity. Again, there is minimal dissection of the dorsal neurovascular structures. 3-0 Prolene sutures are placed and an artificial erection is performed; if straight, ellipses are excised and closed as previously discussed (Fig. 77–4).

Although uncommon, congenital dorsal curvature is usually approached through a circumcising incision. The corpus spongiosum is partially mobilized so that small incisions in the corpora can be placed just lateral to the ventral midline. The techniques used are those previously described and the postoperative course is similar to that of the patient with ventral curve.

Yachia Longitudinal Plication

There are other techniques described for the repair of congenital curvature. Yachia described a plication procedure using longitudinal incisions in the tunica albuginea that are closed transversely (6,7). The long side is therefore plicated without excising tunica. The procedure is similar as previously described with an incision through the previous circumcision scar and complete mobilization (Fig. 77–5).

Multiple Parallel Plication

Multiple parallel plication (MMP) is another technique used in the repair of congenital curvature of the penis without excising any tunica albuginea. In the original descrip-

tion, a pharmacological agent is used to induce an erection. A circumcising incision is performed, the penis is degloved, and the deep dorsal artery and vein are identified. The dorsal neurovascular bundle does not need to be dissected and freed. Multiple deep plication sutures are placed into the tunica albuginea at the point of maximal curvature between the deep dorsal artery and vein using four to six nonabsorbable 3-0 braided sutures. Some of the sutures may not be fully tied down to prevent overcorrection. For patients with lateral or ventral lateral curvature the sutures are placed more laterally using the same vertical orientation. When the patient has dorsal curvature a ventral incision is made and the sutures are placed just lateral to the corpus spongiosum (which does not need to be mobilized).

Penile Disassembly

Perovic and colleagues proposed a penile disassembly technique in hopes of avoiding penile shortening with the plication procedures (5). This technique requires complete disassembly of the penis into its component parts, these being the glans cap with its neurovascular bundle dorsally, the urethra ventrally, and the corporal bodies. Unfortunately, this technique only straightens the penis satisfactorily in 68% of patients and on occasion a plication procedure was required.

Chordee Without Hypospadias

The corpus spongiosum is rarely the limiting factor in these patients even if they appear to have obvious abnormalities. The curvature in these patients is due mainly to the inelasticity of the ventral aspect of the corporal bodies. After the dysgenic tissue is excised, if there is residual chordee a small incision can be made in the ventral midline of the corporal bodies after an artificial erection is obtained. The erectile tissue is not entered with this incision and this allows the ventral tunica to move laterally and noticeably straightens the penis. If this is unsuccessful in correcting the curvature the dorsal neurovascular structures are mobilized and a small ellipse of tunica is excised and closed as discussed earlier (Fig. 77–6).

Some advocate the use of dermal grafts for patients with chordee without hypospadias, especially in those patients with severe chordee or those with a smaller than average penis. This approach does not shorten the penis as a plication procedure would, but there are complications associated with it as well. The major concern with placing a dermal graft is the risk of venoocclusive dysfunction. This is a known complication when using dermis in adult patients with Peyronie's disease. It is thought that the pediatric patient may not develop venoocclusive dysfunction because no tunica is excised and a much smaller graft is used than in the adult. No long-term studies have been published following these patients into adult life to determine the risk.

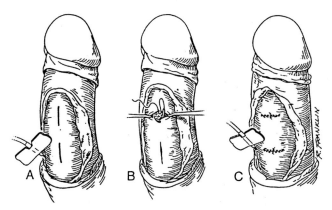

FIG. 77–5. Technique after Yachia for correction of curvature, in this case a patient with congenital lateral curvature. **A:** Buck's fascia is reflected, exposing the lateral tunica albuginea. **B:** Longitudinal incisions are created at the area of maximal curvature as demonstrated by artificial erection. **C:** The longitudinal closures are closed transversely, with artificial erection demonstrating good straightening of the penis.

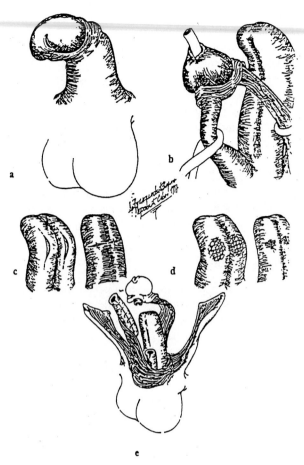

FIG. 77–6.

OUTCOMES

Complications

Surgical complications associated with congenital penile curvature surgery are relatively rare. This is in general a healthy population of patients. The surgical procedure is 85% to 100% successful in reported series. Complications including complaints of penile shortening and penile irregularity from suture sites are heard. There are also complaints of suture granuloma and sometimes pain at the plication site. Temporary loss of glans sensation has been reported in the past and there is one report of a patient with permanent loss of sensation. Postoperative erectile dysfunction is extremely rare and there is one reported case of penile necrosis secondary to a tourniquet; we would not recommend using these.

Results

Eight percent of MMP patients were satisfied with their correction although two of the eight had to undergo a second procedure to correct a residual 15% curvature. All patients did notice the sutures but only one considered them bothersome.

REFERENCES

1. Baskin LS, Lue TF. The correction of congenital penile curvature in young men. *Br J Urol* 1998;81:895–899.
2. Devine CJ, Horton CE. Chordee without hypospadias. *J Urol* 1973; 110:264–271.
3. Kaplan GW, Brock WA. The etiology of chordee. *Urol Clin North Am* 1981;8:383–387.
4. Kramer SA, Aydin G, Kelalis PP. Chordee without hypospadias in children. *J Urol* 1982;128:559.
5. Perovic SV, Djordjevic MLJ, Djakovic NG. A new approach to the treatment of penile curvature. *J Urol* 1998;160:1123–1127.
6. Yachia D. Modified corporoplasty for the treatment of penile curvature. *J Urol* 1990;143:80–82.
7. Yachia D, Beyar M, Aridagon A, Dasc S. The incidence of congenital penile curvature. *J Urol* 1993;150.1478–1479.

SECTION IX

Urinary Diversion

Section Editor: Yrs E. Studer

CHAPTER 78

Ileal Conduit Urinary Diversion

Michael Aleman and Eric A. Klein

Despite the emerging popularity of continent catheterizable and orthotopic voiding urinary diversion techniques, the ileal conduit remains the most common form of urinary diversion performed worldwide. The operation, first described by Bricker in 1950 (1), maintains this popularity in large part because of its applicability to a wide variety of urologic disorders, its tolerability in patients with often significant comorbidities, and its adaptability to almost all patients' anatomic constraints.

DIAGNOSIS

The ileal conduit may be constructed as part of a reconstruction following extirpative pelvic surgery, such as radical or simple cystectomy and pelvic exenteration, or as a diversion with the bladder left *in situ*, such as in cases of neuropathic bladder refractory to conservative management. The clinical evaluation in these patients is therefore directed to their bladder pathology.

INDICATIONS FOR SURGERY

Before choosing an ileal conduit, patients should be counseled on all forms of diversion. Comorbidities such as renal insufficiency (serum creatinine greater than 2.5mg per dL), bowel disease (inflammatory or malignant), extreme obesity, or neurological illness that prevents the ability to perform self-catheterization may make incontinent diversion a wise choice. While it has been suggested in the past that patients with cardiovascular or pulmonary diseases may do better with the shorter, simpler conduit diversions, newer evidence suggests that perioperative morbidity is equivalent with conduit and continent diversions (14).

ALTERNATIVE THERAPY

Continent catheterizable or orthotopic voiding diversions are the most common alternatives to conduit diversion. If the aforementioned concerns make conduit diversion preferable to continent diversion, there still exist options regarding the bowel segment to be used and the type of ureteroenteric anastomosis. Jejunal conduits are associated with a higher incidence of metabolic complications but may be the only viable option in certain patients due to previous surgery, irradiation, or concomitant bowel diseases (9).

Colonic conduits, which are thought to be more protective of kidney function by some surgeons due to their ability to accommodate nonrefluxing anastomoses, may be preferable in children and adults with a longer life expectancy (15). A transverse colon conduit may be wise in patients who have undergone pelvic irradiation due to its higher intraabdominal position. Another use of colon for conduits is the sigmoid conduit diversion in patients who are undergoing pelvic exenteration, with a transverse colostomy that avoids the potential morbidities of a bowel anastomosis.

Other potential urinary diversions include an ileovesicostomy, which can be used in patients undergoing diversion for reasons other than malignancy and avoids the complications associated with ureteral mobilization and ureteroenteric anastomoses. In patients requiring urinary diversion with life expectancies less than several months, percutaneous nephrostomy tubes should be considered.

SURGICAL TECHNIQUE

Most patients can tolerate an at-home preoperative regimen of a clear liquid diet 1 to 2 days before surgery, followed by 4 L of polyethylene glycol on the afternoon before surgery. Broad-spectrum intravenous antibiotics are given at the time of the surgery. The stoma site should be selected after examining the patient in the supine, seated, and standing positions. To best accommodate an appliance the site should not be too near the anterior superior iliac spine, costal margin, umbilicus, surgical scars, or skin folds. The usual ideal location is just medial

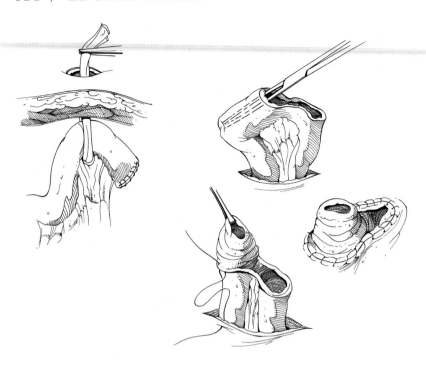

FIG. 78–3. Creation of the end-loop stoma. The defunctionalized limp is positioned cephalad.

78–5. Stents may be passed prior to closure of the anterior wall. This technique allows for the rapid creation of a widely patent ureteroileal anastomosis; its theoretical disadvantage is that a process creating obstruction of one ureter (recurrent malignancy, anastomotic stricture) is more likely to cause bilateral obstruction.

After performing the ureteroileal anastomosis, the proximal end of the conduit is retroperitonealized by sewing the cut edges of the peritoneum to the conduit. Closed-suction drains (Jackson–Pratt type) are placed in the area of the ureteroileal anastomoses and maintained for the first few postoperative days.

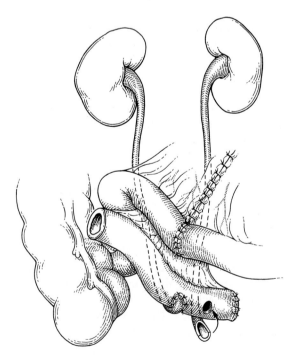

FIG. 78–4. Ideal placement of the vesicoenteric anastomoses using the Bricker technique. The spatulated ureters should pass under the conduit and lie without tension or kinking.

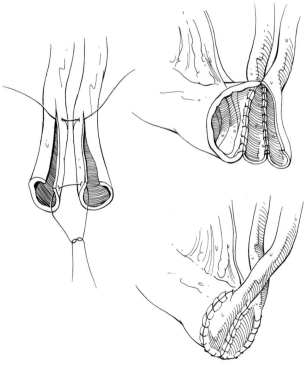

FIG. 78–5. The side-to-side Wallace technique creates a widely patent vesicoenteric anastomosis at the "butt" end of the conduit.

The return of bowel function is the major determinant of the length of the postoperative hospital stay; this is evidenced by similar lengths of hospitalization for urinary diversion procedures with and without cystectomy. Most patients can expect a hospital stay of 6 to 8 days in centers with well-defined clinical pathways (2). Nasogastric decompression is usually maintained for 1 to 2 postoperative days as the initial period of ileus resolves. The conduit also experiences an ileus and its return of peristalsis parallels that of the small bowel; therefore, some surgeons advocate placement of a cut Foley or Rob-Nel catheter to promote conduit drainage in the first few postoperative days. There is no consensus for the optimal length of ureteral stenting (if it is performed at all); the timing of stent removal is left to the discretion of the attending surgeon. Jackson–Pratt drains are left in place until the drainage is negligible; if drainage persists at high levels several days postoperatively, the drain fluid should be sent for creatinine analysis to rule out a urine leak. If a rod is left under the stoma, this may be removed prior to discharge.

Counseling and teaching by the enterostomal therapist should begin in the preoperative period and continue during the hospitalization. The patient or his or her caregivers should be competent in all aspects of stoma care prior to discharge. Follow-up care is tailored to the individual patient; in most cases, a periodic serum renal profile is indicated. In patients undergoing cystectomy for malignancy, urine cytology should be followed. The upper tracts can be assessed via a loopogram, avoiding the toxicity of intravenous contrast agents.

OUTCOMES

Complications

The mortality rate for cystectomy and diversion have steadily decreased over the years since Bricker's initial description; in a recent series a mortality rate of 0.3% was reported (2). Most centers report rates in the 1% to 3% range.

The most common morbidity causing prolonged hospital stay is paralytic ileus (2). These usually resolve quickly with nasogastric decompression; failure to do so after a few days should prompt a diagnostic workup for bowel obstruction. Urine leak at the ureteroileal anastomosis or from the conduit closure and urosepsis are the most common urologic complications of the procedure. Urine leaks can usually be managed successfully with percutaneous nephrostomy diversion.

Late complications of ileal conduits are common but usually are not severe. Stomal stenosis has been reported in up to 29% of ileal conduits (11); proper stoma construction can decrease this incidence. Hyperchloremic metabolic acidosis can occur but is rare in well-functioning conduit; the presence of more than a mild acidosis should prompt an evaluation for obstruction or redundancy of the conduit. Alkalinizing agents or chloride transport blockers (chlorpromazine, nicotinic acid) can effectively treat this acidosis. Ureteroileal anastomotic strictures are also uncommon (about 6% in older series); these can be successfully managed with dilation with a cutting balloon [about a 50% success rate (4)] or with open surgical repair [76% long-term success (5)].

Acute pyelonephritis occurs commonly in patients with ileal conduits (18% of patients). Indeed, bacteriuria can be found in up to three-quarters of ileal conduit urine specimens (13). Most of these can be safely observed without treatment as patients seem to tolerate this chronic colonization well and few progress to acute pyelonephritis. Infections with *Proteus* or *Pseudomonas* are associated with deterioration of the upper tracts and should therefore be treated.

Deterioration in renal function occurs in a significant portion of patients undergoing conduit diversion; over the long term, 7% of patients can develop renal failure requiring dialysis (11). Renal function should be monitored periodically, and declines in function should alert the clinician to examine for correctable causes of renal dysfunction.

Results

The ileal conduit has provided reliable urinary diversion for patients with a variety of underlying illnesses for over 50 years. Continent catheterizable diversions and orthotopic neobladders continue to gain acceptance, and recent studies have focused on quality of life outcomes after continent and incontinent diversions. While some of these studies (7,12) have suggested a significant quality of life advantage to continent diversions, others (6,8) have shown minimal difference. Unfortunately, as younger, thinner, and healthier patients undergo continent diversion while older and more frail patients undergo ileal conduit, a real comparison of the quality of life after these procedures will likely never be possible. Still, it is clear that ileal conduit is a simple form of diversion that is well tolerated by most patients and has fewer contraindications than continent diversions. These factors make it likely that the ileal conduit will continue to play a major role in many urologists' practices.

REFERENCES

1. Bricker EM. Bladder substitution after pelvic evisceration. *Surg Clin North Am* 1950;30:1511.
2. Chang SS, Baumgartner RG, Wells N, Cookson MS, Smith JA Jr. Causes of increased hospital stay after radical cystectomy in a clinical pathway setting. *J Urol* 2002;167:208.
3. Chechile G, Klein EA, Bauer L, Novick AC, Montie JE. Functional equivalence of end and loop ileal conduit stomas. *J Urol* 1992;147:582.
4. Cornud F, Chretien Y, Helenon O, Casanova JM, Correas JM, Bonnel D, Mejean A, Moreau JF. Percutaneous incision of stenotic uroenteric anastomoses with a cutting balloon catheter: long-term results. *Radiology* 2000;214:358.

5. DiMarco DS, LeRoy AJ, Thieling S, Bergstralh EJ, Segura JW. Long-term results of treatment for ureteroenteric strictures. *Urology* 2001;58:909.

6. Dutta SC, Chang SC, Coffey CS, Smith JA Jr, Jack G, Cookson MS. Health related quality of life assessment after radical cystectomy: comparison of ileal conduit with continent orthotopic neobladder. *J Urol* 2002;168:164.

7. Hobisch A, Tosun K, Kinzl J, Kemmler G, Bartsch G, Holtl L, Stenzl A. Life after cystectomy and orthotopic neobladder versus ileal conduit urinary diversion. *Sem Urol Oncol* 2001;19:18.

8. Kitamura H, Miyao N, Yanase M, Masumori N, Matsukawa M, Takahashi A, Itoh N, Tsukamoto T. Quality of life in patients having an ileal conduit, continent reservoir or orthotopic neobladder after cystectomy for bladder carcinoma. *Int J Urol* 1999;6:393.

9. Klein EA, Montie JE, Montague DK, Kay R, Straffon RA. Jejunal conduit urinary diversion. *J Urol* 1986;135:244.

10. Leduc A, Camey M, Teillac P. An original antireflux ureteroileal implantation technique: long-term follow-up. *J Urol* 1987;137:1156.

11. McDougal WS. Use of intestinal segments and urinary diversion. In: Walsh PC, Retik AB, Vaughn ED Jr, Wein AJ, eds. *Campbell's urology*, 7th ed. Philadelphia, W.B. Saunders, 1998.

12. McGuire MS, Grimaldi G, Grotas J, Russo P. The type of urinary diversion after radical cystectomy significantly impacts on the patient's quality of life. *Ann Surg Oncol* 2000;7:4.

13. Middleton AW Jr, Hendren WH. Ileal conduits in children at the Massachusetts General Hospital from 1955 to 1970. *J Urol* 1976;115:591.

14. Parekh DJ, Gilbert WB, Koch MO, Smith JA Jr. Continent urinary reconstruction versus ileal conduit: a contemporary single-institution comparison of perioperative morbidity and mortality. *Urology* 2000;55:852.

15. Stein R, Fisch M, Stockle M, Demirkesen O, Hohenfellner R. Colonic conduit in children: protection of the upper urinary tract 16 years later? *J Urol* 1996;156:1146.

16. Stone AR, Macdermott JPA. The split-cuff ureteral nipple reimplantation technique: reliable reflux prevention from bowel segments. *J Urol* 1989;143:707.

17. Turnbull RB Jr, Fazio V. Advances in the surgical technique of ulcerative colitis surgery: endoanal proctectomy and two-directional myotomy ileostomy. *Surg Annu* 1975;7:315.

CHAPTER 79

Transverse Colonic Conduit

Rudolf Hohenfellner and Margit Fisch

Since the first publication in1969 (10), the transverse colonic conduit has been more and more implemented in patients with urologic or gynecological malignancy and additional radiotherapy (2,9,11,12). With its cranial position outside the irradiation field it fulfills the demand to be nonirradiated, which is of utmost importance for a segment to be used for urinary diversion. Not only the transverse segment but also the ascending and descending colon can be used, which offers an adaptation to the individual patient's situation. The ascending and descending colon are located in a retroperitoneal position as the sigmoid. There are no limitations with regard to short ureters. As a part of the colon, the segments offers the feasability for antirefluxive as well as refluxive ureteral implantation (3,5,8,13) and positioning of the stoma either to the left or right upper abdomen. In addition, colon can be used either in an isoperistaltic or anisoperistaltic way and is less prone to stoma stenosis as ileum when used for creation of a conduit.

In patients with total damage of the ureters by irradiation or retroperitoneal fibrosis and in patients with recurrent urothelial tumor in a single kidney (7), a direct anastomosis of the conduit to the renal pelvis represents an option (pyelotransverse pyelocutaneostomy) (4).

DIAGNOSIS

Preoperatively an intravenous (IV) urograghy should be performed to evaluate the upper urinary tract. An enema with water-soluble contrast medium should be done to exclude diverticula or polyps. The bowel is irrigated with Ringer's lactate solution (8 to 10 L) via a gastric tube or oral intake of 5 to 7 L of Fordtran's solution. The day before surgery, positioning of the stoma should be done. The best position is in the epigastric region; the attached stoma plate has to be checked in sitting, lying, and standing positions of the patient.

INDICATIONS FOR SURGERY

Indications for transverse colonic conduit include urinary diversion in patients with urologic/gynecological malignancies and irradiation damage of bowel and distal ureters. Other indications are urinary incontinence in patients with radiation cystitis, complex vesicovaginal and rectovesicovaginal fistulae after irradiation, recurrent retroperitoneal fibrosis, Crohn's disease, and unsuccessful primary urinary diversion requiring conversion. In patients with recurrent urothelial tumors and a single kidney a direct anastomosis of a conduit to the renal pelvis allows direct endoscopic access to the calices. Absolute contraindications for the transverse colonic conduit are irradiation of the upper abdomen, status postextensive colon resection, and ulcerative colitis.

ALTERNATIVE THERAPY

In young patients a continent transverse pouch (6) represents an alternative.

SURGICAL TECHNIQUE

Instruments required include a basic kidney set with additional instruments for intraabdominal surgery , Siegel's retractor, suction, and a basin containing prepared iodine solution for disinfection. As suture material absorbable monofilament sutures like polyglycolic acid 4-0 are used for closure of the conduit and intestinal anastomosis to reestablish bowel continuity as well as creation of the stoma. The ureters are implanted using 5-0 and 6-0. Intraoperatively, a gastric tube (alternatively gastrostomy), a rectal tube, and a central venous catheter are placed.

Access is gained by median laparotomy. Both ureters are identified at the crossing over the iliac vessels and dissected in the cranial direction. The dissection toward the bladder goes down until the irradiated level is reached. The ureters are cut above the irradiated field where they show good vascularization. There should be capillary arterial bleeding out of the ureteral wall and spontaneous urine efflux. The ureteral stump is ligated and the cranial end is marked by a stay suture. Depending on the remaining length of the ureters it is decided which one can be brought to the opposite side by a retromesenteric pull-through. The retromesenteric entrance should be wide enough and the path of the ureter slightly curved in order not to angle or compress it.

A bowel segment of approximately 15 cm in length in patients with normal weight is selected respecting the course of the vessels (Fig. 79–1). The length of the segment depends on the thickness of abdominal wall. Stay sutures outline the segment. Bowel mobilization differs depending on the segment chosen: If the ascending segment is selected the right colonic flexure is mobilized. The greater omentum is separated from the transverse colon over a distance of 10 to 15 cm starting at the right side. When the descending colon is chosen, the left colonic flexure has to be mobilized and the left part of the omentum has to be separated from the transverse colon. The selection of a transverse colonic segment makes mobilization of both the right and left flexure necessary as well as a complete separation of the greater omentum from the transverse colon.

The mesentery of the selected segment is incised lateral to the supplying artery and the arcade is divided between mosquito clamps and ligated. The fat is dissected from the seromuscularis of the bowel in the area where the segment will be cut and bleeding vessels are coagulated. The segment is isolated without the use of clamps so that the bleeding out of the ends can be seen. The segment is cleaned using moist sponges. Bowel continuity is reestablished by a one-layer seromuscular suture using polyglycolic acid 4-0 and the mesenteric slit is closed by running suture (Fig. 79–2).

One option for ureteral reimplantation uses the Wallace technique (13). Both ureters are resected to an adequate length and spatulated over a distance of 3 cm. A stay suture is placed at the 6-o'clock position and a ureteral stent inserted. The first suture for anastomosis of the medial margins of the ureters is placed at the 12-o'clock position and tied later. The anastomosis is performed by a running suture polyglycolic acid 5-0. The ureteral stents are fixed to the ureteral mucosa (polyglactin 4-0 with short reabsorption time) and subsequently brought out through the conduit. The ureteral plate is then anastomosed to the oral end of the conduit by two running sutures of polyglycolic acid 5-0 (Fig. 79–3a). When the conduit is positioned on the right side and the left ureter is relatively short, it can be implanted antidromically to the right ureter (like the "crossed hands of a ballerina"; Fig. 79–3b).

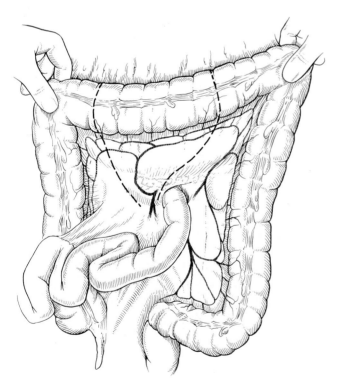

FIG 79–1. A bowel segment of approximately 15 cm in length in patients with normal weight is selected respecting the course of the vessels.

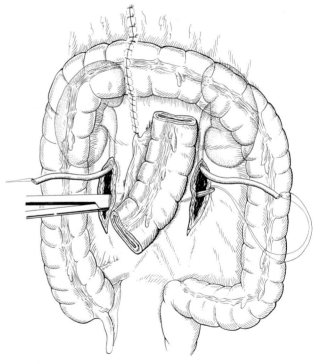

FIG 79–2. Bowel continuity is reestablished by a one-layer seromuscular suture using polyglycolic acid 4-0 and the mesenteric slit is closed by running suture.

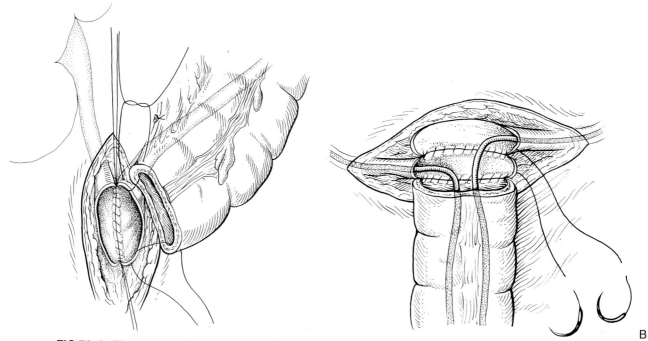

A   B

FIG 79–3. The ureteral plate is then anastomosed to the oral end of the conduit by two running sutures of polyglycolic acid 5-0.

An alternative method of ureteral reimplantation is a direct implantation using a "buttonhole" technique. The conduit is longitudinally opened in the area of the taenia libera over a length of 3 to 4 cm starting at the oral end. Two stay sutures are placed at the backwall of the conduit. The mucosa in between is excised and the seromuscular layer incised to create an entrance for the ureter (Fig. 79–4a). The ureter is pulled through and implanted by two anchor sutures at the 5- and 7-o'clock positions (polyglycolic acid 4-0) and mucomucous sutures (polyglycolic acid 5-0). A stent is inserted, fixed, and led out through the conduit (Fig. 79–4b). The contralateral ureter is implanted in the same manner and the conduit closed (Fig. 79–4c).

Our preferred method for antirefluxive ureteral implantation is the Goodwin–Hohenfellner technique (1). The conduit is longitudinally opened over a length of approx. 4 cm starting from the end chosen for ureteral implantation (proximal end preferable). Four stay sutures are placed to facilitate ureteral implantation. A submucosal tunnel is dissected starting from the end of the conduit (tunnel length, 3 to 4 cm). The bowel mucosa at the end of the tunnel is incised and the ureter is pulled through the respective submucosal tunnel. After spatulation and resection of the ureter to an adequate length, implantation is performed by one anchor suture at the 6-o'clock position, grasping the seromuscularis of the bowel and all layers of the ureter (polyglycolic acid 5-0). The anastomosis is completed by mucomucous single sutures (polyglycolic acid 6-0).

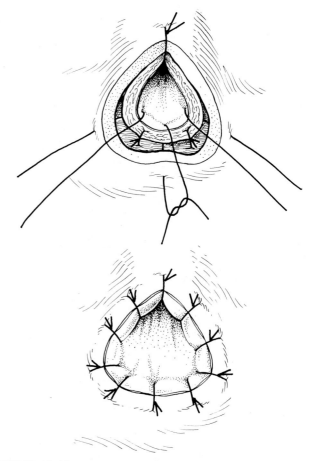

FIG 79–4. The mucosa in between is excised and the seromuscular layer incised to create an entrance for the ureter.

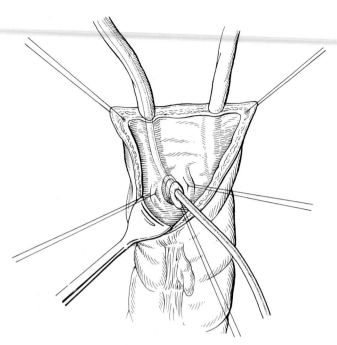

FIG 79–5. For implantation of the second ureter a second tunnel is prepared beside and parallel to the first; the implantation is done in the same way.

To secure the ureteral implantation a 6 Fr ureteral stent is inserted in each ureter and fixed to the bowel mucosa (polyglactin 4-0 with short reabsorption time). For implantation of the second ureter a second tunnel is prepared beside and parallel to the first; the implantation is done in the same way (Fig. 79–5). Both ureteral stents are led out through the aboral end of the conduit. The proximal end of the conduit and of the incision line in the area of the taenia libera are closed (single seromuscular sutures, polyglyconic acid 4-0).

A circular area of the skin (approx. 3 cm in diameter) is excised. The abdominal fascia is crosslike incised and the conduit is pulled through the fascial and the skin opening together with the ureteral stents by means of two Allis clamps after having freed the distal end of the conduit of fat and epiploic appendages. The seromuscularis of the conduit is fixed to the abdominal fascia by circular single stitches of polyglycolic acid 3-0 and the oral end of the conduit is anastomosed to the skin by circular single stitches of polyglycolic acid 5-0 everting the stoma (Fig. 79–6).

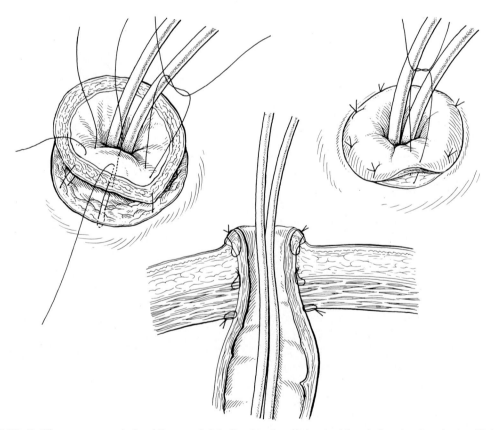

FIG 79–6. The seromuscularis of the conduit is fixed to the abdominal fascia by circular single stitches of polyglycolic acid 3-0 and the oral end of the conduit is anastomosed to the skin by circular single stitches of polyglycolic acid 5-0 everting the stoma.

Pyelotransverse Pyelocutaneostomy

An extensive bowel mobilization is necessary including caecum, root of the mesentry, Treitz's ligament, and the right and left colonic flexures (Fig. 79–7a). The omentum majus is completely dissected from the trans-

verse colon and the bursa omentalis is opened. The bowel is exteriorized out of the abdomen. The ureters are cut at the ureteropelvic junction and the renal pelvis is longitudinally spatulated. A transverse colon segment with a length of 25 to 30 cm and an adequate blood supply is isolated (Fig. 79–7b). After having placed a ureteral stent

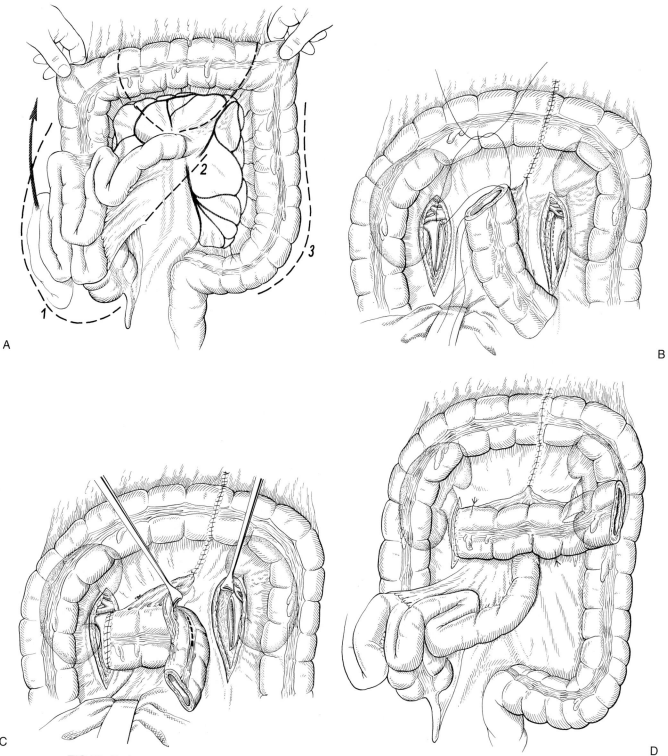

FIG 79–7. An extensive bowel mobilization is necessary including caecum, root of the mesentry, Treitz's ligament, and the right and left colonic flexures.

in a calyx of the right kidney and fixed the stent inside the renal pelvis (polyglactin 4-0 with short reabsorption time) an end-to-end anastomosis of the right renal pelvis and the distal end of the conduit is performed using two running sutures of polyglycolic acid 5-0. The ureteral stent is led out through the conduit before the anastomosis is completed. The conduit is brought to the left renal pelvis without tension (Fig. 79–7c). Also on this side, a stent is inserted into the kidney, fixed, and led out through the conduit later. For anastomosis of the renal pelvis with the conduit, the wall of the conduit is incised at the taenia libera over an adequate length and an end-to-side anastomosis of the renal pelvis and the conduit done by two running sutures of polyglycolic acid 5-0 (Fig. 79–7d). The stoma formation is identical to the standard technique.

Surgical Tips

Transilluminating the mesentry by a fiberoptic light source visualizes the vessels and facilitates the selection of the segment as well as the preparation of the mesenteric slits. When the conduit is positioned on the right side and the left ureter is relatively short, it can be implanted directly to the right ureter (like the crossed hands of a ballerina). This is applicable for the Goodwin–Hohenfellner as well as the Wallace technique. The colonic conduit can be performed so that the urine flow is peristaltic and antiperistaltic so that the stoma can be alternatively positioned in the right or left upper-abdominal quadrant. For an antiperistaltic application, an extensive mobilization of Treitz's ligament and the descending part of the duodenum becomes necessary; otherwise, compression of the duodenum by the conduit may result. An extraperitonealization of the conduit facilitates revisional surgery, as this can be done through a flank incision. Thereby, a transabdominal approach with the need for adhesiolysis can be avoided.

POSTOPERATIVE CARE

Antibiotics are given for 5 days. Parenteral nutrition is continued until bowel contractions appear and then gradually reduced. The gastric tube is removed starting from postoperative day 3 after clamping. The rectal tube stays for 3 days. Ureteral stents are loosened after day 9 and removed after day 10, beginning on one side with a check of the kidney by ultrasonography on day 11. Then, the second stent is removed. An IV urography demonstrates regular kidney function after stent removal.

The acid-base balance should be checked before the patient is discharged. The patient should be taught about all aspects of stoma care.

OUTCOME

Complications and Results

At Mainz University, an incontinent diversion was performed in 679 patients with 1,336 renal units between 1968 and December 1997. Of these, 283 patients with ileal conduit and 336 patients with colonic conduits including 78 transverse conduits could be followed for a mean of 2.7 and 10.7 years, respectively. Indications for urinary diversion were bladder carcinoma in 30%, other malignancies in 12%, and benign disease in 12%. Of these patients, 5.6% with a colonic conduit had complications compared to 10.6% with ileal conduit. Complications were stoma stenosis, urine extravasation, ureteral implantation stenosis, and bowel obstruction. An increase in creatinine was seen in 35% of patients with ileal conduit compared to 17% with colonic conduit. In colonic conduits complications concerning the upper urinary tract were less often observed in patients with refluxive ureteral implantation.

REFERENCES

1. Altwein JE, Jonas U, Hohenfellner R. Long-term follow-up of children with colon conduit urinary diversion and ureterosigmoidostomy. *J Urol* 1977;118:832–836.
2. Altwein JE, Hohenfellner R. Use of the colon as a conduit for urinary diversion. *Surg Gynecol Obstet* 1975;140:33–38.
3. Camey M, Le Duc A. L'enterocystoplastie après cystoprostatectomie totale pour cancer de la vessie. *Ann Urol* 1979;13:114
4. Fisch M, Riedmiller H, Hohenfellner R. Pyelotransverse pyelo-colostomy: An alternative method for high urinary diversion in patients with extended bilateral ureter damage. *Eur Urol* 1991;19:142–149.
5. Leadbetter WF, Clarke BG. Five years experience with ureteroenterostomy by the "combined technique." *J Urol* 1954;73:67–82.
6. Leissner J, Black P, Fisch M, Höckel M, Hohenfellner R. Colon pouch (Mainz pouch III) for continent urinary diversion after pelvic irradiation. *Urology* 2000;56:798–802.
7. Lindell O, Lehtonen T. Rezidivierende urotheliale Tumoren in einzelnieren mit anschluß eines kolonsegmentes an das nierenbecken. *Akt Urol* 1988;19:130–133.
8. Mogg RA. Urinary diversion using the colonic conduit. *Br J Urol* 1967;39:687–692.
9. Morales P, Golimbu M. Colonic urinary diversion: 10 years of experience. *J Urol* 1975;113:302–307.
10. Nelson J H. Atlas of radical pelvic surgery. 1969.
11. Schmidt JD, Buchsbaum HJ, Jacobo EC. Transverse colon conduit for supravesical urinary diversion. *Urology* 1976;8:542–546.
12. Schmidt JD, Buchsbaum HJ, Nachtsheim DA. Long-term follow-up. Further experience with and modifications of the transverse colon conduit in urinary tract diversion. *Br J Urol* 1985;57:284–288.
13. Wallace DM. Ureteric diversion using a conduit. a simplified technique. *Br J Urol* 1966;38:522–527.

CHAPTER 80

Managing the Patient with Orthotopic Bladder Substitution

C. Varol and U.E. Studer

This chapter discusses orthotopic placement of a urinary reservoir fashioned out of small, large, or a combination of the two intestinal segments into the pelvis following a cystectomy. The reservoir is anastomosed to the urethra, allowing for volitional urethral voiding. Although surgeons have used bowel in various ways to substitute a bladder for more than a century, only with better understanding of basic principles of bowel peristalsis, physiology, and applied laws of physics (LaPlace's law) has it been successfully utilized over the last two decades. The keys to success are a good capacity, a low-pressure system made of detuberalized bowel segments with minimal outlet resistance, and preserved sphincter function. A bladder substitute is not a neobladder but attempts to simulate its function.

Several different forms of bladder substitutions have been described and some are presented in the following chapters. Each has its own specific advantages and disadvantages. There are, however, common practical points in the creation and maintenance of a bladder substitute that are important to achieve a good functional outcome. Indeed, the postoperative management of these patients is probably more important than the actual surgical creation. For practical purposes the management phases have been separated into preoperative, intraoperative, postoperative and long-term periods in this chapter. Equal importance must be placed on each phase if satisfactory results are to be obtained.

DIAGNOSIS

The preoperative assessment is identical to a radical cystectomy case in that the exclusion of bone, lung, and lymph node metastases and establishment of operability are of importance. Any major liver, renal, or bowel insufficiency must be excluded.

INDICATIONS FOR SURGERY

Indications for surgery are any patient who has had a cystectomy. The caveats to this diversion, however, are an intense preoperative assessment to maximize the potential outcome. The most important factor that will determine the successful long-term outcome of a bladder substitution is the willingness of the patient to comply with indefinite follow-up. Adequate physical dexterity and a basic comprehension of their new bladder and how it functions are required. Ongoing education is essential for the longevity of the patient and the bladder substitute. If this is not possible an alternative form of treatment should be seriously considered. A dedicated nurse should be involved in the assessment and education prior to surgery and in the aftercare.

Renal Function

The predominant metabolic defects observed after urinary diversion are metabolic acidosis followed by electrolyte abnormalities. The type and severity observed depend on the intestine segment type, length of segment used, time of urine contact with the bowel, and the compensatory reserve of the kidneys. A serum creatinine level of 150 μmol per L is required. Malignant ureteric obstruction or any other reversible causes of renal insufficiency prior to surgery may be taken into account (9,10).

Hepatic Function

Adequate liver function is needed in bladder substitute candidates. The bladder substitute comes into contact with urine where ammonium shifts through the bowel mucosa and enters the circulation. In a urinary tract infection with a urease splitting organism, the ammonium load becomes important. In the presence of liver insufficiency, hyperammonemia results. This phenomenon can lead to neurological decompensation and eventual coma (6).

Bowel Function

Evidence of prior bowel resection, disease, or radiation needs to be elucidated to prevent malabsorption or diarrhea if further bowel resections are used for a bladder substitution. Bowel segment used for a bladder substitute needs to be free of any pathology. An intact ileocecal valve may compensate for a shortened ileum that otherwise would lead to insufficiency. An attempt should also be made to preserve the terminal ileum as this not only minimizes the risk of bowel dysfunction but also interference with vitamin B_{12} and bile salt metabolism. Ileal segments of up to 60 cm can be used in healthy individuals without major repercussions if the ileocecal valve is left intact (4). If more than 60 cm of bowel is used for the reconstruction, the risk of malabsorption increases; it is inevitable when more than 100 cm is used. If the right colon is preserved, an extended length of colon can be used for reconstruction without major malabsorption side effects. This is because fluid reabsorption occurs predominantly in the right colon, while the left colon serves more as a conduit (8).

Paracollicular and Bladder Neck Biopsy

Presence of positive biopsies from the paracollicular region in the prostatic urethra or the bladder neck in women (site of bladder substitution anastomosis) has a high likelihood of a urethral recurrence. These patients should undergo a primary urethrectomy and be considered for an alternative form of urinary diversion. Prostatic infiltration (superficial or stromal) proximal from the paracollicular site, carcinoma *in situ*, and multifocal transitional cancer in the bladder confer a higher chance of urethral recurrence (3). However, these findings are not contraindications to the performance of a bladder substitution.

Continence

The identification of incontinence, especially in females, is essential as it may reflect inadequate rhabdosphincter function. These patients require urodynamic assessment with a urethral pressure profile as it may identify the specific cause and direct treatment. Severe incontinence is a contraindication to bladder substitution (Table 80–1).

TABLE 80–1. *Preoperative checklist*

Patient Agreement to Indefinite Follow-Up
Adequate Mental State, Dexterity, and Mobility
Serum Creatinine of ≤150 mmol/L
Adequate Liver Function
Adequate Bowel Function
No Tumor in the Distal Urethra, Paracollicular, or Bladder Neck Region
Continence Status

ALTERNATIVE THERAPY

There are a variety of urinary diversions that are available including conduits, continent pouches, and tube diversions discussed in other chapters.

SURGICAL TECHNIQUE

The preoperative bowel preparation depends on the bowel segment used for the bladder substitution. Colonic bladder substitutes require a full mechanical bowel preparation with agents such as GlycoPrep. For ileal bladder substitutes, a limited bowel preparation with XPREP and enema are sufficient. Subcutaneous deep venous thrombosis prophylaxis should be implemented the evening before surgery and given in the upper body to prevent pelvic lymphocele formation. In addition, several other pertinent factors in determining a successful outcome need to be contemplated in a bladder substitution.

Nerve Preservation

Preservation of the autonomic nerves to the rhabdosphincter and urogenital diaphragm is controversial, but we feel that it should be attempted on the non–tumor-bearing side as it will increase the chance of potency and aid urinary continence. The nerves from the inferior hypogastric, pelvic plexus, paraprostatic neurovascular bundle, or paravaginal plexus lie dorsal to the bladder in the pararectal/paravaginal area and may indeed be preserved unknowingly. However, they may be injured if the dorsomedial pedicle is transected very dorsally (2,12).

Atraumatic Dissection of the Urethra

Sharp, atraumatic dissection of the urethra with limited use of only bipolar electrocautery at the prostatic apex in men and bladder neck in females is essential. Maximum urethral length must be retained. Preservation of the puboprostatic and pubourethral ligaments and incision of the endopelvic fascia, not at its deepest point but along the bladder neck, in female patients will allow for more urethral stability and improved continence (2).

Ureters

When mobilizing the ureters it is important to maintain the periureteric tissue. This will preserve the blood supply and prevent anastomotic strictures of the ureters. The left ureter needs to be mobilized retrocolic and superior to the inferior mesenteric artery if transposed to the paracaval side, without kinking and free of tension. Ureteric anastomosis should not be obstructive in nature and antireflux ureteric reimplantation is not required in low-pressure ileal bladder substitutes (11). The ureteric stents should be passed through the fatty tissue of the mesentery of the bladder substitute to prevent leakage following their removal (Fig. 80–1).

Bladder Reservoir

If small bowel is used for the reservoir, preservation of the ileocecal valve with the distal 25 cm of ileum is preferable if the risk of accelerated bowel transit time, vitamin B_{12} loss, and bile acid-induced diarrhea is to be minimized. Any intraoperative epidural anesthesia (containing local anesthetics) should be switched off at least 2 hours prior to the measurement of the bowel length as it will result in contraction and shortening of the bowel.

This can eventually lead to longer bowel length measurements and increased reservoir dimensions. This phenomenon can be reversed with an antispasmotic (Buscopan).

For construction of the reservoir, an ileal segment 54 to 60 cm long is isolated approximately 25 cm proximal to the ileocecal valve and bowel continuity is restored (Fig. 80–2). The length of the ileal segment is measured with a ruler in portions of 10 or 15 cm along the border of the mesoileum without stretching the bowel. Irritation of the bowel as well as peridural anesthesia can increase smooth muscle tone and activity and "shorten" the length of the bowel, which will then be too long after muscle relaxation. The distal mesoileum incision transects the main vessels, whereas the proximal mesoileum incision must be short to preserve the main vessels perfusing the future reservoir segment (Fig. 80–2). The mesoileal borders are adapted with a running suture (2-0 polyglycolic acid) in which the mesoileum of the bladder substitute is included (Fig. 80–3). The stitches must be applied superficially, taking care to preserve the blood supply to the bladder substitute. Both ends of the isolated ileal segment are closed by seromuscular running sutures (4-0 polyglycolic acid). The distal end of the ileal segment, approximately 40 to 44 cm long, is opened along its antimesenteric border (Fig. 80–3).

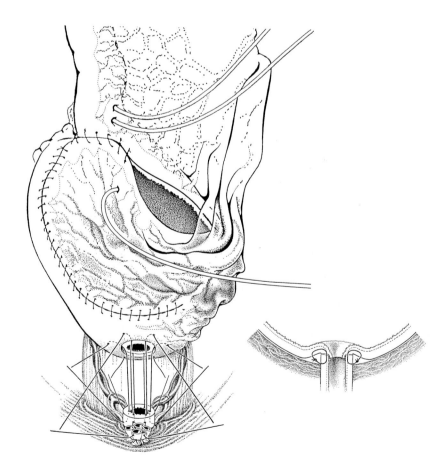

FIG. 80–1. A funnel-shaped reservoir to urethral anastomosis must be avoided because of the risk of subsequent kinking and outlet obstruction.

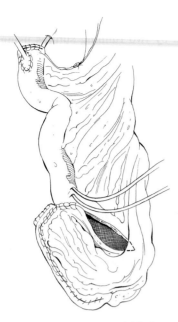

FIG. 80–6. The bottom of the U is folded over between the two ends of the U.

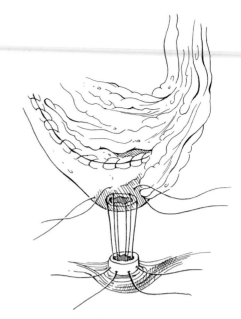

FIG. 80–8. Six polyglycolic acid 2-0 seromuscular sutures are placed between the hole in the reservoir wall and the membranous urethra.

upper half (Fig. 80–6), the surgeon's finger is introduced through the remaining opening to determine the most caudal part of the reservoir. There, a hole, 8 to 10 mm in diameter, is cut out of the pouch wall, outside the suture line (Fig. 80–7). Six polyglycolic acid 2-0 seromuscular sutures are placed between the hole in the reservoir wall and the membranous urethra (Fig. 80–8). An 18 Fr urethral catheter is inserted before tying the six sutures (Fig. 80–9). Before complete closure of the pouch, a 10 Fr cys-

tostomy tube is passed through the wall of the pouch, where it is covered by some mesoileum (Fig. 80–10).

The reservoir to urethral anastomosis must be flat and not funnel shaped to prevent kinking and subsequent hypercontinence (Figs. 80–1 and 80–11). Absorbable suture material should always be used, eliminating any potential nidus for stone formation (Table 80–2).

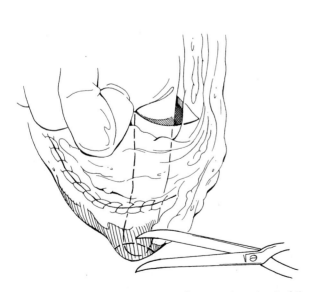

FIG. 80–7. A hole, 8 to 10 mm in diameter, is cut out of the pouch wall, outside the suture line.

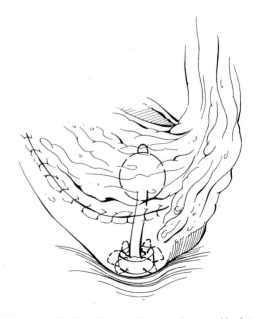

FIG. 80–9. An 18 Fr urethral catheter is inserted before tying the six sutures.

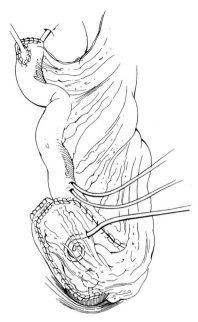

FIG. 80–10. Before complete closure of the pouch, a 10 Fr cystostomy tube is passed through the wall of the pouch, where it is covered by some mesoileum.

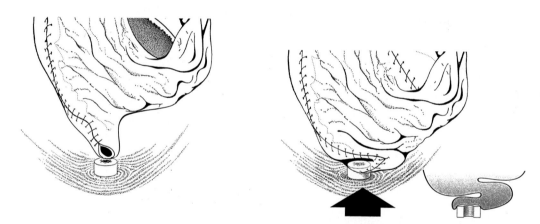

FIG. 80–11. A correct anastomosis of the reservoir to the urethra, which is flat. Placement of cystostomy and ureteric catheters through the fat of the mesentery.

TABLE 80–2. *Intraoperative checklist*

Antibiotics/Compression Stockings
Anatomic Pelvic Exenteration with Attempt of Nerve Preservation on the Non–Tumor-Bearing Side
Atraumatic Dissection with Maximum-Length Preservation of the Urethra
Preservation of Periureteric Tissue
Cease Epidural Anesthesia 2 h Prior to Bowel Length Measurement
Preservation of the Ileocecal Valve and Distal 25 cm of Ileum
Limitation of Small-Bowel Resection to Under 60 cm
Ureterointestinal Anastomosis Should Not Be Obstructive
Low-Pressure Reservoir With Transsected/Opened, Cross-folded Bowel Segments, Spheroidal in Shape
Ureteric Stents and Cystostomy Tubes Placed Through the Fatty Tissue of the Bowel Mesentery
Tension-Free and Flat Anastomosis of the Reservoir to the Urethra

POSTOPERATIVE CARE

The postoperative period is important not only for the management of any fluid and electrolyte abnormalities but also for patient education and adjustment to their bladder substitute. The suprapubic and transurethral catheters need to be flushed and aspirated with saline 0.9% every 6 hours. This is mandatory to prevent any mucus buildup and catheter blockages that may lead to bladder substitution rupture. This risk is highest when bowel activity returns and the catheter is still *in situ*. The prevention of abdominal bloating and return of bowel function can be accelerated with parasympathomimetic medications (e.g., neostigmine 3 to 6×0.5 mg s per cut) and in smokers with nicotine patches. The ureteric catheters should be removed on postoperative day 5 to 7, about the same time as the return of bowel function (Table 80–3).

If the cystogram on postoperative day 10 excludes any urinary extravasations the suprapubic catheter is removed first, followed 48 hours later by the urethral catheter. This allows for the puncture site from the suprapubic catheter in the bladder substitute to seal. A urine sample should be sent for culture when the catheter is removed. Any urinary tract infection must be treated. A quinolone antibiotic is implemented as prophylaxis for 5 days.

The patient is instructed to void in a sitting position every 2 hours during the day and every 3 hours with the help of an alarm clock at night. Voiding needs to occur by relaxation of the pelvic floor, followed by only slight abdominal straining. This may be aided by hand pressure on the lower abdomen and bending forward. Effectiveness of emptying needs to be monitored with in–out catheterization and ultrasound of the reservoir. The voiding interval is gradually increased from every 2 to 4 hours. The patient must not void prior to the allotted time period even if dribble incontinence ensues, aiming for a gradually distended bladder capacity of 500 mL, with subsequent low pressure and enhanced continence. This can be best understood by Laplace's law (pressure = tension/radius) Hence, as the radius of the reservoir increases the pressure in the reservoir decreases.

TABLE 80–3. *Immediate postoperative checklist*

Deep Venous Thrombosis Prophylaxis
Catheters are Flushed and Aspirated Every 6 h
Ureteric Catheters are Removed d 5–7
Cystogram d 10, Withdrawal of Cystostomy Tube if No Leakage
Urethral Catheter is Removed 48 h After Suprapubic Catheter

TABLE 80–4. *Symptoms of metabolic acidosis*

Fatigue
Anorexia
Dyspepsia and Heartburn
Nausea and Vomiting
Weight Loss

OUTCOMES

Complications

Postoperative recovery time to continence depends on good counseling with vigilant sphincter training, the age of the patient, and surgical technique with nerve preservation to the urethra and pelvic floor. Effective sphincter training is taught by performing a digital rectal examination and requesting the contraction of the anal sphincter only. The patient performs this initially 10× hourly, maintaining contraction for 6 seconds, and once continence is achieved on a daily basis. Postmicturition dribble incontinence can be avoided by instructing the patient to milk the urethra at the end of a void (1).

Hypercontinence tends to be a problem primarily with female bladder substitutions. This can be avoided by having an unobstructed outlet with prevention of kinking of the urethra or reservoir (Fig. 80–11). Preserving the autonomic nerve supply to the proximal one-third of the urethra will maintain its tubular shape. If this is denervated, a flaccid, hypotonic urethra results that tends to kink. If in doubt of the innervation, resection of the proximal one-third of the urethra is recommended. However, this may result in dribble incontinence when walking due to a shortened functional urethral length. The pudendal nerve still innervating the distal two-thirds of the urethra and pelvic floor will maintain continence at times of sudden increased abdominal pressure, such as coughing (8).

Following catheter removal, the patient is at increased risk of a metabolic acidosis, in particular in the presence

TABLE 80–5. *Postcatheter removal checklist*

Antibiotic Prophylaxis With a Quinolone Following Catheter Removal for 5 d
All Urinary Tract Infections Must Be Treated
Proper Voiding Technique Must Be Taught
Ensure Reservoir is Emptying Adequately With Ultrasound and In–Out Catheterization
Voids are Gradually Increased From 2 to 4 h (at Night With the Help of an Alarm Clock)
Effective Sphincter Training Must Be Taught and Performed Regularly
Daily Body Weight Measurement and Correct a Negative Base Excess
Oral Fluid Intake of 2–3 L/d for the First 3 mo
Increase Salt Consumption in Ileal Bladder Substitutions Only for the First 3 mo
Lifelong Regular Follow-Up

TABLE 80–6. *Follow-up schema for patients with bladder substitute*

	Months after surgery										
	3	6	12	18	24	30	36	42	48	54	60
Clinical Examination	x	x	x	x	x	x	x	x	x	x	x
Urine Culture	x	x	x	x	x	x	x	x	x	x	x
Body Weight	x	x	x	x	x	x	x	x	x	x	x
Blood Tests[a]	x	x	x	x	x	x	x	x	x	x	x
Folic Acid, Vitamin B_{12}					x		x		x		x
Chest X-Ray		x	x	x	x		x		x		x
Intravenous Ultrasonography			x		x		x				x
Renal Ultrasound	x	x		x		x		x	x	x	
Bone scan (Only if ≥ pT3 and each N+)		x		x							
Pelvic/Abdominal Computed Tomography Scan (Only if ≥ pT3 and Each N+)		x									
Postvoid Residual	x	x	x	x	x	x	x	x	x	x	x
Urethral Lavage		x	x	x	x		x		x		x

[a]Hb, Na^+, K^+, Cl, bicarbonate creatinine, urea, ALP, gamma GT, glutamic-oxaloacetic transaminase, lactate dehydrogenase, venous blood gas analysis.

of residual urine. This is the most frequent undiagnosed complication following a bladder substitution. The urologist as well as the patient need to be aware of the potential symptoms that may arise with a metabolic acidosis (Table 80–4). The base excess can to be monitored with a venous blood gas analysis every second to third day. The base excess needs to be corrected if in a negative parameter. This is usually done with sodium bicarbonate 2 to 6 gm per day in ileal bladder substitution and potassium citrate in colonic bladder substitution. Another cause of metabolic acidosis is hypovolemia due to excess salt loss. These patients have a rapid drop in body weight due to dehydration and anorexia. Daily body weight monitoring becomes essential in the postoperative period. They should consume 2 to 3 L of fluids per day, which needs to be supplemented in ileal bladder substitutes with increased salt intake in their diet to combat any salt-losing syndrome (Table 80–5) (6,7).

Results

Diurnal continence rates of up to 90% and nocturnal over 80% at 12 months should be achieved (5). Meticulous lifelong follow-up is essential for optimal reservoir function and prevention of long-term complications. A suggested schema is illustrated in Table 80–6. A good bladder substitute has no infection, no incontinence, no acidosis, and no or minimal postvoid residual. Uppertract and urethral recurrences can be detected with high sensitivity by performing intravenous ultrasonography and lavage cytology (7). Postvoid residual urine needs to be evaluated and causes such as inguinal or abdominal

hernias identified as they will prevent reservoir emptying. Protruding mucosa or stricture at the urethral–reservoir anastomosis may also be factors that can be managed transurethrally.

REFERENCES

1. Bader P, Hugonnet CL, Burkhard F, Studer UE. Inefficient urethral milking secondary to urethral dysfunction as an additional risk factor for incontinence after radical prostatectomy. *J Urol* 2001;166: 2247–2252.
2. Doherty A, Burkhard F, Holliger S, Studer UE. Bladder substitution in women [Review]. *Curr Urol Rep* 2001;2:350–356.
3. Freeman JA, Thomas A, Esrig D, Stein JP, Donald A, et al. Urethral recurrence in patients with orthotopic ileal neobladders. *J Urol* 1996;156:1615–1619.
4. Hofmann AF. Bile acid malabsorption caused by ileal resection. *Arch Intern Med* 1972;130:597.
5. Madersbacher S, Möhrle K, Burkhard F, Studer UE. Long-term voiding pattern of patients with ileal orthotopic bladder substitutes. *J Urol* 2002;167:2052.
6. Mills RD, Studer UE. Metabolic consequences of continent urinary diversion. *J Urol* 1999;161:1057.
7. Mills RD, Studer UE. Guide to patient selection and follow-up for orthotopic bladder substitution. *Contemp Urol* 2001;Feb:35–40.
8. Proano M, Camilleri M, Phillips SF, Brown ML, Thomford GM. Transit of solids through the human colon: regional quantification in the unprepared bowel. *Am J Physiol* 1990;258(6, Pt 1):G856–G862.
9. Skinner DG, Studer UE, Okada K, Aso Y, Hautmann H, Koontz W, Okada Y. Which patients are suitable for continent diversion or bladder substitution following cystectomy or other definitive local treatment? *Int J Urol* 1995;2[Suppl]:105.
10. Studer UE, Burkhard F, Danuser HJ, Thalmann G. Keys to success in orthotopic bladder substitution. *Can J Urol* 1999;6:876.
11. Studer UE, Siegrist T, Casanova GA, Springer J, Gerber E, Ackermann D, Gurtner F, Zingg EJ. Ileal bladder substitute: antireflux nipple or afferent tubular segment? *Eur Urol* 1991;20:315–326.
12. Turner WH, Danuser H, Moehrle K, Studer UE. The effect of nerve sparing cystectomy technique on postoperative continence after orthotopic bladder substitution. *J Urol* 1997;156:2118.

CHAPTER 81

Orthotopic Urinary Diversion Using an Ileal Low-Pressure Reservoir With an Afferent Tubular Segment

Hansjörg Danuser and Urs E. Studer

This orthotopic bladder substitute offers several significant advantages. One is the ease of surgery, which can be performed by any urologist experienced in performing a radical prostatectomy or a cystectomy and ileal conduit. The short ileum segment, approximately 54 cm long, used to construct this bladder substitute minimizes intestinal malabsorption. The terminal ileum as well as the ileocecal valve is preserved. The reservoir is spherical, achieving a maximum volume:surface area ratio with maximum capacity from a given bowel segment. To avoid metabolic disturbances from reabsorption of urine metabolites a small surface of intestinal mucosa and a short contact time of the urine with the neobladder mucosa is important. On the other hand, according to Laplace's law, a certain reservoir size is mandatory to reduce tension on the neobladder wall and keep intraluminal pressure low. This aids patients to achieve continence.

Another advantage of this bladder substitute is the isoperistaltic tubular afferent segment with the end-to-side ureteroileal anastomosis at its proximal end. It allows resection of the distal ureters including the paraureteral lymphatics at a safe distance from the bladder cancer and reduces the risk of leaving distal ureters behind that may contain carcinoma *in situ*. Further, the shorter the ureters are, the better the blood supply at their distal end and the lower the risk of ischemic stricturing of the distal ureter. The peristalsis of the afferent ileal segments acts as a dynamic antireflux mechanism. In addition, the simple end-to-side technique of the ureteroileal anastomosis and the omission of an additional antireflux mechanism with a potentially high rate of strictures minimizes this risk. Even if a stricture does occur, the distensibility of the afferent tubular segment allows for bridging uni-

lateral ureteral strictures or necrosis by reanastomosis to the more proximal ureter. In case of complicated urethral strictures or urethral tumor recurrence, the afferent tubular segment can easily be transformed into an ileal conduit.

DIAGNOSIS

This procedure is usually performed in patients who have undergone cystectomy. In adults, this is most frequently performed for bladder cancer, which is covered in another chapter.

INDICATIONS FOR SURGERY

Indications for surgery are any patient who undergoes cystectomy and has adequate small bowel and mesenteric length to perform the procedure. This reservoir, with slight modifications, is also useful for bladder augmentation after subtotal cystectomy in patients with a contracted bladder due to neurological disorders or to replace a shrunken bladder and ureter after radiotherapy, in particular in female patients. Patients who want this orthotopic bladder substitute should cooperate and be willing to accept the long-term postoperative education and follow-up. Only then will they achieve urinary continence, void without residual urine, and avoid urinary infections and metabolic disturbances.

ALTERNATIVE THERAPY

These include other types of continent bladder substitutes and pouches, the ureterosigmoidostomy, and the ileal conduit.

SURGICAL TECHNIQUE

All patients receive peri- and postoperative antibiotic prophylaxis consisting of an aminoglycoside and ornidazol for 48 hours and amoxicillin/clavulanate given until all drains are removed 10 to 12 days postoperatively. Heparin is given subcutaneously peri- and postoperatively as thrombosis prophylaxis.

Cystectomy

Pelvic lymphadenectomy and cystectomy are performed according to standard technique (3) with slight modifications. The external iliac vessels, the obturator fossa, and the hypogastric vessels are freed of all lymphatic, fatty, and connective tissue. Having divided the dorsolateral bladder pedicles containing the superior and inferior vesical vessels along the hypogastric arteries, the pelvic floor fascia is incised and Santorini's plexus is ligated. The ureters are divided where they cross the iliac vessels. This allows *en-bloc* removal of the distal ureters and paraureteral lymphatic vessels, together with the cystectomy specimen. The dorsomedial pedicle is resected along the pararectal/presacral plane on the tumor-bearing side. Whenever possible, however, care is taken to preserve the hypogastric fibers and the pelvic plexus situated dorsolaterally to the seminal vesicle on the contralateral non–tumor-bearing side. On this side the dissection along the dorsolateral wall of the seminal vesicle is stopped at the base of the prostate. Santorini's plexus is then divided and the membranous urethra is transected as close as possible to the apex of the prostate by excavating it out of the donut-shaped apex. The neurovascular bundles dorsolateral to the prostate are also preserved on the non–tumor-bearing side.

Preparation of the Ileum Segment for the Bladder Substitute

For construction of the reservoir, an ileal segment approximately 54 cm long is isolated 25 cm proximal to the ileocecal valve and bowel continuity is restored (Fig. 81-1). The length of the ileum segment is measured with a ruler in portions of 10 or 15 cm along the border of the mesoileum without stretching the bowel. Irritation of the bowel as well as epidural anesthesia with local anesthetics should be avoided because this can increase smooth muscle tone and activity and "shorten" the length of the bowel, which will then be too long after muscle relaxation. The distal mesoileum incision transects the main vessels, whereas the proximal mesoileum incision must be short to preserve the main vessels perfusing the future reservoir segment (Fig. 81-1). The mesoileum borders are adapted with a running suture (2-0 polyglycolic acid) in which the mesoileum of the bladder substitute is included (Fig. 81-2). The stitches must be applied super-

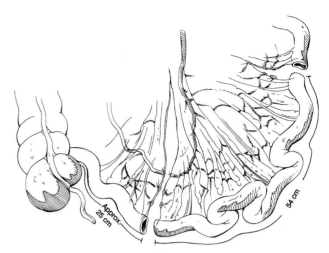

FIG. 81-1. Preparation of the 54-cm long ileal segment for the bladder substitute. Note the different incision depths of the mesoileum proximally and distally to preserve the blood supply.

ficially, taking care to preserve the blood supply to the bladder substitute. Both ends of the isolated ileal segment are closed by seromuscular running sutures (4-0 polyglycolic acid). The distal end of the ileal segment, approximately 40 to 44 cm long, is opened along its antimesenteric border (Fig. 81-2).

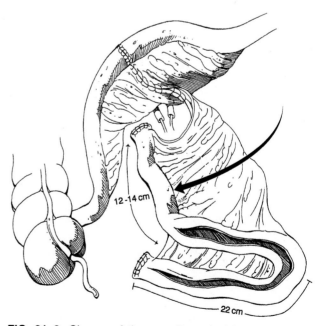

FIG. 81-2. Closure of the mesoileum incision. Avoid deep sutures in the area joining the mesoileum of the terminal ileum to the mesoileum of the bladder substitute so as not to compromise circulation. Transpose the afferent ileal segment according to the arrow.

Ureteroileal End-to-Side Anastomosis

The ureters are split over a length of 1.5 to 2 cm and anastomosed by two running sutures using the Nesbit technique in an open end-to-side fashion to two longitudinal 1.5- to 2-cm long incisions along the paramedian antimesenteric border of the afferent tubular ileal segment, which is 12 to 14 cm long (Fig. 81–3). The ureters are stented with 7 or 8 Fr catheters. To prevent dislocation of the splints, a rapidly absorbable suture (4-0 polyglycolic acid) is placed through the ureter and splint together 3 to 4 cm proximal to the anastomosis. It is tied loosely, not compromising the ureteral blood supply. The most distal periureteral tissue is sutured to the afferent ileal segment to remove tension on the anastomosis and to cover it. The ureteric stents are passed through the wall of the most distal end of the afferent tubular segment, where it is covered by some mesoileum. This provides a "covered" canal in the reservoir wall when withdrawing the ureteric stents 7 to 10 days postoperatively.

Construction of the Bladder Substitute and Anastomosis to the Urethra

To construct the reservoir itself, the two medial borders of the opened U-shaped distal part of the ileal segment are oversewn with a single continuous seromuscular layer 2-0 polyglycolic acid suture (Fig. 81–4). The bottom of the U is folded over between the two ends of the U (Figs. 81–4 and 81–5), resulting in a spherical reservoir consisting of four cross-folded ileal segments. After closure

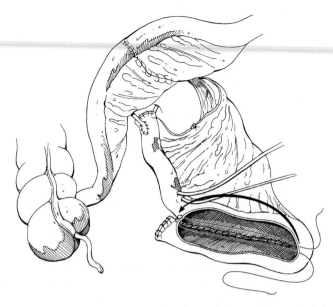

FIG. 81–4. The two medial borders of the antimesenterial opened U-shaped distal ileum segment are oversewn with a single-layer seromuscular running suture. The bottom of the U is folded over and tied between the two ends of the U.

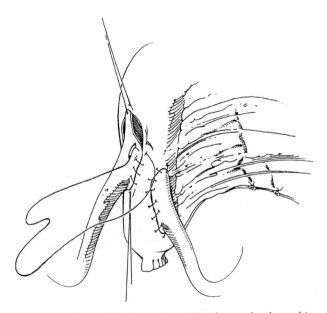

FIG. 81–3. Ureteroileal anastomosis using a simple end-to-side Nesbit technique with a 4-0 running suture assures a low stricture rate.

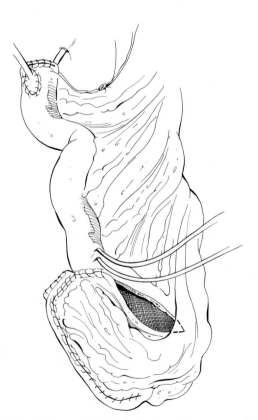

FIG. 81–5. The caudal half of the remaining reservoir opening is closed completely, the cranial half partially by a running seromuscular suture.

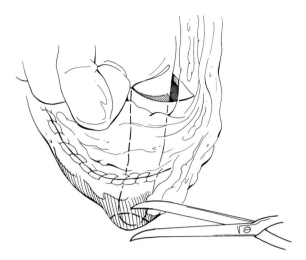

FIG. 81–6. A hole is cut into the most caudal part of the reservoir, close to the mesoileum and 2 to 3 cm away from the edge that resulted from cross-folding the ileal segment.

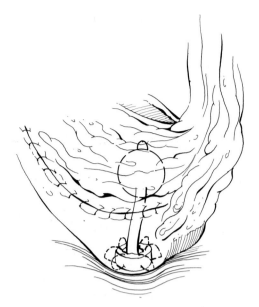

FIG. 81–8. The six prelaid sutures are tied after inserting an 18 Fr urethral catheter.

of the lower half of the anterior wall and part of the upper half (Fig. 81–5), the surgeon's finger is introduced through the remaining opening to determine the most caudal part of the reservoir. There a hole, 8 to 10 mm in diameter, is cut out of the pouch wall, outside the suture line (Fig. 81–6). Six polyglycolic acid 2-0 seromuscular sutures are placed between the hole in the reservoir wall and the membranous urethra (Fig. 81–7). An 18 Fr urethral catheter is inserted before tying the six sutures (Fig.

81–8). Before complete closure of the pouch, a 10 Fr cystostomy tube is passed through the wall of the pouch, where it is covered by some mesoileum (Fig. 81–9). The cystostomy tube is withdrawn 10 days postoperatively after exclusion of any leakage by a "pouchogram." The indwelling catheter is left on continuous drainage for 2 more days before removal to allow for closure of the cystostomy canal in the reservoir wall.

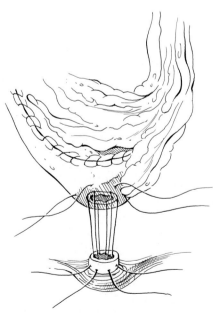

FIG. 81–7. Six seromuscular sutures are placed between the reservoir and the membranous urethra.

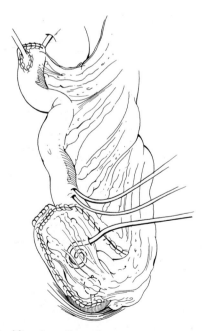

FIG. 81–9. After insertion of a cystostomy tube into the reservoir, the pouch is closed completely.

POSTOPERATIVE CARE

Meticulous postoperative surveillance and teaching of the patient are paramount for good long-term results. In the first postoperative days the bladder substitute should be irrigated and actively aspirated to remove any mucous. The bowel should be stimulated by parasympathomimetics. After catheter removal, a quinolone is given for 5 days. Any persisting bacteriuria is treated until the urine is sterile. Patients are instructed to void every 2 hours, first while sitting, by relaxing the pelvic floor and, if necessary, by abdominal straining (2). Patients are encouraged to drink 2 to 3 L fluid per day and take additional dietary salt. The reservoir will secrete sodium and chloride if the urine is hypoosmolar. The additional salt intake prevents a salt-losing syndrome that may result in hypovolemia and acidosis (4). Therefore, body weight and blood gases are controlled regularly. Patients without metabolic acidosis (negative base excess of more than 2 mmol/L) or with metabolic acidosis compensated by oral intake of sodium bicarbonate are then instructed to retain the urine for 3 and later for 4 hours (even if they become incontinent earlier) until the maximal voiding volume is increased to 500 mL. Patients must understand that when the reservoir is full increased reservoir pressure may cause urinary incontinence but that it is essential to maintain the elevated pressure to expand the reservoir to the desired capacity. If patients void as soon as they become incontinent the reservoir will hardly ever expand and in particular nighttime incontinence will be inevitable due to lack of capacity and the unfavorable pressure characteristics of a low-capacity reservoir. Residual urine is repeatedly ruled out and any bacteriuria is treated.

OUTCOMES

Complications

Early complications are dehydration due to salt-loss syndrome and/or metabolic acidosis and those of extended abdominal surgery (4,5). Specific late complications of the bladder substitute such as intestinal obstruction, pouch necrosis, ureteral strictures, or necrosis are rare.

Results

The median functional capacity of the bladder substitute increases from 120 mL immediately postoperatively to 350 mL after 6 months and 500 mL after 12 months postoperatively by extending the micturition interval from 2 to 4 hours (2,4,5). With the advice to maintain regular voiding intervals of 4 to 6 hours and avoid micturition volumes exceeding 500 mL, overdistension of the reservoir is prevented and its capacity will remain stable for years. Spontaneous voiding with abdominal straining

is possible in 99% of patients. The necessity of intermittent self-catheterization is rare (1%) (4,5).

Urinary continence is poor following removal of the catheter 10 to 14 days postoperatively, but improves within 3 months with the increase of functional bladder capacity. Younger patients and those in whom a nerve-sparing cystectomy was performed achieve continence faster than older patients and patients with previous radiation therapy of the pelvis (9). Daytime continence is achieved in 92% of patients 1 year postoperatively and nighttime continence in 80% of patients 2 years postoperatively (1,2,4,5).

Positive urinary cultures 6 months postoperatively are found in 12% of patients, usually in combination with residual urine. The risk of pyelonephritis within 1 year is less than 2% for patients with this bladder substitute (5).

Ureteral strictures occur in 2% and usually in the left distal ureter (1,5). This low stricture rate is the result of a simple end-to-side anastomosis with short and well-perfused ureters without an antireflux mechanism (6,7).

An antireflux nipple valve in this type of bladder substitute is not necessary for the following reasons:

1. The bladder substitution is a low-pressure reservoir.
2. During voiding abdominal straining simultaneously produces the same pressure increase in the bladder substitute, the abdomen, and the renal pelvis. Without pressure differences retrograde urinary flow is impossible (6,7).
3. The peristalsis of the afferent tubular ileal segment and the peristalsis of the ureter provide a dynamic antireflux mechanism. This could be demonstrated in a video showing simultaneous pressure recordings in the bladder substitute and in the renal pelvis (6,7).
4. The long-term results of a randomized prospective study including 70 patients with either an antireflux mechanism or an afferent isoperistaltic ileal segment support the hypothesis that an antireflux nipple is not necessary. There were no major differences between these two groups except for an increased rate of upper urinary tract obstruction in patients with the antireflux nipples (6).

The incidence of postoperative metabolic acidosis depends mainly on the length of ileum used to construct the reservoir, excluding the length of ileum used for the afferent tubular segment. Metabolic acidosis occurs predominantly within the first 3 months postoperatively. Therefore, prevention by 2 to 6 g sodium bicarbonate per day is recommended. Permanent sodium bicarbonate substitution is only necessary in acidotic patients with reservoirs constructed from ileal segments more than 60 cm long (4,5). A major risk of long-term acidosis would be impaired bone metabolism with osteopenia and/or osteomalacia. However, those patients with a 5- to 8-year follow-up still have bone densities within the normal range (8).

In summary, this orthotopic bladder substitute constructed from 40 to 44 cm ileum and a 14- to 16-cm long afferent tubular ileal segment is a low-pressure urinary reservoir with excellent urodynamic properties providing good day- and nighttime continence. It has a low stricture rate of the ureteroileal anastomosis and an adequate dynamic antireflux mechanism, preventing kidney damage. Further, this urinary diversion is well accepted by patients and promises good results provided that patients are carefully selected, well instructed, and meticulously followed.

REFERENCES

1. Benson MC, Seaman EK, Olsson CA. The ileal ureter neobladder is associated with a high success and low complication rate. *J Urol* 1996; 155:1585.
2. Casanova GA, Springer JP, Gerber E, Studer UE. Urodynamic and clinical aspects of ileal low pressure bladder substitutes. *Br J Urol* 1993; 72:728.
3. Skinner DG. Technique of radical cystectomy. *Urol Clin North Am* 1981;8:353.
4. Studer UE, Danuser H, Hochreiter W, Springer JP, Turner WH, Zingg EJ. Summary of ten years' experience with a ileal low-pressure bladder substitute combined with an afferent tubular isoperistaltic segment. *World J Urol* 1996;14:29.
5. Studer UE, Danuser H, Merz VW, Springer JP, Zingg EJ. Experience in 100 patients with an ileal low pressure bladder substitute combined with an afferent tubular isoperistaltic segment. *J Urol* 1995;154:49.
6. Studer UE, Danuser H, Thalmann GN, Springer JP, Turner WH. Antireflux nipples or afferent tubular segments in 70 patients with ileal low pressure bladder substitutes. Long term results of a prospective randomized trial. *J Urol (in press)*.
7. Studer UE, Spiegel T, Casanova GA, Springer J, Gerber E, Ackermann DK, Gurtner F, Zingg EJ. Ileal bladder substitute: antireflux nipple or afferent tubular segment? *Eur Urol* 1991;20:315.
8. Tschopp AB, Lippuner K, Jaeger P, Merz VW, Danuser H, Studer UE. No evidence of osteopenia 5 to 8 years after ileal orthotopic bladder substitution. *J Urol* 1996;155:71.
9. Turner WH, Danuser HJ, Moehrle K, Studer UE. The effect of nerve sparing cystectomy technique on postoperative continence after orthotopic bladder substitution. *J Urol* 1997;158:2118.

fossa and gently pull out the important nodal tissue and fat, clearly exposing obturator vessels and nerves. Mobilize the peritoneum bluntly in a cephalad direction to expose the anterior surface of the ureter.

Ureteral Mobilization

Do not use the standard vertical incision lateral to the sigmoid mesocolon. Mobilize the peritoneal sac medially on both sides. Continue to locate the ureter extraperitoneally, realizing that it is displaced during exposure because it adheres to the peritoneum (see Fig. 82–1). Mobilize the ureters with sufficient periureteral adventitia in a cephalad direction on both sides. A plane is established between the ureter and the lateral pedicles of the bladder. As the ureter and bladder are retracted medially, the lateral pedicle is exposed. Finally, the ureter is clamped distally. Fine-traction sutures are inserted in the proximal surface of the ureter, and it is divided against the clamps with a scissors. Then, the ureter is dissected proximally so that about 6 to 9 cm is free.

Depending on tumor stage and location, the bladder is completely extraperitonealized and the peritoneum is bisected over the bladder (Fig. 82–1). If this cannot be done safely, an incision in the peritoneum is made high on the base of the bladder, leaving a peritoneal patch on the posterior bladder wall. Approach to the membranous urethra in the male patient.

Urethral preparation with preservation of the continence mechanism is of critical importance when orthotopic diversion is anticipated. Attention to surgical detail is important and deserves special mention. The author believes that the continence mechanism in men may be maximized if dissection in the region of the anterior urethra is minimized. This has led to a slight modification in the technique of the apical dissection in the male patient undergoing orthotopic reconstruction. All fibroareolar connections between the anterior bladder wall, prostate, and undersurface of the pubic symphysis are divided. The endopelvic fascia is incised adjacent to the prostate and the levator muscles are carefully swept off the lateral and apical portions of the prostate (Fig. 82–2A).

With tension placed posteriorly on the prostate, the puboprostatic ligaments are identified and slightly divided just beneath the pubis and lateral to the dorsal venous complex that courses between these ligaments (Fig. 82–2A). Care should be taken to avoid any extensive dissection in this region. The puboprostatic ligaments should only be incised enough to allow for proper apical dissection of the prostate (Fig. 82–2B). The apex of the prostate and membranous urethra becomes palpable. Several methods can be performed to properly control the dorsal venous plexus. An angled clamp may be passed carefully beneath the dorsal venous complex, anterior to the urethra (Figs. 82–3A and 82–3B). The venous complex can then be ligated with a 2-0 absorbable suture and divided close to the apex of the prostate. If any bleeding occurs from the transected venous complex, it can be oversewn with 2-0 polyglycolic acid sutures in a slightly different fashion; the dorsal venous complex may be gathered at the apex of the prostate with a long Allis clamp (Fig. 82–2b).

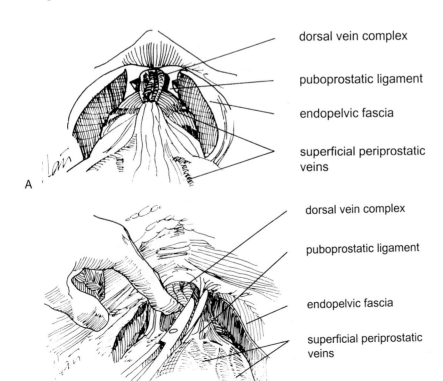

dorsal vein complex

puboprostatic ligament

endopelvic fascia

superficial periprostatic veins

A

dorsal vein complex

puboprostatic ligament

endopelvic fascia

superficial periprostatic veins

B

FIG. 82–2. **A:** The endopelvic fascia adjacent to the prostate is incised. Note that care should be taken not to perform excessive dissection along the pelvic floor levator musculature that could injure the innervation to the rhabdosphincter. The puboprostatic ligaments are slightly divided, providing excellent exposure to the apex of the prostate and the membranous urethra. **B:** Gather the dorsal venous complex with an Allis clamp near the apex of the prostate or with a stitch.

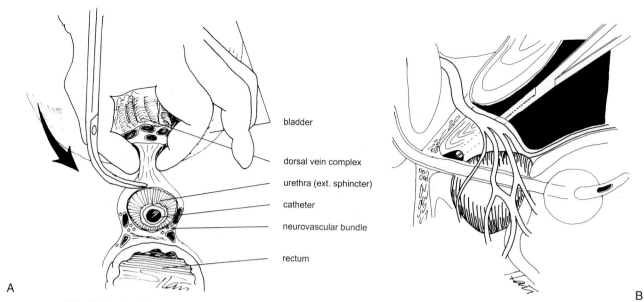

bladder

dorsal vein complex

urethra (ext. sphincter)

catheter

neurovascular bundle

rectum

A

B

FIG. 82–3. A: The dorsal venous complex may be controlled by carefully passing a clamp between the venous complex (anterior) and the urethra (posterior). **B:** A suture is carefully placed anterior to the urethra and around the gathered venous complex.

A 1-0 absorbable suture is then placed under direct vision anterior to the urethra (distal to the apex of the prostate) around the gathered venous complex (Figs. 82–3a and 82–3b). This suture is best placed with the surgeon facing the head of the table and holding the needle driver perpendicular to the patient. This maneuver avoids the unnecessary passage of any instruments between the dorsal venous complex and the rhabdosphincter, which could potentially injure these structures and compromise the continence mechanism.

After the complex has been ligated, it can be sharply divided with excellent exposure to the anterior surface of the urethra (Fig. 82–4). Once the venous complex has been severed, the suture can be used to further secure the complex. The suture is then used to suspend the venous complex anteriorly to the periosteum to help reestablish anterior fixation of the dorsal venous complex and puboprostatic ligaments. This may enhance recovery of continence. The anterior urethra is now exposed. Regardless of the technique, the urethra is then incised 180 degrees, just beyond the apex of the prostate (Fig. 82–5). Six 2-0 polyglycolic acid sutures are placed in the urethra circumferentially, carefully incorporating only the mucosa and submucosa of the striated urethral sphincter muscle anteriorly. The urethral catheter is clamped and divided distally. Two sutures are placed, which should incorporate the rectourethralis muscle posteriorly or the caudal extent of Denonvillier's fascia (Fig. 82–6). Following this, the posterior urethra is divided and the specimen is removed.

puboprostatic ligament

dorsal vein complex

endopelvic fascia

neurovascular bundle

superficial periprostatic veins

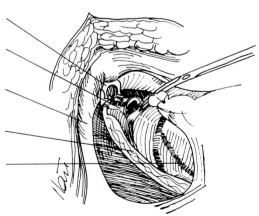

FIG. 82–4. The venous complex is divided. The previously placed suture can then be used to further secure the dorsal venous complex if any bleeding occurs. The complex is then fixed anteriorly to the periosteum.

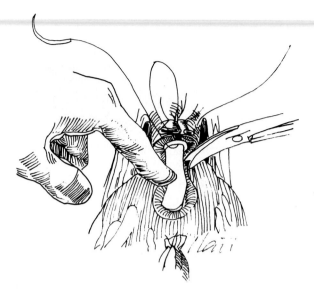

FIG. 82–5. The anterior urethra is incised 180 degrees just beyond the prostate apex.

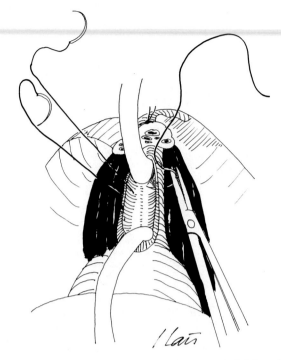

FIG. 82–6. Placement of urethral sutures and division of the posterior urethral wall.

Construction of the Pouch

Adjust the light behind the mesentery and select a 60- to 70-cm long ileal segment 10 to 20 cm proximally from the ileocecal valve (6–8). Spasticity of the bowel or a thick short mesentery may lead to more bowel than necessary, thus increasing the reservoir capacity. It is helpful to place two temporary stay sutures at the intended resection lines. They can be moved several times if necessary. The most dependable part of the segment should be long enough to reach the top of the symphysis pubis in the skin level. Mark that point with a suture. This maneuver guarantees that the reservoir will reach the urethral remnant without difficulty. The distal division of the mesentery along the avascular region

between the ileocolic artery and the terminal branches of the superior mesenteric artery should extend to the base of the mesentery to provide maximum mobility and sufficient length to reach the membranous urethra. The proximal incision of the mesentery is made as short as possible to provide maximum vascular supply to the ileal segment. The ileum is then divided between bowel clamps. A standard bowel anastomosis is performed and the mesenteric trap is closed. The isolated bowel segment is thoroughly cleaned or rinsed with saline or an iodine solution (Fig. 82–7).

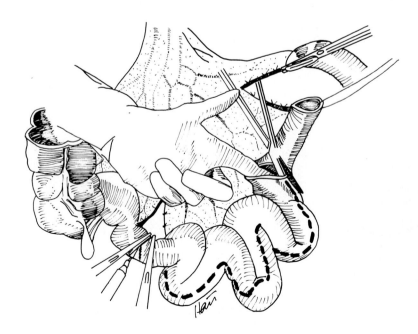

FIG. 82–7. Selection of the ileal segment with an appropriate vascular supply and antimesenteric incision of ileum except for the small chimneys on both sides of the W and the intended site of the ileourethral anastomosis (broken line).

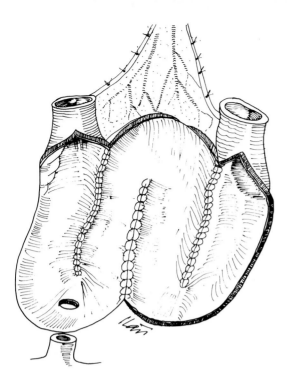

FIG. 82–8. W-shaped reconfiguration of the intestinal segment after detubularization and asymmetrical incision of the ileal wall at the site of the anastomosis to the urethra, forming a U-shaped flap.

Four lengths of ileum are arranged in the shape of a W with 3- to 5-cm long chimneys on each side of the W using five to six Babcock clamps. Other than the two chimneys, the bowel is opened on the antimesenteric border except for a 5- to 7-cm section centered around the marking suture, which is opened to close to the antimesenteric border to create a U-shaped flap. Two centimeters to 3 cm from the tip of that flap, a buttonhole of all layers is excised from the ileal plate. An ileal plate is formed by sewing together the cut edges of the antimesenteric borders of the W using 2-0 synthetic absorbable sutures (SASs) on a straight needle (Fig. 82–8).

A 22 Fr is placed through the buttonhole. For the actual anastomosis, six previously placed double-armed sutures using 3-0 SAS in the urethra are used. The inner sutures are passed through the neobladder outlet in the ileal plate without grasping the ileum, and the corresponding outer sutures grasp the entire ileal wall 5 to 8 mm lateral to the neobladder outlet (Fig. 82–9). This guarantees a wide, ideal, funnel-shaped anastomosis so that mucosa is in direct contact with urethral epithelium. Next, under gentle traction on the transurethral catheter the ileal plate is manipulated down to the urethral remnant and the knots are tied

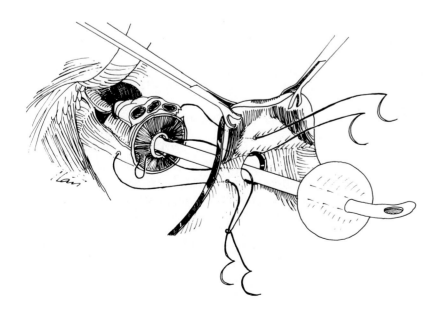

FIG. 82–9. Ileourethral anastomosis, anterior view.

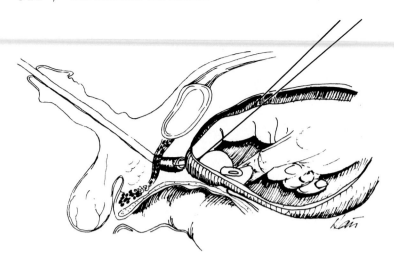

FIG. 82–10. Lateral aspect of the ileourethral anastomosis. The sutures are tied from inside the ileal bladder.

inside the bowel (Fig. 82–10). The cut edges of the 5- to 7-cm U-shaped flap are sewn together over the catheter. The lower third of the anterior wall of the neobladder is closed, beginning inferiorly with interrupted 3-0 SAS (Fig. 82–11).

In 10% of patients, the ileourethral anastomosis may cause some difficulties. In this case, some or all of the following tricks are helpful to overcome this dilemma (Figs. 82–12a and 82–12b): loosening the retractor, straightening the operating table, removing the sacral

cushion, neutralizing the extended position of the patient, bringing up the perineum with a sponge stick, freeing the cecum and descending colon as in retroperitoneal lymph node dissection (RPLND), moving up the neobladder outlet to the tip of the U-shaped flap, or performing an end-to-end anastomosis after tubularization of the U-shaped flap (Fig. 82–13). Any incisions into the mesentery of the neobladder should be avoided. The neobladder mesentery should not be pulled roughly to the pelvic floor.

Refluxing Ileourethral Anastomosis

Controversy exists about the importance of an antireflux mechanism and the benefits are not easy to define in adults undergoing urinary diversion. It is clear that the need for reflux prevention is not the same as in ureterosigmoidostomy conduit or continent diversion. The rationale for implanting the ureters in an antireflux fashion into orthotopic bladder substitutes or continent reservoirs is to prevent the upper urinary tract from retrograde hydrodynamically transmitted pressure peaks and from ascending bacteriuria. However, the routine of antireflux ureter implantation into intestinal urinary reservoirs was born in the era before creation of designated low-pressure reservoirs. Reflux prevention in neobladders is even less important as in a normal bladder because there are no coordinated contractions during micturition and there is a simultaneous pressure increase in neobladder, abdomen, and kidney pelvis during the Valsalva maneuver. Using nonrefluxing techniques the risk of obstruction is at least twice that following a direct anastomosis irrespective of type or bowel segment used and half of these strictures require secondary procedures.

Since 1996 we are using a freely refluxing open end-to-side ureteroileal anastomosis, which is simplest small-bowel surgery that has reduced our stenosis rate from 9.5% to 1.0%. Further advantages of this chimney modification are the extra length to reach the ureteral stump,

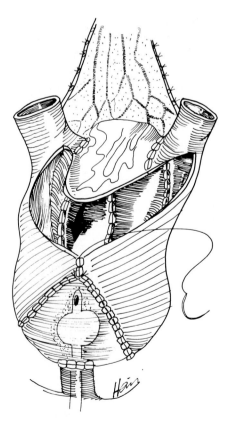

FIG. 82–11. Closure of reservoir.

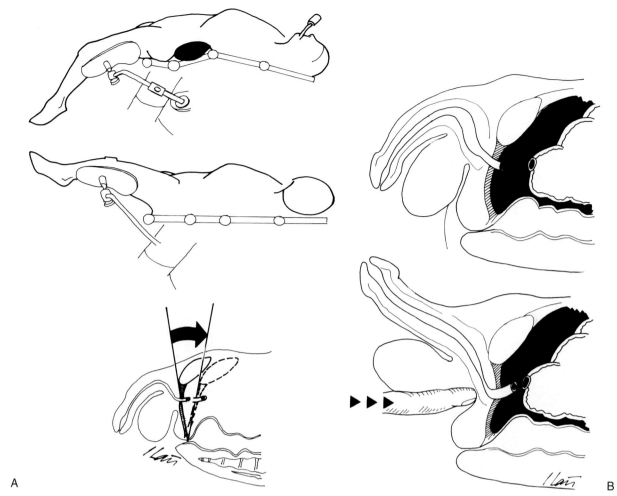

FIG. 82–12. Methods to get the ileal neobladder to the pelvic floor. **a:** Changing the extended position of the patient to slightly supine and removal of the sacral cushion rotate the pelvic floor upward. **b:** Pushing up the perineum with a sponge stick or finger approximates the urethral remnant and neobladder.

the ease of surgery way outside the pelvic cavity, a tension-free anastomosis, no risk of ureteral angulation with neobladder filling, and a simplified flank access for revisional surgery.

On each side, the ureters are trimmed as appropriate for their chimney (Fig. 82–14). The ureterointestinal anastomosis can be done extraperitoneally above the common iliac vessels using a Bricker or Wallace (our choice) technique without competing with the bowel mesentery for an anastomotic site (Fig. 82–14). After placing appropriate ureteral stents, they are brought through the anterior neobladder suture line. The remaining anterior neobladder wall is closed in a T shape with running 3-0 SASs. No cystostomy tube is placed. Two 20 Fr silicone drains are placed into the small pelvis.

Using the two large peritoneal flaps from visceral pelvic peritoneum, this goal can easily been reached (Fig. 82–1). Both flaps are sewn together, except for the por-

tion where the mesentery of the neobladder runs through them. The peritoneal cavity is closed in a standard fashion (Fig. 82–15). Alternatively, the flaps can be sewn to the posterior wall of the neobladder.

Excessive mucus production of the ileal bladder may rarely cause a problem in the postoperative course by obstructing the urethral catheter. Therefore, the ileal bladder is rinsed via the cystostomy with 50 to 100 mL of saline twice a day starting on postoperative day 5. Routinely, the ureteral stents are removed between postoperative days 7 and 14.

As soon as the urine is in contact with the ileal bladder mucosa, reabsorption of urine electrolytes may occur. Therefore, the base excess is checked at weekly intervals for the first 4 weeks and monthly thereafter. Approximately 50% of all patients need temporary alkalinizing therapy.

The urethral catheter is removed between postoperative days 14 and 21, after a cystogram has demonstrated com-

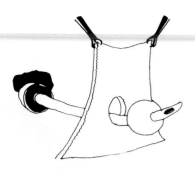

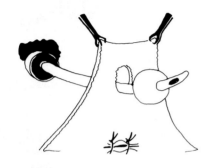

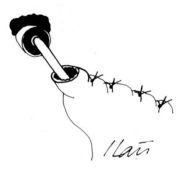

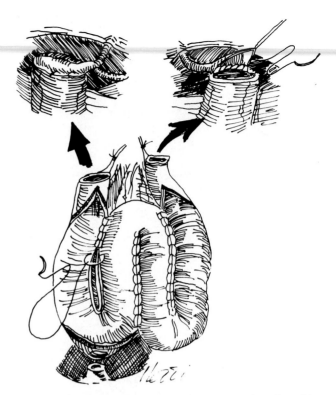

FIG. 82–14. Refluxing ileoureteral anastomosis using chimneys of a 3- to 5-cm afferent limb on each side.

FIG. 82–13. Moving the neobladder outlet closer to the tip of the U-shaped flap of ileal plate. If this still does not allow tension-free anastomosis, one should tubularize the U-shaped form and perform direct (end-to-end) anastomosis.

plete healing of the ileourethral anastomosis. Rarely, there is still leakage from the anastomosis. When this is occurs, it is treated by prolonged catheter drainage until the leak has closed spontaneously.

OUTCOMES

Complications

The complications of both continent catheterizable reservoirs and orthotopic bladder substitutes in the hands of the most experienced surgeons have been considered in detail (4). Reoperation for early complications overall occurred in 3% of continent catheterizable reservoirs and

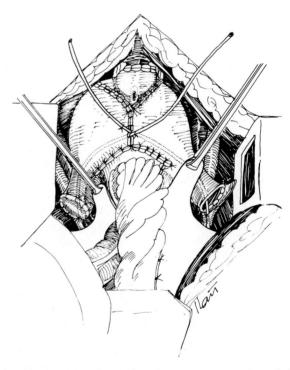

FIG. 82–15. Completely extraperitoneal localization of the neobladder as well as ileourethral and ileoureteral anastomoses.

7% of orthotopic bladder substitutions. Reoperation for late complications overall occurred in about 30% of continent catheterizable reservoirs and 13% of orthotopic bladder substitutions (4). We believe that the morbidity of orthotopic bladder substitutes is actually similar to, or lower than, the true rates of morbidity after conduit formation, contrary to the popular view that conduits are simple and safe.

There are several new complications unknown during the conduit era including incisional hernias, as a consequence of the Valsalva maneuver, neobladder–intestinal and neobladder–cutaneous fistulas, mucus formation, and neobladder rupture. The secretion of mucus can be dramatically increased.

Spontaneous late rupture of neobladders is a rare but potentially life-threatening complication. In the majority of cases is it secondary to acute or chronic overdistension and bacterial infection. Other factors are minor blunt abdominal trauma or urethral occlusion. Chronic ischemic changes of the neobladder's wall, possibly facilitated by detubularization and the variability of the mesenteric circulation, are additional factors that lead to perforation. The rupture site is typically the upper part of the right side of the reservoir. This is the most mobile part of the reservoir, undergoing the most marked distension during overfilling, which may constitute an additional factor for perforation in this location. There is no reliable procedure to establish the diagnosis. Cystography is misleading in three of four patients with neobladder rupture. A high index of suspicion and early aggressive operative treatment in patients suspected of having a neobladder rupture are instrumental in providing a successful outcome. Prevention of neobladder rupture comprises careful monitoring of neobladder emptying. Physicians must be aware of the risk of rupture. Patients must be encouraged to void regularly, especially at bedtime, and perform clean intermittent self-catheterization to avoid chronic reservoir overdistension. In the event of anesthesia proper bladder drainage should be performed.

Results

Perioperative death occurred in 3%. Neobladder-related early and late complications occurred in 15% and 23% of patients, respectively. Neobladder-related early and late abdominal reoperation rates were 0.3% and 4%, respectively. Perioperative neobladder-unrelated early complications were observed in 33% and 12% of patients required operative treatment. Late postoperative complications unrelated to the neobladder occurred in 12% of patients and 5% required open surgical revision. Ninety-six percent of patients void spontaneously, 4% perform clean intermittent catheterization in some form, and 1.7% perform regular intermittent catheterization. Thirty percent to 40% of women require some form of intermittent catheterization to completely empty their neobladder (6). Daytime and nighttime continence was reported as good by 96% and satisfactory by 95% of patients. Unacceptable daytime continence requiring more than one pad per day occurred in only 4% of patients and only 5% are wetting more than one pad per night.

REFERENCES

1. Hautmann RE. The ileal neobladder to the female urethra. *Urol Clin North Am* 1997;24:827–835.
2. Hautmann RE. The ileal neobladder. *Atlas Urol Clin North Am* 2001;9:85–108.
3. Hautmann RE. Review article: Urinary diversion: Ileal conduit to neobladder. *J Urol* 2003;169:834–842.
4. Hautmann RE, de Patriconi R, Gottfried H-W, et al. The ileal neobladder: Complications and functional results in 363 patients after 11 years of followup. *J Urol* 1999;161:422–428.
5. Hautmann RE, Egghart G, Frohneberg D, et al. The ileal neobladder. *J Urol* 1988;139:39–43.
6. Hautmann RE, Paiss T, de Petriconi R. The ileal neobladder in women: 9 years of experience with 18 patients. *J Urol* 1996;155:76–81.
7. Skinner DG, Studer UE, Okada K, et al. Which are suitable for continent diversion or bladder substitution following cystectomy or other definitive local treatment? *Int J Urol* 1995;2[Suppl 2]:105.
8. Studer UE, Hautmann RE, Hohenfellner M, et al. Indications for continent diversion after cystectomy and factors affecting long-term results. *Urol Oncol* 1998;4:172.

CHAPTER 83

The Padua Ileal Bladder

Francesco Pagano and Pierfrancesco Bassi

The Padua ileal bladder ["Vescica Ileale Padovana" (VIP)] was developed as a practical application of the concepts expressed by Camey et al. (3), Bramble (2), Kock (5), and Hinman (4) for the construction of a urinary reservoir employing an intestinal segment: detubularization, reconfiguration, and search for a spherical pouch of adequate capacity. Large- and small-bowel non-detubularized segments used as bladder substitutes have been shown to generate significant intraluminal pressures (4,5) and subsequently cause urinary incontinence and/or renal failure. Disruption of directional peristalsis by opening the antimesenteric border of the bowel (detubularization) and folding (reconfiguration) have been proven to significantly decrease intraluminal pressure by making ineffective the bowel contractions. However, a single folding of the intestinal detubularized segment incompletely suppresses the peristaltic activity as demonstrated by Kock: A double folding is necessary to this aim (5). As a consequence, the double-folding Kock principle is the gold standard in constructing a spherical reservoir from a cylindrical bowel segment.

The capacity and the intraluminal pressure of a reservoir also depend on the geometric configuration as demonstrated by Hinman (4) with geometric considerations: The larger the radius, the larger the volume. From the surgical standpoint, this explains why the double folding produces the largest volume from the same initial intestinal length. Coupling of the double folding with the spherical configuration also offers a relevant feature: At the same endoluminal pressure, the larger diameter accommodates a larger volume, according to Laplace's and Pascal's laws.

According to the above-mentioned principles, the functional requirements of the Padua ileal bladder are adequate capacity (300 to 500 mL), low-pressure storage phase (less than 40 cm of water), no reflux to upper urinary tract, day- and nighttime continence, and voluntary as well as easy and complete voiding "per urethram." An intestinal reservoir respecting these requirements should allow the long-term preservation of renal function and provide a reliable control of continence and voiding with satisfactory patient acceptance.

Further features have also been considered. Because urine absorption throughout the intestinal wall is unavoidable, the shortest intestinal segment must be selected to minimize secondary metabolic disorders. An easy-to-perform and quick procedure with a short learning curve was considered highly desirable. Last but not least, from the oncological standpoint the neobladder must not interfere with the natural history of the disease and the related treatment(s).

The original features of the Padova ileal bladder are the construction of a lower funnel, the spherical reconfiguration, and the close resemblance to the native bladder (the lower funnel resembles an empty prostatic fossa; the ureters lie down in a natural position) and the natural way the reservoir fits into the pelvis.

DIAGNOSIS

This is a reconstructive procedure following the removal of the bladder. Diagnostic studies are dependent upon the underlying disease.

INDICATIONS FOR SURGERY

Any patient who is a candidate for a conduit diversion is potentially suitable for bladder substitution as long as an adequate ileal segment is available. Surgical indications include bladder cancers, neurogenic bladder, congenital abnormalities, and refractory interstitial cystitis, irrespective of the patient age. From the oncological standpoint, the only contraindication is a positive urethral margin biopsy: Patients with locally advanced bladder cancer (T3–T4) with or without nodal involvement or candidates for postoperative systemic chemotherapy are suitable for the procedure. Normal renal function is compulsory: A dilated upper urinary tract(s) does not represent a contraindication to the procedure. To take benefit from the procedure the patient should have intelligence, maturity, and motivation.

SURGICAL TECHNIQUE

The membranous urethra is managed as in radical prostatectomy and is incised as close as possible to the prostatic apex to preserve the distal urethral sphincter. In selected patients, the nerve-sparing cystoprostatectomy can be performed.

A 40-cm ileal segment is isolated, starting at a convenient point 15 to 20 cm from the ileocecal valve (Fig. 83–1). The distal (aboral) mesenteric incision is deepened at the level of the ileocolic artery to obtain better mobility to allow a tension-free urethrointestinal anastomosis. At the contrary, the proximal (oral) mesenteric incision can be short because it does not contribute to the mobility of the reservoir. The intestinal continuity is restored by end-to-end anastomosis with surgical staplers.

The entire ileal segment is split open all along the antimesenteric border (Fig. 83–2).

A lower funnel is created by means of two running sutures, posteriorly and anteriorly, about 5 cm in length, to make the urethrointestinal anastomosis easier and tension free (Fig. 83–3). The ileal anastomotic hole is placed at the lowest edge of the funnel: The eversion of the ileal mucosa in the anastomotic hole is recommended. Medially, the proximal loop is folded on itself in a reversed U shape and the inner opposite borders are sutured side to side to create an upper ileal cup (Fig. 83–4).

The ureteroileal anastomosis with serous-lined extramural reimplantation according to the Abol-Eneim and Ghoneim technique (1) is carried out bilaterally. The edges of two medial intestinal flaps are joined by a running through-and-through suture of 3-0 polyglactin, resulting in the creation of two oblique serous-lined intestinal troughs (Fig. 83–5). The left ureter is brought medially through a suitable mesenteric window in the left mesocolon, providing a downward smooth curve without kinking. Each ureter is then laid into its corresponding trough. A mucosa-to-mucosa anastomosis between the

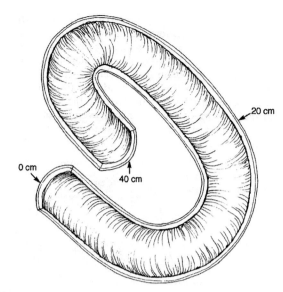

FIG. 83-2. Detubularization and reconfiguration (scheme).

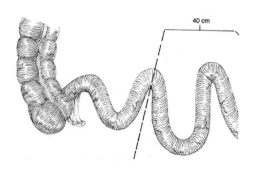

FIG. 83-3. Creation of lower funnel.

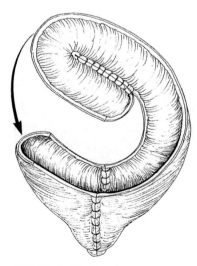

FIG. 83–4. First folding maneuver.

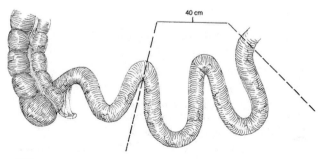

FIG. 83–1. Isolation of a 40-cm segment of distal ileum.

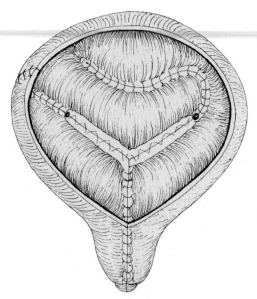

FIG. 83-5. Ureteral reimplantation: serous-lined intestinal troughs.

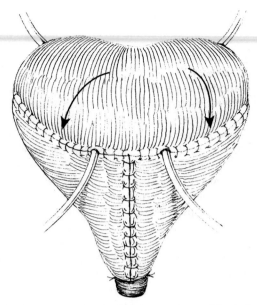

FIG. 83–7. Second folding maneuver and final view.

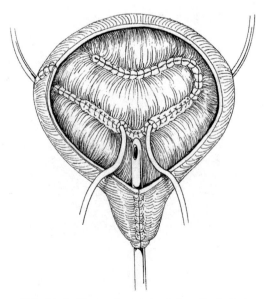

FIG. 83-6. Ureteral reimplantation: final view.

stented (6 Fr) and spatulated end of the ureter and the ileal flaps is performed using 4-0 polyglactin sutures (Fig. 83–6). The implanted ureters are then covered by approximation and an interrupted 3-0 polyglactin suture is inserted. The ureteral stents are fixed to the pouch mucosa close to the ureteral hiatus and secured to their exits (made by stabbing through the anterior wall of the reservoir) using 4-0 gut sutures (Fig. 83–7). The urethroileal anastomosis is performed with six to eight sutures of 3-0 polyglactin.

The closure of the reservoir is completed at the anterior aspect by folding downward the upper edge of the ileal cup to obtain a spherical reservoir. A running suture of 3-0 polyglactin is employed for all sutures of the reservoir. The reservoir is drained by a transurethral 22 Fr Folatex catheter.

Perioperative Care

Bowel preparation is performed by oral administration of 3 to 4 L of electrolyte solution the day before surgery. Parenteral alimentation is supplied until normal bowel function resumes. Wide-spectrum antibiotics are given for 7 days; then, quinolones are administered orally as long as the pouch catheter stays in. The rectal and gastric tubes are left in place for 3 to 4 days or until bowel contractions appear.

The ureters are drained by 6 or 8 Fr stents that are removed after 8 or 9 days. Radiological evaluation of the pouch is performed after 12 days. Special attention is paid to training the patient to empty the reservoir completely by abdominal straining plus simultaneous perineal relaxation and to develop alternatives to the normal voiding desire.

OUTCOMES

Complications

The Padova small-bowel neobladder procedure was first performed in 1987 (6). Since its first applications, some changes have been sequentially introduced to simplify and shorten the procedure. Initially, the sequence was as follows: ileourethral anastomosis, detubularization, lower funnel, ureteral reimplantation according to the Le Duc technique, posterior reconfiguration, and anterior reconfiguration. The length of the ileal segment was progressively reduced from 60 to 50 cm to 40 cm.

Recently, the sequence of maneuvers has been established as follows: detubularization, construction of the lower funnel, posterior reconfiguration, bilateral ureteral reimplantation, incomplete anterior reconfiguration, ileourethral anastomosis, complete reconfiguration, and extraperitonealization of the reservoir. This allows the surgeon to perform the major part of the procedure on the surface of the surgical field, thus reducing the operative time (at present about 2 hours). Because of the unsatisfactory rate of ureterointestinal anastomosis stenoses (7), the Le Duc ureteral reimplantation technique has been abandoned and favorably replaced with the serous-lined extramural reimplantation according to the Abol-Eneim and Ghoneim procedure (1).

Results

Padua ileal bladder is a simple, quick procedure with a short learning curve for the urologist who is accustomed to performing radical prostatectomy, ileal conduit, and antireflux procedures. Functional long-term results (6,7) and complication rates are satisfactory. The procedure provides a good-capacity, low-pressure, nonrefluxing, and continent reservoir by employing only a 40-cm ileal segment.

REFERENCES

1. Abol-Eneim H, Ghoneim MA. A novel uretero-ileal reimplantation technique: the serous lined extramural tunnel. A preliminary report. *J Urol* 1995;151:1193–1197.
2. Bramble FG. The treatment of adult enuresis and urge incontinence by enterocystoplasty. *Br J Urol* 1982;54:693.
3. Camey M, Richard F, Botto H. Bladder replacement by ileocystoplasty. In: King LR, Stone AR, Webster GD, eds. *Bladder reconstruction and continent urinary diversion.* Chicago: Year Book, 1987.
4. Hinman F Jr. Selection of intestinal segments for bladder substitution: physical and physiological characteristics. *J Urol* 1988;139:519–524.
5. Kock NG. The development of the continent ileal reservoir (Kock pouch) and application in patients requiring urinary diversion. In: King RL, Stone AR, Webster GD, eds. *Bladder reconstruction and continent urinary diversion.* Chicago: Year Book, 1987.
6. Pagano F, Artibani W, Ligato P. Vescica Ileale Padovana: a technique for total bladder replacement. *Eur Urol* 1990;17:149–154.
7. Pagano F, Bassi P, Artibani W. The Padua Ileal Bladder (V.I.P., Vescica Ileale Padovana). *Acta Urol Ital* 1996;10(2):79–83, 1996.

CHAPTER 84

The T-Pouch Ileal Neobladder

John P. Stein and Donald G. Skinner

Today, the goals of urinary diversion have evolved from simply diverting the urine and protecting the upper urinary tracts. Contemporary objectives of lower urinary tract reconstruction should also include a form of reconstruction that provides a safe and continent means to store and eliminate urine, with efforts to provide an improved quality of life. Currently, four reasonable options regarding lower urinary tract reconstruction exist: (a) an incontinent cutaneous diversion— including the ileal or colon conduit; (b) a continent cutaneous reservoir—requiring catheterization of a cutaneous stoma; (c) a continent rectal reservoir—with storage and elimination of urine via the rectum; and (d) the orthotopic bladder substitute—with reconstruction to the native intact urethra.

In 1950, Bricker introduced the ileal conduit, which established a simple and reliable form of urinary diversion (2). The concept of a continent cutaneous diversion was eventually popularized in the 1980s at several large institutions. These experiences revolutionized lower urinary tract reconstruction to a continent cutaneous form of diversion. Patients were relieved from the problems of an external collection device; however, they still required catheterization of an abdominal stoma. The continent cutaneous urinary diversion was clearly a step forward and considered an improvement upon the standard ileal or colon conduit.

A natural progression of the continent cutaneous urinary diversion was the orthotopic bladder substitute, which is connected directly to the native intact urethra. The orthotopic neobladder most closely resembles the original bladder in both location and function. The orthotopic neobladder eliminates the need for a cutaneous stoma and a cutaneous collection device. Orthotopic diversion relies on the patients' intact rhabdosphincter continence mechanism (external striated sphincter muscle), eliminating the need for intermittent catheterization in most cases and the often-plagued efferent continence mechanism of most continent cutaneous reservoirs. Void-

ing is accomplished by concomitantly increasing intraabdominal pressure (Valsalva maneuver) with relaxation of the pelvic floor musculature.

Beginning in 1982, the primary form of urinary diversion at our institution was the continent cutaneous ileal reservoir (Kock pouch) as described by Kock and associates (3). The continence and antireflux mechanism of the Kock ileal reservoir required construction of an intussuscepted nipple valve. Throughout this period, significant technical advances and improvements in lower urinary tract reconstruction were made. We have been committed to the principles of the Kock ileal reservoir and reflux prevention in patients undergoing continent urinary reconstruction. Although the principles of the continent Kock ileal reservoir (cutaneous and orthotopic form) are sound, complications can occur. Most complications associated with the Kock ileal reservoir involve the intussuscepted limb: either the antireflux (afferent limb) or the continent catheterizable (efferent limb) nipple.

The most common complications associated with the intussuscepted afferent nipple included the formation of calculi (usually on exposed staples that secure the afferent nipple valve) in 5%, afferent nipple stenosis (thought to be caused by ischemic changes resulting from the mesenteric stripping required to maintain the intussuscepted limb) in 4%, and extussusception (prolapse of the afferent limb) in 1% of patients (6).

The need to improve upon the intussuscepted nipple valve became obvious. Based on reports from Abol-Enein and Ghoneim (1) employing a ureteral extraserosal tunnel, as well as our own experience with the Mitrofanoff appendiceal subserosal tunnel, we subsequently developed and described the novel flap-valve T-mechanism (8). This flap-valve T-mechanism is a versatile technique that can easily be applied as am antireflux mechanism, as well as a continent mechanism in a cutaneous reservoir (9).

The T-mechanism was first successfully incorporated as the afferent antireflux limb of an orthotopic reservoir

(T-pouch) (8) and subsequently into an afferent antireflux and efferent continence limb of a cutaneous reservoir (double-T-pouch) (9). This flap-valve T-mechanism should eliminate the complications associated with the intussuscepted nipple valve while maintaining an effective antireflux or continence mechanism.

DIAGNOSIS

Patients undergoing urinary diversion have either a functional or absolute loss of the bladder. In the United States, diversions are most commonly performed in conjunction with cystectomy. Therefore, any diagnostic studies are related to the underlying disease.

INDICATIONS FOR SURGERY

Any patient who requires a urinary diversion is a candidate for this procedure

ALTERNATIVE THERAPY

Other urinary diversions include intubated (nephrostomy, ureterostomy) and nonintubated (conduits, continent pouches, and orthotopic bladders).

SURGICAL TECHNIQUE

The terminal portion of the ileum is used to construct the orthotopic T-pouch ileal neobladder (Fig. 84–1). The distal mesenteric division is best made along the avascular plane of Treves between the ileocolic artery and terminal branches of the superior mesenteric artery. This division should extend deep into the avascular portion of the mesentery, which is essential for adequate mobility of the reservoir. The proximal mesenteric division, however, is short and provides a broad vascular blood supply to the reservoir. In addition, a small window of mesentery and 5- to 7-cm portion of small bowel most proximal to the overall ileal segment are discarded. This helps ensure mobility to the pouch and small-bowel anastomosis.

The T-pouch reservoir is created from a 44-cm segment of distal ileum placed in an inverted "V" configuration. Each limb of the V measures 22 cm. A proximal 8- to 10-cm segment of ileum (afferent limb) is used to form the afferent antireflux mechanism. Note that if ureteral length is short or compromised, a longer afferent ileal segment (proximal ileum) may be harvested to bridge the ureteral gap.

The ileum is divided between the proximal afferent ileal segment and the 44-cm segment that will form the reservoir portion of the neobladder. The mesentery between these ileal segments is carefully incised for 2 cm with preservation of all major vascular arcades. This mesenteric incision is directed toward the base of the mesentery and provides mobility to the afferent ileal segment, which will ultimately be advanced into the serosal-lined ileal trough formed by the base of the two adjacent 22-cm segments of ileum.

The proximal end of the isolated afferent ileal segment is closed with a running Parker–Kerr suture of 3-0 chromic and a third layer of interrupted 4-0 silk sutures. A standard small-bowel anastomosis is performed to reestablish bowel continuity and the mesenteric trap closed.

The isolated 44-cm ileal segment is then laid out in an inverted V configuration, the apex of the V lying caudally with a suture marking a point between the two 22-cm adjacent segments of ileum (Fig. 84–2). The opened end (base) of the V is directed in a cephalad manner. Note the serosal-lined ileal trough formed at the base of the 44-cm segment.

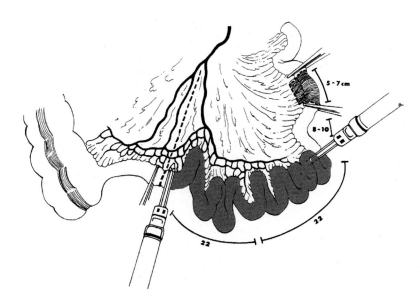

FIG. 84–1. Designated segments of terminal ileum for construction of the orthotopic T-pouch ileal neobladder. Note that the distal mesenteric division is made between the ileocolic and terminal branches of the superior mesenteric artery, which extends into the avascular plane of the mesentery. In addition, a small window of mesentery and a 5- to 7-cm segment of most proximal small bowel is discarded to allow mobility to the pouch and small-bowel anastomosis.

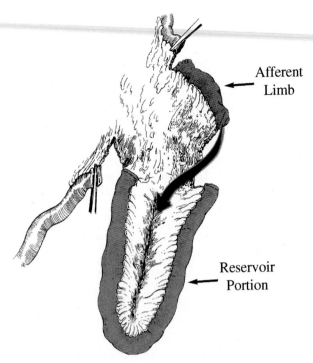

FIG. 84–2. The T-pouch is constructed from an isolated 44-cm ileal segment (laid out in an inverted V configuration) that forms the reservoir portion of the pouch and a proximal 8- to 10-cm segment of ileum to form the antireflux limb. The mesentery between the afferent ileal segment and the proximal portion of the 44-cm ileal segment is carefully incised (2 cm) with preservation of the major vascular arcades. Note the serosal-lined ileal trough created at the base of the two 22-cm ileal segments where the afferent limb will be advanced (arrow).

The antireflux (flap-valve) mechanism is then created by anchoring the distal 4 cm of the afferent ileal segment into the serosal-lined ileal trough formed by the two adjacent 22-cm ileal segments. First, mesenteric Deaver's windows are opened between the vascular arcades (carefully excising mesenteric fat adjacent to the serosa of the ileum, which facilitates the development of these mesenteric windows) for 4 cm proximal to the distal most portion of the isolated afferent ileal segment (Fig. 84–3). Preserving these arcades (blood vessels) maintains a well-vascularized afferent limb and will allow permanent fixation of this portion of the limb into the serosal-lined ileal trough with complete preservation of the mesentery and blood supply. Note that placement of small Penrose drains through each mesenteric window helps identify and facilitates passage of sutures through each.

A series of 3-0 silk sutures are then used to approximate the serosa of the two adjacent 22-cm ileal segments at the base of the V with the sutures being passed through the previously opened Deaver's windows in the afferent ileal limb. This will then anchor the afferent limb into the serosal-lined ileal trough. Specifically, a silk suture is placed into the seromuscular portion of the bowel (adjacent to the mesentery) at the base (most cephalad portion of the V) of one of the 22-cm ileal segments (Fig. 84–4A). The suture is then passed through the most proximal Deaver's windows opened in the afferent ileal limb (Fig. 84–4B) and placed in a corresponding seromuscular site of the bowel (next to mesentery) of the adjacent 22-cm ileal segment (Fig. 84–4C). The suture is brought back through the same Deaver's window and tied down (Fig. 84–4D). In general, two to three silk sutures are placed within each Deaver's window to ensure that the back wall of the reservoir does not separate. This process is repeated through each individual Deaver's window until the distal 4 cm of the afferent segment is permanently fixed in the serosal-lined ileal trough. We have found that placement of small (1/4 in.) Penrose drains through each Deaver's window facilitates passage of the silk suture back and forth through the mesentery without difficulty. The Penrose drains are systematically removed as the afferent limb is fixed within the serosal-lined ileal trough.

Next, the previously anchored portion of the afferent ileal segment (distal 4 cm) is tapered on the antimesenteric (anterior) border over a 30 Fr catheter (Fig. 84–5).

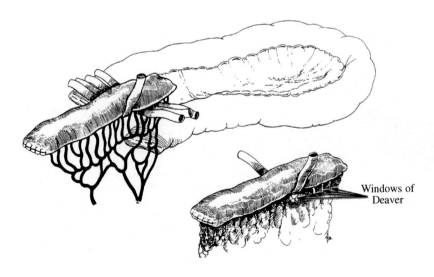

Windows of Deaver

FIG. 84–3. Creation of the antireflux mechanism. First, four mesenteric Deaver's windows are opened (adjacent to the serosa of the ileum) at the distal 4 cm of the isolated afferent ileal segment. Placement of small Penrose drains through each mesenteric window helps identify and facilitates passage of sutures through each (see inset with arrows). The distal 4 cm of the afferent segment will be anchored into the serosal-lined ileal trough formed by the base of the two adjacent 22-cm ileal segments.

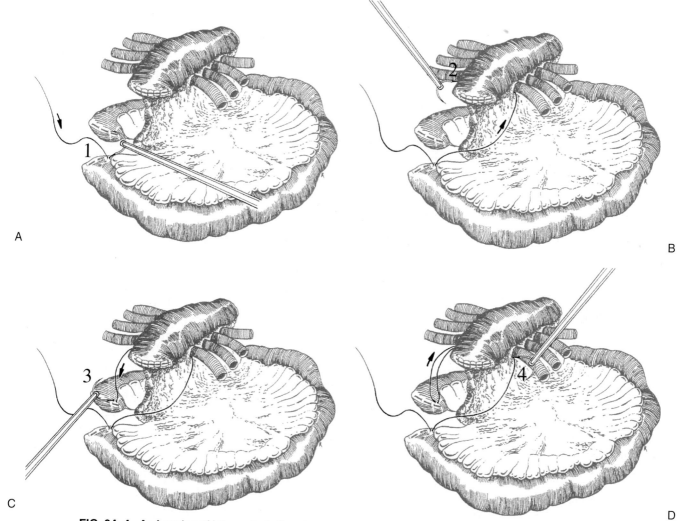

FIG. 84–4. A: A series of interrupted silk sutures are used to approximate the serosa of the base of the two adjacent 22-cm ileal segments. Note that these sutures are brought through the Deaver's windows facilitated by the use of the Penrose drains. **B:** After passing the silk suture through the Deaver's window, it is placed in a corresponding site on the adjacent 22-cm ileal segment. **C,D:** This suture will then be brought back through the same Deaver's window and tied down.

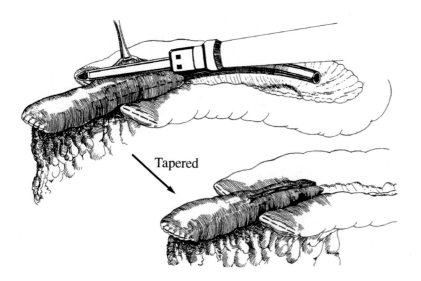

Tapered

FIG. 84–5. The previously anchored distal 4-cm afferent ileal segment is tapered over a 30 Fr catheter on the antimesenteric boarder. Note that the authors prefer to use a GIA-55 stapler to taper this distal 3- to 4-cm afferent segment. The staples will not be exposed as this staple line will be covered by ileal flaps.

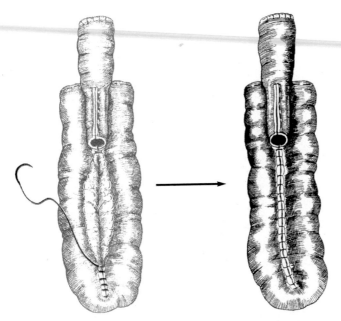

FIG. 84–6. The two 22-cm ileal segments are joined by a running 3-0 polyglycolic acid continuous suture. Note that this suture is placed adjacent to the mesentery and runs from the apex up to the ostium of the afferent ileal segment. The serosa of the two 22-cm ileal segments are reapproximated.

Tapering this portion of the afferent ileal segment reduces the bulk and lumen of the afferent limb and facilitates later coverage of the anchored afferent limb with ileal flaps. In addition, this tapering of the afferent limb will increase the tunnel length:lumen diameter ratio, providing a more effective flap-valve mechanism.

After the distal 4 cm of the afferent ileal segment has been tapered, the remaining portion of the adjacent 22-cm ileal segments are approximated together with a side-to-side 3-0 polyglycolic acid suture. This suture line simply reapproximates the two ileal limbs and is placed adjacent to the mesentery (Fig. 84–6), which can be performed in a running or interrupted fashion.

Starting at the apex of the V, the ileum is then opened immediately adjacent to the previously placed serosal suture line using electrocautery. This incision is carried upward toward the ostium of the afferent limb where the afferent limb is anchored (Fig. 84–7A). Once this incision reaches the level of the afferent ostium, the incision is then extended directly lateral to the antimesenteric border of the ileum and carried upward (cephalad) to the base of the ileal segment. An incision is made in similar fashion on the contralateral 22-cm ileal segment (Fig. 84–7B). Once completed, these incisions provide wide flaps of ileum that will ultimately be brought over and cover the tapered afferent ileal segment to create the antireflux mechanism in a flap-valve technique (Fig. 84–7C).

The previously incised ileal mucosa is then oversewn with two layers of a running 3-0 polyglycolic acid suture starting at the apex and running upward toward the ostium of the afferent limb (Fig. 84–8). Once the ostium of the afferent limb is reached, the running suture is tied. An interrupted mucosa-to-mucosa anastomosis is then performed between the ostium of the afferent ileal limb and the incised intestinal ileal flaps with 3-0 polyglycolic acid sutures (Fig. 84–9). The mucosal edges of the ileal flaps are then approximated over the tapered portion of the afferent ileal limb (4 cm) with a running suture in two layers (Fig. 84–10). This suture line completes the poste-

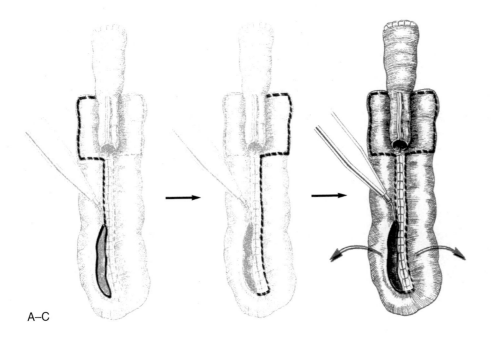

A–C

FIG. 84–7. A,B: The two 22-cm ileal segments are opened immediately adjacent to the serosal suture line beginning at the apex and carried upward to the ostium of the afferent segment. Note that once this incision reaches the ostium it is then directed lateral (to the antimesenteric boarder) and cephalad to the base. The dotted line depicts the incision line. **C:** Completing the incision of the bowel. Note that the incision provides wide flaps of ileum that can easily be brought over and cover the tapered distal afferent ileal segment to form the antireflux mechanism in a flap-valve technique.

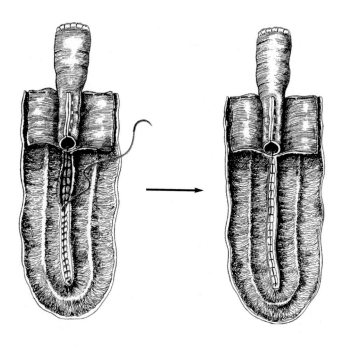

FIG. 84–8. The incised ileal mucosa is oversewn in two layers beginning at the apex and continuing toward (cephalad) the ostium of the afferent ileal segment.

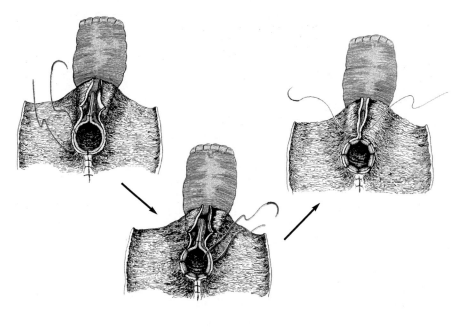

FIG. 84–9. A mucosa-to-mucosa, ileal-to-ileal anastomosis is performed between the ostium of the afferent segment and the edges of the ileal flaps. Note that this is performed with interrupted 3-0 polyglycolic acid sutures with completion of the ileal-to-ileal anastomosis.

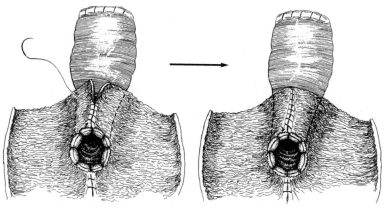

A,B

FIG. 84–10. A: The mucosal edges of the ileal flaps are brought over the tapered distal portion of the afferent ileal segment. **B:** Completion of the posterior suture line covering the afferent segment with the ileal flaps. Note that this will exclude the staple line from the reservoir.

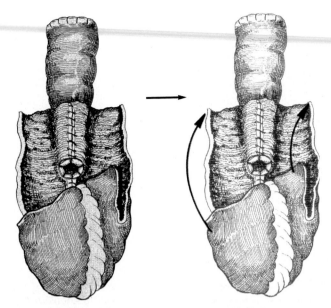

FIG. 84–11. The T-pouch is folded (see arrows) and closed in the opposite direction from which it was opened. This manner of folding will create a low-pressure, large-capacity spherical reservoir.

rior wall of the reservoir and creates the effective flap-valve T-mechanism: the serosal-lined ileal antireflux limb.

The reservoir is then closed by folding the ileum in half in an opposite direction from which it was opened

(Fig. 84–11). This effectively creates a low-pressure, high-capacity urinary reservoir. The anterior wall is closed with a running, two-layer 3-0 polyglycolic acid suture that is watertight (Fig. 84–12). This anterior suture line is stopped just prior to the end of the right side to allow insertion of an index finger. This is the most mobile and dependent portion of the reservoir and will later be anastomosed to the urethra.

Once the pouch has been closed, each ureter is spatulated and a standard, bilateral end-to-side ureteroileal anastomosis is performed to the proximal portion of the afferent limb using interrupted 4-0 polyglycolic acid sutures. These anastomoses are stented with no. 8 infant feeding tubes that are directed from the ipsilateral renal pelvis (kidney), across the ureteroileal anastomosis, through the afferent limb, into the reservoir, and out the neourethra. A 24 Fr hematuria catheter is placed per urethra to provide adequate drainage of the reservoir and the ureteral stents are secured to the end of the urethral catheter with a 3-0 nylon suture. This facilities removal of the stents at approximately 3 weeks, along with the urethral catheter. A tension-free mucosa-to-mucosa urethroileal anastomosis is performed.

OUTCOMES

Complications

From November 1996 through May 2000, 180 patients [142 men (79%)], with a mean age of 67 years (range, 33

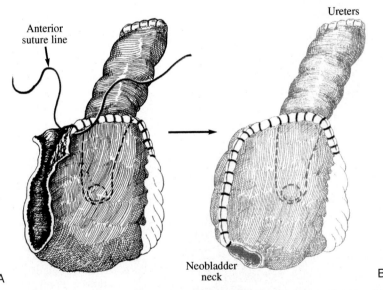

FIG. 84–12. A: The anterior suture line is completed with two layers of a continuous 3-0 polyglycolic acid suture. Note that the anterior suture line is stopped just short of the right side to allow insertion of an index finger, which will be the neourethra. **B:** Completion of the T-pouch. Note that the most mobile and dependent portion of the reservoir will be anastomosed to the urethra following the ureteroileal anastomosis to the proximal portion of the afferent limb.

to 88), underwent an orthotopic T-pouch ileal following cystectomy. All patients had a 4-cm T-limb created to prevent urinary reflux. The indication for cystectomy in this group of patients included bladder cancer in 176 patients (97%): 170 for transitional cell, 3 for squamous cell, and 3 for adenocarcinoma. The median follow-up was 2.8 years (range, 1.4 to 5.3). We analyzed our data according to perioperative mortality, early (within 3 months) and late pouch-related complications (with specific attention to the T-limb), radiographic evaluation, and serum creatinine.

A total of nine (5%) early pouch-related complications occurred, including urine leak in six patients, mucus retention in two, and a pouch-cutaneous fistulae in one. There were no early complications directly related to the T-limb. Eight of the nine early complications were treated conservatively. Late reservoir-related complications occurred in 16 (9%) patients, including ureteroileal stenosis in seven, stones in six, and an ischemic reservoir and pouch-vaginal fistulae in one each. None of these late complications were attributed to the T-limb. The only late complication directly related to the T-limb was stenosis seen in a patient who received adjuvant radiation to the neobladder. A total of 134 patients underwent a gravity pouchogram study with 11 (8%) demonstrating a radiographic abnormality, including 10 patients with urinary reflux into the T-limb and one with a pouch-vaginal fistula. Of 142 patients undergoing an intravenous pyelogram (IVP), a total of 9 (6%) abnormalities were documented, all demonstrating ureteroileal obstruction. The upper urinary tract otherwise remained unchanged or improved in 94% of patients. There have been no episodes of pyelonephritis or worsening renal function in these patients.

Results

The importance of preventing the reflux of urinary constituents following orthotopic reconstruction is a controversial subject and remains a source of much debate. We continue to be strong proponents of reflux prevention in all patients undergoing lower urinary tract reconstruction. We also acknowledge that the complications or risks associated with incorporating an antireflux mechanism (i.e., obstruction) should not outweigh the theoretical advantage of reflux prevention. To meet this end, we have been diligent to critically evaluate our antireflux techniques and continually improve upon existing ideas and methods. This evaluation has subsequently stimulated a change from the intussuscepted nipple in the Kock pouch to the development of the T-mechanism incorporated as an antireflux limb in the T-pouch ileal neobladder (9). This technique provides an effective antireflux mechanism without the complications associated with the intussuscepted nipple.

Many antireflux techniques exist today. The inclusion of an antireflux mechanism in the chronically infected, continent cutaneous reservoir (requiring intermittent catheterization) is critical and not a source of considerable debate. However, consideration of the potential complications of late stenosis from various antireflux techniques could clearly outweigh their theoretical advantage of protecting the upper urinary tract.

Since 1982, we have incorporated the intussuscepted nipple valve as an antireflux mechanism in all forms of urinary diversion and as a continence mechanism in patients undergoing a continent cutaneous Kock ileal reservoir. The basic surgical premise and characteristics of the Kock ileal reservoir are sound: a low-pressure, large-capacity reservoir, employing the intussuscepted antirefluxing and continent nipple valve. The Achilles heel of Kock ileal reservoir, however, remains the intussuscepted nipple valve. Despite several surgical modifications to improve upon the construction of the intussuscepted nipple valve, there remained complications and a relatively high reoperation rate (4–7). The need to improve upon the intussuscepted nipple valve became obvious with time.

The T-mechanism is a flap-valve technique that can be applied as an antireflux and continence mechanism in lower urinary tract reconstruction (8,9). In general, all flap-valve techniques for continence or antireflux rely on the dynamic principle that the channeled segment (appendix, ureter, or intestine) is fixed and tunneled along the inner wall of the reservoir. As reservoir filling occurs, the channel is compressed against the wall of the pouch and continence or reflux prevention is achieved. This technique is based on similar principles for reimplantation of the ureter into the bladder. Keys to success in the flap-valve technique include an appropriate tunnel length:lumen diameter ratio. Further, the wall of the reservoir must be sufficiently capable to allow compression of the tunneled channel as the pouch fills.

The unique aspect of the T-mechanism (antireflux and continence) is the ability to create a reliable and effective flap-valve system (9). Maintenance of the vascular arcades (opening the Deaver's window) provides complete preservation of the mesentery and blood supply to the limb, which should eliminate problems with ischemia or stenosis of the bowel segment. Permanent fixation of the limb into the serosal-lined ileal trough should also eliminate problems associated with prolapse or extussusception of the limb. Importantly, no exposed metallic staples exist within the reservoir, which should reduce the incidence of stone formation typically associated with exposure of metallic foreign bodies to urine. Further, if necessary, the afferent limb can be easily lengthened when there is shortened or compromised ureters. A longer proximal afferent segment may be harvested to bridge any ureteral defect to maintain a tension-free ureteroileal anastomosis.

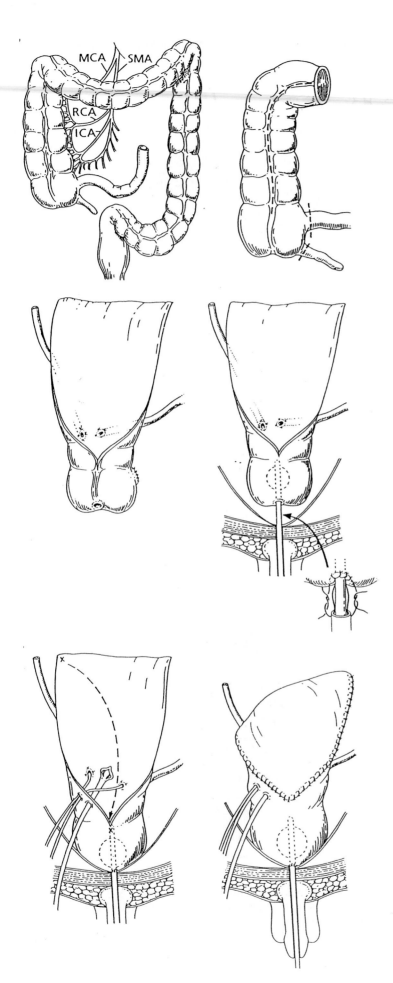

FIG. 85–4. Construction of a right colonic reservoir.
A, B: Isolation of a colonic segment consisting of
cecum, ascending colon, and the right colic flexure.
C, D: Opening of the segment through the taenia libera leaving the cecum intact and anastomosing it to
the urethra. **E, F:** The ureters are anastomosed into
the colonic segment utilizing the so-called "button-
hole" submucous implantation technique. This technique describes the ureters entering the submucosel
tunnel via a hole in the wall of the pouch. Detubularization and reconfiguration is completed by flipping
the upper dorsal half of the segment over to the front
and anastomosing it with the lower ventral half.

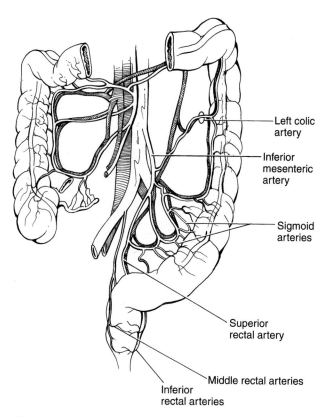

FIG. 85–5. Vascular supply of the left colon and rectum.

Left colic artery

Inferior mesenteric artery

Sigmoid arteries

Superior rectal artery

Middle rectal arteries

Inferior rectal arteries

the other a bowel-derived antireflux mechanism is interposed between ureter and reservoir.

In any case, for implantation of the ureters into the large-bowel segment the left ureter has to be pulled into the right retroperitoneum behind the mesentery of the descending colon as in ileal conduit diversion.

All antirefluxive implantation techniques in which the ureter becomes part of the antirefluxive mechanism have a similar mechanism of action ("flap valve"). They follow the same principle: With an oblique entry of the ureter into the reservoir some length of a "tunnel" is created that allows transmission of the reservoir pressure onto the wall of the ureter, thus creating a force that occludes the ureter progressively with rising reservoir pressures. The most frequently utilized principles to expose the ureter to the reservoir pressure are the submucosal tunnel technique and the seromuscular extramural tunnel technique.

In the submucous tunnel technique, both ureters are implanted into the ascending colon with a 3- to 5-cm submucosal tunnel. Ureters are anchored with 6-0 polyglycolic sutures to the muscle of the bowel wall and the neoorifices are established by 6-0 or 7-0 ureteromucosal sutures.

The most common technique of interposing an antirefluxive device is to take advantage of the ileocecal valve. The cecal side is incorporated in the pouch, while the ureters are anastomosed in an end-to-side (Nesbit) or

spatulated end-to-end (Wallace) technique to the terminal ileum. Thus, the flow of urine is directed from the ureters into the pouch while reflux is prevented by the ileocecal valve.

The ureters are intubated with 6 to 8 Fr stents and a 10 Fr cystostomy catheter and a 22 Fr transurethral Foley balloon catheter are inserted. The anastomosis of the pouch with the anterior bladder wall in bladder augmentation procedures and the anterior wall of the pouch are completed in the same way as described before. However, at the site of submucosal ureteral implantation, the pouch is closed by mucosal sutures only to prevent ureteral obstruction. A 20 Fr gravity drain is placed in the small pelvis and at the ureteral implantation site.

The ureteral stents are removed after 10 days. The transurethral catheter is withdrawn after 3 to 6 weeks after radiographic study of the pouch. Residual urine is checked via the pouchostomy catheter when patients void spontaneously. In neurogenic cases, patients are instructed in intermittent catheterization.

OUTCOMES

Complications

In the early postoperative months, nonperistaltic contractions of the large-bowel segment of a Mainz pouch do occur but subside spontaneously with increasing capacity of the pouch in most cases. For persistent incontinence due to an inadequate low compliance or persistent contractions of the pouch, anticholinergics are administered systemically or topically by installation. If pharmacological therapy fails, the capacity of the pouch has to be enlarged surgically.

About 60% of patients develop postoperatively asymptomatic acidosis as judged by blood gas analyses (base excess < 2.5) that is balanced prophylactically by oral alkali substitution (sodium/potassium citrate/bicarbonate).

In view of a relatively short follow-up period, the risk of secondary malignancies can at present not be assessed finally. Follow-up examinations should include ultrasound of the upper urinary tract, pouchoscopy, and evaluation of serum parameters such as levels of cobalamine and bile acids.

Results

In general, the criteria applied for judgment of the outcome of an orthotopic diversion utilizing intestinal segments are (a) function and morphology of the upper urinary tract, (b) frequency during day and night, (c) continence, and (d) ability for spontaneous micturition. However, one has to keep in mind that especially continence and ability for spontaneous micturition may for a significant part be influenced by the type and quality of surgery preceding the

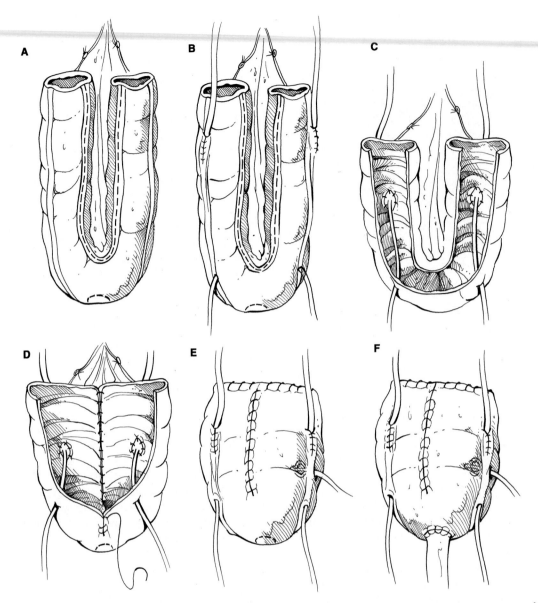

FIG. 85–6. Construction of a sigmoid colon-based reservoir (Reddy). **A:** Isolating a sigma segment of about 30 cm. **B:** Submucosel ureteral implantation. **C, D:** Detubularization and reconfiguration of the segment by antimesenteric opening, folding, and anastomosing the back wall of the pouch. **E, F:** Completion of the anterior wall of the pouch and anastomosis to the urethra.

orthotopic substitution itself. In this respect related factors may be, e.g., preparation of the bladder neck and urethra, sparing of the autonomous nerves, and precautions to prevent pouch displacement. Therefore, functional results attributed to specific kinds of reservoirs rely in fact on more factors than the segment(s) of intestine and geometric model chosen. For ileocecal reservoirs a ureterointestinal stricture rate of 7% is reported. Continence rates for ileocecal reservoirs vary between 75% and 88% during the day and 67% during the night (6,11). Continence rates for sigmoid colon-based reservoirs were significantly less at 50% (11).

REFERENCES

1. Ali-El-Din B, El-Sobky E, Hohenfellner M, Ghoneim M. Orthotopic bladder substitution in women: functional and urodynamic evaluation. *J Urol* 1999;161:1875–1880.
2. Hinman FJ. Selection of intestinal segments for bladder substitution: physical and physiological characteristics. *J Urol* 1988;139:519–523.
3. Hohenfellner M, Black P, Linn J, Dahms S, Thüroff J. Surgical treatment of interstial cystitis in women. *Int Urogynecol J Pelvic Floor Dysfunct* 2000;11:113–119.
4. Hugonnet C, Danuser H, Springer J, Studer U. Urethral sensitivity and the impact on urinary continence in patients with an ileal bladder substitute after cystectomy. *J Urol* 2001;165:1502–1505.
5. Kolettis PN, Klein EA, Novick AC, Winters JC, Appell RA. The Le Bag orthotopic urinary diversion. *J Urol* 1996;156:926–930.
6. Leissner J, Stein R, Hohenfellner R, et al. Radical cystoprostatectomy

combined with Mainz pouch bladder substitution to the urethra: long-term results. *BJU Int* 1999;83:964–970.

7. Light JK, H EU. Le Bag: total replacement of the bladder using an ileocolonic pouch. *J Urol* 1986;136:27–31.

8. Linn J, Hohenfellner M, Roth S, et al. Treatment of intersitial cystitis: Comparison of subtrigonal and supratrigonal cystectomy combined with orthotopic bladder substitution. *J Urol* 1998;159:774–778.

9. Reddy PK. The colonic neobladder. *Urol Clin North Am* 1991;18:609–614.

10. Riedmiller H, Thuroff J, Stockle M, Schofer O, Hohenfellner R. Continent urinary diversion and bladder augmentation in children: the Mainz pouch procedure. *Pediatr Nephrol* 3:68–74.

11. Santucci R, Park C, Mayo M, Lange P. Continence and urodynamic parameters of continent urinary reservoirs: comparison of gastric, ileal, ileocolic, right colon, and sigmoid segments. *Urology* 1999;54:252–257.

12. Stein R, Fisch M, Beetz R, et al. Urinary diversion in children and young adults using the Mainz pouch I technique. *Br J Urol* 1997;79:354–361.

13. Stenzl A, Colleselli K, Poisel S, Feichtinger H, Pontasch H, Bartsch G. Rationale and technique of nerve sparing radical cystectomy before an orthotopic neobladder procedure in women. *J Urol* 1995;154:2044–2049.

14. Thüroff JW, Alken P, Riedmiller H, Jacobi GH, Hohenfellner R. The MAINZ pouch (mixed augmentation ileum and cecum) for bladder augmentation and continent diversion. *J Urol* 1986;136:17–26.

15. Turner W, Danuser H, Moehrle K, Studer U. The effect of nerve sparing cystectomy technique on postoperative continence after orthotopic bladder substitution. *J Urol* 1997 2118–2122.

CHAPTER 86

Continent Catheterizable Reservoir Made From Ileum

Hassan Abol-Enein and Mohamed A. Ghoneim

A substantial number of techniques have been described for creation of continent cutaneous urinary reservoirs. For construction of such systems three elements are required: a low-pressure compliant reservoir, an antirefluxing ureterointestinal anastomosis, and a continent stoma that allows easy catheterization. To create a reservoir with high capacity at low pressure, various segments of bowel have been utilized: the ileum (1), ileocolonic region (2), the ascending colon (3), and transverse colon (4). Regardless of the selected bowel segment, detubularization and double folding are basic prerequisites to achieve this goal.

A reliable antirefluxing ureterointestinal anastomosis is necessary because bacteriuria is a constant feature in these systems, resulting from intermittent catheterization. The technique employed should provide a unidirectional but nonobstructed flow. The antirefluxing mechanism should not be at the expense of a higher incidence of obstructive complications.

Hinman (5) classified continent outlets into four categories according to the mechanism of their action. These included an antiperistaltic ileal segment (6); imbricated or tapered ileal segments resulting in passive tubular resistance (7); outlets using the pressure equilibration principle, including an ileal spout valve (8), flutter valve (9), inkwell hydraulic valve, intussusception nipple (10) or ileal servo mechanism sphincter (11); flap valves that are created by the incorporation of tubular structures within the wall of the reservoir such as the appendix (12), fallopian tubes (13), parts of ileum (14), or tubularized cecal segments (15). Multiplicity of techniques implies that none is optimal. Many of the above techniques rely on an inert or even nonphysiological mechanism, and problems and malfunctions soon appear. In our technique, we utilized the ileum for construction of the low-pressure reservoir and a serous-lined tunnel to provide an antirefluxing mechanism (16) as well as to create a reliable continent outlet (17).

INDICATIONS FOR SURGERY

Any patient who requires bladder replacement is a potential candidate for this operation. The indications of continent cutaneous urinary diversion include the following:

1. *Pelvic malignancies*: In patients for whom cystectomy is indicated for bladder cancer or those requiring an anterior pelvic exenteration for other pelvic malignancies.
2. *Benign indications*: These include neuropathic bladders when conservative measures fail, extensive urethral strictures with damaged urethral sphincter, contracted bladders with compromised urinary continence, complex urinary fistulae affecting the sphincteric mechanism, and some cases of bladder exstrophy with failed attempts of primary repair.
3. *Urinary conversion*: From other types of urinary diversion such as ileal conduits in young healthy patients, patients who develop isolated urethral recurrence following radical cystectomy and orthotopic bladder substitution and in some cases of ureterosigmoidostomy suffering from intractable metabolic acidosis.

PATIENT SELECTION AND EVALUATION

The suitable candidates should have a reasonable manual dexterity. Motivation to carry out clean intermittent catheterization at regular intervals is necessary. Further, a good prognosis might be expected if the indication of diversion was a pelvic malignancy. Patients who are unfit for prolonged surgery and those with a history of previous bowel resection, short-bowel syndrome, and heavily irradiated bowel are among the contraindication for this procedure. Patients with impaired renal function (serum creatinine of 1–8 mg/dL and or creatinine clearance of 40 mL per minute) are unsuitable candidates because metabolic acidosis would be inevitable.

ALTERNATIVE THERAPY

Alternative techniques of urinary diversion should be discussed with the patient when orthotopic bladder substitution or continent cutaneous reservoirs are contraindicated or unfeasible. These include conduit diversion and anal sphincter controlled bladder substitutes. The potential postoperative complications, changes in the future lifestyle, and long-term sequelae should be clearly explained to patients.

SURGICAL TECHNIQUE

Preoperative Preparation

Because the small bowel is utilized, no specific preparation is necessary. Fasting overnight with administration of intravenous fluids to ensure good hydration are required. Patients with histories of thromboembolic disease or varicose veins should receive a prophylactic dose of heparin (5,000 U subcutaneously) the night before the operation and every 12 hours thereafter until ambulation. Compression leg stockings are also advised. Although the intention is to use a concealed umbilical stoma, a stoma therapist should examine the patient and a suitable site of an abdominal stoma is determined. A parenteral broad-spectrum antibiotic is given just before induction of anesthesia and continued postoperatively for 3 days.

SURGICAL TECHNIQUE

The patient is put in the supine position with a Trendelenburg tilt. Slight flexion of the knees would further help in the relaxation of the abdominal muscles, facilitate retraction, and provide wider exposure. If total urethrectomy is planned, the patient is put in a slight lithotomy position for access to the perineum. The surgical area to be sterilized and draped extends from the lower chest down to the upper thighs. A midline incision from the pubis inferiorly to a point halfway between the umbilicus and xyphoid process of the sternum superiorly is in general employed. The incision is encircling the umbilicus by 2 to 3 cm to the left.

The bowel is examined and a 60-cm segment of the terminal ileum is isolated. Backlight transillumination of the mesenteric attachment greatly helps the identification of the arterial arcades supplying the selected segments. The bowel is divided 15 to 20 cm proximal to the cecum in the

avascular window of Treves between the ileocolic artery and the terminal branch of superior mesenteric artery. The ileum is divided proximally in a suitable avascular plane between the superior mesenteric arcades. Continuity of the bowel is reestablished by end-to-end anastomosis. The use of an automatic stapler or handsewn technique is a matter of surgeon's preference. The isolated bowel segment is subsequently subdivided into three parts. The middle 40-cm segment is used for construction of the reservoir, the 10-cm proximal segment is used for creation of the antireflux mechanism, and the distal 10-cm segment is used for creation of the outlet valve (Fig. 86–1). Great attention is paid to preserve an adequate blood supply for the proximal and distal small-bowel segments.

The middle segment is arranged in a "W" configuration and its antimesenteric border is incised by a diathermy knife. The edges of the two medial flaps are joined by a single layer of continuous 3-0 polyglactin sutures. The two lateral limbs are left to serve as serous-lined troughs. The proximal and distal short segments are tapered around a 22 Fr catheter. Bowel tapering could be performed either by simple excision and handsewn technique or by using a one-step technique with automatic gastrointestinal stapler. The proximal one-third of the inlet segment is kept untapered for ureteral anastomosis. Three to four small mesenteric windows close to the mesenteric border are created between the arterial arcades supplying these segments. Each mesenteric window is marked by a small strip of rubber vessel loop. This

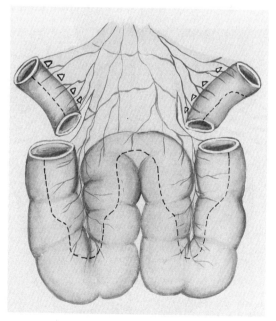

FIG. 86–1. The middle 40-cm segment is used for construction of the reservoir, the 10-cm proximal segment is used for creation of the antireflux mechanism, and the distal 10-cm segment is used for creation of the outlet valve.

POSTOPERATIVE CARE

Parenteral fluids are maintained until bowel habit resumes. Prophylactic antibiotics are given routinely for 5 days. Low-molecular-weight heparin is given for 10 days. The draining tubes are removed when the drainage ceases. The reservoir is irrigated with 30 to 60 mL of normal saline every 8 hours to prevent mucous retention. The ureteric stents are removed after 10 to 12 days postoperatively. The pouch is kept drained for 21 days before training by intermittent catheter clamping. All patients start self-catheterization 2 days before discharge from the hospital. A 2-hour interval is allowed in week 1, which is increased gradually until the pouch matures. By the end of week 6 most patients evacuate the pouch every 4 to 5 hours.

OUTCOMES

Complications

On the basis of our experience in 101 patients, early complications were observed in 15%. These included urinary leakage (2%), pelvic collections (8%), ureteroileal obstruction (1 %), and ileus (3%) and wound complications (3%). Small nonsymptomatic pelvic collections need no treatment. Sizable and/or infected symptomatic ones are usually treated by ultrasound-guided needle aspiration with or without indwelling tube drain. None of these pelvic collections required open drainage. Urinary leakage is infrequent complication in our series (2%). It was due to pouch perforation during catheterization training. Prolonged pouch drainage was required for an additional 2 weeks until healing of the injury occurs. Early evidence of ureteroileal obstruction was observed in one patient. Antegrade fixation of a double-J stent was inserted for 6 weeks. The stent was removed by pouchoscopy carried out through the umbilical stoma. Gastrointestinal and wound complications were similar to other urinary diversion procedures.

Late complications included stomal stenosis at the skin level with catheterization difficulties in 6% of patients. Two-thirds of them had an appendix stoma. Half of these patients required revisional surgery to widen the mucocutaneous stenotic area using wedge skin flap technique. In one child it was impossible to pass a catheter into the pouch due to overdistention resulting in angulation of the outlet tract. Under ultrasound guidance, percutaneous insertion of a pigtail catheter was carried out. Once the pouch became empty, outlet catheterization again was easy. Rupture of the pouch was observed in one patient following blunt abdominal trauma. Laparotomy was necessary and the pouch tear was adequately repaired. Pouch stones were observed in 5% of patients. All of them were amenable for endoscopic manipulations but one patient required open pouchlithotomy. The incidence of upper-tract dilatation due to anastomotic stricture was minimal (1%); the stricture was treated by antegrade balloon dilatation. One patient required left nephroureterectomy 3 years following cystectomy due to renal pelvis tumor. Gravity pouchography demonstrated reflux in three patients (3%). Reflux was asymptomatic in all and patients were kept on prophylactic antimicrobial suppressive therapy. None of the operated patients developed metabolic acidosis. All patients were advised to use oral alkali therapy.

Results

Patients regain their normal lifestyle once healing is completed. Ninety-five percent of our patients are completely dry day and night. Catheterization interval is every 4 to 5 hours during daytime and 1 to 2 hours at night. The average capacity at 6 months postoperative is 550 ± 130 mL. Five patients (5%) had a frequently wet stoma due to failure of continence mechanism. Two patients were revised. One underwent revision of the continent outlet, and augmentation ileopouchoplasty was required to increase pouch capacity in the other. Two patients preferred frequent catheterization to avoid leakage. The remaining patient used to fix a collection device during nighttime and refused further intervention.

Patients have to understand that they have a neobladder constructed from the bowel and this bladder is different from the native one. The usual desire to micturate and the known micturition mechanism no longer exist. However, all patients with dry continent outlet stoma enjoy an excellent lifestyle, normal social activities, accepted body image, and personal satisfaction.

REFERENCES

1. Abol-Enein H, Ghoneim M A. A novel uretero-ileal reimplantation technique: the serous lined extramural tunnel. A preliminary report. *J Urol* 1994;151:1193–1197.
2. Abol-Enein H, Ghoneim MA. Serous-lined extramural ileal valve. A new continent urinary outlet. *J Urol* 1999;161:786–791.
3. Ashken MH. An appliance free ileocecal urinary diversion: Preliminary communication. *B J Urol* 1974;46:631–634.
4. Askhen MH. Urinary reservoirs. In : *Urinary diversion*. Springer-Verlag: Berlin, 1982;112.
5. Benchekroun A. Continent caecal bladder. *Eur Urol* 1987;3:248–251.
6. Bihrlen R, Klee LW, Adams MC, Foster RS. Early clinical experience with the transverse colon-gastric tube continent urinary reservoir. *J Urol* 1991;146:751–753.
7. Gilchrist RR, Merricks JW, Hamlin HH, Rieger IT. Construction of a substitute for bladder and urethra. *Surg Gynecol Obst* 1950;90: 752–760.
8. Goldwasser B, Barrett DM, Benson RC, Jr. Complete bladder replacement using the detubularized right colon. In. King LR, Stone AR, Webster GD, eds: *Bladder reconstruction and continent urinary diversion*. Chicago: Year Book Medical Publishers, 1987;360–366.
9. Hinman F, Jr. Functional classification of conduits for continent diversion. *J Urol* 1990;44:27–30.
10. Kock NG, Nilson AE, Nilsson LO, Narien LJ, Philipson BM. Urinary diversion via a continent ileal reservoir : Clinical results in 12 patients. *J Urol* 1982;128:469–475.
11. Koff A S, Cerulli C, Wise H A. Clinical and Urodynamic features of a new intestinal urinary sphincter for continent urinary diversion. *J Urol* 1989;142:293–296.

12. Lample, A, Hohenfellner M, Schultz-Lample D, Thuroff, J W. In situ tunneled bowel flap tubes: 2 new techniques of a continent outlet for Mainz pouch cutaneous diversion. *J Urol* 1995;153:308–315.
13. Mitrofanoff P. Cystostomie continente trans-appendicularie dans la traitement des vessies neurologiques. *Chir Ped* 1980;21:297–300.
14. Rowland RG, Mitchell ME, Bihrle R. The cecoileal continent urinary reservoir. *World J Urol* 1985;3:185–190.
15. Thuroff JW, Alken P, Riedmiller H. The Mainz pouch (mixed augmentation ileum and cecum) for bladder augmentation and continent urinary diversion. *World J Urol* 1985;3:179–184.
16. Woodhouse CRJ, Malone PR, Cummning J, Reilly T. The Mitrofanoff principle for continent urinary diversion. *Br J Urol* 1989;63:53–57.
17. Zinman L, Libertino JA. Ileocecal conduit for temporary or permanent urinary diversion. *J Urol* 1975;113:317–323.

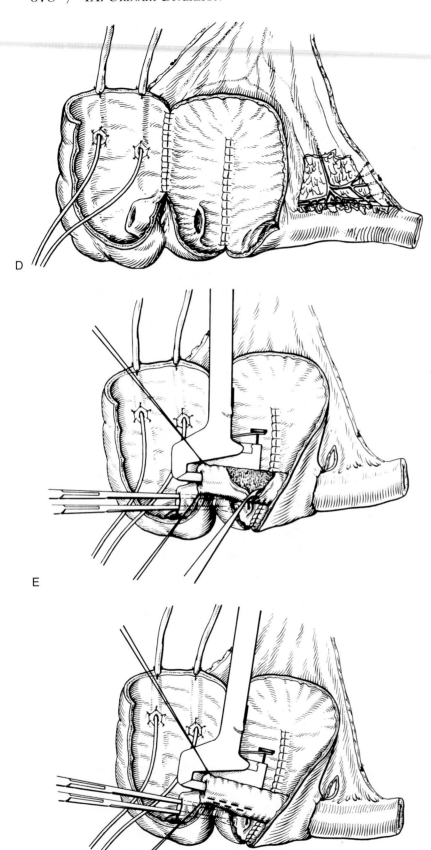

D

E

F

FIG. 87–1. (*continued*) **D:** Removal of mesentery (4 to 5 cm) in the midportion of the oral ileal segment in preparation for intussusception. **E:** Intussusception of the ileal segment and stabilization by applying one row of staples. **F:** The intussuscepted ileal nipple is pulled through the ileocecal valve and two additional rows of staples are used to attach the nipple to the valve. © Thieme Stuttgart, New York.

remaining bowel segment is split antimesenterically. These three opened bowel loops are folded in the form of an incomplete W, and their posterior aspects are sutured to one another to form a broad posterior plate (Fig. 87–1B). Both ureters are implanted into the large-bowel segment of the pouch plate, forming submucosal tunnels for reflux prevention (Fig. 87–1C).

The midportion of the intact ileal segment is freed of its mesentery for a distance of 4 to 5 cm to allow its intussusception (Figs. 87–1D and 87–1E). We apply only one row of staples to stabilize the intussusception itself (Fig. 87–1F). Thereafter, the intussuscepted nipple is pulled through the intact ileocecal valve and two additional rows of staples are applied to attach the nipple to the ileocecal valve. After the mucosa has been removed from the rim of the intussuscepted nipple and the colonic aspect of the ileocecal valve, their circumferences are sewn together with a running suture.

The bowel is then folded on itself in a side-to-side fashion, thus creating a low-pressure and high-capacity reservoir. Ureteral stents (6 or 8 Fr) and a 10 Fr pouchostomy are led through the abdominal wall at separate sites. The entire pouch is rotated so as to bring the efferent limb to the region of the umbilicus. A small button of skin is removed from the depth of the umbilical funnel. The pouch is carefully attached to the posterior fascia with interrupted nonab-

sorbable sutures to prevent the pouch from rotating and kinking. The efferent limb is then connected to the umbilical funnel with interrupted absorbable sutures. If no umbilicus is present (as in the case of exstrophy), it is created by tubularizing a V-shaped cutaneous flap and connecting it to the appendicular stump.

A vigorous washout regimen is started early in the postoperative course. Ureter stents are removed after 10 to 14 days. Clean intermittent catheterization is usually started at the end of postoperative week 3 after leakage and reflux has been ruled out by pouchogram.

Appendix Stoma

If the appendix is present and can be dilated to accommodate a 16 to 18 Fr catheter it is our first choice as ideal efferent segment for construction of a continence mechanism. In this case, a 15-cm segment of cecum and ascending colon is isolated along with two equal-sized limbs of distal ileum (12 to 13 cm each). The lower 5 cm of the cecum (cecal pole) is left tubularized and intact. The seromuscular layer of the intact cecal pole is divided along the tenia down to the mucosa analogous to the Lich–Gregoir procedure for vesicoureteral reflux (Fig. 87–2A). By careful dissection of the seromuscular tissue, a broad submucosal bed (5 cm) is created for the appen-

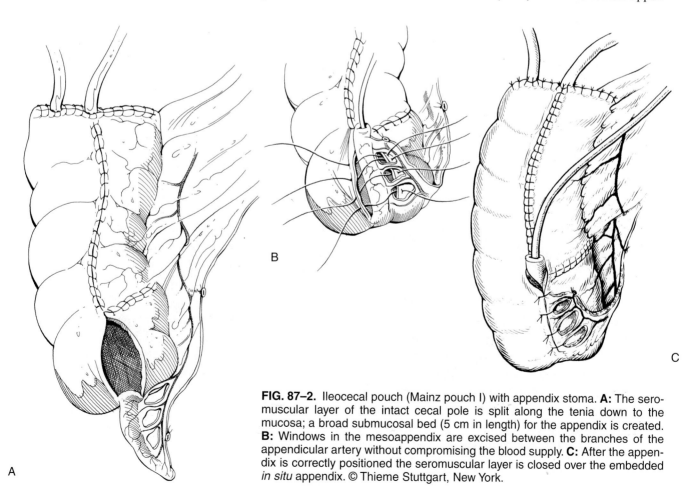

A

B

C

FIG. 87–2. Ileocecal pouch (Mainz pouch I) with appendix stoma. **A:** The seromuscular layer of the intact cecal pole is split along the tenia down to the mucosa; a broad submucosal bed (5 cm in length) for the appendix is created. **B:** Windows in the mesoappendix are excised between the branches of the appendicular artery without compromising the blood supply. **C:** After the appendix is correctly positioned the seromuscular layer is closed over the embedded *in situ* appendix. © Thieme Stuttgart, New York.

dix. The appendicular mesentery is freed of its excessive fatty tissue. Windows in the mesoappendix are excised between the branches of the appendicular artery without compromising the blood supply (Fig. 87–2B). Anatomic variations of the appendicular artery have to be respected and an additional branch of the anterior or posterior cecal artery supplying the base of the appendix should be preserved. After the appendix is correctly positioned the seromuscular layer is closed over the embedded *in situ* appendix with interrupted 4-0 polydioxanone sutures. A short mobile portion of the distal appendix remains for creation of the appendicoumbilical stoma (Fig. 87–2C). Formation of the pouch plate, ureterointestinal anastomosis, and attachment to the umbilicus are identical to the pouch with intussuscepted nipple.

Alternative Techniques for Construction of Continence Mechanism

More recent alternative techniques use a small-caliber conduit fashioned from the cecal wall. One technique uses a full-thickness tube lined by mucosa (Figs. 87–3A and 87–3B) and the other a seromuscular tube lined by serosa (Figs. 87–4A to 87–4C). Other authors have described transversely retubularized ileum (Figs. 87–5A to 87–5C) to create a tunneled access into the right colon (6).

Alternative Techniques for Ureteral Implantation

In dilated, irradiated, or otherwise compromised ureters ureterointestinal anastomosis may be performed according to a technique that has been described by Abol Enein and Ghoneim (serous-lined extramural tunnel) (Figs. 87–6A and 87–6B) (1).

Right Colon Pouches with Intussuscepted or Tapered Terminal Ileum

Several other authors use the ileocecal region in continent cutaneous urinary diversion. In contrast to the Mainz technique, they employ the ileum for construction of the continence mechanism but not for creation of the reservoir itself. Other colon pouches using nipple valve technology for the continence mechanism include modifications from many other centers and differ from one another by only a few features, predominantly related to the technique employed for stabilizing the nipple valve. In the "Tiflis" technique, the continence mechanism is created by tapering and submucosal embedding of terminal ileum (Figs. 87–7A and 87–7B) (2).

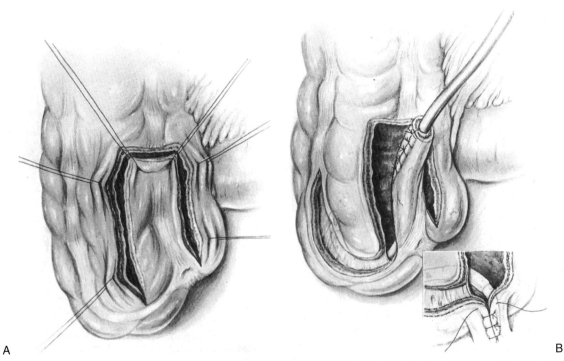

A   B

FIG. 87–3. Full-thickness bowel flap tube. **A:** U-shaped incision (3 × 6 cm) of all layers of bowel wall resulting in pedicled bowel flap at the lower pole of the cecum. **B:** Tubularization of pedicled flap over an 18 Fr Foley catheter and incision of the seromuscularis of the tenia omentalis (5 cm) for submucosal embedding starting at the pedicle of the bowel flap tube. © Thieme Stuttgart, New York.

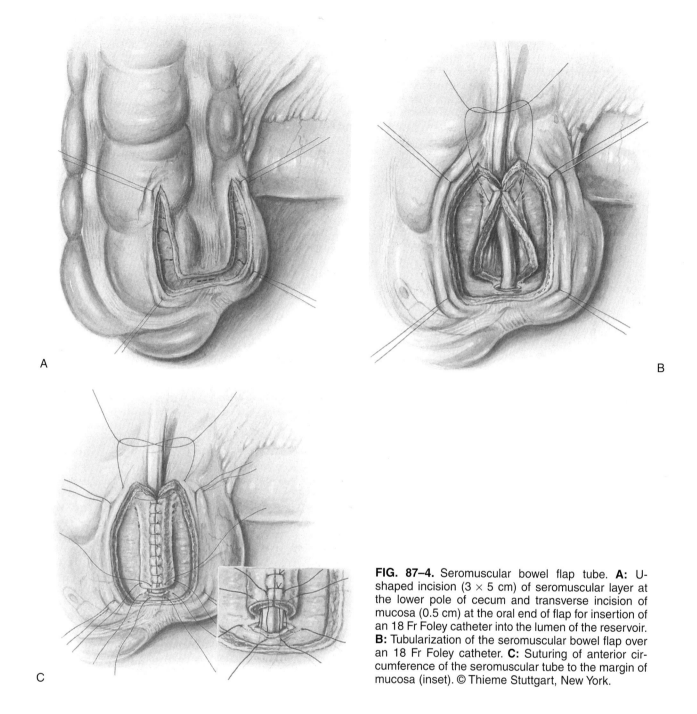

A

B

C

FIG. 87–4. Seromuscular bowel flap tube. **A:** U-shaped incision (3 × 5 cm) of seromuscular layer at the lower pole of cecum and transverse incision of mucosa (0.5 cm) at the oral end of flap for insertion of an 18 Fr Foley catheter into the lumen of the reservoir. **B:** Tubularization of the seromuscular bowel flap over an 18 Fr Foley catheter. **C:** Suturing of anterior circumference of the seromuscular tube to the margin of mucosa (inset). © Thieme Stuttgart, New York.

Indiana Pouch

Between 25 and 30 cm of cecum and ascending colon and 8 to 10 cm of terminal ileum are isolated (9). The entire colonic segment will be detubularized by incising it along its antimesenteric surface. If an appendix is present, it is removed at this time. Reconfiguration of the opened bowel segment by folding the cephalad end down to the apex of the antimesenteric incision allows creation of a spheric reservoir (Fig. 87–8A). For construction of the efferent limb and continence mechanism metal staples are applied sequentially to narrow the efferent limb over a 12 Fr straight catheter (Fig. 87–8B). Excess antimesenteric ileum is removed. The last row of staples is placed at an angle to prevent stapling into the wall of the cecum. After narrowing the efferent limb, the ileocecal valve area is plicated with five to seven Lembert stitches of 3-0 silk suture (Fig. 87–8C). Care is taken to avoid having the sutures enter the lumen of the bowel. Each Lembert suture is progressively wider than the last.

FIG. 87–5. Yang–Monti technique. **A:** Ileal segment 2 to 2.5 cm long is excised and opened longitudinally about 1 cm from mesentery. **B:** Resulting pedicled rectangle (2 × 6 to 7 cm). **C:** Retubularization in transverse direction using interrupted sutures (4-0 chromic catgut or 5-0 polydioxanone) resulting in a small-caliber tube (9neoappendix9) that is divided by mesentery into a short branch (stoma formation, anastomosis with umbilical funnel) and long branch (for submucosal embedding). © Thieme Stuttgart, New York.

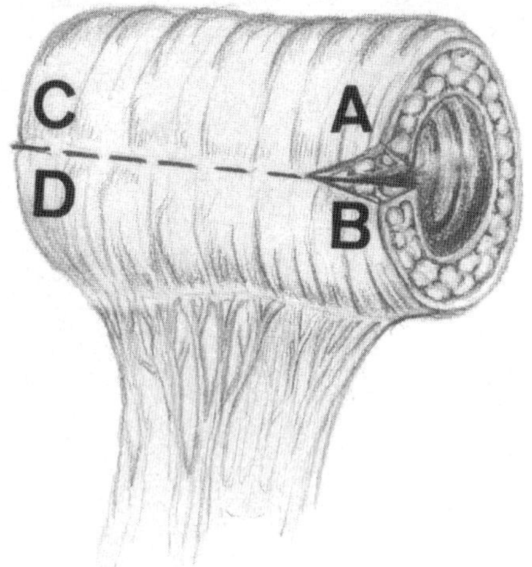

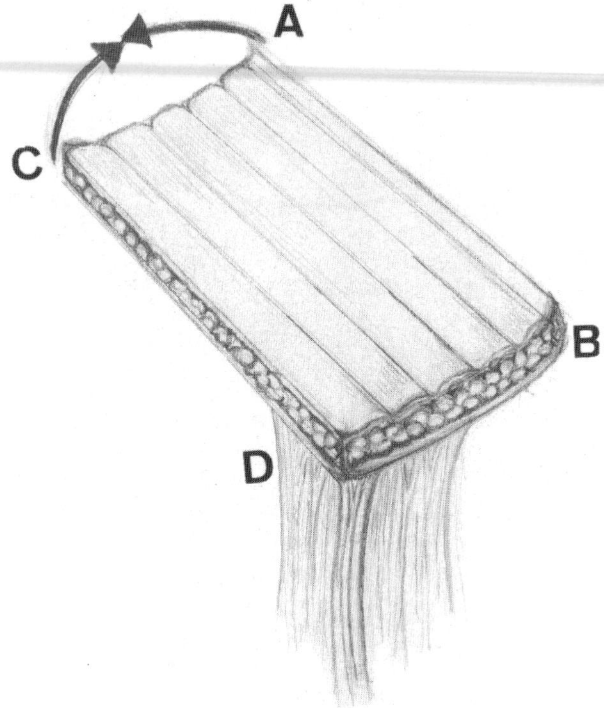

This has the effect of narrowing the ileocecal valve by wrapping cecal wall over the angled staple line. The tightness of the plication sutures is tested by passing an 18 Fr catheter through the efferent limb. Once the efferent limb and continence mechanism have been completed and a Malecot catheter has been placed as cecostomy tube in the dependent portion of the cecum, the reservoir is closed. Both ureters are led in such a manner as to allow alignment with a tenia. A tenial incision is made for each ureter. The ureter is cut obliquely or spatulated and the site for the ureteral orifice is created by incising the bowel mucosa. The ureteromucosal anastomosis is performed with interrupted sutures of 5-0 synthetic absorbable monofile material. The tenia is reapproximated over the ureter with a nonabsorbable 5-0 suture.

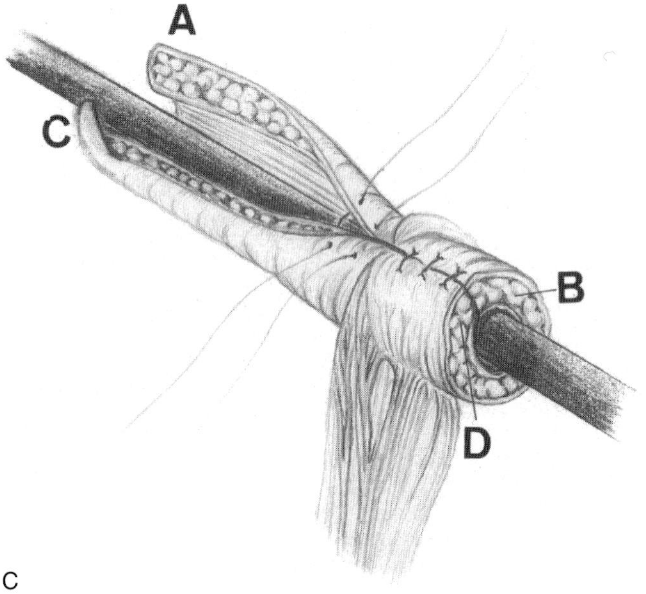

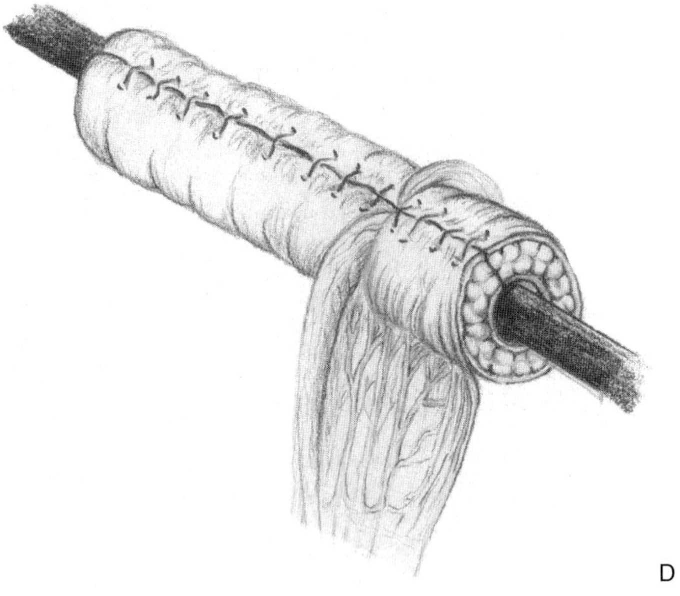

Colon Pouch (Mainz Pouch III)

Between 15 and 17 cm of transverse colon and either ascending [transverse-ascending pouch (TAP)] or descending colon [transverse-descending pouch (TDP)] (Fig. 87–9A) are required to create a pouch of adequate

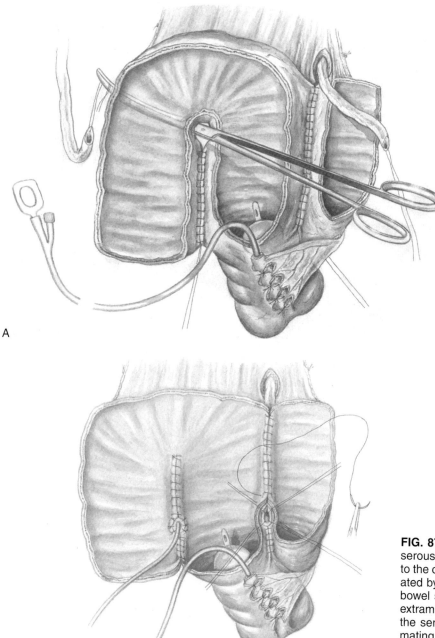

A

B

FIG. 87–6. Ileocecal pouch (Mainz pouch I) with serous-lined implantation of ureters. **A:** In contrast to the original technique the pouch plate is not created by anastomosing the edges of detubularized bowel segments but by creating two serous-lined extramural troughs. **B:** The ureters are placed into the serous-lined tunnels and covered by approximating the margins of the detubularization. © Thieme Stuttgart, New York.

capacity (350 to 400 mL). Complete mobilization of the right or left colic flexure should be performed to gain adequate colon length for the pouch. The greater omentum is dissected from the transverse colon from right to left in the TAP and vice versa in the TDP. The bowel segment is detubularized antimesenterically, leaving 5 to 6 cm of the oral or aboral end intact for construction of the efferent limb. The terminal segment is tapered over an 18 Fr silicone catheter, thus creating a neoappendix (Fig. 87–9B). Mucosa is sewn with polyglycol suture and the seromuscular layer with a nonabsorbable running suture.

Easy insertion of the catheter is important as a shrinkage of approximately 30% has to be reckoned with. After the pouch plate is created antirefluxing ureterointestinal implantation is performed on both sides of the suture line (Fig. 87–9C). For refluxing ureteral implantation about 1 cm² of the bowel mucosa is excised and the seromuscular layer is incised in the shape of a cross. After anchor sutures at the 5- and 7-o'clock positions a watertight anastomosis with 5-0 Monocryl sutures is performed. Ureteral stents and a 10 Fr pouchostomy are led through the abdominal wall at separate sites.

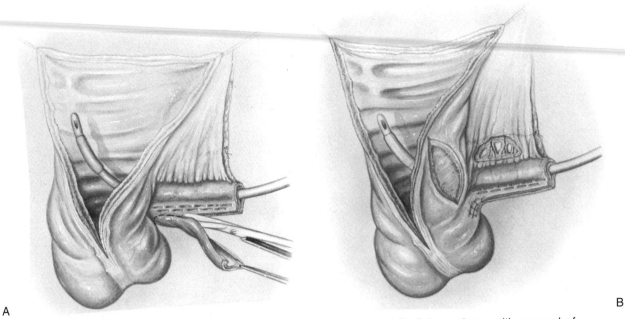

A

B

FIG. 87–7. Tiflis pouch. **A:** Tapering of terminal ileum over an 18 Fr Foley catheter with removal of excessive bowel wall. **B:** Incision of seromuscular layers of the cecum adjacent to the terminal ileum in preparation for submucosal embedding. © Thieme Stuttgart, New York.

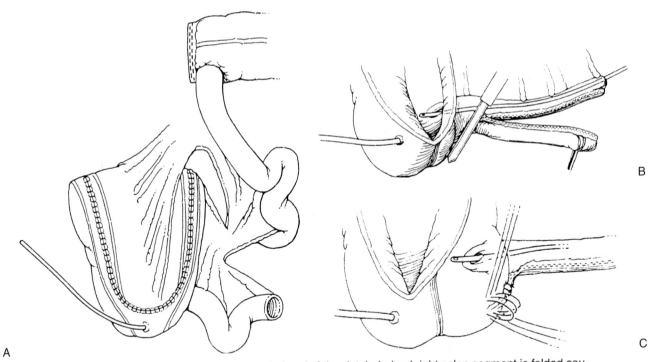

A

B

C

FIG. 87–8. Indiana pouch. **A:** The cephalad end of the detubularized right colon segment is folded caudally to the apex of antimesenteric incision. A Malecot catheter is placed in the dependent portion of the cecum prior to closing the reservoir. **B:** A stapler is used to trim away the excess bowel wall of the ileal segment (tapering). **C:** A total of 5 to 7 Lembert sutures are placed to plicate the ileocecal valve.

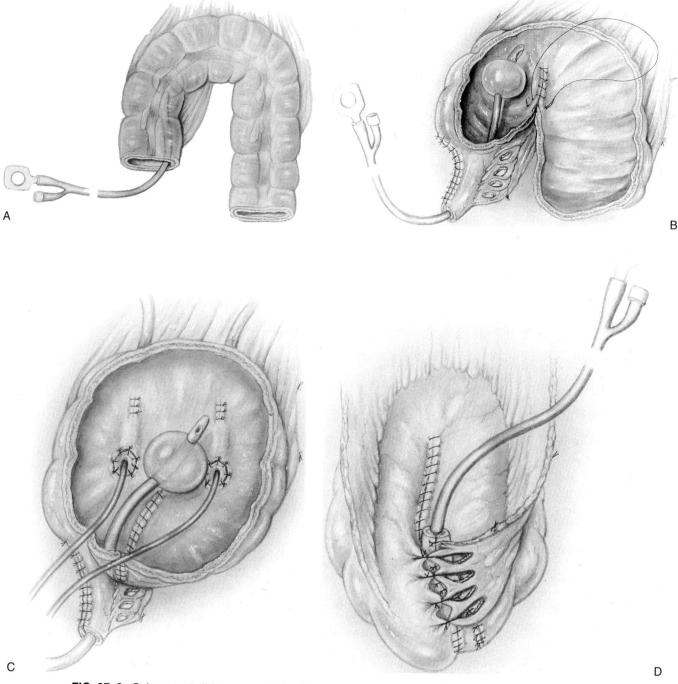

FIG. 87–9. Colon pouch (Mainz pouch III) with tapered colon as efferent limb. **A:** About 15 to 17 cm of nonirradiated large bowel are isolated for reservoir creation. The oral end with a Foley catheter is used for construction of efferent limb. **B:** The colonic segment is detubularized and the pouch plate is formed. The oral end is tapered over an 18 Fr Foley catheter and windows are made in the mesentery. **C:** The ureters are attached to the posterior pouch wall through a submucosal tunnel. **D:** Pouch formation is completed by closing the anterior wall. The efferent segment is embedded serosa-to-serosa by sutures led through mesenteric windows. © Thieme Stuttgart, New York.

The pouch is closed and the efferent segment is established. Windows are dissected in the mesentery of the tapered colon between the vessels. The efferent limb is then placed in the suture line and the seromuscular layer of the anterior wall is approximated through the windows in the mesentery (Fig. 87–9D). Our favorite technique comprises isolation of a short segment of jejunum or ileum, which is tapered over an 18 Fr Foley catheter and embedded submucosally after incising the tenia of a tubularized portion of the colonic segment. Sutures are led

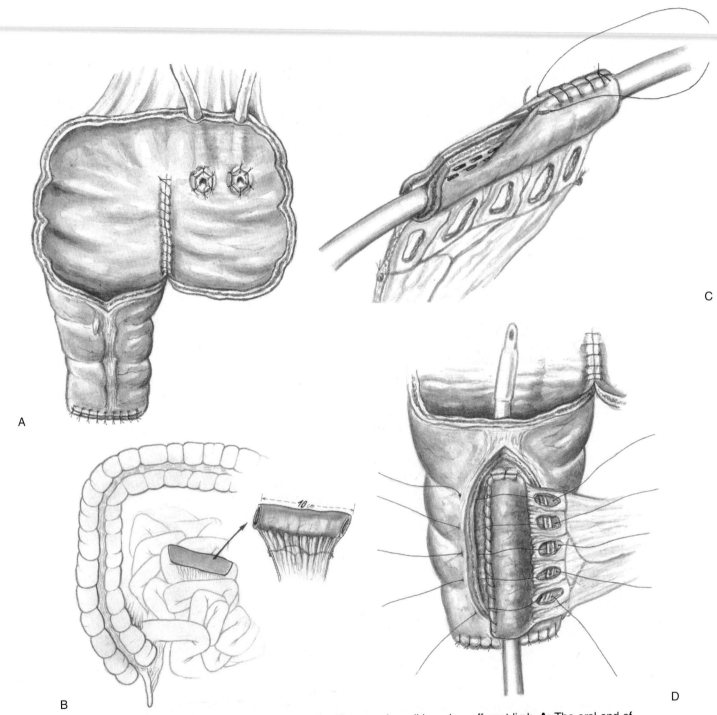

A

B

C

D

FIG. 87–10. Colon pouch (Mainz pouch III) with tapered small bowel as efferent limb. **A:** The oral end of the large-bowel segment is closed and left intact. **B:** A 10-cm jejunal or ileal segment is isolated with careful preservation of its mesenteric pedicle. **C:** The ileal segment is tapered over an 18 Fr Foley catheter, trimming away the excess bowel wall. The tube is formed using a running suture. Windows are created between the vasculature of the mesentery. **D:** Submucosal embedding of tapered ileum after incision of the seromuscular layer of the tenia of the intact colonic segment. Sutures are led through mesenteric windows. © Thieme Stuttgart, New York.

through windows in the ileal mesentery (Figs. 87–10A to 87–10D).

The umbilicointestinal anastomosis is performed in the same fashion as in the ileocecal pouch. Finally, the reservoir is attached to the abdominal wall. The greater omentum is used to cover the pouch and bowel. Ureter stents are removed after 10 to 14 days. Clean intermittent catheterization is started 3 weeks postoperatively.

OUTCOMES

Complications

While continence using the appendix, once established, is durable with late-onset failure of 1% to 2% at about 4 years, stomal stenosis is seen in 8% to 28% of patients depending on the length of follow-up. Although stenosis represents a minor technical problem the subsequent inability to insert the catheter is a distressing complication with potentially serious consequences in patients in whom the Mitrofanoff channel is the only route of evacuation. In these cases the reservoir must be immediately emptied percutaneously, which is facilitated by fixation of the pouch to the abdominal wall.

Skin stenosis may be dilated, incised, or repaired by open surgery, carefully removing fibrotic tissue. According to our experience dilatation alone seldom produces a lasting improvement. We therefore tend to early intervention. Although revisions are usually successful prevention of stenosis is desirable. Stomal stenosis can be avoided by incorporation of a V-shaped flap of umbilical funnel into the spatulated appendix. To prevent recurrence we have developed a cone-shaped metal dilator. Its effective length was designed to cover only the known critical segment of the channel. Directly before inserting the catheter for evacuation of the reservoir, the stoma is gently dilated for a few minutes once or twice daily. A similar effect might be produced by on occasion leaving the catheter in the pouch at night.

Metabolic complications are due to either reduction of the absorptive bowel capacity through functional loss of those segments required for reservoir construction or the highly unphysiological exposure of the reconfigured bowel to urine. Factors that affect solute absorption include the size and segment of bowel used, time of retention of urine, concentration of the solutes in the urine, renal function, and pH and osmolality of the fluid (3,4).

The most common consequence of intestinal urinary diversion is metabolic acidosis. Depending on definition, diagnostic modality, reservoir characteristics, renal function, and length of follow-up, it has been reported in 20% to 100% of patients after ureterosigmoidostomy, bladder substitution, and continent diversion using ileal and/or colonic segments. There is no proven effect on either bone resorption or childhood growth and development.

Intestinal urinary reservoirs have an increased propensity to form urinary calculi, predominantly in the lower tract and with a high tendency to recur with an increasing incidence over time. Risk factors include the presence of foreign material (e.g., staples), recurrent and chronic infection, composition of the urine, mucus production, urinary stasis, and noncompliance with irrigation and catheterization regimens.

Spontaneous rupture or perforation during catheterization has been observed after bladder augmentation, orthotopic ileal and ileocolonic bladder replacement, and in continent cutaneous reservoirs 4 weeks to more than 5 years after surgery.

Hypovitaminosis is a well-studied sequela to resection of bowel, and in particular on vitamin B_{12}, as patients may develop irreversible neurological disease in case of unrecognized deficiency. Substitution of vitamin B_{12} is simple and even less expensive than regular determination. Empirical supplementation may therefore be considered.

Results

Between 1990 and 2002, 765 patients underwent urinary diversion at our department with creation of continent reservoirs in more than 65%. The most common indication for urinary diversion was bladder replacement after anterior exenteration for pelvic malignancies (84.5%). Continent urinary diversion was performed as a primary surgical approach, in conversion procedures, and in salvage maneuvers after failure of previous reconstruction. Three-hundred fifty-eight patients underwent an ileocecal pouch with umbilical stoma (mean follow-up, 63.6 months, 1 to 122). As a continence mechanism the submucosally embedded in situ appendix could be utilized in 159 cases. In 196 cases an ileal intussusception valve was established. The submucosal tunnel was used for most ureteral implants (85%).

Perioperative morbidity was 0.8% in patients with continent diversion. Five major stoma-related complications were observed in patients with in situ appendix (4.4%). Minor complications (outlet stenosis at skin level) occurred in 20 patients (11.3%). Thirty-four patients with intussuscepted ileal nipple (17.3%) required surgical revision of the nipple. All patients with umbilical stoma were completely continent day and night with easy catheterization.

Ureterointestinal stenosis was encountered in 30 patients (8.3%). After disappointing experiences with dilatation and stenting, early reimplantation was performed in most cases, nephrectomy in five due to a significant loss of renal function. Rupture of the continent reservoir occurred in three patients (0.8%), in all cases related to catheter trauma during intermittent self-catheterization.

Whereas no calculi were observed in the appendix group, stones had to be removed from seven patients (2%) with ileal nipple. Although in none of the patients the serum concentration of vitamin B_{12} had dropped below normal, there was a tendency to decrease over time. Mild hyperchloremic metabolic acidosis occurred in 23%, requiring alkalizing medication.

In 12 patients with absent or dysfunctional lower urinary tract, a continent urinary reservoir has been created in preparation for renal transplantation (7). Within a mean follow-up of 26.1 months after kidney transplant renal function was stable, with serum creatinine values ranging from 0.9 to 1.8 mg per dL.

REFERENCES

1. Abol Enein H, Ghoneim MA. A novel uretero-ileal reimplantation technique: the serous lined extramural tunnel. A preliminary report. *J Urol* 1994;151:1193–1197.

2. Chanturaia Z, Pertia A, Managadze G, et al. Right colonic reservoir with sub-mucosally embedded tapered ileum—"Tiflis pouch." *Urol Int* 1997;59:113–118.

3. Gerharz EW, Turner W, Kälble T, et al. Metabolic and functional consequences of urinary reconstruction with bowel. *BJU Int* 2003;91: 143–149.

4. Mills RD, Studer UE. Metabolic consequences of continent urinary diversion. *J Urol* 1999;1057–1066.

5. Mitrofanoff P. Cystostomie continente transappendiculaire dans le traitement des vessies neurologiques. *Chir Pediatr Paris* 1980;21: 297–305.

6. Monti PR, Lara RC, Dutra MA, et al. New techniques for construction of efferent conduits based on the Mitrofanoff principle. *Urology* 1997; 49:112–115.

7. Riedmiller H, Bürger R, Müller S, et al. Continent appendix stoma: a modification of the Mainz pouch technique. *J Urol* 1990;143: 1115–1116.

8. Riedmiller H, Gerharz EW, Köhl U, et al. Continent urinary diversion in preparation for renal transplantation: a staged approach. *Transplantation* 2000;70:1713–1717.

9. Rowland RG. Right colon reservoir using a plicated tapered ileal outlet. In: Webster GD, Goldwasser B, eds. *Urinary diversion,* 1st ed. Oxford, UK: Isis Medical Media, 1995:229–235.

CHAPTER 88

Ureterosigmoidostomy: Mainz Pouch II

Margit Fisch, G. D'Elia, Rudolf Hohenfellner, and Joachim W. Thüroff

Since the introduction of internal urinary diversion 140 years ago by Simon (10) more than 60 modifications of ureterosigmoidostomy have been published. It remained the method of choice for urinary diversion until the late 1950s, when electrolyte imbalance and secondary malignancies arising at the ureteral implantation site were described However, secondary malignancies were later also reported in other forms of urinary diversion (6). The development of new absorbable suture material, modern ureteric stents, antibiotics, and alkalinizing drugs served in solving many of the traditional shortcomings of ureterosigmoidostomy and have rekindled the interest in this technique. Critics of ureterosigmoidostomy tend to quote publications dealing with complications in patients operated on before the 1950s.

After having solved these initial problems, continence began to be the more important issue. Frequency and urgency were often observed and nighttime incontinence was reported to be high (2,8). Urodynamic investigations showed that bowel contractions with a pressure rise in the bowel/reservoir are responsible for the incontinence (5,8). By interrupting the circular contractions (antimesenteric opening of the bowel and 9reconfiguration9) a low-pressure reservoir can be created, thus improving continence rates and protecting the upper urinary tract. Thus, the era of low-pressure anal reservoirs began.

Kock was the first who applied these principles to ureterosigmoidostomy. Utilizing an antimesenteric opening of the rectosigmoid and augmentation by an ileal patch, circular bowel contractions were interrupted and, thereby, a low-pressure reservoir created (9). To avoid metabolic disorders, a valve mechanism cranial to the augmentation was created by invagination of the sigmoid colon. A temporary colostomy was needed to protect the invagination and the advantage of the low-pressure reservoir was tempered by the complexity of the operative procedure. Reports on similar techniques either augmenting the sigmoid segment with ileal (10) or ileocecal (7) segments followed.

At the Johannes Gutenberg University Hospital in Mainz, a more simple but equally effective operative procedure for creation of a low-pressure rectal reservoir was developed, the sigmoid-rectal pouch based upon Kocher's description in 1903 (3,4). Whereas the standard technique for ureteral implantation into the sigmoid-rectal pouch, the submucous tunnel, represents an excellent implantation technique for normal undilated ureters with a low risk of stenosis or reflux, it is associated with an increased complication rate when dilated or thick-walled ureters are present. For these ureters the technique published by Abol-Enein and Ghoneim represents an alternative (1). The technique was described first for the ileal neobladder but is also applicable for the sigmoid-rectal pouch. During the past years modifications of the original technique have been described, showing the increased interest in the procedure. However, the small numbers of patients treated by this modifications or the insufficient follow-up time recently do not allow final judgment. Today the techniques of low-pressure anal reservoirs have completely replaced classic ureterosigmoidostomy.

DIAGNOSIS

The anal sphincter function can be checked by a *water tap enema* (perianal instillation of 200 to 300 mL saline, which the patients should keep at least for 3 hours) and a *rectodynamic investigation* (no incontinence during measurement; anal sphincter profile: resting closure pressure greater than 60 cm H_2O, closure pressure under stress greater than 100 cm H_2O).

INDICATIONS FOR SURGERY

The sigmoid-rectal pouch is suitable for primary urinary diversion, revision of ureterosigmoidostomy, and conversion of incontinent diversion. The procedure is indicated in patients with functional or actual loss of the urinary bladder. Our main indications were urinary diversion in patients with bladder exstrophy or after radical cystectomy for bladder cancer. A competent anal sphincter is a prerequisite for the sigmoid-rectal pouch as it is for ureterosigmoidostomy. There should be no renal insufficiency (creatinine maximum 1.5 mg per dL).

Contraindications are an incompetent anal sphincter, irradiation of the pelvis, diverticulosis of the sigmoid colon, polyposis, and a serum creatinine greater than 1.5 mg%.

ALTERNATIVE THERAPY

Alternatives to the sigmoid-rectal pouch are any other forms of urinary diversion, including bladder substitution, continent cutaneous urinary diversion, and conduit diversion.

SURGICAL TECHNIQUE

For bowel preparation oral administration of 4 to 7 L Fordtan's solution can be used on the day before the operation (alternatively 8 to 10 L of Ringer's lactate solution via a gastric tube). Metronidazole in combination with a cephalosporin (alternatively piperacillin sodium) and an aminoglycoside is given at the beginning of surgery. A gastric tube or gastrostomy and a rectal tube are placed. For parenteral nutrition a central venous catheter has to be inserted.

Classical Ureterosigmoidostomy

After median laparotomy the peritoneum is incised lateral to the descending colon and the left ureter is identified. A peritoneal incision is made on the contralateral site lateral to the ascending colon and the right ureter identified. Both ureters are dissected, respecting the longitudinal vessels running inside Waldeyer's sheet. The dissection is extended caudally to the ureterovesical junction. The ureters are cut as distal as possible and stay sutures are placed at the 6-o'clock position. The ureteral stumps are ligated.

The colon is slightly elevated at the rectosigmoid junction by four stay sutures. After opening of the sigmoid colon over a length of 4 cm by an incision of anterior taenia four mucosal stay sutures are placed in the mucosa of the posterior aspect of the sigmoid (Fig. 88–1). The bowel mucosa is incised between the proximal stay sutures and a buttonhole type of excision of posterior bowel wall is performed. A straight or slightly curved clamp is advanced through the opening and a tunnel is created by blunt dissection below the visceral peritoneum of the mesosigmoid (Fig. 88–2). The ureter is pulled into the lumen of the intestine. After creation of a submucosal tunnel of about 3 cm in length the ureter is threaded through this tunnel, avoiding torsion of the ureter (Fig.

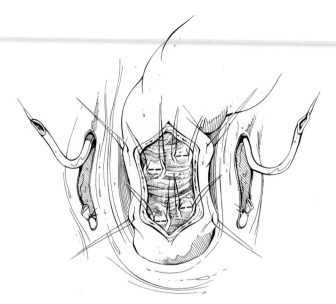

FIG. 88–1. Open transcolonic ureterosigmoidostomy: both ureters have been cut at its entrance into the bladder and mobilized. The site of the planned ureteral implantations in the posterior sigmoid wall are outlined by stay sutures.

88–3). The anterior wall of the ureter is spatulated for a length of 1 cm. For the ureterointestinal anastomosis, an anchor suture is placed at the 6-o'clock position grasping intestinal mucosa and musculature (5-0 polygalactin) and the anastomosis is completed by several ureteromucosal single stitches (6-0 polygalactin). A 6 Fr silastic stent is inserted into the ureter and fixed to the mucosa by a polyglactin 4-0 suture (Figs. 88–4A and 88–4B). The contralateral ureter is implanted about 3 cm lateral and either proximal or distal to the first anastomosis using the same technique (Fig. 88–5). The ureteral stents are

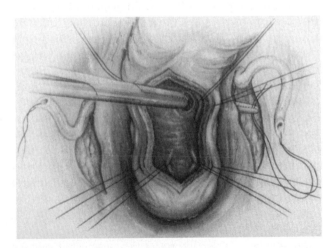

FIG. 88–2. After incision of the mucosa and button-hole type of excision of the posterior bowel wall site the ureter is to be brought through the intestinal wall, a subperitoneal tunnel is modeled bluntly from this point to the left incision in the peritoneum. The curved clamp is advanced precisely below the peritoneum.

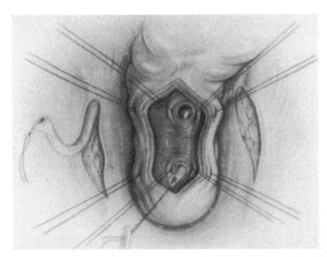

FIG. 88–3. The ureter has been pulled into the bowel and through a submucous tunnel reaching from the proximal to the distal stay sutures.

inserted into the rectal tube and pulled out through the anus. Thereafter, the rectal tube is reinserted.

The anterior sigmoid colon is closed in one layer using interrupted sutures of 4-0 polygalactin or in two layers using running sutures (5-0 polygalactin for the mucosa

and 4-0 polygalactin for the seromuscularis). The peritoneal incisions are closed. At the end of the operation separate fixations of the rectal tube and ureteral stents to the skin of the anus are performed (nonabsorbable material).

Sigmoid-Rectal Pouch (Mainz Pouch II)

Access is gained by a median laparotomy as for ureterosigmoidostomy. The rectosigmoid junction is identified and two stay sutures are placed. The peritoneum is incised lateral to the descending colon and the left ureter is identified. Another peritoneal incision is made lateral to the ascending colon and the right ureter is identified. Both ureters are dissected down to the ureterovesical junction, respecting the longitudinal vessels running inside Waldeyer's sheet. The ureters are cut as distal as possible, stay sutures are placed at the 6-o'clock position and the ureteral stumps are ligated.

For creation of the pouch, the intestine is opened at the anterior taenia starting from the rectosigmoid junction over a total length of 20 to 24 cm distal and proximal of this point (Fig. 88–6). By placing two stay sutures in the middle of the incision at the right side of the opened rectosigmoid the intestine is positioned in a shape of an

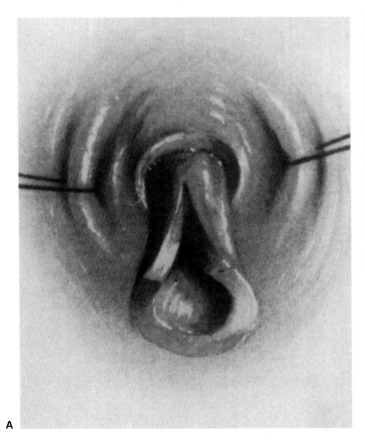

A

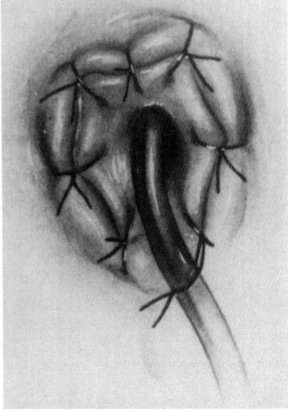

B

FIG. 88–4. Spatulation of the anterior wall of the ureter (a) and uretero-mucosal anastomosis between ureter and intestinal wall. The ureter is stented (b).

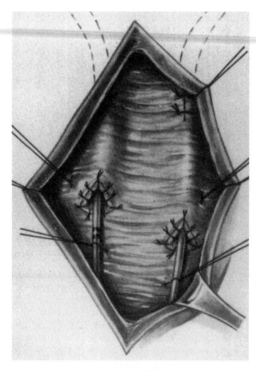

FIG. 88–5. Identical implantation of the right ureter 3 cm lateral and proximal or distal of the first anastomosis.

inverted U. The posterior wall of the pouch is closed by side-to-side anastomosis of the medial margins of the U using two-layer running sutures of 4-0 polygalactin for the seromuscular layer and 5-0 polygalactin for the mucosa (Fig. 88–7).

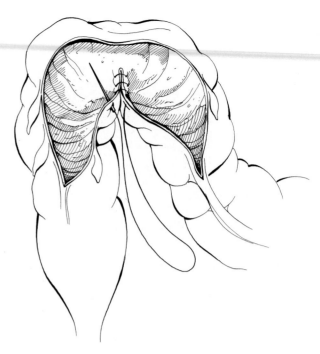

FIG. 88–7. Opening of the rectosigmoid at the anterior taenia starting from the recto-sigmoid junction over a total length of 20 to 24 cm distal and proximal of this point. Side-to-side anastomosis of the medial margins of the cut bowel edges by two- layer closure using running sutures absorbable synthetic suture material 4/0 for the sero-muscular layer and 5/0 for the mucosa.

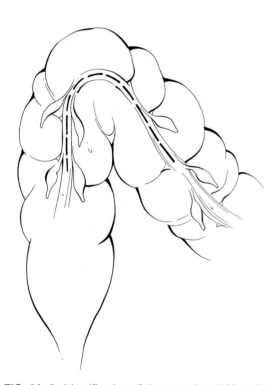

FIG. 88–6. Identification of the rectosigmoid junction.

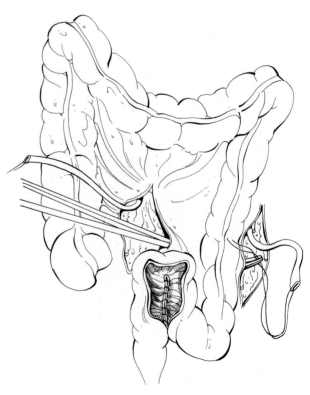

FIG. 88–8. The left ureter is pulled through retromesenterically to the right side.

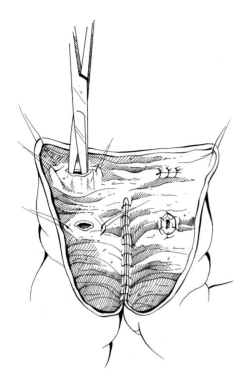

FIG. 88–9. The left ureter is pulled through retromesenterically to the right side.

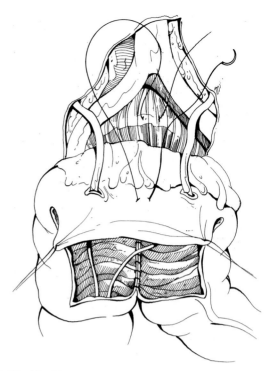

FIG. 88–10. After having inserted a 6 French stent in each ureter, which are pulled out through the anus with the rectal tube, the pouch is fixed to the anterior longitudinal band of the spine in the region of the proximal end of the posterior medial running suture to fixed to the anterior longitudinal cord of the promontory by two Bassini-sutures.

The left ureter is pulled through retromesenterically above the inferior mesenteric artery from the left to the right side (Fig. 88–8). For ureteral implantation, four mucosal stay sutures are placed parallel right and left to the medial running suture. The mucosa is incised and the seromuscular layer is excised between the two cranial stay sutures to create a wide buttonhole type of opening as an entrance of the ureter into the pouch. The dissection of the submucous tunnel starts from this incision downward over a length of 2 to 2.5 cm. The mucosa is incised at the distal end of the tunnel and the ureter is pulled into the tunnel. After having resected the ureter to an adequate length, implantation is completed by placing an anchor suture at the 6-o'clock position (5-0 polygalactin) and several interrupted ureteromucosal sutures (6-0 polygalactin). The cranial mucosal incision is closed by a running suture with polyglactin 4-0, which has a short reabsorption time. The contralateral ureter is implanted in the same manner (Fig. 88–9). Next, 6 Fr ureteral stents are inserted into the ureters and are pulled out through the anus with the rectal tube, which is afterward reinserted. The pouch is fixed to the anterior longitudinal band at the sacral promontory in the region of the proximal end of the posterior medial running sutures by two Bassini sutures with nonabsorbable suture material 3-0 (Fig. 88–10). Closure of the anterior pouch wall is performed in two layer sutures (5-0 polygalactin for the seromuscular and 4-0 polygalactin for the mucosal layer). Alternatively, single-layer closure using interrupted stitches can be used (Fig. 88–11). The peritoneal incisions are closed

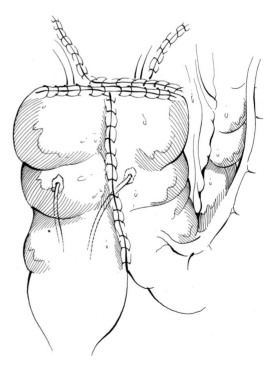

FIG. 88–11. Closure of the anterior pouch wall by seromuscular single stitches with absorbable synthetic suture material 4/0. Closure of the peritoneal incisions.

OUTCOMES

Complications

Of utmost importance for the outcome is patient selection. A functioning anal sphincter is a prerequisite. Also important are technical details such as ureteral implantation, side-to-side anastomosis by two layers, as well as the fixation at the promontory.

Between 1990 and 1999 a sigmoid-rectal pouch was performed in 123 patients (94 adults and 29 children). Mean age was 44 years (10 months to 73 years). Indications were malignancy (N=92), bladder exstrophy and incontinent epispadias (N=26), trauma (N=4), and sinus urogenitalis (N=1). One-hundred and two of the 123 patients were followed with a mean follow-up of 46 months (1 to 9 years). Eight patients died during follow-up due to their primary malignant tumor; another two died unrelated to the underlying disease. Eleven were lost to follow-up. Four early pouch-related complications were encountered: two dislodged ureteral stents requiring temporary nephrostomy and one ileus treated by operative intervention. One patient developed severe complications as a result of anastomotic leakage from a pouch fistula requiring revision and colostomy. Stenosis at the ureteral implantation site was the most common complication (7% or 14 renal units). Eleven renal units required surgical reimplantation. During follow-up, pyelonephritis was observed in 3% of patients. Ninety-nine of the 102 patients were completely continent postoperatively; nighttime continence was 97%. The majority of the patients (70/102 or 69%) use alkalinizing drugs to prevent metabolic acidosis.

Results

Low-pressure rectal reservoirs have replaced classic ureterosigmoidostomy. A classic indication is urinary diversion for bladder malignancies. The technique is excellent for continent diversion in women and is very much accepted in countries in which catheters or stoma bags are difficult to obtain or do not find patient acceptance. Another indication is bladder exstrophy, especially in those patients in whom bladder reconstruction has failed. However, secondary malignancies have to be considered and lifelong surveillance with rectoscopy starting from postoperative year 5 is mandatory. A new indication is laparoscopic cystectomy with removal of the specimen through the rectum during laparoscopic creation of a sigmoid rectal pouch (12).

REFERENCES

1. Abol-Enein H, Ghoneim MA. A novel uretero-ileal reimplantation technique: The serous lined extramural tunnel. A preliminary report. *J Urol* 1994;151:1193–1197.
2. Boyce WH. A new concept concerning treatment of exstrophy of the bladder: 20 years later. *J Urol* 1972;107:476–489.
3. Fisch M, Hohenfellner R. Der sigma-rektum pouch: eine modifikation der harnleiterdarmimplantation. *Akt Urol* 1991;22:I–IX.
4. Fisch M, Wammack R, Müller SC, Hohenfellner R. The Mainz pouch ii (sigma rectum pouch). *J Urol* 1993;149:258–263.
5. Ghoneim MA, Shebab-El-Din AB, Ashamallah AK, Gaballah MA. Evolution of the rectal bladder as a method for urinary diversion. *J Urol* 1981;126:737–740.
6. Kälble T, Tricker AR, Friedl P, Waldherr R, Hoang J, Staehler G, Möhring K. Ureterosigmoidostomy: Long-term results, risk of carcinoma and etiological factors for carcinogenesis. *J Urol* 1990;144:1110–1114.
7. Kato T, Sato K, Miyazaki H, Sasaki S, Matsuo S, Moriyama M. The uretero-ileoceco-proctostomy (ileocecal rectal bladder): early experiences in 18 patients. *J Urol* 1993;150:326–331.
8. Kock NG, Ghoneim MA, Lycke KG, Mahrab MR. Urinary diversion to the augmented and valved rectum: preliminary results with a novel surgical procedure. *J Urol* 1988;140:1375–1379.
9. Miller K, Matsui U, Hautmann R. Functional, augmented rectal bladder: Early clinical experience. *Eur Urol* 1991;19:269–273.
10. Simon J. Ectropia vesica (absence of the anterior walls of the bladder and pubic abdominal parieties); operation for directing the orifices of the ureters into the rectum; temporary success; subsequent death; autopsy. *Lancet* 1852;2:568
11. Stein R, Fisch M, Stöckle M, Hohenfellner R. Urinary diversion in bladder exstrophy and incontinent epispadias: 25 years of experience. *J Urol* 1995;154:1177–1181.
12. Türk I, Deger S, Winkelmann B, Baumgart E, Loening SA. Complete laparoscopic approach for radical cystectomy and continent urinary diversion (sigma rectum pouch). *Tech Urol* 2001;7:2–6.

CHAPTER 89

Palliative Urinary Diversion

Burkhard Ubrig, Michael Waldner, and Stephan Roth

The word palliative derives from the Latin, "palliare," which means to cover with a coat. Palliative therapy acknowledges the impossibility of cure and has as its goal purely the treatment of symptoms. The focus of therapy will change over time as the symptoms change; usually, individualized multimodal treatment rather than one definitive form is necessary. A palliative strategy may occasionally be the appropriate choice for curable disease in the presence of such patient-related factors as high surgical risk, short life expectancy, and lack of will.

Palliative urinary diversion attempts to reduce the sequelae of diseases of the urinary tract (usually cancer), including urgency, pelvic pain, pyocystis, recurrent gross hematuria, and fistulas (e.g., vesicovaginal, vesicorectal, cloacal). In a broader sense, palliative treatment for ureteral obstruction may also be considered here.

DIAGNOSIS

Palliative diversion may be accompanied by cystectomy or be performed as a supravesical diversion. Diagnostic studies are dependent upon the underlying pathlogy.

INDICATIONS FOR SURGERY

In patients with no hope of cure, less invasive means of symptom control should be exhausted. Specific indications include uncontrollable hemorrhage, non-reconstructible injuries to the lower urinary tract, or obstruction.

Whether cystectomy or complete pelvic exenteration is necessary and justifiable must be decided on an individual basis. Cystectomy in locally advanced pelvic cancer may entail a considerable risk of vascular and neural injury. In benign conditions simple cystectomy rather than radical cystectomy may be considered, as it is both less morbid and less time-consuming.

Supravesical diversion without cystectomy may be considered for patients with intractable local symptoms (urgency, infection, fistula formation) and frozen pelvis disease or those at high surgical risk. Indications are infrequent and results of this strategy have rarely been reported in the literature. One possible indication for supravesical cystectomy may be vesicovaginal or vesicovaginorectal fistula, which occurs typically in previously, irradiated carcinoma of the cervix. Quality of life is diminished by incontinence, contamination with feces and urine, and odor. In patients who develop cloacae, an additional colostomy will be needed in most.

It is unclear yet whether bleeding complications from radiation cystitis or locally advanced cancer of the prostate or bladder will be better controlled if the bladder is bypassed by supravesical diversion. Mechanisms involved may include the prevention of bladder distension, which avoids deterioration of fragile tumor vessels and mucosa. Moreover, urine contains natural anticoagulants such as urokinase, which may sustain vesical bleeding. Pomer et al. reported 16 patients with severe hemorrhagic cystitis (two bleeding from tumors) after radiotherapy in whom conservative treatment failed (16). All underwent diversion by cutaneous ureterostomy; 11 were reported to be completely free of gross hematuria and 3 continued to have slight intermittent hematuria. In our own unpublished data from the last 2 years, three of six patients who underwent diversion mainly for recurrent bleeding complications found relief.

ALTERNATIVE THERAPY

Alternatives to palliative treatments are observation, repeated transfusions, or indwelling catheters depending upon the underlying disease process.

SURGICAL TECHNIQUE

Palliative diversion—with or without cystectomy—will usually be performed with the easiest options acceptable. Conduits will usually be preferred. However, even conduits entail major intestinal surgery, and many patients for whom palliation is the goal are poor surgical risks. In many cases less elaborate techniques such as cutaneous ureterostomy or nephrostomy placement may be considered. Continent orthotopic or cutaneous diversion will be considered only in select cases, as it may take 3–12 months before continence with full life quality is attained (8).

Ileal Conduit

Assuming adequate surgical risk and life expectancy, an ileal conduit is the first choice of many urologists. Ostomy care is relatively easy, and patients may return to normal activity soon after discharge. (Figure 89–1) An ileal conduit should not be used in patients with short bowel syndrome or inflammatory small bowel disease and in those who have had high-dose radiation to the ileum. The small intestine and ureters are usually within the radiation portals for treatment of pelvic malignancy and may evidence long-term sequelae. Impaired healing of gut anastomosis and scarring with stricture formation of uretero-intestinal anastomosis may occur.

Sigmoid Colon Conduit

The sigmoid colon is a viable alternative to ileum, if the latter cannot be used for conduit construction (see above). However, it should not be used if diseased, if exposed to radiation, or if the internal iliac arteries have been ligated with the rectum still in place. This latest condition might lead to rectal sloughing because of compromised rectal blood supply (11). The stoma will usually be placed in the lower left abdominal quadrant (Figure 89–1).

Transverse Colon Conduit

The transverse colon is not within the radiation portals commonly used for pelvic malignancies, e.g. cervical cancer. The blood supply via the middle colic artery is usually ample (11). Indications for the use of transverse colon for conduit construction may be marked radiation fibrosis of the ureters or impaired ureteral mobilization because of frozen pelvis or periureteral lymph nodes. The uretero-intestinal anastomosis can be accomplished with very short ureteral stumps. Also, anastomosis with the renal pelvis is feasible. (Fig. 89–1) The perioperative mortality rate has recently been reported at 3% (7).

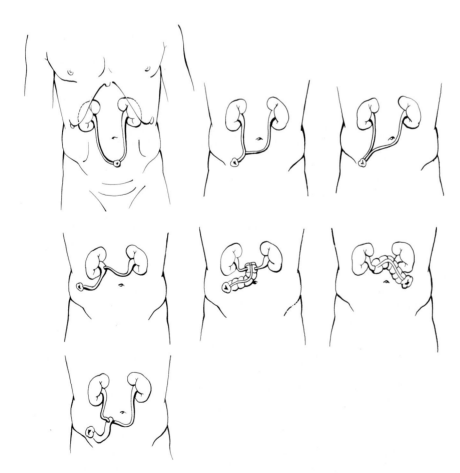

FIG. 89–1. Supravesical urinary diversion. **A–D:** Cutaneous ureterostomy with (A) median or (B) lateral stoma, (C) transureteroureterostomy, and (D) pyeloureteral anastomosis. **E, F:** Transverse colon conduit, with (F) anastomosis to the pyelon; (**G**) ileal conduit.

Bilateral Cutaneous Ureterostomy with Single Stoma

In patients who cannot withstand major gut surgery, cutaneous ureterostomy is an alternative to transintestinal diversion (Figure 89–1): operative time is short and renal function is not a selection factor. Construction of a single stoma in the lateral or midline position is generally feasible and ensures easy care with minimal patient discomfort. Occasionally though, excessive obesity, extensive paraureteral lymph node involvement, or frozen pelvis makes construction of a single stoma impossible.

In cutaneous ureterostomy stoma construction is of critical importance. Stomal stenosis rates of 50% and more have been reported (10). Distal spatulation of the ureteral end and plastic augmentation with a V-shaped skin flap as proposed by Rodeck should be considered (10). Stomal stenosis results mainly from ischemia of the distal ureteral end with consequent sloughing and fibrosis. Also, postoperative tension or hyperplastic epithelium at the uretero-cutaneous anastomosis may play a role. Firm fixation of the anastomosis to the skin and healing by first intention are essential. The following different techniques have been proposed.

Transureteral Cutaneous Ureterostomy

One ureter is led behind the mesentery of the sigmoid to the other side and anastomosed to the contralateral ureter end-to-side (e.g., with 5-0 Monocryl). This ureter will be guided through the abdominal wall and anastomosed to the skin.

Bilateral Cutaneous Ureterostomy

Both ureters are guided to the skin and anastomosed with each other and the stomal skin (Figs. 89–1). This can be done by leading one ureter to the contralateral side behind the sigmoid. Alternatively, the ureters may be mobilized completely extraperitoneally, led around the peritoneal sac, and conjoined in the midline. An infraumbilical stoma will be formed (10).

Transureteropyelocutaneous Ureterostomy

Alternatively, the collecting systems of both renal units have been connected with a high ureteral or pyeloureteral anastomosis (Fig. 89–1). Only one kidney is then diverted either by nephrostomy catheter or unilateral cutaneous ureterostomy. Marx and Laible reported their experience with this technique in 57 patients (5). The surgical approach was via upper-abdominal cross incision; either a pyeloureteral or ureteroureteral anastomosis was performed, and a single nephrostomy was used. Operative mortality was 1.75%; severe late complications occurred in 10.5%. The most frequent problems arose from the nephrostomy and from stenoses of the ureteropelvic or ureteral anastomosis (5).

Transverse Retubularized Colon Segments

In selected patients, transverse reconfigured colon segments may be used successfully to reconstruct extensive ureteral defects (Figs. 89–2 and 89–3). The successful use of a combination of two such segments has been described to divert solitary kidneys in palliative situations (9). In patients with renal insufficiency or a history of irradiation, this technique may be superior to the use of ileum. An advantage of the colon is its immediate proximity to the ureters bilaterally and its position outside the radiation portals for treatment of pelvic malignancy. Nevertheless, unreconfigured colon has not been widely

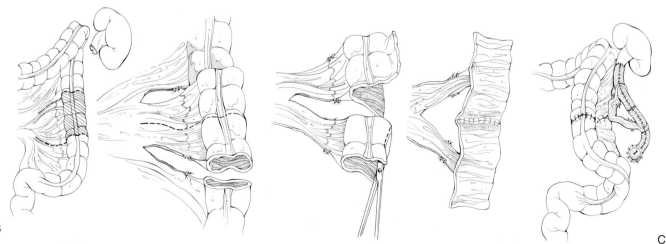

A,B

C

FIG. 89–2. Combined reconfigured colon segments for incontinent diversion of solitary kidney. **A:** A 6-cm segment is excised from the ascending or descending colon. The segment is split in the middle and the rings are opened antimesenterically. When reconfigured, the tube produced will be approximately 18 cm long, suitable for incontinent urinary diversion. **B:** Pyelocolocutaneostomy in a solitary kidney.

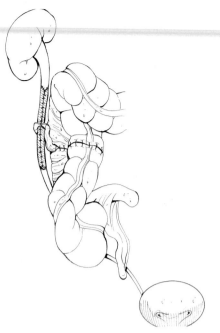

FIG. 89–3. Interposition of a reconfigured colon segment to repair an extensive ureteral defect.

recruited for ureteral replacement because of its wide diameter: its large volume when replacing long defects could result in metabolic or septic complications. Surgical access is via flank or pararectal incision, and intraperitoneal surgery is minimal. The colonic segments are taken immediately proximal to the ureteral defect, necessitating little mobilization of the mesenteric pedicle. Metabolic consequences have not been described and should be absent or low, as only minimal amounts of intestine need be isolated (9).

Percutaneous Nephrostomy

Percutaneous nephrostomy is another alternative for supravesical diversion. The advantages are the relative ease with which these can be placed under local anesthesia, but the drawbacks are the need for continuous replacement due to encrustation as well as the propensity of these to become dislodged. Bilateral nephrostomies are sometimes badly tolerated and usually only the renal unit with better function should be diverted by nephrostomy.

To prevent further flow of urine downstream, additional occlusion of the ureter may sometimes be necessary. Transection and ligation of the ureter with nonabsorbable material may be performed. This may be accomplished by a small flank incision or laparoscopically. If feasible, a unilateral cutaneous ureterostomy may be the better alternative in such cases.

Several percutaneous techniques to obliterate the ureteral lumen have been proposed: butyl-2-cyanoacry-late, detachable balloons, liquid polyacrylonitrile, butyl-2-cyanoacrylate and lipiodol with adjuvant balloon catheter occlusion, electrocautery, and nylon and silicone occlusion devices. Some nephrostomy devices for transient closure of the ureteral lumen have been reported, including modified nephroureteral catheters and balloon occlusion devices. None of these methods has gained wide acceptance.

Defunctionalization of the Contralateral Unit

If only one kidney is diverted and urine continues to flow downstream from the contralateral kidney, it may be necessary to defunctionalize the latter. Many palliative patients are poor candidates for nephrectomy. In a previously obstructed hydronephrotic kidney with significant parenchymal reduction, ligature and transection of the ureter will usually result in long-term success. Postinterventional paralytic ileus and some pain may be expected during the first postoperative days.

However, in unobstructed kidneys, ligature of the ureter should not be done because of significant pain and spontaneous ureteral recanalization. Usually renal arterial embolization will be considered. Excellent results to stop urine production from kidney have been reported with transcatheter ablation (1) with a mixture of ethanol and contrast agent and a combination of sponge and coil plugging of the proximal artery: in 20 patients, urinary flow ceased after two days in 18; two required a second session. The authors propose epidural anesthesia, which may also be used in the first two postoperative days for pain control. Transient postinterventional paralytic ileus and fever may be expected.

Palliative Treatment of Ureteral Obstruction

Common causes of malignant compression of the ureterovesical junction and the prevesical ureter are bladder, prostate, and cervical cancer. Malignant obstruction of the mid- or upper ureter is usually caused by metastatic lymphatic spread as from metastatic breast cancer, lymphatic disease, colon cancer, and cancers of the female internal genitalia. However, even years after radiation therapy, newly arising ureteral obstruction may represent long-term sequelae of radiation and not tumor recurrence.

Indications for treatment should be considered very carefully. Septic episodes, with accompanying persistent pain, are rare in malignant ureteral obstruction if there has been no retrograde endoscopic manipulation. The insertion of a regular double-J stent or a nephrostomy will result in repeated consultations to change the catheters, sometimes under general anesthesia. Any measure carries the risk of infection or dislocation. Many patients are in critical condition, and quality of life should be the main treatment goal.

In patients with unilateral ureteral obstruction and sufficient function of the contralateral kidney, one should generally abstain from therapy; however, if nephrotoxic chemotherapy is planned or life expectancy exceeds 1 to 2 years intervention may be indicated. In patients with bilateral ureteral obstruction and impending renal failure, it is usually sufficient to stent, divert, or bypass only one renal unit (usually the one with better function). In some patients, however, it may be preferable to abstain from any treatment at all. The use of the below-mentioned techniques assumes normal bladder function. Otherwise, supravesical diversion may be discussed.

Retrograde stenting with replaceable double-J stents is often considered the first-line option for relieving ureteral obstruction (Fig. 89–4). Transurethral resection will sometimes be necessary to find the ureteral orifice or intramural ureter hidden in the tumor. In these situations prior antegrade placement of a guide wire or antegrade placement of the stent itself may be very useful. Specific drawbacks of double-J stents are irritative bladder symptoms, stent obstruction and encrustation—necessitating repeated changes (intervals range from 6 weeks to 6 months, but can be much shorter) and stent migration.

Under conditions of extrinsic compression hard polyurethane stents are recommended over soft silicone to ensure patency of the stent lumen. Specially developed "tumor stents" are available.

Two Double-J Stents

Extensive compression from the tumor may lead to malfunction and obstruction of conventional double-J stents. Liu and Hrebinko used two 4.7 Fr double-J stents passed simultaneously over guide wires when drainage with a single ureteral stent had failed (4). The increased stiffness of two stents reduces kinking and luminal compression, and the potential space between the stents likely preserves flow around as well as through them (Fig. 89–4).

Metallic Mesh Stents

Metallic mesh stents such as the Wallstent have been used with limited success. Epithelial hyperplasia and tumor ingrowth through the mesh have been reported to result in recurrent ureteral obstruction. These stents are virtually unremovable. An alternative might be nickel–titanium shape-memory alloy stents that occupy only the obstructed ureteral segment. These are soft and malleable at 10°C and regain their shape when reheated to 55°C. The tendency to form encrustations is apparently low. (3).

OUTCOMES

Complications

In 1992 Desgrandschamps and colleagues introduced their technique of pyelovesical bypass with a composite prosthesis (internal diameter, 18 Fr; external diameter, 28.5 Fr), and Jabbour et al. recently reported long-term results with 35 prosthetic ureters in 27 patients, 22 with malignancies (2). Minor early and late complications were noted in five and three patients, respectively. No encrustations of the inner silicone lumen were noted, although asymptomatic bacteriuria sometimes was. The

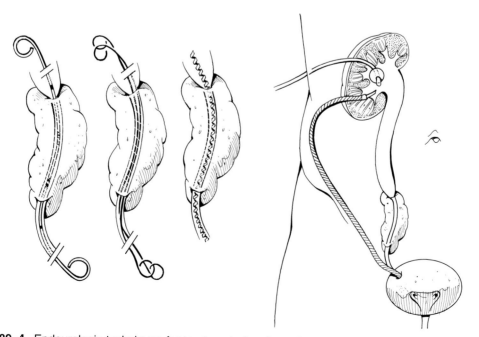

FIG. 89–4. Endourologic techniques for treatment of malignant ureteric obstruction. **A:** Ureteral stent. **B:** Two parallel ureteral stents. **C:** Metal stent. **D:** Nephrostomy tube. **E:** Extraanatomic prosthetic bypass.

CHAPTER 90

Neuroblastoma

Pramod P. Reddy, Brad W. Warner, and Curtis A. Sheldon

Neuroblastoma represents the most common extracranial malignant solid neoplasm of infancy and childhood, and is the most common intraabdominal malignancy in the newborn. The biologic, genetic, and morphological characteristics of this neoplasm demonstrate heterogeneous behavior. These tumors have a varied clinical course, with reports in the literature of spontaneous regression and tumor maturation from malignant to a benign histological form; however, in many cases the disease is progressive (4,7). Neuroblastomas exhibit a wide spectrum of morphological differentiation, ranging from primitive (neuroblastoma) to well differentiated (ganglioneuroma), or between these two extremes the ganglioneuroblastoma.

The clinical incidence of this tumor is approximately 1 in 8,000 to 10,000 children. There are approximately 500 new cases diagnosed each year in the United States; 90% of these cases occur in children less than 7 years old. Cervical and mediastinal lesions tend to present in younger patients less than 1 year of age and tend to have a better prognosis. Neuroblastoma is slightly more common in boys than in girls with a ratio of 1.2:1 and has in some instances been described in familial settings (7).

DIAGNOSIS

Infants presenting with the following four clinical conditions have a higher incidence of neuroblastoma than the general population: Beckwith–Wiedemann syndrome (BWS), Hirschsprung's disease, fetal alcohol syndrome, and fetal hydantoin syndrome.

The clinical presentation of neuroblastoma can be varied and is dependent upon the site of the primary tumor, presence of metastatic disease, age of the patient, and production of metabolically active substances (e.g., catecholamine-producing tumors present with hypertension).

The catecholamine urinary metabolites "vanillylmandelic acid" (VMA) and "homovanillic acid" (HVA) are elevated in more than 80% of patients with a neuroblastoma. An increased VMA/HVA ratio has been shown to be associated with a better prognosis in localized disease. Other metabolic products that might be elevated include lactate dehydrogenase (LDH), serum ferritin, and serum neuron-specific enolase (NSE); all of these products are associated with a poor prognosis.

At least half of children with neuroblastoma will have metastatic disease—in particular to the cortical bone, bone marrow, liver, and skin—at the time of initial presentation. Among the studies in the workup of a child with a suspected neuroblastoma are spot urine for VMA and HVA, chest x-ray, ultrasound of the abdomen, computed tomography (CT) or magnetic resonance imaging (MRI) body scans, radioisotopic bone scan, I[131]-metaiodobenzylguanidine (MIBG) scan, bone marrow aspirate/biopsy from multiple sites, and N-*myc* oncogene copy number of tumor. Serum LDH greater than 1,500 IU per mL and serum ferritin greater than 142 ng per mL are associated with a poor prognosis. Serum NSE greater than 100 ng per mL is seen in patients with metastatic disease.

Staging of Neuroblastoma

Multiple staging systems have evolved in the management of neuroblastoma. The Evans–D'Angio staging system (3) (Table 90–1) consists of a clinical assessment that describes the initial tumor distribution and incorporates whether the tumor crosses the midline. The International Neuroblastoma Staging System (INSS) incorporates many of the important criteria from each of these three staging systems and includes initial tumor distribution as well as its surgical resectability (2) (Table 90–2).

The most useful histological classification is the system described by Shimada (14); this system utilizes the mitosis karyorrhexis index (MKI) of nuclear fragmentation. This system divides the tumors into age-related favorable and unfavorable histological categories based on whether the tumor exhibits a stroma-rich or stroma-poor appearance (14) (Table 90–3).

TABLE 90–1. *Evans staging system*

Stage of tumor	Description of stage
I	Tumor Confined to the Organ of Origin
II	Tumor Extends Beyond Organ of Origin but Does Not Cross the Midline; Unilateral Lymph Nodes May Be Involved
III	Tumor Extends Across the Midline; Bilateral Regional Lymph Nodes May Be Involved
IV	Distant Metastases (Skeletal, Other Organs, Soft Tissues, Distant Lymph Nodes
IV-S	Stage I or II with Remote Disease Confined to One or More of the Following Sites:Liver, Skin, or Bone Marrow, But Without Evidence of Bone Cortex Involvement

From Evans AE, D'Angio GJ, Randolph J. A proposed staging for children with neuroblastoma. Children's Cancer Study Group A. *Cancer* 1971;27:374–378, with permission.

TABLE 90–2. *International Neuroblastoma Staging System*

Stage of tumor	Description of stage
1	Localized Tumor Confined to the Area of Origin. Complete Gross Excision, With or Without Microscopic Residual Disease. Identifiable Ipsilateral and Contralateral Lymph Nodes That Are Microscopically Negative
2-A	Unilateral Tumor With Incomplete Gross Resection. Identifiable Ipsilateral and Contralateral Lymph Nodes That Are Microscopically Negative
2-B	Unilateral Tumor With Complete or Incomplete Gross Excision. Positive Ipsilateral Regional Lymph Nodes. Identifiable Contralateral Lymph Nodes That Are Microscopically Negative
3	Tumor Infiltration Across the Midline With or Without Regional Lymph Node Involvement. Unilateral Tumor With Contralateral Lymph Node Involvement or Midline Tumor With Bilateral Regional Lymph Node Involvement
4	Dissemination of Tumor to Distant Lymph Nodes, Bone Marrow, Bone, Liver, or Other Organs (Except as Defined in Stage 4-S)
4-S	Localized Primary Tumor as Defined for Stage 1 or 2 (Stage 2-A or 2-B), With Dissemination Limited to the Liver, Skin, or Bone Marrow

From Brodeur GM, et al. International criteria for diagnosis, staging, and response to treatment in patients with neuroblastoma. *J Clin Oncol* 1988;6:1874–1881, with permission.

TABLE 90–3. *Shimada pathologic classification*

	Favorable histology	Unfavorable histology
Stroma Rich	Well-Differentiated, Intermixed Appearance	Nodular Appearance
Stroma Poor		
Age <18 mo	Mitosis Karyornhexis Index (MKI) < 200/5,000	MKI < 100/5,000
Age 18–60 mo	MKI > 100/5,000	MKI > 100/5,000
	Differentiating	Undifferentiated
Age >5 yr	None	All

From Shimada H, et al. The International Neuroblastoma Pathology Classification (the Shimada system). *Cancer* 1999;86:364–372, with permission.

INDICATIONS FOR SURGERY

The management of patients presenting with neuroblastoma varies with the extent of disease at the time of diagnosis, the age of the patient, and the staging criteria used. If the patient has stage I or II disease (with favorable histology), then surgical resection alone can be undertaken with reasonable success. A multimodal approach utilizing chemotherapy, radiation, and surgery is used for advanced disease (stages III and IV).

Surgical intervention (second-look laparotomy) is usually performed 13 to 18 weeks after chemotherapy has been administered. During the second-look laparotomy, surgical resection and dissection may appear to be somewhat easier, especially around vital structures and major blood vessels, because chemotherapy usually makes the tumors smaller and firmer. This rubbery consistency also decreases the risk of rupture and spillage of the tumor that might otherwise be encountered. Intraoperative radiation (IORT) may be utilized and is helpful in reducing the exposure to normal adjacent structures. In advanced-stage tumors radiation therapy is delivered to the tumor bed and regional lymph nodes.

Alternative Therapy

There is currently no alternative to surgery in the management of localized disease.

SURGICAL TECHNIQUE

In cases of very large tumors where resection of adjacent organs/intestine might be required a mechanical bowel preparation is reasonable. The procedure is performed with the patient in a supine position. The patient should be given prophylactic antibiotics (broad-spectrum cephalosporin).

Depending upon the location and size of the tumor the surgeon can choose between three different incisions: (a) transverse transperitoneal–supraumbilical incision (for primary tumor of the retroperitoneum), (b) bilateral subcostal chevron incision (for large tumors), or (c) thoracoabdominal incision (for upper abdominal and/or large tumors).

The retroperitoneum is entered by incising the posterior peritoneum along the white line of Toldt. The colon is reflected medially to expose the retroperitoneum. For left-sided tumors the spleen and pancreas are displaced upward and medially. For tumors on the right side the various peritoneal attachments of the liver can be divided to improve exposure. In children with locally metastasizing disease it is sometimes necessary to perform *en bloc* excision of adjacent organs (i.e., ipsilateral kidney, spleen). Neuroblastomas typically have a friable pseudocapsule; therefore, during dissection it is useful to think of the surgery as aimed at dissecting the patient from around the tumor to decrease the risk of tumor spillage. Vascular control should be achieved early in the procedure. These tumors often invade the tunica adventitia of large blood vessels; therefore, special care should be taken to identify and spare the blood supply to important visceral structures such as the branches of the celiac axis and superior mesenteric artery. The venous drainage of these tumors is usually constant, with right-sided tumors draining directly into the inferior vena cava. Left-sided tumors drain into the left renal vein and subdiaphragmatic venous tributaries. Regional lymph nodes should be sampled to complete the surgical staging. Once the tumor has been resected, the margins of the tumor bed should be marked with titanium clips to guide radiation therapy. A liver biopsy is indicated if there is clinical or imaging suspicion of disease within the liver; an effort should be made to biopsy the involved area.

In some instances it is not possible to perform primary resection of the tumor; in these cases a wedge biopsy of the tumor should be obtained for histopathologic and genetic analysis. Neuroblastoma tissue should be rushed to the lab for processing in a fresh state. Following a good response to chemotherapy, the residual tumor may be successfully removed at a second-look procedure (11).

Laparoscopic Procedures (Minimally Invasive) for Neuroblastoma

Recent advances in laparoscopic instrumentation, miniaturization of existing instruments, and improved video capabilities have made minimally invasive surgical (MIS) procedures a safe alternative to open procedures in children. However, the theoretical benefits (i.e., decreased surgical stress, improved postoperative morbidity, reduced time to initiation of enteral nutrition, and improved cosmetic appearance) need to be realized before these techniques can become the mainstay of surgical therapy in this patient group. Because the MIS approach for tumor resection is not routinely practiced, for the purpose of this chapter we will confine our discussion of MIS techniques to laparoscopic tumor biopsy.

General anesthesia is induced and the patient intubated. A nasogastric tube and urethral Foley catheter are placed to decrease the risk of gastroesophageal reflux with possible aspiration of gastric contents or injury to the stomach or bladder. The patient is then positioned in a 45-degree lateral decubitus position. Depending on the surgeon's preference (using the open Hasson technique or the Veress needle technique) the initial trocar is placed and a pneumoperitoneum is created with the pressure maintained between 8 to 10 mm Hg. The anesthesiologist should be requested to maintain relaxation of the abdominal wall; this reduces the need for a high-pressure pneumoperitoneum. The umbilical trocar should be a 12-mm trocar. Two to three 5-mm ports are placed using radially expanding trocar/introducers. The retroperitoneum is then dissected using either electrocautery and/or a harmonic scalpel.

CHAPTER 91

Wilms' Tumor

Robin L. Zagone and Michael L. Ritchey

Wilms' tumor, or nephroblastoma, represents approximately 6% of all childhood cancers in the United States and is the most common primary malignant renal tumor of childhood. The incidence rate of Wilms' tumor is 1 in 10,000 children with a new case rate of 450 to 500 annually in the United States. The mean age at diagnosis for unilateral nephroblastoma is 36.5 months for males and 42.5 months for females. The age of peak incidence for bilateral tumors is lower for both sexes: 29.5 months for males and 32.6 months for females.

Most cases of Wilms' tumor are sporadic; however, there are notable phenotypic syndromes with which 10% of Wilms' tumors are associated. These syndromes have given clues to the genetic basis of the disease. The phenotypic syndromes have been divided into overgrowth and nonovergrowth categories. Examples of overgrowth syndromes are Beckwith–Wiedeman syndrome (macroglossia, omphalocele, and visceromegaly, 10% to 20% tumor incidence), isolated hemihypertrophy (3% to 5% tumor incidence), Perlman syndrome (macrosomia, cryptorchidism, hyperinsulinism, phenotypic facies), Sotos syndrome (acromegaly, cerebral disorders), and Simpson–Golabi–Behemel syndrome (X-linked dysmorphic fascies, macroglossia). Examples of nonovergrowth syndromes are isolated aniridia, trisomy 18, WAGR syndrome (Wilms' tumor, aniridia, genitourinary malformations, mental retardation, 42% tumor incidence), Bloom's syndrome (pre- and postnatal growth deficiency, pigmentation disorders, telangiectasias), and Denys–Drash syndrome (male pseudohermaphroditism and nephropathy). Further, Wilms' tumor is associated with isolated genitourinary anomalies such as hypospadias, cryptorchidism, and renal fusion. Less than 2% of Wilms' tumor cases show patterns of inheritance (3).

The WT1 gene (locus 11p13) encodes a transcriptional factor that serves both tumor suppressive and developmental regulatory functions. It is critical in the early embryogenesis of the genitourinary system. Heterozygous deletion of WT1 in murine models yields complete failure of renal development (3). WT1 mutations are present in a minority of Wilms' tumors (10% to 15%) but are frequently present in cases of Denys–Drash syndrome and Fraser's syndromes (2). This observation suggests multiple potential genetic etiologies for Wilms' tumor.

A second locus at 11p15 has been designated WT2 but the gene has not yet been cloned. Loss of heterozygosity at this locus is associated with Beckwith–Wiedemann syndrome. It is unknown whether this association represents a single gene or set of genes separately responsible for Beckwith–Wiedemann syndrome and Wilms' tumor at the same locus (3). Loss of heterozygosity at 16q is noted in 20% of Wilms' tumors and is associated with poor prognosis. It is speculated that this locus may be important in tumor progression rather than causality.

Nephrogenic rests (NRs) are foci of nephrogenic primitive embryonal tissues that persist in the postnatal kidney but regress by 1 year of age. They are found in 1% of infant postmortem kidneys. The presence of NRs in up to 44% of kidneys removed for Wilms' tumor suggests that they may represent precursor lesions in those genetically predisposed to Wilms' tumor. The radial anatomy of the renal medullary pyramid maps the chronological development of the nephrons within it, the oldest at the medulla and the youngest at the lobar periphery. Therefore, different anatomic distributions of NRs within the renal lobe are important because they may represent events at different stages of organogenesis. For example, peripheral or perilobar NRs are observed in kidneys harboring Wilms' tumors with WT2 locus deletions whereas intralobar NRs are more often observed in those with WT1-associated tumors (1). The presence of multiple NRs, termed nephroblastomatosis, in the nontumoral portion of a Wilms' tumor kidney has been shown to be a risk factor for recurrence (3).

DIAGNOSIS

More than 90% of children with Wilms' tumor present with an abdominal mass found incidentally by a family member or physician. The mass may be extremely large relative to the size of the child and not necessarily confined to one side. Approximately 25% of children will have hematuria at diagnosis, although gross hematuria is less common and warrants further evaluation to rule out tumor extension into the collecting system. Children may present more acutely with abdominal pain, leading to exploration for assumed appendicitis. Tumor rupture into the peritoneal cavity or bleeding within the tumor are the common reasons for presentation with an acute abdomen. A persistent varicocele in the supine position or hepatomegaly may be reflective of inferior vena caval obstruction from tumor thrombus.

The preoperative laboratory evaluation of a child with an abdominal mass should include a complete peripheral blood count, differential white blood cell count, platelet count, liver function tests, and renal function tests. There is an 8% incidence of acquired von Willebrand's disease in newly diagnosed Wilms' tumor patients (4). This defect can be corrected preoperatively with the administration of 1-desamino-8-D-arginine-vasopressin (DDAVP). Serum calcium should also be checked as this can be elevated in both congenital mesoblastic nephroma and rhabdoid tumor of the kidney.

The initial radiographic study that should be obtained in children with abdominal masses is an abdominal ultrasound, which can differentiate between solid and cystic masses. For children with renal tumors, real-time ultrasonography of the inferior vena cava (IVC) is necessary to exclude intracaval tumor thrombus. If this study is inconclusive, magnetic resonance imaging (MRI) is an excellent modality to assess the venous system.

Additional information sought by preoperative imaging is the presence of a functioning contralateral kidney and evidence for extrarenal spread of tumor. The lungs represent the most common site of metastases and chest computed tomography (CT) is currently recommended for evaluation of the lungs. It is unclear how much additional staging information is provided by a CT scan or MRI of the abdomen because local tumor extent and assignment of tumor stage is determined by surgical and pathologic findings.

INDICATIONS FOR SURGERY

The initial management of a child with Wilms' tumor is abdominal exploration. In most cases, a radical nephrectomy can be performed. Histopathology and tumor stage have been demonstrated to be the key determinants of prognosis in patients with Wilms' tumor. Assignment of tumor stage (Table 91–1) is based on intraoperative and pathologic findings.

TABLE 91–1. *Staging system of the National Wilms Tumor Study*

1. Tumor Limited to the Kidney and Completely Excised. The Renal Capsule is Intact and the Tumor was Not Ruptured Prior to Removal. There is No Residual Tumor. The Vessels of the Renal Sinus are Not Involved.
2. Tumor Extends Beyond the Kidney but is Completely Excised. There is regional Extension of the Tumor (i.e., Penetration of the Renal Capsule, Extensive Invasion of the Renal Sinus). The Tumor May Have Been Biopsied or There May be Local Spillage of Tumor Confined to the Flank. Extrarenal Vessels May Contain Tumor Thrombus or be Infiltrated by Tumor.
3. Residual Nonhematogenous Tumor Confined to the Abdomen: Lymph Node Involvement, Diffuse Peritoneal Spillage Either Before or During Surgery, Peritoneal Implants, Tumor Beyond Surgical Margin Either Grossly or Microscopically, or Tumor Not Completely Removed.
4. Hematogenous Metastases (Lung, Liver, Bone, Brain, etc.) or Lymph Node Metastases Outside the Abdominopelvic Region are Present.
5. Bilateral Renal Involvement at Diagnosis.

The International Society of Pediatric Oncology (SIOP) advocates primary chemotherapy for all patients with Wilms' tumor regardless of extent of disease. Preoperative treatment can produce dramatic reduction in the size of the primary tumor, facilitating surgical excision. The SIOP trials have demonstrated that the incidence of tumor rupture is lower after preoperative therapy (11). There is no survival advantage over a primary surgical approach. SIOP investigators use the postchemotherapy stage to determine the amount of postoperative therapy, which may inadequately define the risk of intraabdominal recurrence in unirradiated patients.

The National Wilms' Tumor Study Group (NWTSG) recommends preoperative chemotherapy in children with bilateral tumors, tumors inoperable at surgical exploration, or inferior vena cava extension above the hepatic veins. All other patients should undergo primary excision of the tumor. This allows precise staging of patients with modulation of treatment for each individual, thereby decreasing the intensity of treatment when possible while maintaining excellent overall survival.

ALTERNATIVE THERAPY

Because all children with Wilms' tumor are treated per NWTSG protocol, there is little alternative therapy.

SURGICAL TECHNIQUE

Nephrectomy is routinely performed via a generous transverse abdominal incision. The patient is positioned in a supine fashion with some flexion of the lumbar spine to facilitate the exposure of retroperitoneal structures.

The incision is made approximately 2 finger breadths above the umbilicus. The incision begins in the midaxillary line on the side of the neoplasm. The extent to which the incision is extended across the midline will vary with the size of the tumor and amount of exposure needed. The incision may be extended into a thoracoabdominal approach by continuing through the bed of the ninth or tenth rib, if necessary. The muscle layers are divided sequentially to facilitate exposure. The peritoneal space should be opened very carefully. The tumor will compress the colon and/or small bowel up against the anterior abdominal wall, which can inadvertently lead to enterotomy. A thorough exploration of the abdomen is then performed. The peritoneal cavity is assessed for evidence of preoperative tumor rupture, tumor implants, or drop metastases in the pelvis. The liver is carefully examined, as many of the liver metastases are not identified on preoperative imaging studies, and an assessment of tumor extent is then performed, including palpation of the IVC, assessment of regional lymphadenopathy, perinephric extension, and tumor mobility.

Prior to proceeding with nephrectomy, the contralateral kidney is examined. The colon is reflected medially by incising the white line of Toldt. Gerota's fascia is opened to allow inspection as well as palpation of the anterior and posterior surfaces of the kidney. Any suspicious lesions should be biopsied for frozen section to exclude Wilms' tumor or nephrogenic rests.

The nephrectomy now proceeds by reflection of the colon in a similar fashion as to expose the contralateral kidney. The colonic mesentery is mobilized, with care taken to preserve the colonic vessels that are draped over the tumor. The colon can then be retracted medially to expose the renal vessels (Fig. 91–1). For right-sided tumors, the posterior peritoneum can be incised up to the base of the mesentery. This will allow reflection of the entire colon and small bowel, which provides excellent exposure of the retroperitoneal vessels.

If possible, the renal vessels should be ligated at the beginning of the operation. Once the renal vein has been identified, a vessel loop is placed around the vein. Any nodal tissue around the renal vein may be sent as part of the permanent specimen. The renal vein and IVC should be carefully palpated for the presence of tumor thrombus. The artery can be identified with careful retraction of the vein. Prior to ligation of the vessels, the contralateral renal vessels and superior mesenteric artery are identified to avoid injury to these structures. The renal vessels are then doubly ligated and divided.

An alternative for management of the renal vein is to place a Satinsky clamp on the vena cava just proximal to the insertion of the renal vein. This is of great value when the vein is short or if there is tumor extension through the renal vein. The venous stump in the Satinsky is oversewn with continuous 5-0 Prolene in two layers after the vein is divided (Figs. 91–2A and 91–2B).

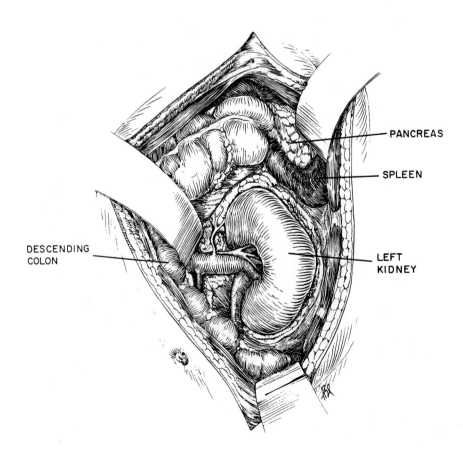

DESCENDING COLON

PANCREAS

SPLEEN

LEFT KIDNEY

FIG. 91–1. Descending colon retracted medially after incising of the line of Toldt and mobilizing of the mesocolon off the anterior surface of the tumor.

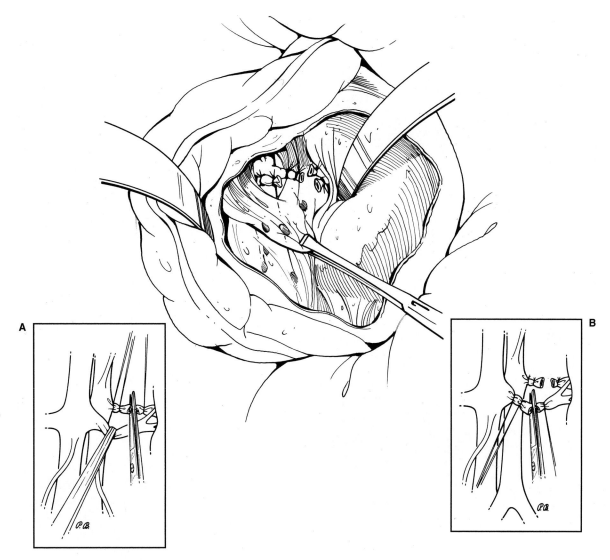

FIG. 91–2. Mobilization of left Wilms' tumor by blunt dissection after ligation and division of the **(A)** renal artery and **(B)** vein.

If a tumor thrombus is present in the IVC, additional surgical exposure is necessary. To extract tumor thrombus from within the vena cava, both proximal and distal vascular control is necessary. For minimal extension below the hepatic veins, the inferior edge of the liver can be retracted to expose the infrahepatic vena cava. For a tumor that extends more cephalad, mobilization of the liver is required. Division of the triangular and coronary ligaments of the liver allows rotation and exposure of the retrohepatic vena cava. Additional exposure can be gained by dividing the lesser hepatic veins. The contralateral renal vein and infrarenal IVC are controlled with vessel loops. The vena cava is then vertically incised just medial to the entrance of the renal vein. If the thrombus is free floating, it may easily be milked out at this point. In many cases, however, the thrombus is adherent to the wall of the IVC. A Fogarty or Foley balloon catheter is passed beyond the level of the hepatic veins

and the balloon inflated and pulled inferiorly, displacing the thrombus into the cavotomy. The vena cava is allowed to fill by releasing the vessel loops on the distal cava and contralateral renal vein. This will displace the air from within the cava. The cavotomy is then clamped with a Satinsky and oversewn in a continuous fashion with a 5-0 Prolene suture (Fig. 91–3).

After the vessels are controlled, a dissection plane is established outside of Gerota's fascia by sharp and blunt dissection. The perforating vessels can be quite large and should be ligated individually. Gentle handling of the tumor is needed to avoid rupture of the tumor during this dissection. Wilms' tumors are very soft and it is easy to enter the tumor, resulting in either local or diffuse tumor spill.

The ureter is divided as low as possible after palpation of the ureter to rule out intraureteral extension. The lymphatic tissue in the renal hilum and adjacent precaval and preaor-

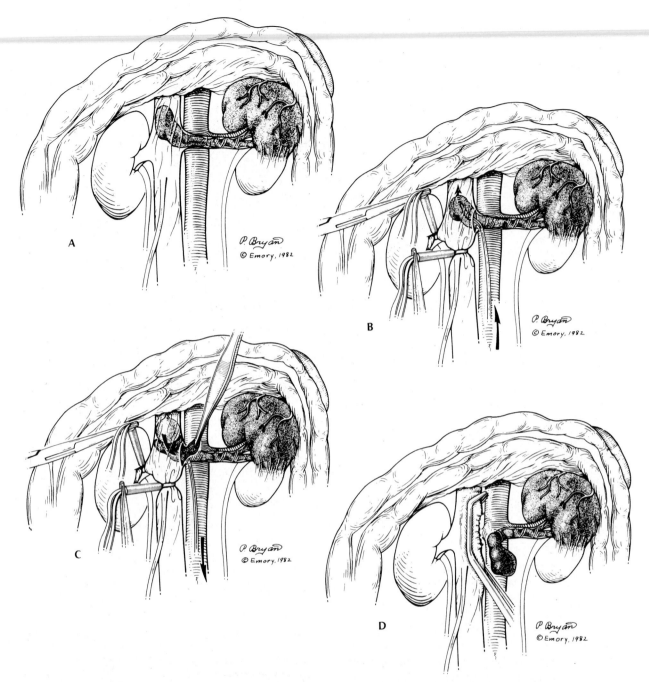

FIG. 91–3. Surgical technique to manage tumor extension through the renal vein. **A:** Into the vena cava (limited to the infrahepatic level). **B:** After exposure of the vessels, the infrarenal vena cava and contralateral renal vein are controlled with vessel loops and the vena cava is incised vertically at the intersection with the renal vein. **C:** A Fogarty catheter is passed superior to the tumor thrombus and the balloon inflated. **D:** The vena cava is flushed of air and a Satinsky clamp is placed to allow closure of the cavotomy

tic area is in general removed with the specimen. Formal lymph node dissection is not required, but all suspicious lymph nodes should be biopsied. After removal of the tumor, the wound is irrigated with saline and hemostasis is assessed. A drain is not routinely left in place unless a portion of the pancreas or liver has been resected. The displaced colon is placed back in the tumor bed.

Bilateral Tumors

Radical nephrectomy should not be performed at the initial operation of a child with bilateral Wilms' tumors. Children treated with preoperative chemotherapy will have more renal units preserved. This is important because the risk of renal failure in patients with bilateral disease approaches 15% at 15 years posttreatment (7). Initial exploration of the abdomen and biopsy of both kidneys are performed to verify the histological type of each tumor, although sampling errors may still occur. Partial nephrectomy or wedge excision can be employed at the initial operation only if all of the tumor can be removed with preservation of the majority of renal parenchyma (greater than 75%) on both sides. Grossly abnormal lymph nodes or other lesions suggestive of extrarenal spread should be biopsied and a surgical stage assigned to each kidney. The patient is given preoperative chemotherapy appropriate to the stage and histology of the tumor.

Tumor response is evaluated with CT after week 5. This can assess the reduction in tumor volume and the feasibility of partial resection. At the time of the second-look procedure, partial nephrectomy or wedge excision of the tumor is performed, but only if it will not compromise tumor resection and negative margins can be obtained. If complete excision of tumor from one kidney can be performed leaving a viable and functioning kidney, then radical nephrectomy can be performed to remove a contralateral kidney with extensive tumor involvement. Enucleation of the tumor should be considered in lieu of a formal partial nephrectomy only if removal of a margin of renal tissue would compromise the vascular supply to the kidney.

If the tumor is not amenable to partial resections, repeat biopsies should be performed. Patients with persistent viable tumor that cannot be resected should be treated with a different chemotherapeutic regimen. The patient should be reassessed after an additional 12 weeks of chemotherapy to determine the feasibility of resection. If there is extensive tumor involvement precluding partial resection in a solitary kidney, radiation therapy can then be instituted to effect tumor shrinkage.

POSTOPERATIVE CARE

Current recommendations for treatment are those utilized in the recently completed NWTS-5 study (Table 91–2). In this study, biologic features of the tumors were assessed in patients not randomized for therapy. This study was done to verify the preliminary findings that loss of heterozygosity (LOH) for chromosomes 16q and 1p are useful markers in identifying patients who will relapse (6). The results of this study have not yet been published. If these variables are found to be predictive of clinical behavior, then this information will be used in subsequent clinical trials to further stratify patients for therapy.

The treatment for patients with stage I or II favorable histology (FH) and stage I anaplastic Wilms' tumor is the same. They should receive a pulse-intensive regimen of vincristine (VCR) and dactinomycin (AMD) for 18 weeks. In NWTS-5, the role of surgery alone for children under 2 years of age with stage I FH tumors weighing under 550 g was examined. This portion of the study was suspended when the number of tumor relapses exceeded the limit allowed by the design of the study and the recommendation was made that all children with stage I tumors receive AMD and VCR. The 2-year survival rate of this cohort of patients with small tumors is 100% with a median follow-up of 1.61 years, and extended follow-up continues (5). Observation of untreated children may yield interesting information on the role of chemotherapy in decreasing the incidence of contralateral relapse in patients with NRs.

Patients with stage III FH and stage II–III focal anaplasia are treated with AMD, VCR, and doxorubicin (DOX) and 1,080 cGy abdominal irradiation. Patients with stage IV FH tumors receive abdominal irradiation based on the local tumor stage and 1,200 cGy to both lungs.

OUTCOMES

Complications

Despite improvements and refinement of surgical technique, the removal of a large nephroblastoma is still prone to intra- and postoperative complications. A marked reduction in complications has been noted in the last 10 years. Chart review yields a complication rate of 19.8% for NWTS-3 (8) and, more recently, 12.7% for NWTS-4 (9). The most common complication was

TABLE 91–2. *Protocol used in National Wilms' Tumor Study—5*

Stage/histology	Radiotherapy	Chemotherapy
Stage I, II FH Stage I Anaplasia	None	EE-4A: *Pulse*-Intensive AMD Plus VCR (18 wk.)
Stage III, IV FH Stage II–IV Focal Anaplasia	1,080 cGy[a]	DD-4A: *Pulse*-Intensive AMD, VCR, and DOX (24 wk)
Stage II–IV Diffuse Anaplasia Stage I–IV CCSK	Yes[b]	Regimen I: AMD, VCR, DOX, CPM, and Etoposide
Stage I–IV Rhabdoid Tumor of the Kidney	Yes[b]	Regimen RTK: Carboplatin, Etoposide, and CPM

AMD, dactinomycin; VCR, vincristine; DOX, doxorubicin; CPM, cyclophosphamide; FH, favorable histology; CCSK, clear-cell sarcoma of the kidney.
[a]Stage IV/FH patients are given radiation based on the local tumor stage.
[b]Radiation therapy is given to all CCSK and RTK patients. Consult protocol for specific treatment.

TABLE 91–3. *National Wilms' Tumor Study—4: Most commonly reported surgical complications after unilateral nephrectomy*

Complication	No. of patients (%)
Small Intestinal Obstruction	27 (5.1)
Extensive Hemorrhage	10 (1.9)
Wound Infection	10 (1.9)
Vascular Injury	8 (1.5)
Splenic Injury	6 (1.1)
Diaphragmatic Tear	2 (0.4)
Incisional Hernia	1 (0.2)
Pneumothorax	1 (0.2)
Chylous Ascites	1 (0.2)

intestinal obstruction (5.1%) secondary to intestinal adhesions or intussusception. This was followed closely by extensive hemorrhage (1.9%), defined as intraoperative blood loss exceeding 50 mL per kg of body weight (Table 91–3).

A mortality rate of 0.5% related to surgical complications was reported from NWTS-3. However, a higher intraoperative mortality rate of 1.5% has been reported from other centers. The latter may reflect that intraoperative deaths may not be reported to the NWTSG. Factors that have been associated with an increased risk for surgical complications are higher tumor stage, tumor size greater than 10 cm, incorrect preoperative diagnosis, thoracoabdominal incision, intracaval tumor extension, and resection of other visceral organs.

Results

The overall survival for children with Wilms' tumor remains in excess of 90% as a result of multimodal therapy. Common sites of recurrence are the lungs, liver, renal fossa, and contralateral kidney. Recurrence is correlated with tumor histology, stage, and margin positivity. Data from NWTS-4 reveal an increased risk for local recurrence in the setting of intraoperative tumor rupture (10). Omission of lymph node biopsy also correlates with recurrence and is attributed to understaging. The average survival at 2 years after recurrence is 43%. Current trials continue to refine chemotherapeutic regimens to improve survival, in particular for higher-risk populations. Finally, basic research continues to widen the understanding of the diverse genetic framework behind this disease.

REFERENCES

1. Beckwith JB. Nephrogenic rests and the pathogenesis of Wilms tumor: Developmental and clinical considerations. *Am J Med Genet* 1998; 79:268–273.
2. Coppes MJ, Liefers GJ, Higuchi M, Zinn AB, Balfe JW, Williams BRG. Inherited WT1 mutations in Denys–Drash syndrome. *Cancer Res* 1992;52:6125–6128.
3. Coppes MJ, Pritchard-Jones K. Principles of Wilms' tumor biology. *Urol Clin North Am* 2000;27:423–433.
4. Coppes MJ, Zandvoort SWH, Sparling CR, et al. Acquired von Willebrand disease in Wilms' tumor patients. *J Clin Oncol* 1993;10:1–7.
5. Green DM, Breslow NE, Beckwith JB, Ritchey ML, et al. Treatment with nephrectomy only for small, stage I/favorable histology Wilms tumor: a report from the National Wilms Tumor Study Group. *J Clin Oncol* 2001;19:3710–3724.
6. Grundy PE, Telzerow PE, Moksness J, Breslow NE. Clinicopathologic correlates of loss of heterozygosity in Wilms tumor: a preliminary analysis. *Med Pediatr Oncol* 1996;27:429–433.
7. Ritchey ML, Green DM, Thomas P, et al. Renal failure in Wilms tumor patients: a report of the NWTSG. *Med Pediatr Oncol* 1996;26:75–80.
8. Ritchey ML, Kelalis PP, Breslow N, et al. Surgical complication following nephrectomy for Wilms' tumor: a report of National Wilms' Tumor Study-3. *Surg Gynecol Obstet* 1992; 175:507–514.
9. Ritchey ML, Shamberger RC, Haase G, et al. Surgical complications after primary nephrectomy for Wilms' tumor: Report from the National Wilms' Tumor Study Group. *J Am Coll Surg* 2001;1:63–68.
10. Shamberger RC, Guthrie KA, Ritchey ML, et al. Surgery-related factors and local recurrence of Wilms' tumor in National Wilms' Tumor Study 4. *Ann Surg* 1999;229:292–297.
11. Tournade MF, Com-Nougue C, Voute PA, et al. Results of the Sixth International Society of Pediatric Oncology Wilms' Tumor Trial and Study: a risk-adapted therapeutic approach in Wilms' tumor. *J Clin Oncol* 1993;11:1014–1023.

CHAPTER 92

Renal Fusion and Ectopia

Ross M. Decter

Abnormalities of renal fusion and ectopia predispose to infection, hydronephrosis, stone disease, and, in some instances, neoplasia. A clear understanding of these anatomic variants and the deviations from standard urologic techniques required to address them is important although clinical problems associated with abnormalities of renal fusion and ectopia present infrequently in urologic practice.

The ureteral bud branches from the wolffian duct and extends toward the metanephric blastema during the fourth and fifth weeks of gestation. The ureteral bud induces the metanephric blastema to form the functioning kidney. The exact mechanism of renal ascent is not known but during normal development the kidneys ascend and rotate. The renal pelvis rotates from an initial anterior position 90 degrees toward the midline until it reaches its final medial position. Migration and rotation occur simultaneously between the fourth and eighth or ninth weeks of gestation. The blood supply to the kidney is derived from successively higher levels of the aorta and its branches during ascent.

The most common anomaly of renal position is malrotation: incomplete rotation of the kidney to its final position. The renal pelvis in a malrotated kidney in general lies anterior to the parenchyma as opposed to its normal medial location. Simple malrotation of a normally positioned kidney is often an incidental finding. The pyelocaliceal systems of malrotated kidneys are morphologically abnormal, but functionally they usually drain without impairment. Malrotation may be seen in kidneys that are otherwise normally positioned and malrotation is commonly observed in ectopic kidneys.

Close approximation of the two proliferating renal blastemas prior to significant ascent is a normal embryological finding (6). If there is any disturbance of separation of the closely approximated renal blastemas, fusion anomalies of the kidneys may develop.

The most common fusion anomaly is the horseshoe kidney. The horseshoe kidney in general ascends until the upper border of the isthmus is at the level of the inferior mesenteric artery. Horseshoe kidney occurs in 1 in 400 to 1 in 1,800 births (9). There is a male predominance for the condition (12). The fusion in horseshoe kidney almost always occurs at the lower poles. Cases of upper pole fusion are recorded rarely (12). The isthmus of the horseshoe kidney lies just below the inferior mesenteric artery at the L4 vertebral level. The blood supply to these kidneys is variable (Fig. 92–1).

Crossed-fused ectopia is the second most common fusion anomaly. This abnormality occurs when the developing kidney crosses from one side to the other during its ascent or when the ureteral bud from one side crosses to the contralateral side and induces abnormal development of that metanephric blastema. Crossed ectopia with fusion may occur in a variety of forms (Fig. 92–2). Although crossed ectopia occurs most frequently with fusion, the anomaly may occur without fusion (Fig. 92–3).

An ectopic kidney lies outside of the normal position in the renal fossa. The kidney, in simple ectopia, in general lies in the ipsilateral retroperitoneal space at a position that is lower than normal (Fig. 92–4). In crossed ectopia, the kidney crosses the midline and is frequently fused to its contralateral mate. The autopsy incidence of renal ectopia is about 1 in 1,000 cases and often is totally asymptomatic (7). Reviews of renal ectopia show that the left and right kidneys are affected with close to equal frequency. Ectopic kidneys occur bilaterally around 10% of the time and the most common position of the ectopic kidney is in the pelvis. Pelvic ectopia was reported in about 55% of patients in

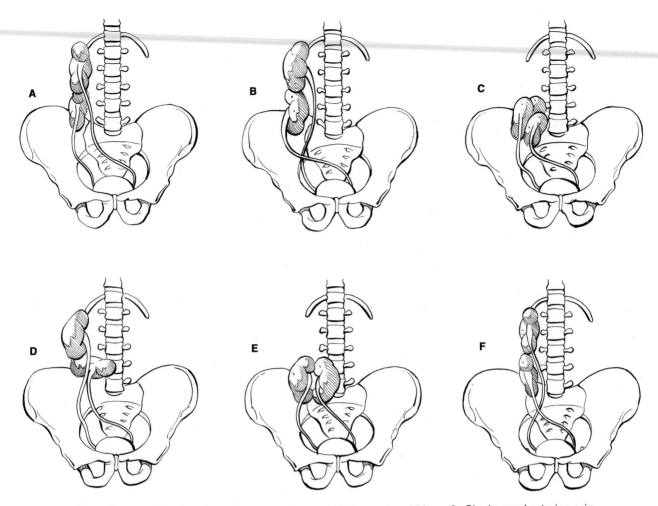

FIG. 92–1. Three common variants of blood supply in horseshoe kidney. **A:** Single renal arteries arising from the aorta. **B:** Multiple aortic arteries. **C:** Multiple aortic and iliac arteries.

one series of ectopic kidneys; crossed-fused ectopia occurred in 27%; lumbar ectopia in 12%; non–crossed-fused ectopia in 5% of patients; and a thoracic kidney was recorded only 1% of the time (7). Rarely, a solitary pelvic kidney occurs. This kidney suffers the risk of injury during pelvic surgical procedures and on occasion has been reported as an unusual cause of giant hydronephrosis.

Ectopic kidneys are smaller than their contralateral mates (4). The blood supply to the pelvic kidney, the most common of the ectopic kidneys, is variable. The arterial supply may arise from the distal aorta or bifurcation, the ipsilateral common iliac, or the hypogastric vessels. In general, the lower the kidney is in its pelvic location, the greater the likelihood that multiple arterial vessels will supply it (5).

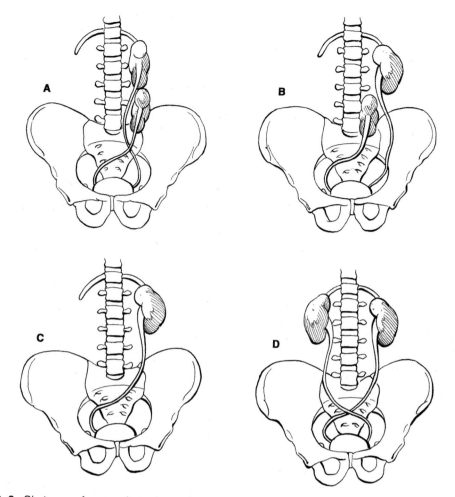

FIG. 92–2. Six types of crossed renal ectopia with fusion. **A:** Ectopic kidney superior. **B:** Sigmoid or S-shaped kidney. **C:** Lump kidney. **D:** L-shaped kidney. **E:** Disk kidney. **F:** Ectopic kidney inferior. (Modified from McDonald JH, McClellan DS. Crossed renal ectopia. *Am J Surg* 1957;93:995, with permission.)

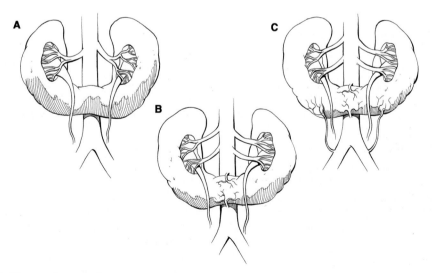

FIG. 92–3. Types of crossed renal ectopia. **A:** Fused. **B:** Nonfused. **C:** Solitary. **D:** Bilateral. (Modified from McDonald JH, McClellan DS. Crossed renal ectopia. *Am J Surg* 1957;93:995, with permission.)

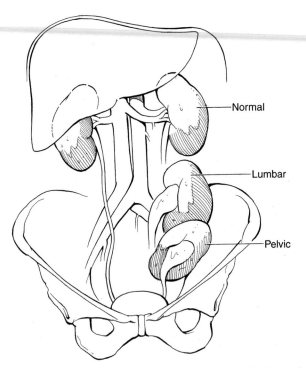

FIG. 92–4. Location of lumbar and pelvic ectopically positioned kidneys in relation to the normally positioned kidney.

DIAGNOSIS

Horseshoe Kidney

Approximately 25% to 33% of patients with horseshoe kidneys who survive beyond the newborn period are asymptomatic (12). Those patients with symptoms will typically present with urinary tract infections (about 50% of the time) or an abdominal mass, hematuria, or abdominal pain (approximately 10% each).

The initial diagnostic evaluation in children is usually an ultrasound and many subsequently have intravenous pyelography (IVP). Most adults have IVP as their initial study. The intravenous pyelographic features of the horseshoe kidney are typical. The renal axis is abnormal, being either vertically orientated or tilted laterally. The renal pelves tend to be located anteriorly and the ureters course ventral to the isthmus. The lower calyces are oriented caudally or even medially as opposed to laterally. Kidneys with fusion anomalies are subject to a high incidence of vesicoureteral reflux, variably reported between 20% and 50%. Voiding cystourethrography (VCUG) is therefore mandated during the evaluation of these patients.

The diagnosis of a ureteropelvic junction (UPJ) obstruction in a horseshoe kidney is straightforward when the patient's symptoms leads to an IVP that reveals significant pyelocaliectasis. In other instances, with less severe dilation and especially when there is coexistent stone disease, we find the diuretic renal scan a valuable aid in assessing the drainage of these systems and deciding whether the hydronephrosis is functionally significant.

Ectopic Kidney

Patients with a symptomatic ectopic kidney frequently present with a urinary tract infection or the ectopic kidney is discovered in the evaluation of abdominal pain. The workup of a palpable abdominal mass or the discovery of the abnormal renal position during the evaluation of other anomalies each account for the diagnosis in about 20% of cases. Hematuria, incontinence, renal insufficiency, and nephrolithiasis are less common presenting complaints. It is important to emphasize that the majority of patients with ectopic kidneys are asymptomatic.

The evaluation in children is usually an ultrasound evaluation, while older patients will in general have an IVP. The ectopic kidney can be difficult to detect on the intravenous pyelogram as the pyelocaliceal system often overlies the bony pelvis. Functional evaluation of the ectopically positioned kidney is routinely performed with a diuretic renal scan. Ectopic kidneys have a high incidence of associated vesicoureteral reflux so a VCUG should be a routine part of the evaluation of these patients.

INDICATIONS FOR SURGERY

The indications for surgical intervention in the ectopic or horseshoe kidney are similar to those in normally positioned kidney. Pyeloplasty is required in patients with symptomatic UPJ obstruction or when the evaluation suggests that the abnormality at the UPJ may impact on ultimate renal function. Symptomatic stone disease needs to be addressed using either open, endoscopic, or extracorporeal techniques. If the evaluation of infections in a horseshoe kidney reveals vesicoureteral reflux operative management, usually ureteral reimplantation may be mandated if the reflux is of high grade, persists, or if prophylaxis fails to prevent infection.

ALTERNATIVE THERAPY

The alternative to surgical intervention for reflux is nonoperative management, usually consisting of observation and antibiotic prophylaxis. Surgery is the only viable option for patients with significant UPJ obstruction, stones, and tumors.

Endopyelotomy has been utilized to treat UPJ obstruction in horseshoe kidneys. The initial results of endopyelotomy performed in adults by experienced surgeons are encouraging; however, we currently prefer pyeloplasty as the initial procedure for UPJ obstructions in children.

SURGICAL TECHNIQUE

Pyeloplasty

Pyeloplasty is the most common open procedure performed on the horseshoe kidney. Division of the isthmus with nephropexy had be considered in the past to be an important part of the procedure, but recent experience suggests that isthmus division or symphysiotomy is rarely necessary in the correction of UPJ obstruction.

The surgical exposure of the horseshoe kidney can be achieved through a midline transperitoneal, anteriorly positioned flank extraperitoneal, or transverse transperitoneal approach. We prefer the transverse transperitoneal exposure as it seems to provide the widest exposure with a cosmetically acceptable scar. The incision extends from the anterior axillary line on the affected side crossing the midline several centimeters below the umbilicus. It can be extended laterally in either direction if necessary. Depending on the position of the affected UPJ, the posterior peritoneum may be incised medial to the inferior mesenteric vein up to Treitz's ligament, inferior and laterally along the small bowel mesentery around the cecum, and up along the line of Toldt on the right side. The small bowel and cecum can then be reflected upward out of the operative field and packed in the upper abdomen. Exposure is maintained with a ring retractor.

Repair of UPJ obstruction in the horseshoe kidney can be performed by a Foley Y–V-plasty or a dismembered pyeloplasty. Although the Foley Y–V repair is nicely suited to the typical high-insertion obstruction seen in horseshoe kidneys (Fig. 92–5), we prefer the dismembered technique because it seems to provide more flexibility. During the conduct of the pyeloplasty care must be taken to avoid inadvertent division of small vessels to the parenchyma and excessive dissection of the ureter or pelvis. As much adventitial tissue is left on the ureter as possible and no vessels to the ureter are sacrificed unless their division is absolutely necessary to provide for adequate mobilization.

After the proximal ureter and renal pelvis are adequately exposed using sharp dissection, two stay stitches of 5-0 chromic are positioned in the ureter just below the UPJ (Fig. 92–5). The ureter is divided between these stitches and carefully mobilized. A pelvic flap is then created by orienting a wide-based inverted V-shaped incision on the renal pelvis with the apex of the inverted V at the UPJ. The flap is designed such that it will provide a dependent portion of pelvis for the anastomosis. It is important that the base of the V be wide to avoid ischemia of the flap. The flap is opened with tenotomy scissors and the tip is trimmed minimally to smooth the point of the V. The ureter is then positioned so the length and position of the spatulation can be judged. The spatulation is positioned on the posterior aspect of the ureter using Potts scissors such that the ureter will not be twisted when it is laid on the dependent pelvic flap. It is critical

that the flap and spatulated ureter are approximated in a tension-free fashion. If the repair is performed under tension an anastomotic stricture may result. It is also important that the upper ureter or anastomosis are not compressed by any of the renal vessels as they may obstruct the repair (3). The anastomosis and dissection are performed with the aid of 2.5× optical magnification. We perform the anastomosis using 7-0 Vicryl in younger children and 6-0 Vicryl in adolescents.

The fact that the ureter is dismembered and freely mobile allows the surgeon to position it so that the ureteral spatulation can extend into a relatively wide portion of the ureter and simultaneously the ureter can be oriented to avoid torsion or redundancy that might kink the ureter distal to the repair. The anastomosis in the dismembered pyeloplasty seems technically easier than the Foley Y–V because the ureter is not fixed at two points.

We begin the anastomosis at the heel, suturing the most dependent portion of the V-shaped incision to the apex of the ureteral spatulation. The initial portion of the anastomosis is performed using interrupted sutures, in general one at the apex and two on either side of the apex. Each stitch must be precisely positioned to avoid postoperative leakage and/or compromise of the lumen. After the apex is anastomosed, the remainder of the pyeloplasty is performed using a running locking 7-0 Vicryl suture up one side of the spatulated ureter and then up the other side. Prior to complete closure, patency of the anastomosis is tested by passing a 5 and 8 feeding tube through the repair. No stent or diversion is in general employed in children. A Penrose drain is positioned near the anastomosis and made to exit through a separate stab wound. The abdominal wall closure is performed using running 3-0 or larger PDS. We close the skin with a subcuticular pull-out stitch of 3-0 Prolene. Most children are discharged the day after surgery. The skin suture is removed between 5 and 7 days postoperatively and the drain is removed at that time if drainage is minimal.

Ureterocalicostomy

A ureterocalicostomy is usually performed to salvage a failed prior pyeloplasty but it should be considered as the primary procedure for UPJ obstruction when there is a small intrarenal pelvis or in other instances when the lower pole parenchyma is extremely thinned (3) (Fig. 92–6). The ureter is carefully separated from the pelvis as described above and if feasible a pyelotomy is performed. We find that a finger inserted into the open renal pelvis and positioned in the lower pole calyx aids in the dissection. The parenchyma over the lower pole calyx is incised with electrocautery; the capsule is peeled back and the parenchyma resected to allow adequate exposure of the calyx. Hemostasis is achieved using cautery and/or sutures of 4-0 chromic through the edge of the resected parenchyma. The ureter is spatulated and the anastomosis

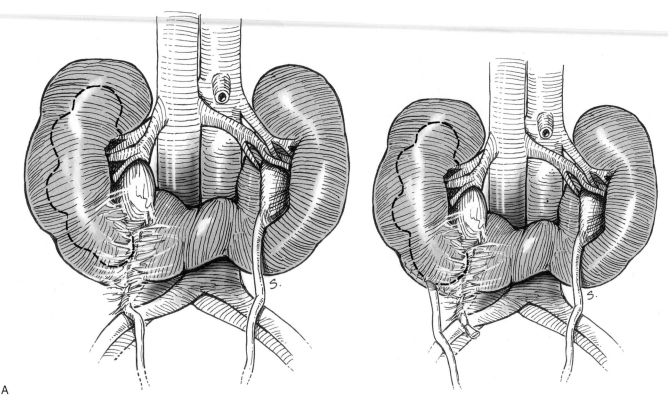

A

B

FIG. 92–7. A: Horseshoe kidney with prior failed pyeloplasty; note the dilated intrarenal collecting system. **B:** After ureterocalicostomy, dependent drainage has been achieved. (Modified from Kay R. Ureterocalicostomy as a salvage procedure. *Urol Times* 2001;April:34, with permission.)

between the ureter and the opened calyx is performed as previously described. It is important to resect enough parenchyma so that it does not impinge upon the anastomosis. The resected edge of the thinned parenchyma will contract during healing. This contraction must be accounted for when the parenchymal resection is performed or the anastomosis will become compressed and obstructed over time. We divert the urine by using either a nephrostomy tube (a 10 or 12 Fr Malecot) and a ureteral stent (usually a 5 Fr feeding tube) or a double-J stent. A ureterocalicostomy as it would appear in a horseshoe kidney is shown in Figure 92–7.

Surgery for Tumors

Wilms' tumor commonly presents in the horseshoe kidney. The involved portion of the kidney and isthmus are in general resected in the course of removal of the tumor. If the tumor occurs in the isthmus, some authors have recommended bilateral lower pole heminephrectomy. If the Wilms' tumor is bilateral at presentation, management is the same as bilateral Wilms' tumors in orthotopically positioned kidneys.

Tumor surgery of the horseshoe kidney deserves special mention because excision of the involved kidney will necessitate division of the isthmus. If the isthmus is composed of a band of fibrous tissue it can be readily divided using cautery; however, if it is functioning parenchyma it must be carefully addressed to avoid excessive blood loss and necrosis of remaining parenchyma with the risk of secondary bleed and urinary fistula. The area must be carefully dissected and arteries to the isthmus sequentially occluded with bulldog clamps to assess the line of demarcation. Once this line is established the capsule is divided sharply and the parenchyma divided. Bleeding from the cut parenchyma is controlled with 4-0 chromic sutures. Any exposed calyces are closed with running locking 4-0 or 5-0 chromic, and the capsule and parenchyma are closed with carefully positioned horizontal mattress sutures of 2-0 chromic (Fig. 92–8).

Stone Surgery in the Horseshoe Kidney

Pyelolithotomy had been utilized in past decades to clear calculi from horseshoe kidneys; currently, percutaneous and extracorporeal techniques are employed almost exclusively. Extracorporeal shock wave lithotripsy (ESWL) in the horseshoe kidney has not enjoyed the success rate that it provides in orthotopically positioned kidneys. Most series note the requirement for an increased number of shocks, the need for increased retreatments, and a somewhat decreased stone clearance rate in horse-

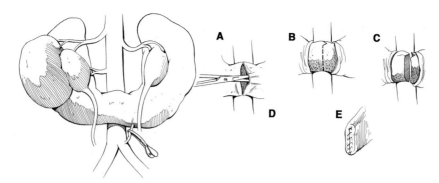

FIG. 92–8. Division of the isthmus of a horseshoe kidney with a right-sided renal tumor. The isthmus blood supply is from the left iliac. **A:** After identification of the line of demarcation an incision is made around the capsule of the isthmus. **B:** The capsule is peeled back. **C:** The parenchyma of the isthmus is transected in a wedge fashion to facilitate closure. **D:** Horizontal mattress sutures of absorbable 2-0 material are used to close the parenchyma for hemostasis. **E:** The capsule is closed over the parenchyma with a continuous absorbable suture.

shoe kidneys compared to stones in normally positioned kidneys. One series recorded a 73% stone-free rate in horseshoe kidneys using ESWL after multiple treatments (10). One of the reasons for difficulties treating stones with ESWL is that the anterior position of the stone makes it harder to position the stone at the F2 focus; often, the surgeon will have to employ the blast path to try to fragment the stone. Some investigators have used prone positioning to overcome this problem.

A percutaneous approach to the horseshoe kidney is readily achieved using an upper- to midposterior calyx to access the kidney. Stones in any calyx can be managed although often a long nephroscope and flexible instrumentation are required (8,11). Reports comparing ESWL of stones in horseshoe kidneys to percutaneous nephrostolithotomy conclude that the percutaneous technique provides superior stone clearance rates (11).

When calculus disease complicates obstruction of the UPJ in a horseshoe kidney the stone is removed at the time of pyeloplasty. In these instances, there may be considerably more reaction around the pelvis and ureter so the use of a nephrostomy tube and ureteral stent is prudent. An antegrade study can be performed 10 to 12 days postoperatively prior to nephrostomy tube removal to confirm drainage through the UPJ and integrity of the repair.

Surgical Options for the Ectopic Kidney

The ectopic kidney can be affected by any of the processes that occur in a normally positioned kidney. Overall, the evaluation and surgical management of these conditions will follow the lines of those discussed with horseshoe kidney. Reflux, if it mandates operative treatment, is addressed by a standard ureteral reimplantation or, alternatively, subureteral injection of a bulking agent.

On occasion, one has to address the problem of a failed pyeloplasty in a patient who has an ectopic pelvic kidney.

Ureterocalicostomy is one alternative in management of this problem; another is the use of a pyelovesicostomy. Pyelovesicostomy has been performed in renal transplant recipients after ureteral loss due to ischemia and/or rejection and has proven to be a viable salvage procedure.

OUTCOMES

Complications

Complications of pyeloplasty, such as prolonged urine leakage and poor anastomotic drainage, occur somewhat more frequently in horseshoe kidneys than in normal kidneys. The risk of renal ischemia caused by damage to an aberrant vessel is increased in the horseshoe or ectopically positioned kidney.

Results

Pyeloplasty in the horseshoe kidney is in general a successful procedure. A higher rate of complications was experienced in the era when division of the isthmus was employed.

REFERENCES

1. Boatman DL, Kolln CP, Flocks RH. Congenital anomalies associated with horseshoe kidney. *J Urol* 1982;107:205.
2. Buntley D. Malignancy associated with horseshoe kidney. *Urology* 1976;VIII:146.
3. Dewan PA, Clark S, Condron S, Henning P. Ureterocalicostomy in the management of pelvi–ureteric junction obstruction in the horseshoe kidney. *Br J Urol Int* 1999;94:366.
4. Dretler SP, Olsson C, Pfister RC. The anatomic, radiologic and clinical characteristics of the pelvic kidney: an analysis of 86 cases. *J Urol* 1971;105:623.
5. Dretler SP, Pfister R, Hendren WH. Extrarenal calyces in the ectopic kidney. *J Urol* 1970;103:406.
6. Friedland GW, DeVries P. Renal ectopia and fusion: embryologic basis. *Urology* 1975;5:698.
7. Gleason PE, Kelalis PP, Husmann DA, Kramer SA. Hydronephrosis in renal ectopia: incidence, etiology and significance. *J Urol* 1994;151: 1660.

8. Jones DJ, Wickham JEA, Kellett MJ. Percutaneous nephrolithotomy for calculi in horseshoe kidneys. *J Urol* 1991;145:481.

9. Kolln CP, Boatman DL, Schmidt JD, Flocks RH. Horseshoe kidney: a review of 105 patients. *J Urol* 1972;107:203.

10. Locke DR, Newman RC, Steinbock GS, Finlayson B. Extracorporeal shock-wave lithotripsy in horseshoe kidneys. *Urology* 1990;35:407.

11. Pearle MS, Traxer OA: Renal urolithiasis: therapy for special circumstances, part II. *AUA Update Ser* 2001;40(20):314.

12. Pitts WR Jr, Muecke EC. Horseshoe kidneys: a 40-year experience. *J Urol* 1975;113:743.

13. Segura JW, Kelalis PP, Burke EC. Horseshoe kidney in children. *J Urol* 1972;108:333.

CHAPTER 93

Transureteroureterostomy

Monisha S. Crisell and H. Gil Rushton

Ureteral surgery and various conditions including trauma, stricture, neoplasm, or previous failed surgical procedure can render a ureter inadequate for successful ureteroureterostomy or ureteroneocystostomy. Transureteroureterostomy (TUU), first described by Higgins (6) in the 1930s, has gained increased prominence in pediatric urology over the past three decades as a method to compensate for a lacking or defective distal ureter. In some cases, bridging the midureter to the contralateral ureter TUU may salvage a renal unit, especially in cases when an ipsilateral psoas hitch and/or Boari flap are insufficient means to accomplish this task. In other situations, TUU can be performed as a salvage procedure following previous failed surgery. More recently, TUU has been employed in complex reconstructive procedures that entail harvesting of the distal donor ureter for alternative purposes.

DIAGNOSIS

In the majority of cases in pediatric urology, TUU is employed as part of a planned reconstruction. The preoperative workup requires thorough assessment of bilateral renal function and drainage, knowledge of the anatomy of both the donor and recipient ureters, and careful evaluation of bladder function. Differential renal function and drainage are the most objectively determined by preoperative 99mTc diethylenetriamine pentaacetic acid (DTPA) or MAG-3 renal scintigraphy. Sonography can aid in determining the presence and severity of hydronephrosis. Contrast imaging with intravenous, retrograde, or antegrade pyelography may be necessary in select cases when detailed anatomic definition of the ureters is required. Contrast voiding cystography is the best modality to assess for the presence of vesicoureteral reflux, which when present may provide a "free" retrograde ureteropyelogram. In cases involving children with abnormal or neuropathic bladder function, preoperative urodynamics is required to evaluate bladder capacity, compliance, and emptying.

Less commonly in children than in adults, initial recognition of a ureteral injury requiring a TUU occurs intraoperatively during resection of a tumor or during exploration for trauma. Fortunately, in the majority of these cases one can usually anticipate a normal recipient ureter and bladder.

INDICATIONS FOR SURGERY

The primary goal of a TUU is to reestablish nonobstructive, nonrefluxing drainage of the ureter. Historically, TUU in children has been performed to either salvage a failed ureteral reimplantation or in conjunction with cutaneous ureterostomy for urinary diversion (4,7,12). Because TUU requires only one ureter for reimplantation, this procedure was commonly employed in the 1980s for urinary undiversion of conduits or in the construction of continent urinary reservoirs (5,10). In the majority of these cases, TUU was used simultaneously with reimplantation of the recipient ureter, many of which required tapering/tailoring frequently with a psoas hitch and/or bladder augmentation. TUU has also been used as an adjunct to reimplant procedures complicated by an abnormal bladder, which precludes reimplantation of more than one ureter. More recently, indications for TUU have been broadened to allow for harvesting the distal donor ureter to construct a continent ureteral conduit for clean intermittent catheterization or for unilateral ureterocystoplasty in cases where there is sufficient ureteral dilatation (8).

Ureteral reconstruction with TUU may not be possible if there is insufficient donor ureter (approximately one-half the original length) for a tension-free anastomosis. Any disease process that has the potential to affect contralateral renal function or drainage is also a contraindication, such as retroperitoneal fibrosis, high-dose radiation therapy, calculus disease, recurrent pyelonephritis, and urothelial malignancy. Although size disparity between ureters has been regarded as a relative contraindication in the past, successful TUU has been accomplished by use of a larger vertical ureterotomy in the recipient ureter to accommodate a larger-caliber donor ureter (5,7,10).

ALTERNATIVE THERAPY

Other procedures to be considered in lieu of TUU include ureteroneocystostomy with a psoas hitch or Boari flap, nephropexy to allow ureteroneocystostomy or ureteroureterostomy, ileal substitution, and autotransplantation. Other alternatives to TUU include mitigating or temporizing procedures such as cutaneous ureterostomy, pyelostomy, nephrostomy drainage, and ureteral stenting. Nephrectomy should also be considered in cases of marginal donor renal function.

SURGICAL TECHNIQUE

The patient is placed supine with such options as kidney rest elevation, retroflexion of the surgical bed, and Trendelenburg positioning to enhance retroperitoneal exposure. A midline vertical incision is usually made in the abdomen, extending from just above the umbilicus to the pubic symphysis. However, in cases of distal TUU following a failed reimplantation a Pfannenstiel incision may be sufficient. A choice of exposure approaches is then available.

Transperitoneal Approach

Wide transperitoneal exposure is indicated in cases that require complex adjunct procedures such as tapered reimplantation of the recipient ureter or bladder augmentation, as well as when there is a long segment of diseased distal donor ureter. This approach would also be preferred when a high TUU is necessary for the distal donor ureter to be used as a continent catheterizable channel or for augmentation of the bladder.

The bowel is packed and retracted superiorly to allow for further dissection. Once the ureters have been visualized as they pass over the iliac vessels, two options for opening the retroperitoneum have been described (2): (a) Two 5-cm vertical incisions may be made over the ureters where they cross the iliac vessels, creating a window on each side (Fig. 93–1); (6) alternatively, wider retroperitoneal exposure can be achieved through a single curved incision that opens the retroperitoneum from over the left distal ureter, extending across the midline along the small-bowel mesentery and cecum, and up the right side along the line of Toldt (Fig. 93–2). This technique allows for more extensive mobilization of the bowel in an upward direction.

Retroperitoneal Approach

This technique provides the benefit of preventing complications associated with intraperitoneal procedures. The authors prefers this approach for a more distal TUU, which requires less mobilization of the donor ureter. Other authors have also described this method as a viable alternative to the transperitoneal approach (1). Most commonly, this approach would be used in salvage procedures for failed ureteral reimplantation.

After the transversalis fascia is incised, the extravesical space is mobilized on each side of the bladder. The ureters are identified crossing beneath the obliterated umbilical arteries. After dividing these vessels with Vicryl ties, the peritoneal sac is retracted superiorly to further expose the retroperitoneum. The peritoneal sac may also be reflected medially to expose the area of interest.

Once adequate exposure has been achieved by either approach, blunt finger dissection is then used to create an ample retroperitoneal tunnel. In cases of a low TUU using a retroperitoneal approach, the tunnel is created beneath the posterior peritoneum just superior to the posterior wall of the bladder and anterior to the sacral promontory. In cases involving a more proximal TUU, the retroperitoneal tunnel should lie beneath the posterior peritoneum, anterior to the great vessels and superior to the IMA. The angle between the aorta and inferior mesenteric artery (IMA) may kink or even obstruct the donor ureter. The position of the IMA should therefore be noted and avoided in calculating the path of the donor ureter to the contralateral retroperitoneum. Rarely, it may be necessary to ligate the IMA to prevent donor ureteral compression.

TUU

Adjunct procedures required for the recipient ureter, such as reimplantation and tapering, should be undertaken prior to the anastomosis of the donor and recipient ureter. For a standard TUU, mobilization of the donor should be sufficient to create a tension-free anastomosis. Because preservation of blood supply is essential for the success of TUU, great care is taken to avoid unnecessary disruption of the adventitia. The ipsilateral gonadal vessel may be tied off with a 3-0 silk suture to provide even greater mobilization with adventitial preservation. If even greater donor ureteral length is necessary, the donor kidney may be gently mobilized, moved inferiorly, and pexed to the psoas muscle using interrupted 3-0 Vicryl or 3-0 polydioxanone sutures.

After dividing the donor ureter as distal as possible, a long tagged 4-0 chromic suture is then placed on the distal-most aspect of the divided donor ureter to allow the ureter to be brought through the retroperitoneal tunnel. A right-angle clamp can then be passed from the recipient

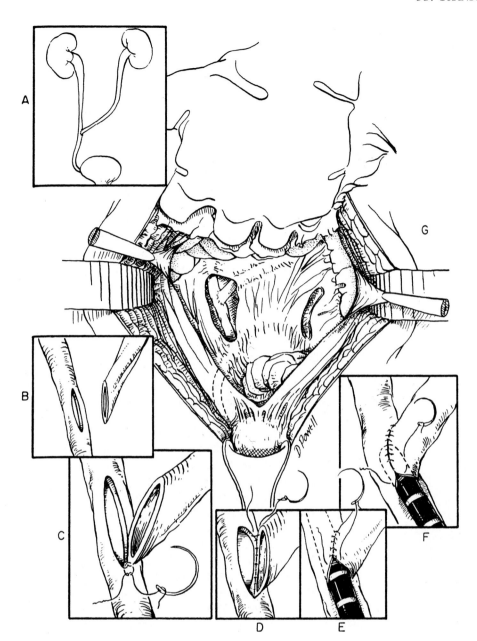

FIG. 93–1. Transureteroureterostomy (TUU) approached by two incisions in the posterior peritoneum. **A:** Schematic diagram of left to right TUU. **B:** The donor ureter is approximated to the vertical ureterotomy on the anteromedial aspect of the recipient ureter. **C, D:** The anastomosis is begun at the apex and is extended to the posterior aspect of the TUU, using either running or interrupted absorbable sutures. **E, F:** The anterior aspect of the anastomosis may be performed over a catheter or feeding tube and removed prior to the last stitch. **G:** Completed TUU *in situ*.

to the donor side to grasp the stay suture on the donor ureter and pull the donor ureter through the tunnel. Care must be taken to avoid twisting or kinking of the ureter, and the ureter should reach easily to the other side without tension.

With respect to the recipient ureter, mobilization should be minimized. To enable touch-free manipulation of the recipient ureter, stay sutures consisting of 4-0 or 5-0 chromic may be placed in the recipient ureteral adventitia, superior and inferior to the intended area of anastomosis. A vertical ureterotomy at least 1.5 cm in length on the anteromedial wall of the recipient ureter is then performed at the site of the anastomosis. The donor ureter is then spatulated to accommodate the recipient ureterotomy. However, spatulation may not necessary if the

donor ureter is sufficiently dilated. The anastomosis is performed using interrupted (Fig. 93–3) or running 4-0 or 5-0 absorbable sutures, beginning with the superior and inferior apices, followed by the approximation of the more posterior wall of the anastomosis. At this juncture, a ureteral catheter or infant feeding tube may be helpful in some cases to facilitate the anterior wall anastomosis. This tube may be removed just prior to the final anastomotic stitch (Fig. 93–1).

The use of an indwelling ureteral stent is mandatory only when the recipient ureter distal to the anastomosis has been altered in some fashion, such as in reimplantation. A 5 or 8 Fr feeding tube or a double-J stent may be used. In addition, nephrostomy drainage of the recipient ureter may be employed if extensive mobilization or

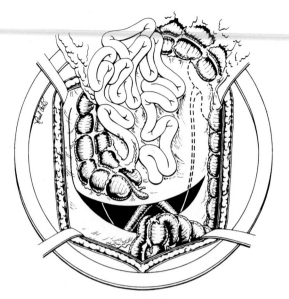

FIG. 93–2. Approach for single curvilinear incision in the posterior peritoneum to mobilize the bowels and mesentery and expose the retroperitoneum.

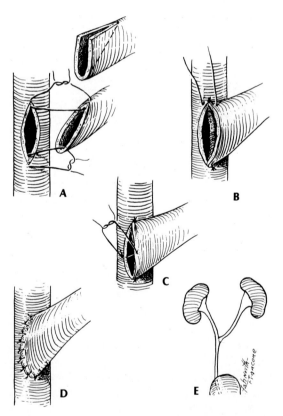

FIG. 93–3. Transureteroureterostomy (TUU) anastomosis performed with interrupted absorbable sutures. **A, B:** After aligning the distal donor ureteral lumen and recipient ureterotomy, apical sutures are placed and tied. **C:** Subsequent intervening interrupted sutures are placed halfway between previously placed sutures. **D:** Completed anastomosis. **E:** Schematic diagram of completed TUU.

tapering of the recipient ureter and/or kidney is required to complete the reconstruction (10). In all cases, it is vital to drain the retroperitoneal space using either a Penrose or closed-suction drain. Further, with the transperitoneal approach it is necessary to close the posterior peritoneum to avoid drainage of urine into the peritoneal cavity. Finally, a suprapubic catheter or urethral catheter should be placed to keep the bladder decompressed, as an overly distended bladder in the early postoperative period may stress the TUU anastomosis.

Approximately 2 months postoperatively the patient should undergo a renal sonogram and/or a diuretic renal scan to assess drainage and/or renal function. Depending on the results, imaging may be repeated in 3 to 9 months until a trend of progression has been established. Renal function by creatinine measurements should also be followed, in particular if these levels were elevated preoperatively.

OUTCOMES

Complications

Postoperative complications include urinoma, pyelonephritis, prolonged anastomotic drainage, and stricture (11). The risk of any of these complications is heightened by tenuous ureteral blood supply from excessive mobilization or from previous radiation (3). Patients with neuropathic bladders may be more at risk for developing new vesicoureteral reflux or distal ureteral stenosis in cases that involve reimplantation of the recipient ureter (9). Early anastomotic obstruction leading to persistent drainage may be initially treated conservatively with placement of a double-J ureteral stent or percutaneous nephrostomy.

Late complications include small-bowel obstruction, but only in cases involving the transperitoneal approach. A TUU performed in the context of neoplasm may suffer from late ureteral obstruction. Subsequent stone disease can potentially obstruct the common segment, rendering the patient anuric and mandating emergent percutaneous nephrostomy drainage. Rarely, compression of the donor ureter by the IMA can develop years after TUU if precautions to avoid the artery during donor ureter tunneling had not been taken. However, despite potential problems and the possible need for reoperation, several series have shown that TUU anastomotic revision is rarely, if ever, necessary. Also, donor renal loss due to chronic infection or obstruction has proven infrequent, ranging from 0% to 6% (7,8,10). Recipient kidney loss is even less common, reportedly occurring only after extensive mobilization required in complex reconstructions (5,10).

Results

Numerous studies have shown excellent results after TUU. Damage to the recipient kidney and ureter has rarely been observed, and successful preservation of both renal units occurs in greater than 90% of cases. TUU performed in the correct setting, with meticulous attention to maintaining ureteral blood supply and a tension-free anastomosis, is clearly an important component of the urologist's repertoire of reconstructive ureteral surgery.

REFERENCES

1. Baert L, Claes H. A retroperitoneal approach for transureteroureterostomy: a neglected and forgotten procedure. *Acta Urol Belg* 1990;58(4):51–58.
2. Casale A. Transureteroureterostomy. In: *Glenn's urologic surgery*, 5th ed. Philadelphia: Lippincott Williams & Wilkins, 1998.
3. Ehrlich RM, Skinner DG. Complications of transureteroureterostomy. *J Urol* 1975;113:467–473.
4. Halpern GN, King LR, Belman AB. Transureteroureterostomy in children. *J Urol* 1973;109:504.
5. Hendren WH, Hensle TW. Transureteroureterostomy: experience with 75 cases. *J Urol* 1980;123:826.
6. Higgins CC. Transuretero-ureteral anastomosis. Report of a clinical case. *J Urol* 1935;34:349.
7. Hodges CV, Barry JM, Fuchs EF, et al. Transureteroureterostomy: 25 year experience with 100 patients. *J Urol* 1980;123:834–838.
8. Mure P, Mollard P, Mouriquand P. Transureteroureterostomy in childhood and adolescence: long-term results in 69 cases. *J Urol* 2000;163: 946–948.
9. Pesce C, Costa L, Campobossa P, et al. Successful use of transureteroureterostomy in children: a clinical study. *Eur J Pediatr Surg* 2001;11: 395–398.
10. Rushton HG, Parrot TS, Woodard JR. The expanded role of transureteroureterostomy in pediatric urology. *J Urol* 1987;138:357–363.
11. Sandoz IL, Paul DP, MacFarlane CA. Complications with transureteroureterostomy. *J Urol* 1977;117:39–42.
12. Weiss RM, Beland GA, Lattimer JK. Transureteroureterostomy and cutaneous ureterostomy as a form of urinary diversion in children, *J Urol* 1966;96:155.

CHAPTER 94

Pyeloplasty

Evan J. Kass and Scott V. Burgess

Ureteropelvic junction (UPJ) obstruction is a common etiology for hydronephrosis in the neonate and young child. UPJ obstruction has been classically divided into intrinsic, extrinsic, and secondary causes. The most common etiology in an infant is an intrinsic adynamic or atretic segment of ureter that inhibits urine exiting from the renal pelvis (3). This restriction to urine flow can lead to varying degrees of renal pelvic dilation and renal damage. Less common causes of intrinsic obstruction include valvular mucosal folds and persistent fetal ureteral convolutions. Extrinsic obstruction is most often the result of periureteral fibrous bands or aberrant lower-pole vessels. Rarely, severe vesicoureteral reflux with periureteral scarring can be a cause of secondary UPJ obstruction.

DIAGNOSIS

Historically, most cases of UPJ obstruction were diagnosed in the older child who presented with symptoms of flank pain, urinary tract infection, hematuria, and abdominal mass. The widespread utilization of prenatal ultrasound has allowed earlier identification of UPJ pathology in the newborn. Children with hydronephrosis persisting on a postnatal ultrasound routinely should have a voiding cystourethrogram to exclude reflux as a possible etiology. When no reflux is present a MAG-3 renogram with Lasix washout allows objective measurement of renal function and drainage. Whitaker antegrade perfusion studies are no longer routinely preformed. The natural history of most children with antenatally detected hydronephrosis is usually benign. Operative intervention is in general reserved for patients demonstrating increasing hydronephrosis, worsening renal function, pain, urinary tract infection, or other symptoms. The role of the Lasix washout half-time remains controversial (2).

INDICATIONS FOR SURGERY

Any procedure for correction of UPJ obstruction must satisfy four criteria first described by Foley in 1937: (a) formation of a funnel at the UPJ, (b) dependent drainage, (c) watertight anastomosis, and (d) tension-free anastomosis (1). The Anderson–Hynes dismembered pyeloplasty is the most widely used procedure today and is in general applicable regardless of the etiology of obstruction. Access to the UPJ can be achieved from several incisions, including anterior extraperitoneal, flank, and dorsal lumbotomy. These approaches allow excellent exposure to the renal pelvis with minimal morbidity to the child. Anterior transperitoneal incisions are rarely used due to the increased morbidity associated with intraperitoneal bowel manipulation and the possibility of secondary bowel obstruction.

ALTERNATIVE THERAPY

Ureterocalicostomy is another option for children with massive hydronephrosis or those who have failed primary pyeloplasty. A Foley Y- or V-plasty is indicated when there is a UPJ obstruction secondary to a high insertion of the ureter, which is often found in patients with horseshoe kidney.

The refinement of more minimally invasive technologies has allowed correction of UPJ obstruction with minimal operative morbidity. Antegrade and retrograde endopyelotomy have been successful in older children with UPJ obstruction (5). This technique is associated with decreased success rates and increased risk of intraoperative and postoperative bleeding. Laparoscopic pyeloplasty is a newly developing technique to correct UPJ obstruction. In expert hands success rates following laparoscopic repairs approach results seen with open pyeloplasty (4). The drawbacks of the laparoscopic techniques include increased operative time, expensive surgical instruments that may not be available at all centers, and proficiency in laparoscopic surgery. Recent advances in the development of needlescopic instrumentation have facilitated laparoscopic pyeloplasty techniques in younger children and may increase the use of such techniques in the future (4). At present, open pyeloplasty with optical magnification is the gold standard with established long-term results.

SURGICAL TECHNIQUE

The patient is placed in the flank position and flexed with the use of rolled towels and/or table flexion with elevation of the kidney rest. We make a transverse incision starting just medial to the angle of the twelfth rib and carry it anteriorly. The subcutaneous tissues and musculofascial layers are opened with electrocautery. The lumbodorsal fascia in then divided, the peritoneum is mobilized medially, and Gerota's fascia is opened.

The lower pole and entire renal pelvis are sharply dissected to identify the UPJ to determine the cause of the obstruction. Care is taken in dissection to preserve the blood supply in the periureteral tissues and ureter. Stay sutures are placed just cephalad to the UPJ and in the ureter to minimize handling of the tissues. The renal pelvis is incised circumferentially, decompressing the obstructed collecting system (Fig. 94–1). The proximal ureter is mobilized using the stay suture distal to the obstructing segment to facilitate handling and the atretic portion is excised. The renal pelvis is trimmed of redundant tissue, the ureter is spatulated for 2 cm, and a 5 Fr feeding tube is placed in the ureter. The ureter is then anastomosed to the most dependent portion of the renal pelvis using 7-0 interrupted PDS sutures and the feeding tube is removed. Optical magnification with a 3.0 to 4.5× loupe facilitates precise suture placement. Alternatively, 7-0 running sutures can be used, but in infants we prefer interrupted sutures to decrease the pursestring effect and subsequent narrowing of the anastomosis. Care is taken to ensure there is no twisting or kinking of the anastomosis. The remainder of the trimmed upper renal pelvis is closed with a running 6-0 polydioxanone suture.

If the UPJ obstruction is secondary to an accessory lower-pole vessel, the divided ureter is brought anterior to the vessel and anastomosed to the pelvis (Fig. 94–2). Pelvic tailoring is often required in this correction as well.

The placement of intraoperative stents and/or nephrostomy tubes remains controversial, and we do not use either routinely. Whereas some of the early pyeloplasty descriptions used both internal and external drainage, many authorities now believe routine stenting is unnecessary. Stents are indicated in children with poor renal function, those undergoing repeat pyeloplasty, those with a solitary kidney, and children requiring extensive renal pelvic tailoring (5). Disadvantages to percutaneous nephrostomy tubes and ureteral stenting include patient discomfort and need for drain removal either in the office or under a second anesthetic. A 0.25-in. Penrose drain is placed in the perirenal space and brought out through a separate, more caudal incision. The musculofascial layers are closed using 3-0 Vicryl. The subcutaneous tissues are closed using 4-0 plain sutures and the skin is reapproximated with 5-0 Monocryl in a subcuticular fashion.

Postoperatively the patient is kept on intravenous antibiotics until the drain in removed, usually on postop-

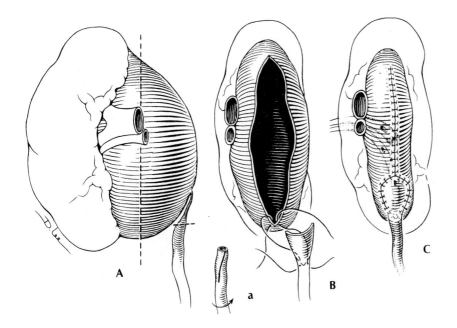

FIG. 94–1. Dismembered pyeloplasty. **A:** The renal pelvis is incised, redundant tissue excised, and the ureter divided distal to the atretic segment. **B:** The ureter is spatulated and brought to the most dependent portion of the pelvis. **C:** The remaining pelvis is closed with running sutures.

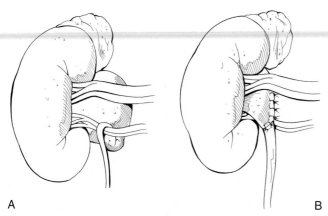

FIG. 94–2. Dismembered pyeloplasty with accessory vessels. **A:** Vessels causing ureteral compression and hydronephrosis. **B:** Anastomosis performed anterior to crossing vessels. Pelvic tailoring as needed.

erative day 1 or 2. We routinely administer ketorolac 0.5 mg/kg intravenously for the first 48 hours. We have found that it provides excellent pain relief, with the majority of children requiring no parenteral narcotic. Children are typically discharged within 24 hours of surgery. A follow-up ultrasound is done at 3 to 4 weeks postoperatively. If a stent was placed at the time of pyeloplasty, it is removed in 4 to 6 weeks.

OUTCOMES

Complications

Most children do very well postoperatively. Significant bleeding, infection, or other morbidity is uncommon. Urinary leakage from the anastomosis can occur and usually resolves spontaneously. When leakage persists or when hydronephrosis increases postoperatively a ureteral stent can be placed in either an antegrade or retrograde fashion.

Results

We have found that dismembered pyeloplasty has been shown to successfully relieve pelvic obstruction in greater than 95% of cases.

REFERENCES

1. Foley F. New plastic operation for strictures at the ureteropelvic junction: report of 20 operations. *J Urol* 1937;38:643–372.
2. Kass E. Pediatric hydronephrosis: my approach to management. *Dialog Pediatr Urol* 2002;25:1–2.
3. Park J. The pathophysiology of UPJ obstruction: current concepts. *Urol Clin North Am* 1998;25:161–170.
4. Tan H. Laparoscopic Anderson–Hynes dismembered pyeloplasty in children using needlescopic intrumentation. *Urol Clin North Am* 2001;28:43–51.
5. Ward A. Ureteropelvic junction obstruction in children: unique considerations for open intervention. *Urol Clin North Am* 1998;25:211–218.

CHAPTER 95

Megaureter

J. Christopher Austin and Douglas A. Canning

Megaureter or wide ureter is a less commonly found but fascinating congenital anomaly of the urinary tract. It is by definition a ureter that is 8 mm or greater in diameter. Megaureter is most easily classified into three categories: (a) refluxing megaureter, (b) obstructed megaureter, and (c) nonobstructed, nonrefluxing megaureter. They can be further subdivided into primary and secondary types, with the secondary types being most commonly due to an abnormality in the bladder such as posterior urethral valves or an acquired condition such as external compression from a mass lesion. Primary megaureters, in contrast, are isolated abnormalities of the ureter or ureterovesical junction.

Prior to the widespread use of screening prenatal ultrasonography, most children with megaureters presented with urinary tract infection, flank pain, urolithiasis, abdominal mass, or hematuria. Today, most are detected without symptoms with hydroureteronephrosis *in utero*. This earlier presentation has led to changes in the approach to management.

The pathophysiology of obstructive megaureters lies not within the dilated segment but in the distal nondilated segment. This segment of ureter fails to effectively propagate the wave of peristasis as it descends down the ureter. This segment is not usually narrowed compared with the normal ureter. When the bolus of urine is propagated to the aperistaltic segment only a portion of the urine passes into the bladder; the remainder is reflected back up the ureter in a yo-yo fashion. This causes the characteristic appearance of the ureter with fusiform dilation affecting the distal ureter more severely. When the amount and force of the bolus is sufficiently large that it dilates the entire ureter and reaches the renal pelvis, hydronephrosis may develop as well.

DIAGNOSIS

Differentiating an obstructed megaureter from a nonrefluxing, nonobstructed megaureter can be difficult. The diagnostic workup depends on the presenting signs and symptoms and may vary from patient to patient. For the child with prenatal hydronephrosis, the usual evaluation includes a voiding cystourethrogram (VCUG), renal/bladder ultrasound, and renal scintigraphy. These studies separate children with refluxing megaureters from those without reflux. Hydroureteronephrosis is identified on the renal ultrasound. The dilated ureter is usually visible in the pelvis and often posterior to the bladder. If the ureter is dilated to the level of the trigone, an ectopic ureter may be present rather than a primary megaureter.

The renal scan, in the newborn, should be performed with mercaptoacetyl triglycine (MAG-3) with diuretic washout. The scan will estimate the relative function of each kidney and measure the clearance of radiotracer from the collecting system. In the past, the $t_{1/2}$ or the time required for one-half of the radiotracer to clear from the renal pelvis had been used as an indicator of obstruction. In practice, the use of the $t_{1/2}$ alone to estimate obstruction is not always fruitful. Because the clearance can be considerably variable based on the patient's prestudy hydration level and the response to the diuretic, we often prefer to follow trends in the relative renal function, reserving surgery for those with increasing $t_{1/2}$ or decreasing relative renal function. The region of interest outlined by the technician when evaluating the clearance of radiotracer should include the ureter.

In children who are symptomatic, the presenting symptom determines the workup. Hematuria, rarely noted in children with megaureter, is normally evaluated initially with a renal/bladder ultrasound. This study can be followed by a renal scan or intravenous pyelogram (IVP). If there is suspicion of renal or ureteral stone, a noncontrast computed tomography (CT) scan should be performed. The renal scan may be required to provide a relative baseline estimate of renal function.

If the anatomy is unclear, magnetic resonance imaging (MRI) may be useful in distinguishing primary megaureters from ectopic ureters. If there is poor renal function on the side of the megaureter and the child is undergoing surgical correction, cystoscopy will demonstrate a normally positioned ureteral orifice in an obstructed megaureter. If an ectopic ureter is present, the trigone on the affected side will be distorted and the ectopic orifice will be located at the bladder neck, prostatic urethra, seminal vesicle, vas, or distal two-thirds of the epididymis in males or within the urethra, introitus, or vagina in females.

INDICATIONS FOR SURGERY

Relative indications to proceed with surgical repair include poor initial relative function (less than 40% of differential renal function by renal scan), progressive dilation, a decreased function (greater than 10%) in serial renal scans, or the development of infections, flank pain, or stones. In infants with a poorly functioning kidney, a staged reconstructive approached with a temporary endcutaneous ureterostomy should be given consideration versus primary surgical repair (8).

Children with a megaureter who present with symptoms of intermittent flank pain or urinary tract infection are usually treated surgically. Prior to surgery, it is imperative to evaluate the child to be sure that the bladder fills with normal compliance and empties normally. A few children will develop a secondary megaureter resulting from high-pressure bladder storage that is transmitted to the ureter and renal pelvis. A significant degree of ureteral dilation can be detected in association with neurogenic bladder dysfunction, posterior urethral valves, or severe voiding dysfunction. Appropriate treatment of the posterior urethral valves or the bladder dysfunction may result in improvement or resolution of ureteral dilation. Failure to recognize bladder dysfunction may lead to increased rates of postoperative reflux.

ALTERNATIVE THERAPY

Because most patients are asymptomatic and identified as part of an *in utero* exam, many children with apparent ureteral dilation do not require surgical correction. Ureteral dilation does not necessarily equal obstruction. Dilation in some boys and girls may represent the residuum of *in utero* obstruction that has resolved. Our experience at the Children's Hospital of Philadelphia has been that the majority of children with megaureter maintain relative renal function and dilation often improves over time. In a series of 25 children with megaureters treated conservatively with a mean follow-up of 7.3 years, hydronephrosis improved in 2 of 3 in those with serial IVP and the differential function remained stable in all followed with serial renal scans (1). Likewise, in a series of 53 patients with 67 megaureters only 17% required surgery for poor initial function or progressive loss of function. In addition, in 34% the dilation completely resolved by ultrasound (2). These two series suggest that the majority of megaureters can be managed conservatively.

SURGICAL TECHNIQUE

The surgical correction is identical for refluxing and obstructed megaureters. Obstructed megaureters have an extravesical segment of variable length with a normal or narrowed caliber that does not contract normally and should be excised. Refluxing megaureters are dilated to the level of the ureterovesical junction. Distal segment excision is not always required.

The child is positioned supine on the operating room table. In males, the lower abdomen and genitalia are fully prepared and draped. Females are placed in a mild froglegged position with gel bolsters under the knees to permit intraoperative access to the urethra. The bladder may be left full during the initial surgical exposure. A Pfannenstiel incision is made in the abdominal skin crease. The rectus fascia is opened along the course of the incision and the flaps of fascia are elevated off the muscle superiorly to just below the umbilicus and inferiorly to the pubis. The rectus muscles are separated in the midline. The space of Retzius is entered.

Intravesical Approach

At this point, depending upon the surgeon's preference, the dissection of the ureter begins either intravesically or through an extravesical exposure. It has been our preference to begin intravesically. The bladder is opened via a midline cystotomy. The bladder dome is packed with damp sponges and a Dennis–Brown retractor is placed to provide exposure of the trigone. A 5 Fr feeding tube is passed up the ureter and secured at the orifice with a 5-0 suture. The urothelium surrounding the orifice is divided using electrocautery. With the mucosa divided circumferentially the ureteral catheter is gently pulled to expose the medial and inferior attachments of the trigonal musculature. These attachments are divided with electrocautery. At this point the dissection proceeds to carefully divide the muscular attachments of the ureter through the plane of Waldeyer's sheath. This dissection will free the distal ureter, which should have a normal or narrowed caliber. The surgeon should recognize the blood supply of the ureter as shown in Figure 95–1. As the dissection proceeds more proximally, the blood supply of the ureter will originate from medial branches of the hypogastric (male) or cervical (female) arteries. These vessels should be preserved, as should the longitudinal blood supply by taking care to prevent dissection too close to the ureteral wall. When the ureter is free from its detrusor attachments the mobilization should proceed extravesically. The ureter at this point can be passed through the bladder wall and the

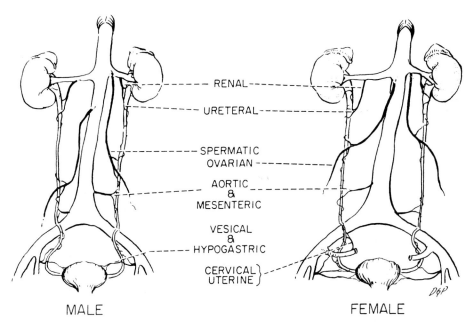

FIG. 95–1. Diagrams of the major arterial supply to the ureter. It is not necessary to sacrifice any medially based blood supply for primary megaureter repair.

dissection proceeds more proximally. When the dilated region of the ureter is reached, dissection should continue until an adequate length for reimplantation has been mobilized, again paying attention to the previous outlined principles for preserving the blood supply. An ischemic distal ureter may lead to fibrosis and obstruction.

At this point the surgeon must decide whether to taper the ureter. In general, if the lumen of the ureter is significantly larger than 12 Fr it should be tapered prior to reimplantation. There are two techniques used to taper the size of the ureter: (a) excisional tapering and (b) tapering by folding. We will review the three most commonly used procedures. The goal of tapering is to provide a distal ureter with a small enough diameter that postoperative vesicoureteral reflux will be prevented with a reasonable length of intramural tunnel. The tapering only needs to extend for a short distance beyond the bladder wall rather than the whole length of the ureter. The dilation of the proximal ureter should improve postoperatively with the relief of obstruction and/or reflux. The decision to perform an excisional versus a folding technique depends on the preference of the surgeon and the size and thickness of the ureter. Folding a very dilated thick wall ureter will create a large amount of bulk, making the creation of the submucosal tunnel difficult. In general, the taper should not be aggressive. In a bladder that functions well, reflux is less hazardous than persistent obstruction.

Excisional tapering (Fig. 95–2) begins with carefully examining the ureter. Without twisting the ureter, the surgeon observes the pattern of blood supply to the ureter. In most cases, the longitudinal ureteral vessels are predominately along the medial aspect of the ureter. Usually, the

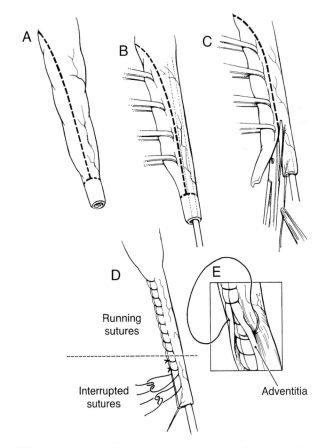

FIG. 95–2. A, B: The wedge of ureter to be excised is secured with Allis or Hendren clamps. C: The outlined segment of ureteral wall is excised sharply. D, E: The ureter is closed in two layers. Distally, interrupted sutures are placed to allow for trimming of the end of the ureter at the time of reimplantation.

excised segment of ureter is taken from the opposite side along the lateral border. The distal nondilated ureteral segment is excised. A 12 Fr catheter is passed up the ureter. With this in place the wedge to be excised is identified and outlined. Aggressive tailoring may result in obstruction. The process of excising and suturing the ureter will result in considerable contraction of the ureteral lumen. The tailored segment should gradually widen as the ureter is reconstructed proximally. The ureter is then closed in one or two layers. The mucosa and the muscularis of the ureter are closed with interrupted or on occasion absorbable running fine sutures. A second layer if desired incorporates the muscularis and adventitia with a series of interrupted absorbable fine sutures. The ureter is then passed back through its original hiatus and reimplanted in a cross-trigonal fashion. The suture line should be positioned facing the detrusor muscle as this will help prevent the development of a ureterovesical fistula. The 12 Fr catheter is replaced with an 8 Fr catheter or double-J stent. The advantage to leaving an open-ended ureteral catheter is that a retrograde ureteral study can be performed postoperatively to demonstrate ureteral drainage and confirm the absence of extravasation. The internal stent is easy to care for and leaves the patient free of external tubes; however, it usually requires a general anesthetic for removal. All tapered reimplants should be stented, regardless of which type of stent is used.

There are two techniques commonly employed for tapering by ureteral folding: (a) Starr plication and (b) the Kaliscinski technique. Both techniques are similar to excisional tapering with regard to the length of ureter to be narrowed and the choice of the segment of the wall based upon the intrinsic blood supply. Starr plication (Fig. 95–3) reduces the diameter of the ureter by infolding the ureteral wall with interrupted Lembert-type

sutures of 5-0 polyglyconate or polydioxan. The tapering begins proximally and gradually reduces the caliber of the ureter until the diameter approaches that of the 12 Fr catheter. Care should be taken to ensure the wedge of folded ureter stays in the same position of the ureteral wall as you proceed distally. In other words, the plication should not spiral from lateral to medial as the sutures are placed more distally. The ureter is reimplanted with the plication sutures facing the detrusor muscle as was described with excisional tapering. The Kaliscinski technique (Fig. 95–4) begins with a running horizontal mattress suture of 5-0 or 6-0 chromic that runs the length of the segment to be tapered, creating a defunctionalized wedge of ureter that is then wrapped around the ureter and secured posterior with interrupted absorbable sutures. The ureter is reimplanted with the imbricated segment against the muscularis. Again, ureteral stents are placed in both repairs as with excisional tapering.

Extravesical Approach

Several authors have reported good results with the extravesical approach to megaureter repair (3,5). In cases of bilateral megaureters, a high rate of voiding dysfunction postoperatively has been reported that may require intermittent catheterizations for a period following surgery. A Foley catheter is placed at the beginning of the procedure. The catheter may be attached with a Y connector to provide for separate irrigation and drainage lines for intraoperative filling and emptying. The ability to regulate the bladder volume aids in the dissection. The incision and initial approach is identical as for the intravesical approach until the bladder is exposed. The dissection then proceeds into the lateral extravesical space. The obliterated umbilical artery is followed to the level of the ureter. The ureter is carefully dissected free and encircled

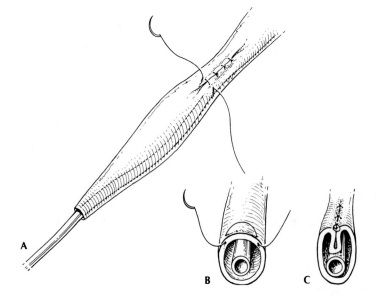

FIG. 95–3. A: Starr plication of the ureter suture to infold the ureter. **B:** Cross section to show placement of Lembert-type sutures. **C:** Cross section after ligation of sutures.

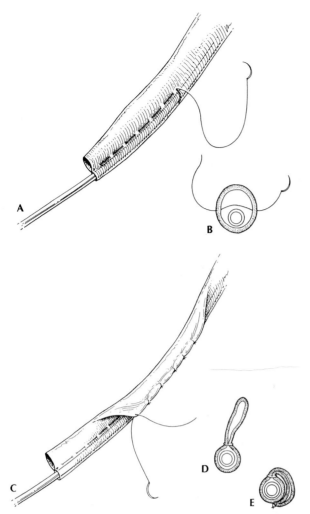

FIG. 95–4. Kaliscinski technique of ureteral imbrication. **A:** Placement of cobbler's stitch to exclude a major portion of the ureteral lumen. **B:** Same in cross section. **C:** After ligation. **D:** Excluded portion of the ureter is folded over and wrapped around the intubated ureter. **E:** Final appearance in cross section.

with a vessel loop. The ureter is dissected distally to the ureterovesical junction. With the bladder full a detrusorotomy is made in a line extending from the bladder neck cephalad and circumscribing the detrusor adjacent to the ureter. The length of the incision should be 3 to 4 cm.

The ureter is freed from all detrusor attachments. The edges of the detrusor are then dissected free of the urothelium to form flaps that can be closed over the ureter. If the urothelium is perforated during the dissection it can be repaired with 6-0 or 7-0 chromic on a tapered needle. In an obstructed megaureter the most distal region is ligated and the ureter divided proximal to the ligature. The aperistaltic segment of the ureter is resected. The dilated ureter is then tapered as necessary. An indwelling stent is placed if the ureter is tapered. The bladder is partially emptied and the ureter is then directly anastomosed to the urothe-

lium at the distal apex of the detrusorotomy using 5-0 absorbable sutures. With this accomplished, the distal ureter is fixed to the detrusor with 5-0 polygliconate horizontal mattress sutures at the apex. The detrusor is then closed over the ureter with 4-0 polydioxan sutures. The hiatus should be approximated, but not closed too tight. A Foley catheter is left indwelling postoperatively.

Staged Approach

Although repair of megaureters has been performed safely in newborns and young infants there is a reasonable concern about reimplanting a markedly dilated ureter into the thin bladder wall of an infant (4,8). In some infants where severe dilation and diminished relative function (less than 20%) exists, end-cutaneous ureterostomy is a good alternative to reimplantation with tapering (4). The infant bladder often empties with high pressure and postponing the definitive reimplant while decompressing the obstructed ureter may reduce complications. In this case an end-cutaneous ureterostomy (technique presented in Chapter 93) is performed and the distal stump is ligated. This provides reliable decompression of the kidney and allows for improvement in the degree of ureteral dilation prior to reimplantation. In some cases the ureterectasis recovers enough to avoid the need for tapering. In addition, if the initial function is poor and the kidney fails to recover following decompression, a nephrectomy rather than reimplantation may be preferred. This temporary measure will allow the reimplant to be delayed until the infant is older. The takedown of the ureterostomy and ureteral reimplantation is usually done when the child is 12 to 18 months old and can be performed intravesically or extravesically.

POSTOPERATIVE CARE

A Foley catheter is usually left in place for 24 to 48 hours. The stent is left in place for 10 to 14 days. Children are discharged from the hospital on prophylactic antibiotics. Injection of external stents at low pressure by gravity infusion with antibiotic coverage is performed to document drainage. If there is not prompt drainage around the stent, it is left for another 10 to 14 days and the study repeated. Patients are evaluated with a renal ultrasound 1 month after surgery or stent removal. If hydronephrosis is not improved a renal scan should be obtained. A VCUG and renal scan is performed 3 months after surgery and the ultrasound is repeated at 1 year.

OUTCOMES

Complications

The most common complication related to surgery for megaureters is new or persistent reflux. This complication is more common when the surgery is performed for refluxing megaureters than for obstructed megaureters. Management options include observation with prophylaxis, endoscopic injection, and surgical revision. Obstruction is a rare complication with reported rates of 0% to 4% (2–4). It should be initially evaluated endoscopically as on occasion a synechia has been reported to narrow the orifice. Strictures can be assessed by retrograde pyelography. Initial management with dilation and stenting may be successful, but failures will require an open revision.

Results

Most series report success rates greater than 90% (4,7,8). In a series of infants treated with reimplantation, 20% had reflux postoperatively; however, with time a few patients had spontaneous resolution of their reflux, lowering the rate to 12.5% (6). Extravesical reimplants had rates of postoperative reflux similar to intravesical rates (12%). When performed bilaterally for megaureters, two-thirds of patients required intermittent catheterization for a period of 1 to 4 months (3).

REFERENCES

1. Baskin LS, Zderic SA, Snyder HM, Duckett JW. Primary dilated megaureter: long term follow-up. *J Urol* 1994;152:918–921.
2. Liu HY, Dhillon HK, Young CK, et al. Clinical outcome and management of prenatally diagnosed primary megaureter. *J Urol* 1994;152: 914–917.
3. McLorie GA, Jayanthi VR, Kinaham TJ, et al. A modified extravesical technique for megaureter repair. *Br J Urol* 1994;74:715–719.
4. Perdzynski W, Kalicinski ZH. Long-term results after megaureter folding in children. *J Pediatr Surg* 1996;31:1211–1217.
5. Perovic S. Surgical treatment of megaureters using detrusor tunneling extravesical ureteroneocystostomy. *J Urol* 1994;152:622–625.
6. Peters CA, Mandell J, Lebowitz RL, et al. Congenital obstructed megaureters in early infancy: diagnosis and treatment. *J Urol* 1989;142: 641–645.
7. Rabinowitz R, Barkin M, Schillinger JF, et al. The influence of etiology on the surgical management and prognosis of the massively dilated ureter in children. *J Urol* 1978;119:808–813.
8. Vereecken RL, Proesmans W. A review of ninety-two obstructive megaureters in children. *Eur Urol* 1999;36:342–347.

CHAPTER 96

Prune Belly (Triad) Syndrome

David B. Joseph

Triad syndrome—the clinical association of a thin flaccid abdominal wall, undescended testes, and bladder hypertrophy with hydroureters—was originally described in 1895 by Parker (10). Shortly thereafter, Osler presented a similar constellation of findings in a child he described as having the appearance of a wrinkled prune (11). From that point, prune belly has unfortunately become synonymous with this syndrome. This clinical manifestation is also known as the Eagle–Barrett syndrome and the abdominal muscular deficiency syndrome. By classic description, the triad syndrome occurs in boys. However, 5% are girls presenting with similar physical findings with the obvious exception of the gonadal abnormality. The incidence of triad syndrome occurs in 1 of every 30,000 to 50,000 live births. Most cases are sporadic, although a familial occurrence has been described.

Approximately three-quarters of children with classic triad syndrome will have other associated anomalies. Urethral abnormalities including atresia and megalourethra have been reported but they are not required as part of the triad. When atresia is present there is often an associated patent urachus. The most common skeletal abnormality is a thoracic deformity resulting in a protruded upper sternum, depressed lower sternum, and splayed ribs. Other less frequent skeletal deformities include talipes equinovarus, congenital hip dislocation, calcaneus valgus, polydactyly, syndactyly, arthrogryposis, scoliosis, and lordosis. Intestinal malformations are noted in approximately one-third of children and most often due to defective fixation or malrotation of the midgut. Cardiac atrial or ventricular septal defects have been reported in approximately 15% of children.

DIAGNOSIS

Using fetal sonography, the diagnosis of a child with the triad syndrome can be established *in utero*. However, similar findings are seen in a fetus with posterior urethral valves or the megacystis–megaureters syndrome. Close inspection of the abdominal wall musculature should hedge the differential diagnosis to that of the triad syndrome. *In utero* diagnosis allows for a planned neonatal investigation. At birth, the diagnosis of triad syndrome is often obvious with the pathognomonic physical findings of a loose, lax, wrinkled abdominal wall, flared chest, and undescended testes.

Several classifications of the triad syndrome have been established based on severity and initial clinical presentation. There is no single classification system that incorporates the total spectrum of this syndrome. For practical purposes, children can be grouped into severe, moderate, or mild presentations. With a severe presentation, survival is often limited by significant respiratory compromise due to pulmonary immaturity and dysplasia, as well as extensive renal dysplasia, resulting in a Potter-like syndrome. Children described with moderate involvement have combined renal and respiratory insufficiency mandating close observation and early intervention to minimize the sequelae of pulmonary and renal compromise. The combination of increased bilateral renal echogenicity on sonography, chronic urinary tract infections (UTIs), and a nadir serum creatine of greater than 0.7 mg per dL are prognostic for renal failure (8). Monitoring of the urinary system is necessary to prevent progressive renal deterioration due to stagnation of urinary flow, UTIs, and possible urinary tract obstruction. Urinary tract reconstruction may play an important role in limiting long-term morbidity. Children with mild involvement do not suffer from respiratory or renal compromise. While long-term follow-up is necessary, operative intervention is often limited to orchiopexy and abdominal wall reconstruction.

A team approach consisting of a pediatric urologist, neonatologist, nephrologist, pulmonologist, and cardiologist is required to maximize the outcome. The initial cardiorespiratory status of the neonate must be established. The baby should undergo a chest x-ray and, when indicated, cardiac sonography. Urologic evaluation commences with abdominal sonography and a baseline chemistry profile. Both the upper and lower urinary tract should be assessed. Attention should be placed on the degree of hydronephrosis, the volume of renal parenchyma, and its echogenicity. Often, there will be a disproportionate degree of lower ureteral and urinary tract dilation when compared to the proximal ureter and kidney. On occasion, a marked transition of ureteral dilation is noted. If the infant is clinically stable with normal renal function and voiding per urethra or draining through a patent urachus, further diagnostic testing can be placed on hold.

Children with renal insufficiency should undergo further imaging to differentiate renal dysplasia and stagnant urine flow from true obstruction. While the MAG-3 renal scan has limitations in the newborn it still provides the most objective data. The voiding cystourethrogram can assess vesicoureteral reflux and the effectiveness of bladder emptying. It is of utmost importance that any invasive lower urinary tract imaging be performed in a sterile environment with the child receiving pre- and postprocedural antibiotics. The neonate with triad syndrome and hydroureteronephrosis is susceptible to bacteriuria and can quickly become symptomatic. Persistent bacteriuria is often difficult to clear.

Megalourethra has been classified as two varieties, scaphoid and fusiform (Fig. 96–1). With the more common scaphoid defect the abnormal urethral segment is confined to the penile portion of the corpus spongiosum, resulting in a variable length of massively enlarged ventral, anterior urethra similar in appearance to a saccular diverticulum. The fusiform variety encompasses not only a defect of the corpus spongiosum but also deficiency of one or both corpus cavernosum, resulting in circumferential ballooning of the urethra and generalized penile flaccidity. Megalourethra is usually an isolated defect but can present with upper urinary tract changes including hydronephrosis, vesicoureteral reflux, and renal dysplasia. As previously discussed, it has been reported to occur with the triad syndrome, which may represent a continuation of the abnormal mesodermal theory of development related to the triad syndrome.

INDICATIONS FOR SURGERY

Each child presents with a unique constellation of problems resulting in its own set of considerations and requires individualized care. Therefore, no one treatment plan is appropriate for all children. In general, operative management can be divided into three broad areas:

1. Reconstruction of the urinary system.
2. Reconstruction of the abdominal wall.
3. Transfer of the intraabdominal testes to the scrotum.

Urinary Tract Reconstruction

Controversy surrounds the need for aggressive urinary tract reconstruction. Early aggressive operative intervention for all children is countered by the fact that renal dysplasia may be inherent, thus preventing any intervention from improving the functional status. In addition, imaging studies depicting significant hydroureteronephrosis do not always correlate with obstruction or the potential for symptoms and hydroureteronephrosis by itself does not mandate reconstruction. Urinary tract reconstruction is beneficial in a child who has a component of obstructive uropathy and has been shown to have improved renal function with decompression of the urinary system. Reconstruction is also of benefit in the child who has progressive hydroureteronephrosis associated with increasing renal compromise and in the child who has recurrent symptomatic UTIs due to stagnant urine flow.

Urinary diversion plays a temporary initial role in the management of acute renal failure or sepsis. Often, children with urethral atresia or obstruction will present with a patent urachus, effectively emptying their lower tract. Infants with associated posterior urethral abnormalities resulting in obstruction or poor bladder decompression, who are not candidates for intermittent catheterization, benefit from a vesicostomy. A vesicostomy, however, may not adequately drain the upper urinary tract due to a relative obstruction of the ureter at the level of the bladder or

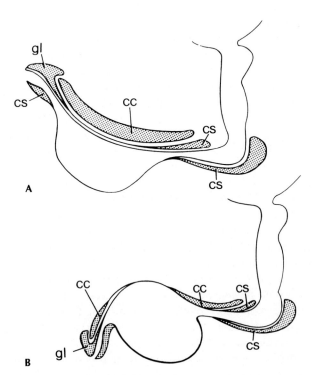

FIG. 96–1. A: Scaphoid megalourethra. Corpora spongiosum (CS) is deficient throughout the ventral aspect of penile urethra. Corpora cavernosum (CC) is normal. **B:** Fusiform megalourethra. Both corpora spongiosum and cavernosum are deficient. Note that glans (gl) is normal in both variants.

poor urinary transport secondary to a highly compliant adynamic ureter. Vesicostomy should only be undertaken when bladder catheterization has been shown to be effective. Otherwise, temporary diversion of the upper urinary tract will be required. Nephrostomy tube drainage is helpful to stabilize an acute problem but its long-term effectiveness is limited, resulting in a need for a more formal upper urinary tract diversion. There is a theoretical advantage in performing upper tract diversion as proximal as possible. This should maximally relieve stress to the kidney and limit stagnation of urine in a dilated tortuous ureter. However, there is often a disproportionate degree of distal versus proximal ureteral dilation that can prevent easy access of the proximal ureter.

It is compelling to preform a reduction cystoplasty during urinary reconstruction in a child with triad syndrome. However, long-term follow-up has not shown an objective advantage (1,6). With time, the bladder will often regain its large size, lose its tone, and result in inadequate emptying. For these reasons, it is not practical to proceed with reductive cystoplasty as the primary indication for urinary reconstruction. If a large, poorly contracting bladder results in inadequate urinary emptying, intermittent catheterization would be a more appropriate form of management. However, when formal urinary reconstruction is required for upper tract reconstruction and ureteral tailoring reductive cystoplasty can be performed and may provide limited improved bladder emptying.

Reconstruction of the Abdominal Wall

Several techniques have been devised to maximize the cosmetic benefits of abdominal wall reconstruction in children with triad syndrome. There is evidence indicating that the muscular defect is more pronounced centrally and caudally. Initial reconstructive efforts were based on removal of this abnormal tissue. While the appearance of the abdomen was improved, it was not ideal and resulted in a transverse incision and loss of the umbilicus. Monfort described preservation of the umbilicus and others have added various modifications (2,4,7). Based on this approach, abdominal wall reconstruction now allows for an excellent cosmetic and functional outcome. The benefit of abdominal wall reconstruction is dependent on the degree of abdominal wall laxity. The timing for this procedure should be based on the need for other operative intervention. If it is obvious that the child will not require upper urinary tract reconstruction, abdominal wall reconstruction can be undertaken at any time. If, however, there is the potential for upper urinary tract reconstruction, abdominal wall reconstruction should be deferred until the time of that intervention.

Orchiopexy

The timing for orchiopexy can be individualized based on the child's need for urinary reconstructive surgery. If urinary reconstructive surgery is required, orchiopexy can be performed at the same time. If urinary reconstructive surgery is not required, then timing and approach are variable. Placement of the testes within the scrotum is important for psychological and hormonal factors but, unfortunately, fertility is not improved. Biopsies of testes have shown a Sertoli-cell-only feature prohibiting future fertility.

Urethral Reconstruction

Correction of the megalourethra is dependent on presenting symptoms of urinary dribbling and/or urinary infections. Most often operative correction is undertaken because of the unusual appearance of the megalourethra. Urethral tapering is an appropriate treatment.

ALTERNATIVE THERAPY

There is no effective alternative to surgical reconstruction.

SURGICAL TECHNIQUE

Vesicostomy

A vesicostomy is placed between the symphysis and umbilicus. A 2- to 3-cm incision is made down to the rectus fascia. A triangular segment of fascia is removed, which will help limit problems of stenosis. The rectus is separated, the space of Retzius is entered, and the dome of the bladder is identified along with the urachus and umbilical ligaments. The bladder is opened in this region to decrease the risk of prolapse. The bladder wall is secured to the rectus fascia with 4-0 polyglactin sutures and the bladder epithelium is approximated to the skin.

Distal Cutaneous Ureterostomy

When there is minimal proximal dilation, a low distal cutaneous ureterostomy provides adequate decompression with relief of stagnated urine flow and stabilization of renal function. The ureter can be approached from a small (2.5-cm) incision placed in a lower inguinal location. The muscles are split to enter the retroperitoneum. The ureter may have the appearance of bowel due to its large size. When in doubt, a 21-gauge needle should be passed, aspirating contents to confirm urine. Once confirmed, the ureter is opened at the level of the obliterated umbilical artery. The size of the ureter usually prevents postoperative stenosis, allowing for either an end or loop ureteral anastomosis. An advantage of distal diversion is noted at the time of definitive urinary reconstruction. The proximal urinary system will have remained uncompromised, allowing for easier mobilization and greater flexibility when tailoring the ureter.

Ureteral Reconstruction

When definitive primary urinary reconstruction is necessary, the initial approach to the ureter can be extravesical. The ureter is isolated at the level of the bladder and proximal dissection ensues. If there is an obvious transitional phase noted on imaging between the dilated distal ureter and the normal proximal ureter, the dissection should be continued proximal to the transition point. During dissection, the adventitial tissue surrounding the ureter is preserved to prevent devascularization. All of the distal ureter is excised when there is adequate length for the proximal ureter to be reimplanted in the bladder in a standard fashion or with the assistance of a psoas hitch.

If total proximal and distal ureteral tailoring is necessary due to massive dilation, full mobilization of the ureter will be required. This can be accomplished via a retroperitoneal approach but in most children it is helpful to enter the peritoneum and reflect either the descending or ascending colon along the white line of Toldt. The dilated ureter is often exceedingly redundant and tortuous. Straightening of the ureter without devascularization is required. The functional capability of the ureter for peristalsis and transmission of urine into the bladder parallels the degree of hydroureter. Therefore, ureteral tapering may enhance urinary flow into the bladder. Multiple techniques exist for ureteral tailoring, including ureteral imbrication and formal ureteral excision as with any megaureter (Fig. 96–2). Ureteral imbrication is appropriate for marginally dilated ureters. But, when massive ureteral dilation is present, which is usually the reason for reconstruction, formal excision is preferred, eliminating the bulky tissue that results from the large imbricated ureter.

The ureter is tapered loosely over either a 10 or 12 Fr catheter depending on the child's age and size. The excised ureteral segment may need to take an unconventional course to preserve adequate blood supply to the tailored ureter. If a large, redundant, renal pelvis is present in association with a dilated proximal ureter, a reduction pyeloplasty should be performed inline with the ureteral excision. Preservation of the proximal ureteral blood supply is mandatory.

After excision, the ureter and renal pelvis is closed in a two-layer technique using absorbable sutures. The first running suture line is 5-0 or 6-0 chromic gut, polydioxanone, or polyglactic acid directly opposing the mucosa and muscularis of the ureter. The second layer reapproximates the adventitial tissue using the same suture material. Both running layers are discontinued a few centimeters from the distal end of the ureter. The very distal portion of the ureter is closed with interrupted sutures. This allows for excision of the distal ureter without interruption of the running suture line. Enough ureteral length should be preserved to allow for a tunneled antirefluxing ureteroneocystostomy in all cases. A ureteral stent will remain for 5 to 10 days postoperatively.

Reduction Cystoplasty

Reductive cystoplasty should include the urachus and majority of the dome of the bladder (Fig. 96–3). A 2- to 3-cm strip of mucosa is removed from one side of the bladder wall, allowing for a reinforced overlapping suture line. The bladder is closed in three independent layers

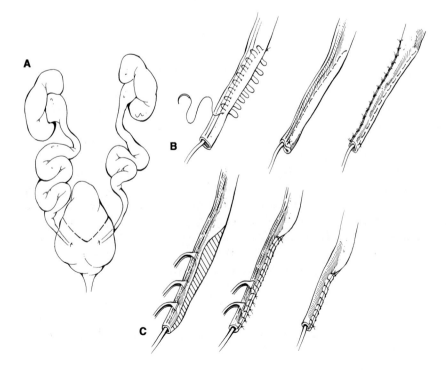

FIG. 96–2. A: The tortuous dilated ureter is carefully straightened without compromising blood supply. The redundant portion is excised and the remaining distal segment tapered if necessary. **B:** Ureteral folding over a 10 or 12 Fr ureteral catheter. **C:** Formal ureteral tapering with excision and closure. *Note:* The continuous running closure stops 1 to 2 cm from the end of the segment, followed by interrupted suture placement, allowing for excision of the distal end of the ureter without compromise of the running closure.

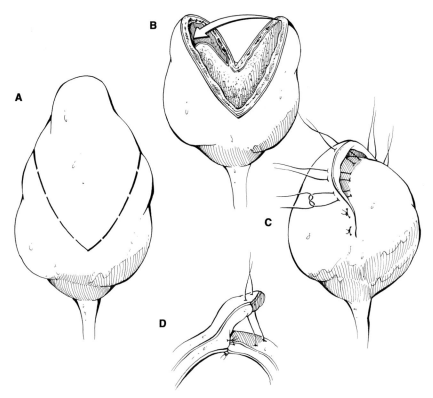

FIG. 96–3. Reduction cystoplasty. **A:** The dome of the bladder, including any urachal remnant, is removed. A 2- to 3-cm mucosal strip is then removed from one portion of the bladder. **C,D:** The bladder is closed with overlapping suture lines.

using a running suture of 3-0 chromic gut, polydioxanone, or polyglactic acid. A suprapubic tube is inserted for postoperative monitoring regarding the effectiveness of bladder emptying.

Abdominal Wall Reconstruction

The Monfort approach begins with a midline incision from the tip of the xyphoid process carried inferiorly, circumscribing the umbilicus, leaving an adequate umbilical island of tissue, and ending at the symphysis pubis (Fig. 96–4). A full-thickness skin flap is created bilaterally, elevating the subcutaneous fat from the underlying fascia. The dissection is continued laterally to the anterior axillary line. Often, there will be variability and asymmetry of muscular development. Care must be taken not to enter the peritoneum while mobilizing the skin flaps, in particular in areas where the fascia is relatively thin. An incision is then made lateral to the superior epigastric artery through the fascia entering the peritoneum. The incision is continued lateral and parallel to the course of the superior and inferior epigastric arteries from the costal margin to the symphysis pubis. The fascia is then elevated and the contralateral superior and inferior epigastric arteries are identified. A second parallel incision is made lateral to these arteries. The central fascial bridge with the umbilical island is now supported by both sets of epigas-

tric arteries. The two lateral incisions provide excellent exposure for orchiopexy and major urinary tract reconstruction when required.

At the time of abdominal closure, the lateral fascia wall is secured to the central fascial strip with a running 2-0 or 3-0 polyglactin suture. The lateral fascia can be scored with the cautery along the intended suture line to enhance adherence. The edge of the lateral fascia is then overlapped and secured in the midline with figure-of-8 suture placement using 2-0 or 3-0 polyglactin sutures. This pants-over-vest closure provides additional ventral support. Two flat 7 Fr suction drains are placed between the fascia and the subcutaneous space. The skin flaps are then tailored, removing the excess, allowing for a midline and periumbilical closure. The skin flap is closed in multiple layers, securing the subcutaneous tissue with 4-0 plain gut sutures. The epithelial edge is reapproximated with a running subcuticular suture of 4-0 or 5-0 polyglactin. The drains remain in place for 2 or 3 days for decompression of the dead space.

Orchiopexy

With an open approach, the gonad is usually closely associated with a dilated distal ureter. To determine whether the testicle can be delivered into the scrotum without sacrifice of the gonadal artery, the testicle should be released from the ureter. An incision is made in the

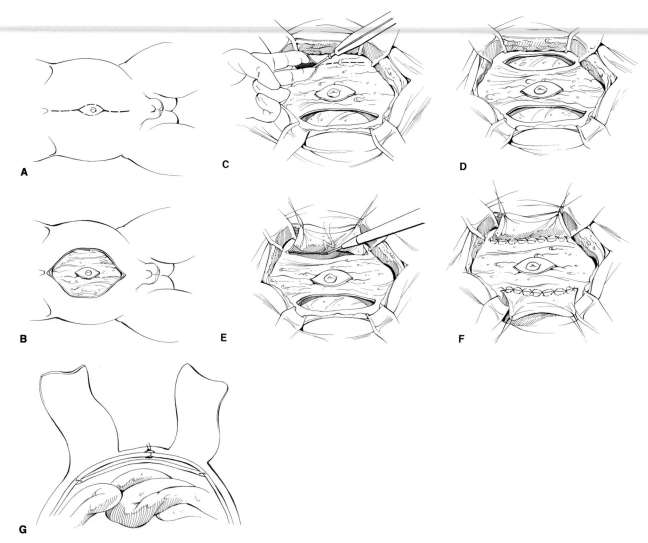

FIG. 96–4. A: An incision is begun at the xyphoid, circumscribing the umbilicus, and carried down to the pubis. **B:** Skin flaps are then elevated, dissecting between the subcutaneous fat and the fascial layer. The lateral extension is the anterior auxiliary line. **C, D:** The umbilicus is supported by the central fascial bridge. Incisions will be made into the peritoneum lateral to the epigastric vessels. The central fascial bridge is easily manipulated to allow for excellent intraabdominal exposure. **E:** At the time of closure, a line is scored on the peritoneal surface of the fascia. **F:** The central fascial strip is then secured laterally to the scored fascia line with a running suture of 2-0 or 3-0 polyglactin. **G:** The lateral fascia is then secured in the midline above and below the umbilicus with 2-0 or 3-0 polyglactin. Centrally, the fascia is secured directly to the umbilicus. This allows for an overlapping reinforced fascial wall closure. Subcutaneous tissue is closed with 3-0 or 4-0 plain gut and the skin with a running subcuticular 4-0 or 5-0 polyglactin suture.

peritoneum lateral to the gonadal artery taken to the internal ring. In a proximal location of the gonadal vessels, the overlying peritoneum is incised and the incision is continued medial and caudally along the course of the vessels and vas deferens. It is important to not disrupt the vascular supply of the peritoneal pedicle running on both sides of the vas deferens. If it becomes apparent that the testes will not reach into the scrotum after mobilization, the gonadal artery is sacrificed to obtain adequate length for the testicle to be delivered in the scrotum as described by Fowler and Stephens (5). The blood supply to the

testes is maintained by the vasal artery and small anastomotic channels within the peritoneal flap. A tunnel is then made into the scrotum and an incision placed inferiorly in the scrotum to create a dartos pouch. A clamp is passed from the scrotum to the inguinal canal. The testicle is grasped, pulled down through the tunnel, and delivered to the scrotum. Care must be taken not to twist or place the peritoneal pedicle on tension. If desired, the testicle can be secured to the dartos tissue with 5-0 polydioxanone. If orchiopexy is undertaken early, in particular within the first 6 months of life, there is often adequate vascular length to deliver the testicle directly into the scrotum without transection of the testicular artery. When the orchidopexy is approached as an independent procedure it can be undertaken laparoscopically.

Urethral Reconstruction

Urethral reconfiguration is most effectively undertaken by formal excisional tapering as described by Nesbitt (Fig. 96–5). An incision is made inline with the previous circumcision or beneath the coronal sulcus if uncircumcised. The penile shaft skin is then mobilized to the base of the penis. The anterior urethral wall is usually thin and poorly supported and care needs to be taken to prevent inadvertent entrance into the urethra. The urethra is split in the midline ventrally. The redundant portion of the urethra is excised and the urethra is reapproximated over a 10 or 12 Fr catheter depending on the child's age. The urethra is closed in two layers using a 6-0 or 7-0 polydioxanone or polyglactic acid sutures. The glanular urethra is usually patent and the reconstruction is limited to the penile shaft. Because of poor development of the spongiosum it may be difficult to achieve additional tissue for a second layer of coverage. The penile shaft skin is then secured to the coronal tissue with 6-0 chromic sutures. A urethral stent or catheter is placed for 7 days. The penis is dressed with the personal technique used for a hypospadias repair.

A variant of megalourethra is the "megameatus with an intact prepuce" (MIP) (3). This is corrected using standard hypospadias techniques (Fig. 96–6). The glans is infiltrated with a mixture of 1:200,000 epinephrine for hemostasis. Parallel incisions are made lateral to the urethral plate and extended into the glans, creating two glanular wings. The incisions are continued along the shaft of the penis and connected beneath the urethral meatus. The urethra is then tubularized over an 8 or 12 Fr catheter using 6-0 or 7-0 polyglactic or polyglycolic acid sutures. The glans is closed in the midline, reapproximating the deep tissue with 6-0 Vicryl and the epithelium with 6-0 chromic. The penile shaft skin is brought up and the excess excised and then reapproximated to the coronal ring. A urethral stent or catheter can be positioned for 7 days depending on the length of the defect. The penis is dressed as above.

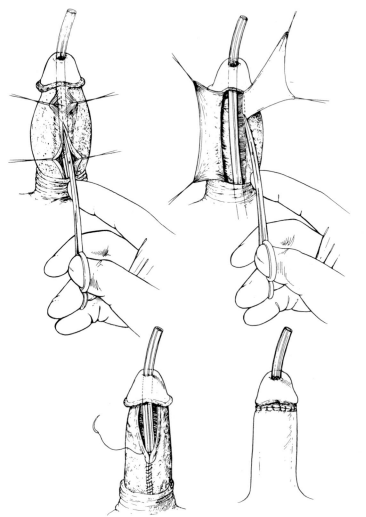

FIG. 96–5. Nesbitt reduction urethroplasty for megalourethra. **A:** The urethra is opened vertically in the midline, **B:** followed by excision of the lateral redundant tissue. **C:** Reconstruction is carried out over a 12 Fr catheter using two layers of running suture. **D:** The penile skin is reapproximated to the coronal margin circumferentially.

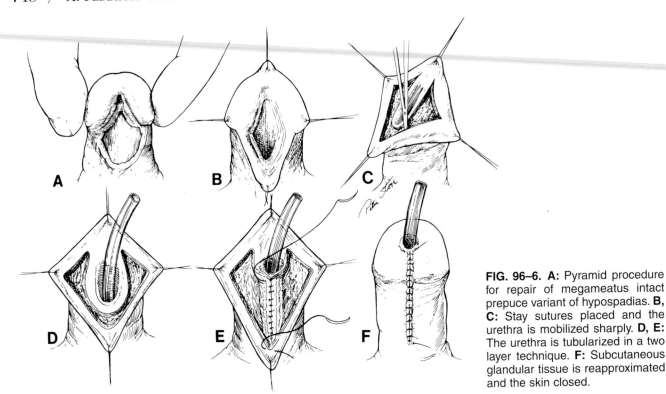

FIG. 96–6. A: Pyramid procedure for repair of megameatus intact prepuce variant of hypospadias. **B, C:** Stay sutures placed and the urethra is mobilized sharply. **D, E:** The urethra is tubularized in a two layer technique. **F:** Subcutaneous glandular tissue is reapproximated and the skin closed.

OUTCOMES

Complications

Ureteral devascularization resulting in ischemia and subsequent obstruction can occur if attention has not been paid to the ureteral blood supply. The risk of bowel obstruction is present as in any intraabdominal procedure. Testicular ischemia and atrophy due to a single-stage Fowler–Stephens procedure has been reported to occur in 30% of children. This can be decreased with a staged approach.

The cosmetic appearance following urethral tapering is good and only limited by any residual corpora cavernosa deficiency. Postvoid dribbling can be abolished and the risk of urinary infections due to stagnant urine can be diminished. The most common complication is that of a urethral fistula due to limited spongiosum tissue for a multiple-layer closure. The circumferential degloving of the penis with subsequent reapproximation of the penile shaft skin to the corona will limit fistula formation. The greatest risk for a fistula is located at the level of the ventral coronal sulcus.

Results

The results of urologic reconstruction can be very gratifying in the initial postoperative period, in particular the cosmetic appearance of the abdomen and improvement in upper urinary tract drainage. Voiding function may become more effective due to the benefits of abdominal wall reconstruction and reduction cystoplasty (9). However, with time there can be an increase in both bladder size and ureteral dilation. This is often due to ineffective voiding and is inde-

pendent of bladder reduction. For those reasons, long-term follow-up of the urinary tract is required. Patients should be prepared for the potential need for intermittent catheterization. Because of normal sensation, children are often unwilling to cooperate with urethral catheterization. If catheterization appears to be a realistic possibility at the time of urinary reconstruction, placement of an appendicovesicostomy should be considered. This provides excellent access to the bladder in a normally sensate child.

REFERENCES

1. Bukowski TM, Perlmutter AD. Reduction cystoplasty in the prune-belly syndrome: a long term follow up. *J Urol* 1994;152:2113–2116.
2. Bukowski TM, Smith CA. Monfort abdominoplasty with neoumbilical modification. *J Urol* 2000;164:1711–1713.
3. Duckett JW, Keating MA. Technical challenges of the megameatus intact prepuce hypospadias variant: the pyramid procedure. *J Urol* 1989;141:1407–1409.
4. Ehrlich RM, Lesavoy MA, Fine RN. Total abdominal wall reconstruction in the prune-belly syndrome. *J Urol* 1986;136:282–285.
5. Fowler R, Stephens FD. The role of testicular vascular anatomy in the salvage of high undescended testis. *Aust NZ J Surg* 1959;29:92–106.
6. Kinahan TJ, Churchill BM, McLorie GA, et al. The efficiency of bladder emptying in the prune-belly syndrome. *J Urol* 1992;148:600–603.
7. Montfort G, Guys JM, Boccoardo A, et al. A novel technique for reconstruction of the abdominal wall in the prune belly syndrome. *J Urol* 1991;146:639–640.
8. Noh PH, Cooper CS, Winkler AC, Zderic SA, Snyder HM, Canning DA. Prognostic factors for long-term renal function in boys with the prune-belly syndrome. *J Urol* 1999;162:1399–1401.
9. Smith CA, Smith EA, Parrott TS, Broecker BH, Woodard JR. Voiding function in patients with the prune-belly syndrome after Monfort abdominoplasty. *J Urol* 1998;159:1675–1679.
10. Oster W. Congenital absence of the abdominal muscles with distended and hypertrophied urinary bladder. *Bull Johns Hopkins Hosp* 1901;12:331–335.
11. Parker RW. Absence of abdominal muscles in an infant. *Lancet* 1895;23:1252.

CHAPTER 97

Childhood Rhabdomyosarcoma

Hsi-Yang Wu and Howard M. Snyder III

The management of rhabdomyosarcoma (RMS) remains the most controversial topic in pediatric urologic oncology. While all agree that a combination of surgery, chemotherapy, and radiotherapy is best, the optimal timing and extent of the three treatment modalities remains unclear. It is useful to remember three key points:

1. Chemotherapy cures microscopic disease.
2. Residual mass does not equal disease.
3. Radiotherapy renders pathology very difficult to read.

Twenty percent of RMS involves the bladder, prostate, vagina, or paratesticular area. RMS peaks between ages 2 to 4 and ages 15 to 19. The tumor is nonencapsulated, grows rapidly, and spreads to regional lymph nodes as well as hematogenously. The Intergroup Rhabdomyosarcoma Study Group (IRSG) has been conducting studies in the United States since 1972 to achieve better survival with less morbidity, and is currently conducting IRS V to investigate new chemotherapeutic options. Patient survival, which was only 40% to 73% prior to chemotherapy, has improved to 86% in IRS IV with VAC (vincristine, dactinomycin, cyclophosphamide) (3). During the same time, the surgical approach has changed from initial exenterative surgery to organ-preserving surgery following chemotherapy. The functional bladder salvage rate has risen from 25% to 60% with this change in management.

RMS consists of small, blue, round cells, arising from undifferentiated mesoderm, with a microscopic appearance of spindle cells resembling fetal skeletal muscle. Embryonal pathology accounts for 90% of genitourinary RMS. Embryonal pathology is more favorable than alveolar pathology, which tends to occur in extremities. Sarcoma botyroides ("bunch of grapes") is a polypoid form of embryonal pathology. Current lab efforts have found genetic translocations between chromosomes 1;13 (favorable) and 2;13 (very high risk) to be prognostic

markers in patients with alveolar tumors with metastatic disease (13).

DIAGNOSIS

Bladder and prostate primaries present with urinary retention and gross hematuria and tend to be located at the trigone and bladder neck. Often, determining which organ from which the tumor arose can be difficult. Vaginal primaries present with vaginal bleeding or an introital mass and tend to occur on the anterior vaginal wall. Paratesticular primaries present with a painless scrotal mass. The preoperative evaluation can be carried out with ultrasound, computed tomography (CT), or magnetic resonance imaging (MRI) (T2 weighting). The retroperitoneum is best evaluated with CT or MRI. Metastatic workup is completed with a chest x-ray, liver function tests, bone scan, and bone marrow biopsy.

The IRS study includes both preoperative staging and postoperative grouping (3) (Tables 97–1 and 97–2). The IRS I–III studies grouped patients based on completeness of resection, introducing biases (shifting patients from group 1 to group 3) that are not seen with the use of the tumor–node–metastasis (TNM) system in IRS IV–V.

TABLE 97–1. *Preoperative staging*

T1: Confined to Organ of Origin, a: $\leq$ 5 cm, b: > 5 cm
T2: Extension or Fixed to Surrounding Tissue, a: $\leq$ 5 cm, b: > 5 cm
No: Regional Nodes Clinically Negative
N1: Regional Nodes Clinically Positive
Nx: Unknown
M0: No Distant Metastasis
M1: Metastasis Present
Stage I: Vaginal and Paratesticular RMS, any T, any N, M0
Stage II: Bladder/Prostate RMS, T1a or T2a, No or Nx, M0
Stage III: Bladder/Prostate RMS, (T1a or T2a) and N1, M0, OR (T1b or T2b), any N, M0
Stage IV: Any Tumor with M1

TABLE 97–2. *Postoperative grouping*

Group 1: Localized Disease, Completely Excised, No
    Microscopic Residual
    A: Confined to Site of Origin, Completely Resected
    B: Infiltrating Beyond Site of Origin, Completely Resected
Group 2: Total Gross Resection
    A: Gross Resection with Microscopic Local Residual
    B: Regional Disease with Involved Lymph Nodes,
Completely Resected with No Microscopic Residual
    C: Microscopic Local and/or Nodal Residual
Group 3: Incomplete Resection or Biopsy with Gross
    Residual
Group 4: Distant Metastases

INDICATIONS FOR SURGERY

During the initial procedure, adequate tissue for a definitive diagnosis should be obtained and, if possible, one should remove the tumor without removing the affected organ (with the exception of paratesticular RMS, where the testis is removed with the tumor inguinally). If excision is not possible, primary chemotherapy should be given. In follow-up staging, a biopsy is needed during the second-look operation because residual mass does not always represent tumor. The cancer can involute more rapidly than the supporting stroma. Definitive surgery aims to do a good radical but pelvic organ-sparing operation if possible. If microscopic residual disease is found, it is treated with brachytherapy or external beam radiotherapy. Exenteration is reserved for patients who fail this protocol of chemotherapy, conservative surgery, and radiotherapy. In Europe, the approach is to give primary chemotherapy without initial local control (radiotherapy or surgery) and offer local therapy based on the initial chemotherapy response (4,6).

ALTERNATIVE THERAPY

The use of surgery or radiotherapy as definitive local control remains a difficult choice. In favor of radiotherapy, it has been remarkably successful in decreasing the need for radical surgery to achieve a cure. However, the difficulty with radiotherapy and bladder rhabdomyosarcoma is that because the tumors tend to be located at the bladder neck even the lowest dose (41 Gy) that the radiation oncologists are willing to deliver may significantly risk urinary continence. Current attempts at limiting radiation toxicity to adjacent organs involve both conformal radiotherapy and brachytherapy. The long-term risk of radiation vasculitis, which is inevitably progressive, as well as possible bony pelvis deformity in these children is another issue to consider. Therefore, one must sometimes weigh whether preserving a bladder without an outlet is better than removing the bladder entirely (5,12). The final issue is that postradiation artifact makes subsequent biopsy very difficult to interpret, so it would make sense to delay radiation until the patient is free of gross disease.

SURGICAL TECHNIQUE

For bladder and prostate RMS, we will summarize the surgical options available after the initial biopsy has shown RMS, the patient has received chemotherapy, and the choice has been made to use surgery to achieve local control. For vaginal and paratesticular RMS, we will review the overall surgical approach starting with the initial resection.

Bladder

The approach to partial or total cystectomy is similar to that for muscle-invasive transitional cell carcinoma (see chapters 23, 24). We will highlight the technical points that are unique to the management of bladder RMS.

The initial step after opening the abdomen is to examine the retroperitoneum. While we do not perform a full retroperitoneal lymphadenectomy because there is no therapeutic benefit, any suspicious lymph nodes along the vessels between the obturator fossa and the renal veins are removed. The next step is to properly stage the tumor by obtaining multiple frozen section biopsies of the bladder around the area of the tumor. If these are negative and the tumor is amenable to partial cystectomy with a 2- to 3-cm margin, then the bladder does not need to be entirely removed. RMS is a nonencapsulated, infiltrative tumor, so adequate margins are necessary.

If the tumor extends down the urethra, then the symphysis should be split to gain better access. After completing distal dissection of the urethra, the symphysis is closed with long-term absorbable sutures. With this improved exposure, it is also possible to perform a nerve-sparing dissection (see chapter 33), although follow-up potency data is not yet available. The placement of brachytherapy catheters for afterloading (to treat microscopic positive margins if needed) should be considered.

Following cystectomy, we have often placed Dexon mesh across the abdomen to hold the intestines out of the pelvis at the level of the sacral promontory. This is done by attaching it to the sacral promontory and wrapping it around the sigmoid. This serves to prevent adhesion of the bowel to the raw surface of the pelvis until it has reepithelialized, and if postoperative radiation is necessary for microscopic residual disease it limits the exposure of the bowel to the radiation field. Currently, pelvic exenteration is reserved for patients who have failed both chemotherapy and radiotherapy and who have tumors that invade both the bladder and the rectum.

The final surgical decision is whether to proceed with continent urinary reconstruction at the same time. We have taken the approach that it is not necessary to perform the reconstruction at the same time unless the patient is both motivated and able to perform clean intermittent catheterization to drain a urinary reservoir. For younger patients who are not ready to manage a urinary reservoir, we have either brought up the remaining bladder plate with ureterovesical junctions intact as a vesicostomy or performed low end-cutaneous ureterostomies, with the ureters placed side by side as a single stoma on the abdomen.

Prostate

The approach is similar to that for localized prostatic adenocarcinoma (see chapter 33). Again, no follow-up on nerve-sparing procedures is yet available. Splitting the symphysis is useful as it is essential to remove the urethra to the midbulbar level, and the placement of brachytherapy catheters for afterloading (to treat microscopic positive margins if needed) should be considered.

Vagina

The patient is placed in the lithotomy position and the pelvis and vagina are prepped. For the initial resection, vaginoscopy is helpful in defining the limits of the tumor. Stay sutures and a small weighted vaginal speculum are helpful for exposure, as is a headlight for vision. Sharp excision of the tumor is carried out, staying away from the external sphincter, urethra, and bladder neck. The vaginal mucosa is closed with interrupted absorbable sutures. Hysterectomy is rarely carried out because uterine tumors are rare and tend to present in older females (greater than 10 years old).

Paratestis

The testis and adnexa are removed via inguinal orchiectomy (see chapter 62). Frozen section of the proximal cord should reveal no tumor. The key step is to avoid making a scrotal incision for a solid paratesticular mass because, while chemotherapy often cures residual disease, some cases have required hemiscrotectomy due to tumor infiltration. Retroperitoneal lymph node dissection is carried out for all boys with stage I disease older than age 10, regardless of findings on abdominal CT. The technique is identical to that used for retroperitoneal involvement by testicular tumors (see chapter 63) Again, sympathetic nerve-sparing techniques can be used to maintain ejaculation, but no follow-up data are currently available. For boys under age 10, the retroperitoneum is imaged by CT or MRI, and if there is no gross disease then retroperitoneal lymph node dissection is not performed. Chemotherapy has been shown to adequately clear microscopic disease (30% to 40% incidence).

Postoperative Decisions

Review of the pathology may reveal persistent rhabdomyoblasts in a patient who has received as much chemotherapy as can safely be given. Currently, there is debate concerning the malignant potential of these cells, which represent matured rhabdomyoblasts (7,9). Normally, resection of the involved organ is carried out. If this would require destruction of a functional bladder, observation with frequent radiological follow-up may be an option to consider.

OUTCOMES

Complications

The majority of patients have acute toxicity from the chemotherapy: Ninety percent developed myelosuppression, 55% developed significant infections, and renal toxicity was seen in 2% (3). Most relapses occur within 3 years of initial diagnosis (11). Late recurrences can occur in patients who are treated with chemotherapy alone. Of 883 patients, 10 developed a secondary cancer. Patients with preexisting renal abnormalities were at a higher risk of death (5% vs. 1%). Relapse in group 3 (incomplete resection) patients was associated with a 22% chance of 3-year survival, compared to 41% in group 1 or 2 patients (localized disease or total gross resection) (3). The experience from IRS I–II suggests a 27% long-term urinary complication rate, with incontinence being the major issue. Twenty-nine percent required sex hormone replacement and 11% were shorter than expected (12). If radiotherapy has been used, there is an increased risk of a secondary neoplasm, often another sarcoma, in the radiation field.

Results

Bladder and Prostate

Bladder and prostate RMS has a 2.5/1 male predominance. IRS III included intensified chemotherapy (dactinomycin, Etopside) and 6 weeks of radiotherapy, increasing the functional bladder salvage rate from 25% to 60%. The initial procedure consists of percutaneous, endoscopic, or transrectal biopsy of the mass, followed by chemotherapy. In IRS IV, VAC was shown to be as effective as two other three drug regimens (VIE/VAE: ifosfamide, etoposide) (3). On second look, half of patients were managed with biopsy, 37% had partial cystectomy, and 13% had prostatectomy. For persistent disease, group 2 was treated with 41 Gy and group 3 was treated with 50 Gy. At 24 weeks, a third operative evaluation was performed with consideration for exenteration. Patients with embryonal pathology had an 83% 3-year failure-free survival, compared to 40% in those with alveolar pathology. All patients with group 4 (metastatic) prostate disease died. Bladder function (as assessed by questionnaire) was normal in 73%, whereas 8% had incontinence and 9% had frequency and nocturia. Renal function as assessed by serum blood urea nitrogen and creatinine was normal in 95%, although 29% of patients had abnormal renal scans (10).

Vagina

Surgery and chemotherapy cure most cases of vaginal RMS. In the overall IRS I–IV experience, 42% of patients were treated with surgery and chemotherapy, 19% required additional radiotherapy, 21% were treated with biopsy and chemotherapy alone, and 12% were managed with biopsy, chemotherapy, and radiotherapy (2). In IRS IV, only 19% of patients required wide excision of the tumor. Primary treatment with VAC chemotherapy is usually successful, and a biopsy 8 to 12 weeks after chemotherapy is recommended. Pelvic lymph node dissection is not necessary. Rhabdomyoblasts on biopsy are evidence of chemotherapy response, and therefore further chemotherapy, instead of resection, is the proper treatment. Radiotherapy should only be used for persistent disease or relapse (1).

Paratestis

Paratesticular RMS has two peak incidences: in the 3- to 4-month-old boy and in the teenager. Scrotal ultrasound will confirm the paratesticular primary, which should then be resected along with the testis in a radical inguinal orchiectomy. Serum β-human chorionic gonadotropin and α-fetoprotein should be obtained to confirm that the mass is not a testicular primary. Thirty percent to 40% will have metastases to the retroperitoneum. The biologic activity of the tumor is different between the neonate and the teenager (90% vs. 63% failure-free survival at 3 years). In previous studies, all patients underwent retroperitoneal lymph node dissection (RPLND) (3). However, Olive et al. showed in 1984 that of 19 patients with clinical stage I disease 17 were cured with adjuvant chemotherapy alone. This showed that chemotherapy can clear microscopic retroperitoneal disease, making RPLND unnecessary (8). In IRS IV, RPLND was not recommended, leading to a significant understaging of disease and a decrease in failure-free survival because patients with negative CT scans did not receive radiation. Thirty percent of those patients who were clinically stage I and over at 10 years of age required retreatment. Because the outcome for stage I disease in those under 10 years of age was so good in IRS IV, those patients who are less than 10 years old and have stage I disease and negative abdominal/pelvic CT are treated with VA (vincristine, dactinomycin) only in IRS V, whereas all patients with stage I disease who are 10 years or older undergo RPLND regardless of CT findings. Group 2 tumors (positive lymph nodes on pathology) are treated with radiotherapy and VAC. Three-year failure-free survival is 81% for group 1 tumors overall, but those patients more than 10 years old only had a 63% survival (3).

REFERENCES

1. Andrassy RJ. Modern approach to rhabdomyosarcoma of the vagina and uterus. Presented at the Section on Surgery, American Academy of Pediatrics meeting, Chicago, 2000.
2. Arndt CAS, Donaldson SS, Anderson JR, et al. What constitutes optimal therapy for patients with rhabdomyosarcoma of the female genital tract? *Cancer* 2001;91:2454–2468.
3. Crist WM, Anderson JR, Meza JL, et al. Intergroup Rhabdomyosarcoma Study—IV: Results for patients with nonmetastatic disease. *J Clin Oncol* 2001;19:3091–3102.
4. Flamant F, Rodary C, Rey A, et al. Treatment of non-metastatic rhabdomyosarcoma in childhood and adolescence. Results of the second study of the International Society of Paediatric Oncology: MMT84. *Eur J Cancer* 1998;34:1050–1062.
5. Hays DM, Raney RB, Wharam MD, et al. Children with vesical rhabdomyosarcoma (RMS) treated by partial cystectomy with neoadjuvant or adjuvant chemotherapy, with or without radiotherapy. *J Pediatr Hem/Oncol* 1995;17:46–52.
6. Koscielniak E, Harms D, Henze G, et al. Results of treatment for soft tissue sarcoma in childhood and adolescence: A final report of the German cooperative soft tissue sarcoma study CWS-86. *J Clin Oncol* 1999;17:3706–3719.
7. Leuschner I, Harms D, Mattke A, et al. Rhabdomyosarcoma of the urinary bladder and vagina. *Am J Surg Pathol* 2001;25:856–864.
8. Olive D, Flamant F, Zucker JM, et al. Paraaortic lymphadenectomy is not necessary in the treatment of localized paratesticular rhabdomyosarcoma. *Cancer* 1984;54:1283–1287.
9. Ortega JA, Rowland J, Monforte H, et al. Presence of well-differentiated rhabdomyoblasts at the end of therapy for pelvic rhabdomyosarcoma: Implications for the outcome. *J Pediatr Hem/Oncol*, 2000;22:106–111.
10. Paidas CN. Results of rhabdomyosarcoma of the bladder and prostate: Is bladder preservation successful? Presented at the Section on Surgery, American Academy of Pediatrics meeting, Chicago, 2000.
11. Pappo AS, Anderson JR, Crist WM, et al. Survival after relapse in children and adolescents with rhabdomyosarcoma: A report from the Intergroup Rhabdomyosarcoma Study Group. *J Clin Oncol* 1999;17:3487–3493.
12. Raney B, Heyn R, Hays DM, et al. Sequelae of treatment in 109 patients followed 5 to 15 years after diagnosis of sarcoma of the bladder and prostate. *Cancer* 1993;71:2387–2394.
13. Sorenson PH, Lynch JC, Qualman SJ, et al. PAX3-FKHR and PAX7-FKHR gene fusions are prognostic indicators in alveolar rhabdomyosarcoma: a report from the Children's Oncology Group. *J Clin Oncol* 2002;20:2672–2679.

CHAPTER 98

Vesicoureteral Reflux

Mark R. Zaontz

Considering that vesicoureteral reflux (VUR) was first recognized during the time of Galen (150 AD), not much progress was noted until the beginning of the 20th century

Young (16) and later Sampson (12) noted that those patients with both normal ureterovesical junction and ureteral path through the bladder did not have VUR. It was not until the 1950s that the strong relationship between VUR and pyelonephritis was recognized by Hutch (7). His work demonstrated the pathologic anatomy that underlies VUR which led to successful surgical correction of this entity. His pioneering work was also instrumental in making the voiding cystourethrogram (VCUG) part of the evaluation in patients with urinary tract infection as well as hydronephrosis.

Until the 1980s, the treatment for reflux was largely surgical, with cure rates approaching 98%. However, multicenter studies have shown that the lower grades of reflux had high spontaneous resolution rates and could be followed at least initially by medical management using prophylactic antibiotics and yearly reassessment. Higher grades of reflux are associated with a higher incidence of renal scarring and lower rates of spontaneous resolution.

Surgical correction of reflux may not prevent progression of reflux nephropathy when present, although corrected reflux in general prevents new renal scarring. Reflux in the presence of sterile urine in general does not cause renal damage, although reflux in the presence of urinary tract infection (UTI) can lead to renal scarring.

Boys in general present with higher reflux grades than females of the same age, but also have a higher spontaneous resolution rate than females. Studies showing that circumcised boys with low grades of reflux rarely get UTIs or related morbidity has led to a nonoperative algorithm in this group of patients.

Reflux is commonly linked with voiding dysfunction in children. Recent evidence using urodynamics and biofeedback techniques have shown high spontaneous cure rates for refluxing children with concomitant voiding dysfunction. Conversely, children with significant voiding dys-

function have higher failure rates from conventional surgery than those with normal bladder function.

Sampson (12) in the early 1900s proposed a flap valve mechanism for the ureterovesical junction that was corroborated by Gruber (6), who found that those ureters with shorter intravesical segments were more prone to have reflux and therefore have a defective flap valve mechanism. Stephens and Lenahan (14) added that the deficiency of the intravesical ureter's longitudinal muscle with or without a deficiency in ureteral tunnel length was also responsible for the reflux phenomenon. From a surgical perspective we have learned that a 5:1 ureteral tunnel length:ureteral lumen diameter ratio is necessary to prevent reflux.

While most cases of reflux are congenital in nature and considered primary reflux, increased intravesical pressure due to anatomic bladder outlet obstruction or functional causes such as neuropathic bladder/voiding dysfunction may lead to what is termed secondary reflux.

DIAGNOSIS

Today, thanks in great part to common antenatal screening, reflux is often diagnosed prior to the development of a urinary infection and, as a result, pyelonephritis may be avoided by promptly beginning prophylaxis just after delivery. Presenting symptoms in neonates may include malaise, fever, vomiting, diarrhea, or failure to thrive. Toddlers and young children may have more typical symptoms such as fever, frequency, urgency, dysuria, foul-smelling urine, incontinence, or abdominal and/or back discomfort.

It is critical that a urine culture be obtained in all cases of suspected UTI. A urinalysis alone is unacceptable as it only alludes to the presence of UTI and at best is only 80% accurate in diagnosis. Radiographic evaluation is indicated after the first UTI in boys of any age and in all preadolescent girls. Further, any girl with a febrile infection or recurrent UTIs should be studied regardless of her

GRADE OF REFLUX

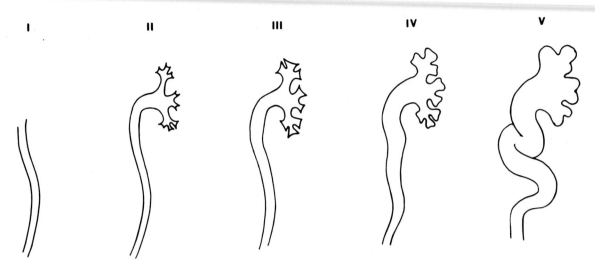

FIG. 98–1. International classification of vesicourethral reflux. Grade I, into the nondilated ureter; grade II, into the pelvis and calyces without dilation; grade III, mild to moderate dilation of the ureter, renal pelvis, and calyces with minimal blunting of the fornices; grade IV, moderate ureteral tortuosity and dilation of the pelvis and calyces; grade V, gross dilation of the ureter, pelvis, and calyces and loss of papillary impressions and ureteral tortuosity.

age. Workup for UTI should include an ultrasound of the kidneys and bladder as well as a voiding cystourethrogram (VCUG). In cases where screening is needed for siblings or children of known refluxers, a renal ultrasound and nuclear cystogram (NVCUG) for girls and a fluoroscopic VCUG for boys is recommended.

Once reflux is diagnosed, it is graded according to the International Study Classification (Fig. 98–1) (8). This system is based on the radiographic appearance of the ureter and collecting system during a VCUG. Follow-up studies are in general done using nuclear cystography at yearly intervals to assess the resolution or progression of reflux.

Ultrasound appears to be relatively accurate in determining the presence or absence of renal scars in low-grade reflux patients. However, in those with higher-grade reflux a "normal" renal ultrasound may miss significant renal scarring. The ^{99m}Tc-labeled dimercapto-succinic acid (DMSA) scan is to date the best available study to access focal pyelonephritis and renal scarring.

Cystoscopy has little value in predicting the presence or cessation of reflux based on ureteral orifice configuration or location. Factors such as tunnel length or the presence of incomplete versus complete duplication anomalies will guide the surgeon to choose an appropriate technique, open or endoscopic.

INDICATIONS FOR SURGERY

Indications for surgical correction of vesicoureteral reflux include an older patient, higher grade of reflux, presence of renal damage, noncompliance with prophy-

laxis, and the family's concerns with respect to repeated invasive testing and long-term prophylaxis. Findings from the International Reflux Study lends support toward surgical intervention in grade III and IV refluxers, with the majority of these patients failing to resolve their reflux (15). Other studies have supported these findings with rates of resolution of reflux ranging from 10% to 33% in patients with grade IV reflux (3,13). Surgery is in general recommended for grade V reflux because of the low likelihood of spontaneous resolution.

Females should not be allowed to go into puberty with reflux due to the increased risk and morbidity of pyelonephritis during pregnancy. Recurrent breakthrough urinary infection while on adequate antibiotic prophylaxis is the *sine qua non* for surgical intervention because otherwise these children are at high risk for renal damage.

ALTERNATIVE THERAPY

There are several factors that must be taken into consideration for appropriate management: reflux grade, presence/degree of renal scarring, patient age, presence or absence of bladder outlet obstruction, compliance of the patient/family on prophylactic antibiotics, ability to remain infection free while on prophylaxis, and presence/absence of associated voiding dysfunction. Reflux may spontaneously resolve and the peak time for resolution is between 5 and 7 years of age. The lower the grade of reflux the higher is the likelihood for spontaneous resolution. Unilateral reflux is statistically more likely to resolve than bilateral reflux. Medical management consists of antibiotic prophylaxis, usually a sulfa-based compound or nitrofurantoin at bedtime. In addition to antibiotics, bladder training in cases of dysfunctional voiding is instituted. This is designed to improve bladder emptying at regular intervals, obviate bladder–sphincter dyssynergia, and have minimal postvoid residual. This may require a variety of teaching aids and the use of pharmacotherapy such as anticholinergics. In addition, urodynamics and biofeedback may be used in selected cases. Equally important is to improve bowel function/evacuation in the presence of constipation.

SURGICAL TECHNIQUE

Once the decision is made for surgical intervention, there are a myriad of operative procedures available depending on one's preference and comfort level. The existing techniques are divided into endoscopic, extravesical, intravesical, a combination of intravesical and extravesical approaches, and laparoscopic correction.

Endoscopic Surgery

Teflon was the first bulking agent used for endoscopic correction of reflux. Although the results were encouraging, later studies showed that there was migration of the Teflon particles to the lung, lymph nodes, and brain as well as the finding of granuloma formation; this resulted in the search for more biocompatible bulking agents (1). These have included both autologous agents (fat, blood, human collagen, bladder muscle cells, and chondrogel) and nonautologous agents (silicone, bioglass, polyvinyl alcohol, and dextronomer microspheres). Deflux (dextronomer microspheres) is at present approved by the US Food and Drug Administration for use as a bulking agent.

In performing this procedure, the patient is placed in the lithotomy position after anesthesia is induced and then prepped and draped for a standard cystoscopic procedure. My preference for cystoscopes is the offset lens variety with a straight working channel that can accommodate a 5 Fr instrument. Once cystoscopic evaluation reveals a ureteral orifice with enough of a submucosal tunnel to allow needle placement, a 23-gauge needle is connected to a 1-cc syringe containing the Deflux. The needle is first flushed with sterile saline to allow for greater ease of injecting Deflux, following which the needle is primed so that the Deflux can be seen at the needle's end. It is important that the bladder is only partially filled to allow for easier subureteric injection. The needle is then inserted through the working channel and is carefully advanced with the bevel in the up position about 5 mm from the ureteral orifice under the mucosa at the 6-o'clock position. The needle is advanced further until it sits directly below the orifice itself in the submucosal plane (Fig. 98–2). I like to jiggle the needle gently to confirm its proper location just prior to injection. The Deflux is slowly injected, raising and compressing the ureteral orifice until it sits flattened on the top of a mound created by the bulking agent. In general, the average injection is between 0.4 and 0.7 cc. The needle is removed within 15 seconds of completing the injection to allow for sealing of the material. Single injections are preferable to avoid multiple sticks and extravasation of the bulking material. The bladder is then emptied, the endoscope removed, and the procedure terminated. Postoperatively I obtain a renal/bladder ultrasound at 1 month to rule out occult hydronephrosis and hydroureter and a VCUG/NVCUG in 3 months to assess the results of the procedure. Antibiotic prophylaxis is continued until reflux has been deemed a cure.

Extravesical Approach

Lich and Gregoir in the 1960s separately developed the extravesical approach to correct reflux (5,9). Further

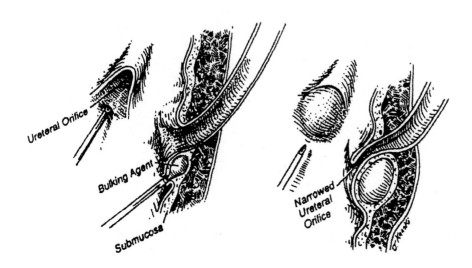

FIG. 98–2. Principle of endoscopic treatment of reflux. Bulking agent is injected beneath ureteral orifice with needle. The buttress that is provided helps coapt distal ureter. (From Atala A, Keating M. Vesicoureteral reflux. In Walsh PC, Retick AB, Wein A, Vaughan ED, Eds. Cambell's urology. Vol. 2. Philadelphia: WB Saunders, 1997)

Ureteral Orifice

Bulking Agent

Submucosa

Narrowed Ureteral Orifice

modifications of this approach have yielded success equal to that of the intravesical techiques (17). The benefits of this procedure are several: (a) The surgery is performed outside of the bladder mucosa and as such avoids gross hematuria and irritable postoperative voiding problems such as urgency symptoms and bladder spasms, (b) catheter drainage of the bladder is brief, (c) wound drains are avoided, and (d) ureteral stents are eliminated. A further advantage of this technique is that hospital stay is brief, averaging 1.5 days in my hands, thus decreasing overall hospital costs.

Prior to incision, after the patient is prepped and draped, the bladder is catheterized and the bladder filled to about one-third to one-half of its estimated capacity with sterile saline. This allows for easier dissection when separating the detrusor muscle from the mucosa. The bladder may be further filled or emptied depending on the surgeon's preference during the procedure. The surgical procedure for detrusorrhaphy begins similarly to the intravesical approach with a Pfannenstiel incision. A Dennis–Browne retractor is then placed over moistened gauze pads and the bladder is carefully mobilized and rotated anteromedially, exposing the appropriate perivesical space. Care should be taken to avoid entering the peritoneum during this maneuver. Placing an appropriate sized Deaver retractor to help keep the rotated bladder in place will greatly facilitate locating the obliterated hypogastric vessel. This vessel is tied off with 3-0 polyglycolic acid suture and the lateral most tie is clamped to help expose the ureter, which lies just beneath this vessel. In cases of bilateral detrusorrhaphy, the obliterated hypogastric vessel need not be tied off but simply recognized for ease of finding the underlying ureter. This minimal dissection technique as well as limiting the dissection of the extravesical submucosal tunnel may help prevent significant nerve denervation and avoid postoperative urinary retention.

The ureter is carefully mobilized and encircled with a vessel loop (Fig. 98–3). The ureter is freed up its entry point into the bladder. During this maneuver the Deaver retractors may need to be reset such that the ureter is in the middle of the operative field throughout the procedure. A tennis racket incision is made around the ureteral detrusor hiatus and deepened until the ureter is only attached to its connection with the mucosa. The incision is then extended such that a 3- to 5-cm trough is created. All vessels encountered during this dissection are tied off with 4-0 or 3-0 polyglycolic acid suture. Dissection carefully proceeds down to the mucosa and great care is exercised to avoid making a rent in the bladder (Fig. 98–4). If this occurs, immediately close the defect with the 6-0 chromic catgut. Place stay sutures of 3-0 polyglycolic acid on the detrusor edges to facilitate dissection of the mucosa off of the detrusor muscle. The mucosal dissection should be generous enough to allow the ureter to easily sit in the newly created trough and permit the detrusor muscle to be closed over the ureter without tension. Prior to this step, further dissection is performed toward the bladder neck beyond the distal most detrusor incision to allow placement of the advancement sutures. Once completed, the ureteral orifice is advanced on the trigone toward the bladder neck with a pair of "vest-type" sutures of 4-0 chromic catgut (Fig. 98–5). The first limb of the sutures is through the detrusor (outside/in). The sutures enter the detrusor at the distal limit of the trigonal musculature and exit in the plane between the mucosa and detrusor. The second limb of the suture is through the ureteral muscle and the final limb of the suture is back through the detrusor (inside/out). Tying the pair of vest sutures advances and anchors the ureteral orifice distally and creates a new longer submucosal tunnel. The remaining detrusor defect is closed over the ureter in two layers; the first is a running layer and the second is an interrupted Lembert suture, both using 4-0 polyglycolic acid suture. Care must be exercised to avoid making the

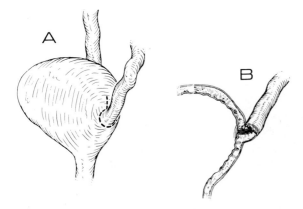

FIG. 98–3. A: After ureteral mobilization detrusor is incised (dotted lines) at level of ureteral hiatus. **B:** Sagittal section demonstrates ureteral hiatus.

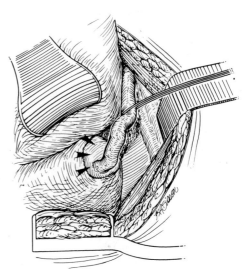

FIG. 98–4. Ureter contiguous with detrusor mucosa (arrowheads).

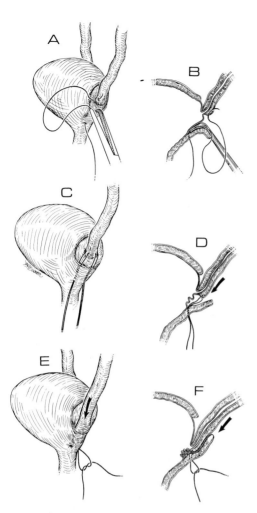

FIG. 98–5. A: Bladder mucosa is elevated off of bladder wall muscle and vest-type sutures are placed. **B:** Sagittal section shows suture passing between undermined mucosa and detrusor. **C:** Alignment of vest sutures after placement. **D:** Sagittal section demonstrates appropriate positioning of sutures. **E:** Tying vest sutures advances and anchors ureter onto trigone. **F:** Sagittal section of ureteromeatal advancement.

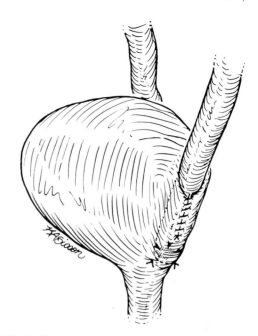

FIG. 98–6. Closure of detrusor flaps over ureter allows for long submucosal tunnel and completes detrusorrhaphy.

ureteral hiatus too snug. The exit point for the ureter should be able to admit a hemostat between the detrusor and the ureter easily (Fig. 98–6). No perivesical drains or ureteral stents are used and the Foley catheter is removed the following morning.

Complete and incomplete ureteral duplication may also be approached extravesically. Cystoscopy at the time of surgery is recommended to visualize the ureteral orifice location with respect to location and proximity to each other as well as distance to the bladder neck. This information will aid in determining if detrusorrhaphy is feasible or if another technique is more appropriate.

Intravesical Approach

One of the earlier and still highly popular and successful techniques to correct reflux is the Politano–Lead-

better approach (11). This procedure is performed entirely intravesical and avoids mobilization of the bladder as seen in the extravesical approach. Once the bladder is exposed via the technique described for the extravesical approach, it is opened in the midline between 3-0 chromic catgut stay sutures. The bladder is packed with moist 4 × 8-inch gauze pads to allow superior retraction of the bladder and easier exposure of the ureteral orifices. This is further facilitated with the placement of a Dennis–Browne retractor with the curved blades actually within the bladder over moist sponges. The ureteral orifice is identified and intubated with a 5 Fr feeding tube and secured with 4-0 or 5-0 silk sutures to allow tenting of the ureter by pulling on the feeding tube. As with all intravesical repairs the ureter is mobilized in similar fashion (Fig. 98–7). An incision is made to score the mucosa around the orifice. This can be done with a scalpel, tenotomy scissor, or, as I prefer, the cutting current of the bovie, which provides a precise incision. Carefully, using long tenotomy scissors, vascular forceps, Kittner dissector, a right-angle clamp, and judicious use of the cautery unit, the muscular attachments to the ureter are taken down. As the dissection proceeds proximally, I have employed the use of a number 3 Freer elevator along the posterior surface of the ureter, which further aids in mobilization. It is critically important to stay outside of the adventitia of the ureter to avoid devascularization during its dissection. As the peritoneum is encountered, it is generously swept back off the ureter to avoid injuring the bowel during the relocation of the ureter. A hernia retractor or a very thin Deaver helps to better expose the peritoneum and extravesical attach-

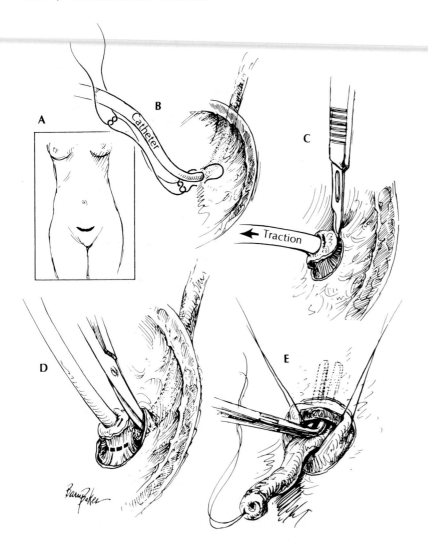

FIG. 98–7. Intravesical mobilization of ureter. **A:** Low transverse incision. **B:** A 3.5 or 5.0 Fr polyethylene tube and traction suture. **C:** Incision around meatus with mucosal cuff using long-handled knife. **D:** Cutting and blunt dissection of muscle of superficial trigone. **E:** Extravesical mobilization with right-angle clamp and Kittner dissector.

ments to the ureter. Take care in the male to avoid injury to the vas deferens.

After completion of ureteral mobilization, the surgeon may choose one of several procedures to complete the ureteral reimplantation. The Politano–Leadbetter repair employs a suprahiatal approach (Figs. 98–8 and 98–9). A submucosal tunnel is created from the old hiatus superiorly, long enough to achieve a 5:1 ratio of submucosal tunnel to ureteral diameter. I like to use a 135-degree blunt-tip Metzenbaum scissors to facilitate this maneuver and avoid tearing the bladder mucosa. Once the desired tunnel length is achieved, the new hiatus is developed by making a small incision directly on top of a right-angle clamp. Using a stay suture or the feeding tube, the mobilized ureter is passed from the old hiatus to the new hiatus, care being taken to avoid twisting, kinking, or angulating the ureter as well as avoiding the peritoneum. The old hiatus is repaired with 4-0 chromic catgut. The ureter is then brought through the new tunnel. The old meatus is then trimmed up and spatulated if necessary. The distal and posterior lip of the ureter is anchored first with a deep suture of 4-0 or 5-0 chromic catgut to the mucosa

and muscular layers of the bladder. The remaining anastomosis is performed with the same suture for a mucosal-to-mucosal approximation. Leaving a ureteral stent is at the surgeon's preference. In general, I assess how the urine output appears from the reimplanted ureteral orifice. If there is copious drainage, I do not leave a stent. If I am uncomfortable with urine drainage or there is significant edema at the orifice, a stent is left and brought out through a separate stab wound in the bladder and secured there with a chromic catgut suture. Then, a separate stab wound is made to bring the stent out through the skin and secured there with 4-0 nylon. Likewise, if I have to taper the ureter a stent is left in place for 4 to 7 days postoperatively. I close all bladders in three layers using running 4-0 chromic catgut for the mucosa, muscularis, and seromuscular layers. This has allowed me to avoid leaving any perivesical drains when the ureters are not stented. A Foley catheter remains in the bladder for 1 or 2 postoperative days.

The Glenn–Anderson procedure (Fig. 98–10) (4), in comparison to the Politano–Leadbetter, is an infrahiatal repair and develops a submucosal tunnel toward the blad-

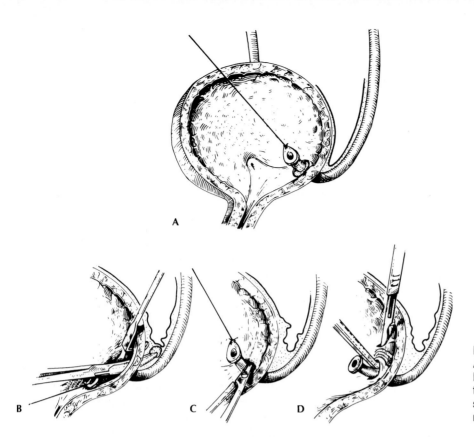

FIG. 98–8. Politano–Leadbetter repair. **A:** Mobilization of intravesical ureter. **B:** Dissection of peritoneum with Kittner dissector. **C:** Development of submucosal tunnel. **D:** Creation of the new hiatus.

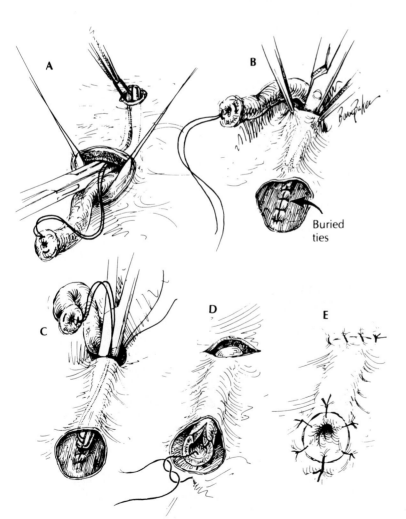

Buried ties

FIG. 98–9. Politano–Leadbetter repair and details of ureteral reimplant. **A:** The ureter is brought through the new hiatus, and the old hiatus is closed with interrupted absorbable suture. **B:** The ureter is brought through the new tunnel (**C**), spatulated if necessary (**D**), and sewn in place with interrupted absorbable suture (**E**).

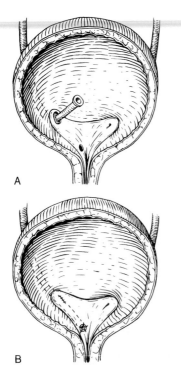

FIG. 98–10. Glenn–Anderson repair. (From Walker RW. Vesi-coureteral reflux. In: Gillenwater JY, Grahhack JR, Howards SS, Duckett JW Jr, eds. *Adult and pediatric urology*, vol 2. St. Louis: Mosby–Year Book, 1996, with permission.)

der neck (Fig. 98–11). It is in particular advantageous when there is good distance between the native ureteral orifice and the bladder neck such that an appropriate tunnel length can be obtained. Adequate mobilization of the ureter is paramount to achieve satisfactory success rates. If the tunnel length appears too short on initial inspection, moving the hiatus more superiorly will allow for satisfactory tunnel creation. Advantages of the Glenn–Anderson technique are that the entire procedure is done under direct vision and creates a relatively straight tunnel with an easily catheterized ureter.

The transtrigonal approach (Cohen) (2) is similar to the Glenn–Anderson procedure with the exception that the ureter is transposed across the trigone (Fig. 98–12). This is in particular useful in small-capacity and neurogenic bladders where an appropriately long tunnel is critical to success. The ureteral course created is an extension of the natural direction of the ureter; thus, it carries a low risk of ureteral kinking and obstruction. If bilateral reimplant is necessary, it is important to create separate tunnel paths for each ureter. Always remember to close the hiatus with absorbable 4-0 chromic catgut. Leave enough room for a hemostat or right-angle clamp to be interposed between the ureter and the approximated detrusor muscle to avoid obstruction at the hiatus. A potential disadvantage of the Cohen technique is the dif-

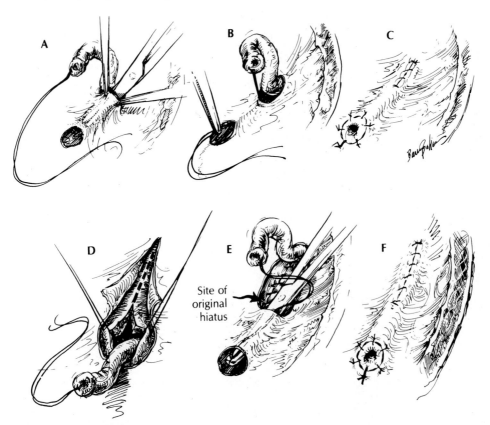

FIG. 98–11. Glenn–Anderson repair: Details of ureteral reimplantation. **A:** Tunnel made toward bladder neck. The ureter is brought through the tunnel (**B**) and sewn in place (**C**). An alternative, similar to the Mathison technique, allows enlargement of hiatus (**D**) and results in longer (**E, F**).

duplication can be approached extravesically as well as intravesically. The key to intravesical surgery is to mobilize the duplicated ureters as one unit because their blood supply at the bladder level is intertwined within a common sheath (Fig. 98–13). This will avoid unnecessary devascularization. The technique chosen for reimplant can be any of the intravesical repairs mentioned. In cases of a low-lying incomplete duplication, an ipsilateral ureteroureterostomy is an attractive alternative. In situations where there is an associated ectopic ureter with a salvageable renal moiety, separate ureteral tunnels should be created.

One tip that I have found useful to aid in freeing up the ureter and also with submucosal dissection for all of the intravesical techniques is the use of 1% lidocaine (Xylocaine) with a 1:100,000 epinephrine solution. This is injected periureterally at the orifice and along the proposed subepithelial tunnel using a 26-gauge needle. This minimizes bleeding and provides ease of dissection in a readily defined plane.

Intra–Extravesical Approach

The Paquin technique (Fig. 98–14) (10) is a commonly used repair and has the advantage over the Politano–Leadbetter approach of doing the complete procedure under direct vision, thus avoiding the potential risk of peritoneal injury. The approach to the ureter is extravesical, similar to that described in detrusorrhaphy. When the ureter is mobilized to the level of the detrusor hiatus, a right-angle clamp is used to clamp the ureter and then oversew the distal stump after the ureter has been divided using polyglycolic acid suture. Alternatively, the bladder may be opened in the midline and the ureteral orifice circumscribed and mobilized from within the bladder. The ureter should be intubated with a 5 or 8 Fr feeding tube and secured with a suture prior to mobilization. The ureter is then passed extravesically, taking care to avoid the peritoneum, which should be swept off of the posterior lateral bladder wall. If ureteral tailoring is warranted, it is performed at this point of the procedure. If a longer tunnel is needed and ureteral length is suspect, consider a psoas hitch at this time as well (Fig. 98–15). Using two fingers inside the bladder, bring the bladder up to the psoas muscle tendon where it should sit under no tension. Place interrupted figure of eight sutures of heavy chromic or polyglycolic acid from the tendon of the psoas to the bladder wall just lateral to where the new ureteral hiatus will be situated. Avoid the genitofemoral nerve running along the psoas muscle during this maneuver. Likewise, the vas deferens in boys and the fallopian tubes in girls must be protected.

A submucosal tunnel is created as described for the Politano–Leadbetter repair. The ureter is brought through the new hiatus, under the subepithelial tunnel, and secured its the new location. Care is taken to avoid twist-

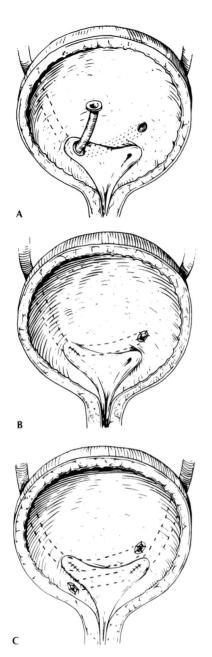

FIG. 98–12. Cohen technique of ureteral reimplantation. Cross-trigonal tunnel, with the stippled area (**A**) sewn in place with interrupted sutures (**B**). **C:** Bilateral reimplants easily accomplished. (From Walker RW. Vesicoureteral reflux. In: Gillenwater JY, Grayhack JT, Howards SS, Duckett JW Jr, eds. *Adult and pediatric urology*, vol 2. St. Louis: Mosby–Year Book, 1996, with permission.)

ficulty of ureteral access postoperatively. These patients may need percutaneous access for any future procedures.

Ureteral Duplication

Determining whether the ureteral duplication is complete or incomplete guides operative considerations. In the absence of a ureterocele, an intravesical complete

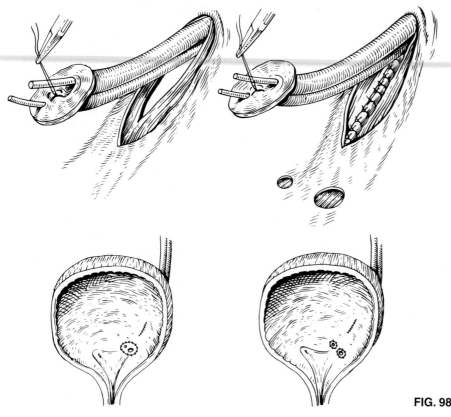

FIG. 98–13. Reimplantation of duplex ureters.

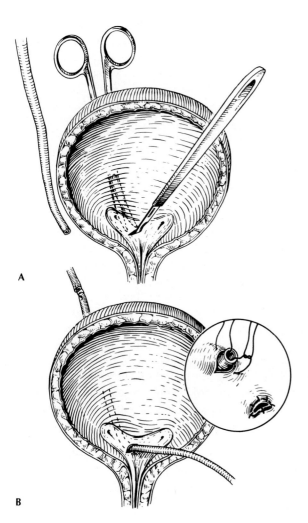

A

B

FIG. 98–14. Paquin repair.

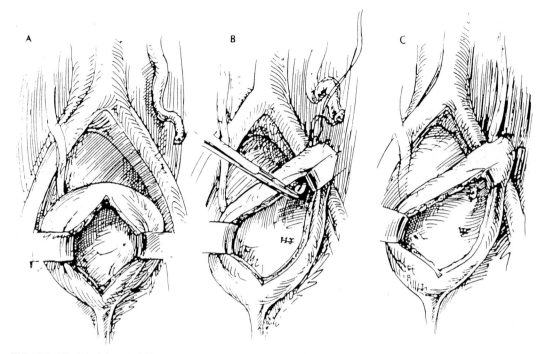

FIG. 98–15. Bladder mobilized and sutured to psoas over iliac vessels by psoas hitch. **A:** Blunt dissection and exposure of psoas tendon and iliac vessels. **B:** Psoas hitch with interrupted absorbable sutures. **C:** Completed reimplant. Long submucosal tunnel to prevent reflux is shown. (From Ehrlich RM, Melman A, Skinner DG. The use of the vesicopsoas hitch in urologic surgery. *J Urol* 1978;119:324, with permission.)

ing or kinking the ureter as it is brought back intravesically. As with all of the intravesical techniques, after the final ureteral anastomosis is complete, a 5 Fr feeding tube should easily pass up through the reimplanted ureter to the kidney.

Laparoscopic Repair

The modern era of laparoscopy has brought forth many new and innovative techniques. These new procedures have been designed to decrease morbidity and hospital costs as well as speed patient recovery. Among these is the laparoscopic extravesical ureteral reimplant. Designed to emulate the Lich–Gregoir repair, this repair is at present utilized in few centers specializing in laparoscopic technique. This particular repair requires two surgeons and can be performed intraperitoneally or retroperitoneally. The technique for intraperitoneal access has been well described. In the pediatric population, access to the peritoneum should be performed using an open technique. I do this using the 10-mm Hassan trocar to avoid intraperitoneal injury. Once the pneumoperitoneum is created, three other trocars are placed. A second 10-mm trocar (instruments) is placed 1 to 5 cm above the infraumbilical site(camera) on the opposite side of the refluxing ureter in the midclavicular line. Two 5-mm trocars are placed in the left and right midclavicular lines at the level of the anterior superior iliac spine for dissecting

instruments and retraction. The operating room table is rotated away from the refluxing side to shift the peritoneal contents and bladder away from the operative location. The peritoneum is incised over the iliac vessels, where the obliterated hypogastric artery is recognized. The ureter is identified (Fig. 98–16), grasped with a Babcock-type instrument, and tented up to allow dissection and mobilization of the ureter for 3 or 4 cm proximal to its detrusor insertion. This will allow placement of the ureter within a trough that is to be created. Next, using electrocautery the muscle layer of the bladder is incised for approximately 3 cm proximal to the ureterovesical junction. Spreading carefully with scissors will expose the mucosa. Dissection continues for the length of the tunnel until the mucosa bulges throughout the incision. The ureter is placed in the trough and the detrusor edges are approximated and the ureter advanced with a fixation suture at the distal most part of the trough. The remaining detrusor defect is closed over the ureter with either absorbable polydioxanone suture or staples. A Foley catheter is left overnight.

At present, laparoscopic correction of reflux takes longer then traditional repairs and the incisions made are actually more unsightly than the single lower-abdominal incision done for open surgery. The instruments used are more costly. As a whole, the laparoscopic repair is not yet as cost effective as either open surgery or endoscopic correction.

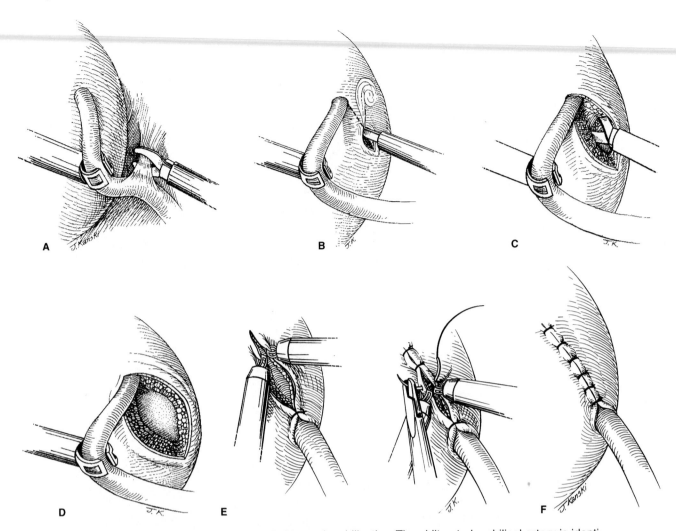

FIG. 98–16. Laparoscopic reimplant. **A:** Ureteral mobilization. The obliterated umbilical artery is identified and traced distally until the ureter is seen. The ureter is grasped gently and the periureteral tissue dissected bluntly toward the ureterovescial junction. **B–D:** Creation of bladder wall trough. Bladder wall is incised with electrocautery 3 cm proximal to the ureterovesical junction. Muscle fibers are gently cut and spread. Dissection is complete when mucosal tissue bulges outward. **E:** After placing the ureter in the trough-grasping instruments, the superior aspect of the bladder wall is wrapped around the ureter and a suture placed proximally, immobilizing the ureter in the trough (left). Remaining sutures are placed throughout the length of the tunnel (right). **F:** Completed repair. (From Atala A, Keating M. Vesicoureteral reflux. In: Walsh PC, Retik AB, Wein A, Vaughan ED, eds. *Campbell's urology*, vol 2. Philadelphia: WB Saunders, 1997, with permission.)

POSTOPERATIVE CARE

The patient stays on prophylactic antibiotics until reflux has been shown to be resolved. An ultrasound of the kidneys and bladder is usually done 4 to 6 weeks after surgery to assess for occult hydronephrosis and hydroureter. Assuming the ultrasound is normal, a follow-up voiding cystourethrogram or nuclear cystogram is performed 3 months later to assess the surgical result. If reflux is no longer present, I routinely repeat a renal ultrasound 1 year later to make sure that anatomically all is well. Should known renal scarring be present, then yearly urinalysis, blood pressure measurements, and periodic ultrasounds are recommended.

OUTCOMES

Complications

Fortunately, the success rates for open surgery to correct reflux approach 98% for nondilated ureters and those with normal bladder function. In cases with dilated ureters, significant voiding dysfunction, neuropathic bladder, and anatomic conditions such as prune belly syndrome and posterior urethral valves, the success rates diminish somewhat. Previously unrecognized bladder and bowel dysfunction are the most common causes of postoperative problems and need to be vigorously addressed. The most common complication is persisting reflux on the operative side or contralateral reflux of a previously nonrefluxing ureter. In most cases observation is the treatment of choice as the vast majority of these patients will have spontaneous resolution of reflux within 1 year. Always look for voiding or bowel dysfunction in any case of persistent reflux. If the recurrent reflux is high grade then most likely there was a technical failure such as not creating a long enough tunnel or insufficient ureteral mobilization. These cases frequently require reoperation. Always treat any voiding problems first.

Ureteral obstruction is a fortunately a rare complication of reflux surgery and frequently is transient in nature, resulting from postoperative bladder spasms, edema, or blood clots. Hence, it is not unusual to see some mild renal or ureteral dilatation in the first few weeks after surgery on sonography. Should problems persist ureteral stenting or percutaneous nephrostomy will help temporize the situation until resolution occurs spontaneously or surgical reimplantation is performed. Higher-grade obstructions usually present with a variety of symptoms such as flank pain, fever, nausea, vomiting, and ileus. These are due to angulation, obstruction at the hiatus, extravasation (of a tapered ureter), or ureteral ischemia with resultant stricturing. Urinary diversion or stenting is paramount in these situations and redo reimplantation required. If the remaining ureter is too short to reimplant in the standard fashion, consider a psoas hitch or a transureteral ureterostomy.

Bladder diverticula are usually the result of a defect in the closure of the muscular hiatus at the original procedure. If the diverticula is wide mouthed and drains well in the absence of obstruction or reflux, then observation is all that is needed. In the presence of ureteral pathology or poor drainage of the diverticula, surgical correction is necessary.

Conclusions

Surgical management of vesicoureteral reflux is a highly successful if performed for the right indications and one adheres to the proper principals of good surgical technique. There are a myriad of corrective techniques available, each with their respective advantages and disadvantages. It is up to the individual surgeon to decide what works best in his or her hands after analyzing the available information on their respective patients.

REFERENCES

1. Aaronson IA, Rames RA, Greene WB, et al. Endoscopic treatment of reflux: migration of Teflon to the lungs and brain. *Eur Urol* 1993;23: 394.
2. Cohen SJ. The Cohen reimplantation technique. *Birth Defects* 1977;13: 391.
3. Duckett JW. Vesicoureteral reflux: a conservative analysis. *Am J Kidney Dis* 1983;3:139–144.
4. Glen JF, Anderson EE. Technical considerations in distal tunnel ureteral reimplantation. *J Urol* 1978;119:194.
5. Gregoir W, Van Regemorter GV. Le reflux vesico-ureteral congenital. *Urol Int* 1964;18:122.
6. Gruber CM. A comparative study of the intravesical ureters (ureterovesical valves) in man and in experimental animals. *J Urol* 1929;21:567.
7. Hutch JA. Vesicoureteral reflux in the paraplegic: Cause and correction. *J Urol* 1952;68:457.
8. International Reflux Study Committee. Medical versus surgical treatment of primary vesicoureteral reflux. *Pediatrics* 1981;67:392–400.
9. Lich R Jr, Howerton LW, Davis LA. Recurrent urosepsis in children. *J Urol* 1961; 86:554.
10. Paquin AJ. Ureterovesical anastomosis. The description and evaluation of a technique. *J Urol* 1959;82:573.
11. Politano VA, Leadbetter WF. An operative technique for the correction of vesicoureteral reflux. *J Urol* 1958;79:932–941.
12. Sampson JA. Ascending renal infection with special reference to the reflux of urine from the bladder into the ureters. *Johns Hopkins Hosp Bull* 1903;14:334.
13. Skoog SJ, Belman AB, Majd M. A nonsurgical approach to the management of primary vesicoureteral reflux. *J Urol* 1987;138:941.
14. Stephens FD, Lenaghan D. The anatomical basis and dynamics of vesicoureteral reflux. *J Urol* 1962;87:669.
15. Weiss R, Duckett J, Spitzer A, on behalf of the International Reflux Study in Children. Results of a randomized clinical trial of medical vs. surgical management of infants and children with grades III and IV primary vesicoureteral reflux (United States). *J Urol* 1992;148: 1667.
16. Young HH, Wesson MB. The anatomy and surgery of the trigone. *Arch Surg* 1921;3:1.
17. Zaontz MR, Maizels M, Sugar EC, Firlit. Detrusorrhaphy: extravesical ureteral advancement to correct vesicoureteral reflux in children. *J Urol* 1987;138:947–949.

CHAPTER 99

Ureteroceles

Chester J. Koh and David A. Diamond

Ureteroceles are congenital cystic dilations of the intravesical submucosal ureter. They are more commonly found in female children and are almost exclusively diagnosed in Caucasians. Approximately 10% of these children have bilateral ureteroceles. Ureteroceles may be "orthotopic" and contained entirely within the bladder or "ectopic" and partially situated at the bladder neck or urethra. An orthotopic ureterocele is typically associated with a single collecting system, while an ectopic ureterocele is usually associated with the upper-pole moiety of a kidney with complete ureteral duplication.

DIAGNOSIS

Increasingly, ureteroceles are diagnosed by prenatal ultrasonography, which can demonstrate both the intravesical cystic dilation as well as the corresponding hydronephrosis. These patients should undergo a comprehensive postnatal urologic evaluation and be placed on prophylactic antibiotics, which may help to prevent future urinary tract infections (UTIs) (9).

However, for many children the diagnosis of ureterocele is only made after a UTI or urosepsis. Ureteroceles can also present as a palpable abdominal mass usually representing a hydronephrotic kidney, or as a vaginal mass, which represents prolapse of an ectopic ureterocele. Large ureteroceles may even lead to obstruction of the bladder neck or of the contralateral ureteral orifice, which may result in bilateral hydronephrosis.

Ultrasonography is, in general, the first radiological study obtained in diagnosing ureteroceles. In addition to the intravesical cystic dilation, ureteroceles are usually seen with duplex collecting systems, with the ureterocele being associated with hydronephrosis of the upper-pole moiety.

A voiding cystourethrogram (VCUG) is essential in the evaluation of the patient with a ureterocele because of the high incidence of concomitant ipsilateral vesicoureteral reflux. In addition to the reflux, VCUG can demonstrate the size and location of the ureterocele.

Currently, the dimercapto succinic acid (DMSA) renal scan provides the most precise estimates of the differential renal function between each kidney, as well as of the associated upper pole's contribution to the overall renal function. DMSA scans may even detect lower moiety abnormalities that may not have been demonstrated by ultrasonography (2).

Intravenous urography (IVU) is less commonly used in the modern evaluation of ureteroceles. However, in cases of unusual urinary tract anatomy IVU may be helpful in the delineation of previously undefined anatomy. Severe hydroureteronephrosis associated with a ureterocele may lead to lateral deviation of the upper pole away from the spine.

INDICATIONS FOR SURGERY

The goals of surgical treatment should be the preservation of renal function, elimination of obstruction and reflux, prevention or elimination of infection, and maintenance of urinary continence (8) while minimizing surgical morbidity. The main factors to consider in developing an individual treatment plan should be patient age, patient's clinical presentation, ureterocele size and anatomy, presence of reflux and UTI, and function of the involved renal segments.

ALTERNATIVE THERAPY

The anatomy and clinical presentations of children with ureteroceles vary widely. Therefore, each child should have an individualized treatment plan as no single method of surgical repair is appropriate for all cases. Table 99–1 lists some therapeutic options for patients with ureteroceles.

TABLE 99–1. *Ureterocele therapeutic options*

Upper-Pole Preservation
  Endoscopic Incision of the Ureterocele
  Complete Lower-Tract Reconstruction (Excision of
    Ureterocele with Ureteral Reimplantation)
  Ureteroureterostomy/Ureteropyelostomy
Upper-Pole Ablation
  Upper-Tract Approach (Upper-Pole Nephrectomy and
    Partial Ureterectomy)
Complete Reconstruction

SURGICAL TECHNIQUE

Techniques that preserve functional upper-pole moieties are listed below. However, in many instances the upper pole has little to no contribution to the overall renal function and upper-pole ablative techniques, also described below, may be indicated.

Upper-Pole Preservation

Endoscopic Incision of the Ureterocele

The goal of endoscopic incision of ureteroceles is to decompress the ureterocele in a minimally invasive manner while minimizing the risk of postincision vesicoureteral reflux and the need for further urinary tract reconstruction (4). This technique can be used in infants if infant-sized endoscopic equipment is available and should be used to drain obstructive urinary systems in any ureterocele patient with urosepsis. Blyth and coauthors recommended the use of a 3 Fr Bugbee wire electrode (using the cutting current) to incise the roof of the ureterocele through its full thickness near its base and proximal to the bladder neck (1). A new unobstructed intravesical ureteral orifice will be created, and the roof of the collapsed ureterocele can act as a flap-valve mechanism to prevent reflux. While the Bugbee electrode has been a widely utilized instrument for ureterocele puncture, it has limitations, primarily that following initial decompression enlargement of the puncture site is difficult. Therefore, we prefer to use the pediatric resectoscope and the right-angle hook electrode with the cutting current, which allows one to make a clean transverse incision and enlarge it by placing the hook into the original incision and withdrawing under vision (Fig. 99–1). Magnification with the use of video projection helps improve the accuracy of the incision. Making the incision as distal and as close to the bladder neck as possible should reduce the risk of postoperative reflux into the corresponding ureter. The adequacy of the incision can be confirmed by the presence of a jet of urine from the ureterocele or by visualization of the urothelium inside the ureterocele. The major advantage of the endoscopic incision is that it can be done on an outpatient basis, without the need for hospitalization.

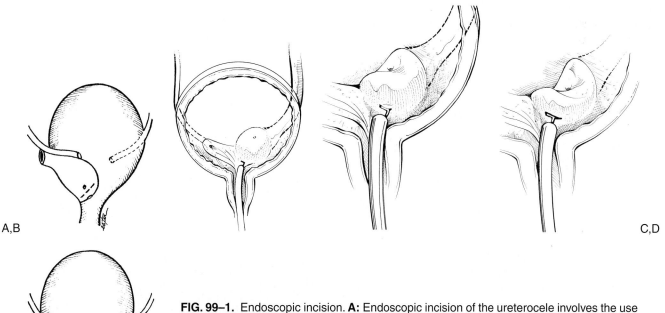

A,B

C,D

E

FIG. 99–1. Endoscopic incision. **A:** Endoscopic incision of the ureterocele involves the use of the pediatric resectoscope and the right-angle hook electrode with the cutting current to create a small transverse incision proximal to the bladder neck. **B:** The right-angle hook electrode in position for the initial decompression. **C:** The ureterocele after the initial decompression. **D:** The right-angle hook electrode in position for enlarging the incision. **E:** After drainage, the ureterocele collapses and acts as a flap valve to prevent reflux; the lower-pole ureter lies over the collapsed ureterocele.

Complete Lower-Tract Reconstruction (Excision of Ureterocele with Ureteral Reimplantation)

For excision of the ureterocele and common sheath reimplantation of upper- and lower-pole ureters, a Pfannenstiel incision is made and the bladder is opened (Fig. 99–2). The lower pole and contralateral ureters are intubated with 5 Fr feeding tubes and multiple circumferential stay sutures are placed. A circumferential incision is made around the perimeter of the ureterocele with electrocautery and the wall of the ureterocele and its associated upper-pole ureter are dissected away from the thinned posterior muscular wall of the bladder, incorporating the lower-pole ureter in the dissection. All attempts should be made to avoid injury to the sphincteric mechanisms at the bladder neck during the distal dissection of the ureterocele. The upper- and lower-pole ureters are dissected as a common sheath to avoid injury to the blood supply of both ureters. After excising the distal ureterocele, the dilated upper-pole ureter often requires tapering. The thin posterior bladder wall is repaired by imbrication of adjacent muscle with running 3-0 absorbable sutures to provide sufficient muscle backing for the reimplanted ureters. An unoperated portion of the bladder floor is selected and the ureters are reimplanted as a common sheath into a generous ureteral tunnel.

Ureteroureterostomy/Ureteropyelostomy

In upper urinary tract anastomotic techniques, the dissection of the upper tracts should be kept to a minimum, and mobilization should be directed toward the upper-pole ureter, so that distortion of the adjacent lower-pole ureter can be avoided. Because the upper-pole ureter is usually larger than the lower-pole ureter, generous spatulation of the ureters during ureteroureterostomy may be necessary for an optimal end-to-side anastomosis. Furthermore, a feeding tube should be passed distally into the ureterocele to decompress it.

Upper-Pole Ablation

Upper-Tract Approach (Upper-Pole Nephrectomy and Partial Ureterectomy)

In many cases, the upper pole associated with the ureterocele has minimal or no contribution to the overall renal function. The upper-tract approach (upper-pole nephrectomy and partial ureterectomy) should lead to the relief of obstruction, prevention of recurrent infection, and resolution of the reflux that is present in about half of these patients. This approach should result in the decompression

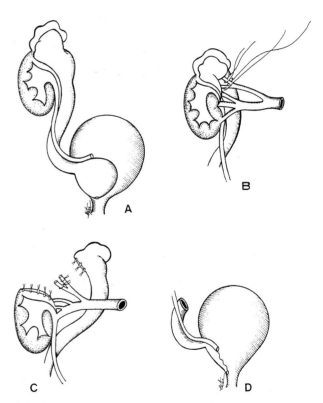

FIG. 99–3. Upper-pole partial nephrectomy and partial ureterectomy. **A:** This procedure is commonly used for a duplex system with a nonfunctioning upper pole and minimal or absent ipsilateral reflux. **B:** The upper-pole ureter is transected early after a stay suture has been placed proximally. Upward traction on the proximal portion of the transected ureter assists in the manipulation of the upper pole during the partial nephrectomy. **C:** After removal of the upper pole, the wedge-shaped kidney defect is repaired with 3-0 chromic sutures in a vertical mattress fashion. **D:** This approach should result in the decompression of the ureterocele, with the return of the trigone to a more normal configuration.

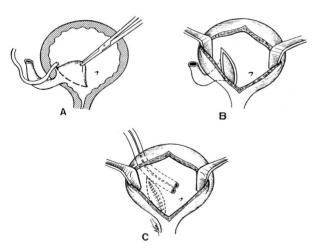

FIG. 99–2. Complete lower-tract reconstruction. **A:** After the bladder is opened, multiple circumferential stay sutures are placed around the ureterocele to assist with the excision. **B:** All ureters should be intubated with 5 Fr feeding tubes for identification of the ureters during the dissection. **C:** After excising the ureterocele, the posterior bladder wall is repaired with running 3-0 absorbable sutures and the ureters are reimplanted into a generous tunnel.

of the ureterocele, hopefully with resolution of the ipsilateral lower-pole reflux, because the trigone will be returned to a more normal configuration. This usually eliminates the need for lower-tract reconstruction with a potentially difficult bladder neck and urethral dissection (8).

For the upper-pole heminephrectomy, we suggest the use of the flank approach, which offers superior access to the upper-pole vessels. Care should be taken to avoid excessive retraction upon the kidney to avoid damage to the viable lower pole. In many cases, the upper pole resembles a dysplastic nubbin, and early division of the upper-pole ureter and upward traction on the proximal portion of the transected ureter usually helps in the definition and manipulation of the upper pole (Fig. 99–3). After the upper-pole vessels are sequentially ligated, demarcation of the upper-pole parenchyma should become apparent. We recommend the use of a no. 15 blade or electrocautery around the upper-pole parenchyma, which usually results in a wedge-shaped defect. During the dissection of the upper-pole parenchyma, the plane of dissection should remain as close to the upper-pole ureter to avoid injury to the vascular supply of the lower-pole ureter. After the upper-pole nephrectomy, the wedge-shaped defect is closed with interrupted 3-0 chromic sutures in a vertical mattress fashion, which achieves effective hemostasis.

Complete Reconstruction

In certain instances, a complete reconstruction may be indicated where both an upper-tract repair and a lower-tract reconstruction are performed via separate incisions in a single stage. These situations include the presence of high-grade reflux into the ipsilateral lower-pole ureter or the presence of lower-pole reflux associated with a large, everting ureterocele and a nonfunctioning upper pole. Depending on the amount of upper-tract function, either an upper-pole nephrectomy with partial ureterectomy or a ureteropyelostomy (as described above) are performed for the upper-tract repair. Lower-tract reconstruction is also performed, which involves the excision of the ureterocele with reimplantation of the ureters as a common sheath, as previously described.

OUTCOMES

Complications

Excision of the ureterocele with ureteral reimplantation achieves the goal of upper-tract drainage. However, the disadvantage of this approach is the morbidity associated with bladder surgery, including hematuria, bladder spasm, and catheter drainage. Extensive distal dissection also carries the risk of bladder neck and sphincteric injury, which may jeopardize urinary continence (3).

Results

Endoscopic incision of the ureterocele may be the only surgical procedure required for many patients. For infants, endoscopic incision may be used as a temporizing measure that achieves early decompression. Secondary surgery, if necessary, can be performed electively when the child is older. If the ureterocele is orthotopic, one can expect high rates of decompression and low rates of de novo reflux and the need for secondary procedures (5). On the other hand, ectopic ureteroceles are associated with a high rate of secondary surgery and a significant incidence of postoperative reflux after endoscopic incision. Therefore, patients with ectopic ureteroceles may be best served by more definitive reconstruction, even those less than 1 year of age (6).

The upper-tract approach, which includes upper-pole nephrectomy and partial ureterectomy, is usually reserved for the patient with an upper pole that provides little or no contribution to the overall renal function and mild or absent ipsilateral reflux. This approach has the advantage of avoiding the lower-tract complications noted above.

For patients who are at significant risk for requiring a second procedure with some of the approaches detailed above, such as those patients with large, ectopic ureteroceles or high-grade ipsilateral reflux, complete upper- and lower-tract reconstruction in a single stage has the advantage of expediency (7).

REFERENCES

1. Blyth B, Passerini-Glazel G, Camuffo C, Snyder HM III, Duckett JW. Endoscopic incision of ureteroceles: intravesical versus ectopic. J Urol 1993;149:556–559; discussion 560.
2. Connolly LP, Connolly SA, Drubach LA, Zurakowski D, Ted Treves S. Ectopic ureteroceles in infants with prenatal hydronephrosis: use of renal cortical scintigraphy. Clin Nucl Med 2002;27:169–175.
3. Coplen DE, Duckett JW. The modern approach to ureteroceles. J Urol 1995;153:166–171.
4. De Filippo RE, Bauer SB. New surgical techniques in pediatric urology. Curr Opin Urol 2001;11:591–596.
5. Hagg MJ, Mourachov PV, Snyder HM, et al. The modern endoscopic approach to ureterocele. J Urol 2000;163:940–943.
6. Husmann D, Strand B, Ewalt D, Clement M, Kramer S, Allen T. Management of ectopic ureterocele associated with renal duplication: a comparison of partial nephrectomy and endoscopic decompression. J Urol 1999;162:1406–1409.
7. Scherz HC, Kaplan GW, Packer MG, Brock WA. Ectopic ureteroceles: surgical management with preservation of continence—review of 60 cases. J Urol 1989;142:538–541; discussion 542–543.
8. Schlussel RN, Retik AB. Ectopic ureter, ureterocele, and other anomalies of the ureter. In: Walsh PC, ed. Campbell's urology, 8th ed. Philadelphia, WB Saunders, 2002:2022–2034.
9. Upadhyay J, Bolduc S, Braga L, et al. Impact of prenatal diagnosis on the morbidity associated with ureterocele management. J Urol 2002; 167:2560–2565.

CHAPTER 100

Urachal Anomalies and Related Umbilical Disorders

Leslie D. Tackett and Anthony A. Caldamone

During bladder development, the urogenital sinus is initially contiguous with the allantois. When the lumen of the allantoic duct becomes obliterated, the urachus remains connecting the bladder to the umbilicus (Figs. 100–1A and 100–1B). It continues to elongate as the fetus grows. The urachus is a muscular tube, with a length ranging from 3 to 10 cm and a diameter of approximately 8 to 10 mm, that extends from the dome of the bladder to the umbilicus. It has three distinct tissue layers: (a) an epithelial-lined lumen with cuboidal or transitional epithelium, (b) an intermediate connective tissue layer, and (c) an outer smooth muscle layer. In the adult, the urachus lies between two layers of umbilicovesical fascia along with the umbilical ligaments and the remnants of the obliterated umbilical arteries. This fascial investment tends to contain the spread of urachal disease between the peritoneum and transversalis fascia (Fig. 100–1C).

The urachus normally closes or involutes at approximately 32 weeks gestation, and urachal anomalies in general represent an abnormality in this process. These anomalies are characterized as patent urachus, urachal cyst, urachal sinus, and urachal diverticulum (Fig. 100–2) (1,2).

DIAGNOSIS

In general, the diagnosis of urachal anomalies requires clinical suspicion and a thorough physical examination. Further evaluation in patients with periumbilical drainage should include a sinogram, and those with a periumbilical mass should undergo ultrasonographic imaging. A voiding cystourethrogram may only be required in selected patients (4,8).

Complete failure of the urachal lumen to close results in an open connection between the bladder and the umbilicus. Patients present with umbilical leakage of urine and often a protruding tissue mass (Fig. 100–3). The leakage may be more obvious during times of increased intraabdominal pressure such as crying, coughing, or straining. The fluid may be analyzed for urea and creatinine to confirm its urinary quality. Two factors thought to contribute to a persistent patent urachus are bladder outlet obstruction and failure of the bladder to descend into the pelvis (5,6,9). With regard to bladder outlet obstruction, distal urinary obstruction is thought not to be the only causative factor because normally the urachus closes developmentally before the urethra becomes tubularized (11). In addition only 14% of patients with patent urachus demonstrate bladder outlet obstruction clinically, and it is uncommon for a patent urachus to be associated with posterior urethral valves. The diagnosis may be confirmed with a sinogram although a voiding cystourethrogram may be more useful because it may rule out bladder outlet obstruction concurrently. Alternatively, methylene blue or indigo carmine may be instilled in either the bladder or the umbilical opening and detected in the umbilicus or bladder, respectively. The differential diagnosis for patent urachus includes patent omphalomesenteric duct, urachal sinus, omphalitis, granulation of a healing umbilical stump, and infected umbilical vessel.

Segmental or incomplete closure of the urachal lumen may result in the formation of a urachal cyst (Fig. 100–4). The cyst usually forms in the proximal or lower third of the urachal remnant near the bladder (10). Usually, the cyst is lined with transitional epithelium and filled with serous fluid, but mucinous contents have been described. In general, urachal cysts are small and asymptomatic. Symptoms such as pain, redness with localized swelling, and tenderness below the umbilicus may occur with infection and may be accompanied by chills, fever, irritative voiding symptoms, hematuria, and pyuria. Alterna-

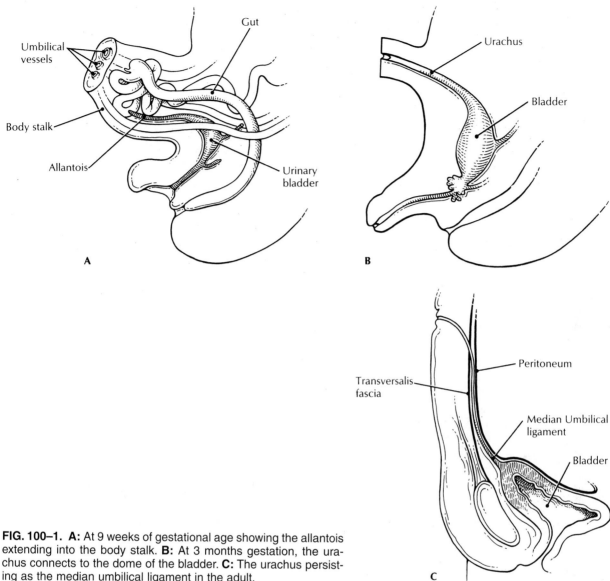

FIG. 100–1. A: At 9 weeks of gestational age showing the allantois extending into the body stalk. **B:** At 3 months gestation, the urachus connects to the dome of the bladder. **C:** The urachus persisting as the median umbilical ligament in the adult.

tively, symptoms may arise as the result of mass effect due to a large urachal cyst. These patients present with a sensation of abdominal fullness or pain, a mass, or irritative voiding symptoms due to compression of the bladder. Diagnosis is most easily confirmed by ultrasound or computed tomography (CT).

Incomplete closure of the urachus may also result in a urachal sinus. This may be the result of a urachal cyst that extended either to the bladder or to the skin for drainage. Some urachal sinuses may alternate and at first drain at the umbilicus and then later into the bladder. Presenting symptoms may include periumbilical redness and tenderness with intermittent drainage, umbilical irritation or granulation tissue, or symptoms of urinary tract infection. Clinical suspicion of a urachal sinus may be confirmed by a sinogram or ultrasound. A cystogram may show an irregular area at the dome of the bladder. Cystoscopy may demonstrate an inflamed area at the dome that may extrude purulent drainage.

A urachal diverticulum results from failure of closure of the urachus adjacent to the bladder, leaving a wide-mouth diverticulum at the dome of the bladder. Most commonly, the urachal diverticulum may or may not be associated with bladder outlet obstruction as has been often reported in patients with prune belly syndrome. In general, aside from treatment for any coexisting bladder outlet obstruction, the urachal diverticulum requires no specific management as it usually drains well.

Omphalomesenteric disorders may be confused with urachal anomalies. The omphalomesenteric duct is a fetal structure that connects the yolk sac and the gut. Incomplete closure of this tubular structure may lead to a patent

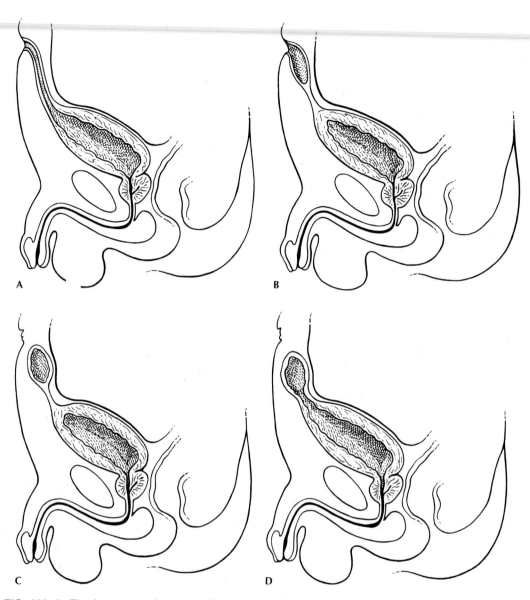

FIG. 100–2. The four types of abnormalities involving the urachus. **A:** Complete patency to the umbilicus. **B:** A blind-ending urachal sinus open at the umbilicus but not complete to the bladder. **C:** A urachal cyst without communication to either the umbilicus or the bladder. **D:** Simple diverticulum from the dome of the bladder.

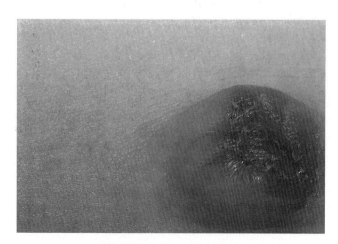

FIG. 100–3. Patent urachus.

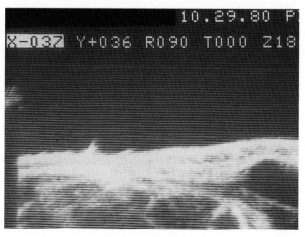

FIG. 100–4. Abdominal ultrasound that demonstrates an infected urachal cyst.

omphalomesenteric duct, an omphalomesenteric sinus, or an omphalomesenteric cyst. A patent duct may be characterized by the drainage of intestinal fluid or fecal material. A sinogram should demonstrate a connection to the gastrointestinal tract.

Malignant lesions of the urachus are rare. The most common sign of urachal cancer is hematuria. Patients may also present with a suprapubic mass, abdominal pain, irritative voiding symptoms, or mucus in the urine. The diagnosis may be made by identification of a filling defect at the dome of the bladder with calcifications on intravenous urogram or cystogram, CT, and cystoscopy with transurethral biopsy. Adenocarcinoma is the most common malignancy; however, sarcoma and transitional cell carcinoma have been reported (12).

INDICATIONS FOR SURGERY

Surgical management is central to the treatment of urachal anomalies with the exception of the patent urachus in the neonate, which may close spontaneously in the absence of bladder outlet obstruction, and the wide-mouth diverticulum, which in general requires no treatment. In the patient with a persistently patent urachus, surgical excision is recommended because of the risk of recurrent infections, stone formation, and persistent umbilical drainage, excoriation, and pain.

Urachal cysts that are symptomatic due to size or infection also merit surgical treatment. Incidentally discovered small, asymptomatic urachal cysts may be excised at the time of discovery or watched for the development of symptoms or progressive enlargement. With infected cysts, initial drainage followed by delayed excision may be required. Similarly, in the case of the urachal sinus initial treatment should focus on the eradication of any infection before excision is undertaken.

Treatment of urachal malignancy follows the principles of treatment for any malignancy of the bladder and is discussed elsewhere in this book.

SURGICAL TECHNIQUE

For the patent urachus, urachal cyst, alternating urachal sinus, or urachal diverticulum requiring correction, the patient is placed in a supine position. If possible, a small catheter, guide wire, or probe is placed through the patent urachus (Fig. 100–5). If nothing will pass, the tract may be stained with methylene blue for later identification. A Foley catheter should be placed in the bladder and the bladder distended with sterile saline to bring the anterior bladder wall up to the abdominal wall and, in doing so, push the peritoneum cephalad.

The urachus may be approached via a vertical midline incision or a transverse infraumbilical incision one-half to two-thirds the distance from the symphysis pubis to the umbilicus. Although the transverse infraumbilical incision will result in excellent exposure, alternatively a vertical midline incision along the course of the urachus may be more direct and can allow for extension to the umbilicus in a cosmetic fashion, should this be required because of difficulty in procuring the umbilical end of the urachus or for any additional necessary procedures. The rectus fascia is opened and the dome of the bladder is identified. The urachus is identified and isolated. Once the proximal portion of the urachus is delineated, it is resected along with a small cuff of bladder to prevent a residual diverticulum. The bladder is then closed in two layers. Dissection then proceeds toward the umbilicus. The operation is facilitated by identifying the proper plane of dissection between the peritoneum posterior to the urachus and the posterior rectus fascia, which is anterior to the urachus. In this same plane will lie the obliterated umbilical arteries, which may be ligated proximally on the bladder wall or distally at the umbilicus.

Infected urachal remnant structures, such as urachal cyst or sinus, may present a more challenging dissection. In fact, it is sometimes advisable to drain a large infected urachal cyst initially percutaneously and allow a period for antibiotic therapy to reduce the local inflammation. Smaller infected urachal cysts or sinuses, however, can be managed safely as a single procedure. With these infected remnants, it may be impossible to dissect the urachus away from contiguous structures. For instance, a larger portion of the bladder may need to be removed with the infected urachal cyst. Similarly, one may find it impossible to separate the infected cyst or sinus from the underlying peritoneum. One should be extremely careful in identifying adherent loops of bowel that may have been involved in the inflammatory process and could easily be injured.

Once the urachus is completely dissected distally it is excised or ligated at its obliterated point. The goal is to remove all urachal tissue and leave the umbilicus intact. If an umbilical hernia is present, it may be corrected concurrently. A catheter may be left in the bladder and a drain in the prevesical space postoperatively at the surgeon's discretion.

For the urachal sinus draining at the umbilicus, dissection is begun by circumscribing the sinus, again with the goal of preserving as much of the umbilicus as possible. The obliterated umbilical arteries are ligated as they are encountered. The tract is dissected to its termination, excised, and the area is drained because the sinus tract is usually infected.

An alternative to open surgical treatment is laparoscopic treatment. Laparoscopic treatment has been reported in both children and adults using the same principals as open surgical treatment (3,7).

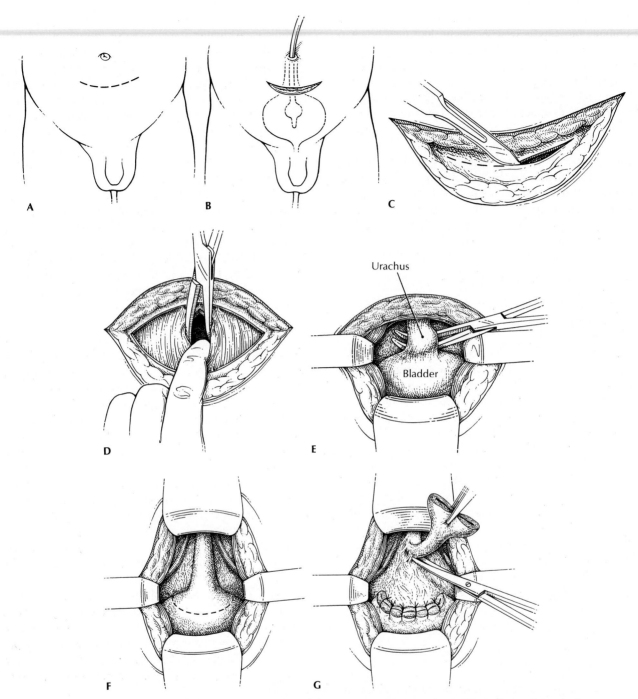

FIG. 100–5. A, B: Typical transverse infraumbilical approach to the urachus. The catheter through the urachus can aid in identification of a patency. **C, D:** The fascia is divided transversely and the rectus muscle is parted in the midline, remaining preperitoneal. **E:** The urachus or urachal remnant can be separated from the peritoneum and identified in its proximal and distal extent. **F, G:** The urachus is resected with a cuff of bladder and the bladder closed in a watertight fashion. The urachus is removed completely out to the umbilicus if necessary.

OUTCOMES

Complications

Postoperative complications include persistent urinary drainage, which can be managed by prolonged bladder catheter drainage, and infection, which is in general superficial and responds well to antibiotic therapy.

REFERENCES

1. Bauer SB, Retik AB. Urachal anomalies and related umbilical disorders. *Urol Clin North Am* 1978;5:195.
2. Blichert-Toft M, Koch F, Nielson OV. Anatomic variants of the urachus related to clinical appearance and surgical treatment of urachal lesions. *Surg Gynecol Obstet* 1973;137:51–54.
3. Caddedu JA, Boyle KE, Fabrizio MD, et al. Laparoscopic management of urachal cysts in adulthood. *J Urol* 2000;164:1526–1528.
4. Cilento BG, Bauer SB, Retik AB, et al. Urachal anomalies: defining the best diagnostic modality. *Urology* 1998;52:120–122.
5. Herbst WP. Patent urachus. *South Med J* 1937;30:711–719.
6. Hinman F. Surgical disorders of the bladder and umbilicus of urachal origin. *Surg Gynecol Obstet* 1961;113:605–614.
7. Khurana S, Borzi PA. Laparoscopic management of complicated urachal disease in children. *J Urol* 2002;168:1526–1528.
8. Mesrobian HGO, Zacharias A, Balcom AH, et al. Ten years of experience with isolated urachal anomalies in children. *J Urol* 1997;158:1316–1318.
9. Nix JT, Menville JG, Albert M, Wendt DL. Congenital patent urachus. *J Urol* 1958;79:264.
10. Persutte WH, Lenke RR, Kropp K, Ghareeh C. Antenatal diagnosis of fetal patent urachus. *J Ultrasound Med* 1988;7:399–403.
11. Schreck WR, Campbell WA III. The relation of bladder outlet obstruction to urinary–umbilical fistula. *J Urol* 1972;108:641–643.
12. Sheldon CA, Clayman RA, Gonzalez R, Williams RD, Fraley EE. Malignant urachal lesions. *J Urol* 1984;131:1–8.

CHAPTER 101

Vesical Neck Reconstruction

Mark C. Adams and John C. Pope IV

Prior to toilet training, the functions of the lower urinary tract include storage of urine at low pressure and good emptying. The result is protection of the upper tract and avoidance of urinary tract infection. Adequate outflow resistance is not necessary during that time but is eventually critical to achieve urinary continence, another ultimate function of the lower tract. Congenital anomalies resulting in inadequate outflow resistance, and thus failure to achieve urinary continence, can in general be divided into two groups based on pathophysiology. In the first group there is an anatomic or developmental abnormality where the bladder outlet is malformed and incapable of providing adequate resistance. This group would include patients with bladder exstrophy, bilateral single ectopic ureters, persistent cloaca, and rarely an extensive ureterocele. In the second, more common, group involving neurogenic dysfunction, the outlet is normally developed from an anatomic standpoint but abnormal neurological control results in inadequate function.

DIAGNOSIS

When urinary continence is not achieved in children, the critical evaluation is video urodynamic study of the bladder and outlet. Parameters that need to be evaluated include sphincteric function, outflow resistance, detrusor function, and bladder compliance.

Monitoring of external urinary sphincter activity is helpful during studies of storage and emptying. Perineal surface electrodes are most widely used to evaluate the activity; however, in children with neurogenic dysfunction who tolerate placement a concentric needle electrode or dual electrodes placed through a 25-gauge needle increase accuracy.

The functional length and pressure of the external sphincter is important and can be measured with urethral pressure profilometry. This measurement is technically challenging in a small child and there are no adequate standard nomograms for urethral pressure profilometry to use in pediatric patients. Continuous monitoring of the urethral pressure during filling in the area of maximum resistance may demonstrate an etiology of incontinence. Some surgeons also use leak point pressure to evaluate outflow resistance during passive filling and performance of Valsalva maneuvers. Simultaneous fluoroscopic observation is advantageous.

Detrusor function should be evaluated by the cystometrogram, synergistic relaxation of the external sphincter on electromyography, urinary flow rate, and measurement of postvoid residual urine. Bladder compliance should also be evaluated with the detrusor pressure measured as the bladder is filled with warm saline or contrast (37°C) at a rate equal to or less than 10% of estimated or known bladder capacity. Such filling minimizes irritation of the bladder that may artifactually increase bladder pressure. Other artifacts that affect the measurement of compliance such as urinary infections or low urethral resistance should be eliminated to obtain the best results.

Before reconstructive surgery on the bladder is considered, the status of the patient's upper urinary tract should also be evaluated. Standard evaluation includes renal ultrasonography and serum electrolytes including creatinine. If hydronephrosis is present, renography should be obtained to rule out obstruction. Vesicoureteral reflux should be sought on voiding cystourethrography, often at the time of video urodynamic evaluation. Any upper-tract obstruction or reflux should be corrected at the time of lower urinary tract reconstruction.

Unfortunately, no test ensures that a patient will be able to void spontaneously and empty well after outlet reconstruction with or without bladder augmentation. All patients must be prepared to perform clean intermittent catheterization before considering reconstruction. The native urethra should, therefore, be examined for the ease and discomfort of catheterization.

INDICATIONS FOR SURGERY

If urinary continence is not achieved at an appropriate age in patients with congenital anomalies, and the patient has failed behavioral regimens such as timed voidings, had urodynamics, and failed all medical regimens and other conservative therapies (e.g., intermittent catheterizations), then surgical intervention should be considered. It is critical to ensure that the bladder is a compliant storage reservoir prior to any reconstructive procedure on the lower urinary tract. Increasing outflow resistance in the presence of inadequate bladder capacity would put the patient at significant risk for upper-tract deterioration and febrile urinary tract infection. Determining the commitment of the patient and family to achieve a good result with reconstructive surgery, including a willingness to perform intermittent catheterization if necessary, is critical.

ALTERNATE THERAPY

In few areas of reconstructive urology are there as many choices to consider as for bladder neck repair and as little consensus as to which repair is appropriate for a given patient or setting. One reason for the variety of choices is the wide range of patients and problems for which the procedures are used. In some cases, the procedure to increase outflow resistance may logically be chosen based on particular patient considerations, but the experience and confidence of the surgeon with a given technique also may play a significant role in the choice.

Conceptually, techniques to increase outflow resistance may be considered as one of two general types. The first set of repairs is used to improve the function of the native outlet while the second set is designed to repair the anatomy and functionally alter the outlet. Several procedures that may provide benefit and are occasionally used include urethral suspensions, injection of bulking agents, artificial sphincters, and obliteration of the bladder neck.

One of the first bladder neck repairs to function in such a manner was the urethral suspension described by Marshall–Marchetti–Krantz and since modified by numerous surgeons. While these procedures have been successful in treating stress urinary incontinence among neurologically normal females, they have had minimal effect and are rarely indicated for pediatric patients with congenital anatomic anomalies of the outlet or neurogenic dysfunction.

Recently, transurethral injection of bulking agents has been tried to improve the function of the existing outlet. Injection therapy is relatively simple, avoids any incision, but has met with limited results for significant outlet anomalies (7). Injection therapy may be useful after primary repairs in patients who have some persistent incontinence.

The most definitive procedure to improve the function of the outlet as it exists is placement of an artificial urinary sphincter. This group of procedures would seem appropriate for patients with a normal or near normal outlet from an anatomic standpoint and to have little role for patients with significant anatomic anomalies such as bladder exstrophy or bilateral single ectopic ureters.

The ultimate procedure to increase outlet resistance is division of the bladder neck. Effective closure requires extensive mobilization of the bladder and bladder neck away from the urethra with interposition of omentum between. It must be accompanied by construction of a continent abdominal wall stoma for bladder catheterization and effectively moves the reconstruction into the realm of continent urinary diversion. Division of the bladder neck has in general been reserved for complex patients who have failed multiple prior procedures to effectively increase outflow resistance.

SURGICAL TECHNIQUE

Fascial Sling for Bladder Neck Suspension

In adults, fascial slings may be performed transvaginally, and a small patch of fascia is secured with suspension sutures. In pediatric patients with congenital anomalies, fascial slings have in general been placed from above often at the time of bladder augmentation. Before placement, the pelvic floor is cleared of overlying fatty tissue and a 2-cm incision made through the endopelvic fascia on either side of the bladder neck and proximal urethra (Fig. 101–1A). This area may be identified by palpation of a transurethral catheter and balloon seated at the bladder neck. Using blunt dissection, a plane is developed between the bladder neck and vagina in girls or rectum in boys (Fig. 101–1B). This plane may at times be more easily developed from the cul-de-sac by dissecting behind the bladder and ureters from above. With a difficult dissection it may be useful to open the bladder, in particular if bladder augmentation is planned.

Once the proper plane is developed and the appropriate length of graft determined, a rectus abdominus fascial strip 1 cm in width and appropriate in length is harvested. The fascia may be taken in either a vertical or horizontal fashion depending on the initial incision. Fascia from other sites has been utilized but require a second incision. Autologous cadaveric tissue or biodegradable scaffolds may also be used.

All of the grafts are in general brought though the rectus muscle and anterior rectus fascia on either side and approximated to the anterior rectus fascia using permanent sutures (Fig. 101–1C). If long enough, the two limbs of the sling may also be approximated to each other superficial to the fascia. In patients with stress incontinence, the sling is placed tightly enough to maintain the proximal urethra and bladder neck in the appropriate

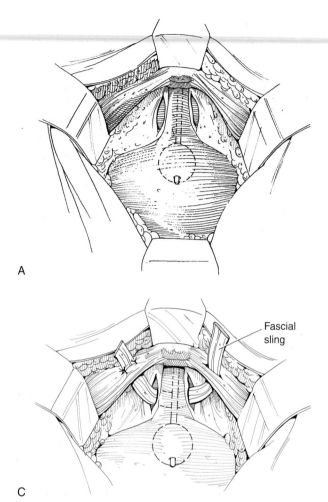

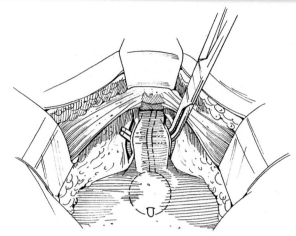

FIG. 101–1. Pubovaginal sling. **A:** The endopelvic fascia is cleared of fatty tissue and a 2-cm incision made on either side of the urethra. A Foley catheter through the urethra may be palpated for identification of the urethra and bladder neck. **B:** The plane between the posterior urethra and anterior vagina is carefully developed using a right-angle clamp. **C:** A fascial strip 1 cm wide is passed through the anterior rectus fascia and rectus muscle lateral to the midline incision. It is secured on the left to the anterior fascia. The sling is then passed behind the bladder and will be brought through the right rectus muscle and fascia to be secured at the proper tension.

anatomic position. Too snug of placement in such a setting may impede spontaneous voiding. When used for patients with neurogenic dysfunction who will not rely on spontaneous voiding, the sling may be pulled up more tightly to improve compression of the bladder neck and proximal urethra. If intermittent catheterization postoperatively will be performed through the native urethra, intraoperative catheterization should be repeated frequently to make sure the fascial sling is not placed so tight as to impede catheterization.

Young–Dees–Leadbetter Bladder Neck Repair

Often done after bladder exstrophy closure, the procedure is typically performed through a lower midline incision. For patients with epispadias who do not require augmentation, the reconstruction may be done through a Pfannenstiel incision. The anterior bladder is opened. This incision is carried as far distally into the proximal urethra as possible. Splitting of the intersymphyseal band with subsequent closure may allow closure and tapering of the proximal urethra. Virtually all exstrophy patients require antireflux surgery, and typically the ureteral hia-

tus is initially quite low in the bladder. The ureters are mobilized and reimplanted into the bladder 3 to 4 cm more cephalad in location. Typically, the ureters are reimplanted with a cross-trigonal technique, although the tunnels may even be angled upward in a cephalad direction from the new hiatus. A 12- to 15-mm wide strip of mucosa is preserved in the posterior midline of the urethra and bladder trigone for reconstruction of the neourethra. Parallel incisions through mucosa are made on either side of this strip and the triangles of trigone mucosa on either side excised (Fig. 101–2A). Submucosal infiltration of dilute epinephrine in those two areas may aid in excision and decrease bleeding. The midline strip of mucosa and subsequent neourethra are typically made 4 to 6 cm long depending on how much proximal urethra is exposed and reconstructed. The midline strip is tubularized over an 8 Fr catheter using absorbable sutures to approximate the edges. This tubularization may be done with interrupted or running absorbable sutures but should be tension free (Fig. 101–2B). Small purchases of the adjacent superficial muscle of the trigone may be included with the mucosa for strength. The closure is easier to begin distally and finished cephalad. The lateral

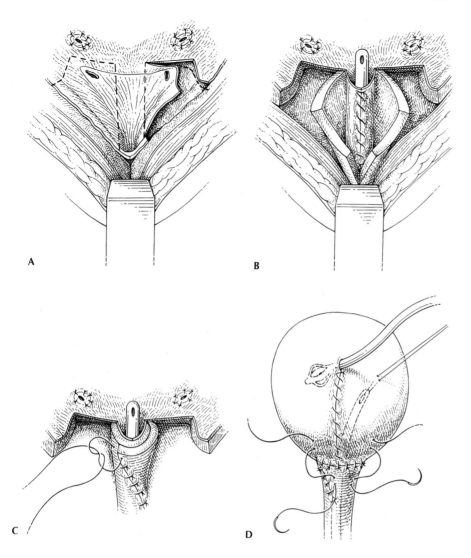

FIG. 101–2. Young–Dees bladder neck repair. **A:** The trigone mucosa is incised to leave a posterior, central strip of mucosa 15 mm wide. The triangles of mucosa on either side are excised. The ureters have previously been reimplanted in a more cephalad position. **B:** The central mucosa strip is tubularized using a running absorbable suture. **C:** The lateral trigone muscle flaps are closed in an overlapping fashion around the neourethra. **D:** After completion of the bladder and urethral closure, several pairs of suspension sutures secure the urethra and bladder to the underside of the intersymphyseal band and lower abdominal wall.

flaps of trigone muscle are then wrapped over the neourethra in an overlapping fashion. To do so without tension, the muscle must be incised transversely at the cephalad margin of the mucosal excision. One flap of muscle is wrapped over the neourethra and approximated to the underside of the other muscle flap using interrupted, absorbable mattress sutures. The second flap of muscle is then wrapped over the first and approximated to the outside of the muscle, again with absorbable sutures (Fig. 101–2C). A soft urethral catheter is left in place during healing but should be secured so as to avoid tension on the neourethra. Ureteral stents or catheters are often left in place because of potential edema. The bladder is closed in two layers.

If bladder augmentation is required, the bladder should be closed to itself for a short distance from the urethra prior to applying the bowel segment. A clear demarcation between the neourethra and bladder can often be seen after closure. Care should be taken that there is effective closure of the urethra and bladder at this junction. The bladder may tend to kink over the urethra at that level, and the neourethra and new bladder neck should be suspended to the undersurface of the intersymphyseal band and lower abdominal wall using several pairs of sutures as described for the Marshall–Marchetti–Krantz procedure (Fig. 101–2D).

Alternatively, Leadbetter described full-thickness, parallel incisions through the trigone mucosa and muscle on either side of the central strip. These incisions, again, made 12 to 15 mm apart, are started distally at the old bladder neck and continued in a cephalad direction for 4 to 5 cm (Fig. 101–3A). The central strip of mucosa is tubularized with interrupted or running absorbable sutures. The muscle of the central strip is closed as a second layer. If the incision through the muscle is made slightly wider than on the mucosa, the muscle may be approximated in an overlapping manner but to a lesser degree than that described by Young and Dees. The lateral triangles of full-thickness trigone are left in continuity with the bladder and included in that closure (Fig. 101–3B).

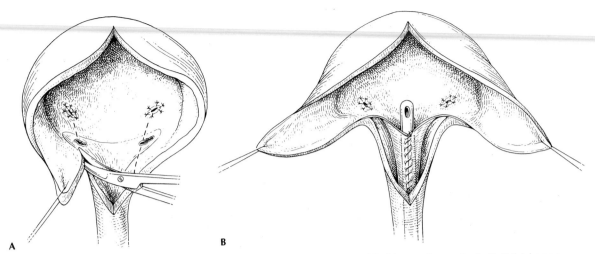

FIG. 101–3. Leadbetter modification of Young–Dees–Leadbetter bladder neck repair. **A:** Full-thickness parallel incisions are made through the trigone mucosa and muscle, leaving a central strip 15 mm wide. **B:** The mucosa of the neourethra is tubularized using a running absorbable suture. The muscle is then closed. The lateral flaps of trigone are left in continuity with the bladder.

Kropp Urethral Lengthening Procedure

The bladder is exposed through a lower midline incision and the bladder neck is identified by palpation of a catheter placed through the urethra. A rectangular, full-thickness strip of anterior bladder is marked and incised. This strip is based at the bladder neck and should be left in continuity with the urethra (5). The incised strip measures 6 cm in length and 2 cm in width (Fig. 101–4A). Stay sutures placed at the cephalad corners of the strip aid in mobilization. The bladder cephalad to the strip is open in the midline. After anterior incision, the catheter is pulled over the pubis to expose the posterior bladder neck. This allows identification of the ureteral orifices, which are catheterized. If reflux is not present and the space between the orifices is adequate for urethral tunneling, ureteral reimplantation may not be necessary. The ureteral stents are often left in place for 4 to 5 days due to edema. Posterior incision of the mucosa at the bladder neck is performed using cutting current with the electrosurgical cautery to completely separate the neourethra from the bladder at the mucosal level. Further dissection through the posterior muscle in the midline is performed to allow smooth tubularization of the neourethra. Posterolateral musculoadventitial tissue at the 5- and 7-o'clock positions is left intact so that the bladder remains anchored in a caudal position. This eventually ensures that the tubularized neourethra reaches well into the bladder lumen to achieve an effective flap valve.

The anterior bladder flap in continuity with the urethra is tubularized by approximating the mucosa and then muscle with continuous absorbable sutures (Fig. 101–4B). This closure is again begun distally and continued in a proximal or cephalad direction.

A submucosal tunnel is developed from the posterior bladder neck to a position several centimeters above the interureteric ridge (Fig 101–4C). The more cephalad portion of this tunnel is easily developed from above and the more distal or caudal portion typically from the bladder neck (Fig. 101–4D). This tunnel must be made wide enough that the neourethra can be brought through in a nice smooth course. Care must be taken that there is no kink whatsoever at the entrance of the neourethra into the bladder at the area of the old bladder neck. Any kinking at that level will result in difficult catheterization.

Alternatively, the mucosa in the posterior midline may be incised for the entire length for the proposed tunnel. The mucosa on either side is then mobilized to create a wide trough into which to place the urethra. The mucosa from either side is then approximated to the adventitia of the neourethra and will eventually grow to cover it completely. The tubularized neourethra should not be redundant in length relative to the submucosal tunnel to minimize the risk of difficult catheterization. If necessary, excess length may be excised. The proximal end of the neourethra is approximated to the bladder mucosa at its orifice with interrupted absorbable suture (Fig. 101–4E). Distally, the lateral and anterior bladder is securely approximately to the adventitia and muscle of the urethra (Fig. 101–4F). This closure should be performed as distally as possible on the urethra to avoid foreshortening of the tunnel within the bladder. Ease of catheterization through the neourethra should be tested at each step of reconstruction and any problems addressed when noted. If augmentation of the bladder is necessary, the incision is extended and the peritoneal cavity entered. A short segment of distal bladder should be closed to itself up from the urethra prior to placing the segment for augmentation. A soft urethral catheter is left in place per urethra during healing. The catheter should be secured so as to avoid any pressure on the reconstructed urethra. The catheter is usu-

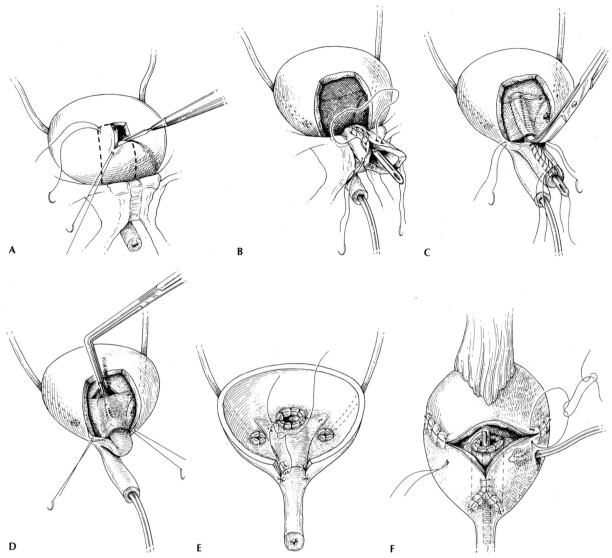

FIG. 101–4. Kropp procedure for urethral lengthening. **A:** A 6 × 2 cm flap of anterior bladder is mobilized in continuity with the urethra. **B:** The flap is tubularized. **C:** The posterior mucosa is incised transversely at the bladder neck and a tunnel created for the neourethra from the old bladder neck to a position above the interureteric ridge. **D:** The neourethra is brought through the tunnel, taking care that it does not kink. Note that the posterolateral musculoadventitial tissue is intact and keeps the bladder anchored distally. **E:** The proximal end of the neourethra is trimmed flush with its orifice in the bladder. The end is approximated to the vesical mucosa circumferentially. **F:** The bladder is carefully closed distally by approximating the bladder muscle and mucosa to the adventitia of the neourethra. The neourethra extends well into the lumen of the bladder to create an effective flap valve. Bladder augmentation is performed when necessary.

ally left in place for 4 to 6 weeks during healing, often with a suprapubic cystotomy tube as well. After a static cystogram demonstrates no leakage and good healing, self-catheterization may begin.

Pippi Salle Urethral Lengthening Procedure

In an effort to achieve the effective flap valve created with the Kropp procedure while decreasing the risk for problems with catheterization, Salle et al. (9) described a modification for urethral lengthening. The anterior bladder wall flap is used as an onlay and eventually contributes half of the circumference of the neourethra. Therefore, a full-thickness anterior bladder flap 5 × 1 cm is mobilized in continuity with the bladder neck (Fig. 101–5A). One millimeter of mucosa on either side is excised to avoid overlapping suture lines. Two parallel incisions through the mucosa of the trigone are made so

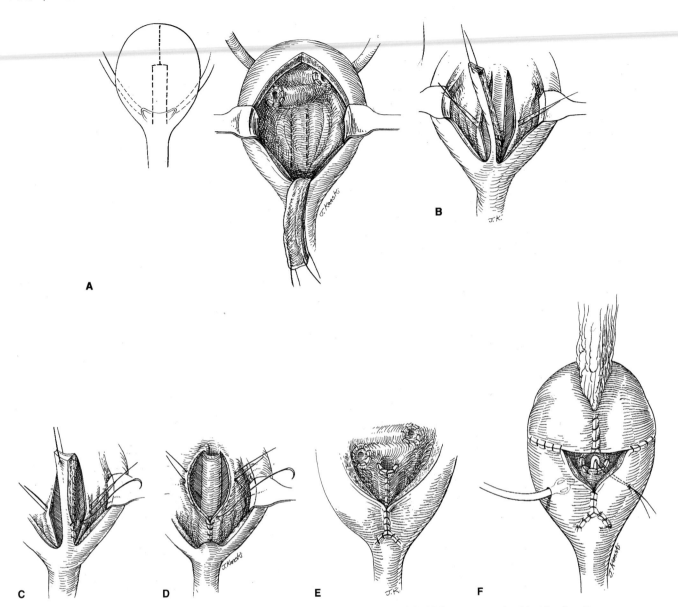

FIG. 101–5. Pippi Salle procedure for urethral lengthening. **A:** A full-thickness, anterior bladder flap 5 × 1 cm is marked and incised. Parallel incisions through the trigone mucosa posteriorly leave a central strip of similar length and width. **B:** The lateral trigone mucosa is mobilized to cover the neourethra. The mucosa of the anterior flap is approximated to the edge of the central mucosal strip using a running absorbable suture. **C:** The muscle of the anterior flap is approximated to the superficial trigone muscle on either side of the mucosal closure. **D:** The lateral mucosa is closed over the neourethra. **E:** The distal bladder is closed to itself and carefully to the urethra. **F:** Bladder augmentation is performed when necessary.

as to leave a central strip of mucosa 8 to 10 mm in width and 5 cm in length. The lateral trigone mucosa on either side is mobilized to eventually close over the neourethra. The mucosa of the anterior flap is approximated to the midline strip of trigone mucosa using a running absorbable suture started distally (Fig. 101–5B). The muscle of the anterior flap is approximated to the superficial muscle on either side of the central mucosa (Fig. 101–5C). The trigone muscle on either side of the poste-

rior mucosal strip may be incised superficially to provide an edge to which to sew the muscle of the anterior flap. Closure of the lateral mucosa of the trigone over the reconstructed neourethra creates a flap valve and a neourethra with an intact posterior wall (Fig. 101–5D,E). Distally, the muscle and mucosa of the bladder neck are approximated to the lateral and anterior adventitia and muscle of the neourethra as distally as possible. Proximally, the neourethra should extend well into the lumen of the bladder to create an effective flap-valve mechanism for continence. The neourethra and ureters are often stented temporarily in a manner similar to that described for the Kropp procedure (Fig. 101–5F).

OUTCOMES

Complications

Relatively common clinical problems after bladder neck reconstruction include urinary tract infection and bladder stones. Both may occur in exstrophy patients after Young–Dees–Leadbetter bladder neck repair due to poor emptying (13) but are even more common among patients with neurogenic dysfunction requiring intermittent catheterization, in particular if bladder augmentation has been performed. It is important to perform routine surveillance for hydronephrosis of the upper urinary tract with ultrasonography after bladder neck repair. This is in particular true among patients with neurogenic dysfunction if they have not undergone bladder augmentation. Even if the bladder appeared adequate prior to outlet reconstruction, up to one-quarter of patients may develop bladder hostility after an increase in outlet resistance, which may silently threaten the kidneys (1).

Results

In the pediatric population, fascial slings have been used most extensively in patients with neurogenic sphincter incompetence. Long-term success with slings in that population has varied greatly, from 40% to 100%. Success rates have varied so much that it is not clear that any particular modification of the sling configuration results in any difference in terms of continence. Fascial slings have been used more extensively and with better results in girls with neurogenic dysfunction in whom the continence rate may reach 75% (8). The primary factor predictive of success has been concomitant enterocystoplasty to ensure a compliant bladder. Placement does not in general interfere with the ability to perform intermittent catheterization, which is usually necessary in the patient population.

The Young–Dees–Leadbetter bladder neck repair has been used most commonly in the classic staged reconstruction for bladder exstrophy. Continence with spontaneous voiding has been achieved in up to 80% of patients with exstrophy and may be even higher for patients with epispadias (4). Other authors have reported a lower continence rate, and even among patients considered dry clinical and urodynamic problems related to poor emptying may exist (13). When used for patients with neurogenic dysfunction and denervated sphincter muscle, the procedure initially resulted in continence in approximately 25% of patients but can be improved to almost 70% if combined with bladder augmentation (3,6). Due to the high percentage of additional procedures required, the repair has in general fallen out of favor for patients with neurogenic dysfunction. Reliable catheterization through the urethra after a Young–Dees–Leadbetter repair may be difficult.

The urethral lengthening procedures have primarily been used in boys with neurogenic bladder dysfunction. Using the technique described by Kropp, continence has been achieved in 75% to 90% of such patients (2,5). Difficulty with catheterization has been reported in 40% of male patients in some series, although that incidence may be lowered when the posterior urethra is not totally transected (2). Because of concerns about the potential problem with catheterization, some surgeons prefer routine construction of a continent catheterizable stoma (12). A significant incidence of new reflux has been apparent in some series using the Kropp technique (12). Using Salle et al.'s modification, less trouble with catheterization in males has been noted, although continence rates have not been quite as high (10,11). Urethrovesical fistula and partial necrosis of the intravesical neourethra have on occasion resulted in incontinence after the repair, and widening the base of the anterior flap at the level of the bladder neck may decrease those problems.

REFERENCES

1. Bauer SB, Reda EF, Colodny AH, Retik AB. Detrusor instability: A delayed complication in association with the artificial sphincter. *J Urol* 1986;135:1212.
2. Belman AB, Kaplan GW. Experience with the Kropp anti-incontinence procedure. *J Urol* 1989;141:1160.
3. Donnahoo KK, Rink RC, Cain MP, Casale AJ. The Young–Dees–Leadbetter bladder neck repair for neurogenic incontinence. *J Urol* 1999; 161:1946–1949.
4. Gearhart JP, Jeffs RD. Exstrophy–epispadias complex and bladder anomalies. In: Walsh PC, Retik AB, Vaughan ED, Wein AJ, eds. *Campbell's urology*, 7th ed. Philadelphia: WB Saunders, 1998:1939–1990.
5. Kropp KA, Angwafo FF. Urethral lengthening and reimplantation for neurogenic incontinence in children. *J Urol* 1986;135:533.
6. Leadbetter GW. Surgical reconstruction for complete urinary incontinence: A 10 to 22 year follow-up. *J Urol* 1985;133:205.
7. Perez LM, Smith EA, Parrott TS, Broecker BH, Massad CA, Woodard JR. Submucosal bladder neck injection of bovine dermal collagen for stress urinary incontinence in the pediatric population. *J Urol* 1996; 156:633–636.
8. Perez LM, Smith EA, Broecker BH, Massad CA, Parrott TS, Woodard JR. Outcome of sling cystourethropexy in the pediatric population: A critical review. *J Urol* 1996;156:642–646.
9. Pippi Salle JL, deFraga JCS, Amarante A, et al. Urethral lengthening with anterior bladder wall flap for urinary incontinence: A new approach. *J Urol* 1994;152:803.
10. Rink RC, Adams MC, Keating MA. The flip-flap technique to lengthen the urethra (Salle procedure) for treatment of neurogenic urinary incontinence. *J Urol* 1994;152:799.
11. Salle JL, McLorie GA, Bagli DJ, Khoury AE. Urethral lengthening with anterior bladder wall flap (Pippi Salle procedure): Modifications and extended indications of the technique. *J Urol* 1997;158:585–590.
12. Snodgrass W. A simplified Kropp procedure for incontinence. *J Urol* 1997;158:1049–1052.
13. Yerkes EB, Adams MC, Rink RC, Pope JC IV, Brock JW III. How well do patients with exstrophy actually void? *J Urol* 2000;164(3, Pt 2):1044.

CHAPTER 102

Surgery for Posterior Urethral Valves

Rosalia Misseri and Kenneth I. Glassberg

A posterior urethral valve (PUV) is the most common cause of congenital bladder outlet obstruction in boys. It is associated with a dilated posterior urethra, poor urinary stream, and incomplete bladder emptying. Bilateral hydroureteronephrosis of varying degrees is almost always present and frequently accompanied by vesicoureteral reflux and/or bladder diverticuli.

DIAGNOSIS

With the widespread use of antenatal ultrasound, PUVs are often diagnosed prenatally. The condition is suspected *in utero* when a male fetus undergoes sonography and bilateral hydroureteronephrosis is identified along with a thick-walled bladder that does not empty completely. In severely affected fetuses, oligohydramnios, pulmonary hypoplasia, and Potter's syndrome may occur. Newborns may present with abdominal masses representing a distended bladder or hydronephrotic kidney, dry diapers, nonspecific gastrointestinal symptoms, respiratory distress, or urinary ascites. Younger boys usually present with urinary tract infection, respiratory distress, abdominal distension, sepsis, and azotemia, while older boys may present with hematuria, dysfunctional voiding symptomatology, incontinence, poor urinary stream, and urinary tract infections.

If a PUV is suspected in an infant, prophylactic antibiotics should be initiated and the bladder should be drained with a 5 or 8 Fr feeding tube taped in place with a clear transparent dressing. The feeding tube is left in place until a voiding cystourethrogram (VCUG) is obtained to make the diagnosis. In patients with severe hydroureteronephrosis and/or azotemia, the catheter should be left in place until the azotemia resolves/stabilizes and hydroureteronephrosis improves.

The VCUG of a boy with a PUV will reveal a posterior urethra that appears dilated, often taking on a "shield shape" or squared-off appearance. The bladder neck is often clearly demarcated and may appear as a thick collar and the urethra distal to the obstruction will appear less full than normal.

INDICATIONS FOR SURGERY

Today, most valve ablation is accomplished transurethrally. Controversy still exists as to what to do once the bladder has been drained with a catheter (Fig. 102–1). For severe hydronephrosis, some report better long-term outcomes when these infants are temporarily diverted, while others feel that primary valve ablation is the treatment of choice (2). For those who believe temporary diversion is best, many methods of diverting the obstructed bladder exist.

ALTERNATIVE THERAPY

There is no effective alternative therapy.

SURGICAL TECHNIQUE

Transurethral Valve Ablation

Valve ablation is most commonly accomplished transurethrally. The size of the infant's fossa navicularis usually limits the size of cystoscope that may be used. Typically, a 7.5 or 8.5 Fr scope is used in infants, while a 10 Fr scope is used in older children. Cystoscopes as small as 6 Fr with 4 Fr working channels are available. The cystoscope should be well lubricated and advanced under direct vision. Gentle dilation of the distal urethra may be required to advance the cystourethroscope. With the bladder full and applying gentle suprapubic pressure, the valve leaflets are more easily seen coming off the verumontanum and extending distally to fuse anteriorly (Fig. 102–2). The goal of valve ablation is to disrupt the leaflet, hence destroying the obstruction.

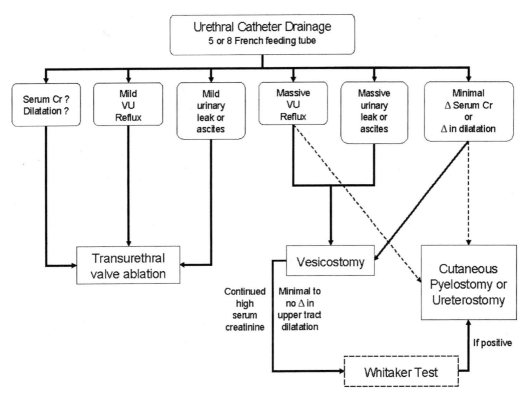

FIG. 102–1. Management of posterior urethral valves. Solid lines represent our treatments of choice; broken lines indicate possible alternatives. (Modified from Glassberg KI, Horowitz, M. Urethral valves and other anomalies of the male urethra. In: Belman AB, King LR, Kramer SA, eds. *Clinical pediatric urology*, 4th ed. London: Martin Dunitz Ltd, 2002, with permission.)

A posterior urethral valve may be ablated or incised in several ways. It may be ablated using a 3 Fr Bugbee electrode through a cystoscope. Alternatively, the wire insert of a 3 Fr ureteral catheter with the distal end connected to

Posterior Urethral Valve

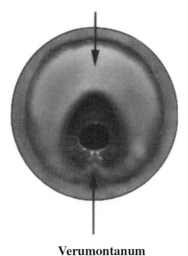

Verumontanum

FIG. 102–2. Cystoscopic appearance of type 1 posterior urethral valve.

electrocautery may be used. Once in position the wire is advanced and pushed into the valve at the 5- and 7-o'clock positions while employing a cutting current of 20 to 25 W. (Note that power settings may vary from machine to machine.)

Using a small pediatric resectoscope, the valves are incised with a right-angle hook, loop electrode, or hook-shaped cold knife. When using a loop electrode, a narrow, more oblong loop is preferable to a wider, more circular loop. Some debate exists as to the best location for valve incision. Williams and colleagues preferred incising at the 12-o'clock position, while Gonzales advocates cutting at the 4-, 8-, and 12-o'clock position (3,6). However, most prefer incising at the 4- to 5-o'clock and 7- to 8-o'clock positions with the cutting current set at 20 to 25 W pure cut.

Lasers such as the neodymium:YAG have also been employed for posterior urethral valve ablation. Additional methods of PUV ablation have also been described for use in patients with small-caliber urethras. With the advent of smaller scopes, perineal urethrostomy is now rarely necessary for valve ablation. Zaontz and Firlit have described percutaneous antegrade ablation of PUV as well as antegrade incision of PUV in infants with small-caliber urethras (7).

Once the valves are endoscopically ablated the bladder should be cystoscoped to evaluate for diverticuli, trabeculations, and the appearance of the ureteral orifices. A full stream should be noted at the end of the procedure while applying gentle pressure to the suprapubic area. A small urethral catheter is left in place for 1 to 2 days following the procedure. A VCUG may be performed after the catheter is removed to assess the success of the procedure. Timing of the VCUG is often determined by the surgeon based on his/her confidence in the adequacy of ablation. A VCUG and urodynamics or preferably videourodynamics should be delayed no more than 6 to 8 weeks after ablation. If bladder dynamics are found to be abnormal, e.g., diminished compliance or detrusor hyperactivity, anticholinergic therapy should be considered. Anticholinergic therapy may also be instituted immediately after valve ablation or prior to closure or reversal of vesical or supravesical diversion.

Vesicostomy

With the patient in the supine position the lower abdominal skin is prepared and draped in the typical fashion. The procedure is more easily performed with a full bladder. A 2-cm transverse incision is then made midway between the pubic symphysis and umbilicus. The rectus fascia is exposed and a 2 × 2 cm cruciate incision is made. Alternately, a triangle or circle of rectus fascia measuring 2 cm may be excised. One must remember that the size of the fascial opening ultimately determines the caliber of the stoma. The rectus muscles are then retracted laterally, exposing the bladder. A 3-0 suture is placed near the dome of the bladder and used for traction. Using the traction suture the bladder is mobilized superiorly. The peritoneum is gently swept off of the superior aspect of the bladder. Additional cephalad sutures may be placed in a stepwise fashion to help bring the dome into the surgical field. Care is taken to avoid the peritoneal contents. With gentle traction one should be able to visualize the urachus or obliterated hypogastric artery.

The vesicostomy may be created in one of two ways. In the first method, a stay suture is placed proximal to the urachus. The urachus is then transected and excised. In the second method, the portion of the bladder cephalad to the urachal remnant is used as the site for the vesicostomy. The bladder is incised and the fascial edges are sewn to the outer bladder wall using 4-0 polyglactin sutures approximately 0.5 to 1 cm from the opening created in the bladder. The vesicostomy should be calibrated to 24 Fr. If the fascial defect is too large, interrupted 3-0 polyglactin sutures may be used to narrow the opening. The edges of the detrusor are then sewn to the skin using 4-0 polyglactin sutures in an interrupted fashion. If the skin incision is wider than the stoma created, the skin is approximated with a suture of choice (Fig. 102–3).

The decision to close a vesicostomy should be made only once bladder dynamics have been assessed and a plan for permanent therapy has been devised. Ultimately, the timing of closure is dictated by the surgeon's philosophy. Some believe an empty bladder becomes a contracted bladder, while others close vesicostomies just prior to the expected time of potty training.

An adequate size balloon catheter is placed into the stoma of the vesicostomy. With the balloon inflated an elliptical skin incision is made around the stoma. The subcutaneous and perivesical tissues are dissected circumferentially around the vesicostomy. Next, 3-0 chromic stay sutures are placed through the bladder wall approximately 1 cm cephalad and 1 cm caudad to the stoma. The skin and protruding portion of the bladder are excised. The previously placed catheter is removed and a urethral catheter is placed for bladder drainage. The bladder defect is then closed in two layers: A running 3-0 chromic suture is used to reapproximate the bladder mucosa followed by interrupted 3-0 polyglactin sutures as a second layer. The remainder of the wound is closed in a standard fashion.

Supravesical Diversion

Cutaneous Pyelostomy

To safely perform a cutaneous pyelostomy, the renal pelvis should be sufficiently dilated to avoid tension on the renal pelvis as it is pulled toward the abdominal wall. A dilated renal pelvis also ensures that dissection can be carried out away from the ureteropelvic junction.

The renal pelvis may be approached in several ways including dorsal lumbotomy or subcostal midline extraperitoneal approach. A surgeon may use the approach he/she is most comfortable with; however, the dorsal lumbotomy incision is quite advantageous in the pediatric population. Despite the limited exposure that this incision affords, it is excellent for visualization of the renal pelvis and upper ureter. The procedure avoids a muscle-splitting incision and, therefore, incurs less postoperative pain.

After the patient is intubated, he should be placed in the prone position on the operating room table. Cushions should then be placed under the chest and just superior to the anterior superior iliac spines. The landmarks include the twelfth rib superiorly, the iliac crest inferiorly, and the lateral border of the sacrospinalis medially. A vertical incision with a slight curve at its distal end is made approximately one-third to one-half the distance between the twelfth rib and the iliac crest. Alternatively, an oblique incision may be made along Langer's lines (Fig. 102–4). Care should be taken to avoid injuring the subcostal neurovascular bundle. The lumbodorsal fascia is exposed by elevating the skin and subcutaneous tissues for about 3 cm on either side of the incision so that a vertical fascial incision may be comfortably made. The posterior layer of

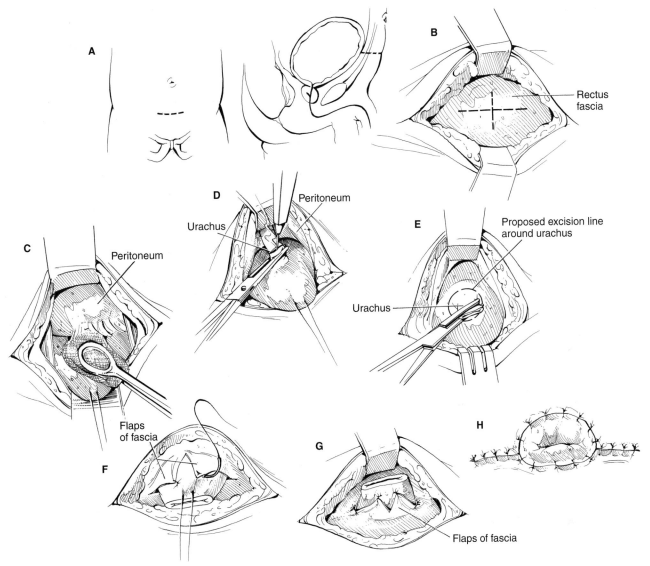

FIG. 102–3. Blocksom vesicostomy. **A:** A 2-cm transverse incision is made midway between the pubic symphysis and umbilicus. **B:** A 2 × 2 cm cruciate fascial incision is made. **C:** Using the traction suture the bladder is mobilized superiorly. The peritoneum is gently swept off of the superior aspect of the bladder. **D:** The urachus is incised and the bladder is further mobilized. **E:** The urachus is excised. **F, G:** The outer bladder wall is sewn to the edges of the incised rectus fascia. **H:** The edges of the detrusor are sewn to the skin. (Modified from Belman AB, King LR. Vesicostomy: useful means of reversible urinary diversion in selected infant. *Urology* 1973;1:208–213, with permission.)

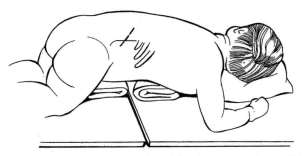

FIG. 102–4. Positioning for dorsal lumbotomy and possible skin incisions. The solid line represents our incision of choice; the broken line represents a suitable alternative.

the lumbodorsal fascia is incised vertically 2 cm lateral to the midline. The sacrospinalis muscle is then retracted medially. This exposes the middle layer of the lumbodorsal fascia, which is incised at the lateral border of the quadratus lumborum. Retracting the quadratus lumborum medially, the anterior layer of the lumbodorsal fascia is exposed (Fig. 102–5). This layer and the transversalis fascia is then incised between the subcostal and iliohypogastric nerves. The perinephric fat should then be in view. The kidney should be located in the superomedial part of the wound.

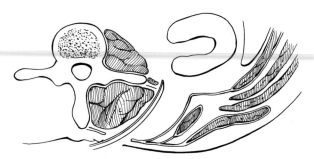

FIG. 102–5. Fascial incision through lumbodorsal fascia lateral to the sacrospinalis and quadratus lumborum, avoiding the division of muscles.

Once Gerota's fascia is entered, the dilated renal pelvis is identified and rotated anteromedially. The surgeon must assess if the pelvis can comfortably reach the skin. If not, a very proximal portion of the ureter may be brought out to serve the same purpose. Care should be taken to avoid dissection near the ureteropelvic junction (UPJ) so as to avoid the possibility of a future UPJ obstruction. Two 3-0 chromic traction sutures are placed on the posterior aspect of the renal pelvis away from the UPJ. Using a scalpel a 3-cm incision is made. The full thickness of the renal pelvis is sutured to the posterior corner of the skin incision using multiple interrupted 4-0 polyglactin sutures (Fig. 102–6). The pyelostomy should be calibrated to approximately 20 Fr to avoid future stenosis or prolapse. Once the planned procedure has been performed, the posterior layer of the lumbodorsal fascia is reapproximated with 3-0 polyglactin sutures and the skin is then closed with either a subcuticular suture or skin staples.

High Cutaneous Loop Ureterostomy

This method is typically employed when the renal pelvis is not large enough for a cutaneous pyelostomy to be performed. The initial steps for a high cutaneous ureterostomy are similar to that for a cutaneous pyelostomy. The ureter is brought to skin level. Two 3-0 polyglactin sutures are placed in the upper ureter approximately 5 mm from each other. Using a scalpel a 2-cm vertical ureterotomy is created. The abdominal musculature is closed on either side and behind the loop of ureter. Care is taken to avoid strangulating the ureter. The incised ureteral margins are sewn to the skin using interrupted 4—0 polyglactin sutures. The final product is a double-barreled ureteral stoma (Fig. 102–7).

Loop ureterostomies maintain continuity of part of the ureter, therefore decreasing the likelihood of disruption of ureteral blood supply and possibly making closure of the ureterostomy simpler.

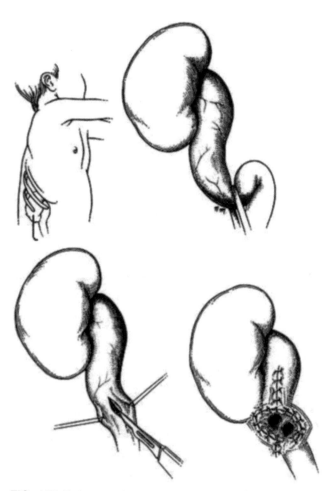

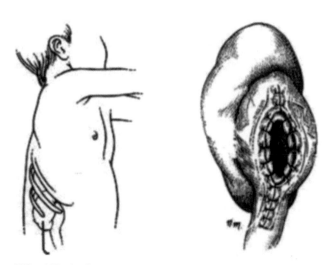

FIG. 102–6. Cutaneous pyelostomy (sutures at the skin level).

FIG. 102–7. Loop cutaneous ureterostomy (sutures at the skin level).

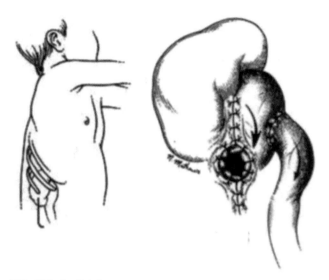

FIG. 102–8. Pelvioureterostomy-en-Y (Sober ureterostomy).

Pelvioureterostomy-en-Y (Sober Loop Ureterostomy)

The Sober Y ureterostomy allows some urine to drain into the bladder, thus avoiding a completely defunctionalized bladder that may eventually become contracted (5). It is not the procedure of choice in critically ill patients as it is more extensive and time consuming than other forms of diversion and is best used in patients with redundant tortuous ureters. The ureter is mobilized from the level of the kidney to the level of the true pelvis. The ureter is divided at a point where the lower ureteral segment comfortably reaches the renal pelvis. The upper ureter that remains in continuity with the renal pelvis is brought out to the flank caudad to the flank incision. The proximal end of the lower portion of the transected ureter is anastomosed to the renal pelvis. This is done in an end-to-side fashion after creating a pelviotomy at a point that will not cause ureteral kinking. The anastomosis is performed using a 5-0 or 6-0 polyglactin suture in a running fashion (Fig. 102–8). The flank incision is closed in the standard fashion. A small Penrose drain may be temporarily placed. Initially, most urine will drain via the ureterostomy. Overtime, increasing amounts of urine will drain into the bladder.

End Cutaneous Ureterostomy

To successfully perform a cutaneous ureterostomy, the ureter must be sufficiently thick walled and dilated. Preservation of the ureteral blood supply is essential. The ureter should be approached extraperitoneally via either a low abdominal incision or a Gibson incision. The ureter should be carefully dissected from the level of the sacral promontory to the bladder with care to avoid stripping the ureter's

adventitia. Once dissected, a thick vessel loop or Penrose drain should be placed around the ureter. One should estimate whether the ligated ureter will comfortably reach the anterior abdominal wall at the right or left lower quadrant. Once satisfied with this, the ureter is clamped and cut. The distal segment is ligated using a 3-0 polyglactin suture. A 3-0 polyglactin stay suture is placed on the cut end in order to avoid the ureter's medial blood supply.

The cutaneous stoma is then created. Stomas should be placed in the right or left lower quadrant for ease of stomal fit in the event an appliance will be used. Once the site of the stoma has been determined, a V-shaped incision is made and taken down through the subcutaneous tissues and rectus sheath. Using the previously placed stay suture, the ureter is gently brought through the incision. If the ureter seems stretched, additional mobilization may be necessary. The ureter is then spatulated medially to avoid its blood supply. The apex of the spatulated ureter is then sewn to the apex of the skin incision using a 3 or 4-0 polyglactin suture. The ureter is then sewn to the other angles of the skin incision and additional sutures are placed circumferentially.

Bilateral end ureterostomies may be brought to the midline or either lower quadrant. The medial wall of each ureter is incised approximately 3 cm. The apex of the incised ureters are sewn to each other using a two-armed 5-0 polyglactin suture. The incised walls of the ureters are then sewn to each other in a running fashion.

Closure of Supravesical Diversions

To close a cutaneous pyelostomy, an elliptical skin incision is made around the stoma. The portion of pelvis that has been exteriorized is trimmed so that healthy renal pelvic edges may be approximated. Using a 6-0 polyglactin suture in a running fashion the renal pelvis is closed in a transverse fashion. The UPJ should be inspected to ensure that no kinking has occurred secondary to pyelostomy closure.

To close a loop ureterostomy, an elliptical skin incision is made in the skin surrounding the stoma. The proximal and distal ureteral segments are mobilized. The fibrotic exposed portions of the ureter are excised, maintaining the continuity of the ureter's back wall. The remaining ureteral margins are then spatulated and closed in a transverse fashion using a 6-0 polyglactin suture (Fig. 102–9). Again, one must ensure that no angulation or narrowing of the ureter has occurred.

A Sober ureterostomy may be reversed by excising the stoma at the skin level along with the limb of ureter used to create the cutaneous ureterostomy. The dissection is taken down to the level of the renal pelvis. The defect in the renal pelvis is closed using a 6-0 polyglactin suture in a running watertight fashion.

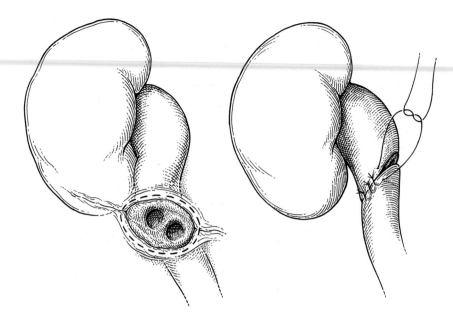

FIG. 102–9. Takedown of loop cutaneous ureterostomy.

OUTCOMES

Complications

Cutaneous vesicostomies may be complicated by early or late prolapse of the dome or posterior bladder wall, which is the most frequent complication. To prevent prolapse the most cephalad portion of the bladder or the urachus should be used as the site for the vesicostomy. By employing this portion of the bladder, the peritonealized part of the dome becomes immobilized, and decreases the risk of prolapse. The stomal opening itself should be no larger than 2 cm. The final stoma should calibrate to 24 Fr. Excessive mucosal eversion should not be mistaken for prolapse. Despite its appearance, no intervention is necessary for excessive eversion.

If the vesicostomy does not appear to be draining well and there is evidence of large amounts of residual bladder urine, the suspicion of stomal stenosis should be raised. Stomal stenosis rates of 3% to 12% have been reported (4). The stenosis may be secondary to a small fascial opening or excessive tension on the vesicocutaneous anastomosis. Continuous drainage of urine into a diaper commonly may lead to parastomal dermatitis. Prolonged, severe dermatitis may ultimately lead to stomal stenosis. This can be prevented by air drying the skin or applying topical ointments used for diaper rash. Fungal superinfection may occur and may be treated with antifungal creams and powders.

Some infants, in particular those with persistent vesicoureteral reflux, may have recurrent urinary tract infections even with small bladder residuals and without stomal stenosis. These children may benefit from intermittent catheterization through their vesicostomies.

The most common complication associated with pyelostomy is chronic skin irritation and dermatitis. As in other forms of diversion, chronic bacteriuria is also common. Less common complications of pyelostomy include stomal stenosis and prolapse of the renal pelvis. Chronic bacteriuria has been found in approximately two-thirds of patients with ureterostomies and is the most common complication in this group. Stomal stenosis occurs in 11% to 70% of patients undergoing end cutaneous ureterostomies (1). The incidence of stenosis and obstruction is related to the caliber of the ureter used as well as the type of stoma created. Chronic skin irritation may also result in scarring and stenosis.

Results

Despite the ease of performing a vesical diversion and its effectiveness in relieving bladder outlet obstruction, controversy exists regarding both its necessity and ultimate effects on bladder function (2,3).

ANTERIOR URETHRAL VALVES

Anterior urethral valves occur 10 times less frequently than posterior urethral valves and may be located anywhere along the anterior urethra. In most cases, an anterior urethral valve is actually a congenital urethral diverticulum with the lip of the diverticulum preventing antegrade flow of urine. The bulging diverticulum may further obstruct the urethra by compressing the lumen. These children present with symptoms similar to those with a posterior urethral valve including varying degrees of hydroureteronephrosis; however, many also present with penile ballooning. As with PUV, the diagnosis is also made on VCUG. A renal ultrasound should be performed to complete the evaluation. Cystourethroscopy may miss the valve due to the retrograde flow of fluid during the procedure.

The obstruction is relieved endoscopically. The distal lip is incised using a hook or right-angle wire electrode. If unsuccessful, the diverticulum may be excised and the urethra reconfigured. Staged urethroplasty may be the best treatment option when faced with a large urethral diverticulum. Management of the hydro-ureteronephrosis would be similar to that in a patient with a PUV.

REFERENCES

1. Burstein JD, Firlit CF. Complications of cutaneous ureterostomy and other cutaneous diversion. *Urol Clin North Am* 1983;10:433–443.

2. Glassberg KI. The valve bladder syndrome: 20 years later. *J Urol* 2001; 166:1406–1414.

3. Gonzales ET Jr. Posterior urethral valves and other anomalies. In: Walsh PC, Retik AB, Vaughan ED Jr, Wein AJ, eds. *Campbell's urology*, 7th ed. Philadelphia: WB Saunders, 1998:2069–2091.

4. Skoog SJ. Pediatric vesical diversion. In: Graham SD, Glenn JF, eds. *Glenn's urologic surgery*. 5th ed. Philadelphia: Lippincott Williams & Wilkins, 1998:871–878.

5. Sober I. Pelvioureterostomy-en-Y. *J Urol* 1972;107:473–475.

6. Williams DI, Whitaker RA, Barratt TM, Keeton JE. Urethral valves. *Br J Urol* 1973;45:200–205.

7. Zaontz MR, Firlit CF. Percutaneous antegrade ablation of posterior urethral valves in infants with small caliber urethras: an alternative to urinary diversion. *J Urol* 1986;136:247–248.

ACKNOWLEDGMENTS

The authors acknowledge the assistance of Ivan Colon, MD.

CHAPTER 103

Hypospadias

A. Barry Belman

Hypospadias, one of the most common of the congenital urogenital abnormalities, continues to be one of our most challenging and gratifying problems. Significant advances have occurred over the past several years that have raised the bar of expectations for success. The current challenge is to create a normal appearing penis in a single operation with only a small risk of a complication. Duckett aptly applied the name hypospadiology to the study of this subject.

Although inheritance plays a role in approximately 20-25 percent, hypospadias is most frequently a spontaneous occurrence without an obvious underlying cause. In siblings there appears to be about a 10-fold risk for the abnormality, but the exact mode of inheritance remains unclear. Penile development is stimulated by the effects of testosterone produced by the fetus on androgen sensitive structures including the wolffian structures, the genital tubercle and labio-scrotal folds. It has been postulated that a reduced response to testosterone stimulation or a reduction or delay in testosterone production may be responsible for hypospadias (2).

The genital tubercle is first seen at about six weeks gestation. It enlarges under the stimulation of fetal testosterone. The urethral groove that ultimately becomes the urethra lies between parallel folds along the undersurface of the tubercle. The scrotum forms from swellings on either side of the urethral groove. The urethral folds unite over the urethral groove from proximal to distal forming the urethra. Any arrest in development will cause hypospadias. The glanular urethra distal to the fossa navicularis is formed by an ingrowth of tissue that cores through the glans to meet the more proximal urethra. Blind ending glans pits are failed attempts to form this most distal part of the urethra.

Hypospadias is almost always associated with a hooded prepuce. The exception being the megameatal variant. The fact that the meatus is abnormally located is often not recognized when the foreskin is complete until circumcision is carried out or, in the uncircumcised, when the foreskin retracts. However, circumcision does not usually interfere with correction as this form is, most often, quite mild.

The prevalence of hypospadias in the entire United States doubled between 1970 and 1993, increasing to 39.7 per 10,000 births (approximately .78 per 100 male births). This increase has not been attributed to better recognition or reporting since the incidence of severe hypospadias increased at an even higher rate, from three- to fivefold. The cause for this increase is unknown.

DIAGNOSIS

The penis should be described anatomically noting both the meatal location and severity of chordee (Figure 103–1). For example, a boy may have a mid-shaft hypospadias without chordee or penoscrotal hypospadias with mild, moderate or severe chordee. Meatal position can best be identified by lifting the ventral skin away from the shaft, exaggerating the meatal opening. (Figure 103–2) The presumed newborn male with hypospadias who does not have two gonads clearly palpable should be evaluated for a chromosomal abnormality prior to hospital discharge to rule out adrenogenital syndrome.

Chordee occurs more frequently in those with more severe hypospadias but can also be found independent of hypospadias. Chordee without hypospadias may simply be a consequence of short ventral skin. However, abnormal development of the distal urethra or ventral corporeal fascia may also play a role.

INDICATIONS FOR SURGERY

Indications for surgery is the presence of hypospadias and timing of the repair is usually as early as is feasible. Manley and Epstein reported reduced anxiety when repairs were carried out prior to 18 months of age (9). Belman and Kass found no increased incidence of surgical complications when surgery is performed from 2-11 months of age (3).

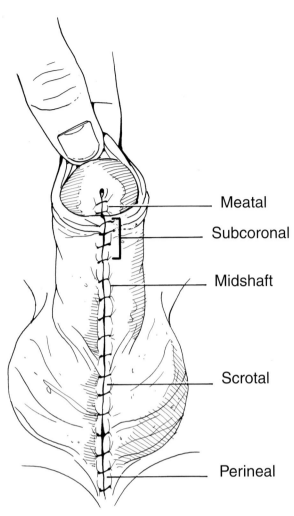

FIG. 103–1. Stages of hypospadias.

Meatal

Subcoronal

Midshaft

Scrotal

Perineal

ALTERNATIVE THERAPY

There is no alternative to surgical repair. There are, however, multiple procedures that can be performed depending upon the degree of hypospadias.

SURGICAL TECHNIQUE

The current success of hypospadias repair can be attributed to the contributions of many of our predecessors. Devine and Horton stressed tissue handling, more extensive use of vascular flaps was advanced by Hodgson and Duckett, and better coverage of suture lines by Smith. Smith utilized a de-epithelialized flap of ventral tissue at the second stage of his standard two-stage hypospadias repair to cover the urethra and prevent crossing suture lines. Subsequently, this application was applied to single stage repairs. Modifications include use of tunica vaginalis and scrotal dartos as a second layer to achieve the same purpose.

Chordee

Correction of chordee is an integral part of hypospadias repair and is generally accomplished at the time of urethroplasty. Occasionally a two-stage procedure becomes necessary with chordee correction as the first step. The most popular method of correcting chordee is by dorsal placation as originally described by Nesbit. (Figure 103–3) The fascial edges are then reapproximated with buried suture. A modification of this technique, tunica albuginia plication, does not require excision of fascia but, instead, parallel transverse incisions are approximated with non-absorbable 5-0 Prolene (polypropelene) over a buried strip of fascia. Suture that is slowly absorbed, such as PDS (polydiaxanone), may be prefer-

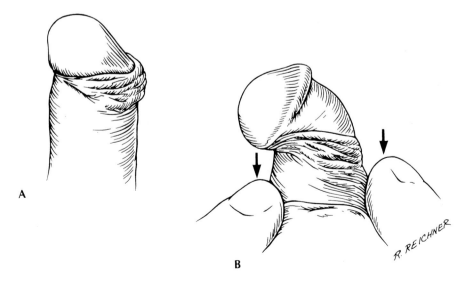

R. REICHNER

FIG. 103–2. (A) Distal hypospadias with dorsal hood of prepuce. **(B)** Traction of the skin toward the base causes ventral tilt of the glans.

A

B

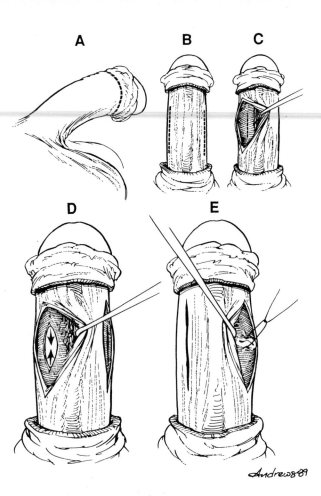

FIG. 103–3. Correction of persisting chordee. The plane between Buck's fascia and the tunica albuginea is established ventrolaterally (**C**) to avoid beginning the dissection at the edge of the neurovascular bundle. The incision in the tunica albuginea is superficial, care being taken not to enter the vascular tissue of the corpora casvernosa (**D**). A repeat artificial erection is essential after plication is complete.

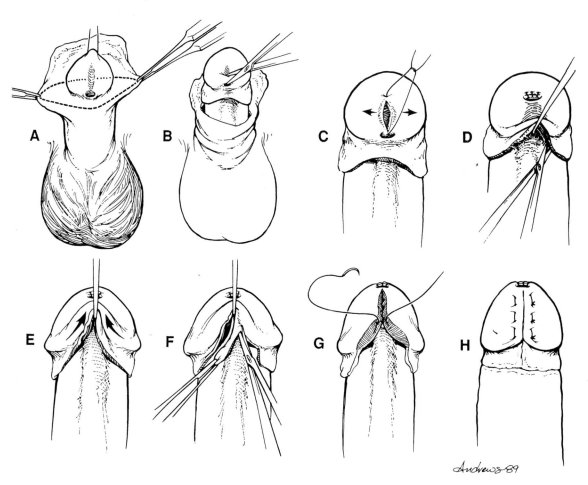

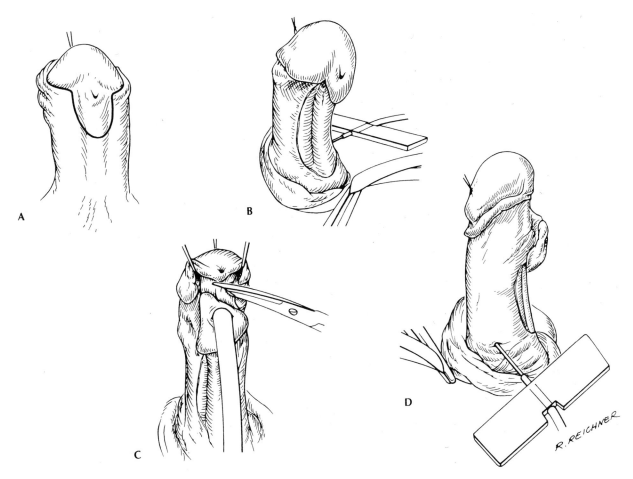

FIG. 103–5. Distal hypospadias with urethral mobilization. (**A**) Incisions for flip flop operation are outlined. The glans incisions have not yet been marked. (**B**) After completion of mobilization of penile skin, the chordee is still present. (**C**) A dysgenetic band deep and distal to the meatus is dissected out and excised. (**D**) An artificial erection now reveals the penis to be straight.

able to avoid persistent foci of subcutaneous irritation. More recently, Baskin et al, after studying nerve distribution in the human fetus, have recommended midline plication for correction (1).

MAGPI

The MAGPI (meatal advancement, glanuloplasty) procedure changed attitudes regarding ultimate meatal position with only 1.2 percent of patients requiring a second procedure. However, meatal regression can occur. Originally described as applicable to the subcoronal meatus, when applied to coronal hypospadias a 35 percent failure rate was reported by Unluer, et al. (11) Variants of this procedure have been described (Figure 103–4).

Coronal Hypospadias

Urethral advancement: Introduced in the late 1800's by Beck, this procedure employs proximal urethral dissection and mobilization distally to advance the meatus to the ideal location. (Figure 103–5).

FIG. 103–4. MAGPI (meatal advancement, glanduloplasty). Note the proximal location of the initial circumcising incision in relation to the urethral meatus (**A**). The dorsal meatotomy is as shown (**B and C**). The glans is then detached from the lateral margin of the corpus spongiosum and side of the corpora cavernosa (**D**). The edge of the glans on either side that will be approximated ventrally is identified (**E**). The triangle of skin between these two points and the urethral meatus is excised completely (**F**). Dissection must stay right on the skin because the urethra here is usually thin and easily entered. Excising this skin, though, allows glans to be reapproximated to glans and affords a much more reconstruction (**G and H**).

>103. Hypospadias / 795

Rolled Midline Tube

Based on the historic contributions of Duplay, with modifications, the rolled midline tube has gained renewed popularity. King applied this maneuver to distal hypospadias. Subsequently, complications have been reduced with application of a de-epithelialized flap to cover the urethral closure. Snodgrass introduced a further modification that has gained popularity. An incision is made in the midline of the urethral plate disrupting its continuity. This allows the two halves to hinge together upon vertical closure (Figure 103–6). The incidence of fistula or meatal stenosis is very low with this procedure. To increase success rate, a de-epithelialized flap was also applied to this procedure. The technique has also been applied to reoperative hypospadias surgery as well as to more proximal repairs (Figure 103–7). When applied to complex hypospadias the proximal urethra may have to be constructed with a pedicle tube while the distal urethra is formed by tubularizing the incised urethral plate. Dorsal plication is necessary for chordee correction.

Megameatal Hypospadias Repair

As previously noted, a variant of hypospadias with an intact foreskin exists. Although the enlarged meatus may be glanular in location, often it is found at the corona or subcorona. The distal urethra also tends to be extremely wide. This abnormality is easily repaired because of the width of the urethral plate, the broad flat glans, and abundant ventral skin and can be readily accomplished even if

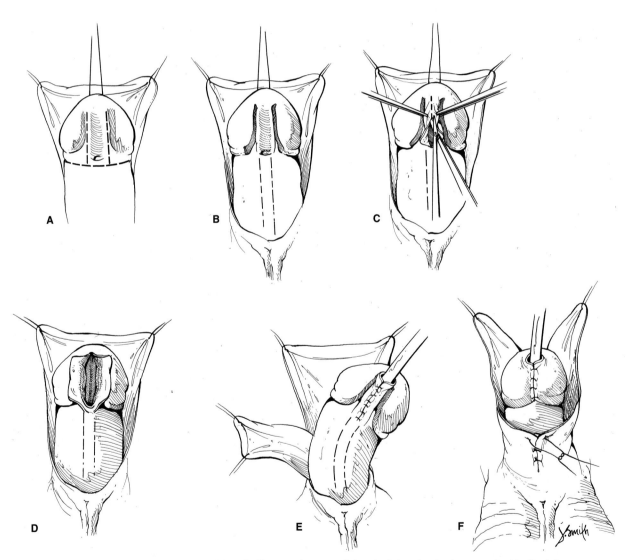

FIG. 103–6. TIP: **(A)** Horizontal line indicates circumscribing incision to deglove penis. Vertical lines show junction of urethral plate and the ventral glans. **(B)** Parallel incisions separate urethral plate from glans. **(C)** Midline incision of urethral plate from meatus to granular tip. **(D)** Incision has widened and deepened the urethral plate. **(E)** Plate tubularized over 6-Fr stent. Dorsal subcutaneous tissues are rotated ventrally to cover the repair. **(F)** Midline closure of glans wing, mucosa collar, and ventral shaft skin.

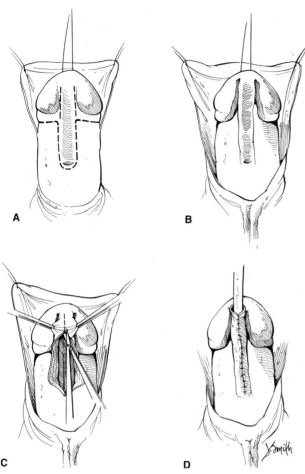

the patient has been circumcised. Incisions are made on either side of the urethral plate into the distal glans and the wide urethral plate is rolled into a tube (Figure 103–8). The plate itself does not need to be incised to gain circumferance. To avoid crossing suture lines and reduce complications, prior to glans closure subcutaneous tissue from the ventral penile shaft can be advanced over the urethra.

Meatal-Based Flap Procedures

These operations are based on the method introduced by Ombredanne in the early part of the 1900's. The most popular and enduring meatal based flap repair was introduced by Mathieu (Figure103–9). A rectangle of ventral urethral skin proximal to the hypospadiac meatus is outlined, the length determined by the distance from the meatus to the end of the glans. The flap and its subcutaneous tissue is dissected from the remainder of the ventral skin. Incisions are carried distally on either side of the urethral plate into the glans. The flap is flipped distally and anastomosed to the urethral plate with running 7-0 subcuticular stitches that invert the skin edges. A layer of subcutaneous tissue can be brought directly over these suture lines to minimize complications. The glans is approximated with one or two buried mattressed 6-0 Vicryl while interrupted 7-0 Vicryl closes the glanular epithelium. Penile skin is ideally closed in the midline with excess skin excised to give a normal, circumcised appearance. Hakim, et al reported a complication rate of 2.63 percent in a group of 114 boys when a urethral stent was used post operatively as compared to a complication rate of 3.6 percent in a group of 222 in whom a stent was not utilized (6).

FIG. 103–7. Proximal TIP repair. (**A**) U-Shaped circumscribing incision preserves the proximal aspect of urethral plate. (**B**) Distal urethral plate separated from glans. (**C**) Entire urethral plate divided in the midline to widen and deepen it. (**D**) Plate tubularized over catheter.

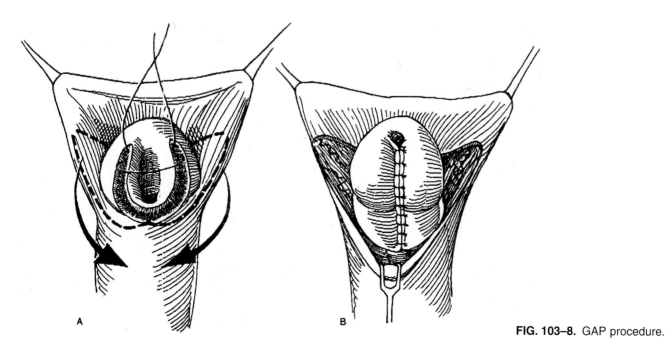

FIG. 103–8. GAP procedure.

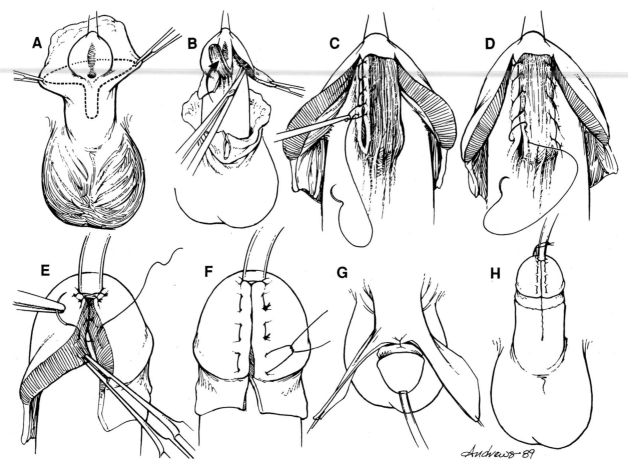

FIG. 103–9. Mathieu hypospadias repair (flip-flap). As the initial skin incision is made (**A**), a sheet of dartos fascia wider than the flap is preserved (**B**). This will be used to cover the suture lines of the neourethra. Spongy tissue of the glans is excises from beneath the distal end of the glans strip. The neourethra is closed in two layers (**C and D**). The glans is closed in two layers. Deeper sutures bring a thick layer of flans around the neourethra, reestablishing the normal relation of the glans to the urethra (**E**). Care is taken to be sure the coronal sulcus is reapproximated (**F**). The laterally placed mucosal collars are repositioned ventrally. A midline closure of the transposed foreskin is accomplished on the ventrum (**H**).

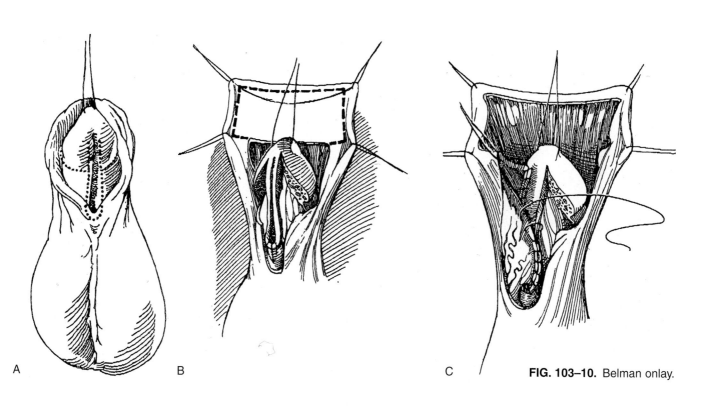

FIG. 103–10. Belman onlay.

Onlay Flap Repairs

Onlay flap repairs have become very popular and can be applied to all patients without penile chordee. The procedure as originally described utilized a transverse pedicle flap of inner preputial skin. An alternative is to split the foreskin, deepithelialize the outer skin and applying the inner foreskin as an island pedicle onlay (Figure 103–10). This results in the island flap being served by the blood supply of one-half of the prepuce. After anastomosing the pedicle flap to the urethral plate, the broad vascular pedicle is sutured on each side to the depths of the glanular incisions to completely cover the new urethra. That procedure is called the split-prepuce in-situ onlay repair and, in a series of 100 consecutive cases reported by Rushton and Belman, fistulae occurred in only 4 percent (10).

Correcting Hypospadias with Chordee

Historically, chordee was first released by transection of the urethral plate along with aggressive dissection of the ventral fascia, freeing abnormal connective tissue from this region. The tubularized urethra was then formed from grafts, flaps or at a second stage. However, chordee release by dorsal plication. has led to greater use of onlay flaps and an extended tubularized incised urethral plate approach.

After the surgeon is satisfied that the penis is straight, the width and length of skin required is measured and marked appropriately. The undersurface of the foreskin is separated from the remainder of the prepuce along these lines. Adequate length of the pedicle is required to swing the skin ventral without tension. The tube is constructed over a catheter with running suture. The anastomosis should be spatulated to prevent stenosis (Figure 103–11).

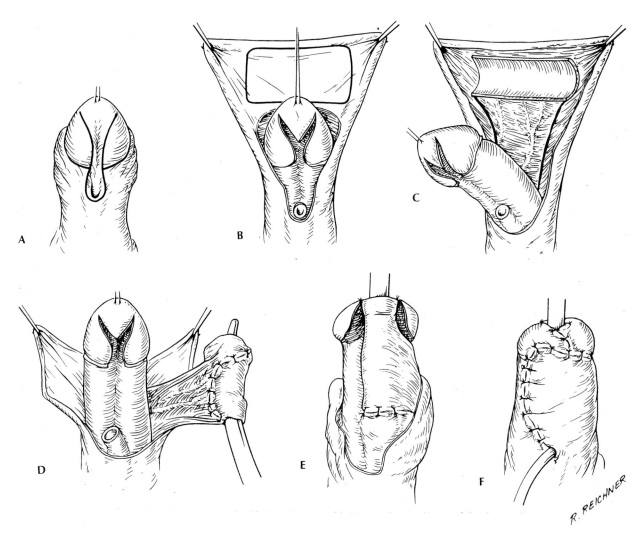

FIG. 103–11. Transverse preputial island flap. (**A**) Incision is marked to mobilize the skin and urethra and release the chordee. (**B**) Dissection is complete and the penis is straight. There is a measured area of innerface. Preputial skin is marked for incision. (**C**) Transverse flap of prepuce is isolated on its vascular pedicle. The rest of the prepuce is supplied with blood by vessels in the skin. (**D**) The flap has been formed into a tube lumen and transferred to the ventral surface on its pedicle. (**E**) The tube has been attached to the urethra at is proximal end and to the glans flap distally. (**F**) The glans wings have been closed over the neourethra and the slin of the prepuce has been brought ventrally to cover the penis.

The glans is split and dissected laterally from the deep penile fascia (glans wings) to allow closure over the new urethra without tension. This is very important as glanular disruption is the consequence of failure to provide a tension-free closure. A second layer of deepithelialized skin or tunica vaginalis is brought over the entire neourethra to reduce risks of fistula formation and to add vasculature to the distal urethra.

Scrotal and Perineal Hypospadias

There is rarely sufficient preputial skin to form the entire urethra when the hypospadiac meatus is severely proximal. Preoperative testosterone administration may be helpful to both gain skin and increase glanular size. In some, particularly those with penoscrotal transposition (Figure 103–12) a planned two-stage repair should be considered. When that is elected chordee is corrected and skin brought to the ventral surface during the first stage. Urethral construction, generally achieved by rolling a midline tube, is accomplished at the second stage 4-6 months later.

Free Graft Repairs

Urethroplasy utilizing a free graft of tissue from the foreskin was popular until pedicle flaps became so successful. When non-penile tissue was utilized, results were often complicated by hair growth or contraction. Memmelaar introduced the bladder mucosa graft in 1947, the use of which became popular in the 1980's. Bladder mucosa was particularly applicable for patients with

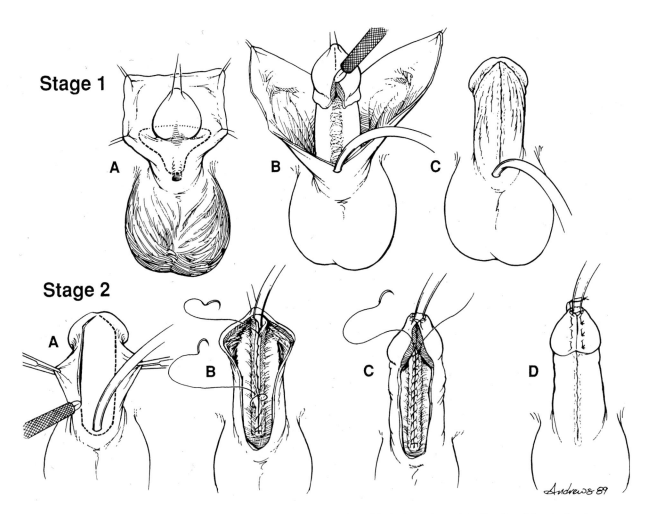

FIG. 103–12. Two-stage repair. *Stage 1*: The unfolded foreskin is brought out to the tip of the incised and mobilized glanular wings (**B**). Delicate sutures reapproximate the skin in the midline and fix the skin to the corpora cavernosa (**C**). *Stage 2*: A sufficient strip of skin is outlined (**A**). Dissection of the shaft skin is lateral and away from the neourethra. Two layers of inverting sutures are used to close the neourethra (**B**). If the prepuce has been positioned sufficiently distal at the first stage, a normally positioned meatus with good ventral glandular support can be achieved (**C**). Any excess shaft skin is excised, but the dartos layer is preserved (deepithelialization) to drape across the neourethral suture line (**D**).

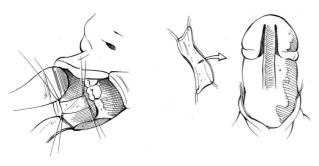

FIG. 103–13. Buccolmucosa harvested from check and used as free graft onlay repair.

complex problems, such as those who had failed hypospadias repair in whom adequate penile skin was lacking for further correction. However, bladder mucosa tolerates surface exposure poorly. Meatal stenosis and meatal prolapse were reported in 68 percent of a group when the urethra was constructed from bladder mucosa to the tip of the glans (8).

On the other hand, buccal mucosa tolerates exposure to air and may be better adapted to penile use (Figure 103–13). The risk of meatal stenosis is low. The sub-basement membrane vascularity appears to be more abundant in buccal as compared to bladder mucosa and the epithelial layer is thicker. These qualities appear to enhance its success. Buccal mucosa can be applied both as an onlay or formed into a tube.

OUTCOMES

Complications

Urethrocutaneous fistula continues to be the most common postoperative problem following hypospadias repair. However the incidence is quite low, particularly with the increasing popularity of applying a second complete covering over the neourethra. The risk of fistula for a distal onlay repair is less than 5 percent when a second layer is used to cover the neourethra (5). For more complex repairs the risk is significantly higher.

Repair of small urethrocutaneous fistulae is a simple matter done most often as an outpatient procedure without use of a urethral stent. Prior to fistula closure, the urethra should be calibrated to assure the absence of distal stenosis. The secret to successful closure is similar to achieving success with the original repair: optical magnification, the use of fine sutures, careful technique and covering the suture line completely with a second layer best obtained by de-epethilializing adjacent tissue.

Urethral meatal stenosis is a consequence of loss of blood supply to the distal urethra. If the problem is simply that of a web at the meatus, dilation or a ventral inci-

sion may resolve the problem. Occasionally a parent is sent home with a urethral dilator, which, if inserted on a daily basis, may resolve the more mild problems. Most often, however, distal reconstruction becomes necessary as dilation alone is rarely effective in the face of a devascularized scar.

Loss of vascularity to the new urethra is the usual etiology for strictures. Contraction of a circular anastomosis may also be the cause. The risk for contraction can be reduced by spatulating the anastamosis between the original hypospadiac meatus and the newly constructed urethra. Incise the meatus proximally for a few millimeters to create a fish-mouth appearance prior to attaching the new urethra. Treatment of strictures generally requires an open procedure, however a trial of either dilation or visual urethrotomy may be worthwhile. Hsaio et al had success with one or the other of these methods in 46 percent of patients when the attempt was carried out within the first 3 months following the hypospadias repair (7). However, cure was achieved in only 16 percent when treatment was initiated 3 months after the original procedure. Duel et al reported a 21 percent resolution with direct vision urethrotomy in a group of 29 patients (4). In the older patient, daily self-dilation with a soft catheter for 6-12 weeks may be successful. In the young child failure after a single dilation under anesthesia indicates that open repair is probably required for resolution.

Urethral diverticula may be either the result of increased intraurethral pressure secondary to distal narrowing or distensability of the newly constructed urethra. Indications for surgical excision are recurrent urinary tract infections or significant post-void urinary dribbling. As is true for fistulae, the urethra should first be calibrated to rule out distal stenosis. If the diverticulum is not adherent to the overlying skin the repair may be facilitated by retracting the penile skin (degloving), rather than incising the skin over the diverticulum. After diverticular resection and urethral closure the skin is then brought back over the repair. This avoids crossing suture lines. Occasionally, following a tubularized urethroplasty a large saccular dilatation occurs even in the absence of infection or distal narrowing. This may be a consequence of poor tissue support over the urethra or having tubularized too wide a pedicle flap at the time of initial repair. These saccules are repaired by incising along the midline and excising the redundant mucosa. The submucosa of the diverticulum is preserved and brought together in overlapping layers after closure of the urethra. This both prevents leaks and offers tissue support to prevent recurrence. If coexisting urethral stenosis is discovered, the stenotic area is incised and a portion of the redundant tissue making up the diverticulum is appropriately swung to repair the narrowing.

Results

Success with hypospadias surgery has made great advances over the past two decades. Distal hypospadias is being repaired with a complication rate of less than 5% and the penis appears near normal. Even most complex problems are amenable to style stage repair with only 1 in 5 needing additional surgery.

Part can be attributed to a greater concentration of these children being managed by pediatric urologist. However, we must also give credit to better suture material and instrumentation.

REFERENCES

1. Baskin LS, Erol A, Li YW, Cunha GR Anatomical studies of hypospadias. *J Urol.* 1998 Sep;160(3 Pt 2):1108–15
2. Baskin LS, Sutherland LS, DiSandro SJ, Haywood SW, Lipschultz J, Cunha GR The effect of testosterone on androgen receptors and penile growth *J Urol* 158: 1113, 1997.
3. Belman AB Kass EJ Hypospadias repair in children less than 1 year old. *J Urol.* 1982 Dec;128(6):1273–4.
4. Duel BP, Barthold JS, Gonzalez R. Management of urethral strictures after hypospadias repair. *J Urol.* 1998 Jul;160(1):170–1.
5. Gonzalez R, Smith C, Denes ED Double onlay preputial flap for proximal hypospadias repair. *J Urol.* 1996 Aug;156(2 Pt 2):832–4.
6. Hakim S, Merguerian PA, Rabinowitz R, Shortliffe LD, McKenna PH Outcome analysis of the modified Mathieu hypospadias repair: comparison of stented and unstented repairs. *J Urol.* 1996 Aug;156(2 Pt 2):836–8.
7. Hsiao KC, Baez-Trinidad L, Lendvay T, Smith EA, Broecker B, Scherz H, Kirsch AJ Direct vision internal urethrotomy for the treatment of pediatric urethral strictures: analysis of 50 patients. *J Urol.* 2003 Sep;170(3):952–5.
8. Kinkead TM, Borzi PA, Duffy PG, Ransley PG Long-term followup of bladder mucosa graft for male urethral reconstruction. *J Urol.* 1994 Apr;151(4):1056–8.
9. Manley CB, Epstein ES Early hypospadias repair. *J Urol.* 1981 May;125(5):698–700.
10. Rushton HG, Belman AB The split prepuce in situ onlay hypospadias repair. *J Urol.* 1998 Sep;160(3 Pt 2):1134–6.
11. Unluer ES, Miroglu C, Ozdiler E, Ozturk R Long-term follow-up results of the MAGPI (meatal advancement and glanuloplasty) operations in distal hypospadias. *Int Urol Nephrol.* 1991;23(6):581–7.

CHAPTER 104

Single-Stage Reconstruction for Exstrophy

Richard W. Grady and Michael E. Mitchell

Because bladder exstrophy is a congenital anomaly that has characteristic external physical manifestations, the diagnosis of exstrophy is usually not subtle. The anterior portion of the bladder and/or urethra and abdominal wall structures are apparently deficient and the pubis symphysis is widely separated from the midline (Fig. 104–1). The exstrophic defects are typically found in isolation; other organ systems are only infrequently affected.

DIAGNOSIS

In some situations, the diagnosis may be made antenatally although many affected fetuses are not detected

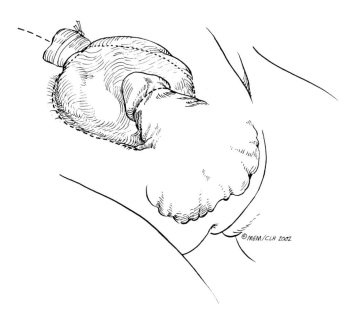

FIG. 104–1. Initial dissection—inferior view. Broken lines indicate lines of dissection. Note that the lines of dissection proceed around the umbilicus and superior to it. The lines of dissection also extend subcoronally around the ventral aspect of the penis. See Figure 104–2 for another view of the initial lines of dissection

before birth. Ultrasonography can reliably detect exstrophy before the twentieth week of gestation. Potential ultrasonographic findings of exstrophy include a semi-solid mass protruding from the abdominal wall, an absent bladder, a lower-abdominal protrusion, an anteriorly displaced scrotum with a small phallus in male fetuses, normal kidneys in association with a low-set umbilical cord, and an abnormal iliac crest widening.

Antenatal diagnosis also allows parents the opportunity to discuss early management of the patient. The overall prognosis of these children is excellent if initially treated at medical centers with physicians experienced in the treatment of this disorder.

INDICATIONS FOR SURGERY

Exstrophy anomalies are nonlethal, so children with exstrophy can survive untreated. Before the modern era of surgery and anesthesia, some patients with bladder exstrophy survived untreated into adulthood. Reports exist of such patients with classic bladder exstrophy living into their eighth decade (9). However, significant morbidity exists with these conditions if they are left untreated, including bladder and kidney infection, skin breakdown, and tumor formation in the bladder plate. The surrounding skin around the exposed exstrophic bladder is often inflamed secondary to urine contact dermatitis, loss of skin integrity from constant wetness, and secondary infection. When these patients receive effective surgical and medical treatment, they can lead productive, healthy lives with minimal morbidity from their underlying urologic abnormality.

Inguinal hernias are commonly associated with exstrophy in both male and female patients and are a consequence of enlarged internal and external inguinal rings combined with compromised fascial support and lack of obliquity of the inguinal canal (2,10). In a review of patients from Toronto Sick Children's Hospital 56% of classic male exstrophy patients and 15% of classic female exstrophy patients developed inguinal hernias over a 10-year period. These should be repaired at the time of primary bladder closure to prevent incarcerated hernias that could affect up to 50% of these patients in the first 2 years of life (1). Reinforcement of the transversalis and internal oblique fascia during hernia repair decreases the incidence of later direct inguinal hernias.

ALTERNATIVE THERAPY

There is no alternative therapy other than surgery that may be performed in a series of operations (staged approach) (3).

SURGICAL TECHNIQUE

The primary goals for exstrophy reconstruction include preservation of kidney function, urinary continence, low-pressure urine storage reservoir, volitional voiding, and functionally and cosmetically acceptable external genitalia. Secondary goals for reconstruction include minimization of urinary tract infections, adequate pelvic floor support, minimization of the risk for malignancy associated with the urinary tract, minimization of the risk for urinary calculi, and adequate abdominal wall fascia.

Surgical reconstruction of exstrophy and epispadias represents one of the most significant challenges for physicians who specialize in the urologic care of children. Over the last decade, a novel single-stage surgical reconstructive approach has been developed for the exstrophy–epispadias complex. This operation evolved out of a technique developed for the treatment of epispadias—the complete penile disassembly technique (8). By employing this technique, the surgeon permits the tissue deformation in exstrophy to return most closely to an anatomically normal position. We have used this approach—the disassembly technique with complete primary exstrophy repair (CPER)—exclusively for the surgical treatment of newborns with exstrophy since 1990 (5). This operation or its principles may also be employed in reoperative repairs or delayed repairs for exstrophy.

After delivery, the umbilical cord is ligated with silk suture rather than a plastic or metal clamp to prevent trauma to the exposed bladder plate. A hydrated gel dressing may be used to protect the exposed bladder from superficial trauma. This type of dressing is easy to use, keeps the bladder plate from desiccating, and stays in place to allow handling of the infant with minimal risk of trauma to the bladder. Plastic wrap is an acceptable alternative. Dressings should be replaced daily and the bladder should be irrigated with normal saline with each diaper change. A humidified air incubator may also minimize bladder trauma (1).

We routinely use intravenous antibiotic therapy in the pre- and postoperative periods to decrease the risk for infection following reconstruction. We also perform preoperative ultrasonography to assess the kidneys and establish a baseline examination for later ultrasonographic studies. Preoperative spinal sonographic examination should be considered if sacral dimpling or other signs of spina bifida occulta are noted on physical examination.

In the newborn period, we perform primary exstrophy closure using general inhalation anesthesia. Nitrous oxide during primary closure may cause bowel distension, which decreases surgical exposure during the operation and increases the risk of wound dehiscence. We ask our anesthesiologists to avoid using it when possible. Some advocate the use of nasogastric tube drainage to decrease abdominal distension in the postoperative period (3). We do not use nasogastric suction in most patients but do routinely use a one-time caudal block to reduce the inhaled anesthetic requirement during the operation.

For patients older than 3 days, or newborns with a wide pubic diastasis, in conjunction with our orthopedic surgery colleagues, we perform anterior iliac osteotomies at the time of CPER. Osteotomies assist closure and enhance anterior pelvic floor support, which may improve later urinary continence. Forcing a primary closure without osteotomies in a child with a wide pubic diastasis and abdominal defect can lead to increased abdominal pressures. This increased pressure can compromise vascular circulation to the intestines, kidneys, and genitalia.

CPER Surgical Technique: Boys

After standard preparation of the surgical field, we place traction sutures transversely into each of the hemiglans of the penis and the lines of dissection are marked. (Figs. 104–1 and 104–2). Next, 3.5 Fr umbilical artery catheters are placed into both ureters and sutured

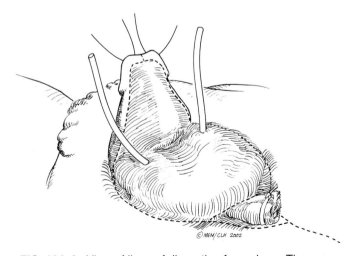

FIG. 104–2. View of lines of dissection from above. The urethral dissection is carried along the lateral aspect of the urethral plate.

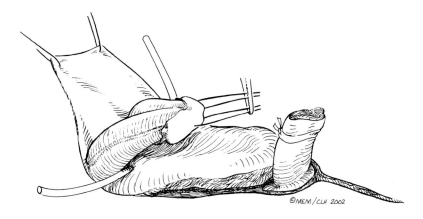

FIG. 104–3. Ventral dissection is initiated most easily below the glans with a circumcising incision. The dissection may be carried proximally.

in place with 5-0 chromic sutures. Initial dissection begins superiorly and proceeds inferiorly to separate the bladder plate from the adjacent skin and fascia. We use tungsten fine-tip electrocautery (Colorado tip®) during this dissection. The umbilical vessels may be ligated if necessary but are preferentially preserved as a vascular pedicle for the umbilicus. We also incise the periumbilical skin circumferentially at this time. The umbilicus will be moved superiorly to a more anatomically normal location.

The penile dissection begins along the ventral aspect of the penis as a circumcising incision (Fig. 104–1). This step precedes dissection of the urethral wedge from the corporal bodies because it is easier to identify the plane of dissection above Buck's fascia ventrally (Fig. 104–3). Buck's fascia is deficient or absent around the corpora spongiosum and thus as the dissection progresses medially to separate the urethra from the corpora cavernosa the plane shifts subtly from above Buck's fascia to just above the tunica albuginea. Failure to adjust the plane of dissection will carry the dissection into the corpora spongiosa; this will result in excessive bleeding during the deep ventral dissection of the urethral wedge from the corporal bodies.

We apply methylene blue or brilliant green to the urethra to help identify the demarcation of urothelium and squamous epithelium. Injection of the surrounding tissues with 0.25% lidocaine and 1:200,00 U per mL epinephrine also improves hemostasis and assists the dissection. The margins of the dorsal urethra can be delineated because the urothelium is smooth and shiny because it is not keratinized. Shallow incisions are made laterally to begin the urethral dissection (Fig. 104–4). Sharp dissection is required to develop the plane between the urethral wedge and the corporal bodies, taking care to preserve urethral width. Careful lateral dissection of the penile shaft skin and dartos fascia from the corporal bodies will avoid damaging the laterally located neurovascular bundles on the corpora of the epispadic penis. The paired neurovascular bundles are always lateral to the margins of the urethral wedge and the lateral dissection on the penis should be superficial to Buck's fascia to avoid injury to the neurovascular bundles.

Once a plane is established between the corpora cavernosa and the urethral wedge (Fig. 104–5), the penis may be disassembled into three components—the right and left corporal bodies with their respective hemiglans and the urethral wedge (urothelium with underlying corpora

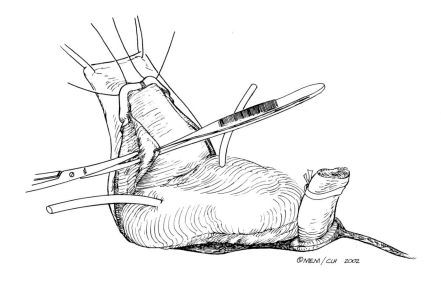

FIG. 104–4. The urethra is dissected from the corporal bodies. This plane of dissection is developed from both a ventral and lateral perspective using sharp dissection.

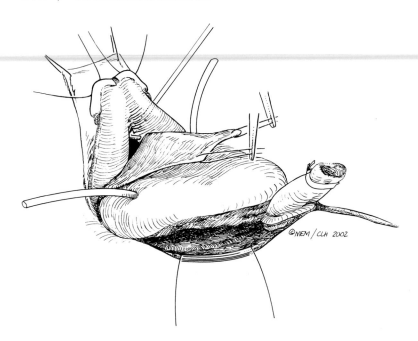

FIG. 104–5. Disassembly of the corporal bodies from the urethra and corpora spongiosa (the urethral wedge) can often be most easily begun at the position depicted here. The dissection is carried distally to completely separate the glans penis.

spongiosa) (12). We have found the easiest plane of dissection between the corporal bodies to be proximal and ventral (Fig. 104–6). The plane of dissection should be carried out at the level of the tunica albuginea of the corpora cavernosa. After a plane is established between the urethral wedge and the corporal bodies, this dissection is carried distally to separate the three components from each other (Fig. 104–7). Complete separation of the corporal bodies increases exposure to the pelvic diaphragm for deep dissection. The corporal bodies may be completely separated from each other because they exist on a separate blood supply (Figs. 104–6 and 104–7). Note that

it is important to keep the underlying corpora spongiosa with the urethra; the blood supply to the urethra is based on this corporal tissue, which should appear wedge-shaped after its dissection from the adjacent corpora cavernosa. The urethral/corpora spongiosa component will later be tubularized and placed ventral to the corporal bodies. Also note that paraexstrophy skin flaps *cannot* be used with this technique because this maneuver will devascularize the distal urethra; and, because the bladder and urethra are moved posteriorly in the pelvis as a unit (with a common proximal blood supply), division of the urethral wedge is never considered. In some cases, a male

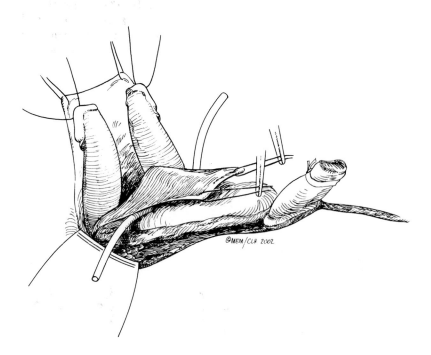

FIG. 104–6. The urethra and corporal bodies are separated distally to allow deep dissection of the pelvic floor musculature.

patient will be left with a hypospadias that will require later surgical reconstruction.

After separating the components distally (Fig. 104–6), the urethral dissection is carried proximally to the bladder neck. Exposure to the pelvic diaphragm is optimized by complete separation of the urethra and corporal bodies, creating surgical exposure for the deep incision of the intersymphyseal band (Fig. 104–6). When dissecting the urethral wedge from the corporal bodies medially, the dissection plane is on the tunica albuginea of the corpora cavernosa (Fig. 104–7) and should be carried down to the intersymphyseal band (the condensation of anterior pelvic fascia and ligaments and the anterior portion of the pelvic diaphragm) (Fig. 104–8 inset). Deep incision of the intersymphyseal band posterior and lateral to each side of the urethral wedge is absolutely necessary to allow the bladder to achieve a posterior position in the pelvis. This dissection should be continued until the pelvic floor musculature becomes visible. Failure to adequately dissect the bladder and urethral wedge from these surrounding structures will prevent posterior movement of the bladder neck in the pelvis and create anterior tension along the urethral plate.

Once the intersymphyseal band is adequately incised and the bladder and urethral wedge are adequately dissected from the surrounding tissues, both these structures should be easily positioned deep in the pelvis. The bladder can be closed and the urethra tubularized. This portion of the repair is straightforward and anatomic if the previous dissection is performed adequately. To provide urinary drainage, we place a suprapubic tube and bring it out through the umbilicus. The bladder is closed in three

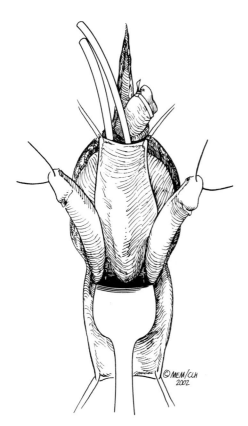

FIG. 104–7. Perineal view of complete disassembly. Note depth of dissection.

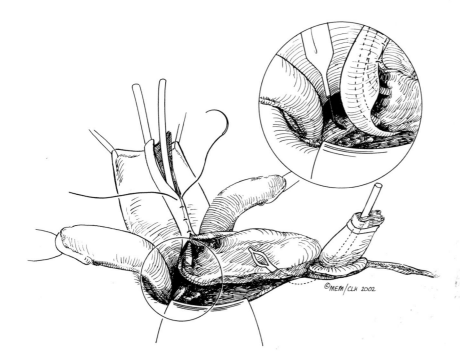

FIG. 104–8. The exposure for deep dissection is optimal after complete separation of the corporal bodies. It is crucial to adequately divide the intersymphyseal band (inset) to allow the bladder and urethra to move posteriorly.

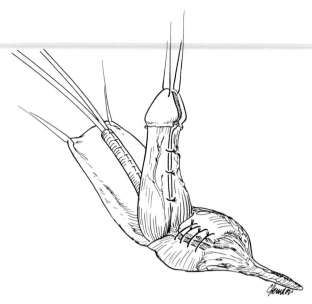

FIG. 104–9. The urethra and bladder are reapproximated in a two-layer closure.

proximated using an interrupted or running 2-0 polydiaxonone suture. We also place interrupted sutures along the dorsal aspect of the corporal bodies to reapproximate them (Fig. 104–11). We provide penile skin coverage by using either a primary dorsal closure or reversed Byars flaps if needed. Skin covering the abdominal wall is reapproximated using a two-layer closure of absorbable monofilament suture.

Penile reconstruction is not initiated until the abdominal wall fascia and symphyseal closure is complete. The corporal bodies will rotate medially with abdominal wall closure when the lateral margins of Buck's fascia of each corpora cavernosa are approximated, which will assist in correcting the dorsal deflection (Fig. 104–10). On occasion, significant discrepancies in the dorsal and ventral lengths of the corpora will require dermal graft insertion. This is rarely, if ever, needed in newborn closures.

If there is adequate urethral length, the urethra may be brought up to each hemiglans ventrally to create an orthotopic meatus (Fig. 104–11). We reconfigure the glans using interrupted mattress sutures of polydiaxonone followed by horizontal mattress sutures of 7-0 monofilament to reapproximate the glans epithelium. The neourethra is matured with 7-0 braided polyglactin suture similar to our standard hypospadias repair. When needed, we also will perform glans tissue reduction to create a conical-appearing glans. Tacking sutures are placed ventrally and dorsally to prevent penile shaft skin from riding over the corporal bodies and "burying" the penis (Figs. 104–12 and 104–13).

In our hands, the urethra lacks enough length to reach the glans in about half the cases. In this situation we mature the urethra along the ventral aspect of the penis to create a hypospadias. This can be corrected at a later date as a second-stage procedure. We often leave redundant shaft skin ventrally in these patients to assist in later penile reconstructive procedures.

layers with monofilament absorbable suture (i.e., Monocryl and Vicryl). The urethra is tubularized using a two-layer running closure with monofilament and braided absorbable suture (Fig. 104–9). Because of the previous deep dissection, we can position the tubularized urethra ventral to the corpora in a tension-free fashion. If the urethra cannot be positioned ventrally without creating tension, it is likely that a deeper incision is required into the intersymphyseal band and pelvic diaphragm.

We reapproximate the pubic symphysis using 0-0 polydiaxonone interrupted figure-of-eight sutures with the knots left anteriorly to prevent suture erosion into the bladder neck (Fig. 104–10). The rectus fascia is reap-

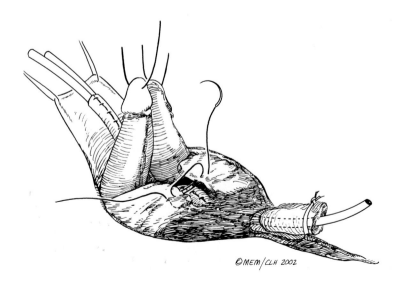

FIG. 104–10. After the bladder and urethra are reconstructed, these structures will move posteriorly. The urethra will assume a more normal anatomic position. The pubis symphysis is reapproximated with two figure-of-eight sutures.

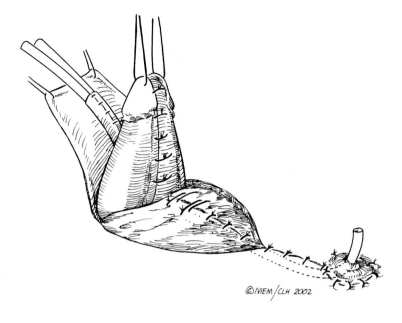

FIG. 104–11. The corporal bodies will rotate medially so that the neurovascular bodies are located medially. The suprapubic tube can be brought out through the umbilicus. The umbilicus is moved superiorly to a more normal anatomic location.

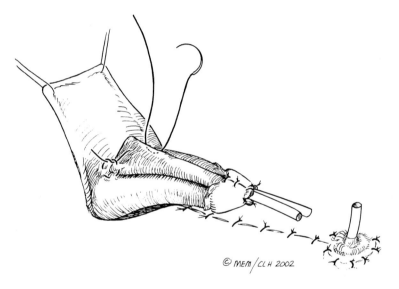

FIG. 104–12. The ventral shaft skin is secured to the base of the penis to prevent the penile shaft skin from riding over the body of the penis. The ureteral catheters are brought out through the urethra.

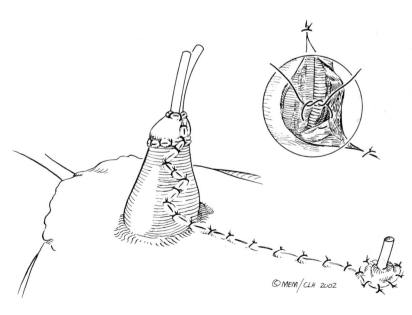

FIG. 104–13. To adequately cover the penis dorsally, Z-plasty incisions may be necessary. We also employ tacking sutures dorsally (inset) as well.

CPER Technique: Girls

The principles of this single-stage technique are similar in boys and girls. After preoperative antibiotic therapy is given and the patient is prepared and draped in a sterile field, we mark the planned lines of incision (Fig. 104–14). The bladder neck, urethra, and vagina are mobilized as a unit using a tungsten-tip electrocautery (Colorado tip®) to minimize tissue damage while achieving hemostasis. The appropriate plane of dissection is found anteriorly along the medial aspect of the bifid clitoris and proceeds posteriorly along the lateral aspect of the vaginal vault (Fig. 104–15). The vagina is mobilized with the urethral plate and bladder neck, noting that the urethra and bladder neck should not be dissected from the anterior vaginal wall as this will compromise the blood supply to the urethra. During the posterior lateral dissection, the intersymphyseal bands will be encountered and should be deeply incised to allow the vagina, urethra, and bladder neck to move posteriorly. The posterior limit of the dissection is reached when the pelvic floor musculature is exposed. The proximal urethra can be lengthened

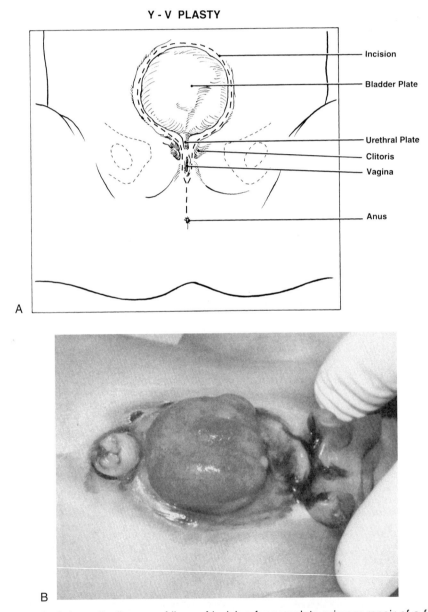

Y - V PLASTY

Incision

Bladder Plate

Urethral Plate

Clitoris

Vagina

Anus

A

B

FIG. 104–14. A: Schematic diagram of lines of incision for complete primary repair of a female infant with bladder exstrophy. Note how this concept has been applied to the repair of female epispadias in the adjacent photograph (**B**) demonstrating lines of incision for an infant girl with epispadias. Note the posterior extent of dissection to allow movement of the vagina, bladder neck, and urethra as a unit posteriorly.

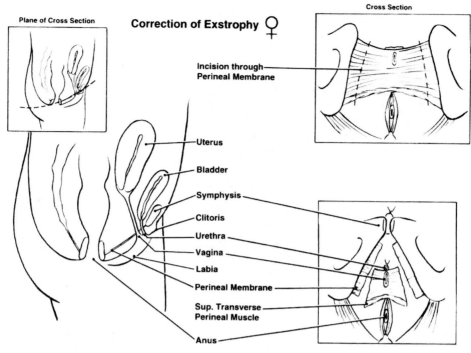

Correction of Exstrophy ♀

Plane of Cross Section

Cross Section

Incision through Perineal Membrane

Uterus

Bladder

Symphysis

Clitoris

Urethra

Vagina

Labia

Perineal Membrane

Sup. Transverse Perineal Muscle

Anus

FIG. 104–15. The plane of dissection lies adjacent to the urethra and vaginal vault (broken lines in upper right cross-sectional view).

to some degree with parallel incisions in the bladder plate to the trigone.

Following adequate dissection the vagina and urethra are moved posteriorly in the perineum with a Y–V-plasty (Fig. 104–16). The urethra is then tubularized using a two-layer closure of absorbable sutures. Prior to the urethral closure, we routinely place a suprapubic tube to provide postoperative urine drainage. The bladder, bladder neck, and urethra should be positioned deeply in the pelvis and traverse the pelvic diaphragm and the pubis symphysis is reapproximated using two 0-0 polydiaxanone (PDS) figure-of-eight sutures (Fig. 104–17). Osteotomies may be

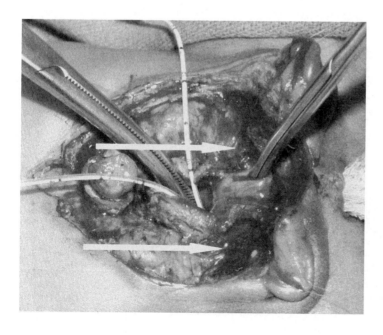

FIG. 104–16. The intersymphyseal band is incised laterally (white arrows) to allow the urethra, bladder, and vaginal vault to move posteriorly as a unit.

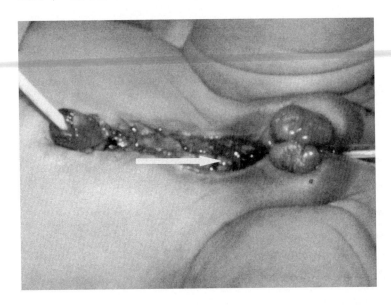

FIG. 104–17. The pubis symphysis is reapproximated (arrow). With adequate dissection, the pubis symphysis can be reapproximated with minimal compressive effects on the urethra and bladder.

necessary when a wide pubic diastasis prevents a low-tension reapproximation of the pubic symphysis. We use anterior iliac osteotomies in these situations. The rectus fascia can then be closed in the midline. We mature the neourethra with 5-0 Vicryl sutures and reapproximate the already denuded bifid clitoris medially so that they fuse together after suturing with 7-0 Maxon suture (Fig. 104–18). The labia majora should be advanced posteriorly to the perineum at this time as well using a Z-plasty skin closure.

Postoperatively, the patient must be immobilized to decrease lateral stresses on the closure after any primary reconstructive procedure for exstrophy. We prefer to use a spica cast for 3 weeks to prevent external hip rotation and optimize pubic apposition, which can facilitate early discharge and home care (Fig. 104–19). Other alternatives include modified Buck's traction or external fixation devices. Internal fixation may be necessary in older patients.

Because of the high incidence of vesicoureteral reflux, we prescribe low-dose suppressive antibiotic therapy for all newborns after bladder closure. This is continued until the vesicoureteral reflux is corrected or resolves spontaneously. Postoperative factors that appear to directly impact the success of initial closure include postoperative immobilization, use of postoperative antibiotics, ureteral stenting catheters, adequate postoperative pain management, avoidance of abdominal distension, adequate nutritional support, and secure fixation of urinary drainage catheters (7).

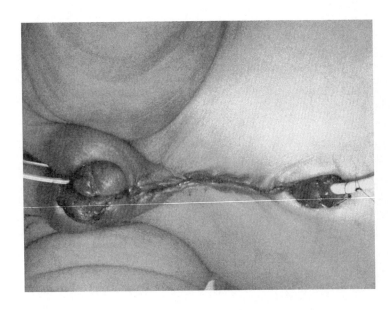

FIG. 104–18. Final reconstruction demonstrates apposition of the labia and clitoral bodies. Denuding the epithelium on the clitoris medially improves the cosmetic results postoperatively.

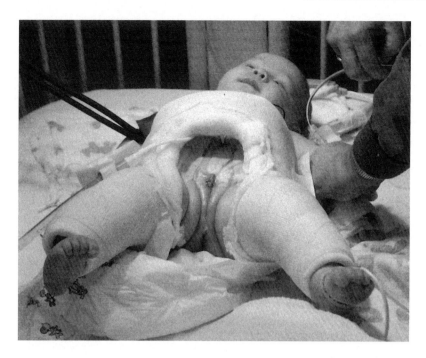

FIG. 104–19. Use of a spica cast postoperatively to immobilize the pelvis and prevent hip abduction.

OUTCOMES

Complications

The most commonly reported complication of single-stage exstrophy closure is urethrocutaneous fistula formation (at the penopubic angle dorsally). These fistulas will often close spontaneously. They may initially be managed conservatively by providing urinary diversion via catheter drainage. If the fistula does not close after conservative management, the bladder and urethra should be examined cystoscopically for the possibility of obstruction.

Other complications of CPER include atrophy of the corpora cavernosa and urethra. These complications can occur if the blood supply to the corporal bodies or urethral wedge are damaged during dissection but are unusual and underscore the importance of involving surgeons experienced in the surgical management of these patients in their care (4).

If a child develops chronic bladder and kidney infections following exstrophy closure, he or she should be appropriately evaluated for possible outlet obstruction. We routinely maintain our patients on suppressive antibiotic therapy if they have vesicoureteral reflux.

Results

To date, our single-institution experience with this technique includes 37 children (29 with classic bladder exstrophy and 8 with cloacal exstrophy). The majority of these children underwent reconstruction in the newborn period. Because this operation does not address vesicoureteral reflux, the majority of children in this series (n=20) have documented reflux following closure. Seventeen of these children have undergone ureteral reimplantation. In contrast to previous experience with reported single-stage closure techniques in the 1970s, the majority of children in our series do not have hydronephrosis following reconstruction (n=27). In those children with hydronephrosis, most was transient and disappeared within the first year of life. This is a marked change from previous single-stage repair series that reported rates of hydronephrosis and renal damage as high as 90% (1,11).

Daytime continence rates in this series are currently over 80%. Primary continence without the need for further bladder neck reconstruction was achieved in 16% of boys and 23% of girls. Following bladder neck reconstruction (using the Mitchell technique) 83% of boys and 85% of girls with classic exstrophy or epispadias have achieved daytime urinary continence with volitional voiding (6).

REFERENCES

1. Churchill B, Merguerian PA, Khoury AE, Husmann DA, McLorie GA. Bladder exstrophy and epispadias. In: O'Donnell, Koff, eds. *Pediatric urology.* Oxford, UK: Reed Elsevier, 1997:495–508.
2. Connolly JA, et al. Prevalence and repair of inguinal hernias in children with bladder exstrophy. *J Urol* 1995;154:1900–1901.
3. Gearhart JP. Bladder exstrophy: staged reconstruction. *Curr Opin Urol* 1999;9:499–506.
4. Gearhart JP. Complete repair of bladder exstrophy in the newborn: complications and management. *J Urol* 2001;165(6, Pt 2): 2431–2433.
5. Grady RW, Mitchell ME. Complete primary repair of exstrophy. *J Urol* 1999;162:1415–1420.
6. Grady RW, Mitchell ME. An update of the complete primary exstrophy repair. In: Grady RW, Joyen BD, Roedel M, et al., eds. *Proceedings of the Second International Symposium of the Exstrophy–Epispadias Complex.* American Academy of Pediatrics 2003 National Conference, New Orleans, LA Oct. 2003 p. 102.

7. Husmann DA, McLorie GA, Churchill BM. Closure of the exstrophic bladder: an evaluation of the factors leading to its success and its importance on urinary continence. *J Urol* 1989;142(2, Pt 2):522–524; discussion 542–543.

8. Mitchell ME, Bagli DJ. Complete penile disassembly for epispadias repair: the Mitchell technique. *J Urol* 1996;155:300–304.

9. O'Kane HO, Megaw JM. Carcinoma in the exstrophic bladder. *Br J Surg* 1968;55:631–635.

10. Stringer MD, Duffy PG, Ransley PG. Inguinal hernias associated with bladder exstrophy. *Br J Urol* 1994;73:308–309.

11. Williams DI, Keeton JE. Further progress with reconstruction of the exstrophied bladder. *Br J Surg* 1973;60:203–207.

CHAPTER 105

Bladder Exstrophy and Epispadias

Dominic Frimberger and John P. Gearhart

Bladder exstrophy is a rare and complex urogenital malformation with an incidence that varies between 1:10.000 to 1:50.000 live births, affecting males five to six times more often than females (5).

Until the middle of the 19th century, bladder exstrophy was treated primarily nonsurgically. Early forms of repair focused on abdominal wall closure using skin flaps for partial reconstruction, leaving a fistula to attach a urinal for dryness. Trendelenburg first stated that pubic reapproximation would not only prevent prolapse of the reconstructed bladder but also be crucial to achieve continence. Although his theoretical assumptions were correct, his surgical efforts were not successful. In 1942 Hugh Hampton Young performed the first successful primary closure of a female exstrophy patient. Although similar reports about continent, primary closures were published in the same area, the numbers were small and most surgeons were not able to reproduce these favorable results. Both Jeffs et al. (8) and Cendron (2) published their description about successful staged reconstruction in the mid-1970s and their pioneering work set the standard for modern exstrophy treatment today.

Derived from the earlier surgical approaches are the primary objectives of the modern surgical management of classic bladder exstrophy:

1. Secure initial abdominal, bladder, and posterior urethra closure.
2. Reconstruction of a functional and cosmetically acceptable penis in the male and external genitalia in the female. In special circumstances the epispadias repair can be combined with the first step at time of initial closure.
3. Urinary continence with the preservation of renal function.

Classic bladder exstrophy involves an open abdominal wall, bladder, and urethra and a wide diastases of the symphysis pubis, which is caused by a 30% bony deficit of the anterior pubic rami in combination with a 12- and 18-degree external rotation of the posterior and anterior aspects of the pelvis, respectively. The subsequent malrotation of the pubic bones adds up to an increased distance between the triradiate cartilages of 131%. A further characteristic of bladder exstrophy is the shortened distance between the umbilicus and the anus, with an altogether short and broad perineum. Associated omphaloceles and umbilical or inguinal hernias are usually not severe and are repaired at time of closure. In addition, girls present with a bifid clitoris and a short vagina that often has a stenotic orifice. The genital defect in males is much more severe and characterized by a 50% shortening of the anterior corpora cavernosa and an upward deviation of the penis. Therefore, the general mean penile length of 3.5 cm at full term cannot be reached; however, erectile function is almost always intact (4).

The upper urinary tract is usually unaffected in its development. But, because anomalies are described, a preoperative ultrasound evaluation is mandatory. However, the lower parts of the ureters have a more lateral course in the true pelvis and enter the bladder with little or no obliquity, resulting in ureteral reflux in almost 100% of cases.

Newborn bladder exstrophy patients present with an increased collagen to smooth-muscle ratio, which normalizes after successful closure, and a reduced number of myelinated nerves in the bladder muscle (9,10). Therefore bladder exstrophy is thought to represent a maturational delay in overall development involving several organ systems.

DIAGNOSIS

The definite diagnosis is made after examining the newborn at birth; however, the malformation can be discovered during routine prenatal ultrasound. Despite the magnitude of the defect, it can be mistaken for an omphalocele or gastroschisis. Bladder exstrophy is suspected during prenatal ultrasound in the absence of bladder filling on repeated examinations, a low-set umbilicus, widening of the pubis ramus, diminutive genitalia, and a lower abdominal mass, increasing in size throughout the pregnancy (6,13).

INDICATIONS FOR SURGERY

Once bladder exstrophy is suspected, arrangements should be made for the mother to deliver the child in a specialized center to ensure immediate postnatal, professional closure and reconstruction. The delicate bladder mucosa has to be protected until surgery by sterile saline irrigations and application of a plastic wrap to prevent metaplasia and the formation of polyps. The fragile mucosa as well as detrusor function is best preserved by closing the bladder in the newborn period.

ALTERNATIVE THERAPY

To reduce the numbers of procedures required for complete reconstruction and improve results, complete single-stage reconstruction or a combination of procedures has been suggested. Grady and Mitchell proposed the one-stage closure in the newborn period without reimplanting the ureters, reconstructing the bladder neck, or performing osteotomies (7). Initial results using the penile disassembly technique for epispadias repair left some children with a residual hypospadias, necessitating later repair. Moreover, 50% of children presented with urinary breakthrough infections despite antibiotic prophylaxis, subsequently requiring ureteral reimplantation. Schrott performs bladder closure, ureteral reimplantation, epispadias repair, and bladder neck reconstruction in the newborn period, using the same technique even for older children without osteotomies (16). Combining newborn exstrophy closure with later bladder neck reconstruction and epispadias repair has been described by Baka-Jakubiak (1). A completely different approach is the creation of a ureterosigmoidostomy as proposed by Stein and associates as an initial procedure after bladder and abdominal wall closure in one procedure (17).

The size and the functional capacity of the detrusor muscle are important considerations for the outcome. Therefore, in the rare presence of a small, fibrotic bladder patch without elasticity or contractility the operation should be deferred until adequate growth of the bladder template took place. If sufficient size is not reached 4 to 6 months after birth, alternative options like creation of a colon conduit or ureterosigmoidostomy have to be employed.

SURGICAL TECHNIQUE

Care has to be taken to create a latex-free operation because many children with bladder exstrophy are prone to latex allergies.

Timing and Staging

The original description of the staged closure has been significantly modified in the last decade, leading to a dramatic increase in success of the procedure. Modern staged closure has defined strict criteria for the selection of patients suitable for this approach. The technique includes early bladder, posterior urethra, and abdominal wall closure, usually with pelvic osteotomy in the newborn period, subsequently followed by an early epispadias repair at 6 months to 1 year of age after local testosterone stimulation. Around age 4 to 5 years a competent bladder neck is reconstructed along with bilateral ureteral reimplantation, when adequate bladder capacity is reached and the child is maturationally ready to participate in a postoperative voiding program (5).

Successful initial bladder and posterior urethral closure is the most important factor for achieving urinary continence and sufficient bladder capacity. The primary objective in initial, functional closure is to convert the bladder exstrophy into a complete epispadias with incontinence with balanced posterior outlet resistance that preserves renal function but stimulates bladder growth.

The role of pelvic osteotomy performed at time of initial closure ensures a tension-free approximation of the bladder, posterior urethral, and abdominal wall, placement of the urethra deep within the pelvic ring, enhancing bladder outlet resistance, and finally aligning the large pelvic floor muscles to support the bladder neck. Usually, osteotomies are not needed in the patient less than 72 hours old, with malleable pubic bones that are easily brought together in the midline by medial rotation of the greater trochanters, However, if the pubic bones are more than 4 cm apart or in cases of doubt of a tension-free closure osteotomies are key to prevent dehiscence or bladder prolapse.

Osteotomy

The bilateral anterior innominate and vertical iliac osteotomy has been used in our institution because it has numerous advantages to the posterior approach. The patient is placed in a supine position, preparing and draping the lower body below the costal margins and placing soft absorbent gauze over the exposed bladder. The pelvis is exposed from the inferior wings inferiorly and the pectineal tubercle and posteriorly to the sacroiliac joints. The periosteum and sciatic notch are carefully elevated and a Gigli saw is used to create a transverse innominate osteotomy exiting anteriorly at a point halfway between the anterosuperior and the anteroinferior spines (Fig. 105–1). This osteotomy is created at a slightly more cranial level than that described for a Salter osteotomy to allow placement of external fixator pins in the distal segments. Also, the posterior ileum may be incised from the anterior approach in an effort to correct the deformity

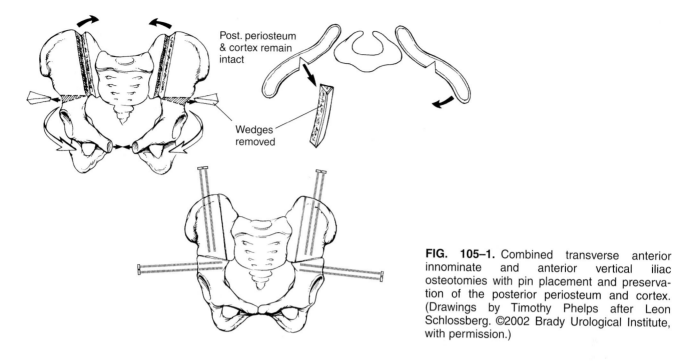

Post. periosteum
& cortex remain
intact

Wedges
removed

FIG. 105–1. Combined transverse anterior innominate and anterior vertical iliac osteotomies with pin placement and preservation of the posterior periosteum and cortex. (Drawings by Timothy Phelps after Leon Schlossberg. ©2002 Brady Urological Institute, with permission.)

more completely. This is important because anatomic studies have shown that the posterior portion of the pelvis is also externally rotated in patients with exstrophy, and as patients age they lose the elasticity of their sacroiliac ligaments. An osteotome is used to create a closing wedge osteotomy vertically and just lateral to the sacroiliac joint. The posterior iliac cortex is kept intact and used as a hinge (Fig. 105–2). Two fixator pins are placed in the inferior osteotomized segment and two pins are placed in the wing of the ileum superiorly. Radiographs are obtained to confirm pin placement, soft tissues are closed, and the urologic procedure is performed.

External fixators are applied between the pins to hold the pelvis in a correct position.

Radiographs are taken 7 to 10 days postoperatively. If the diastasis has not been completely reduced, the right and left sides can be gradually approximated using the fixator bars over several days. Light longitudinal Buck's skin traction is used to keep the legs still. The patient remains supine in traction for approximately 4 weeks to prevent dislodgment of tubes and destabilization of the pelvis. The external fixator is kept on for approximately 6 weeks, until adequate callus is seen at the site of osteotomy. The pins are removed under light sedation at the bedside. Postoperatively, newborns undergoing closure without osteotomy are immobilized in modified Bryant traction for 4 weeks with the hips in 90 degrees of flexion.

The use of spica casts or mummy wraps are associated with multiple failures of the closure and lower-extremity complications (12).

Bladder, Posterior Urethral, and Abdominal Wall Closure

The various steps in primary bladder closure are illustrated in Figure 105–2. A strip of mucosa 2 cm wide, extending from the distal trigone to below the verumontanum in the male and to the vaginal orifice in the female, is outlined for prostatic and posterior urethral reconstruction (Fig. 105–2A). With the advent of the modified Cantwell–Ransley epispadias repair, the urethral plate should not be incised unless the length of the urethral groove from the verumontanum to the glans is so short that it interferes with eventual penile length and produces dorsal angulation. If so, then the urethral groove is lengthened. Figures 105–2B to 105–2D show marking of the incision from just above the umbilicus down around the junction of the bladder and the paraexstrophy skin to the level of the urethral plate. The appropriate plane is entered just above the umbilicus and a plane is established between the rectus fascia and the bladder (Figs. 105–2E and 105–2F). The umbilical vessels are doubly ligated and incised and allowed to fall into the pelvis. The peritoneum is taken off the dome of the bladder, to be deeply placed into the pelvis at the time of closure. The plane is continued caudally down between the bladder and rectus fascia until the urogenital diaphragm fibers are encountered bilaterally. With electrocautery, these urogenital diaphragm fibers between the bladder neck, the posterior urethra, and the pubic bone are taken sharply down to the pelvic floor in their entirety (Fig. 105–2F). A double-pronged skin hook can be inserted into the pelvic

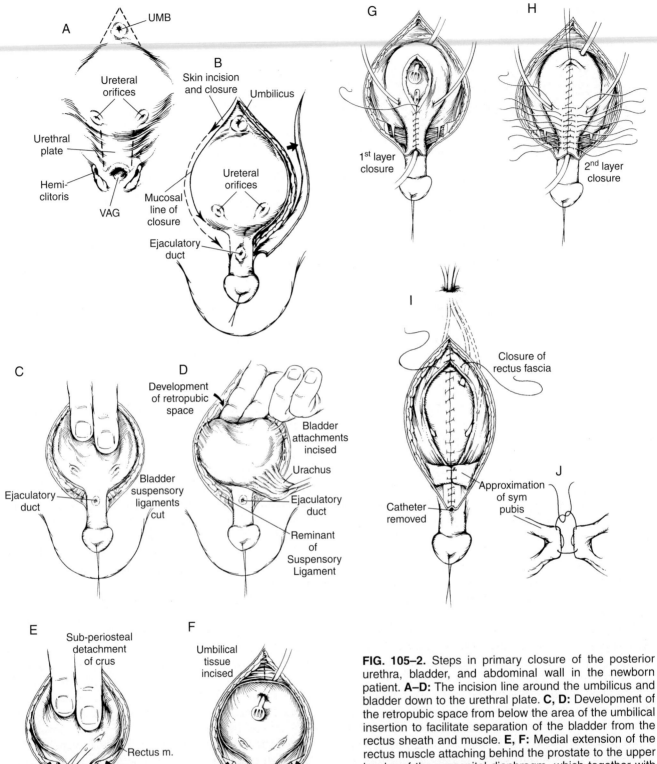

FIG. 105–2. Steps in primary closure of the posterior urethra, bladder, and abdominal wall in the newborn patient. **A–D:** The incision line around the umbilicus and bladder down to the urethral plate. **C, D:** Development of the retropubic space from below the area of the umbilical insertion to facilitate separation of the bladder from the rectus sheath and muscle. **E, F:** Medial extension of the rectus muscle attaching behind the prostate to the upper border of the urogenital diaphragm, which together with the anterior corpus is freed from the pubis by deep incision. **G, H:** Ureteral stent placement and layered closure of the bladder wall. **I, J:** A horizontal mattress suture is tied on the external surface of the pubic symphysis and exit of the ureteral and suprapubic tube at the site of the neoumbilical opening. (Drawings by Timothy Phelps after Leon Schlossberg. ©2002 Brady Urological Institute, with permission.)

bone and pulled laterally to accentuate the urogenital diaphragm fibers. If this maneuver is not performed adequately, the vesicourethral unit will be brought anteriorly with pelvic closure in an unsatisfactory position for later reconstruction.

If the decision is made to transect the urethral groove, then it is cut distal to the verumontanum with continuity maintained between the thin, mucosa-like non–hair-bearing skin adjacent to the posterior urethra and bladder neck and the skin and mucosa of the penile glans. Flaps in the area of thin skin are subsequently moved distally and rotated to reconstruct the urethral groove, resurfacing the penis dorsally. The corporal bodies are not brought together because later Cantwell–Ransley epispadias repair requires the urethral plate to be brought underneath the corporal bodies. If the urethral plate is left in continuity, it must be mobilized up to the level of the prostate to create as much urethral and penile length as possible. Apparent penile lengthening is achieved by exposing the corpora cavernosa bilaterally and freeing the corpora from their attachments to the suspensory ligaments. After the urogenital diaphragm is completely incised bilaterally, freeing the bladder neck and urethra well from the pubis, the mucosa and muscle of the bladder and the posterior urethra well onto the penis are closed in the anterior midline (Fig. 105–2G). The resulting orifice should be easy passed by a 12 to 14 Fr sound, creating enough resistance to aid in bladder adaptation and prevent prolapse but not too much to cause outlet resistance altering the upper tracts. A second layer is closed if possible (Fig. 105–2H)). Bladder drainage is achieved using a suprapubic nonlatex Malecot catheter for 4 weeks. The urethra is not stented to prevent necrosis. Ureteral stents are left in place for 10 to 14 days, until swelling goes down.

By applying gentle pressure over the greater trochanters bilaterally, the pubic bones are approximated in the midline. A horizontal mattress suture of no. 2 nylon is placed between the fibrous cartilages of the pubic rami and tied anteriorly to the pubic closure to avoid the neourethra (Figs. 105–2I and 105–2J). A second stitch is placed caudal to the insertion of the rectus fascia if possible for added support. Should the sutures work loose or cut through the tissues during subsequent healing, the anterior placement of the knot of the horizontal mattress suture ensures that it will not erode through into the urethra. A V-shaped flap of abdominal skin at a point corresponding to the normal position of the umbilicus is tacked down to the abdominal fascia, and the drainage tubes exit this neoumbilicus.

Postoperatively, before suprapubic tube removal the bladder outlet is calibrated to ensure free passage of urine. Repeated ultrasound examinations are obtained before discharge and every 3 months to check for upper-tract dilatation and residual urine. Continuous, prophylactic antibiotic therapy is advised to prevent upper-tract infection from ureteral reflux. Yearly gravity cystograms under anesthesia are performed to receive quality information about reflux and, more importantly, bladder capacity. For successful continent procedures a minimal bladder capacity of 85 cc is needed. An increase in bladder capacity is seen after epispadias repair, which is why the bladder neck procedure is performed after the urethral reconstruction.

Epispadias Repair

Four key concerns have to be addressed: (a) a functional and cosmetically pleasing penis, (b) correction of dorsal chordee, (c) urethral reconstruction, and (d) penile skin closure and glandular reconstruction. In patients undergoing delayed repair or reclosure, a combined epispadias/exstrophy closure using the modified Cantwell–Ransley repair is possible.

The modified Cantwell–Ransley repair is begun by placing a nylon suture through the ventral glans for traction. A metal advancement and glanuloplasty incorporated (MAGPI) incision is made in the urethral plate distally and closed with 6-0 polyglycolic sutures in a transverse fashion to flatten the distal urethral plate and advance the urethra to the tip of the phallus (Fig. 105–3A). The reconstructed neourethra will be in excellent glandular position once the wings a closed. Next, incisions are made over two parallel lines marked previously over the dorsum of the penis that outline a 18-mm wide strip of urethral mucosa extending from the prostatic urethral meatus to the tip of the glans (Fig. 105–3A). Triangular mucosal areas of the dorsal gland are excised adjacent to the urethral strip, and thick glandular flaps are constructed bilaterally. Lateral skin flaps are mobilized and undermined.

A Z-incision of the suprapubic area permits exposure and division of the suspensory ligament and old scar tissue from the initial exstrophy closure. The ventral skin is taken down to the level of the scrotum (Fig. 105–3B). Care is taken to preserve the mesentery to the urethral plate, which arises proximally and extends upward between the corpora as a blood supply to the urethral plate. The corpora are dissected ventrally on the surface of Buck's fascia. The plane is followed closely bilaterally until one exits on the dorsum of the penis between the corpora spongiosum and the corporal body (Fig. 105–3C).

After placement of loops, the urethral plate is dissected just on the corporal bodies to the level of the prostate and the glans, respectively (Fig. 105–3D). Care is taken to leave the most distal 1-cm attachment of the mucosal plate to the glans intact. The neurovascular bundles (NVB) are dissected free from the corporal bodies only if rotating the corpora over the urethra does not straighten the penis. The urethral strip is closed in a linear manner from the prostatic opening to the glans over an 8 Fr silicone stent with 6-0 polyglycolic sutures. Afterward, the corporal bodies are incised at the point of maximal curvature, leaving a diamond-shaped defect (Fig. 105–3E). The corpora are then

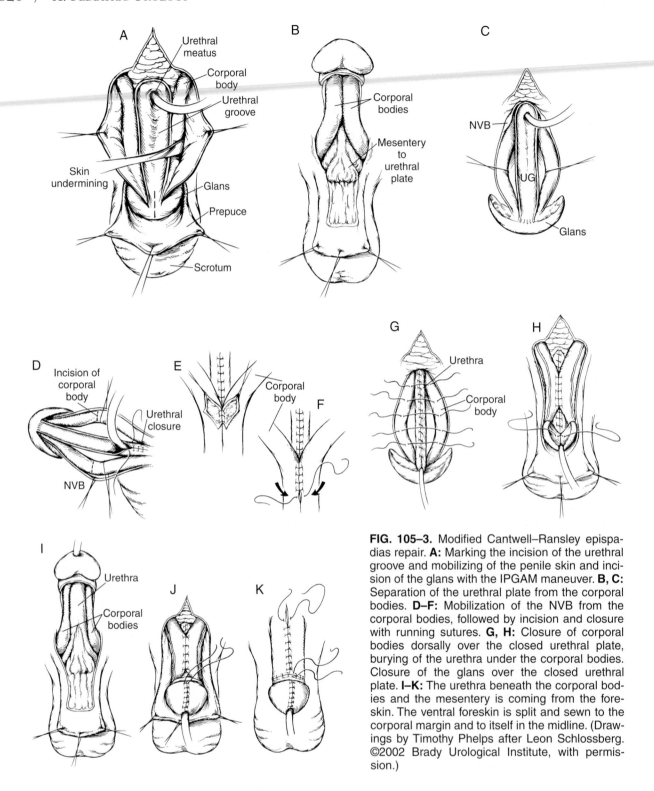

FIG. 105–3. Modified Cantwell–Ransley epispadias repair. **A:** Marking the incision of the urethral groove and mobilizing of the penile skin and incision of the glans with the IPGAM maneuver. **B, C:** Separation of the urethral plate from the corporal bodies. **D–F:** Mobilization of the NVB from the corporal bodies, followed by incision and closure with running sutures. **G, H:** Closure of corporal bodies dorsally over the closed urethral plate, burying of the urethra under the corporal bodies. Closure of the glans over the closed urethral plate. **I–K:** The urethra beneath the corporal bodies and the mesentery is coming from the foreskin. The ventral foreskin is split and sewn to the corporal margin and to itself in the midline. (Drawings by Timothy Phelps after Leon Schlossberg. ©2002 Brady Urological Institute, with permission.)

closed over the neourethra with two running sutures of 5-0 polydioxanone (PDS), with the adjacent areas of the diamond sutured to each other (Fig. 105–3F). The now ventrally placed urethra is secured in place with further 5-0 polyglycolic acid sutures between the corpora, especially at the coronal level (Figs. 105–3G to 105–3I). The glans wings are subcuticulary closed with 5-0 and the glans epithelium with 6-0 polyglycolic acid. Finally, the ventral skin is brought up and sutured to the ventral edge of the corona, while the flaps provide coverage of the dorsum. The skin as well as the Z-plasty at the base of the penis is reapproximated with interrupted 5-0 or 6-0 polyglycolic acid sutures (Figs. 105–3J and 105–3K). The silicon stent is secured and left for 10 to 12 days.

In females the mons and external genitalia are reconstructed at time of initial exstrophy closure. The bifid clitoris is denuded medially and brought together in the midline, along with labia minora reconstruction, creating a fourchette.

Postoperatively it is critical to control pain and bladder spasms to prevent urine extravasation and fistula formation. This is best achieved by preoperative placement of a caudal epidural catheter and the administration of oxybutynin medication. At time of discharge, the postoperative plastic occlusive dressing is left intact and the patient supplied with oral broad- spectrum antibiotics, pain medications, and antispasmodics.

Continence and Antireflux Procedure

The bladder is opened through a transverse incision at the bladder neck with a vertical incision (Fig. 105–4A). Figure 105–4 depicts a Cohen transtrigonal ureteral reimplantation or a cephalotrigonal reimplantation for either moving the ureter across the bladder above the trigone or, if the ureters are too low, moving them on the upper aspect of the trigone (Fig. 105–4B). The modified Young–Dees–Leadbetter procedure is begun by selecting a posterior strip of mucosa 15 to 18 mm wide and 30 mm long that extends from the midtrigone to the prostate or posterior urethra (Fig. 105–4C). The bladder muscle lateral

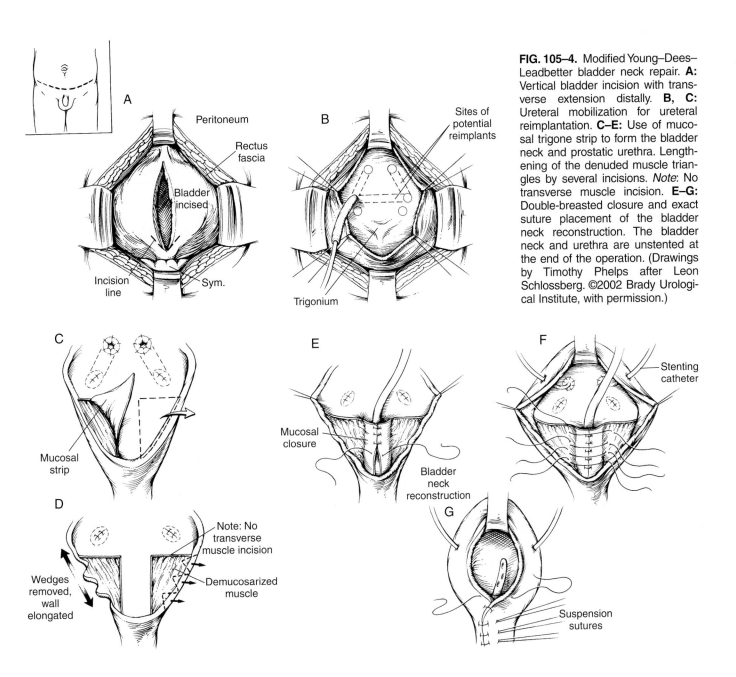

FIG. 105–4. Modified Young–Dees–Leadbetter bladder neck repair. **A:** Vertical bladder incision with transverse extension distally. **B, C:** Ureteral mobilization for ureteral reimplantation. **C–E:** Use of mucosal trigone strip to form the bladder neck and prostatic urethra. Lengthening of the denuded muscle triangles by several incisions. *Note*: No transverse muscle incision. **E–G:** Double-breasted closure and exact suture placement of the bladder neck reconstruction. The bladder neck and urethra are unstented at the end of the operation. (Drawings by Timothy Phelps after Leon Schlossberg. ©2002 Brady Urological Institute, with permission.)

to the mucosal strip is denuded of mucosa and sponges, soaked in 1:200,000 epinephrine, are applied to control bleeding for better visualization. Tailoring of the muscle triangles is aided by multiple small incisions on the free edge bilaterally that allow the area of reconstruction to assume a more cephalic position (Fig. 105–4D). A transverse, full-thickness muscular incision is not performed as described in the original Young–Dees–Leadbetter procedure because there is a significant risk of denervation and ischemia for the bladder neck. The edges of the mucosa and underlying muscle are closed with interrupted sutures of 4-0 polyglycolic acid (Fig. 105–4E). The adjacent denuded muscle flaps are overlapped and sutured firmly in place with a 3-0 polydioxanone to provide reinforcement of the bladder neck and urethral reconstruction (Figs. 105–4F and 105–4G). Two to three of the overlapping sutures are left long, brought through the rectus fascia, and tied as bladder suspension to elevate the bladder neck (Fig. 105–4G). An 8 Fr urethral stent may be used during construction but is removed afterward. Exposure is essential for the creation of a continent bladder neck. Therefore, if visualization of the posterior urethra is problematic the intrasymphyseal bar has to be cut and afterward approximated with 0 PDS nylon sutures. In this case the child should be immobilized postoperatively.

The ureteral stents are removed after 10 to 12 days and the suprapubic catheter is clamped after 3 weeks, for no longer than 1 hour for the first time. After residual free voiding is achieved, the suprapubic catheter is removed. The patient is followed-up with frequent bladder and renal ultrasounds in the first few months.

OUTCOMES

Complications

The two most common complications of primary closure are bladder prolapse and dehiscence. Both of these are serious complications requiring reclosure and mandatory osteotomy. In addition, after primary closure, patients have to be monitored for adequate urinary drainage. In case of upper tract dilation, recurrent infections or inadequate bladder drainage, the bladder outlet has to be evaluated. If the outlet is too tight, upper tract decompensation might occur. After epispadias repair, in 12%–15% of patients' fistulas can develop and are usually easily repaired as an outpatient procedure. The biggest challenge of the child and the parents after the continence procedure is the initiation of the voiding trial. If the child can not void, an 8 French catheter is placed under anesthesia and left in place for 5 days and the voiding trial is initiated again (5). If the child is not dry for a period of 3 hours during the day by one year after surgery, the bladder neck reconstruction has failed. Multiple options are available for these children to achieve future continence.

Results

Several series have shown the success and applicability of the staged functional method for the treatment of bladder exstrophy (11,14,15). Our current data from 65 patients, treated totally at our institution, with bladder exstrophy that underwent initial modern staged functional closure show 77% to be continent day and night with 91% being socially dry (3). Continence is correctly defined as being dry for more than 3 hours. Socially continent patients achieve that goal during the day but have bed-wetting incidences during nighttime. The risk of bladder neck failure is higher for the group with smaller bladder capacities (under 85 cc). Careful evaluations of patients, especially considering bladder capacity and function, will help define more accurate guidelines to improve the rate of continent patients.

REFERENCES

1. Baka-Jakubiak M. Combined bladder neck, urethral and penile reconstruction in boys with exstrophy–epispadias complex. Br J Urol Int 2000;86:513–518.
2. Cendron J. La reconstruction vesicale. Ann Chir Infant 1971;12:371.
3. Chan YD, Jeffs RD, Gearhart JP. Determinants of continence in the bladder exstrophy population: Predictors of success? Urology 2001;57: 774–777.
4. Feldman KW, Smith DW. Fetal phallic growth and penile standards for newborn males. J Pediatr 1975;86:395–398.
5. Gearhart JP. The bladder exstrophy–epispadias–cloacal exstrophy complex. In: Gearhart JP, Rink RC, Mouriquand PDE, eds. Pediatric urology. Philadelphia: WB Saunders, 2001:511–546.
6. Gearhart JP, Ben-Chaim J, Jeffs RD. Criteria for the prenatal diagnosis of classic bladder exstrophy. Obstet Gynecol 1995;85:961–964.
7. Grady R, Mitchell ME. Complete repair of bladder exstrophy. J Urol 1999;162:1415–1420.
8. Jeffs RD, Charrios R, Mnay M, Juransz AR. Primary closure of the exstrophied bladder. In: Scott R, ed. Current controversies in urologic management. Philadelphia: WB Saunders, 1972:235.
9. Lee BR, Pearlman EJ, Partin AW, et al. Evaluation of smooth-muscle and collagen subtypes in normal newborns and those born with bladder exstrophy. J Urol 1996;156:2034–2036.
10. Mathews RI, Wills M, Pearlman E, et al. Neural innervation of the newborn exstrophy bladder: An immunohistological study. J Urol 1999; 162:506–508.
11. McMahon DR, Kane MP, Husmann DA, et al. Vesical neck reconstruction in patients with the exstrophy–epispadias–complex. J Urol 1996;155:1411–1413.
12. Meldrum KK, Baird AD, Gearheart JP. Pelvic and extremity immobilization after bladder exstrophy closure: complications and impact on success. J Urol 2003;62:1109–1113.
13. Mirk M, Calisti A, Feleni A. Prenatal sonographic diagnosis of bladder exstrophy. J Ultrasound Med 1986;5:291.
14. Mollard P, Mouriquand PE, Buttin X. Urinary continence after reconstruction of classic bladder exstrophy (73 cases). Br J Urol 1994;73: 298–302.
15. Perlmutter AD, Weinstein MD, Rademan C. Vesical neck reconstruction in patients with the bladder exstrophy complex. J Urol 1991;146: 613–615.
16. Schrott KM. Komplette einzeitige Aufbauplastik der Blasenekstrophie. In: Schreiter F, ed. Plastisch-rekonstruktive chirurgie in der urologie. Stuttgart: Georg Thieme-Verlag, 1999:430–438.
17. Stein R, Fisch M, Black P, Hohenfellner R. Strategies for reconstruction of unsuccessful or unsatisfactory primary treatment of patients with bladder exstrophy or incontinent epispadias. J Urol 1999;161: 1934–1941.

CHAPTER 106

Congenital Anomalies of the Scrotum

David R. Roth

Isolated congenital anomalies of the scrotum, including inclusion cysts, the bifid or hypoplastic scrotum, penoscrotal transposition, and webbed penis, are unusual. Most often these anomalies are found in association with other abnormalities: penoscrotal transposition and bifid scrotum with hypospadias, bifid scrotum and scrotal ectopia with exstrophy, and scrotal hypoplasia with cryptorchidism. When these anomalies occur in conjunction with other genital abnormalities, the scrotum can be surgically repaired with excellent results at the time of the procedure to correct the primary anomaly. It is important, however, that neonatal circumcision be avoided in boys with genital anomalies because the prepuce may be required for reconstruction of the penis and its presence will allow greater flexibility for the surgeon.

DIAGNOSIS

The diagnosis of scrotal congenital anomalies is made by physical examination. Rarely do these anomalies occur as solitary lesions, and the patient should be appropriately evaluated for associated anomalies. The physician should examine the scrotum for its relative position to the penis, rectum, and median raphe. The appearance of the scrotum should be noted with attention to symmetry and distribution of its rugations. The testes, penis, urethra, and rectum should be inspected to ensure that they are normal.

INDICATIONS FOR SURGERY

Timing of the surgical repair of urogenital anomalies is important with regard to feasibility of the surgery, safety of the surgery to the patient, and the psychological impact of the anomaly and surgery. Because congenital scrotal anomalies do not interfere with urinary function, repair can be scheduled at the time that is most appropriate for the infant and most convenient for parents and physi-

cians. Technically, from the surgeon's point of view, there is little to be gained by delaying surgery beyond the child's fourth to sixth month because by that time the genitalia have developed to sufficient size for easy reconstruction. With optical magnification and the standardization of fine sutures, excellent results can be expected even in the very young child. In addition to the degree of scrotal development, the safety of anesthetics has always been a concern in determining the minimum age at which an operation seems appropriate. However, as a result of the proliferation of specially trained and dedicated pediatric anesthesiologists, the anesthetic complication rate has reached a nadir at approximately 3 months of age. To delay repair beyond that time is no longer necessary in centers dedicated to pediatric surgery.

Psychological concerns limit the opposite end of the time spectrum (7). The child's anxiety concerning hospitalization, gender identity, and subsequent sexual development must be considered. If genital surgery is performed before the child is 18 months of age, he neither remembers the surgery nor associates the experience with an abnormality of his penis or scrotum. Therefore, a window (4 to 18 months) exists for surgery, limited on the younger side by both anesthetic and technical concerns and on the older side by memory and psychological issues. Parents need to determine a time during that 14-month period that is best for their schedules. Because most of these surgical repairs require only external relocation of skin, they usually can be performed on an outpatient basis and only rarely with a hospital stay of a single night. A further consideration is that it is easier for parents to care postoperatively for a boy who is younger and not yet walking.

Certain technical points are relevant to all of these operations and warrant mentioning. For instance, optical magnification has proved to be very useful. Several companies now make loupes in powers of 2.5 to 4.5× that practitioners have found to be invaluable when performing delicate surgery on the genitalia. Also helpful are the fine (6-0 to 8-0) absorbable (plain, chromic) sutures, which are excellent materials with which to repair a child's scrotum. They do not have to be removed and are absorbed quickly, so skin tracks are unlikely to form. Prophylactic antibiotics are seldom necessary in uncomplicated cases with the prepubertal child.

ALTERNATIVE THERAPY

There are no alternatives to surgical correction of the congenital anomaly. On the other hand, nontreatment is an option and reconstructive surgery can be delayed until the boy can participate in the decision to proceed. The psychological advantage of earlier surgery would need to be weighed against the importance of allowing the youngster to be involved in the decision-making process.

SURGICAL TECHNIQUE

Bifid Scrotum

Isolated bifid scrotum is rare. When it occurs, the corpus spongiosum appears to be continuous with a prominent median raphe of the scrotum: a fibrous band that separates and divides the scrotum into two individual parts. Surgical reapproximation of the two hemiscrotums can be achieved after excision of the fibrous midline band. The underlying urethra must be preserved and allowed to fall away from the dense band. This requires mobilization of each hemiscrotum to the extent that it can be elevated and moved medially to the midline. Closure is accomplished in at least two layers. Deep absorbable sutures allow fixation and reconstruction of the midline. Fine absorbable sutures should be used to close the skin. In general, interrupted simple sutures are used, but a running subcuticular closure may also be utilized.

Penoscrotal Transposition

Various degrees of penoscrotal transposition exist, ranging from the complete form, in which the scrotum is actually anterior and cephalad to the base of the penis, to incomplete forms, in which the penis emerges from the center of the scrotum, and the milder forms, in which only the superior edges of the scrotum lie anterior to the penis. For correction of the anomaly, the two hemiscrotums are mobilized, swept inferiorly and medially, and sutured together. It may be necessary to transpose the penis cephalad to the scrotum. This can be achieved by using a skin bridge (Fig. 106–1) or by dividing the abnormal scrotum in its midline cephalad and caudal to the phallus and swinging both halves below the penis (Fig. 106–2) (2). Some authors suggest leaving a segment of skin intact cephalad to the penis to avoid jeopardizing the vascularity and lymphatic drainage of the penile shaft

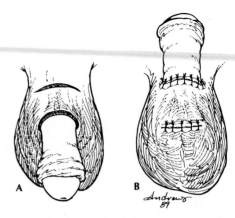

FIG. 106–1. A: In the moderately severe case of penoscrotal transposition, the phallus is circumscribed and freed of supporting tissue. An incision is made cephalad to the base of the phallus. **B:** The penis can then be brought back through the new opening and the skin sutured about it. The original opening is then sewn closed.

skin. For less severe cases of penoscrotal transposition, the wedge of ectopic scrotal skin is removed and the resultant defect closed, thereby eliminating the problem (6). This approach is most appropriate when there is incomplete mild penoscrotal transposition (Fig. 106–3).

Scrotal Hypoplasia

Scrotal hypoplasia is almost always restricted to boys with cryptorchidism. A limited course of androgen stimulation (testosterone enanthate 2 mg per kg intramuscu-

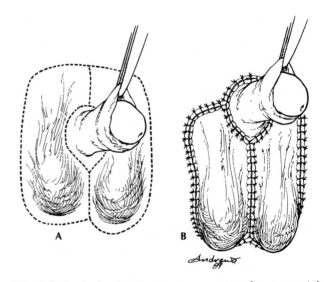

FIG. 106–2. A: In the more severe case of penoscrotal transposition, each hemiscrotum is circumscribed. **B:** Once each side is freed to rotate caudally and medially the two portions are sewn together. Some authors suggest leaving a bridge of skin cephalad to decrease the possibility of a vascular insult.

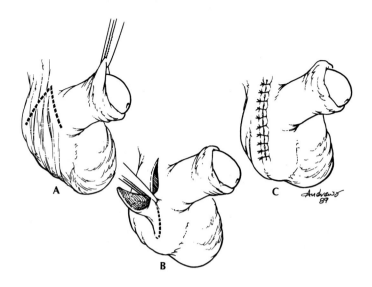

FIG. 106–3. A, B: In the mild case of penoscrotal transformation, a V-shaped wedge of ectopic scrotal skin is excised. **C:** The defect is then closed, thereby eliminating the ectopic scrotal skin.

larly) will induce scrotal development and enlargement (1). This allows easier surgical placement of either a testis or prosthesis in the poorly developed scrotum at the time of inguinal surgery for the undescended testis. The hormonal treatment should be undertaken only in conjunction with either an orchiopexy or placement of a testicular prosthesis because the effects of the testosterone are temporary; if the scrotum is not distended, it may revert to its hypoplastic appearance.

Scrotal Ectopia

Although less common than either scrotal transposition or a bifid scrotum and usually associated with cloacal exstrophy, scrotal ectopia on occasion is found in the otherwise normal child (4). The ectopic scrotal tissue can be found on the inner aspect of the thigh or caudal and inferior to the external inguinal ring. Often, the ipsilateral testis can be found within the ectopic tissue. Correction is accomplished by relocating the ectopic tissue, by way of a flap or graft, or by utilizing the normally positioned contralateral hemiscrotum as a reservoir for both gonads and discarding the ectopic tissue (8). The latter can be accomplished by stretching local tissue either primarily or after pretreatment with parenteral testosterone enanthate (2 mg per kg intramuscularly). The ectopic scrotal tissue in that case can then be excised.

Webbed Penis

In boys with a webbed penis, scrotal skin is tethered to the ventrum of the penile shaft. This tethering produces a web of skin stretching from the penis to the scrotal base. The webbed penis causes no problem during childhood. However, as the scrotal skin is hair bearing future intercourse could be difficult or uncomfortable. Therefore, a

webbed penis should be corrected during infancy. A modified circumcision can often correct the defect. The circumcision incision is brought more distal than normal on the ventrum, thereby preserving all penile shaft skin possible in that location. After the inner preputial skin is excised, the additional length on the ventrum allows the scrotum to fall away from the glans and penis. If necessary, skin from the dorsum can be mobilized and swept ventrally to provide additional shaft skin (Fig. 106–4). A second type of repair can be performed by incising the web transversely and closing it longitudinally, thereby separating the penis from the median raphe of the scrotum. A circumcision should be considered at the same time because it facilitates the approximation of the skin (Fig. 106–5).

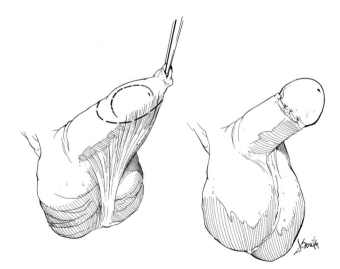

FIG. 106–4. In the mildly webbed penis, a modified circumcision may be all that is required. With the ventral incision made at the phimotic band, the ventral skin can be repositioned to cover the penile shaft appropriately.

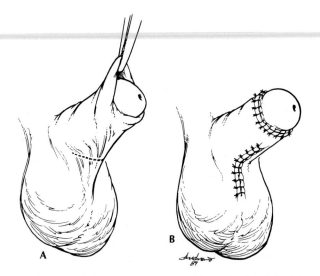

FIG. 106–5. In the moderately webbed penis, the defect can be repaired by **(A)** transversely incising the web and **(B)** closing it longitudinally. As in the mild cases, a modified circumcision incision with preservation of all the ventral skin can be helpful in recovering the penile shaft.

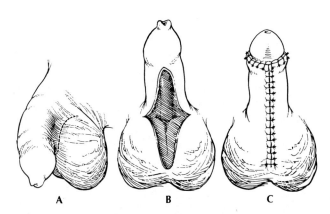

FIG. 106–6. A: In a severely webbed penis, an incision is made between the penis and scrotum. **B:** Skin flaps are elevated in all directions so that the surgical defect can be closed. **C:** A two-layer closure is used to stabilize and approximate the skin and underlying tissues.

In more severe cases of webbed penis, a U-shaped incision is made about the phallus (5). This releases the penis from the dependent scrotum. Flaps are developed to allow ventral closure of the penis with fine absorbable sutures. The scrotum is closed in a side-to-side manner (Fig. 106–6).

Scrotal Inclusion Cysts

Midline scrotal inclusion cysts are in general dermatoid in origin and can be managed by local excision (3). However, care must be taken not to confuse these with the sinus associated with an imperforate anus. Both are located in the median raphe and can be multiple. Because cysts can lead to calculi formation or infection, local excision should be considered.

OUTCOMES

Complications

Complications from these surgeries are in general uncommon. Superficial infections can be treated with antibiotics.

Results

The cosmetic results of this surgery are usually excellent.

REFERENCES

1. Gearhart JP, Jeffs RD. Use of parenteral testosterone therapy in genital reconstructive surgery. *J Urol* 1987;138:1077–1078.
2. Glenn JF, Anderson EE. Surgical correction of incomplete penoscrotal transposition. *J Urol* 1973;110:603–605.
3. Hamada Y, Sakiyama H, Nakashima K, Oka M. Median raphe cysts and canal of the penis. *Eur Urol* 1982;8:312–313.
4. Lamm DL, Kaplan GW. Accessory and ectopic scrota. *Urology* 1977;9:149–153.
5. Perlmutter AD, Chamberlain JW. Webbed penis without chordee. *J Urol* 1972;107:320–321.
6. Redman JF. The surgical correction of incomplete scrotal transposition associated with hypospadias. *J Urol* 1983;129:565–567.
7. Schultz JP, Klykylo WM, Wacksman J. Timing of elective hypospadias repair in children. *Pediatrics* 1983;71:342–351.
8. Spears T, Franco I, Reda EF, Hernandez-Graulau J, Levitt SB. Accessory and ectopic scrotum with VATER association. *Urology* 1992;40:343–345.

CHAPTER 107

Pediatric Cryptorchidism, Hydroceles, and Hernias

Christopher S. Cooper and Steven G. Docimo

Between 3% and 5% of full-term boys are born with an undescended testicle. Often associated with the undescended testicle is a patent process vaginalis that predisposes to hydrocele and hernia formation. The urologist treating the infant with an undescended testicle must therefore be familiar with the anatomy and operative techniques employed in treating this common condition (Fig. 107–1). This familiarity assists with orchidopexy, hydrocele, and hernia repair.

CRYPTORCHIDISM

Cryptorchidism includes the strict definition of a hidden or nonpalpable testicle as well as a testicle that is undescended but palpable in the inguinal canal. True undescended testicles stop along the normal path of descent into the scrotum. They may remain in the abdominal cavity (least common) or in the inguinal canal or just outside the external ring [canalicular and suprascrotal (most common), respectively]. The incidence of undescended testicles increases from 3% to 5% in full-term infants to 30% in premature infants. Most of these testicles descend within the first 6 months of life and by 1 year of age the prevalence is slightly less than 1%. Although the left testicle is affected more often, 10% of children with cryptorchidism will have both testicles affected. Twenty percent of boys who present with cryptorchidism have at least one nonpalpable testis. Of non-

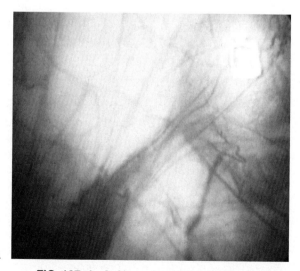
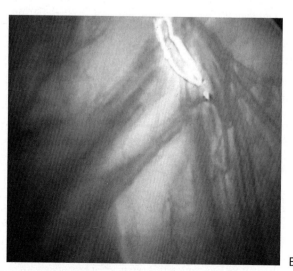

FIG. 107–1. A: Normal anatomy. **B:** The presence of blind-ending spermatic vessels indicates absence of the testicle and laparoscopy is terminated at this time. (From Matthews R, Docimo SG. Laparoscopy for the management of the undescended testis. In: *Atlas of the Urologic Clinics of North America*, vol. 8. Philadelphia: WB Saunders, 2000:91–102, with permission.)

palpable testes, 40% are atrophic or absent, 20% are intraabdominal, and 40% are canalicular, scrotal, or ectopic testes.

Diagnosis

The diagnosis of cryptorchidism relies on the physical examination. Absence of an identifiable testicle with ultrasound, computed tomography, or magnetic resonance imaging does not guarantee testicular agenesis and therefore does not alter the need for surgical exploration. The testicular examination in the infant and young child requires two hands and patient relaxation. One hand is placed near the anterior superior iliac spine and the other on the scrotum. The first hand is swept from the anterior iliac spine along the inguinal canal to gently express any retained testicular tissue into the scrotum. A true undescended or ectopic inguinal testis may slide or "pop" under the examiner's fingers during this maneuver. A low ectopic or retractile testis will be felt by the second hand as the testis is milked into the scrotum by the first hand. To distinguish a retractile testicle, the testicle is brought into the scrotal position; holding it in place for at least 1 minute fatigues the cremaster muscle. After this maneuver, a retractile testicle remains in the scrotum whereas an ectopic or undescended testis immediately springs out of the scrotum. If a testis cannot be palpated in the inguinal canal or the scrotum, or in the typical ectopic sites, evaluation for a nonpalpable testis must be performed.

An older child with bilateral nonpalpable testes should undergo hormonal evaluation for testicular absence (6). Elevations in luteinizing hormone (LH) and follicle-stimulating hormone (FSH) and absence of detectable müllerian inhibiting substance (MIS) suggest testicular absence (8). Testicular absence is confirmed by a negative human chorionic gonadotropin (HCG) stimulation test and elevated gonadotropins. The HCG stimulation test is performed by the administration of intramuscular HCG (2,000 IU per day for 3 to 4 days) (4). Raised gonadotropin levels (FSH and LH) *and* a lack of a testosterone rise from HCG indicate bilateral absent testes and a formal surgical exploration is not necessary. When one or both components are lacking or there is detectable MIS, surgical exploration is warranted.

Indications for Surgery

Treatment of the undescended testicle offers the possibility of improved fertility, decreased incidence of malignancy, correction of patent processus vaginalis, prevention of testis torsion, and improvement in body image. Because changes related to fertility occur in the undescended testicle as young as 1 year of age and spontaneous descent rarely occurs after 6 months of age, the optimal time for surgical correction is around 6 months of age.

Almost 90% of undescended testes have an associated patent processus vaginalis. If a patient presents with an incarcerated or strangulated inguinal hernia, repair at the time of presentation along with orchiopexy should be undertaken. Otherwise, the hernia should be repaired at the time of orchiopexy. Occult inguinal hernia in patients with untreated undescended testis can present at any time with the typical symptoms or complications, including incarceration.

Alternative Therapy

Hormonal therapy is an option in the treatment of cryptorchidism because the condition may be related to hypogonadotropic hypogonadism. HCG is the only hormone approved for use in the treatment of cryptorchidism in the United States. Side effects of administration of HCG include enlargement of the penis, growth of pubic hair, increased testicular size, and aggressive behavior during administration. The likelihood of success with hormonal therapy is greatest for the most distal undescended testes or for testes that have been previously descended (7). Some suggest that hormonal therapy is effective only for retractile and not truly undescended testes (11). Although hormonal therapy may not be effective in achieving testicular descent, it may improve fertility in cryptorchid boys (2).

Surgical Technique

Prior to any surgical intervention, the patient is reexamined while under anesthesia because on occasion a retractile testicle descends under anesthesia or a previously nonpalpable testicle becomes palpable. A bimanual examination with a finger in the rectum may permit detection of an intraabdominal testicle. For a palpable testicle an open inguinal approach is performed. For the nonpalpable testicle, either a laparoscopic or an open inguinal approach may be performed.

Inguinal Orchidopexy

An incision is made in a groin crease along Langer's lines and carried through Scarpa's fascia to the level of the anterior aspect of the inguinal canal. The anterior aspect of the inguinal canal is incised, taking care to identify and protect the underlying ilioinguinal nerve. The spermatic cord is identified and elevated and dissected free of the anterior cremaster fibers. If no cord structures are identified attention is turned to the level of the internal ring and by retraction in the internal ring frequently a testicle may be identified just inside the internal ring. If no testicle is identified the peritoneum is opened and a search is made for either a testicle or a blind-ending vas and vessels. Blind-ending spermatic vessels must be identified to confirm absence of a testicle.

After identification of the spermatic cord in the canal, division of the gubernaculum with a hemostat on the proximal end provides a means of manipulating the testicle and cord structures safely. Care must be taken at this point to avoid a long-looped vas deferens that sometimes extends distally. Elevation of the cord permits blunt sweeping dissection of the inferior cremaster fibers to the level of the internal ring. By placing a retractor in the internal ring and pulling the cord and attached peritoneum medially the surgeon gains access to the retroperitoneal space along the lateral aspect of the internal ring, which is enveloped in the endopelvic fascia. The cord and peritoneum may then be swept anterior and medial with blunt dissection in the retroperitoneal space.

To free the remaining anterior and medial retroperitoneal attachments to the spermatic vessels and vas deferens, the internal spermatic fascia is divided, allowing separation of the processus and contiguous peritoneum from the vas and vessels and complete access to the retroperitoneum (Fig. 107–2). With a nonpatent processus vaginalis, a hemostat providing anterior traction on the tip of the peritoneal reflection permits dissection of the underlying cord from the internal spermatic fascia binding it to the peritoneum. With a patent processus vaginalis, the posterior cord is exposed, the internal spermatic fascia is swept off the cord structures, and the processus vaginalis is freed to the level of the peritoneum. The processus is ligated with a 3-0 Vicryl suture. At this time, the anterior and medial retroperitoneal attachments to the cord may be approached by placing a retractor anterior to the vessels in the internal ring, allowing the bands of the retroperitoneal fascia to be bluntly dissected from the vessels to obtain increased cord length. The dissection of the vas and vessels can be extended in the retroperitoneum up to the level of the renal hilum if the need arises.

With an absent testicle blind-ending vas and vessels may be encountered in the inguinal canal. The tubular structures in the canal must be traced proximally to the internal ring, where the divergence of the vas and vessels

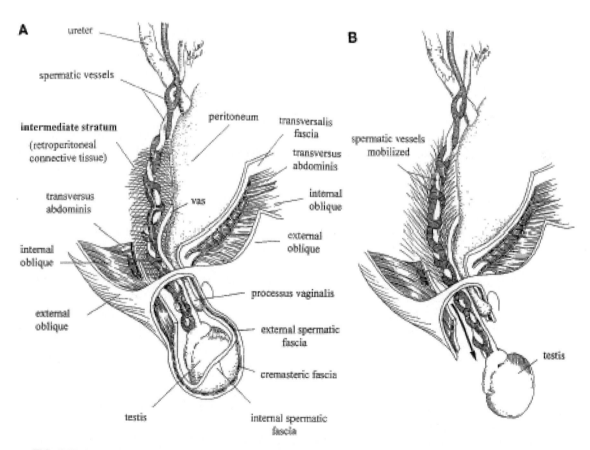

FIG. 107–2. Anatomy of inguinal orchiopexy. **A:** Relationship of the vas deferens, spermatic vessels, and processus vaginalis to investing fascial layers. The transversalis fascia is contiguous with internal spermatic fascia. **B:** With tension applied to the cord (arrow), orientation of the fibers of the intermediate stratum investing the retroperitoneal spermatic cord is changed so that fibers become parallel to cord structures. Freeing the vas and vessels from this investing fascia is the most important step in achieving distal testicular displacement. (From Hutcheson JC, Cooper CS, Snyder HM III. The anatomical approach to inguinal orchidopexy. *J Urol* 2000;164:1702–1704, with permission.)

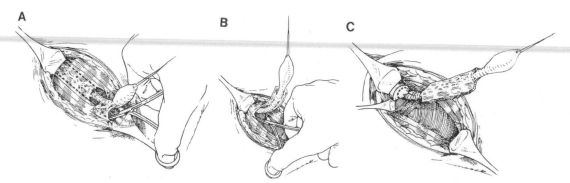

FIG. 107–3. Reoperative orchidopexy demonstrating external oblique fascial incisions lateral and medial to the cord structure. The adherent scar tissue is dissected with the spermatic cord and no attempt is made to dissect the spermatic cord from the scar. (From Cartwright PC, Velagapudi S, Snyder HM III, Keating MA. A surgical approach to reoperative orchiopexy. *J Urol* 1993;149:817–818, with permission.)

helps the surgeon positively identify the latter as spermatic vessels. With identification of blind-ending spermatic vessels no further exploration for a testis is indicated. However, a blind-ending vas deferens is not sufficient reason to stop the exploration because there are patients with a wide separation of the vas and an intraabdominal testis. When no spermatic cord structures are identified in the inguinal canal the dissection is carried to the internal ring and into the retroperitoneum. If no structures are identified the peritoneum is opened and the testicle or blind-ending spermatic vessels are sought.

Repeat inguinal exploration for a failed orchidopexy is associated with scar tissue surrounding the testicle and spermatic cord. Following the inguinal incision the testicle should be identified and freed from surrounding scar tissue. Once this is accomplished the cord can usually be freed along its posterior aspect extending through the inguinal canal. No attempt is made to dissect the cord from the scar extending along its anterior surface and the overlying external oblique fascia. By cutting the fascia along the medial and lateral sides of the cord and then connecting these incisions above the internal oblique muscle a strip of fascia is left attached to the cord (Fig. 107–3). The peritoneum may then be opened and the spermatic vessels freed as described above. At this level there is rarely any significant scar tissue.

Scrotal Fixation (Subdartos Pouch)

Multiple methods have been described for fixing the testis to the scrotum, although the subdartos pouch is our preferred method. Following a transverse incision in the hemiscrotum a pocket for the testicle is created by dissecting the scrotal skin from the adherent underlying dartos. Care must be taken not to develop the pouch too lateral or too inferior because this could result in an ectopic testis. Once adequate cord length has been obtained the testicle is brought through the dartos and placed in the pouch. The cord is inspected for torsion. For additional security, the inlet into the pouch may be narrowed with a single polyglycolic acid suture at a diameter less than that of the testis but not so narrow as to compromise the blood supply of the testis. A small portion of the parietal tunica vaginalis is incorporated into this stitch for further fixation. The use of an absorbable suture may heighten the inflammatory reaction around the testis and create a greater degree of scarring.

Transperitoneal Orchidopexy

An incision is made transversely or in the midline with subsequent intraperitoneal exploration. The spermatic vessels may be dissected free from their attachments cephalad to the level of their origin/insertion. With intraabdominal testicles, this dissection should leave a broad leaf of peritoneum attached to the vas deferens along the medial aspect in case transection of the spermatic vessels is required (see below). A new external inguinal ring is created lateral to the pubic tubercle to provide the most direct route into the scrotum.

Despite a high retroperitoneal dissection, some testicles may not reach a scrotal location due to short spermatic vessels. Often, these testicles can be identified after opening the peritoneum by applying traction to the testicle and observing minimal caudal displacement and no redundancy in the spermatic vessels. In this case the surgeon must consider either bringing the testicle down as low as possible with an anticipated reoperative orchidopexy in 6 to 12 months or transection of the spermatic vessels with immediate or secondary orchidopexy. A Fowler–Stephens test involves occluding the spermatic vessels with atraumatic bulldog clamps and then incising the tunica albuginea and watching for testicular bleeding. If there is adequate bleeding a Fowler–Stephens orchidopexy is performed by ligating the vessels and a broad-based medial pedicle of peritoneum and the vas deferens are mobilized. This procedure should not be done for a failed previous inguinal orchidopexy because the collateral blood supply along the vas deferens will have been compromised and is unreliable. An alternative is the staged testicular vessel transection orchiopexy, which involves ligation at the initial stage without mobilization to provide time for vasal collateral blood supply hypertrophy. After several months at the second stage the vessels are divided and the testicle brought into a scrotal location after a dissection similar to that described above.

Scrotal Orchidopexy

The high transscrotal incision for testicular mobilization including ligation of an associated inguinal hernia has been applied to primary and secondary cryptorchidism, although the technical difficulty of inguinal herniorrhaphy through this approach has limited its popularity. The scrotal approach may be especially suited to ectopic or ascended testes, including those that have failed prior orchidopexy. An alternative procedure is a low scrotal incision, with addition of an inguinal incision if a patent processus is encountered. A scrotal incision is made and blunt dissection is used to expose the processus vaginalis. The processus is opened, the testis is delivered, the processus is probed, and, if patent, an inguinal incision is made.

Laparoscopic Orchidopexy

Laparoscopy has been applied most commonly to the nonpalpable testis, although laparoscopic orchidopexy for palpable testes has been described. Many techniques for laparoscopic access to the abdomen have been described, but the authors prefer open access using a radially dilating trocar via a small incision in the superior fold of the umbilicus. A 3-mm transverse incision is made and stay sutures are placed on the anterior fascia. This layer is opened vertically and the peritoneum identified and opened under direct vision. The sleeve of the trocar is inserted and then dilated to 3, 5, or 10 mm, depending on the procedure to be performed. Diagnostic laparoscopy will reveal one of three findings: (a) blind-ending spermatic vessels proximal to the internal ring, proving a vanishing testis; (b) vas and vessels exiting the internal ring, proving that there is no intraabdominal testicle; or (c) an intraabdominal testicle (Fig. 107–1).

If vas and vessels exit the internal ring, it is controversial whether inguinal or scrotal exploration needs to be carried out to remove an atrophic testis, should one exist. This aspect of the procedure takes little time, and in general we recommend exploration. If an intraabdominal testis is found, there are three main options for management:

1. If the testis appears abnormal, laparoscopic orchiectomy versus open orchiectomy may be performed.

2. If the testis appears to be high with short vessels, a first-stage Fowler–Stephens operation can be performed laparoscopically, dividing the vessels in anticipation of orchidopexy 6 months later.

3. If it appears that the testis can be brought to the scrotum without dividing the vessels, a laparoscopic or open orchidopexy can be performed.

If it is elected to proceed with a laparoscopic orchidopexy, two accessory ports need to be placed in the anterior axillary line just below the level of the umbilicus bilaterally (Fig. 107–4). Dividing the spermatic vessels as a first-stage Fowler–Stephens procedure can be accomplished in several ways. Using vascular clips allows a landmark for the second-stage procedure, and also gives secure ligation. Electrocautery and laser have also been used, allowing one to avoid the 5-mm sized trocar. To use

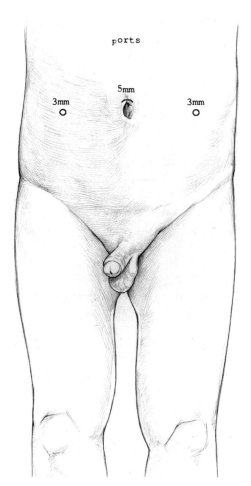

FIG. 107–4. Port sites used for laparoscopic orchidopexy. A 5-mm trocar is used through a curved incision in the upper edge of the umbilicus. Two 3-mm ports are inserted in the anterior axillary line just inferior to the umbilicus. (From Matthews R, Docimo SG. Laparoscopy for the management of the undescended testis. In: *Atlas of the Urologic Clinics of North America*, vol. 8. Philadelphia: WB Saunders, 2000:91–102, with permission.)

clips, the peritoneum is incised medial to the vessels and the plane of dissection behind the cord is developed. At least two clips are then applied to complete the procedure.

Laparoscopic orchidopexy is performed with the same port arrangement as orchiectomy. An initial peritoneal incision is made lateral to the spermatic vessels and carried as high as exposure will allow and distally to the vas deferens (Fig. 107–5). Rarely is it necessary to mobilize the ipsilateral colon, although one should be prepared to do so. The retroperitoneal dissection lifts the gubernaculum, which is divided after the course of the vas deferens is determined, making sure to remain distal to the caudal most portion of the vas. If the vas extends into the inguinal canal, the anterior wall of the processus vaginalis can be opened to advance the processus and gubernaculum into the peritoneum until a safe site for division is found. Once the gubernaculum is divided, the testis can be retracted toward the opposite internal ring to more completely free the vessels. The distal peritoneal triangle between the vessels and vas deferens is preserved to enhance collateral blood supply and to allow a Fowler–Stephens orchidopexy if vascular length is insufficient at the end of the procedure. The peritoneum above this triangle can be divided and stripped off of the proximal vessels to achieve more length. The testis should easily reach the opposite internal ring before attempting to pass it into the scrotum.

A horizontal scrotal incision is made and a subdartos pouch is created. Next, a straight grasper is passed through the ipsilateral port and then advanced through the abdominal wall either medial or lateral to the inferior epigastric vessels, depending on the need for extra length. The instrument is advanced anterior to the pubis and through the scrotal incision. The sleeve of the radially

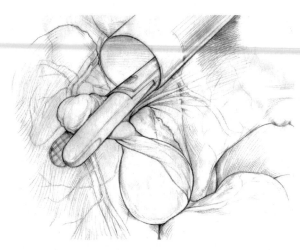

FIG. 107–6. The testis in transferred to the hemiscrotum using a grasper on the gubernaculum. (From Matthews R, Docimo SG. Laparoscopy for the management of the undescended testis. In: *Atlas of the Urologic Clinics of North America*, vol. 8. Philadelphia: WB Saunders, 2000:91–102, with permission.)

dilating trocar is passed into the abdomen from the scrotum using the shaft of the grasper as a guide. The instrument is withdrawn, and a 5- or 10-mm insert is used to dilate the sleeve, depending on the size of the testis. A locking grasper (i.e., Allis clamp) is introduced through the scrotal trocar and used to draw the testis into the scrotum (Fig. 107–6). The vessels are observed laparoscopically during this maneuver to avoid avulsion. The testis is fixed in the scrotum using usual methods.

Outcomes

Complications

Retraction is the most common complication of orchidopexy and usually occurs secondary to an incomplete initial dissection. It is possible that some cases of retracted testicle after an orchidopexy occur because of dislodgement of the testis from the scrotum. To prevent this possibility, straddle toys are avoided for at least 3 weeks following the operation.

The most significant complication is testicular atrophy, which occurs in 1% to 2% of cases of orchidopexy. The dissection of the testicular vessels and/or postoperative swelling and inflammation can result in ischemic injury that leads to testicular atrophy. The failure rate with orchidopexy is 8% for distal undescended testes and 26% for intraabdominal undescended testes (3). Other potential complications include ascent of the testis (requiring reoperative orchiopexy), infection, and bleeding.

Results

Successful therapy as defined by a viable testis positioned in the scrotum is dependent on the preoperative

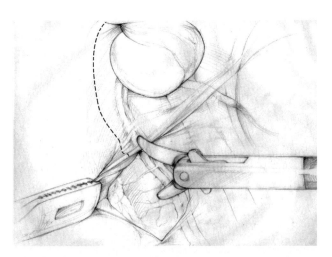

FIG. 107–5. Dissection begins lateral to the spermatic vessels and is directed toward the internal ring. (From Matthews R, Docimo SG. Laparoscopy for the management of the undescended testis. In: *Atlas of the Urologic Clinics of North America*, vol. 8. Philadelphia: WB Saunders, 2000:91–102, with permission.)

anatomic position of the testis. Success rates are 74% for the abdominal testis, 87% for canalicular, and 92% for those distal to the external ring. Success rates for various operative techniques are 89% for the standard "inguinal" orchidopexy, 67% for Fowler–Stephens, 77% for staged Fowler–Stephens, 81% for transabdominal, 73% for two stage, and 84% for microvascular (5). A recent multiinstitutional review of laparoscopic orchidopexy yielded success rates of 97.2% for primary laparoscopic orchidopexy, 74.1% for the single-stage laparoscopic Fowler–Stephens approach, and 87.9% for staged laparoscopic Fowler–Stephens procedures (1). All of these results suggest an advantage to maintaining intact vessels where possible.

Paternity rates among men who had attempted to father children were 65%, 90%, and 93% in men with bilateral cryptorchidism, unilateral cryptorchidism, and normally descended testicles, respectively (9). If only one testis is undescended, the sperm count will be subnormal in 25% to 33% and the serum FSH concentration will be slightly elevated (10,12). The presence of these abnormalities suggests that both testes are abnormal, perhaps congenitally, although only one fails to descend. If both testes are undescended, the sperm count usually will be severely subnormal and the serum testosterone may be reduced (12).

HYDROCELE/HERNIA

A hydrocele consists of a collection of fluid in the tunica vaginalis around the testicle. In children this is almost always found in association with a patent processus vaginalis that permits flow of peritoneal fluid into the tunica vaginalis (communicating hydrocele). An indirect inguinal hernia forms when bowel or any other tissue from the abdominal cavity protrudes into the patent processus vaginalis. Between 0.8% and 4.4% of newborns and up to 30% of premature infants have an inguinal hernia. Boys are six times more likely than girls to have a hernia and right-sided hernias occur twice as frequently as left-sided hernias, with bilateral hernias occurring about 10% of the time.

Diagnosis

Children with a hydrocele or hernia present with swelling in the groin and scrotum/labia. This swelling may be persistent or intermittent and may not be observed by the physician. Often, it is noted only by the parents when the child is crying or straining and the intraabdominal pressure is elevated. In this case, the diagnosis depends on a reliable history from the parents describing the intermittent groin and scrotal swelling. Older children may be examined while standing and performing a Valsalva maneuver to increase the intraabdominal pressure.

With increasing size of the hydrocele, the testicle becomes more difficult to palpate and often is not palpa-

ble. Usually, a hydrocele becomes narrow at the level of the internal ring and the examiner is able to detect this narrowing and get above the swelling. With a hernia, the swelling extends through the internal ring. The fluid in a hydrocele sac will transilluminate; however, bowel can also be transilluminated, making this a nonspecific finding for either a hydrocele or a hernia. Ultrasonography may help define the testicle and rule out any testicular pathology, as well as help differentiate a hydrocele from a hernia.

Indications for Surgery

The majority of infant hydroceles resolve by 18 months of age as the patent processus obliterates. If a hydrocele persists beyond 18 months, then it is unlikely to undergo spontaneous resolution and surgical treatment is indicated. When the fluid in a hydrocele sac is easily reduced, it suggests the size of the patent processus vaginalis is larger than with a hydrocele that does not have easily reducible fluid. This exam finding and a history of waxing and waning size of the hydrocele may serve as an indication for surgical correction before 18 months of age.

A healthy child presenting with an incarcerated hernia should undergo attempts at manually reducing the hernia. This may require sedation and placement of the child in the Trendelenburg position. Once the hernia is reduced, surgical correction should be performed within the next several days because an inguinal hernia will not resolve spontaneously and the child is at risk for repeat incarceration. If the hernia is not reducible an emergent operation should be performed. Preterm infants with a reducible hernia may be observed during their stay in the intensive care unit until they are thought to be medically stable enough to undergo a surgical procedure.

Because of the high incidence of a contralateral patent processus some surgeons routinely explore the contralateral groin during hernia surgery. Others site only a 20% chance of developing a clinical contralateral hernia and suggest that routine contralateral surgery should not be performed. Some physicians will perform laparoscopy through the hernia sac and examine the contralateral inguinal ring to determine if a contralateral groin exploration and hernia repair is required and others will perform a pneumoperitoneum and feel for crepitance in the contralateral groin as an indication to operate on this side.

Alternative Therapy

There are no alternative therapies.

Surgical Technique

A similar incision is made for hernias or hydroceles as previously described. After the inguinal canal is opened, the cremaster fibers may be spread off the anterior aspect of the spermatic cord. The hernia sac or patent processus vaginalis is identified and grasped with a hemostat. By elevation of the hernia sac the cord is brought up and may be freed from surrounding cremaster attachments, permitting the surgeons' finger to be placed beneath the entire spermatic cord and hernia sac. The sac may then be teased off the underlying cord by breaking apart the internal spermatic fascia that encases the cord structures and the hernia sac. As this is done, the cord structures may be separated from the hernia sac. When the cord structures are completely free the sac is transacted and then dissected up to the internal inguinal ring. It is important to identify the internal spermatic fascia and break this down so that when the sac is twisted and ligated the cord structures will not become incorporated. The hernia sac is doubly ligated with an absorbable suture. The distal sac or hydrocele is then delivered along with the testicle into the wound and opened, taking care not to injure the cord structures. The authors routinely sew the sac behind the cord or testis with an absorbable suture to prevent the possibility of reformation of the hydrocele. Repair of the dilated internal inguinal ring may be required and is accomplished by approximation of the transversalis fascia to itself at the level of the internal ring, taking care not to strangulate the cord. The conjoined tendon may also be sutured to the shelving edge of the inguinal ligament. The external oblique aponeurosis and wound is then closed with absorbable suture.

Outcomes

Complications

Recurrence or persistence of the hernia or hydrocele may occur if the patent processus is not well ligated. Injury to the underlying vessels and/or vas deferens may result in testicular atrophy. Displacement of the testicle to an extrascrotal location may occur after surgery. To prevent this complication every hydrocele and hernia repair should be concluded by confirmation of the testis location in its normal dependent scrotal position.

REFERENCES

1. Baker LA, Docimo SG, Surer I, et al. A multi-institutional analysis of laparoscopic orchidopexy. *Br J Urol Int* 2001;87:484–489.
2. Demirbilek S, Atayurt HF, Celik N, et al. Does treatment with human chorionic gonadotropin induce reversible changes in undescended testes in boys? *Pediatr Surg Int* 1997;12:591–594.
3. Docimo SG. The results of surgical therapy for cryptorchidism: a literature review and analysis. *J Urol* 1995;154:1148–1152.
4. Grant DB, Laurance BM, Atherden SM, et al. hCG stimulation test in children with abnormal sexual development. *Arch Dis Child* 1976;51:596–601.
5. Hutcheson JC, Cooper CS, Snyder HM III. The anatomical approach to inguinal orchiopexy. *J Urol* 2000;164:1702–1704.
6. Jarow JP, Berkovitz GD, Migeon CJ, et al. Elevation of serum gonadotropins establishes the diagnosis of anorchism in prepubertal boys with bilateral cryptorchidism. *J Urol* 1986;136:277–279.
7. Kaleva M, Arsalo A, Louhimo I, et al. Treatment with human chorionic gonadotropin for cryptorchidism: clinical and histological effects. *Int J Androl* 1996;19:293–298.
8. Lee MM, Donahoe PK, Silverman BL, et al. Measurements of serum müllerian inhibiting substance in the evaluation of children with nonpalpable gonads. *N Engl J Med* 1997;336:1480–1486.
9. Lee PA, Coughlin MT. Fertility after bilateral cryptorchidism. Evaluation by paternity, hormone, and semen data. *Hormone Res* 2001;55:28–32.
10. Lipshultz LI, Caminos-Torres R, Greenspan CS, et al. Testicular function after orchiopexy for unilaterally undescended testis. *N Engl J Med* 1976;295:15–18.
11. Rajfer J, Handelsman DJ, Swerdloff RS, et al. Hormonal therapy of cryptorchidism. A randomized, double-blind study comparing human chorionic gonadotropin and gonadotropin-releasing hormone. *N Engl J Med* 1986;314:466–470.
12. Werder EA, Illig R, Torresani T, et al. Gonadal function in young adults after surgical treatment of cryptorchidism. *Br Med J* 1976;4:1357–1359.

CHAPTER 108

Urogenital Sinus and Cloacal Anomalies

Richard C. Rink

Anomalies of the urogenital sinus occur on a spectrum, ranging from a distal communication between the urethra and vagina to a complex confluence between the urethra, vagina, and rectum. A distal common channel for these structures drains to a single perineal opening. The latter clinical presentation results from persistence of the cloaca and is essentially a severe urogenital sinus abnormality with high imperforate anus. In addition to a more bizarre and diverse internal anatomy, patients with cloacal anomalies have a high incidence of other serious midline congenital anomalies. Important elements of baseline evaluation and surgical management of urogenital sinus and cloacal anomalies are discussed in detail in this chapter.

Urogenital sinus abnormalities in general occur in one of two forms: pure urogenital sinus anomalies and females with intersex conditions. The latter group is much more common. In these children surgical management must not only address the urinary and vaginal communication but also the masculinization of the clitoris and labia.

DIAGNOSIS

The majority of children with urogenital sinus abnormalities are detected at birth due to genital ambiguity. The initial evaluation in this group of children requires a team approach to gender identification with appropriate rapid chromosomal and endocrinologic studies. The history and physical exam are often helpful in establishing a correct diagnosis. Congenital adrenal hyperplasia (CAH) secondary to 21-hydroxlaste deficiency is most common. Some children may be identified antenatally on ultrasound by noting a fluid-filled mass (distended vagina) posterior to the bladder. Persistence of the cloaca is suspected *in utero* when a large fluid-filled pelvic structure, bilateral hydroureteronephrosis, oligohydramnios, and ascites are seen with a 46 XX karyotype. Hydrometro-

colpos due to retention of urine and secretions results in upper-tract distension, and ascites occurs due to retrograde flow through the genital tract into the peritoneum.

Prematurity and multiple congenital defects are common in children with cloacal anomalies. Initial evaluation of these children should therefore include medical stabilization and evaluation for midline abnormalities. Abdominal distension is common and may result in respiratory embarrassment. Cardiac, renal, and upper gastrointestinal anomalies and spinal dysraphism are frequently identified. Although these infants are uniformly female, ambiguity of the genitalia may occur and should be investigated. A single perineal opening is noted anteriorly and the anus is absent. The perineum is in general flat with variable amounts of labial tissue mounded around the anterior orifice. The buttocks are often poorly developed and the sacrum is deficient on abdominal plain film.

Renal ultrasound anomalies of number and fusion occur. A genitogram confirms magnetic resonance imaging (MRI) clarifies the complex pelvic relationships, evaluates the structural quality of the sphincter complex, and defines the anatomy of the lumbosacral spine and distal cord. After gender identification and stabilization of the child, radiographic evaluation is begun. Genitography is of utmost importance to help determine the anatomy (i.e., length of common sinus, location of vaginal confluence, status of bladder, presence or absence of vesicoureteral reflux, or vaginal duplication). Patients with cloacal anomalies will show communication between the urogenital tract and rectum and vesicoureteral reflux is commonly identified. Ultrasonography of the pelvis and kidneys is also of help to identify the uterus, ovaries, and any vaginal distention or in the case of cloacal anomalies may reveal hydronephrosis or increased echogenicity suggestive of renal dysplasia. The adrenal glands in CAH may be prominent with a cerebriform appearance. MRI of the pelvis is an excellent tool to determine pelvic anatomy and note the presence of lumbosacral spinal cord anomalies that may be present.

Pure urogenital sinus anomalies are in general not detected early because of normal external genitalia. These patients are usually found at puberty with hydrometrocolpos or difficulty with tampon insertion. Some children are identified earlier with incontinence and urinary tract infection (UTI) from urine pooling within the vagina.

INDICATIONS FOR SURGERY

It is important for the reader to understand that there is a great deal of controversy surrounding feminizing genitoplasty. There are proponents of (a) very early neonatal reconstruction, (b) delayed postpubertal reconstruction (this usually involves vaginoplasty), and (c) no surgery unless the patient requests it. There are obvious advantages and disadvantages to each of these approaches. All children with genital ambiguity should be evaluated promptly by a gender assignment team consisting of a neonatologist, geneticist, endocrinologist, pediatric urologist, and psychiatrist who are all working with and for the child and family. For the purposes of this presentation we will assume that the family and gender assignment team agree to proceed with surgery. It is our belief that early reconstruction is most appropriate with all three steps (clitoroplasty, vaginoplasty, and labioplasty) completed in a single stage (3). Delayed postpubertal vaginoplasty, however, could easily be done by the same techniques described in this chapter.

ALTERNATIVE THERAPY

Due to the complex nature of cloacal anomalies and the high incidence of other congenital defects, some children will not go on to formal reconstruction. Certainly, temporary diversion of the gastrointestinal tract and decompression of the urinary tract are required. Not all patients are candidates for a functional rectal pull-through. Those with deficient colonic length or inadequate sphincteric function may be best served by permanent colostomy.

SURGICAL TECHNIQUE

All children receive a polyethylene glycol electrolyte solution bowel preparation and prophylactic parenteral antibiotics preoperatively. Endoscopy is performed with the child in the lithotomy position. This is one of the most important steps in reconstruction as it defines the level of vaginal confluence and allows identification of any other lower genitourinary pathology such as vaginal duplication, ectopic ureter, etc. The distance of the vagina from the bladder neck is the most critical aspect and dictates the type of vaginoplasty. Endoscopy also allows place-

ment of a Fogarty catheter into the vagina, which is left indwelling with the balloon inflated. Correct placement is confirmed by repeating endoscopy. The Fogarty balloon will aid in identification of the vagina during the reconstruction. A separate small Foley catheter is passed into the bladder.

Historically, urogenital sinus surgery has been performed with the child in the lithotomy position. While this position is acceptable, we have found it much easier to prepare the entire lower portion of the body circumferentially to allow access to the abdomen and perineum and to allow the child to be supine or prone. Further, it dramatically improves visualization for the surgical assistants.

Clitoroplasty

In cases of genital ambiguity the operation begins with placement of a traction suture in the glans clitoris. Using a skin scribe, the proposed incisions are outlined as shown in Figure 108–1. Historically, a very wide-based inverted "U"-shaped perineal flap has been created. Improved cosmesis occurs, however, if the flap has a narrower base, avoiding the appearance of a triangular introitus. After injecting 0.5% lidocaine with 1:200,000 epinephrine subcutaneously along the proposed suture lines, the clitoroplasty is begun. The entire clitoris is degloved by creating a plane between Buck's fascia and the dartos circumferentially. Ventrally, the incision is carried around

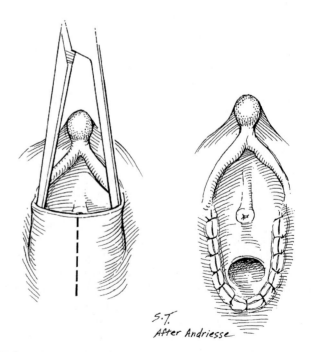

FIG. 108–1. Flap vaginoplasty. **a:** Proposed incision lines are outlined. **b:** Perineal flap developed and clitoroplasty completed with proposed incision to open the urogenital sinus.

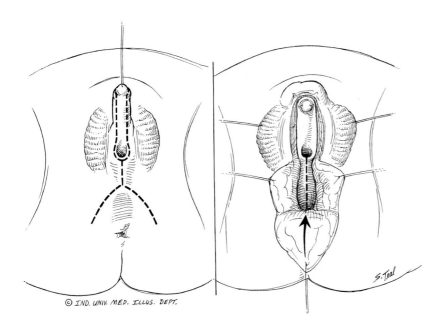

FIG. 108–2. Clitoris degloved. Proposed incision for excision of erectile tissue.

the urogenital sinus meatus. The rounded apex of the perineal flap should extend to near the meatus. This flap is elevated with its underlying subcutaneous and adipose tissue to expose the urogenital sinus (Fig. 108–1b). Dorsally, the suspensory ligament is divided and the bifurcation of the corporal bodies is exposed ventrally. With the entire clitoris now exposed, a tourniquet is placed at its base. A vertical ventromedial incision is made (very near the midline ventrally) along the entire corporal body to the glans (Fig. 108–2). The erectile tissue is exposed and excised with care not to injure Buck's fascia, the tunica albuginea, the neurovascular bundle, or glans. This is performed bilaterally to the level of the bifurcation. The proximal end of each corporal body is oversewn with 4-0 polyglycolic acid sutures to prevent bleeding. With Buck's fascia folded, the glans is now secured to the corporal stumps with 4-0 PDS sutures. We had previously sutured the glans to the pubis but found that this technique prevents appropriate concealment of the glans. At times the glans is quite large but one should resist aggressive glans reduction. If any reduction is done, it should only occur on the ventral aspect of the glans to prevent loss of sensation.

Vaginoplasty

The most complex component of reconstruction of the urogenital sinus is the vaginoplasty. While multiple techniques of vaginal reconstruction have been described, they all fall in general into four types: (a) cut-back vaginoplasty, (b) flap vaginoplasty, (c) pull-through vaginoplasty, and (d) vaginal replacement. The type of vaginoplasty is determined by the location of the confluence between the vagina and the common urogenital sinus.

The *cut-back vaginoplasty* is applicable only for minor labial fusion and is in fact contraindicated for any true urogenital sinus anomaly. In this procedure the sinus is opened with a midline vertical incision that is then closed transversely in a Heineke–Mikulicz fashion. It is of historical significance only and will not be addressed further.

Low Vaginal Confluence

For the low confluence a *flap vaginoplasty* is performed (Figs. 108–1a and 108–1b). This procedure leaves the vagina in the same anatomic location but opens the sinus to provide a larger common opening for the urethra and vagina. It is contraindicated in patients with a high vaginal confluence. The previously elevated perineal flap must be long enough to allow a tension-free anastomosis to the normal-caliber proximal vagina. Redundancy of the flap, however, will create a lip of tissue at the introitus. The exposed ventral aspect of the sinus is opened in the midline and the incision is carried through the narrowed distal one-third of the vagina into the normal-caliber proximal vagina. This is very important and prevents later vaginal stenosis. It is also noteworthy that the flap vaginoplasty does not change the vaginal location or confluence but merely exposes the vagina by widely opening the introitus. Because the anterior and lateral aspect of the vagina is untouched, stenosis is uncommon.

High Vaginal Confluence

If the vaginal confluence is near the bladder neck, a flap vaginoplasty is contraindicated as it will result in severe female hypospadias with urine pooling. Deep spatulation of the sinus and posterior vagina may permanently open and injure the sphincteric mechanism. Therefore, a *pull-through vaginoplasty* is required (Figs. 108–3a and 108–3b), which allows a complete separation of the vagina from the sinus. The sinus is closed to create a urethra and the vagina is brought to the perineum. In this technically demanding procedure the vagina is completely separated from the sinus. The dissection of the anterior wall of the vagina from the urethra and bladder neck is the most difficult, and if not done with care and excellent exposure it may result in injury to the urethra or sphincteric mechanism. The initial portion of this procedure is identical to the flap vaginoplasty. It is important to expose the entire posterior wall of the vagina by dividing the bulbospongiosus muscle and sweeping the rectum posteriorly. The sinus is opened in the midline until the Fogarty balloon is exposed in the vagina. At this time we rotate the patient to the prone position and elevate the posterior wall of the vagina with a malleable retractor, providing excellent exposure of the anterior wall of the vagina and its confluence with the urethra (Fig. 108–3b) (4). Stay sutures on the vagina are very helpful. With the vagina separated from the urethra and sinus, the opened sinus is closed in layers over a catheter, allowing the sinus to become the urethra. Unfortunately, "pull-through" is at times a misnomer: Even following complete circumferential vaginal mobilization; the vagina may not reach the perineum. In these situations the perineal flap will create the distal posterior vaginal wall and the anterior wall can be created by either a preputial or labial flap. In extreme situations, bowel interposition may be required to create the distal vagina. A Penrose drain is left in the vagina and the Foley remains in the urethra.

Labioplasty

Having completed the clitoroplasty and vaginoplasty, only the labial reconstruction remains. The phallic skin is unfurled and divided in the midline longitudinally (similar to Byar's flaps), stopping short of the base to allow a clitoral hood. These skin flaps are now sutured in place inferiorly along either side of the vagina to create labia minora. The anteriorly displaced labia majora are mobilized posteriorly by making lateral incisions in a Y–V fashion. The mobilized labia majora are now sutured to the labia minora and to the apex of the perineal flap. This step moves the labia posteriorly to their normal location on either side of the vagina.

Cloacal Anomalies

Surgical management of children with cloacal anomalies occurs in several important steps, but the formal reconstruction is best performed in a single stage. Neonates require early diverting colostomy. Hendren prefers a right colostomy to leave adequate distal length and intact blood supply for subsequent rectal pull-through (1). A long distal colonic segment, however, can allow persistent retention of urine in the mucus fistula and result in refractory hyperchloremic metabolic acidosis. Preliminary mapping of the anorectal sphincter complex provides prognostic information for future rectal pull-through.

Decompression of the genitourinary tract is performed during endoscopic investigation of the cloacal anatomy. Inspissated mucus and meconium debris are drained.

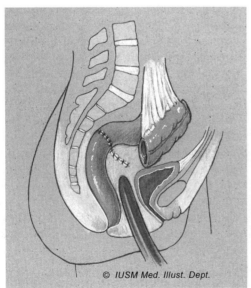
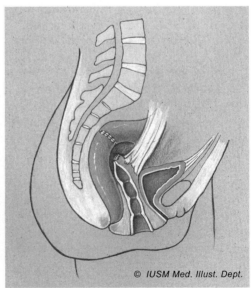

A   B

FIG. 108–3. Pull-through vaginoplasty, prone approach. **a:** Proposed midline incision to open the urogenital sinus with the rectum elevated by a retractor. **b:** Sinus opened into the back wall of the vagina with exposed by placing a retractor. **c:** Proposed incision for vaginal separation.

Because the bladder neck and vagina are often closely related, the vagina passively retains voided urine. If vaginal voiding is a problem, intermittent catheterization of the common channel will allow decompression, with the catheter most likely entering the vagina rather than the bladder. Poor emptying is suspected in children with persistence of hydronephrosis postnatally. Alternatively, if the common channel is narrow it can be opened distally to facilitate voiding. If the above measures fail, cutaneous vesicostomy is performed. Cutaneous vaginostomy allows free drainage but tethers the vagina anteriorly and complicates the subsequent vaginoplasty.

Severe anomalies of other organ systems should be corrected early. Other urinary tract abnormalities that may compromise long-term renal function should be addressed. Colonization of the urinary tract is common but symptomatic infections mandate aggressive therapy. Assuming that all other congenital issues have been satisfactorily addressed, formal repair of the cloaca with Pena's posterior sagittal anorectovaginourethroplasty (PSARVUP) is planned for 6 to 12 months of age. This demanding procedure should be completed in a single stage, capitalizing on the virgin tissue planes for both anorectal and urogenital reconstruction.

The initial preparations for repair of the persistent cloaca are similar to that described above for the high-confluence urogenital sinus. After a circumferential lower-body preparation and endoscopic placement of Fogarty catheters, the patient is placed prone on chest and pelvic rolls. The sphincter complex is stimulated and the optimal positions for the anus, perineal body, vagina, and urethra are marked. The perineum is incised in the mid-line from the tip of the spine to the posterior margin of the single perineal orifice. The sphincteric muscles are split in the midline and tagged to facilitate subsequent reconstruction. The rectal communication is sharply dissected off the common channel and the distal colon is mobilized for pull-through. Urethroplasty and vaginoplasty then proceed as in repair of the urogenital sinus described above. Currently, we prefer the technique of total urogenital mobilization. Even if this maneuver cannot bring the vagina to the perineum, it does improve exposure to the confluence for completion of a pull-through vaginoplasty. Duplicate vaginas are often encountered and are combined by division of the vertical septum. Vaginal agenesis or atresia requires bowel interposition for vaginoplasty (Fig. 108–4), and again this is best performed at the time of rectal pull-through and urethroplasty.

Total Urogenital Mobilization

Total urogenital mobilization (TUM), described by Pena in 1997, entails complete circumferential dissection of the intact urogenital sinus, urethra, and vagina from the pubis (2). This was originally proposed for cloacal anomalies but has since been often applied to those with a urogenital sinus only. TUM allows the midlevel vagina to be moved to the perineum easily, and while the high-confluence vagina may still require a pull-through vaginoplasty it is much more easily performed.

The initial incisions are similar to those described above but the urogenital sinus is mobilized intact off the corporal bodies to their bifurcation (Figs. 108–5a and

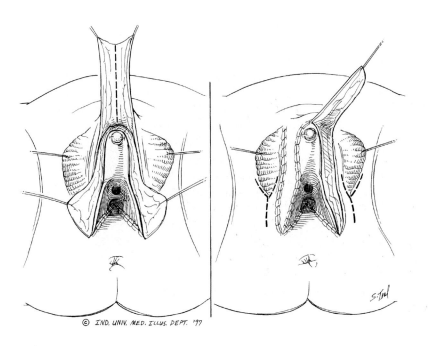

FIG. 108–4. Colon replacement vaginoplasty. **a:** Colonic segment isolated, perineal dissection for the vagina. **b:** Completed vaginoplasty.

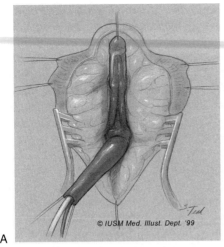
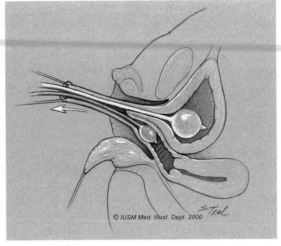

A

B

FIG. 108–5. Complete circumferential mobilization of the intact sinus.

108–5b). At this time the dissection is continued posteriorly in the midline, separating the rectum from the posterior wall of the vagina. The Fogarty balloon within the vagina is palpated and an incision is made into the vaginal wall posteriorly near the confluence. If the vagina reaches the perineum no further dissection is performed. In Pena's original description the mobilized sinus was amputated, but Rink et al. have shown that this is important tissue to save for the reconstruction. If the vagina does not reach the perineum, then the sinus is mobilized between the corporal bifurcation and off the pubis. When these avascular attachments from the pubis are divided, the sinus moves toward the perineum. If the sinus is near the perineum, a flap vaginoplasty can be accomplished by sewing in the perineal flap. The redundant sinus is then split ventrally to create a mucosa-lined vestibule (Figs. 108–6a and 108–6b) (5). Recently, we described splitting the sinus laterally to create a posterior vaginal wall (Figs. 108–7a and 108–7b). This is also a form of flap vaginoplasty. If the vagina is high following the TUM, then the vagina is separated from the sinus as described above for a pull-through vaginoplasty. This vaginal separation is again more easily achieved by placing the patient prone over chest rolls. The mobilized sinus is split dorsally and the opened sinus is rotated to create an anterior vaginal wall (Figs. 108–8a and 108–8b).

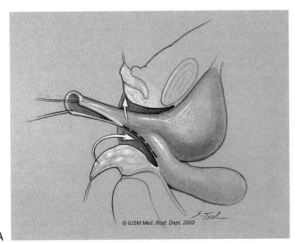
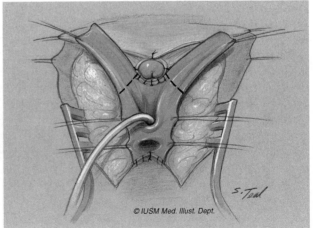

A

B

FIG. 108–6. A: Mobilized sinus open on ventral aspect to expose the vagina. **B:** Sinus used to create mucosal-lined vestibule.

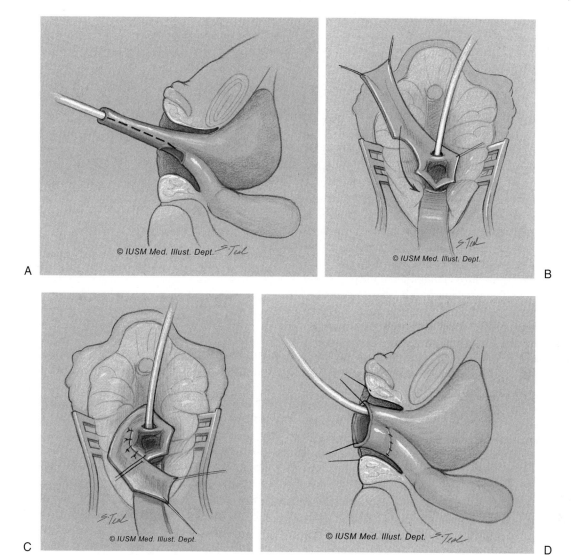

FIG. 108–7. The mobilized sinus is split laterally to allow rotation of the flap to create a posterior vaginal wall.

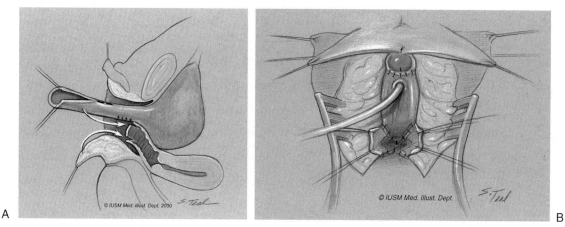

FIG. 108–8. The sinus is opened dorsally for a pull-through vaginoplasty and rotated to create an anterior vaginal wall.

OUTCOMES

Complications

Results

This is a time of widespread evaluation of all aspects of feminizing genitoplasty. There is little agreement on any component, including timing of the procedure or even the necessity of some aspects such as clitoroplasty. While virtually all surgical reports note excellent cosmetic results, little data is available on long-term results. There is debate about both the psychological aspects of having genital surgery and the psychological aspects of not having the surgery and growing up with genital ambiguity. Clitoroplasty is controversial as no one knows if it is a clinical problem to have an enlarged clitoris. Should the parents make the decision about early surgery or should it be postponed until the patient can decide? If the latter, then what are the social implications of having ambiguous genitalia? Virtually all agree that the vagina must be exposed to allow egress of menstrual fluid but when this should be done remains controversial. TUM results are far too short term, and while the procedure is technically easier the long-term results may show that sphincteric injury with incontinence or stress incontinence from moving the bladder neck inferiorly occur with unacceptable frequency. The issues are complex and will only be solved by long-term prospective multiinstitutional studies.

From an anatomic and cosmetic standpoint, surgical reconstruction of cloacal anomalies is now satisfactory in the majority of cases (Fig. 108–9). Unfortunately, the functional success of the urinary and rectal elements of the reconstruction also depends upon sacral nerve function and the quality and innervation of the sphincteric complexes. The bladder neck and intrinsic sphincter are inherently deficient with a high confluence. No natural plane exists between the bladder neck or trigone and vagina, and the continence mechanism may be further compromised as the vagina is dissected off the bladder neck. The external sphincter may also be congenitally deficient or may be injured during reconstruction. Due to abnormal sacral nerve function, these patients may require intermittent catheterization or further reconstruction, such as outlet resistance enhancement or augmentation cystoplasty, to achieve continence.

Outcomes of vaginoplasty are as reported with the high-confluence urogenital sinus. Total urogenital mobilization appears to reduce the incidence of stenosis,

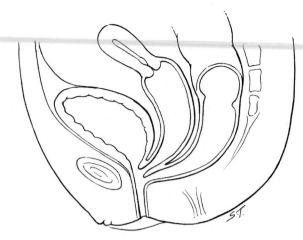

FIG. 108–9. Cloacal anomaly. The vagina and rectum may vary from relatively normal caliber to quite distended.

although long-term pubertal follow-up is pending. Introital revision may be required at puberty after bowel interposition vaginoplasty in infancy.

The most important issue in functional outcome after repair of a persistent cloaca is the long-term preservation of renal function. Many of these children have congenital renal dysplasia related to vesicoureteral reflux and/or *in utero* infravesical urinary tract obstruction. Persistent postnatal hydronephrosis is aggressively addressed with diversion if necessary. Chronic renal failure also occurs, however, in the fortunate subset of patients who achieve a normal nadir creatinine in infancy (6). Even after apparently successful lower urinary tract reconstruction, these patients require urodynamic evaluation and high vigilance to prevent upper urinary tract deterioration due to silent bladder dysfunction.

REFERENCES

1. Hendren WH. Cloacal malformations: Experience with 105 cases. *J Pediatr Surg* 1992;27:890–901.
2. Pena A. Total urogenital mobilization—an easier way to repair cloacas. *J Pediatr Surg* 1997;32:263–268.
3. Rink RC, Adams MC. Feminizing genitoplasty: State of the art world. *J Urol* 1998;16:212–218.
4. Rink RC, Pope JC, Kropp BP, et al. Reconstruction of the high urogenital sinus: Early perineal prone approach without division of the rectum. *J Urol* 1997;158:1293–1297.
5. Rink RC, Yerkes EB. Surgical management of female genital anomalies, intersex (urogenital sinus) disorders and cloacal anomalies. In: Gearhart JP, Rick RC, Mouriquand PDE, eds. *Pediatric urology.* Philadelphia: WB Saunders, 2001.
6. Warne SA, Wilcox DT, Ledermann SE, Ransley PG. Renal outcome in patients with cloaca. *J Urol* 2002;167:2548–2551.

CHAPTER 109

Surgery to Correct Ambiguous Genitalia

Anthony J. Casale and C.D Anthony Herndon

Ambiguous genitalia or intersex are terms used to describe a congenital condition where the appearance of the genitalia is neither classically male nor female. The condition affects both external genitalia (phallus, labia, scrotum, and introitus) and internal reproductive structures (vagina, urethra, urogenital sinus). In these cases there is usually a conflict between the genetic sex, gonadal sex, and apparent gender as based on genital appearance.

The historic goal of surgery for ambiguous genitalia is to provide the child with genitalia that have the appearance of and are functional as either male or female gender and are consistent with their genetic and gonadal sex when possible. Society dictates that the appearance of the infant's genitals and therefore apparent gender is the subject of great and immediate interest for the immediate and extended family and friends, making ambiguous genitalia a cause of intense concern and confusion for all. It is this powerful interest that has driven physicians and families to treat the condition as an emergency even if there are often no additional health risks. The historical approach to this issue has been to assign gender based on several factors, including the potential for reproduction, the technical limits of surgical reconstruction (i.e., our limited ability to create a male phallus without adequate corpora), and the belief that gender was determined by genital appearance and role assignment in childhood.

DIAGNOSIS

The first task for the physician faced with a child with intersex is to correctly diagnose the underlying condition responsible for the appearance of the genitalia. A team including pediatric urologist, pediatric endocrinologist, neonatologist, and either pediatric psychologist or psychiatrist provides the best approach for this complex process.

The first step in diagnosis is a thorough physical exam. The initial caregivers in the nursery are usually alerted to the possibility of gender ambiguity if the phallus is small or curved and if the labioscrotal folds are partially fused (Fig. 109–1). The pediatric urologist should then document the length and diameter of the phallus and the position and number of external perineal openings, including the position of any potential urogenital (UG) orifices as well as the rectum. The state of fusion of the labioscrotal folds and their location is important, as is the presence or absence of palpable gonads. The presence of a palpable gonad almost always is consistent with male gender. Hyperpigmentation of the labioscrotal skin is common in cases of congenital adrenal hyperplasia (CAH). The

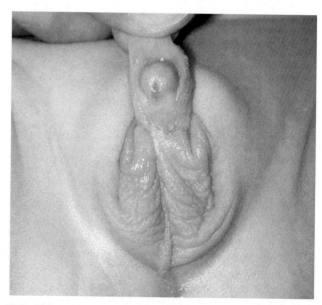

FIG. 109–1. This intersex female demonstrates labial/scrotal fusion and a hypertrophied phallus with a distal urogenital sinus opening.

843

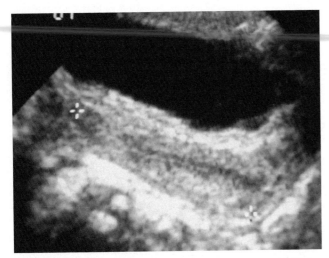

FIG. 109–2. Pelvic ultrasound demonstrates the uterus in the midline position posterior to the urinary bladder.

blood pressure should be measured carefully because of the threat of hypertension with CAH.

Chromosomal studies should be sent immediately. In the immediate newborn period the presence of functioning testicular tissue can be determined by measuring serum testosterone, which is elevated in the first few days of life. CAH is diagnosed by finding elevated plasma levels of 17-hydroxyprogesterone and androstenedione and urine levels of pregnanetriol and 17-ketosteroids.

Imaging studies of the infant should include a pelvic ultrasound looking for the presence of a uterus and retrograde injection of contrast into the UG sinus (genitogram) to identify the presence of a vagina and uterus. The uterus can usually be identified on pelvic ultrasound of the newborn as a 1-cm solid midline mass just posterior to the bladder (Fig. 109–2). The uterus can often be identified on genitogram with a cervical impression outlined by the contrast in the vagina.

INDICATIONS FOR SURGERY

Genital ambiguity is a result of an abnormality in sexual determination resulting from a defect in genetic, gonadal, or genital tissue differentiation and is classified into four categories: female psuedohermaphrodite, male psuedohermaphrodite, mixed gonadal dygensis, and true hermaphrodite. Female genital reconstruction, also called feminizing genitoplasty, is restricted to female psuedohermaphrodite, mixed gonadal dygensis, and true hermaphrodite individuals who have the potential to have normal female sexual function. CAH is a form of female psuedohermaphrodite and is by far the most common condition causing ambiguous genitalia. CAH is responsible for over 70% of ambiguous genitalia and the vast majority of patients treated with feminizing genitoplasty.

Candidates for feminizing genitoplasty have two distinct problems: the fusion of their internal reproductive system with the urinary tract as a UG sinus with a single external orifice and the virilization of the external genitalia with fused labioscrotal folds and clitoral enlargement. The internal anatomy can cause problems by pooling of urine within the vagina and uterus and inadequate vaginal drainage for secretions and menses. There is no adequate external vaginal orifice for sexual intercourse.

During the initial investigation the family is advised not to delay naming the child until gender is established and to delay reporting the child's gender to others, stating only that the child had some developmental problems that need to be investigated. It is during this period that the gender assignment team should carefully educate and council the family with the nature of their child's problem and the limitations and potential inherent in the exact condition. There are actually two decisions to be made by the parents: the gender of the child and whether to have reconstructive surgery. Gender decisions have always been considered urgent while surgical reconstruction decisions may be made later as long as there is not a health concern because of inadequate drainage of urine.

ALTERNATIVE THERAPY

There is no alternative to surgery

SURGICAL TECHNIQUE

Once the decision for feminizing genitoplasty has been made the timing of the procedure is of some importance. In cases of CAH glucocorticoid and mineralocorticoid replacement therapy will diminish androgen production by the adrenal and lead to partial reversal of the clitoral hypertrophy. For this reason the external genital surgery should be delayed until at least 6 months of age. Some surgeons prefer to delay reconstruction of the internal structures until adolescence if the child does not have problems with urine retention and urinary tract infection because historically patients who have reconstruction early in life require a secondary procedure at adolescence to correct vaginal stenosis. On the other hand, those children who have early reconstruction need only dilations or simple revisions of the vagina at adolescence in contrast to the child who delays the major reconstruction to later in life. We prefer to do a complete reconstruction at 6 months of age and explain to the family that a second minor procedure may be needed later.

A comprehensive definition of the anatomy is imperative in planning for and accomplishing the reconstruction. The upper urinary tract should be imaged with ultrasound and if the kidneys are not normal lasix renal scan. The lower urinary tract should be imaged with a retrograde genitogram (Fig. 109–3), which gives the surgeon important information about the length of the UG sinus,

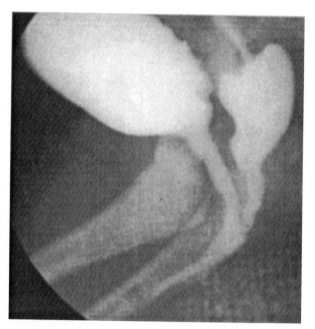

FIG. 109–3. Genitogram demonstrates confluence of the urethra anteriorly and vagina posteriorly. Note cervical impression at the apex of the vagina and contrast within the cervix.

the point of confluence of the vagina and urethra, and their relative lengths and position within the pelvis. The level of this confluence, either high (UG sinus greater than 3 cm) or low (UG sinus less than 3 cm), ultimately determines the surgical approach. Further imaging of the pelvic organs may be necessary in complex cases and can be done with magnetic resonance imaging or computed tomography scanning with good visualization.

Finally, an examination under anesthesia is needed including cystoscopy and vaginoscopy. It is often easier to measure the length of the UG sinus and determine the height of the confluence with the scope than with imaging. The length of the UG sinus can be measured by placing the tip of the scope at the point of confluence and marking the scope at the level of the external meatus. When the scope is withdrawn the length of the UG sinus is estimated by measuring the distance from the mark on the barrel to the tip of the scope. These measurements of the UG sinus, vagina, and urethra along with the position of the confluence of all three are important to plan what techniques may be necessary for repair.

Surgical Position

Most of the surgery for ambiguous genitalia can be performed in the lithotomy position. We follow Hendren and Atala's recommendations to prep the patient circumferentially while applying sterile wrapping to the lower legs to allow the patient to be turned from the lithotomy to the prone position as necessary during the operation (4).

Cliteroplasty

The goal of cliteroplasty is to reduce the size of the enlarged clitoris to one that is within the range of normal for females. The glans clitoris must be preserved for sensation but the corpora should be shortened. A circumferential incision is made on the clitoris just proximal to the coronal sulcus and the clitoris is degloved from skin and subcutaneous tissue. The urethral plate and rudimentary corpus spongiosum may be divided distally and dissected with the subcutaneous tissue or just mobilized from the corpora cavernosa while leaving it attached both proximally and distally. We prefer to divide the urethral plate from the glans during this dissection. Incisions are made in the tunica albuginea of the corpora at the 2- and 10-o'clock positions using needle point electrocautery. These incisions are extended and joined across the ventral aspect of the corpora at the subcoronal level distally and 0.5 cm above the pubis proximally (Fig. 109–4). The dorsal tunica albuginea (including the enclosed neurovascular bundle) is dissected from the erectile tissue and remaining tunica of the corpora. The erectile tissue bodies and their ventral and lateral fascia can be dissected from the dorsal fascia and excised. A 4-0 polyglycolic acid suture can be used to ligate each corporal body at its base. The rim of fascia on the glans can be sewn to the fascia on the stumps of the corpora with 4-0 sutures to reseat the glans and stabilize it. The dorsal fascia, which contains the neurovascular bundle, is allowed to fold under the skin cranial to the glans. The urethral plate, which was previously separated from the glans, can now be shortened and partially split in the midline to flatten the introitus and shorten the distance from the vagina to the clitoris (Fig. 109–5).

The glans clitoris is often quite large and several procedures have been described to reduce its size. We have preferred not to decrease the overall size of the glans but instead to conceal some of the dorsal glans with the glans hood. A small patch of the dorsal glans epithelium at the base can be excised leaving the erectile tissue intact and the glans hood can be sewn to this area and allowed to fold over the remainder of the glans. This leaves the glans with its full erectile capability, leaves it accessible, and covers it appropriately with a skin hood.

Labioplasty

The goal of labioplasty is to create a normal appearing and functioning female perineum and introitus. The shaft skin and dorsal prepuce of the clitoris can be utilized to form the labia minora and fashion a clitoral hood. The original skin incision had degloved the clitoris and left all skin based on the dorsal pedicle. This skin can then be split in the midline for approximately two-thirds of its length (Fig. 109–6). At the proximal end of the incision a transverse incision is made and curved proximally at each

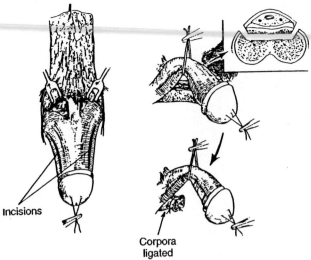

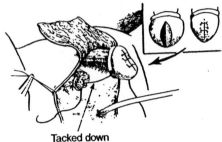

Incisions

Corpora
ligated

Tacked down

FIG. 109–4. Coroporotomy incisions are extended from the 10- and 2-o'clock positions laterally from just below the corona to 0.5 cm above the pubis. The corporal bodies are ligated at their base and the bodies excised, leaving the dorsal strip of fascia including the neurovascular bundles preserved with the glans.

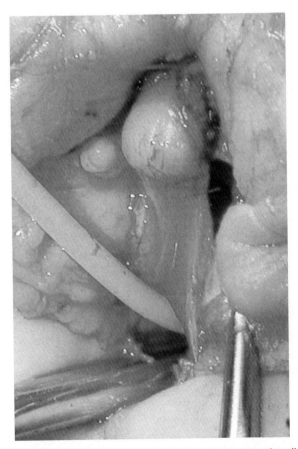

FIG. 109–5. The urethral plate is used to shorten the distance between the clitoris and the vagina, producing a more normal introitus.

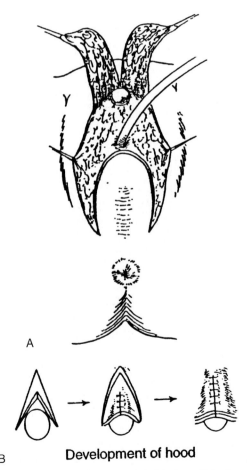

A

B

Development of hood

FIG. 109–6. The dorsal preputial skin is split in the midline and reconfigured to create a clitoral hood.

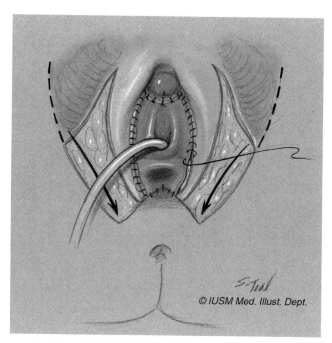

FIG. 109–7. The dorsal preputial skin flaps are mobilized laterally and advanced toward the vagina. There, they are sewn to the lateral edge of the urethral plate as a labial flap. The labial–scrotal folds are then sewn to the lateral edge of the labia minora to form labia majora.

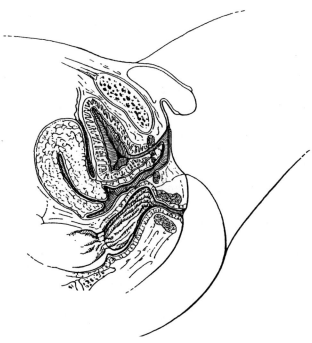

FIG. 109–8. This illustration demonstrates a low-confluence urogenital sinus with a short common urogenital sinus channel draining the urinary bladder and vagina.

end for a few millimeters to develop a flap that is used for the clitoral hood. The two long sides of the shaft skin are folded to form long thin vertical two-sided flaps that will form the labia minora. The horizontal central flap is folded under itself to form a two-sided hood for the clitoris. The clitoral hood is sewn to the base of the dorsal aspect of the clitoris and around each side to the approximate 3- and 9-o'clock positions. Each of the three flaps is sewn into shape using 5-0 absorbable sutures.

The labia minora are created with the two lateral strips of shaft skin. They are dissected on their pedicles to allow them to extend to the vagina or midperineum (Fig. 109–7). They are then sewn to the lateral aspect of the urethral plate, which now lies in the midline between the vagina and clitoris. A three-way stitch is used to fasten the labia minora to the introitus and narrow their base so that they maintain their character and their base does not spread and flatten (Fig. 109–8). The labioscrotal folds are then sewn to the labia minora to form the labia majora. All sutures are absorbable 4-0 and 5-0 and while some suture lines can be a running 5-0 any point of potential tension such as corners should be fixed with an interrupted 4-0 skin suture.

Low-Confluence UG Sinus

The goal of UG sinus reconstruction is to create separate functional openings for the urinary and genital tracts. The low-confluence UG sinus has a long urethra and vagina that join near the perineal surface, resulting in a short common channel or sinus (Fig. 109–9). There are two good options for managing these anomalies. John Lattimer introduced the posterior flap vaginoplasty in 1964 and it is still a useful technique.

A U-shaped incision is made in the perineum with the open end facing caudally and the proximal point at the orifice of the UG sinus. This incision isolates a posteriorly based skin flap (Fig. 109–10). This flap was originally designed to be wide based but it needs to be no wider than half of the circumference of the proposed vagina (a 1- to 1.5-cm flap in infants). The excellent blood supply of the tissue allows a narrower flap, which results in a more normally functional and cosmetic introitus.

Once the skin flap is isolated it is mobilized from the deeper tissue and folded back to expose the caudal wall of the UG sinus (Fig. 109–11). A fine-tipped hemostat can be placed in the orifice and the sinus split using electrocautery in the midline to the level that exposes the confluence of the sinus vagina and urethra. The vagina is split further and as deep as the apex of the poster skin flap will reach. With a catheter in the urethra the posterior skin flap is sewn in position starting at the apex and using interrupted absorbable 4-0 sutures. This advancement of the flap into the sinus and vagina both widens the introitus and the vagina and reorients the vagina into a more

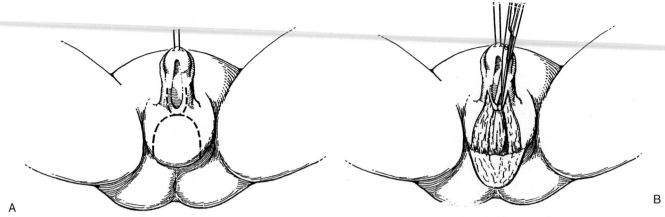

FIG. 109–9. Inverted U incision produces a posterior-based perineal skin flap used to reconstruct the posterior wall of the vagina.

vertical position, improving passive drainage (Fig. 109–12).

The other option for the low UG sinus is a limited total urogenital mobilization (TUM) technique as described originally by Pena (8). This is a relatively simple technique and is initiated by a circumferential incision around the UG sinus orifice (Fig. 109–13). This dissection is continued around the sinus while providing constant traction on the sinus with multiple stay sutures. The entire sinus vagina and urethra can then be mobilized caudally, delivering the confluence of the urethra, vagina, and sinus to the level of the perineal skin (Fig. 109–14). Pena originally described this technique for use in cloacal reconstruction and stressed that the dissection must extend

high in the pelvis but this is not always necessary in the low-confluence UG sinus. The dissection can be considered complete when the confluence is at the level of the perineum.

If the vagina and urethra reach the appropriate level and are wide enough to be functional then the distal UG sinus can be amputated and discarded. If the vagina is too narrow the posterior wall of the vagina can be split and a posteriorly based perineal skin flap can be inserted to widen it.

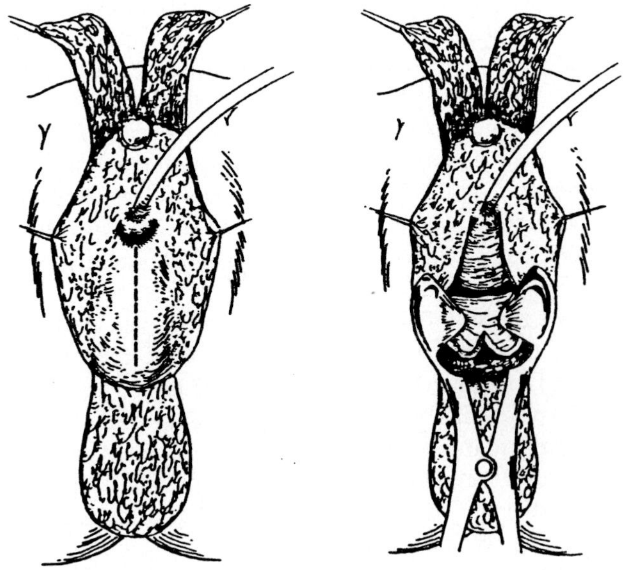

High-Confluence UG Sinus

The high-confluence UG sinus with a short urethra and vagina and a long common UG sinus channel is much more of a challenge to reconstruct because of the position of the confluence high within the pelvis and the relative lack of suitable tissue for reconstruction. In this condition the urethra and vagina are short and tethered far from the introitus by soft-tissue attachments within the pelvis.

Early attempts to repair these children were made using the techniques that were more suitable for low-confluence variants and this fact may explain many of the poor surgical results now apparent in older patients. Pena's TUM is a perineal-based approach that is based on circumferential dissection of the UG sinus, vagina, and urethra and advancement of these structures toward the perineal surface. This approach leaves the child with a urethra of normal length by lowering the bladder and vagina in the pelvis. The TUM also lowers the proximal vagina and uterus in the pelvis, allowing the vagina to be reconstructed with less outside tissue. The TUM has become an important tool in the reconstruction of children with UG sinus, in particular those with a high confluence.

The initial circumferential dissection around the UG sinus is performed just as with the lower-confluence variant. Multiple stay sutures are placed and the dissection

FIG. 109–10. The caudal portion of the urogenital sinus is exposed by deflecting the perineal skin flap inferiorly. The sinus can then be mobilized intact or split in the midline ventrally to the level of the vagina in very low-confluence cases.

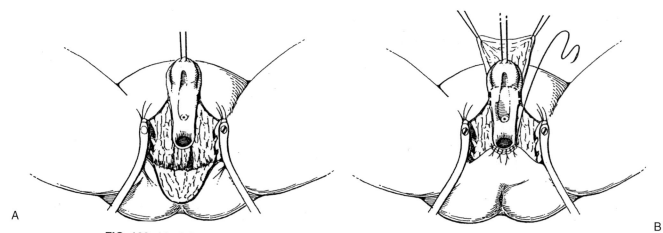

FIG. 109–11. Advancement of the perineal skin flap widens the posterior wall of the introitus and reorients the vagina in a more vertical plane.

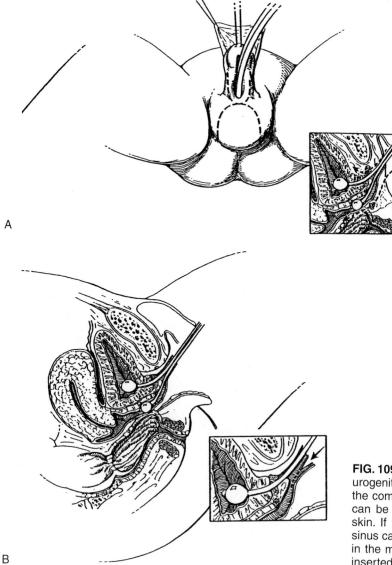

FIG. 109–12. Total urogenital sinus mobilization (TUM) for the urogenital sinus begins by circumferential dissection around the common channel. With cranial dissection the entire sinus can be mobilized and delivered to the level of the perineal skin. If the vagina reaches the perineum easily the excess sinus can be amputated. If the vagina is narrow it can be split in the midline posteriorly and the posterior perineal skin flap inserted as part of the posterior vaginal wall.

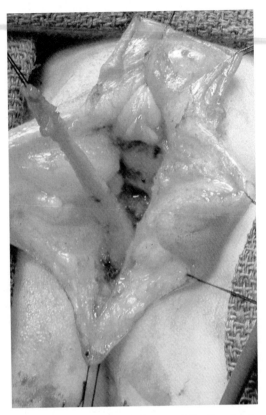

FIG. 109–13. Total urogenital sinus mobilization for the high urogenital (UG) sinus requires a more extensive circumferential cranial dissection that takes down all the attachments to the pubic bone.

can be performed in the lithotomy position. Unlike the lower-confluence UG sinus those who have a high confluence need much more extensive dissection to allow the vagina to come close enough to the perineum for satisfactory reconstruction. The dissection usually must reach the level of the pubis both anterior and posterior to the UG.

If the vagina and urethra reach the appropriate level and are wide enough to be functional then the distal UG sinus can be amputated and discarded. This is usually not the case, however, and the distal vagina is usually too narrow. In this case the vagina can be divided from the sinus and dissected away from the urethra and bladder and split in the midline dorsally. The mobilized sinus can also then be split in the midline dorsally and the sinus can be folded back on itself ventrally and advanced into the vagina as a flap to widen the vagina. If the vagina is still too narrow the posterior vaginal wall can be split as well and a posteriorly based perineal skin flap can be inserted. The TUM has allowed UG sinus reconstruction and minimized the need to perform the difficult dissection between bladder and vagina.

We prefer to approach the child with high UG sinus as an individual who may need various techniques for successful repair. The options are TUM, mobilization of the vagina from the urethra/bladder, and various flaps to augment the vagina from either the UG sinus tissue or perineal skin. The less severe cases may only need TUM and a posterior skin flap while the most severe cases need all techniques to have a successful outcome.

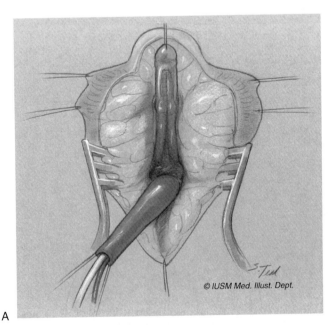
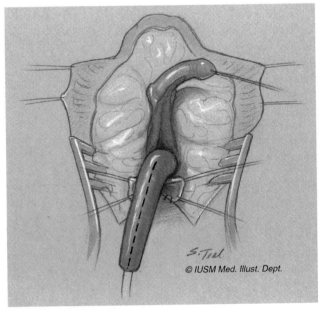

A   B

FIG. 109–14. If the vagina does not reach the introitus easily additional length can be obtained by splitting the urogenital sinus wall dorsally and folding the sinus mucosa back onto itself and inserting it as part of the anterior vaginal wall.

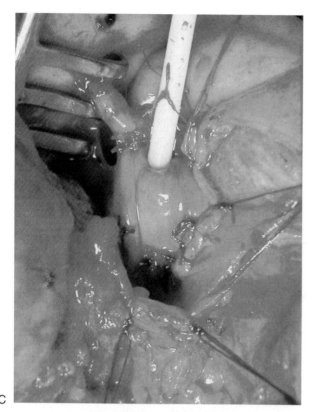

C

FIG. 109–14. (*Continued*)

OUTCOMES

Complications

The most common complication of genitoplasty is bleeding, both immediate and delayed. The tissue is very vascular and the use of injected dilute epinephrine during the procedure may be helpful. Late bleeding may originate from the corpora cavernosa or vaginal wall and can usually be controlled with pressure dressing. Pressure dressing must be carefully applied because it is possible to cause vascular compromise of the glans clitoris in the immediate postsurgical period.

The neurovascular pedicle of the glans clitoris can be injured during the original dissection. This potential injury is minimized by leaving the entire dorsal fascia, including the bundles, intact during and after dissection. Infections in the urine or wound are also possible but uncommon. It is not unusual to find a small dehiscence of the wound at the posterior apex of the labial incisions due to tension from movement. These heal without surgical intervention. They can be bathed normally and dressed with antibiotic ointment. The skin stress in this area is the prime reason to close with longer-lasting absorbable sutures.

Results

At this time surgical results are consistently good in terms of appearance and potential for function. There is, however, little long-term outcome data for feminizing genitoplasty and the studies that have been done are, by necessity, evaluating the surgical technique that was in fashion 25 years ago. The techniques have improved and while we can see superior cosmetic and functional results in young children and adolescents treated more recently we still need to observe and evaluate these patients as they mature.

The question of gender assignment is one of great importance and intense study at this time. While it is necessary to learn from our patients we must learn from all of them and not focus on only those who have been dissatisfied with their treatment. We now know that gender identity is much more complex than to be dependent on genital appearance and gender roles. While we must continuously reevaluate our management of these difficult problems we should not lose faith in the ability of surgery to create urogenital structures that can function normally and have an appearance consistent with the classic norm of the human body. Feminizing genitoplasty, like all surgery, has demonstrated that the most difficult question remains the choice of the correct procedure for the proper patient.

REFERENCES

1. Aaronson IA. The investigation and management of the infant with ambiguous genitalia: a surgeon's perspective. *Curr Prob Pediatr* 2001; 31:168–194.
2. Fortunoff S, Lattimer JK, Edson M. Vaginoplasty technique for female pseudohermaphrodites. *Surg Gynecol Obstet* 1964;118:545.
3. Gonzalez R, Fernandes ET. Single-stage feminization genitoplasty. *J Urol* 1990;143:776–778.
4. Hendren WH, Atala A. Repair of high vagina in girls with severely masculinized anatomy from the adrenogenital syndrome. *J Pediatr Surg* 1995;30:91–94.
5. Ludwinkowski B, Oesch Hayward I, Gonzalez R. Total urogenital sinus mobilization: expanded applications. *Br J Urol Int* 1999;83:820–822.
6. Mollard P, Juskiewenski S, Sarkissian J. Cliteroplasty in intersex: a new technique. *Br J Urol* 1981;53:371–373.
7. Passerini-Glazel G. A new one-stage procedure for cliterovaginoplasty in severely masculinized female pseudohermaphrodites. *J Urol* 1989; 142:565–568.
8. Pena A. Total urogenital mobilization: an easier way to repair cloacas. *J Pediatr Surg* 1997;32:263–268.
9. Rink RC, Adams MC. Feminizing genitoplasty: State of the art. *World J Urol* 1998;16:212–218.
10. Schober JM. Long-term outcomes and changing attitudes to intersexuality. *Br J Urol Int* 1999;83:39–50.

CHAPTER 110

Circumcision

Irene M. McAleer and George W. Kaplan

Circumcision, in the United States, is probably the most commonly performed surgical procedure on men. In 1995, 64% of all newborns in the United States were circumcised (3). The incidence of circumcision in other countries is lower; for example, in Canada the circumcision rate is 48% and even lower in Europe, Asia, and South America (4).

DIAGNOSIS

No diagnostic studies are needed preoperatively. The history should rule out comorbidities or bleeding diatheses. The physical examination should rule out congenital abnormalities of the penis that mitigate against circumcision.

INDICATIONS FOR SURGERY

Circumcision may also be performed after the newborn period for the presence of diseases such as phimosis, paraphimosis, balanoposthitis, or condylomata. It may be performed in the neonatal period, infancy, or childhood for cultural or religious reasons. Although there are medical benefits that accrue to the male circumcised in infancy—reduction in the incidence of urinary infections (9), reduction in the incidence of sexually transmitted disease (6), marked reduction in the incidence of penile carcinoma (7)—these benefits are at least in part outweighed by the risks of the procedure: bleeding, infection, and poor outcome (2).

The American Academy of Pediatrics, after careful review of the extant medical literature, has concluded that there are benefits to be had from neonatal circumcision but these are not so compelling as to warrant universal routine circumcision (3). Conversely, there are some opponents who feel that neonatal circumcision is never warranted (8).

Because circumcision is so common, there are a number of misguided ideas and practices that have crept into American medical practice and these sometimes lead to circumcision for reasons that are not completely medically sound. At birth the prepuce, in over 90% of infants, is fused to the glans and is not retractable. Over the first several years of life the prepuce and the glans gradually separate from each other so that the prepuce becomes retractable. It may not be fully retractable until puberty and still may fall within the limits of normalcy. In the normal process of separation, cystic spaces that become filled with smegma form (1,5). It is not necessary for parents or physicians to retract the prepuce so that retractability occurs. Forcible retraction of the prepuce causes the child pain and can produce paraphimosis, often necessitating a dorsal slit. The encysted smegma eventually becomes spontaneously discharged from under the prepuce and does not need to be removed. These collections of smegma on occasion become infected and produce a balanoposthitis, which will then resolve by spontaneous discharge of purulent material from the preputial sac. Such episodes are not a mandatory indication for circumcision as the prepuce in that area of the penis is now permanently separated from the glans and should not produce recurrences of balanoposthitis.

ALTERNATIVE THERAPY

Alternatives include observation, medical management of the balanoposthitis, and dorsal slit. One problem that is related to circumcision, in that it often leads to the need for circumcision, is paraphimosis. This occurs when the prepuce is retracted behind the glans penis and, because the preputial orifice is tight, becomes trapped in this position. There is then swelling of the glans that prevents its reduction. Untreated paraphimosis can lead to infection and tissue loss. The edema can often be reduced by injecting hyaluronidase into the edematous tissue, thereby allowing for easier reduction of the paraphimosis. Another way to effect resolution of the edema is to place

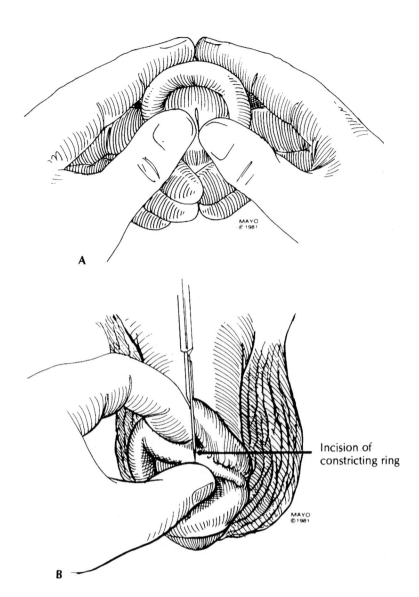

FIG. 110–1. A. A manual reduction of paraphimosis. **B.** Dorsal slit.

granulated sugar over the edematous tissue so the osmotic gradient pulls fluid out. The paraphimosis is reduced by grasping the penis between the second and third fingers of both hands and pulling the shaft skin distally while simultaneously applying cephalad pressure with both thumbs (Fig. 110–1). If this maneuver is unsuccessful, a dorsal slit is necessary to open the phimotic constriction ring. After the inflammation and edema have subsided circumcision can be performed as a secondary procedure. It is inadvisable to perform urgent circumcision at the time the paraphimosis is reduced as the marked edema that is present leads to an unsatisfactory long-term result.

SURGICAL TECHNIQUE

Circumcision, whether in an infant or an adult, has certain basic principles and goals. The goal of the operation is to remove an adequate amount of the prepuce such that the glans is exposed and balanoposthitis, phimosis, and paraphimosis are prevented. Neither too much nor too little skin should be removed as the former can tether the penis and on occasion produce chordee while the latter may produce problems with phimosis or paraphimosis. These goals should be achievable in most instances while observing asepsis, achieving hemostasis, and simultaneously protecting the glans so that it is not injured.

Outside the newborn period anesthesia in children is best accomplished with a general anesthetic. In adolescents and adults either local or general anesthesia can be used depending on the preference of the patient and surgeon.

After the penis is cleansed and draped, it is helpful to mark the area of the coronal ridge (as seen through the shaft skin) in ink to identify the incision circumferentially about the shaft skin. The prepuce should be retracted and all adhesions between the glans and the inner preputial epithelium should be lysed bluntly. If phimosis prevents the retraction of the glans a dorsal slit may be necessary as a preliminary maneuver. To perform a dorsal slit it is helpful to place one blade of a straight clamp inside the preputial sac in the dorsal midline (ensuring that the blade is not within the urethral meatus) while the other blade is placed on the outer skin. The clamp is closed and left in place for a few minutes to crush tissue and produce temporary hemostasis, after which the crushed area is incised with scissors. In the adult or older child it may be helpful to mark the proposed line of incision in the inner preputial sac with ink. This should be 3 to 4 mL below the coronal sulcus.

A common method of excising the prepuce at this point is performed by incising the two previously marked lines of incision circumferentially about the penis and dividing the tissue between the layers. Hemostasis is secured in general with cautery although vessels can be individually ligated. Previous teaching had been that use of electrocautery on the penis was hazardous but experience with modern electrosurgical units has shown conclusively that this is not a valid concern. The skin and the inner preputial epithelium are then coapted with fine absorbable sutures (Fig. 110–2).

An alternative (and older) method is accomplished by putting the prepuce on stretch by applying a hemostat to the dorsal and ventral aspects of the preputial orifice The area of the shaft skin previously marked as overlying the coronal ridge is pulled forward beyond the tip of the glans and a straight clamp is applied, taking care to ensure that the glans is not included in the clamp. The prepuce distal to the clamp is amputated with a knife, the clamp is removed, hemostasis is secured, and the skin edges are coapted.

Neonatal Circumcision

In newborns, it was customary in the past to perform circumcision without anesthesia. However, current studies suggest that infants do experience pain and techniques are now available to safely provide anesthesia to newborn infants just as in older children and adults. Local anesthesia is best provided using a local anesthetic such as lidocaine or bupivacaine as a dorsal penile block or as a ring block at the base of the penis. The anesthetic dose must be adjusted for the weight of the patient.

In newborns, circumcision is in general accomplished using some type of device. The goals and principles involved are the same as in the above-described methods. The common devices in use in the United States are the Gomco clamp, the Plastibell, and the Mogen clamp. The

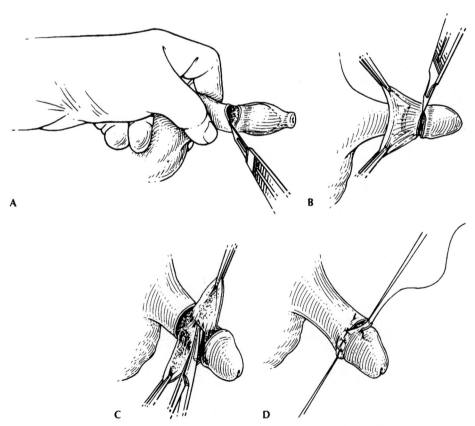

FIG. 110–2. A. An incision is made on the shaft. **B.** A second incision is made below the coronal sulcus. **C.** The skin between the incisions is excised. **D.** The wound edges are coapted.

methodology for the Gomco clamp and Plastibell is similar. After local anesthesia has been provided, and the skin cleansed, the area of the coronal ridge is marked as described above. A dorsal slit is then made. The Gomco device has three parts—a bell (available in varying sizes) that fits over the glans, a plate, and a screw to complete the assembly. After the dorsal slit is performed and the bell has been placed over the glans, it is helpful to place a safety pin through the distal corners of the prepuce to keep them aligned. The plate is now placed over the glans and the shaft skin pulled up until the marked area can be seen emerging from the hole in the plate. The screw is then placed and tightened. The device is left *in situ* for several minutes and the prepuce distal to the plate is the excised with a knife. It is imperative that electrocautery not be applied to the Gomco device as this can result in total necrosis of the penis. The device is then removed in the reverse order from which it was applied. The screw is

loosened such that the plate can be disengaged from the bell and removed. The cut edges of the penile skin are then gently teased over the edge of the bell so that it can be removed. In general, there is no need for sutures as hemostasis is complete and the edges are coapted (Fig. 110–3).

The Plastibell follows the same principles as the Gomco device. After the bell is applied, a heavy string is tied over a groove at the base of the bell at the level of the previously marked area on the shaft. The distal prepuce is then excised. The distal part of the bell is snapped off, leaving a plastic ring under the inner preputial epithelium. In roughly 1 week the skin distal to the ligature sloughs and the ring comes off spontaneously.

The Mogen clamp is a clothespin-like device and the methodology of its application is akin to one of the open surgical methods described above. After the skin is cleansed and the area of the coronal ridge as seen through

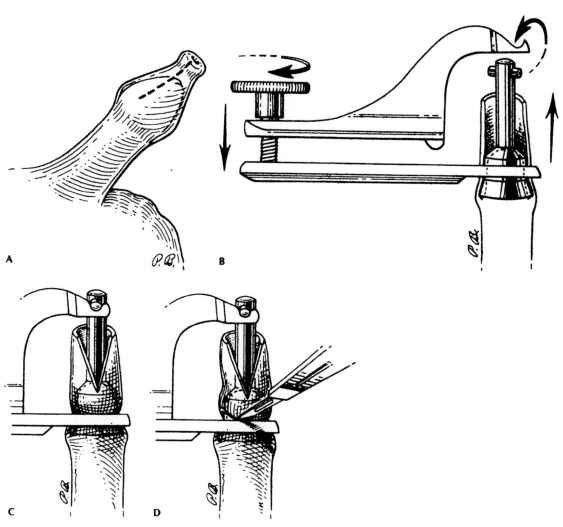

FIG. 110–3. Gomco circumcision. **A.** Line of incision for dorsal slit. **B,C.** Application of the device. **D.** Excision of the prepuce.

the shaft skin marked with ink, the adhesions between the glans and the inner prepuce are lysed with a blunt probe. It is usually not necessary to perform a dorsal slit when using the Mogen clamp. The prepuce is pulled distally and the clamp applied, taking care to ensure that the glans is not included in the clamp. The clamp is closed and left *in situ* for a few moments. The prepuce distal to the clamp is excised and the clamp is removed.

OUTCOMES

Complications

As is true with any operation, there are certain complications that are inherent risks. Bleeding is the most frequent and occurs in approximately 0.1% of cases. Most episodes of bleeding are minor and respond to pressure alone. Some are more persistent and require cautery or suture for control. Infection is the next most frequent complication seen. Such infections are in general minor and superficial; they manifest by redness and purulence at the circumcision site that in general responds to local wound care. Serious complications, which fortunately are rare, include recurrent phimosis, wound separation, major tissue loss, concealed penis, skin bridges between the shaft and the glans, inclusion cysts, urethrocutaneous fistula, and loss of some of the glans or, extremely rarely, all of the penis.

Results

A circumcision should remove a sufficient amount of the prepuce so that the glans is exposed, thereby significantly reducing the risk of developing phimosis, paraphimosis, or balanoposthitis. This is the result achieved in almost all instances but complications do occur in a small number of cases and can rarely portend a bad result.

REFERENCES

1. Gairdner D. Fate of the foreskin: A study of circumcision. *Br Med J* 1949;2:1433.
2. Kaplan GW. Complications of circumcision. *Urol Clin North Am* 1983;10:543.
3. Lannon CM, Bailey AGD, Fleischman AR, et al. Circumcision policy statement. *Pediatrics* 1999;103:686.
4. Leitch IO. Circumcision: A continuing enigma. *Aust Pediatr J* 1970;6:59.
5. Oster J. Further fate of the foreskin. *Arch Dis Child* 1968;43:200.
6. Parker SW, Stewart AJ, Wren MN, et al. Circumcision and sexually transmissable disease. *Med J Aust* 1983;2:228.
7. Persky L, deKernion J. Carcinoma of the penis. *CA Cancer J Clin* 1986;36:258.
8. Schoen EJ. The status of circumcision of newborns. *N Engl J Med* 1990;322:1308.
9. Wiswell TE, Hackey WE. Urinary tract infection and the uncircumcised state: An update. *Clin. Pediatr* 1993;32:130.

CHAPTER 111

Augmentation Cystoplasty in Children

Hans G. Pohl

Neuropathicity, bladder outlet obstruction, or embryological abnormalities may result in a bladder too small or too hypertonic to provide normal storage and evacuation of urine. The goal of augmentation cystoplasty in the pediatric patient is to provide a sufficiently capacious reservoir that stores urine at low pressure and as a result improves urinary continence and prevents upper urinary tract deterioration.

DIAGNOSIS

Evaluation should include imaging of the upper tracts, urodynamic evaluation and evaluation of the bladder outlet, and urine culture (9). In the child with no prior history of bowel resection or gastrointestinal comorbidity, it is in general not necessary to evaluate the intestinal tract. However, radiological imaging is essential in patients with intestinal atresia, intestinal malrotation, and imperforate anus because it is likely that anatomic abnormalities or prior surgical intervention would obviate the use of specific bowel segments.

INDICATIONS FOR SURGERY

The majority of pediatric patients requiring augmentation cystoplasty have small-capacity, noncompliant, or hypertonic bladders as a result of neuropathicity, from myelodysplasia or traumatic spinal cord injury, or myogenic failure, from posterior urethral valves. On occasion, augmentation cystoplasty is required to provide adequate bladder volume in cases of classic exstrophy, cloacal exstrophy, and cloacal malformations. Bladder dysfunction should initially be treated with anticholinergic medications and clean intermittent catheterization

(CIC) in an effort to diminish neurogenic detrusor overactivity, improve compliance, and provide regular and effective bladder emptying. When urodynamic evidence exists that nonoperative measures have failed, augmentation cystoplasty is indicated. Intravesical storage pressure greater than 40 cm H_2O is the most robust indication for augmenting the bladder. Incontinence and urinary tract infections (UTIs), with or without vesicoureteral reflux, are associated symptoms that may benefit from enterocystoplasty. However, a thorough evaluation is warranted to ascertain what type of augmentation to perform and whether a secondary procedure is indicated in addition to enterocystoplasty to provide continence and/or prevent upper-tract deterioration. Because the combination of urinary infection, detrusor overactivity, and vesicoureteral reflux poses a significant risk for renal scarring, antireflux surgery should be considered at the time of augmentation cystoplasty when reflux is high grade or recurrent symptomatic urinary infection has occurred. If bladder outlet surgery is entertained in conjunction with enterocystoplasty, the incontinence procedure should be performed prior to opening the peritoneal cavity to minimize insensible fluid loss.

ALTERNATIVE THERAPY

Alternatives are either medical management or urinary diversion.

SURGICAL TECHNIQUE

Preoperative preparation must include a thorough review of the anticipated goals of the surgery with the parent(s) and patient. During this meeting, the family's ability to comply with the postoperative care of a bladder augmented with bowel must be assessed. When CIC has been performed preoperatively, the postoperative catheterization and irrigations are more readily adhered

This chapter is dedicated to W. H. Hendren, whose creative use of intestine in urologic reconstruction I have been honored to observe.

TABLE 111–1. *Types of complications following pediatric augmentation cystoplasty*

Preoperative counseling and informed consent
Bleeding (Pelvic Hematoma)
Infection (More Common After Colonic Than Ileal Anastomosis)
Small-Bowel Obstruction
Urinary Leak
Ureteral Stricture
Vesicoureteral Reflux
Bladder Calculi
Metabolic Abnormalities
Poor Somatic Growth
Hematuria–Dysuria Syndrome
Excoriation Around Stoma Site

to, reducing the incidence of urinary infections, bladder calculi, or bladder perforation. Table 111–1 outlines the most common complications of augmentation cystoplasty in the early and late postoperative periods.

There is no ideal segment of bowel for augmentation cystoplasty; each has a set of characteristics that are advantages or liabilities depending on the clinical scenario. It should be noted that none of these complications are seen following ureterocystoplasty, making it the ideal tissue for bladder augmentation. However, it is a procedure ideally performed in a patient with a severely dilated ureter that subtends a nonfunctioning kidney.

Bowel cleansing is performed prior to augmentation cystoplasty (Table 111–2).

The patient is positioned supine on the operating table. General anesthesia with endotracheal intubation is mandatory; however, if no spinal abnormality exists that contraindicates the use of an epidural catheter consideration should be given to regional anesthesia as well. The surgical field is prepared and draped from the xyphoid process inferiorly, including the genitalia. A Foley catheter is inserted urethrally. A midline incision is created beginning at the symphysis pubis and extending superiorly toward the umbilicus.

TABLE 111–2. *Commonly utilized bowel cleansing performed prior to augmentation cystoplasty*

	GoLytely®-based bowel prep	
Weight (kg)	Vol. infused every 10 min (cc)	Total vol. infused (cc)
<10	80	1,100
10–20	100	1,600
20–30	140	2,200
30–40	180	2,900
40–50	200	3,200
> 50	240	4,000

Neomycin Base 25 mg/kg × 3
Erythromycin Base 20 mg/kg × 3
Saline Enemas Until Clear

When a continent diversion is not planned, a midline cystotomy suffices to prepare the bladder for augmentation. Ureteral reimplants can be easily performed at this point (Fig. 111–1). However, when a continent catheterizable stoma is planned either a paramedian or transverse cystotomy should be considered because these incisions create bladder flaps that facilitate the creation of a long submucosal tunnel for the appendix or ileal tube. Regardless of the bladder incision created, it must be sufficiently long to open the bladder widely. If the cystotomy is too short, the augmented segment may behave as a diverticulum, thus facilitating urinary stasis and stone formation. Once the bladder has been prepared, the midline incision is carried above the umbilicus and the peritoneum is entered. Retraction at this point is provided by a Bookwalter retractor.

Ileocystoplasty

Ileum is by far the most popular segment used for bladder augmentation (Table 111–3). The segment, 20 to 25 cm long, is based on a pedicle that is supplied by branches of the superior mesenteric artery and that is sufficiently mobile to be brought into the pelvis (Fig. 111–2). On occasion, an abnormally thick, fatty, or short mesentery can limit mobility of the vascular pedicle, thus necessitating extensive division of the mesentery posteriorly. The terminal 15 to 20 cm of ileum, as measured from the ileocecal valve proximally, is spared to retain bile salt absorption, thus preventing steatorrhea and vitamin B_{12} deficiency (Fig. 111–3). The portion of ileum to be used is measured and 5-0 silk sutures used to mark the proximal and distal limits of resection. Prior to dividing the mesentery, the vascular supply to the isolated segment should be observed by transillumination and the proposed incisions in the mesentery marked. Beginning at the mesenteric border of the bowel, the mesentery is divided between pairs of fine hemostats and the vascular arcades are ligated with 5-0 silk suture ties. The bowel is then divided between atraumatic bowel clamps that have been applied at the proximal and distal limits of resection. Once the ileal segment reaches into the pelvis without tension on the vascular pedicle, no further mesenteric division is needed. An ileoileal anastomosis is performed cephalad to the isolated ileal segment and the mesenteric trap is closed. The bowel clamps are removed and a thorough lavage of the ileal segment is performed with sterile saline. The segment is folded 180 degrees and the adjoining serosal surfaces are sutured with 4-0 PGA. The antimesenteric border of the ileal segment can then be opened using scissors or the cutting current with little concern for bleeding, which usually ceases spontaneously. A second suture line is created by placing 4-0 polyglycolic acid (PGA) through the full thickness of the bowel wall in a continuous fashion. Once the ileal cap has been formed, it is anastomosed to the opened bladder

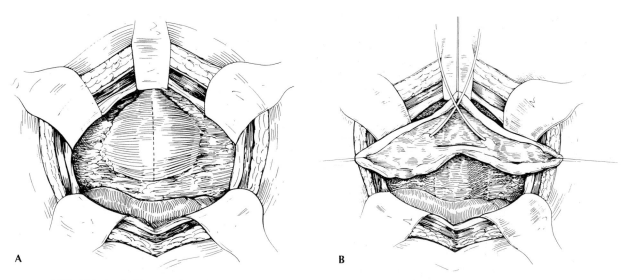

FIG. 111–1. A: Preparation of the bladder for clam augmentation enterocystoplasty. **B:** A sagittal incision is made to create two bladder flaps.

beginning at the most posterior portion of the bladder incision. Hemostatic clamps may be left on the short ends of the tied sutures to identify the most posterior limit of the anastomotic line, thus facilitating placement of the second, reinforcing suture layer between the serosal surfaces of the bladder and ileum. A suprapubic catheter is placed through the bladder wall prior to completion of the first anastomotic closure.

Right Colocystoplasty and Mainz Enterocystoplasty

Enterocystoplasty with a segment of ascending colon is based on vascular supply from the ileocolic artery (Fig. 111–2). Dissection begins at the inferior edge of the

cecum and progresses cephalad along the line of Toldt, the peritoneal reflection lateral to the right colon. At the hepatic flexure, the hepatocolic ligament must be divided. Next, the omental attachments to the colon are divided and the omentum is packed into the left upper quadrant with moist lap sponges. The ascending colon is divided at the watershed between the ileocolic and right colic arteries, approximately midway between the cecum and hepatic flexure. The ileum is divided close to the ileocecal valve. An ileocolonic anastomosis is performed and the mesenteric trap is closed. If the appendix will not be used to create a continent catheterizable stoma, an appendectomy is performed at this point. The bowel is folded 180 degrees and the serosal surfaces sutured with 4-0

TABLE 111–3. *Comparison of gastrointestinal segments in pediatric augmentation cystoplasty*

	Advantages	Disadvantages
Ileum	Most Compliant Less Mucus	Diarrhea Vitamin B_{12} Deficiency Short Mesentery Hyperchloremic Acidosis Poor Muscle Backing
Sigmoid	Readily Mobilized Easily Implanted Good Muscle Backing	Unit Contractions Lower Compliance Mucus Hyperchloremic Acidosis Perforation Risk
Ileocecal	Valve as Antireflux/Continence Mechanism Good Capacity Reservoir Constant Blood Supply	Diarrhea Not Always Available Contractile
Stomach	Short Gut/Radiation Chloride Pump Minimal Mucus Fewer Infections Ease of Implantation Good Muscle Backing	Hypochloremic Alkalosis Rhythmic Contractions Hematuria/Dysuria

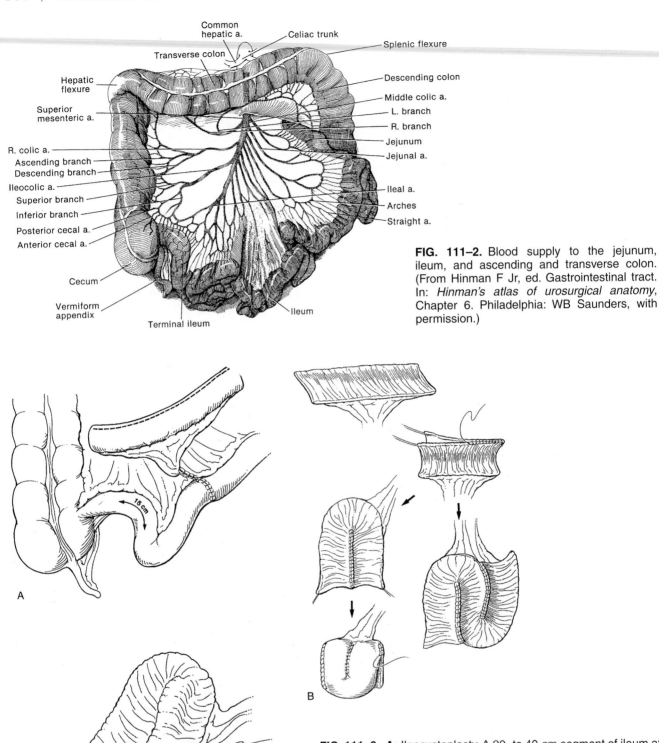

FIG. 111–2. Blood supply to the jejunum, ileum, and ascending and transverse colon. (From Hinman F Jr, ed. Gastrointestinal tract. In: *Hinman's atlas of urosurgical anatomy*, Chapter 6. Philadelphia: WB Saunders, with permission.)

FIG. 111–3. A: Ileocystoplasty. A 20- to 40-cm segment of ileum at least 15 cm from the ileocecal valve is removed and opened on its antimesenteric border. Ileoileostomy reconstitutes the bowel. **B:** The opened ileal segment should be reconfigured. This can be done in a U, S, or W configuration. It can be furthered folded as a cup patch. **C:** The reconfigured ileal segment is anastomosed widely to the native bladder. (From Adams MC, Joseph DB. Urinary tract reconstruction in children. In: Walsh et al., eds. *Campbell's urologic surgery*, 8th ed. Chapter 71. Philadelphia: WB Saunders, with permission.)

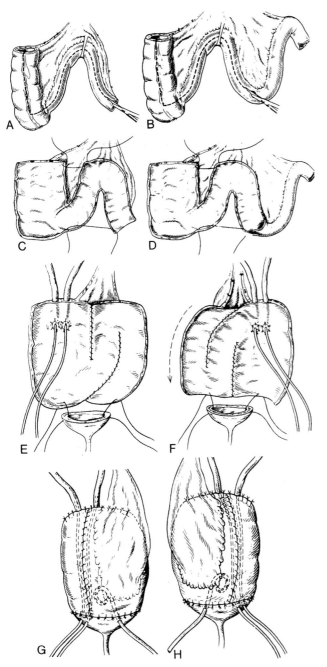

FIG. 111–4. The Mainz ileocecocystoplasty. **A, B:** The ileal segment is twice the length as the cecal segment. **C, D:** It is opened on the antimesenteric border. **E, F:** The ureters can be opened into the opened cecal segment if necessary. **G, H:** The ileocecal segment is anastomosed to the native bladder. (From Thuroff JW, et al. The Mainz Pouch. In: King LR, et al., eds. *Bladder reconstruction and continent urinary diversion.* Chicago: Year Book, 1987, with permission.)

PGA. The bowel is incised along its antimesenteric border and the edges are sutured full thickness with 4-0 PGA placed in a continuous fashion. The resulting colonic plate is folded once again. This time the full-thickness suture line is placed first and reinforced with a second

continuous line of 4-0 PGA. The resulting cup is inverted and anastomosed to the bladder opening as described for the ileocystoplasty. An alternative approach that has gained wide popularity is the Mainz augmentation, in which 15 to 30 cm of terminal ileum are isolated in continuity with the right colon and detubularized, anastomosed to each other, and sutured to the cystotomy (Fig. 111–4).

Sigmoidocystoplasty

Because the diameter of the sigmoid is much greater than that of the ileum, a shorter segment is necessary to perform a successful augmentation cystoplasty. The isolated segment derives its blood supply from the sigmoid branches of the inferior mesenteric artery (Fig. 111–5). A mesenteric incision is created proximally and distally and bowel clamps applied to minimize fecal soiling. The sigmoid is divided and a sigmoidosigmoidostomy performed lateral to the mesentery of the isolated segment (Fig. 111–6). Two methods are available for anastomosing the bowel segment to the bladder: (a) The proximal and distal ends of the segment are closed and the bowel is opened along its antimesenteric border and sutured to the bladder opening; (b) the bowel is opened along its antimesenteric border first, then folded 180 degress into a U shape prior to suturing it to the bladder. The latter method likely disrupts the high unit contractions of the sigmoid more than the first; however, it requires that a greater length of sigmoid be isolated.

Gastrocystoplasty

The bladder may be augmented with a gastric segment derived from either the antrum or the body of the stomach. When antral gastrocystoplasty is performed, the enteric stream is reconstructed using a Billroth I anastomosis (gastroduodenostomy). This procedure is now rarely performed in children because resection of the antrum has been associated with delayed gastric emptying, gastric dumping syndrome, and feeding difficulties. Currently, most surgeons prefer the use of the stomach body instead. A segment between 10 and 20 cm is marked along the greater curvature of the stomach and drawn as a rhomboid that extends toward the lesser curvature, ending 1 cm from the edge so as not to interrupt branches of the vagus nerve. Two arterial supplies exist to the greater curvature of the stomach: (a) the right gastroepiploic artery, derived from the right gastric artery; and (b) the left gastroepiploic artery, from the splenic artery (Fig. 111–7). If the right gastroepiploic artery is chosen, the gastric segment should be obtained from higher on the greater curvature or lower if based on the left (Fig. 111–8). The gastroepiploic arteries supply the stomach with anterior and posterior branches that must be divided before the segment can be excised from the stomach.

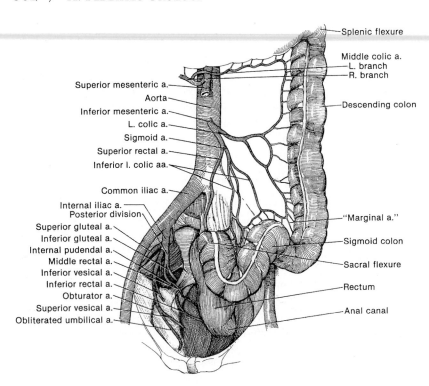

FIG. 111–5. Blood supply to the descending and sigmoid colon and rectum. (From Hinman F Jr, ed. Gastrointestinal tract. In: *Hinman's atlas of urosurgical anatomy.* Philadelphia: WB Saunders, with permission.)

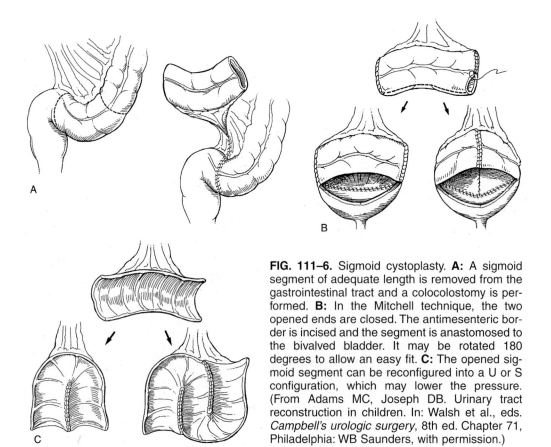

FIG. 111–6. Sigmoid cystoplasty. **A:** A sigmoid segment of adequate length is removed from the gastrointestinal tract and a colocolostomy is performed. **B:** In the Mitchell technique, the two opened ends are closed. The antimesenteric border is incised and the segment is anastomosed to the bivalved bladder. It may be rotated 180 degrees to allow an easy fit. **C:** The opened sigmoid segment can be reconfigured into a U or S configuration, which may lower the pressure. (From Adams MC, Joseph DB. Urinary tract reconstruction in children. In: Walsh et al., eds. *Campbell's urologic surgery*, 8th ed. Chapter 71, Philadelphia: WB Saunders, with permission.)

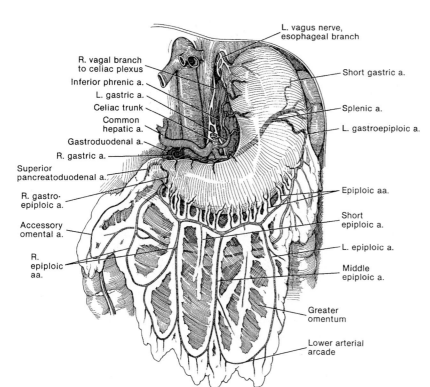

FIG. 111–7. Blood supply to the anterior aspect of the stomach and greater omentum. (From Hinman F Jr, ed. Gastrointestinal tract. In: Hinman F Jr, ed. *Hinman's atlas of urosurgical anatomy*, Chapter 6. Philadelphia: WB Saunders, with permission.)

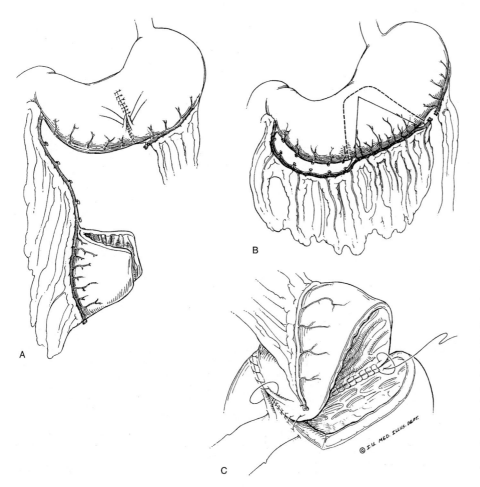

FIG. 111–8. Gastrocystoplasy using body. **A:** A gastric segment of body is mobilized on the right gastroepiploic artery. The left vessel may also be used; neither vessel as a pedicle should be free floating through the peritoneum. **B:** A longer gastric segment along the greater curvature with a wider apex provides more surface area for augmentation. **C:** The gastric segment is anastomosed to the bivalved bladder with the mucosa inverted. (From Adams MC, Joseph DB. Urinary tract reconstruction in children. In: Walsh et al., eds. *Campbell's urologic surgery*, 8th ed. Chapter 71, with permission.)

Atraumatic intestinal clamps are applied in parallel at the proposed incision sites on the stomach. Alternatively, an intestinal stapling device can be used to divide the stomach; however, the staples must be removed later. The vascular pedicle must be retroperitonealized to prevent internal hernia formation. A window is created in the transverse mesocolon that accepts the gastric augment and its vascular pedicle. The segment is passed posterior to the mesocolon and exits a second window that has been created in the small-bowel mesentery inferiorly. If the vascular pedicle is too short, additional branches between the gastroepiploic artery and the stomach must be divided. The stomach is sutured to the bladder beginning along the posterior aspect of the cystotomy.

Ureterocystoplasty

Unlike enterocystoplasty, ureterocystoplasty does not require a midline transperitoneal incision. The entire procedure can be performed retroperitoneally through a flank incision, to perform the nephrectomy and harvest the proximal portion of the ureter, and a Pfannenstiel incision, through which the augmentation is performed. Only a midline incision should be considered when two functioning kidneys exist because a transureteroureterostomy will be required to reestablish continuity of the upper urinary tract after distal ureter has been harvested (Fig. 111–9). Following the nephrectomy, careful mobilization of the ureter from its retroperitoneal location includes dissection of all surrounding adventitia away from the peritoneal lining toward the ureter itself. The ureter is then passed into the pelvis. A midline cystotomy is created such that the posterior portion of the incision includes the ureterovesical junction. The ureter, too, is incised along its anterior aspect. A spherical reservoir can be created by folding the proximal end of the ureter toward the cystotomy in an inverted U and suturing the adjoining edges of the ureter to itself. The remainder of the anastomosis between the ureter and the bladder is performed as in enterocystoplasty, beginning at the posterior aspect of the cystotomy and proceeding in an anterior fashion. Drainage tubes are placed through the native bladder muscle tissue.

Urinary and Abdominal Drainage Following Augmentation Cystoplasty

If an incontinence procedure has not been performed, an appropriately sized urethral Foley catheter is used. However, because the retention balloon can cause pressure necrosis of the bladder neck following incontinence procedures, some surgeons would instead use a Rob-Nel

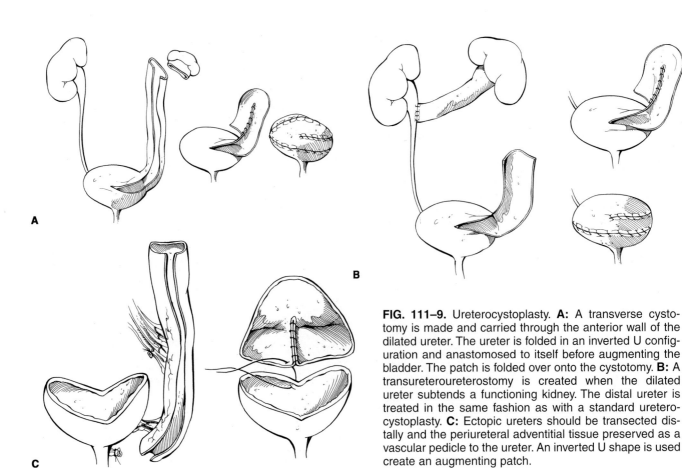

FIG. 111–9. Ureterocystoplasty. **A:** A transverse cystotomy is made and carried through the anterior wall of the dilated ureter. The ureter is folded in an inverted U configuration and anastomosed to itself before augmenting the bladder. The patch is folded over onto the cystotomy. **B:** A transureteroureterostomy is created when the dilated ureter subtends a functioning kidney. The distal ureter is treated in the same fashion as with a standard ureterocystoplasty. **C:** Ectopic ureters should be transected distally and the periureteral adventitial tissue preserved as a vascular pedicle to the ureter. An inverted U shape is used create an augmenting patch.

catheter or silastic feeding tube that may be secured with 3-0 silk sutures passed through the bladder and abdominal wall and tied over a cotton bolster. In addition, a suprapubic Malecot catheter should be placed through a separate incision in the native bladder and brought out through the anterior abdominal wall. It is advised that this tube in particular be secured with 3-0 nylon sutures because it will remain until after a cystogram has demonstrated a healed anastomosis and the patient is successfully catheterizing the reconstructed bladder, 4 weeks at the least. Irrigation with sterile saline should be instituted on postoperative day 3 in an effort to cleanse the newly augmented bladder free of the often copious amounts of mucus that the enteric segments produce. Jackson–Pratt closed-system vacuum drains are employed briefly following surgery and removed when minimal peritoneal drainage exists. In patients with ventriculoperitoneal shunts, cerebrospinal fluid can be confused for persistent peritoneal drainage. In particular in these patients, the surgeon should resist the temptation to maintain these drains for an extended period of time.

OUTCOMES

Complications

The two most likely gastrointestinal complications following augmentation cystoplasty in children are diarrhea and vitamin B_{12} deficiency (each in up to 23%). Diarrhea is most often found following the use of the ileocecal valve. Vitamin B_{12} deficiency can be avoided by limiting the length of small bowel harvested and in particular by preserving the terminal 20 cm of ileum, the major site of B_{12} absorption.

Despite the incorporation of intestine into the urinary tract, its absorptive and secretory capacity is retained: Chloride, ammonium, hydrogen ions, and organic acids are readily absorbed and bicarbonate ions are secreted into the urine. The resultant hyperchloremic metabolic acidosis is driven by the absorption of ammonium ions, which are followed by chloride in an attempt to maintain electroneutrality. The amount of bowel used, length of time that bowel mucosa is in contact with urine, and degree of underlying renal impairment contribute to the severity of the metabolic disturbance. Acidosis is rarely seen in patients with normal renal function, and any measurable increase in serum chloride and decrease in serum bicarbonate is subtle. Mild cases of metabolic acidosis can be managed with oral sodium bicarbonate (1 to 3 mEq per kg per day), with the goal being an increase in serum bicarbonate to a value greater than 20 mEq per L. Severe acidosis requires intravenous administration of bicarbonate usually as Dextrose 5% with 0.25 normal saline and 50 mEq per L of sodium bicarbonate. Hyperchloremic metabolic acidosis is most common following sigmoidocystoplasty.

Use of jejunum is associated with a unique metabolic derangement, a hypochloremic, hyponatremic, hyperkalemic metabolic acidosis. For this reason, it is recommended that jejunum not be used in pediatric augmentation cystoplasty, especially when renal function is poor.

As a consequence of the net secretion of chloride and hydrogen ions across the gastric mucosa, augmentation with stomach results in a hypochloremic metabolic alkalosis in 3% to 24% of patients (6,10). This effect can be used to advantage in patients with renal dysfunction and acidemia, who will demonstrate decreased serum chloride and increased serum bicarbonate following gastrocystoplasty (1,8).

The immediate goal of augmentation cystoplasty should be that intravesical storage pressure decreases well below the threshold of 40 cm H_2O, thus averting progressive upper-tract deterioration. Although any gastrointestinal segment can provide a sufficiently compliant augment if it is very long and fully detubularized, most authors agree that, for a given length of bowel, ileum provides the greatest compliance of any segment (5,7,13). Of 323 patients who had undergone enterocystoplasty in one large review, 6% required an additional augmentation because of persistently elevated intravesical pressure.

Regardless of the segment chosen, persistent bacteriuria is common following augmentation cystoplasty, occurring in up to 95% of patients. Symptomatic cystitis, defined as incontinence, suprapubic pain, foul-smelling urine, and perhaps increased mucus production, may be more likely when CIC is performed sporadically and incompletely or when mucus and stones serve as a nidus for colonizing bacteria. Any patient with symptoms suggestive of UTI should be considered for antimicrobial therapy irrespective of the form of augmentation performed.

The reported incidence of bladder calculi has ranged between 8% and 52% of patients following augmentation cystoplasty, yet the occurrence of bladder calculi may be more a result of poor patient compliance with CIC, colonization with urea-splitting bacteria, and the presence of mucus to serve as a nidus for the aggregation of salts (2).

Perforation is the most serious complication of augmentation enterocystoplasty and patients may present critically ill despite few localizing signs and symptoms. The condition should immediately be suspected when an augmented patient presents with fever and abdominal pain no matter how mild the symptoms: Shoulder pain secondary to diaphragmatic irritation from urine in the peritoneal cavity has also been reported. Which gastrointestinal segment carries the greatest risk of perforation is debatable. Therefore, any child is potentially at risk irrespective of the segment used. The underlying etiology for all perforations is believed to be ischemia within the bowel wall as a consequence of either overdistension from infrequent emptying or high-pressure contractions or even reconfiguration by detubularization.

Patients suspected of having bladder perforation should undergo fluid resuscitation and receive intravenous broad-spectrum antibiotics and Foley catheter drainage while the evaluation is underway. A standard cystogram may miss up to 33% of bladder perforations; therefore, computerized tomography cystograms are advocated (11). While some have successfully employed nonoperative management, surgical exploration with resection of necrotic tissue and primary closure of the defect should be performed in a gravely ill patient or when the patient fails to improve during nonoperative management (12).

Hematuria–dysuria syndrome occurs in 9% to 70% of patients who have undergone a gastrocystoplasty; it presents with perineal pain, dysuria, hematuria, and skin excoriation around either the urethral meatus or the stoma of a catheterizable channel. A recent study of 10 children with hematuria–dysuria syndrome identified a positive correlation between the presence of infecting *Helicobacter pylori*, reduced urine pH, and the presence of symptoms following gastrocystoplasty. The authors recommend evaluating all patients who are under consideration for a gastric augment for the presence of *H. pylori* and treating the infection before performing surgery (3,4). Oral therapy with histamine-2 or H+/K+ adenosine triphosphatase blockers should be helpful in symptomatic patients. If prolonged catheterization is anticipated, then bladder irrigations should be performed with a sodium bicarbonate-containing solution.

REFERENCES

1. Adams MC, Mitchell ME, Rink RC. Gastrocystoplasty: an alternative solution to the problem of urological reconstruction in the severely compromised patient. *J Urol* 1988;140:1152–1156.
2. Barroso U, Jednak R, Fleming P, Barthold JS, Gonzalez R. Bladder calculi in children who perform clean intermittent catheterization. *Br J Urol Int* 2000;85:879–984.
3. Celayir S, Goksel S, Buyukunal SN. The relationship between *Helicobacter pylori* infection and acid–hematuria syndrome in pediatric patients with gastric augmentation—II. *J Pediatr Surg* 1999;34:532–535.
4. Celayir S, Goksel S, Unal T, Buyukunal SN. *Helicobacter pylori* infection in a child with gastric augmentation. *J Pediatr Surg* 1997;32:1757–1758.
5. Hinman F Jr. Selection of intestinal segments for bladder substitution: Physical and physiological characteristics. *J Urol* 1988;139:519(abst).
6. Hollensbe DW, Adams MC, Rink RC. Comparison of different gastrointestinal segments for bladder augmentation. In: *Proceedings of the Annual Meeting of the American Urological Association*. Washington, DC, 1992(abst).
7. Koff SA. Guidelines to determine the size and shape of intestinal segments used for reconstruction. *J Urol* 1988;140:1150(abst).
8. Kurzrock EA, Baskin LS, Kogan BA. Gastrocystoplasty: long-term followup. *J Urol* 1998;160:2182–2186.
9. Lytton B, Green DF. Urodynamic studies in patients undergoing bladder replacement surgery. *J Urol* 1989;141:1394–1397.
10. Plaire JC, Snodgrass WT, Grady RW, Mitchell ME. Long-term followup of the hematuria–dysuria syndrome. *J Urol* 2000;164:921–923.
11. Pope JC, Albers P, Rink RCea. Spontaneous rupture of the augmented bladder: From silence to chaos. In: *Proceedings of the Annual Meeting of the European Society of Pediatric Urology*. Istanbul, 1999(abst).
12. Slaton JW, Kropp KA. Conservative management of suspected bladder rupture after augmentation enterocystoplasty. *J Urol* 1994;152:713–715.
13. Studer UE, Zingg EJ. Ileal orthotopic bladder substitutes. What we have learned from 12 years' experience with 200 patients. *Urol Clin North Am* 1997;24:781–793(abst).

CHAPTER 112

Mitrofanoff Procedure in Pediatric Urinary Tract Reconstruction

Mark P. Cain

The Mitrofanoff principle offered a major advancement to continent urinary reconstruction for children and young adults. Earlier innovations—including clean intermittent catheterization (CIC), bladder augmentation, and a variety of bladder neck tightening procedures—made continent bladder reconstruction possible. The technically difficult problem was creating a bladder outlet that was tight enough to ensure continence but wide enough to allow reliable catheterization over a lifetime. The concept of a continent catheterizable abdominal channel was introduced by Paul Mitrofanoff in 1980 (11) and has since been adopted as the ideal alternate urinary continence mechanism in most pediatric centers worldwide. This principle involves creation of a flap valve continence mechanism for a conduit that is tunneled into a low-pressure urinary reservoir that can then be catheterized and emptied via an abdominal stoma (Fig. 112–1).

There are multiple surgical options for creating the Mitrofanoff channel. Appendicovesicostomy has by tradition been used due to the reliable blood supply, adequate lumen for catheterization, and supple muscular wall. Long-term follow-up has shown that appendicovesicostomy provides a durable channel with minimal late complications (8,9). In the absence of a suitable appendix, or in conditions where the appendix is used for an alternate procedure [such as for a Malone antegrade continence enema (MACE channel)], there are multiple options that have been described. The most reliable alternatives have been the Monti–Yang ileovesicostomy, ureterovesicostomy, and continent bladder tube.

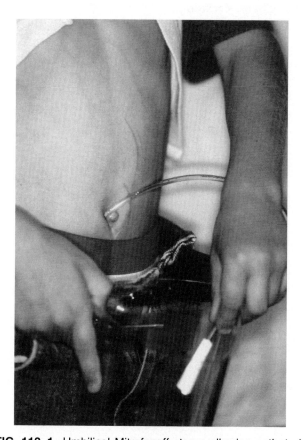

FIG. 112–1. Umbilical Mitrofanoff stoma allowing catheterization in the sitting or standing position.

DIAGNOSIS

The Mitrofanoff procedure can be performed with essentially any underlying bladder pathology. The most frequent diagnosis for children undergoing the procedure is neuropathic bladder, usually due to myelomeningocele. This procedure has also been described for reconstruction in patients with exstrophy-epispadias, cloacal anomalies, prune belly syndrome, posterior urethral valves, and other conditions. Although many of these children will require a bladder outlet procedure to provide urinary continence, some will have an intact and continent bladder outlet and the Mitrofanoff channel will provide an alternate to urethral catheterization. This is especially useful in wheelchair-bound patients who cannot access their perineum independently and also in patients with normal urethral sensation where catheterization can be traumatic both physically and psychologically.

INDICATIONS FOR SURGERY

In the past, the primary indication for bladder reconstruction was for upper urinary tract preservation. In the era of aggressive use of anticholinergics and intermittent catheterization in young patients, the more common indication for a Mitrofanoff channel is for urinary continence and convenient, independent bladder management for the patient. All patients should undergo a trial of CIC to demonstrate that they are reliable and able to comply with a daily routine prior to bladder reconstruction.

ALTERNATIVE THERAPY

The most common alternative to continent bladder reconstruction with a Mitrofanoff stoma is anticholinergic therapy with clean intermittent urethral catheterization. With careful attention to catheterization schedules and fluid intake, social dryness can be achieved in many patients with neuropathic bladder and other underlying bladder pathology.

Less frequently used alternatives are long-term incontinent vesicostomy and conduit urinary diversion. Although these are both considered suboptimal in the era of continent urinary reconstruction, there will be a subset of patients who are unable to care for themselves because of physical, mental, or psychosocial problems, and the

incontinent diversion provides a safer long-term option for these patients.

In the rare patient with a completely nonusable bladder, a continent urinary reservoir with a continent catheterizable channel is another alternative.

SURGICAL TECHNIQUE

All patients are admitted the day before surgery for intravenous antibiotics to sterilize the urinary tract and for a mechanical and antibiotic bowel preparation. This is in particular important for patients with ventriculoperitoneal shunts, who have a risk of shunt infection. Potential sites for stomal location should be determined preoperatively, with the patient in the sitting and supine position.

Surgical exposure is usually obtained through a midline transabdominal incision that is carried around the umbilicus to leave enough fascia to close the abdomen without compromising an umbilical stoma. A lower transverse Pfannenstiel incision will also allow adequate exposure for both bladder augmentation and the Mitrofanoff stoma in thin patients. Laparoscopic mobilization of the right colon and isolation of the appendix has been described, which allows a smaller lower-abdominal incision without the concern of inadequate exposure.

Appendicovesicostomy

The right colon is mobilized beyond the hepatic flexure to allow maximal freedom of the appendiceal mesentery. If the appendix is retrocecal in location it is mobilized carefully from the cecal attachments with extra caution to avoid injuring the appendiceal artery, which is a branch of the ileocolic artery (Fig. 112–2). In some

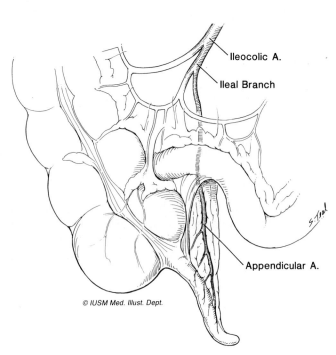

Ileocolic A.

Ileal Branch

Appendicular A.

© IUSM Med. Illust. Dept.

FIG. 112–2. Vascular anatomy of appendicular artery.

cases there is significant inflammation due to the presence of a ventriculoperitoneal shunt, and the peritoneal incision must be carried medially to adequately mobilize the appendix. When the length of appendix is inadequate, it can be extended by incorporating a segment of distal cecum as described by Cromie et al. (5). Prior to detaching the appendix, the bladder is mobilized to ensure that the bladder and appendix can easily reach the chosen site for the abdominal stoma without tension. The bladder is then opened to the left of the midline for a right lower-quadrant appendicovesicostomy or in a wide U-shaped anterior bladder incision for an umbilical stoma. The appendix is detached from the cecum either sharply or with a stapling device, and the cecum is closed with absorbable and permanent sutures. The mesentery to the appendiceal artery can be freed from the cecal mesentery to allow complete mobilization of the appendix if needed (Fig. 112–3). The terminal end of the appendix is then opened, and a 12 Fr catheter is passed to ensure that the appendix has an adequate lumen. If necessary the appendix can be gently dilated with serial sounds. If bladder augmentation is to be performed, the segment of bowel is isolated, harvested, and reconfigured appropriately. If an additional segment of intestine is required for the Mitrofanoff (e.g., Monti–Yang) channel it can be harvested simultaneously. The site of the bladder hiatus is then selected, again ensuring that it can easily reach the posterior abdominal wall fascia without tension. The site of the hiatus is opened wide enough to allow the appendix to pass without any tension and a vessel loop is passed through the hiatus for traction. A submucosal bladder tunnel is then created using sharp dissection. Placing sev-

eral traction sutures on the bladder to flatten out the posterior bladder wall facilitates this dissection. The orientation of the tunnel should be directed away from the bladder outlet and trigone to prevent painful catheterization postoperatively. The tunnel length should be at least 2.5 cm in length. It is sometimes helpful to inject 1:200,000 epinephrine along the path of the submucosal tunnel to facilitate the dissection and minimize bleeding. The terminal end of the appendix is then passed through the bladder hiatus and submucosal tunnel. The appendix is spatulated and secured distally with two 4-0 absorbable sutures incorporating full-thickness bites of the appendix and detrusor muscle and mucosa. The remainder of the anastomosis is completed using 4-0 or 5-0 absorbable sutures, securing the bladder mucosa to the appendix. The appendix is also secured at the level of the bladder hiatus using several 4-0 absorbable sutures. The channel is catheterized with a 12 or 14 Fr catheter to ensure that it passes easily across the hiatus and submucosal tunnel. The stomal site is then selected, taking care to ensure that the bladder hiatus can reach the posterior fascia without tension. A U-shaped (umbilical) or V-shaped skin incision is made at the stomal site, and the flap is freed sharply to the level of the fascia. A cruciate incision is made in the fascia and widened to allow passage of an index finger. The appendix is then brought through the fascial opening and the appendiceal/bladder hiatus is secured to the posterior fascial wall using 3-0 absorbable sutures, taking care to not angulate or compress the appendiceal mesentery (Fig. 112–4). This maneuver ensures a short, straight extravesical appendix channel. The cecal end of the appendix is then spatulated on the antimesenteric side, and if there is redundant appendix it is amputated. The stomal anastomosis is secured using interrupted 4-0 absorbable sutures (Fig. 112–5). The stoma is then catheterized multiple times with the bladder both distended and empty to ensure that there is no angulation in the channel. A 12 Fr catheter is left indwelling for 3 weeks before initiating intermittent catheterization.

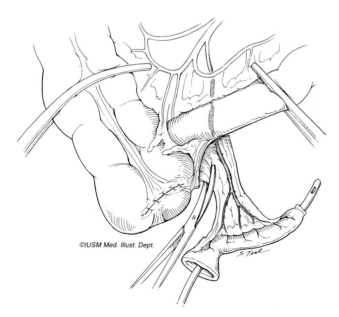

FIG. 112–3. The mesentery to the appendix can be mobilized carefully, taking care to not injure the appendicular artery.

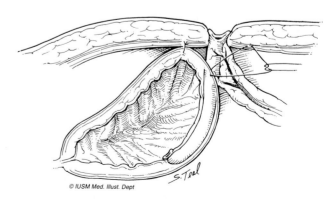

FIG. 112–4. The bladder is secured to the posterior abdominal fascia to avoid redundancy in the extravesical channel, which can be a source of late catheterization problems.

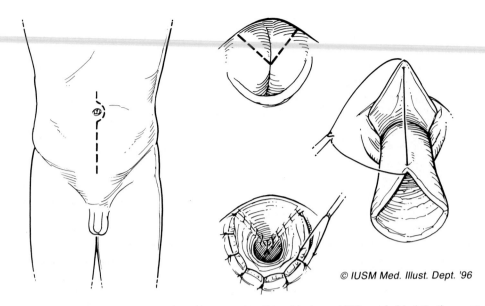

© IUSM Med. Illust. Dept. '96

FIG. 112–5. The skin stoma is completed by securing the wide-based V-flap of skin into the spatulated channel.

Monti–Yang Ileovesicostomy

The concept of retubularized ileum as a replacement for the appendicovesicostomy was introduced in 1997 (2,7,12), and has quickly become the procedure of choice for the Mitrofanoff channel. The growing indications and use of the MACE channel (10,14) has led to preservation of the appendix for the appendicocecostomy stoma and the need for alternatives for a bladder channel. Because many of the children will also undergo bladder augmentation at the time of reconstruction, the Monti–Yang channel can be easily constructed from a segment of the bowel harvested for augmentation.

A 2.5- to 3-cm segment of intestine is harvested with a well-vascularized segment of mesentery (Fig. 112–6). If ileal augmentation is planned, the Monti–Yang segment can be easily harvested from the distal end of the segment with a shared mesentery. The ileal segment is opened on the antimesenteric side (Fig. 112–7). It can be opened slightly off the midline to provide a longer segment for implanting into the bladder. The opened segment is then retubularized transversely in two layers over a 14 Fr catheter. The bowel mucosa is approximated with running 5-0 or 6-0 absorbable sutures and the muscular layer is closed with running or interrupted 4-0 absorbable sutures (Figs. 112–8A and 112–8B). The stomal end is not closed initially, providing wide spatulation of the antimesenteric side of the tube for later stomal anastomosis. The technique of implanting the tube into the bladder and creating a stoma is identical to that for appendicovesicostomy

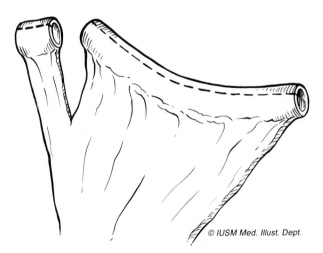

© IUSM Med. Illust. Dept.

FIG. 112–6. A 2.5- to 3-cm segment of ileum is harvested, distal to the segment of intestine to be used for augmentation (if indicated).

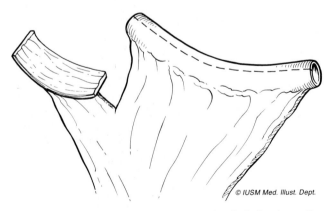

© IUSM Med. Illust. Dept.

FIG. 112–7. The Monti segment is detubularized on the antimesenteric side. This incision can be between the 9- and 12-o'clock positions depending on the desired length of intravesical tunnel.

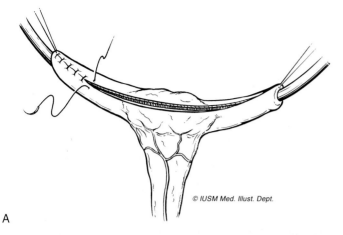

© IUSM Med. Illust. Dept.

A

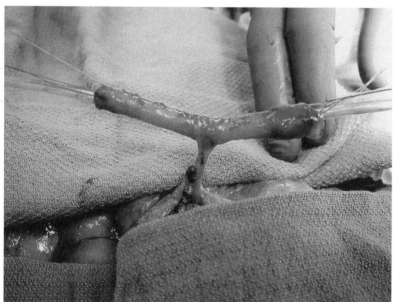

B

FIG. 112–8. **A:** The channel is closed in two layers of absorbable sutures. The stomal end is either closed with interrupted sutures or not closed to allow adequate spatulation at the skin stoma. **B:** Operative photo of completed Monti channel.

(Fig. 112–9). The Monti–Yang tube can be created out of any segment of intestine with good results. If there is inadequate bladder volume for creation of a submucosal tunnel, the tube can be implanted into a segment of bowel using an extravesical technique, but care must be taken to secure the entire tunnel length to the posterior fascia to prevent breakdown of the muscular backing of the tunnel and subsequent late incontinence. The Monti channel can also be used for the MACE channel, with two channels created side by side (Fig. 112–10). A 12 Fr catheter is left across the channel for 3 weeks before initiating intermittent catheterization.

When the Monti channel does not provide adequate length to reach the abdominal stomal site, then two Monti tubes can be reconfigured and connected (the "double Monti"). This can provide a longer limb to reach the skin stoma but also introduces additional postoperative complications of diverticulum, angulation, and perforation at the anastomosis of the two channels. To avoid this com-

plication, Casale described a long ileovesicostomy technique using a single piece of bowel to create a channel 10 to 14 cm in length (4). This technique involves a 3.5- to 4-cm segment of bowel that is isolated on its mesentery and divided into two equal segments for approximately 80% of the bowel circumference, leaving the two segments attached on the antimesenteric side. The two loops of intestine are opened close to the mesentery on opposite sides, allowing the bowel to unfold in opposite directions, creating a long flat plate of intestine that can be retubularized after trimming the redundant lateral edges.

Continent Vesicostomy

Small subsets of patients only require creation of a catheterizable bladder channel without bladder augmentation or other intraabdominal procedures. These patients are good candidates for extraperitoneal continent vesicostomy. The largest reported experience is using the pro-

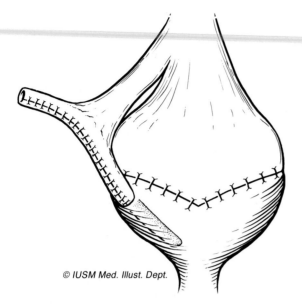

FIG. 112–9. The Monti channel can be brought out to either a lower-abdominal stoma or to the umbilicus. The mesentery is mobilized from the pedicle of the bladder augmentation to provide a tension-free skin anastomosis.

cedure described by Cain et al. (3), utilizing an intravesical submucosal–mucosal lined tunnel to create the continence mechanism.

This procedure has been successfully used with a variety of underlying bladder pathologies. The bladder is

opened to allow creation of either a midline or lateral full-thickness bladder flap (Fig. 112–11A). Incisions are extended intravesically, leaving a 2.5-cm plate of mucosa. The mucosa is sharply dissected off the underlying detrusor muscle laterally (Fig. 112–11B). The intra- and extravesical mucosal tube is created over a 14 Fr catheter with running 6-0 absorbable suture (Fig. 112–11C). The detrusor muscle of the extravesical portion of the tube is then closed with 4-0 absorbable sutures (Fig. 112–11D). The continence mechanism is then created by closing the lateral edges of the bladder mucosa over the mucosal tube using running 5-0 absorbable suture (Fig. 112–11E). The stoma can be created either in the lower abdomen or umbilicus. An indwelling 12 Fr catheter is left in place for 3 weeks.

Ureterovesicostomy

The ureter can be used as a catheterizable channel but has been less popular than bowel channels due to the additional upper urinary tract reconstruction required and the higher risk of skin stenosis and stomal leakage (13). When there is a unilateral nonfunctioning kidney with a nonrefluxing distal ureter a ureteral channel should be considered, but this unfortunate situation should be avoidable in the present era of careful management of these patients from early in life. Several reports have documented successful distal ureteral reimplantation at the time of the ureterovesicostomy. Obviously, careful mobilization of the ureter to prevent proximal and distal stenosis is an important technical factor.

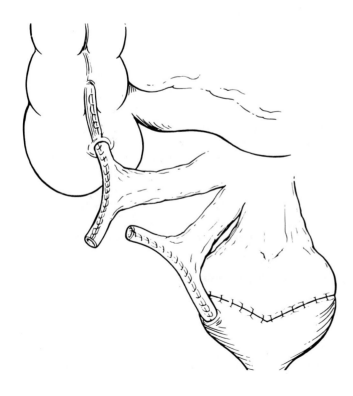

FIG. 112–10. The "double Monti," utilizing a Monti channel for both the Malone antegrade continence enema and Mitrofanoff channels.

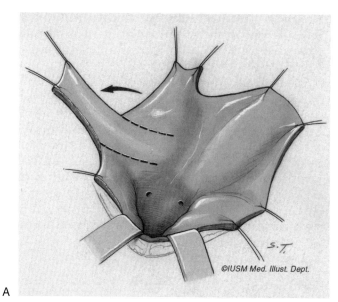

A

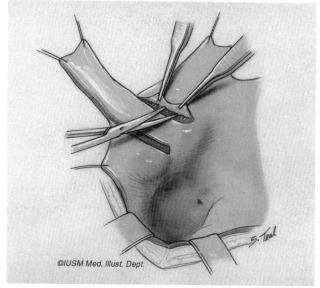

B

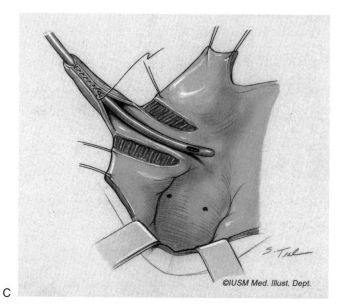

C

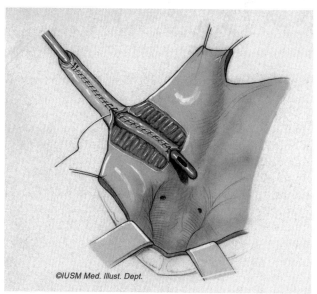

D

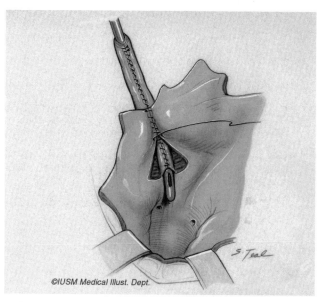

E

FIG. 112–11. A: A 2.5-cm full-thickness bladder tube is harvested with adequate length to reach an abdominal stomal site. **B:** Intravesical mucosal incisions are made, leaving a 2.5-cm mucosal strip. The mucosal incisions should extend approximately 2.5 cm into the bladder. The lateral mucosal edges are mobilized sharply. **C:** The mucosal channel is closed using running 6-0 suture. **D:** The detrusor muscle of the extravesical portion of the bladder tube is closed with running 4-0 suture. **E:** The lateral mucosal edges are closed over the intravesical mucosal tube to create the continence mechanism.

TABLE 112–1. *Complications of mitrofanoff channel*

Stomal Stenosis
Stomal Incontinence
Difficulty Catheterizing Channel
Intraabdominal Adhesions
Shunt Infection
Abdominal Abscess
Painful Catheterization
Prolapsed Stomal Mucosa
Peristomal Hernia
Wound Dehiscence/Infection

OUTCOMES

Complications

Potential complications of the Mitrofanoff channel are listed in Table 112–1. The most common complication is stomal stenosis, occurring in 10% to 20% of channels in most series. The continent vesicostomy has a much higher rate of stenosis than either appendix or Monti–Yang channels. A short period of catheter dilation will avoid the need for surgical intervention in some patients. If necessary, revision of the stoma with a well-vascularized flap of skin is usually successful to manage significant stenosis.

Difficulty catheterizing the channel can occur secondary to angulation, perforation/false passage, or stenosis of the channel. Initially this should be treated conservatively with placement of an indwelling catheter for 1 to 2 weeks. On occasion reoperation will be necessary, and the patient and surgeon should be prepared to replace the entire tube if required.

Complications can occur many years after construction of a Mitrofanoff channel, and long-term follow-up with these patients is mandatory, especially when the Mitrofanoff channel is the sole means to empty the bladder.

Results

Most recent series have reported long-term success in up to 96% to 98% of Mitrofanoff channels (1,8). Because appendicovesicostomy has been used since the initial description of the procedure, there is better long-term data for this specific procedure, which has been shown to be durable over long periods of intermittent catheterization. We recently reported our results using the Monti–Yang channel in 112 consecutive patients, achieving 97% success with an average of 2-year follow-up (6).

Because of the short continence zone required with the mucosal flap valve technique for continent vesicostomy, there has been nearly 100% success with this procedure with respect to stomal continence.

Failure to obtain continence can be due to an inadequate submucosal tunnel, a fistula into the Mitrofanoff tube, breakdown of the muscular backing to the submucosal tunnel (especially when implanted into a bowel segment), or poor compliance/high intravesical pressure. In many instances, the underlying problem will be the bladder, and any patient with a failed Mitrofanoff should undergo repeat urodynamic studies of the bladder and a trial of anticholinergics. We have had good success with reimplanting a previously constructed channel at the time of secondary bladder augmentation when the initial Mitrofanoff channel has failed because of changing bladder dynamics.

REFERENCES

1. Cain MP, Casale AJ, King SK, Rink RC. Appendicovesicostomy and newer alternatives for the Mitrofanoff procedure: Results in the last 100 patients at Riley Childrens's Hospital. *J Urol* 1999;162:749.
2. Cain MP, Casale AJ, Rink RC. Initial experience using a catheterizable ileovesicostomy (Monti procedure) in children. *Urology* 1998;52:870.
3. Cain MP, Rink RC, Yerkes EB, Kaefer M, Casale AJ. Long-term follow up and outcome of continent catheterizable vesicostomy using the Rink modification. *J Urol* 2002;168:2583–2585.
4. Casale AJ. A long continent ileovesicostomy using a single piece of bowel. *J Urol* 1999;162:1743–1745.
5. Cromie WJ, Barada JH, Weingarten JL. Cecal tubularization: lengthening technique for creation of catheterizable conduit. *Urology* 1991; 37:41–42.
6. Gitlin JS, Cain MP, Lawrence P, Casale AJ, Kaefer M, Rink RC. The Riley Hospital experience with 112 Monti catheterizable channels. Presented at the American Academy of Pediatrics Annual Meeting, Section on Urology, Boston, 2002(abst 2).
7. Gosalbez R, Wei D, Gousse A, Castellan M, Labbie A. Refashioned short bowel segments for the construction of catheterizable channels (the Monti procedure): Early clinical experience. *J Urol* 1998;160: 1099–1102.
8. Harris CF, Cooper CS, Hutcheson JC, Snyder HM. Appendicovesicostomy: The Mitrofanoff procedure—a 15 year perspective. *J Urol* 2000; 163:1922–1926.
9. Liard A, Seguier-Lipszyc E, Mathiot A, Mitrofanoff P. The Mitrofanoff procedure: 20 years later. *J Urol* 2001;165:2394–2398.
10. Malone PS, Ransley PG, Kiely EM. Preliminary report: the antegrade continence enema. *Lancet* 1990;336:1217–1218.
11. Mitrofanoff P. Cystostomie continent trans-appendiculaire dans le traitement des vessies neurologiques. *Chir Ped* 1980;21:297.
12. Monti PR, Lara RC, Dutra MA, de Carvalho JR. New techniques for construction of efferent conduits based on the Mitrofanoff principle. *Urology* 1997;49:112–115.
13. Mor Y, Kajbafzadeh AM, German K, Mouriquand PD, Duffy PG, Ransley PG. The role of ureter in the creation of Mitrofanoff channels in children. *J Urol* 1997;157:635–637.
14. Wedderburn A, Lee RS, Denny A, Steinbrecher HA, Koyle MA, Malone PS. Synchronous bladder reconstruction and antegrade continence enema. *J Urol* 2001;165:2392–2393.

Laparoscopic Surgery

Section Editor: Leonard G. Gomella

CHAPTER 113A

Basic Laparoscopy

Leonard G. Gomella, Paul K. Pietrow, and David M. Albala

Increasingly, traditional open urologic surgical procedures are being performed laparoscopically through either a trans- or extraperitoneal approach (2–4). Chapters 113–132 include laparoscopic procedures commonly performed by urologists in the United States. This chapter provides the foundation for any laparoscopic procedure and describes techniques to enter the intra- or extraperitoneal space, insufflate, place viewing and access ports (including hand-assist devices), and the steps necessary to exit the abdomen. This chapter outlines the basic laparoscopic approaches used for the other laparoscopic procedures described in this edition.

INDICATIONS FOR SURGERY

Laparoscopy provides a minimally invasive approach to many standard open surgical procedures. Benefits to laparoscopic intervention may include decreased hospitalization and recovery time, less pain, and enhanced cosmetics.

Contraindications to transperitoneal laparoscopy include inability to tolerate general anesthesia or pneumoperitoneum (i.e., severe cardiac or pulmonary disease), extreme obesity, intestinal obstruction and/or substantial distention, massive hemoperitoneum, generalized peritonitis, extensive prior abdominal surgery, abdominal wall infection, uncorrectable coagulopathy, large abdominal wall hernias, or advanced intraabdominal malignancy. This list, in general, also applies to hand-assisted laparoscopic procedures. Hand-assisted laparoscopy may allow patients who have had extensive abdominal surgery to be considered for this approach due to the more reliable visualization of adhesions. Contraindications to extraperitoneal laparoscopy include most contraindications as above, plus prior surgery or inflammation in the extraperitoneal space.

ALTERNATIVE THERAPY

Patients should be informed of the alternate approaches available, including open surgery, and the team's experience with the specific procedure. The patient must also be informed that the procedure may be terminated or converted to an open approach due to inability to complete the procedure or complications. Patients often view laparoscopic surgery so favorably that they may expect to have no discomfort and immediately return to full activities. The patient must understand that interventional laparoscopy is still a surgical procedure with some of the inconveniences associated with any operation.

SURGICAL TECHNIQUE

Basic Laparoscopy

The majority of laparoscopic procedures are performed through the transperitoneal approach. The peritoneal cavity can be reliably entered and distended and provides a large working space. The patient preparation is standard for most interventions.

Patient Preparation

Routine bowel preparation, such as magnesium citrate the day before and enemas the day of surgery, will help decompress the lower intestine, which is desirable during procedures such as nephrectomy and prostatectomy. General endotracheal anesthesia is essential for interventional laparoscopy. Nitrous oxide anesthesia is discouraged because some surgeons believe it may cause bowel distension. Patients should be positioned with adequate padding and secured to the table to allow table repositioning during the procedure. The arms should be tucked at the side after large-bore intravenous access is completed or may padded upon arm boards if in the flank or semiflank position. A beanbag is useful for procedures such as transperitoneal nephrectomy that require the patient to be rolled to a lateral position.

Orogastric and urinary catheters lessen the risk of visceral injury and facilitate visualization, and should be used in all urologic laparoscopic procedures. Perioperative broad-spectrum antibiotics [e.g., 1 gm cefazolin (Ancef)] are employed in the event of inadvertent bowel injury. The field should always be prepped widely should there be need to convert to an open procedure. For pelvic laparoscopy, such as prostatectomy or lymphadenectomy in males, the genitalia should be prepped into the field so that there is access to the urethra for instrumentation or to decompress pneumoscrotum. For procedures such as bladder neck suspension in females, the patient should be in the lithotomy position with the vagina prepped.

Detailed information on laparoscopic instrumentation is available elsewhere and specific instrumentation may be needed for the growing list of specialized procedures (1). The positioning of monitors should be determined based on the procedure. For pelvic surgery, a single monitor at the foot is usually sufficient; for procedures such as nephrectomy and adrenalectomy, monitors on either side of the bed are recommended.

Establishing the Pneumoperitoneum

Initial pneumoperitoneum is established for most standard laparoscopic approaches and for many hand-assisted techniques. Entry into the abdominal cavity with the Veress needle is most commonly performed at the inferior or superior margin of the umbilicus. The umbilicus is the central point of the peritoneal cavity, making it an ideal observation site. Here, the abdominal wall is only two layers thick (fascia and peritoneum) and easy to traverse percutaneously (Fig. 113A–1). Placement of the needle into the abdominal cavity is a blind procedure with potential for injury to the underlying structures. If the patient has undergone prior surgery, open entry using the Hasson technique is considered the safest method (see below).

The patient should be placed in the 10- to 20-degree Trendelenburg position to help drop the intestines out of the pelvis. The Veress needle type has a spring-loaded, blunt-tipped obturator to help prevent injury. A small incision is made at the inferior or superior border of the umbilicus. The abdominal wall can be elevated by grasping the periumbilical area with a sponge or with towel clamps. These maneuvers *may* raise the umbilicus up and away from the intestines but, more importantly, stabilize the abdominal wall. The needle is grasped like a dart along the shaft to limit its excursion into the abdominal

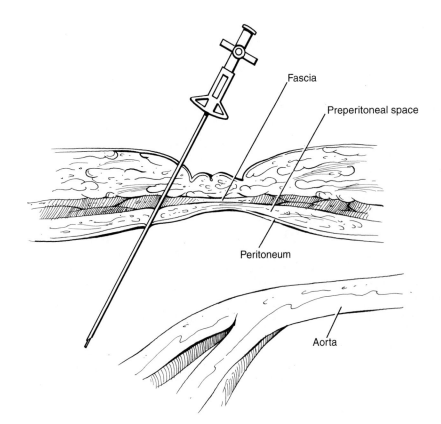

Fascia

Preperitoneal space

Peritoneum

Aorta

FIG. 113A–1. The Veress needle is most often placed at the inferior or superior aspect of the umbilicus. The needle is directed into the hollow of the pelvis, below the bifurcation of the great vessels.

cavity with the angle of entry directed slightly caudad into the pelvis. Two distinct "pops" are felt as the needle passes through the fascia and peritoneum. It is important to traverse the layers of the abdominal wall in a near perpendicular fashion to avoid bouncing off" of the peritoneum and remaining in the preperitoneal space. The umbilicus lies directly over the right iliac vessels, just below the aortic bifurcation at L4–L5 (Fig. 113A–1). Deep penetration with the needle directly posteriorly could produce vascular injury.

Once the needle is in the peritoneal cavity, confirmatory tests are performed prior to insufflation, although none are foolproof. These include:

1. "*Color test*". Aspiration of colored (red, yellow, green, brown) or malodorous fluid suggests improper placement.
2. "*Drop test.*" Apply a drop of saline inside the hub of the needle and lift the abdominal wall. If in proper position, the drop will enter the abdomen due to the negative intraperitoneal pressure.
3. *Modified Palmer test.* Inject 10 mL of saline into the needle and attempt to aspirate. Inability to aspirate the fluid suggests the fluid has dispersed into the abdomen and the needle is in correct position.
4. *Initial pressure reading* less than 8 mm Hg. The insufflator is turned on with no flow to obtain a pressure reading.
5. *A decrease in pressure* with elevation of the abdominal wall.

If perforation of a viscus occurs, the needle should be removed and discarded. A new needle may then be inserted at another location or the surgeon may choose to obtain open access using the Hasson technique (see below). Once insufflation has been completed and the primary trocar has been introduced, the injury can be examined with the laparoscope and a decision made as to the appropriate management.

If blood appears, the Veress needle should be withdrawn slightly. Its positioning should be retested, the pneumoperitoneum established, and the injury inspected for possible repair. Because of the small size of the Veress needle, the majority of these injuries do not require open operative intervention.

CO_2 insufflation should be started at a "low" flow rate, which should initially maintain an intraabdominal pressure of less than 8 mm Hg. A high initial intraabdominal pressure with a low flow suggests improper needle placement. Once insufflation is underway, the abdomen should be observed to assure that a symmetrical pneumoperitoneum is developing. It is useful to monitor the insufflation by percussion over the liver, noting the characteristic dull echo tone that indicates proper insufflation.

If the distention appears correct, the rate of flow of CO_2 may be increased to "high flow" (usually greater than 6 L per minute). Initially, the abdomen is insufflated to 15 to 20 mm Hg to provide maximum distention of the abdominal cavity and assist with atraumatic placement of the early trocars. An adult abdomen will typically require 5 to 6 L of CO_2 to create an adequate pneumoperitoneum, while children may require as little as 1 to 1.5 L. The working pressure should be decreased to 12 to 15 mm Hg after all trocars are placed to prevent complications of barotrauma.

If preperitoneal insufflation occurs, an attempt can be made to open the peritoneum with laparoscopic scissors and guide the tip of the trocar beneath it. CO_2 gas is then insufflated into the true peritoneal cavity, compressing the preperitoneal gas. Alternatively, evacuation of the preperitoneal space with a needle and syringe and reinsertion of the needle at the same or other site (i.e., superior umbilical position) may be attempted. In no case should compression of the abdomen occur as this will disperse the CO_2 gas within the preperitoneal space. Open access (Hasson technique) can be used if these techniques are unsuccessful.

Primary Trocar Placement

Once the pneumoperitoneum is established, the Veress needle is removed and the primary (laparoscope) trocar is inserted. A 10- or 10/11-mm trocar is used in adults to allow passage of the laparoscope. (*Note*: The trocar designation refers to the size of the instrument that can be inserted into the trocar and not the overall diameter of the trocar.) The incision site used for the Veress needle should be enlarged and the subcutaneous tissue spread to the fascia using a hemostat. The skin incision should be sufficient to allow the trocar to pass without resistance. It is helpful to press the end of the trocar on the skin to create an impression that serves as a guide for the size of the incision.

The proper technique to insert a trocar is to apply firm, steady pressure with a gentle, twisting movement. A finger can be held along the shaft to serve as a brake from pushing the trocar in too far (Fig. 113A–2). Pressure should be applied using the arm and elbow and not the weight of the shoulder and upper body. The trocar should be directed toward the site of interest within the peritoneum to avoid torque from the abdominal wall during the rest of the case (Fig. 113A–2). The abdominal wall can be lifted and stabilized with hemostats (Fig. 113A–3). Entry into the peritoneum is usually indicated by a sudden decrease in resistance and the characteristic "clicks" made by the trocar safety shield locking in place. Most disposable trocars have a "safety shield" that covers the sharp tip after peritoneal entry to limit injury. The sharp obturator is removed and a quick check will determine if the trocar has entered the peritoneal cavity. The stopcock on the trocar can be left open during insertion, causing a rush of gas to escape ("whoosh test"), suggesting intraperitoneal placement.

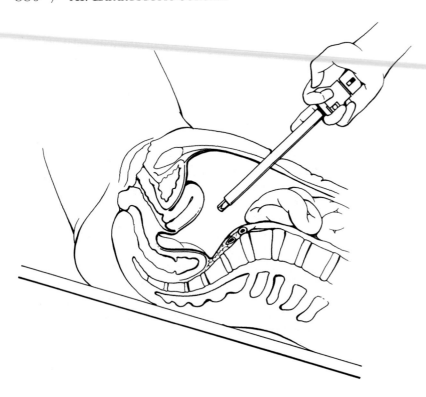

FIG. 113A–2. Primary shielded trocar is held with a finger along the shaft to limit the depth of entry of the trocar.

Visualizing trocars are available from various manufacturers (Optiview, Ethicon Endosurgery, Cincinnati, OH) that enhance the safe entry into the abdomen and have largely replaced the shielded metal trocars. After the initial skin incision is made, the laparoscope is placed into one of the visualizing trocars that has a plastic cutting tip. The trocar is the inserted and, using pressure, gently twisted back and forth to penetrate the layers of the

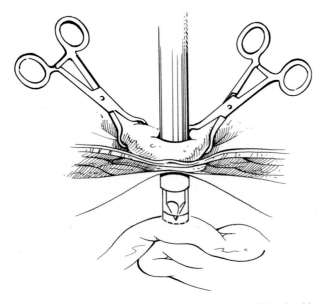

FIG. 113A–3. The abdominal wall can be stabilized with towel clips placed on either side of the umbilicus during primary trocar insertion.

abdominal wall. This process is monitored under direct visualization of the tip of the trocar through the laparoscope. After the peritoneal cavity is entered, the obturator is removed and the laparoscope is placed into the trocar. New trocars are available that coaxially dilate the abdominal wall and do not create the tears in the fascia associated with standard "blade" trocars. These devices (Versaport, US Surgical, Norwalk, CT) employ a Veress neddle that is passed through an expandable, mesh sheath. Once entry is obtained into the peritoneal cavity, the needle is extracted and a trocar is passed through the sheath and into the abdomen. These trocars are available in multiple sizes and can be large enough to accommodate 12-mm instruments. The primary advantage of the coaxially dilating trocars is that the abdominal wall does not require formal closure of the fascia because the dilated fascia is able to contract and prevent bowel excursion.

The chance of a serious injury at the time of the insertion of the primary trocar is much greater than with the Veress needle because of its larger size and the greater force required to penetrate the abdominal wall. Although the ideal working pressure of the pneumoperitoneum is 10 to 12 mm Hg, an initial pressure of 15 to 20 mm Hg is needed until the all trocars are placed to ensure a "tense" pneumoperitoneum.

The CO_2 insufflator is connected to the stopcock on the trocar and insufflation is resumed. The laparoscope, attached to a high-resolution video camera, should be white balanced and introduced for exploration of the abdomen. Visual inspection of the abdomen is necessary to assess for possible injury by the Veress needle or trocar.

Lens fogging is caused by passage of the room-temperature laparoscope into the warm, humid abdomen. As the laparoscope warms during the procedure, fogging becomes less problematic. To deal with fogging, the following techniques are useful: heating the laparoscope before insertion in sterile heating blocks or in warmed sterile saline and the application of antifogging solutions. Limiting the amount of time the scope is removed from the abdomen during the procedure will prevent cooling of the lens. If fogging or debris cover the lens, it can be gently wiped on a clean piece of bowel; touching fat or a blood-tinged surface may leave a film on the end of the laparoscope. Limit the contact time on the tissue, however, because the laparoscope tip can become quite warm.

Hasson Technique (Open Access)

Many surgeons use this as the primary access for all patients and do not use the Veress needle pneumoperitoneum and initial blind primary trocar placement. Open access (Hasson technique) is also useful both for correcting preperitoneal insufflation with the Veress needle and in the patient at high risk for multiple adhesions. The advantage is that entry into the peritoneal cavity is under direct vision, minimizing the risk of injury.

An infraumbilical incision is made and two stay sutures (such as 0 Prolene) are placed through the fascia on either side. The fascia and peritoneum are directly visualized and opened (Fig. 113A–4A). The Hasson style trocar has a blunt tip and different features based on the manufacturer. Some trocars have a tapered end that seals in the pneumoperitoneum while others rely on retention balloons or grips to maintain the trocar in the peritoneal cavity. The stay sutures are either attached to the cannula to hold it in position (Fig. 113A–4B), if needed, or secured with hemostats for use during closure of the fascia. The insufflation tubing is attached to the Hasson-style trocar and immediately "high flow" can be selected. The pneumoperitoneum should develop rapidly.

Secondary Trocar Placement

The placement of secondary or "working" trocars can be carefully monitored externally and internally to reduce the risk of injury. In addition to trocars with safety shields, newer plastic-tipped safety trocars are available. Checking that there is full pneumoperitoneum before trocar insertion, spreading subcutaneous tissue with a hemostat, using an adequate skin incision, verifying anatomic landmarks, and directing the trocar under direct visualization with a laparoscope will limit trocar injuries.

The room is darkened and the light from the laparoscope is used to transilluminate the anterior abdominal wall to identify the epigastric vessels. Trocar sizes and sites are selected according to the procedure to be performed, the patient's anatomy, and the surgeon's preference. At least one larger secondary trocar (10 or 10/11 mm) is usually placed to allow the passage of larger instruments such as clip appliers and to allow removal of specimens. Linear stapling devices are passed through 12-mm trocars. Extended-length trocars are available if patients have particularly thick abdominal walls. Trocar placement for specific procedures is noted in the appropriate chapters that follow.

The selected site for the secondary trocar is gently pushed with the index finger while the site is observed through the laparoscope. The site is evaluated to confirm that there are no underlying vessels or bowel. A skin inci-

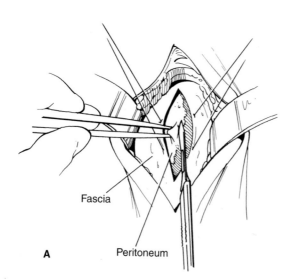

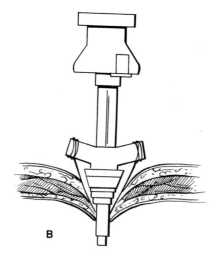

FIG. 113A–4. A: Open laparoscopy using the Hasson technique. The peritoneum is entered under direct vision. **B:** A blunt-tipped Hasson style is secured using the stay sutures.

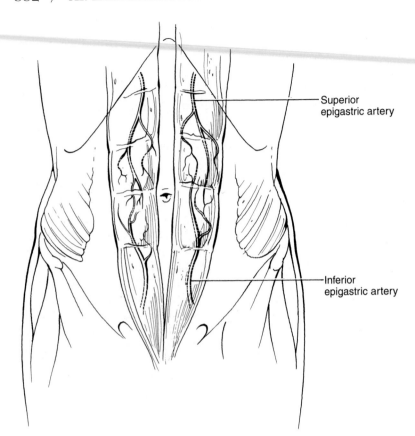

Superior
epigastric artery

Inferior
epigastric artery

FIG. 113A–5. Secondary trocars should be placed in the midline (linea alba) or at least 8 cm from the midline to avoid injury to the rectus or the epigastric vessels.

sion of appropriate diameter to accommodate the trocar is made. Skin incisions should be sufficient to remove the skin as a point of resistance during trocar insertion but not large enough to allow gas leakage. It is useful to spread the subcutaneous tissue down to fascia with a clamp until the impression of clamp tip is visible on the peritoneum. The hemostat is removed and the trocar is introduced with the same technique described for the primary trocar except that the progress into the abdomen is followed on the monitor. Newer trocars have intrinsic stability threads that limit accidental removal. Suturing trocars to the skin using a heavy silk tether to prevent accidental removal during the case may on occasion be needed.

The secondary trocars are oriented toward the surgical site. This configuration minimizes the side-to-side excursion required of the trocars and the "crossing swords" problem is avoided. A general rule is to place secondary trocars in the midline or at least 8 cm from the midline in adults to avoid the rectus sheath (Fig. 113A–5). If the rectus muscle is penetrated by the trocar, there is an increased risk of bleeding from the muscle or epigastric vessels.

Trocar Removal

At the end of the procedure, the pneumoperitoneum should be lowered to 5 mm Hg or less to observe for any bleeding that may be tamponaded by the elevated work-ing pressure. A brief survey of the abdomen should verify that there was no injury outside the operative field.

Trocar sites should be examined prior to and after removal of the sheaths for bleeding or herniation. During trocar removal and fascial closure, bowel can become trapped along the trocar pathway. Trocar removal and suturing should be observed laparoscopically with 10 mm and larger trocars requiring fascial suturing in adults. If the Hasson technique was used, the umbilical port can usually be closed by tying the preplaced sutures together.

Before the final trocar is removed, as much CO_2 as possible should be expelled by compressing the abdomen with the flapper valve or stopcock in the open position. This will reduce postoperative shoulder pain due to diaphragmatic irritation from the CO_2 gas. If pneumoscrotum is present, this should also be manually decompressed at this time.

If standard placement of the initial 10-mm port was used, the following procedure is useful. All secondary 10-mm sites are sutured while the umbilical camera is in position. A cystoscope or 5-mm laparoscope is placed in a 5-mm trocar site and the closure of the umbilical site is observed intraabdominally. The pneumoperitoneum is evacuated by holding down the flapper valve and manually compressing the abdomen, and the final 5-mm port is removed.

Fascial closure can be accomplished by a variety of techniques. Typically, 0 or 2-0 absorbable suture (i.e.

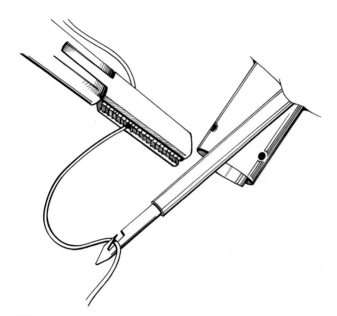

FIG. 113A–6. One technique to close the trocar site uses a device such as the Endoclose fascial closure needle. Here, the 2-0 absorbable suture has been passed into the abdomen alongside the trocar. The suture is grasped and the needle is withdrawn and passed on the opposite side of the trocar.

Vicryl) on a small curved needle (i.e., CT-3 or UR-5) is used. Fascial edges are grasped with either a toothed forcep or Scanlon clamps. Army–Navy retractors help facilitate exposure.

Laparoscopic closure needles (i.e., Endoclose, US Surgical) are also available that are similar to a Stamey style needle. A free 0 or 2-0 absorbable suture is engaged and passed percutaneously along the side of the trocar, through the fascia, and into the abdominal cavity using laparoscopic guidance. (*Note:* If stability threads were used to secure the trocar, they may interfere with passage of the closure device. Release the thread and slide it out of the incision while maintaining the trocar in the abdominal cavity.) The end of the suture is held with a laparoscopic grasper while the spring-loaded end is depressed to release the suture (Fig. 113A–6). The closure device is then passed on the opposite side of the trocar, the free end of the suture placed in the end of the needle using laparoscopic guidance. Once engaged, the device is withdrawn with the attached end of the suture. The trocar is removed and the ends of the suture tied from the outside using laparoscopic control. Another closure method utilizes the Inlet Closure Kit (Carter–Thomason suture-passing device and Pilot suture guide, Inlet Medical, Eden Prairie, MN). A suture guide (10 to 12 or 5 mm) device is placed into the trocar site and the suture-passing device is loaded with a 2-0 absorbable suture and the suture passed inside. The suture is released and the needle placed in the opposite hole and the suture retrieved and removed through the opposite guide hole. The guide is removed and the suture tied from outside the body. If coaxially dilating trocars are used, the abdominal wall may not require formal closure as noted above.

The skin site should be thoroughly irrigated prior to closure. Herniation is most often associated with trocars larger than 10 mm and when it does occur is often due to a wound infection rather than improper fascial closure. Skin sites are closed with staples, subcutaneous suture reinforced by steristrips, or skin adhesive.

REFERENCES

1. Goldstein DS, Winfield H. Laparoscopic instrumentation. In: Gomella LG, Kozminski M, Winfield H, eds. *Laparoscopic urologic surgery.* New York: Raven Press, 1994:21.
2. Gomella LG, Albala DM. Laparoscopic urological surgery—1994. *Br J Urol* 1994;74:267–273.
3. Hedican SP. Laparoscopy in urology. *Surg Clin North Am* 2000;80: 1465–1485.
4. Jackson CL. Urologic laparoscopy. *Surg Oncol Clin North Am* 2001;10: 571–578.

Advanced Laparoscopy: Extraperitoneal and Hand-Assisted Laparoscopy and Pediatrics

Leonard G. Gomella, Paul K. Pietrow, and David M. Albala

Traditional laparoscopy approaches the target organs through the peritoneum in contrast to open urologic surgery, which is frequently in the extraperitoneal (pre- and retroperitoneal) space. The use of transperitoneal laparoscopic techniques for a variety of procedures is widely accepted. However, significant complications, such as bowel or vascular injuries, can occur when utilizing the transperitoneal approach.

The extraperitoneal approach has been investigated for a variety of procedures, including lymphadenectomy, bladder neck suspension, and ureteral, renal, and adrenal procedures. There are several potential advantages to the extraperitoneal laparoscopic approach. By avoiding the peritoneal cavity, the risk of visceral and vascular injury may be reduced and preperitoneal landmarks, such as Cooper's ligament and the iliac vessels, can be visualized directly. Intestinal retraction may be easier because the "peritoneal envelope" surrounds the intestines and individual bowel loops need not be retracted. Prolonged ileus appears to be less with this approach. Herniation through trocar sites, postoperative ileus, and adhesions may be reduced compared to the transperitoneal approach. Limitations to the extraperitoneal approach include prior surgical procedures or inflammatory processes that may obliterate this potential space. Excessive fat in the extraperitoneal space may obscure the anatomy, in particular in the retroperitoneum. However, the more obese patient may be better suited for an extraperitoneal pelvic lymphadenectomy than with the transperitoneal approach. The limited retroperitoneal working area may make placement of trocars more difficult as well as limiting the removal of large masses, such as renal tumors. There is data to suggest that there may be more CO_2 absorption in the extraperitoneal space; however, this can be in general managed by aggressive ventilation (6).

DEVELOPING THE EXTRAPERITONEAL SPACE

Simple extraperitoneal insufflation will cause the CO_2 gas to track along fascial planes and will not develop the extraperitoneal space. Balloon dissection of this space is key to performing any procedure in this area.

Gaur was the first to describe balloon distention of the extraperitoneal space using a simple device consisting of a surgical glove finger mounted on a red rubber catheter secured with a silk tie (3). The catheter was connected to a blood pressure bulb insufflator and the balloon inflated to 110 mm Hg intermittently until a visible bulge was seen in the abdomen. Workers at the University of Iowa have replaced the glove finger with a more durable finger cot from an O'Connor-style drape or recommend using two glove fingers tied over each other to limit rupture. Instead of using air, saline can be used to distend these self-made balloons (12).

Several commercially available trocar mounted balloons are available. The Spacemaker (US Surgical, Norwalk, CT) is trocar mounted and designed to be filled with air. An advantage of this device is that the inflation and distention of the space can be laparoscopically monitored through the clear balloon. Since the initial descriptions of these techniques, many authors have now reported on their success and versatility (4).

PELVIC EXTRAPERITONEAL LAPAROSCOPY

Bladder neck suspension, hernia repair, and pelvic lymph node dissection can be approached through the pelvic extraperitoneal space. Patient preparation and positioning are identical to transperitoneal laparoscopy.

A vertical skin incision is made 1 to 2 cm below the inferior umbilical crease to avoid the confluence of the anterior and posterior rectus sheaths at the umbilicus. The skin incision should be large enough to accept a 10/11-mm trocar. The tissues are spread with a clamp to the anterior rectus sheath. Two absorbable 0 (i.e., Vicryl) stay sutures are placed in each side of the midline. Next, the anterior rectus sheath is incised along the linea alba between the sutures. The two bellies of the rectus muscle are separated by blunt dissection and a finger is passed behind the rectus and above the posterior fascia. Blunt finger dissection is used to create the access space between the rectus and the posterior sheath.

A balloon device of choice is lubricated with sterile jelly and passed behind the rectus but above the posterior sheath. This enters the preperitoneal space at the level of the arcuate line (Fig. 113B–1) and is a reliable means of avoiding entry into the peritoneum. The balloon can be passed inferiorly with external manual guidance down to the pubis. The balloon is inflated to approximately 300 mm Hg with air using an inflation bulb. The balloon is left inflated for several minutes, deflated, and inflated a second time.

The balloon is removed and a 10-mm Hasson-style cannula is placed. The CO_2 insufflator is attached and set on high flow at 8 to 10 mm Hg. Inspection of the preperitoneal space usually confirms adequate dissection of the prevesical space. The right side typically dissects more completely than the left. However, a minimal amount of blunt dissection will expose the external iliac vessels on the left side if needed.

Additional trocars are placed under direct vision. The pressure is briefly increased to 15 mm Hg to facilitate secondary trocar placement. Prolonged pressure at this level may cause tracking of the gas into the subcutaneous tissues. Trocar insertion is identical to the transperitoneal approach (transillumination, visual inspection for ves-

sels, etc.). It is critical to ensure that the lateral trocars do not traverse the peritoneal cavity and they are beyond the peritoneal reflection. After the trocars are placed, the pressure can be decreased to 10 mm Hg, which is maintained throughout the procedure.

As an alternative approach, especially for procedures such as bladder neck suspension where lateral exposure at the level of the iliac vessels is not needed, a small vertical incision is made in the midline about one-third the distance below the umbilicus, between the umbilicus and pubis. Under vision, the rectus fascia is incised and stay sutures are placed on the fascia. The extraperitoneal space is developed with an index finger. The balloon device is inserted and inflated as above.

RETROPERITONEAL LAPAROSCOPY

This form of laparoscopy is often called "retroperitoneoscopy" and is used most often for renal and adrenal procedures. Studies have demonstrated that the peritoneum is never more posterior than the posterior axillary line and that placing the patient in the lateral position further moves the peritoneum anteriorly (2). Finger dissection can then free up the anterior lip of the peritoneal reflection and allow more anterior trocar placement.

Stenting of the ipsilateral ureter preoperatively is often helpful. Following the usual preparation for transperitoneal laparoscopy, the patient is placed in a standard flank position. A beanbag on the operating table is helpful for this position. A 2-cm transverse skin incision is made just anterior to the tip of the twelfth rib. An alternate site for the skin incision is Petit's triangle approximately two finger breadths above the anterior superior iliac spine (Fig. 113B–2). The posterior layer of the thoracolumbar fascia is identified and two stay sutures are

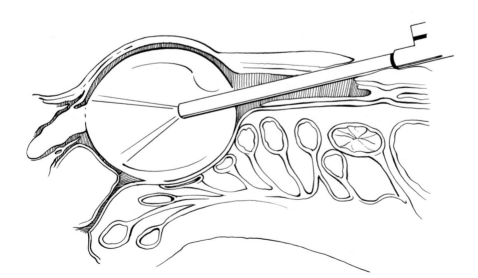

FIG. 113B–1. Technique of trocar-mounted balloon dissection of the preperitoneal space.

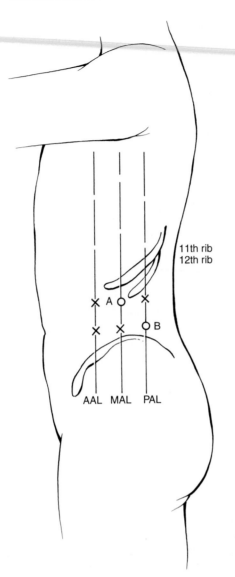

FIG. 113B–2. For retroperitoneal procedures, the initial trocar is placed (**A**) 1 to 2 cm from the tip of the twelfth rib or (**B**) in Petit's triangle, 1 to 2 cm above the anterior superior iliac spine. Additional ports can be placed as needed between the posterior and anterior axillary lines.

positioned. The flank muscles are split to the anterior thoracolumbar fascia; two additional stay sutures are positioned.

The anterior layer of thoracolumbar fascia is incised and the retroperitoneal space is entered. To enter the retroperitoneum, an index finger should be used to develop the space initially and sweep the peritoneum away anteriorly.

If a renal procedure (i.e., cyst excision, renal biopsy) is planned, it is helpful to place the balloon directly into Gerota's fascia to facilitate the procedure. The index finger is introduced into the retroperitoneum in a cephalad direction to palpate the lower pole of the kidney. In a thin patient, Gerota's fascia can be pierced with a finger and the perirenal space entered. Finger dissection within

Gerota's fascia creates an adequate space for placement of the balloon adjacent to the renal parenchyma. In obese patients, abundant retroperitoneal fat may preclude localization of the lower pole with finger dissection. Here, Gerota's fascia can be grasped with two Scanlon or Allis clamps and delivered into the skin incision. Gerota's fascia is incised under vision and the balloon dilator is visually placed within Gerota's fascia. The retroperitoneal approach for laparoscopic nephrectomy in obese patients is considered a relative contraindication.

A commercially manufactured or self-made balloon, as noted above, is inserted in the retroperitoneum. The passage of the self-made balloon can be facilitated by backloading into a large Amplatz dilator sheath. The degree of balloon dilation varies with the patient's body habitus: One to 1.2 L of normal saline or room air is average in adults (Fig. 113B–1). The balloon is kept inflated for 5 minutes to facilitate hemostasis.

Following balloon removal, a Hasson blunt-tipped trocar is inserted into the retroperitoneum and secured with the preplaced stay sutures or with the trocars' retention mechanism. Visualization of the psoas muscle confirms proper balloon dilation of the retroperitoneum (or the lower pole of the kidney if the dilator was placed inside Gerota's fascia). The peritoneal envelope may be further mobilized with sweeping motions of the laparoscope. If difficulty is encountered mobilizing the peritoneum, an operating laparoscope can be used to pass a blunt-tipped dissector into the retroperitoneum.

The insertion of secondary trocars under manual, rather than laparoscopic, control has been described to minimize trocar injury to the peritoneum (5). The laparoscope and the Hasson cannula are removed and the index finger of the left hand (for a right-handed surgeon) is introduced into the retroperitoneum. An "S-shaped" retractor is inserted into the retroperitoneum in such a manner that it lies immediately in front of the finger (i.e., the retractor is cradled by the finger). The fingertip mobilizes and retracts the peritoneum away from the abdominal wall; the S-retractor prevents inadvertent trocar injury to the surgeon's finger. With the surgeon's right hand, the secondary trocars are inserted under bimanual control, with the aim being to introduce the trocar onto the S-shaped retractor. Secondary trocars are placed based on the procedure to be performed. Typical placement for retroperitoneal procedures are demonstrated in Figure 113B–2. No trocars are positioned behind the posterior axillary line.

BASIC HAND-ASSISTED LAPAROSCOPY

Hand-assisted laparoscopy has now been applied to many surgical scenarios and has been reported to provide many of the same advantages as "pure" laparoscopy in terms of patient recovery and morbidity (7,8,10,13,14). The hand-assisted approach can offer some benefits over pure laparoscopic techniques:

1. It allows the surgeon to maintain tactile feedback during the operation.
2. The human hand provides a more facile retractor and dissector than standard rigid instruments.
3. Surgical specimens can be easily removed intact, avoiding morcellation.
4. It helps bridge the gap between standard open skills and advanced laparoscopic skills. This can be helpful for surgeons new to laparoscopy.
5. The ability to perform rapid hand exchanges can provide a safer environment in which to train other surgeons and to manage potential complications such as bleeding.

Drawbacks of hand-assisted laparoscopy include the creation of a more noticeable (albeit small) incision, the potential for a slower recovery than pure laparoscopy, and the risk of wound dehiscence that exists with any open incision.

Recent advances in hand-assist devices have made these instruments easier to place and more comfortable for the surgeon. The first-generation devices in general relied upon adhesive materials to affix the device. The newer devices rely on compression against the peritoneal surface and body wall to remain in position. These newer devices permit rapid hand exchanges, allowing a more experienced surgeon easy entrance into the abdomen in the event of a complication.

Use of most of the second-generation devices begins with the creation of an open incision that is approximately equal in length to the surgeon's glove size, avoiding the use of a "blind" Veress needle access. Based on body wall thickness, the skin incision is approximately the surgeon's glove size (e.g., 7.5-cm skin incision for a size 7.5 glove).

The exact positioning of the incision depends upon the planned procedure, the body habitus of the patient, and surgeon preference (see subsequent chapters for details). Most often, the hand port is inserted in a midline incision. Once the peritoneal cavity has been entered, the inside surface of the anterior abdominal wall is inspected for the presence of adhesions, which can be taken down sharply. The GelPort (Applied Medical, Rancho Santa Margarita, CA) employs an inner sleeve that is passed into the abdominal cavity and pulled out through the incision. An inner ring holds the sleeve in place. The sleeve is then secured with a base plate that lies on the anterior abdominal wall. The GelPort covering is then attached to the base plate. The entire three-piece system (Fig. 113B–3) is relatively easy to assemble once the incision has been established in the abdominal wall.

The Lap Disc (Ethicon Inc, Cincinnati, OH) consists of three rings connected by a silicone membrane (Fig. 113B–4). The lower and middle rings bridge the abdominal wall, while the upper ring rotates on the middle, acting as an iris to seal the device around the surgeon's hand.

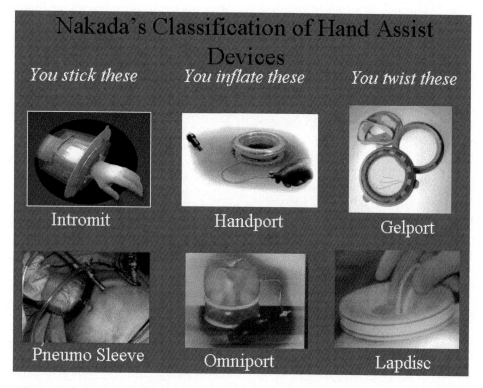

FIG. 113B–3. Classification of laparoscopic hand-assist devices. Positioning relies on either adhesives, inflated collars, or mechanical compression. (Courtesy of Stephen Nakada, MD.)

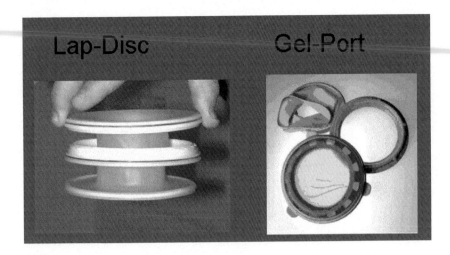

FIG. 113B–4. The authors' devices of choice for hand-assisted laparoscopy. The Lap Disc consists of three rings connected by a silicone membrane. The lower and middle rings bridge the abdominal wall, while the upper ring rotates on the middle, acting as an iris to seal the port around the surgeon's hand. Two sizes are now available for abdominal wall less than 5 cm thick or form 5 to 9 cm thick. The three-piece GelPort is relatively easy to assemble and provides an adequate seal around the surgeon's wrist while minimizing fatigue.

This device is also applied to the abdominal wall after an open incision is established into the peritoneal cavity. Use of a sterile, water-soluble lubricant on the surgeon's hand is recommended to ensure smooth entry and exit through the Lap Disc.

At this point, an empty trocar can be passed into the abdominal cavity through the hand device and the abdomen can be insufflated at a high-flow rate. The surgeon's nondominant hand is then passed into the abdomen and secondary trocars are placed. Skin incisions are made in appropriate locations and the first trocar can be passed between the surgeon's fingers while lifting up on the abdominal wall. Insufflation should then continue through this trocar and additional trocars are placed under direct laparoscopic vision. As always, the insufflation should then be changed to any trocar that does not contain the laparoscope to minimize fogging difficulties. Alternatively, the laparoscope with an accompanying trocar can be passed through the hand-assist device. In this case, the abdomen can be insufflated through the trocar in the hand-assist device and the secondary trocar can be placed under direct vision.

Prior to beginning the dissection, laparotomy pads can be preplaced into the abdominal cavity and used to blot any bleeding during the dissection. It is, of course, imperative to remove these pads prior to exiting the abdomen and a helpful reminder system should be created with the rest of the operating room staff instead of relying solely upon sponge counts.

Exiting the abdomen should be carried out with the secondary sites being closed under direct visualization through a port placed in the hand-assist device. The hand site is closed in the standard fashion.

POSTOPERATIVE MANAGEMENT

Depending on the procedure, clear liquids can be given after the effects of anesthesia have cleared. Diets can then be advanced as tolerated. For procedure such as pelvic lymphadenectomy, discharge is typically within 24 hours. For more extensive procedures (i.e., nephrectomy), it may be necessary to advance the diet more slowly. The requirement for postoperative analgesics is usually minimal; excessive pain should raise the suspicion of a complication. Patients should be advised that delayed postoperative bruising is on occasion encountered. Return to full activities is more rapid than with the equivalent open procedure.

PEDIATRIC LAPAROSCOPY

Most principles of adult laparoscopy can be applied to the pediatric population with the following exceptions:

1. In younger children, the bladder is an intraabdominal structure requiring more care with lower abdominal trocar placement.
2. The peritoneal membrane is loosely attached to the abdominal wall, making it potentially difficult to pass a Veress needle. Many authors advocate an open access technique for *all* children.
3. The total CO_2 to insufflate the abdomen is in general 1 to 3 L. Pressures should be kept lower than in adults (8 to 10 mmHg).
4. The 5mm trocars are commonly used in children and the sites *must* be sutured at the end of the case.
5. Many standard laparoscopic instruments will be either too large or long for pediatric procedures, thereby requiring specialized equipment.

OUTCOMES

Complications

Open laparoscopy using the blunt-tipped Hasson trocar or hand-assisted approaches offer the opportunity to minimize the risk of trocar injury. Significant perforation of a major blood vessel, bladder, or gastrointestinal tract with a trocar should be managed by immediate laparotomy and repair. If this injury is encountered, the trocar and sheath should be left in place while opening the abdomen to minimize further contamination or bleeding. In selected instances, laparoscopic repair may be appropriate but often requires significant advanced skills.

Vascular injury within the abdominal wall, especially the inferior epigastric vessels, is sometimes seen. If there is a vascular injury to the anterior abdominal wall, a through-and-through suture can be placed on a bolster using a Stamey-style needle or laparoscopic closure device and removed after 24 to 48 hours.

Anesthetic problems can be caused by the absorption of CO_2 or the physiological effects of the pneumoperitoneum. Both the intra- and extraperitoneal surfaces can readily absorb CO_2 and may cause hypercarbia. End tidal CO_2 monitoring by the anesthesia team can often identify this problem before it becomes clinically significant. Increasing the minute ventilation can usually keep the blood CO_2 levels in a safe range. Barotrauma can be minimized by keeping the insufflation pressures in general less than 12 mm Hg. High intraabdominal pressure (prolonged periods above 15 to 20 mm Hg) can interfere with cardiac output and respiration. High pressures can also result in subcutaneous emphysema that can exacerbate hypercarbia, and on occasion cause pneumomediastinum and pneumothorax. Oliguria may occur in patients with increased intraabdominal procedures. This is usually transient, however, and the urge to aggressively hydrate the patient should be avoided.

Life-threatening gas embolism is rare and most often caused by direct insufflation of CO_2 gas into a vessel by the Veress needle. Subtle collection of CO_2 gas in the venous system through an open vessel can rarely occur. The use of an esophageal Doppler monitor of the right atrium can detect free intravascular gas. Detailed information of the management of laparoscopic complications is available (1).

Results

In a recent review of over 1,085 diverse urologic laparoscopic procedures, the current overall complication rate was 7%. Transfusions were required in less than 1% of procedures, while open conversion was necessary in only 2% (11). Vascular (n=7) and bowel (n=11) complications made up a significant percentage of the 75 total complications. Proper patient selection, formal training, surgeon's experience, and working with others who are involved with laparoscopic surgery appear to be the best determinants for a successful outcome in urologic laparoscopy (9).

Laparoscopic surgery can be more technically demanding and time consuming than open surgical intervention. However, it is the patient who ultimately benefits from this minimally invasive technique with shorter hospital stay, less postoperative pain, a more cosmetic result, and more rapid return to full activities.

REFERENCES

1. Abdel-Meguid TA, Gomella LG. Complications of laparoscopy: Prevention and management. In: Smith AD, ed., *Smith's Textbook of Endourology*. St. Louis, MO: Quality Medical Publishers, 1996:851–857.
2. Capelouto CC, Moore RG, Silverman SG, Kavoussi LR. Retroperitoneoscopy: anatomical rationale for direct retroperitoneal access. *J Urol* 1994;152:2008.
3. Gaur DD. Laparoscopic operative retroperitoneoscopy: Use of a new device. *J Urol* 1992;148:1137.
4. Gaur DD, Rathi SS, Ravandale AV, Gopichand M. A single-centre experience of retroperitoneoscopy using the balloon technique. *BJU Int* 2001;87:602–606..
5. Gill IS, Grune MT, Munch LC. Access technique for retroperitoneoscopy *J Urol* 1996;156:1120.
6. Mullet CE, Viale JP, Sagnard PE, et al. Pulmonary CO_2 elimination during surgical procedure using intra- or extraperitoneal CO_2 insufflation. *Anesth Analg* 1993;76:622.
7. Nakada SY, Fadden P, Jarrard DF, Moon TD. Hand-assisted laparoscopic radical nephrectomy: comparison to open radical nephrectomy. *Urology* 2001;58:517–520.
8. Pietrow PK, Albala DM. Hand-assisted urological laparoscopy. *Curr Opin Urol* 2002;12:233–237.
9. See WA, Cooper CS, Fisher RJ. Predictors of laparoscopic complications after formal training in laparoscopic surgery. *JAMA* 1993;270:2689.
10. Shalhav AL, Dunn MD, Portis AJ, Elbahnasy AM, McDougall EM, Clayman RV. Laparoscopic nephroureterectomy for upper tract transitional cell cancer: the Washington University experience. *J Urol* 2000;163:1100–1104.
11. Soulie M, Salomon L, Seguin P, Mervant C, Mouly P, Hoznek A, Antiphon P, Plante P, Abbou CC. Multi-institutional study of complications in 1085 laparoscopic urologic procedures. *Urology* 2001;58:899–903.
12. Winfield H, Lund GO. Extraperitoneal laparoscopic surgery: Creating a working space. *Contemp Urol* 1995;7:17–22.
13. Wolf JS Jr, Merion RM, Leichtman AB, Campbell DA Jr, Magee JC, Punch JD, Turcotte JG, Konnak JW. Randomized controlled trial of hand-assisted laparoscopic versus open surgical live donor nephrectomy. *Transplantation* 2001;72:284–290.
14. Wolf JS Jr, Seifman BD, Montie JE. Nephron sparing surgery for suspected malignancy: open surgery compared to laparoscopy with selective use of hand assistance. *J Urol* 2000;163:1659–1664.

CHAPTER 114

Laparoscopic Pelvic Lymph Node Dissection: Transperitoneal and Extraperitoneal Approaches

Pasquale Casale and Leonard G. Gomella

First described in the early 1990s, laparoscopic pelvic lymph node dissection (LPLND) was considered a breakthrough in the surgical staging of prostate cancer. Throughout the mid-1990s, this was the most frequently performed laparoscopic urologic procedure. Historically, LPLND provided an entrée into the field of laparoscopy and provided an opportunity for the urologic surgeon to master the laparoscopic skills necessary for more advanced procedures such as nephrectomy and pyeloplasty. With the introduction of laparoscopic radical prostatectomy, there is renewed interest in laparoscopic pelvic lymphadenectomy.

The dramatic changes in the demographics of prostate cancer has led to a decline in the clinical application of LPLND for staging prostate cancer. However, there remain clinical scenarios where LPLND is a useful surgical technique. When combined with laparoscopic radical prostatectomy, LPLND may be used depending on the patient's risk factors. Laparoscopic node dissection can also be used in situations where knowing the exact histological status of the pelvic nodes might alter treatment (i.e., decisions to perform brachytherapy or external beam radiation therapy, cryoablation of the prostate, penile and urethral cancer staging, melanoma staging, etc.). The technique of both trans- and extraperitoneal LPLND techniques will be described.

DIAGNOSIS

LPLND is in itself a diagnostic procedure.

INDICATIONS FOR SURGERY

The most common indication for LPLND is the need to assess the pelvic lymph nodes in patients with prostate cancer who have a significant risk of metastatic disease and where the determination of node status histologically may impact the treatment plan. Those patients at highest risk of nodal involvement based on guidelines such as the Partin tables may benefit the most (2). In general, LPLND is potentially most useful for any patient with a Gleason score of 7 or higher, prostate-specific assay (PSA) greater than 20 ng per mL, and advanced clinical T stage, independently or in combination.

LPLND may be performed prior to radical perineal prostatectomy to accurately assess nodal status. Laparoscopic mobilization of the seminal vesicles has been described in association with node dissection and the most difficult part of the perineal dissection can be completed by this approach. LPLND may be implemented prior to cryoablation of the prostate depending upon the patient's risk factors. Other malignancies may also be staged with LPLND, including bladder, penile, and urethral carcinomas. Patients with transitional cell carcinoma of the bladder and radiological evidence of pelvic lymphadenopathy that is inaccessible to computed tomography (CT)-guided biopsy may have LPLND to correctly stage their disease. Patients with adenocarcinoma or squamous cell carcinoma may also benefit.

Penile cancer metastasizes to the superficial and deep inguinal lymph nodes, with metastases to the iliac lymph nodes suggesting a worse prognosis. Some authors recommend bilateral pelvic lymphadenectomy as the initial staging procedure for all patients with invasive penile cancer and palpably enlarged inguinal lymph nodes. Positive nodes from an LPLND might eliminate the need for an inguinal dissection with its associated morbidity. Urethral cancer often presents in advanced stages, more commonly in women. The proximal urethral lymphatics drain to the external and internal iliac lymph nodes, as well as the obturator nodes, which can be sampled with LPLND when indicated prior to radical exenteration. In the case of melanoma, LPLND has become an excepted technique. Both intra- and extraperitoneal approaches are used in the diagnosis of malignant melanoma. It was found useful in stage I with high risk of metastasis (Clark I–IV; Breslow greater than 0.76 mm), stage II, and stage III to evaluate efficacy of systemic treatment (7).

Contraindications to transperitoneal lymphadenectomy potentially include the inability to tolerate a general anesthetic or pneumoperitoneum (due to heart or lung disease), extreme obesity, large intraabdominal masses, ileus or obstruction, extensive lower-abdominal surgery, aneurysmal disease, previous vascular graft surgery, history of peritonitis, bleeding dyscrasias, and diaphragmatic hernia, to name a few.

For the extraperitoneal approach, in addition to being unable to tolerate a general anesthetic, previous lower-abdominal surgery may obliterate the space of Retzius to make exposure to the preperitoneal space difficult. Bleeding dyscrasias may lead to pelvic hematomas after development of the space of Retzius. There may be increased CO_2 absorption during extraperitoneal LPLND, but this point is not clear. While this can in general be managed with increased respiratory rate and tidal volume by the anesthesiologist, it may become a more serious problem in those patients with poor cardiopulmonary reserves. Compromised cardiopulmonary function should serve as a relative contraindication to the extraperitoneal approach.

ALTERNATIVE THERAPY

Open pelvic lymphadenectomy is considered the standard for lymph node sampling. Percutaneous needle biopsy can be considered to confirm the presence of enlarged lymph nodes due to prostate cancer metastasis.

SURGICAL TECHNIQUE

Transperitoneal Lymphadenectomy

Adequate preoperative counseling should include the risks and benefits of LPLND, as well as the alternative approaches. This discussion should include the commonly recognized injuries and the possibility of conversion to an open procedure. The patient undergoes routine preoperative evaluation, including a type and screen for blood products. A mechanical bowel preparation cleanses the bowel in case of a bowel injury and serves to decompress the bowel to improve laparoscopic exposure. Patients are given milk of magnesia the afternoon before and a Fleet's enema the morning of the procedure. Patients are encouraged to avoid dairy products 2 days prior to the procedure to help control intestinal gas. Broad-spectrum antibiotics (such as ceftriaxone) are given preoperatively and for several doses postoperatively.

The basic laparoscopic technique has been well described previously in chapter 113A. General endotracheal anesthesia is administered and an orogastric tube and Foley catheter are placed. The patient is positioned supine on the operating table with a roll of towels under the buttocks and the table is flexed slightly to allow easier access to the pelvis. The entire abdomen is prepped from pubis to the subcostal area. Gentle Trendelenburg positioning will displace the small intestine out of the operative field. Rolling the table to the opposite side of the dissection also helps improve visualization. Wide adhesive tape is used across the thighs and chest to secure the patient to the operating table during the procedure. Ensure that the tape does not have direct contact with the skin. Intermittent pneumatic compression stockings are applied to help prevent deep venous thrombosis.

The abdomen is prepared and draped widely in the event that a laparotomy needs to be performed. Include the external genitalia in the prep field because manual decompression of the scrotum is sometimes necessary in cases of pneumoscrotum. The pneumoperitoneum is established by using a Veress needle or by the open Hasson technique, based on surgeon's preference and the patient's risk factors. Initial insufflation pressure is 15 to 18 mm Hg. A 10-mm laparoscopic port is placed through the initial incision in the infra- or supraumbilical crease. This incision is in general made longitudinal in the event that it needs to be extended for laparotomy. Next, a 10-mm, 0- or 30-degree laparoscope is inserted. The abdominal cavity is examined for laparoscopic access injury or evidence of any pathology. Adhesions may need to be lysed prior to placement of the other ports. For most patients, three additional ports are sufficient, placed in a diamond configuration (Fig. 114–1A). The 10/11-mm suprapubic port is placed 3 to 5 cm above the symphysis pubis and the two 5-mm lateral ports are placed midway between the umbilicus and the anterior superior iliac spine off the lateral border of the rectus abdominis muscle. For more obese patients, five ports can be used, resulting in a horseshoe configuration (Fig. 114–1B). The additional port is often useful for retraction. After ports are placed, the pressure is decreased to 12 to 15 mm Hg.

Place the patient in a 30-degree Trendelenburg position with the table rolled laterally 15 to 30 degrees, resulting in the elevation of the operative side. This position allows the bowel to be displaced by gravity toward the head and the contralateral side, thus enhancing exposure. The sigmoid and cecum may be somewhat adherent to the pelvic sidewall and must be mobilized before the exposure is suitable. This is accomplished by incising along the white line of Toldt and moving the large bowel medially.

The key laparoscopic landmarks for LPLND are the obliterated umbilical artery, the internal inguinal ring, and the vas deferens. The external iliac and gonadal vessels are often identified coursing beneath the posterior peritoneum. Incise the peritoneum high up over the pubis midway between the obliterated umbilical artery and the

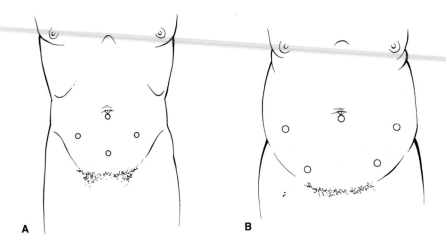

FIG. 114–1. A: The standard diamond configuration for trocar placement with the laparoscope placed in the subumbilical position. **B:** The horseshoe configuration is useful for obese patients.

internal inguinal ring. The incision in the peritoneum extends cephalad, medial to the external iliac vein to just proximal to the bifurcation of the iliac vessels (Fig. 114–2). Tactile identification of the pubic ramus is initially performed and then gentle stripping of the loose areolar tissue allows its visualization. The vas deferens usually crosses in the middle of the incision and is divided with electrocautery or cut and clipped if it is obstructing the dissection.

Next, the lateral aspect of the node package is developed by sweeping the fibroadipose tissue from the medial and anterior surfaces of the external iliac vein using sharp

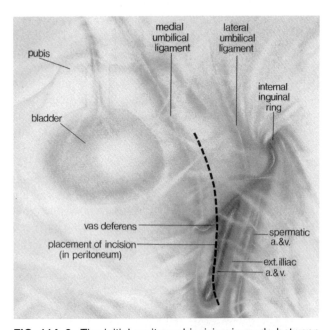

FIG. 114–2. The initial peritoneal incision is made between the obliterated umbilical artery (medical umbilical ligament) and the internal inguinal ring. (From Gomella LG, et al., eds. *Laparoscopic urologic surgery*, 1st ed. Philadelphia: Raven Press, 1994:117, with permission.)

and blunt dissection as needed (Fig. 114–3). Begin this maneuver at the pubis and work proximally toward the bifurcation of the iliac vessels. An accessory obturator vein branching from the external iliac vein near the pubis is seen in up to 40% of patients and can be clipped or spared depending on how readily the distal node package can be mobilized. Caution is needed proximally where the ureter crosses the iliac vessels, usually at the common iliac bifurcation.

The medial aspect of the nodal package is developed by gentle medial retraction of the obliterated umbilical artery and blunt dissection of the underlying tissue toward the iliac vessels. The obturator nerve should come into view and can be bluntly cleared of lymphatic tissue. As the medial aspect is freed, the distal nodal tissue can be thinned and lifted upward. Near the pubis there frequently are venous variations that can be easily injured. Careful use of cautery and hemoclips allows the node package to be freed while obliterating the transected lymphatics. The obturator nerve must be identified, with any nodes stripped carefully away from the nerve. Caution is needed because the obturator artery and/or vein can be injured at this point. The nodal package is grasped at its distal extent and retracted anterior and cephalad. The dissection is then completed to the level of the iliac vessel bifurcation, where the proximal lymphatic vessels are clipped or cauterized. Once completely free, the nodal tissue is grasped with laparoscopic Russian or spoon forceps and delivered through a 10/11-mm port with a gentle twisting motion. The port valve must be manually opened to avoid shredding the tissue. The specimen can also be placed in a laparoscopic specimen retrieval pouch and delivered through the 10/11 port.

The obturator fossa should resemble the configuration seen after standard open pelvic lymphadenectomy. The fossa is inspected for residual lymphatic tissue and persistent bleeding. The table is rolled laterally in the opposite direction and the procedure repeated on the contralateral side. Frozen section evaluation may be useful

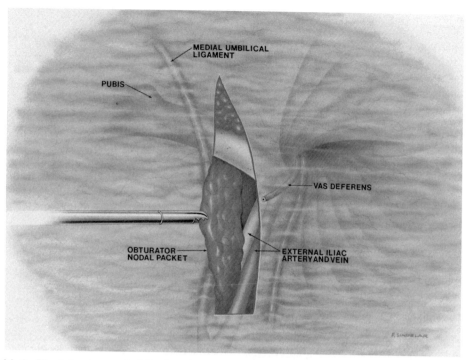

FIG. 114–3. The lateral aspect of the lymph node package is carefully dissected from the external iliac vein using medial retraction on the package. (From Gomella LG, et al., eds. *Laparoscopic urologic surgery*, 1st ed. Philadelphia: Raven Press, 1994:118, with permission.)

depending on the intraoperative findings and the indications for surgery. When both sides have been completed, the entire abdominal cavity is again inspected for inadvertent injury and persistent bleeding. The intraabdominal pressure is lowered to 5 mm Hg to identify any bleeding previously tamponaded by the pneumoperitoneum. The ports are removed and the incisions closed according to the surgeon's preference (see Chapter 113A).

Extraperitoneal Lymphadenectomy

Preliminary experience with LPLND approached the target organs through the peritoneum in contrast to open urologic surgery, which is confined mostly to the extraperitoneal (pre- and retroperitoneal) spaces. While early reports have supported the use of laparoscopic techniques for a variety of procedures, significant complications, such as bowel or vascular injuries, can occur when utilizing the transperitoneal approach. As a result, an extraperitoneal approach has been investigated for a variety of procedures, including pelvic lymph node dissection, urethral, and renal procedures. A number of factors support the extraperitoneal approach. Open extraperitoneal pelvic lymphadenectomy has been shown to be superior to the transperitoneal approach in terms of patient tolerance, reduced morbidity, and fewer postoperative complications (3). In addition, adhesions in the pelvis as a result of transperitoneal surgery could contribute to bowel injury from subsequent radiation therapy.

Principles of extraperitoneal laparoscopy are reviewed in Chapter 113A.

Several authors have reported on the extraperitoneal LND technique (1,12). The procedure can also be performed as part of an extraperitoneal laparoscopic radical prostatectomy. After the space is developed as described in Chapter 113A, the balloon is deflated and the trocar removed. Next, a 10-mm Hasson style cannula is placed. The CO_2 insufflator is attached and set on high flow at 8 to 10 mm Hg pressure, which is maintained throughout the actual procedure. Inspection of the preperitoneal space usually confirms adequate dissection of the iliac vessels and the pubic arch with minimal bleeding. The right side typically dissects more completely than the left. However, a minimal amount of blunt dissection will expose the vessels on the left side.

Additional trocars are placed under direct vision. The pressure is briefly increased to 15 to 20 mm Hg to facilitate secondary trocar placement. Prolonged pressure at this level may cause tracking of the gas into the subcutaneous tissues. A diamond configuration similar to transperitoneal lymphadenectomy is used: two 10-mm ports laterally and a 5-mm port in the midline. The lateral ports are placed approximately one-third of the way between the anterior superior iliac spine and the umbilicus and the midline port is placed approximately 2 to 3 cm above the pubis, using the same precautions (transillumination, visual inspection for vessels, etc.) as for standard laparoscopic techniques. It is critical to ensure that the lateral ports do not traverse the peritoneal cavity and they are beyond the peritoneal reflection. The right lower quadrant is typically placed first to allow easy blunt dissection of the left side of the pelvis prior to the placement of the left lower-quadrant trocar. After the trocars are placed, the pressure can be decreased to 10 to 12 mm Hg.

The anatomic landmarks for preperitoneal lymphadenectomy are identical to those of a standard open modified pelvic lymphadenectomy. The symphysis pubis and bladder can be identified in the midline and pubic bone can be followed laterally on each side to identify the deep inguinal rings. The external iliac artery pulsations are also easily identified. A modified obturator pelvic lymph node dissection through the extraperitoneal approach is used that is familiar to most urologic surgeons. The limits of the dissection are proximally the bifurcation of the iliac vessels, distally the circumflex iliac vein, and inferomedially the obturator nerve.

The operating surgeon is positioned on the contralateral side of the area of dissection. The patient is placed in slight Trendelenburg position and rotated toward the surgeon. The procedure is started by an incision in the fibroareolar tissue along the medial side of the external iliac artery. Blunt medial dissection identifies the external iliac vein and defines the lateral edge of the nodal package. The vas deferens is typically seen crossing obliquely across the incision and can be clipped and divided if needed. Dissection is carried out along the external iliac vein, developing the lymph node package both proximally and distally. At the distal edge of the packet, careful dissection is carried out to identify any accessory obturator vessels.

The obturator nerve is identified at the posteromedial border of the dissection. The nodal package is dissected proximally, as one piece, off the obturator fossa and nerve. The exposure can be optimized by the use of a laparoscopic vein retractor on the external iliac vein. At the intersection of the obturator nerve and the iliac vein, blunt and sharp dissection are used to develop the proximal extent of the nodal package, with clips used to seal the proximal lymphatics. Removal of the package is accomplished by the use of large grasping forceps or a laparoscopic specimen retrieval pouch through a 10-mm trocar sheath. The obturator fossa is irrigated and carefully inspected for hemostasis. The identical procedure is repeated on the left side.

At the end of the procedure, the trocar sheaths are removed under direct observation and the port sites closed as described for the transperitoneal approach. The scrotum is manually compressed if there is evidence of pneumoscrotum before the last trocar is removed. A drain may be placed in the space of Retzius and brought out through the 5-mm port site if needed. Postoperative management is identical to the transperitoneal laparoscopic approach, with the diet rapidly advanced and discharge within 24 hours.

POSTOPERATIVE CARE

All patients are admitted to the hospital for a brief (less than 24 hours) observation and receive two more doses of prophylactic antibiotics. The orogastric tube is removed prior to extubation and the diet is advanced as tolerated. The Foley catheter is removed once the patient is alert and oriented. If a drain is placed, it can be removed once the output has decreased. Routine postoperative nursing care is important for detecting any complications (e.g., delayed bleeding). Patients are in general discharged within 24 hours and return to normal activity within 1 week.

OUTCOMES

Complications

Complications of LPLND include all of the problems encountered in general laparoscopic surgery, including vascular and visceral injuries (5,6,9,11). In addition, there are certain problems that are more specific to this procedure. In working near the bladder, there is increased risk of bladder injury if the dissection is carried too far medial to the obliterated umbilical artery. The ureter is at risk for injury (especially thermal injury) while dividing the lymphatic branches near the bifurcation of the iliac vessels. Troublesome bleeding may occur from the accessory obturator veins, the obturator vessels (if dissecting below the obturator nerve), or the iliac vein itself. Postoperatively, there is the expected risk of lymphocele formation, although this does not seem to be higher than in open PLND. The extraperitoneal approach minimizes the risk of bowel injury.

In the large series, the rate of conversion to open PLND ranges from 3% to 5%, with factors such as obesity and history of previous surgery or radiation contributing to the need for laparotomy. In a multicenter study of 372 patients undergoing LPLND, there were 55 complications (15%). Laparotomy was required in 13 of these patients, 7 at the initial operation and 6 at a later date (9). All authors agree that there is a steep learning curve and the majority of problems and conversions occur early in each surgeon's experience. With increased skill in laparoscopic suturing techniques, some repairs (e.g., closure of a small enterotomy) may be undertaken without laparotomy and the rate of laparotomy and complications will fall further.

Results

There are several large series published that demonstrate LPLND is a safe and effective procedure (4,8,10,13). A mean laparoscopic retrieval of 4.6 and 4.5 nodes from the right and left sides, respectively, is typical. The time for the procedure is now in general less than 90 minutes and patients are usually discharged within 24 hours. Blood loss and postoperative analgesic requirements are minimal.

LPLND has been demonstrated to be a safe and effective procedure in the hands of many urologists at different institutions. While the indications for LPLND have declined somewhat, we believe this procedure will continue to play a significant role in the staging of urologic malignancies.

REFERENCES

1. Abdel-Meguid TA, Gomella LG. Extraperitoneal laparoscopic lymphadenectomy: Insufflative and gasless techniques. In: Eden C (ed.), *Extra-peritoneal laparoscopic surgery*. Oxford, UK: Blackwell Scientific, 1997:31–45.
2. Blute ML, Bergstralh EJ, Partin AW, Walsh PC, Kattan MW, Scardino PT, Montie JE, Pearson JD, Slezak JM, Zincke H. Validation of Partin tables for predicting pathological stage of clinically localized prostate cancer. *J Urol* 2000;164:1591–1595.
3. Freiha FS, Salzman J. Surgical staging of prostate cancer: transperitoneal versus extraperitoneal lymphadenectomy. *J Urol* 1977;118:616.
4. Glascock JM, Winfield HN. Pelvic lymphadenectomy: intra- and extraperitoneal access. In: Smith AD, et al., eds. *Smith's textbook of endourology*. St. Louis, MO: Quality Medical Publishing, 1996:870.
5. Gomella LG, Lotfi MA, Ruckle H. Management of laparoscopic complications. In: Gomella LG, Kozminski M, Winfield H, eds. *Laparoscopic urologic surgery*. New York: Raven Press, 1994:257–266.
6. Gomella LG, Taha-Meguid TA, Lotfi MA, Hirsch IH, Albala D, Manyak M, Kozminski M, Sosa E, Stone NN. Laparoscopic urologic surgery: Continued improvement in outcome. *J Laparoendoscop Surg* 1997;7(2):77–86.
7. Jones WO, Cable RL, Gilling PJ. Laparoscopic pelvic lymphadenectomy for malignant melanoma. *Aust NZ J Surg* 1995;65:765–767.
8. Kava BR, Dalbagni G, Conlon KC, Russo P. Results of laparoscopic pelvic lymphadenectomy in patients at high risk for nodal metastases from prostate cancer. *Ann Surg Oncol* 1998;5:173–180.
9. Kavoussi LR, Sosa E, Chandhoke PS, et al. Complications of laparoscopic pelvic lymph node dissection. *J Urol* 1993;149:322.
10. Kerbl K, Clayman RV, Petros JA, Chandhoke PS, Gill IS. Staging pelvic lymphadenectomy for prostate cancer: a comparison of laparoscopic and open techniques. *J Urol* 1993;150:396.
11. Lotfi MA, Kozminski M, Gomella LG. Complications of laparoscopy: Prevention and management. *AUA Update Series* 1993;XII:lessons 31 and 32.
12. Raboy A, Adler H, Albert P. Extraperitoneal endoscopic pelvic lymph node dissection: a review of 125 patients. *J Urol* 1997;158:2202–2204; discussion 2204–2205.
13. Rukstalis DB, Gerber GS, Vogelzang NJ, Haraf DJ, Straus FH, Chodak GW. Laparoscopic pelvic lymph node dissection: a review of 103 consecutive cases. *J Urol* 1994;151:670.

CHAPTER 115

Laparoscopic Varix Ligation

James F. Donovan and Bradley W. Anderson

Treating varicoceles laparoscopically has waxed and waned in popularity since first reported in 1988. Recent advances in technology (improved lighting and optic transmission) and instrumentation (small 3- to 5-mm trocars and 3-mm instruments) have made laparoscopic varix ligation a modality that is unquestionably less invasive than all other surgical approaches and equal in efficacy.

DIAGNOSIS

Grade III (grossly visible) and grade II (palpable without special maneuvers) varicoceles are the most easily detected and are relevant in settings of both infertility and discomfort. Grade I varicoceles (palpable impulse on performance of the Valsalva maneuver) are more subtle and are relevant in the setting of infertility only. The significance with regard to infertility of the so-called "subclinical" varicocele (detectable only by ultrasonography, thermography, or other radiological techniques) is more controversial. Arguments for and against repair have been made, and as yet no consensus exists.

INDICATIONS FOR SURGERY

The indications for varix ligation are the same irrespective of intended treatment modality (laparoscopic or open surgery or transvenous ablation). Patients with palpable varicoceles who fulfill the following criteria can be offered varicocelectomy:

1. Scrotal pain not attributable to other pathology.
2. Male factor infertility manifested by some degree of oligoasthenospermia and/or failure to impregnate a female who is free of demonstrable female factor infertility during 1 year of unprotected intercourse.
3. Adolescent testicular growth retardation.
4. Grades II and III varicoceles in the prepubescent male. While prophylactic ligation of varicoceles in the postpubertal male is not recommended, Richter and associates suggest prophylactic repair in the prepubertal male may improve testis growth and future fertility (12).

The incidence of varices is approximately 15% in the adult male population, but the majority of these men will suffer neither male factor subfertility nor pain due to varicocele. Therefore, prophylactic ligation of varices is not recommended in the adult male. In general, the repair of subclinical varicoceles is not recommended in any patient group, although Pianalto and associates assert that subfertile males undergoing ligation of a palpable varix may benefit in terms of improved seminal fluid measures and pregnancy by simultaneous repair of contralateral subclinical varix (10). Perhaps the only contraindication to the laparoscopic repair of varicoceles is a prior high varix ablation (open or laparoscopic). Laparoscopic and high retroperitoneal (Palomo) varix ligations expose the spermatic veins just above the internal ring; second surgeries in this location would encounter scar and adhesions, making the operation more difficult and possibly increasing the probability of complication. Further, scarring and fibrosis would make the identification of collateral spermatic veins missed in the first attempt unlikely.

Obesity or prior abdominal surgery are considered relative contraindications by some but are not insurmountable impediments to an experienced and diligent laparoscopist. One exception is prior laparoscopic inguinal hernia repair with mesh. Adhesions are dense following placement of mesh in the retroperitoneal space behind the internal ring and Hasselbach's triangle. These patients should avoid secondary procedures in close proximity to prosthetic mesh.

ALTERNATIVE THERAPY

Alternate approaches to varicocele management include subinguinal–microscopic (Marmar–Goldstein)

(4,7), inguinal (Ivanissevitch) (5), open retroperitoneal or high ligation (Palomo technique) (9), and transvenous embolization (8).

SURGICAL TECHNIQUE

A general anesthetic is administered and the patient placed in the supine position with arms adducted. The abdomen is prepped from xiphoid to genitalia. Having access to the genitalia is helpful, allowing manual traction on the involved testis to visually identify the extent of the spermatic vessels, which tend to be fanned out somewhat under the peritoneum. If one sees an unexpectedly distended bladder upon entry to the abdomen, access to the genitalia can also allow simple in-and-out catheterization.

Access to the peritoneum for insufflation may be performed by Veress needle puncture or open insertion of a Hasson cannula. These techniques are reviewed elsewhere. Both novice and veteran laparoscopists advocate the use of the Hasson cannula for reasons of safety in the direct visual approach. We prefer the Veress needle in the majority of cases in part because we wish to use 5-mm rather than the 10.5-mm laparoscope; thus, the Hasson cannula is overkill. We do consider the Hasson technique in patients who have undergone previous abdominal surgery.

After insufflation and insertion of the subumbilical trocar, we insert the laparoscope and thoroughly inspect the peritoneal contents with special attention to the viscera underlying the site of Veress needle insertion. Optimal sites for right and left lateral trocars are identified and local anesthetic instilled along the path of trocar insertion. The recommended locations are two symmetrical sites just outside the rectus muscle and slightly inferior to the umbilicus (Fig. 115–1). Placing the lateral trocars too far cephalad may put the point of varix ligation beyond the reach of available instruments while trocar sites too far caudad may impede the use of graspers and scissors trapped within the trocar sheath.

The instruments most useful in dissection are a curved-tip scissors and a curved-tip (Maryland) grasper. A blunt probe can on occasion be used to sweep vessels together into a single package or lift and stabilize the vessel package. While suture ligation of the vessels is possible, a 5-mm disposable clip applier makes the procedure go more quickly. Careful note should be made of the means of operation of the clip applier used because some have an open end that allows partial ligation of a large packet of veins (e.g., US Surgical, Norwalk, CT) while others have a wraparound design (e.g., Ethicon) that can only be used on packets sufficiently small. Other useful instruments include a 5-mm laparoscopic Doppler probe (Meadox, MedSonic) to identify and locate the testicular artery. Advanced coagulation and dissecting systems such as a harmonic scalpel, LigaSure, and Gyrus bipolar cautery

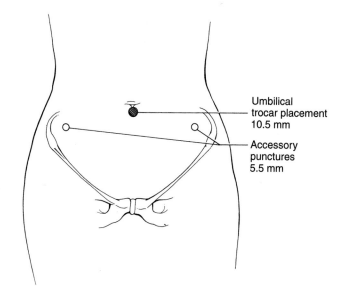

FIG. 115–1. Appropriate position of trocars for varix ligation. The array of trocars is used in either left or bilateral varix ligation. The subumbilical trocar is either a Hasson cannula for open laparoscopy or a standard trocar inserted following Veress needle insufflation. The operating trocars are 5.5 mm when a 5-mm clip applier is available or 10 mm when one must rely upon a 10.5-mm hemoclip applier.

(manufacturer?) have been used as the sole means of dividing the spermatic vessels, but these disposable instruments increase the cost of the operation and are rarely, if ever, necessary in the absence of extensive adhesions.

After placement of the trocars, the spermatic vessels are identified. Looking through the peritoneal membrane, the spermatic vascular bundle traverses the internal ring, joining the vas deferens. When necessary, we will lyse adhesions and mobilize the sigmoid colon to gain exposure just cephalad to the internal ring. The Trendelenburg position can be a useful maneuver to achieve optimal exposure. Gentle intermittent traction on the affected testis allows the surgeon to delineate the lateral and medial extent of the spermatic vessels. We make a 3- to 5-cm peritoneal incision just lateral and parallel to the vascular bundle, with a caudal limit of 3 cm above the internal ring (Figs. 115–2 and 115–3). With the contralateral hand, one grasps the medial edge of the peritoneal incision, raising it medially and anteriorly. Using the ipsilateral hand, the closed tips of the scissors gently sweep the vessels off the undersurface of the peritoneal flap. This medial flap is then bisected perpendicular to the lateral incision, leaving a "T-shaped" defect that completely exposes the underlying vascular bundle (Fig. 115–4). Testicular traction confirms the limits of the spermatic vascular bundle, and blunt instruments are used to sweep all the vessels together into a single packet. The iliac arteries, genitofemoral nerve, vas deferens, and inferior epi-

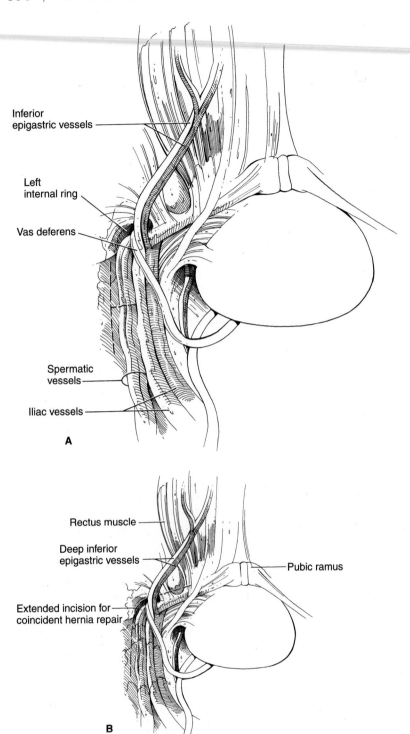

Inferior
epigastric vessels

Left
internal ring

Vas deferens

Spermatic
vessels

Iliac vessels

A

Rectus muscle

Deep inferior
epigastric vessels

Extended incision for
coincident hernia repair

Pubic ramus

B

FIG. 115–2. A: A 3- to 5-cm incision through the peritoneum is made lateral to the spermatic vascular bundle and extends cephalad from a point 3 to 5 cm above the internal ring. **B:** When a coincident laparoscopic inguinal hernia repair is planned, the peritoneal incision extends anterior and lateral to the internal ring and continues anterior and medial to reach the lateral edge of the rectus muscle.

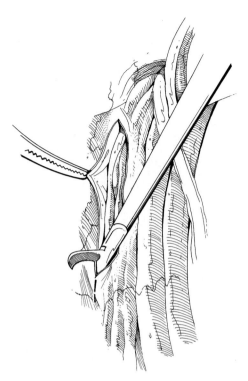

FIG. 115–3. Incision through the peritoneum lateral to the spermatic vascular bundle. Traction upon the testis will define collateral vessels traversing the internal ring, which should be ablated. The extent of planned varix ligation should be determined prior to performing the initial peritoneal incision.

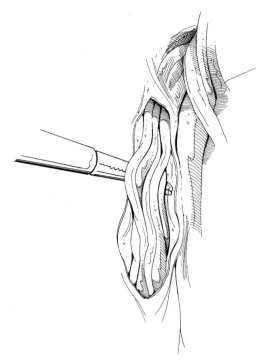

FIG. 115–5. The entire spermatic vascular bundle is mobilized from the underlying psoas muscle. A combination of sharp and blunt dissection facilitates separation of the spermatic vessels from surrounding tissues. One should avoid deep dissection to spare the underlying genitofemoral nerve crossing anterior to the psoas muscle.

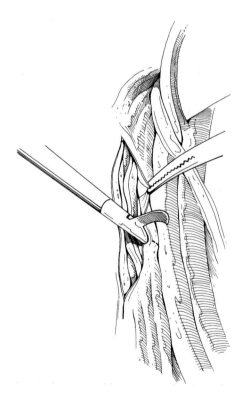

FIG. 115–4. The medial peritoneal flap is lifted and the spermatic vessels swept from the underlying surface. A medial incision bisects the peritoneal flap and provides exposure of the underlying spermatic vascular bundle.

gastric vessels are close enough to be theoretically at risk, but strict attention to the limits of dissection described should render such injuries exceedingly rare.

The entire spermatic vascular bundle is then freed from the underlying psoas muscle using gentle blunt dissection (Fig. 115–5). At this point, either an artery-sparing technique or a mass ligation technique is used.

Artery-Sparing Technique

The spermatic vascular bundle is first bluntly and gently separated into medial and lateral bundles. Adequate length on the separation of the two bundles is necessary, usually at least 2 cm. Close inspection will reveal the pulsation of the spermatic artery in one of the bundles. An instrument must be used to lift the spermatic vessels off the underlying iliac artery to dampen transmission of the adjacent iliac artery pulse. Once the bundle containing the artery is identified, the vascular bundle not containing the artery is divided between clips or ligatures (Fig. 115–6). The laparoscopic Doppler probe can also assist in the process of identification.

The remaining vascular bundle is divided into two smaller bundles and the location of the spermatic artery pinpointed. The process is repeated until the spermatic artery is skeletonized (Fig 115–7). This process can be

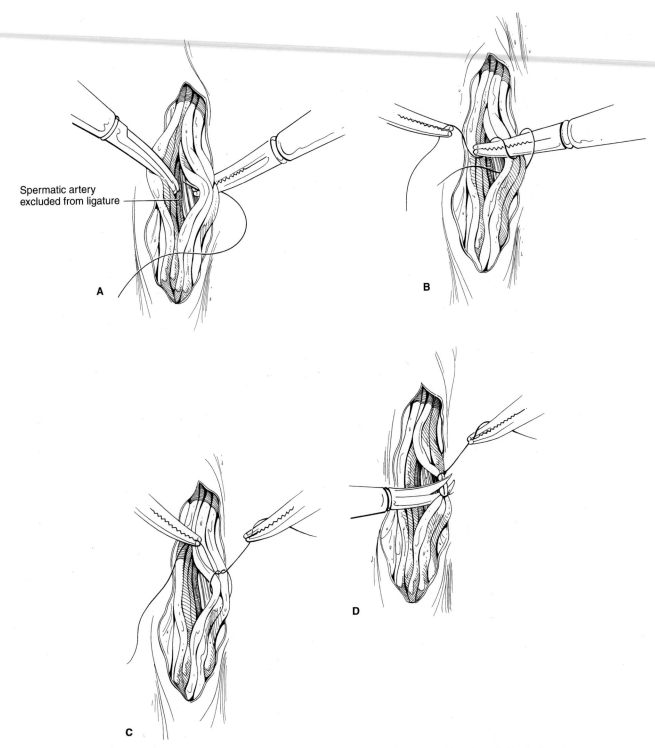

Spermatic artery
excluded from ligature

A

B

C

D

FIG. 115–6. A: The vascular bundle that does not contain spermatic artery is ligated and then divided. For small venous aggregates or single spermatic veins, the 5-mm reusable clip applier is utilized. Otherwise, we prefer suture ligature. A 5- to 10-cm ligature is passed into the abdominal cavity. One end is passed from right to left under the vessels to be ligated, extending only 1 cm beyond the vessels. The other end is long to facilitate instrument tie. **B:** The long end is grasped by the left-hand instrument, allowing sufficient slack to permit easy wrapping around the tip of the right-hand instrument. The instrument tie can be accomplished with two curved dissectors with tips rotated up. Alternatively, instruments specifically designed for laparoscopic suture and ligation may be used. **C:** The nonarterial vascular bundle is ligated. **D:** The spermatic veins are divided between ligatures.

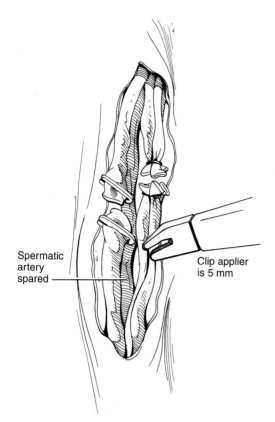

FIG. 115–7. Upon completion of the procedure, all spermatic veins have been ligated and divided by either clip or suture. Only the spermatic artery(ies) remain and arterial patency is documented by Doppler.

tedious due to the small caliber of the artery and the presence of adherent venules. Preservation of the artery should not distract from the primary objective, which is ablation of all spermatic veins. In some cases, the artery will be sacrificed to complete the varix ligation. Finally, we inspect the operative field while retracting the testes to identify any spermatic veins that have escaped ablation. Cautery may be used with appropriate care to protect adjacent structures.

Mass Ligation Technique

Alternatively, the surgeon may prefer mass ligation of the spermatic vessels (laparoscopic Palomo technique.) This approach sacrifices the spermatic artery intentionally, anticipating adequate collateral arterial supply from the artery to the vas deferens and/or the cremasteric artery. While the testicular artery is not a contributing cause of subfertility in the male with varicocele, preservation of the testicular artery does not appear to improve outcome with regard to restoration of fertility following varix ligation. We would exercise caution in patients whose collateral circulation may be compromised by prior inguinal or scrotal surgery (e.g., herniorrhaphy or vasectomy).

The procedure is similar to that described above with the exception of segregation of artery and nonartery vascular bundles. Once the packet of spermatic veins is mobilized, splitting into several smaller bundles is performed without any attempt to identify the spermatic artery. The entire spermatic vascular envelope may be mass ligated with 2-0 silk intracorporeal ties or smaller vascular bundles can be clip ligated and divided. This process is quick in comparison to arterial preservation.

An orderly exit from the abdomen requires a reduction of insufflation pressure and inspection of the field for bleeding. The lateral trocars are removed under direct laparoscopic vision, inspecting for bleeding. After complete desufflation of the abdomen, the camera and umbilical trocar are slowly removed, inspecting for bleeding on the way out. If a 10-mm trocar has been used, a 5-mm 45-degree laparoscope is inserted through one of the lateral trocars and the 10-mm defect closed with 2-0 PDS suture using a Carter trocar; sites 5 mm and smaller do not require fascial closure. We close skin incisions 5 mm in size with subcuticular 4-0 absorbable sutures and steristrips or close with Dermabond. If scrotal emphysema is present, we eliminate with brief compression.

Needlescope Technique

A needlescope technique can be used to further minimize the invasiveness of the procedure. The above general procedure is used with few modifications. It is possible to do the entire procedure through three needlescopic ports (2- or 3-mm working ports), ligating the veins with suture. The advantages of being able to use a 5-mm clip applier are considerable, so we continue to use a 5-mm port at the umbilicus but prefer an Interdyne trocar system, which uses a radially expanding sheath that leaves a fascial defect of approximately 4 mm rather than the 6- to 7-mm defect resulting from standard trocars with a 5-mm inner working diameter.

All trocar sites are anesthetized with Marcaine 0.5% with epinephrine. We make a 4-mm incision through the inferior umbilicus. Gentle blunt dissection exposes the linea alba. We place a 2-0 absorbable suture on either side of the midline followed by a punctate incision just long enough to accept the Veress needle, which is inserted while retracting upward on the midline sutures. After CO_2 insufflation to a pressure of 15 mm Hg, the Veress needle is removed and reinserted after loading an Interdyne sheath. A 5-mm trocar is inserted to radially expand the Interdyne outer sheath. Following insertion of the 5-mm laparoscope, lateral needlescope trocars are placed. There are disposable 2-mm ports and instruments (e.g., US Surgical) available, but we have found that Storz 3-mm reusable trocars and instruments are more sturdy and usable. Only small skin incisions are necessary.

If performing artery-sparing ligation with needlescope instruments, it is necessary to grasp the vascular packet to gain circumferential control. Because the artery is usually found in the medial portion of the spermatic vessel complex, grasping the lateral edge of the packet and retracting lateral and upward is considered safe. So, gently grasping a fine lateral edge of the vascular bundle and retracting it anteriorly is quite safe. Close inspection of the bundle prior to picking up an edge prevents unintentional arterial injury.

To perform a non–artery-sparing ligation of the entire bundle, the bundle is freed from the underlying psoas in the usual fashion. Through the ipsilateral needlescope port, a blunt instrument or probe lifts the bundle anteromedially. Using a 5-mm hemoclip (US Surgical) inserted through the subumbilical port, we double-clip the distal and proximal spermatic vascular bundle and divide the tissue. Typically, 5-mm clips will not enclose the entire vascular bundle, necessitating repeated sequences of clip ligation and division stepwise to complete the transection. The 5-mm camera is replaced at the umbilicus, and final inspection and exit are performed as described above. The inner sheath of the Interdyne trocar is removed, collapsing the outer expandable sheath, which is then gently removed after assuring complete desufflation. The two traction sutures can be tied to each other, although fascial closure of a 5-mm Interdyne port is unnecessary. The needlescopic ports require only a small sterile adhesive strip or skin cement. A single subcuticular suture and a sterile adhesive strip suffice for closing the umbilical port.

Our experience has been that 2- and 3-mm lateral ports cause virtually no discomfort at any time postoperatively. The 5-mm Interdyne umbilical trocar causes discomfort for only a couple of days.

OUTCOMES

Complications

Due to the age group involved, perioperative complications are rare. Potential complications include bleeding, a need to convert to an open procedure, infection, testis atrophy or loss, and failure to correct the varicocele. Even with successful correction of the varicocele (i.e., absence of a palpable varix at 6 months following surgery), signs and/or symptoms that prompted the operation (orchalgia, oligoasthenospermia) may persist. Operative times vary based upon extent of operation (unilateral or bilateral), complexity of repair (artery sparing > artery sacrifice),

and laparoscopic experience (novice > expert). With experience, non–artery-sparing procedures will last 15 to 30 minutes and artery-sparing procedures will last 45 to 60 minutes. Patients are discharged on the day of surgery without restrictions in physical activity.

Results

A recent large randomized trial comparing open to laparoscopic varix ligation revealed similar outcomes in terms of efficacy and complications but clear advantages in terms of pain and recovery time (11), and other nonrandomized large series corroborate these findings; further, results indicate that spermatic arterial ligation did not influence response and did not result in testicular atrophy (1,3).

The controversy regarding laparoscopic varix ligation (2,6) is moot now that 5-mm expandable sheath trocars and/or needlescopes and needle trocars have replaced the large 10-mm trocars used during the early days of laparoscopic repairs. The relative cost of laparoscopy has also plummeted with the increase in laparoscopic applications and the advent of more sophisticated reusable instruments. As a safe, effective, and minimally invasive procedure, laparoscopic varix ligation is an important part of the urologist's laparoscopic arsenal.

REFERENCES

1. Bebars GA, Zaki A, Dawood AR, El-Gohary MA. Laparoscopic versus open high ligation of the testicular veins for the treatment of varicocele. JSLS 2000;4:209–213.
2. Donovan JF Jr. Laparoscopic varix ligation [Editorial]. Urology 1994;44:467–469.
3. Esposito C, Monguzzi G, Gonzalez-Sabin MA, et al. Results and complications of laparoscopic surgery for pediatric varicocele. J Pediatr Surg 2001;36:767–769.
4. Goldstein M, Gilbert BR, Dicker AP, et al. Microsurgical inguinal varicocelectomy with delivery of the testis: an artery and lymphatic sparing technique. J Urol 1992;148:1808.
5. Ivanissevich O. Left varicocele due to reflux: experience with 4470 operative cases in forty-two years. J Int Coll Surg 1960;34:742.
6. Jarow JP. Varicocele repair: low ligation. Urology 1994;44:470–472.
7. Marmar JL, DeBenedictis TJ, Praiss D. The management of varicoceles by microdissection of the spermatic cord at the external inguinal ring. Fertil Steril 1985;43:583.
8. Murray RR Jr, Mitchell SE, Kadir S. Comparison of recurrent varicocele anatomy following surgery and percutaneous balloon occlusion. J Urol 1986;135:286.
9. Palomo A. Radical cure of varicocele by a new technique: preliminary report. J Urol 1994;61:604.
10. Pianalto B, Bonanni G, Martella S, et al. Results of laparoscopic bilateral varicocelectomy. Ann Ital Chir 2000;71:587–591.
11. Podkamenev VV, Stalmakhovich VN, Urkov PS, et al. Laparoscopic surgery for pediatric varicoceles: randomized controlled trial. J Pediatr Surg 2002;37:727–729.
12. Richter F, Stock JA, LaSalle M, et al. Management of prepubertal varicoceles—results of a questionnaire study among pediatric urologists and urologists with infertility training. Urology 2001;58:98–102.

CHAPTER 116

Standard Laparoscopic Nephrectomy and Nephroureterectomy

David I. Lee, Jaime Landman, and Ralph V. Clayman

Laparoscopic nephrectomy is commonly being applied in most cases of benign renal disease and in a growing percentage of patients in whom a radical nephrectomy is indicated for renal cell cancer. A natural extension of this technique has been the development of laparoscopic nephroureterectomy for upper-tract transitional cell carcinoma (TCC) or, less commonly, benign disease. This chapter describes the indications, technique, postoperative management, complications, and results of laparoscopic nephrectomy and nephroureterectomy.

LAPAROSCOPIC NEPHRECTOMY: TRANSPERITONEAL AND RETROPERITONEAL

Diagnosis

Renal masses are commonly discovered as incidental findings on screening radiological imaging. Computed tomography (CT) scans or magnetic resonance imaging (MRI) are sufficient in characterization of the local extent of the mass. Prior to the procedure, a chest radiograph and CT scan (with and without contrast) are obtained as part of a metastatic evaluation. The CT scan is examined for liver metastases, lymphadenopathy, and renal vein or vena caval involvement and to assess the adrenal glands. Preoperative blood work includes a serum creatinine, liver function studies, alkaline phosphatase, and calcium levels. If the last two values are elevated or the patient complains of site-specific bone pain, a bone scan is obtained. Nuclear medicine renography is usually performed to evaluate function in a kidney that is expected to be poorly functioning

Indications for Surgery

Laparoscopic nephrectomy for a renal tumor was introduced by Clayman et al. (9) in 1990; in experienced hands, this approach has become an accepted alternative to traditional open radical nephrectomy for small and midsized renal masses without evidence of renal vein or inferior vena caval involvement (i.e., T1 and T2 renal tumors). Also, nearly any nonfunctioning kidney that requires removal can be approached in this fashion. Further, at many institutions the laparoscopic approach has become the standard for performing donor nephrectomy. Recently, it has also been successfully applied to the removal of polycystic kidneys. The only relative contraindication is xanthogranulomatous pyelonephritis (3).

Alternative Therapy

Open radical nephrectomy is the preferred alternative therapy. Recent experience in nephron-sparing procedures has validated partial nephrectomy as a viable alternative in patients with renal masses 4 cm or smaller in size. Ablative technologies such as cryotherapy, radiofrequency (RF) ablation, and high-intensity focused ultrasound (HIFU) are being utilized and are under close investigation.

Nephrectomy: Patient Preparation and Positioning

A formal bowel preparation is not routinely performed, but a clear liquid diet is advised for the day prior to the procedure and a Dulcolax suppository is given on the day prior to surgery. One gram of cefazolin (Ancef) is administered preoperatively. In the obese patient or the individual with a history of deep venous thrombosis, 5,000 U of heparin are administered subcutaneously 2 hours prior to the procedure and continued on a 12-hour basis postoperatively until the patient is ambulatory. At the outset of the procedure, just prior to any skin incision, 30 mg of ketorolac (Toradol) is given intravenously.

General endotracheal anesthesia is induced and the patient's stomach and bladder are decompressed with an orogastric tube and Foley catheter, respectively. Pneumatic compression stockings are applied to both legs. The patient is carefully positioned in a 70-degree flank position with the affected kidney on the upside. The operating table is fully flexed and the kidney rest is fully raised beneath the iliac crest. Use of orthopedic table braces to support the patient at the shoulder and hip are helpful for maintaining the patient securely in the flank position. The downside leg is flexed at the knee and separated from the extended upside leg by pillows; the upside leg is placed on a sufficient number of pillows until it is level with the flank, thereby precluding any strain on the upside leg when the table is flexed and the kidney rest raised. The downside heel, hip, and knee are cushioned. The downside arm is padded and an axillary roll is carefully positioned. The upside arm is placed on a well-padded armboard; the armboard is positioned such that there is no tension on the brachial plexus. Once the patient has been properly positioned, he/she is secured to the operating table by *padded* safety straps that are passed over the chest, hip, and knee.

Surgical Technique

Transperitoneal Radical/Total Nephrectomy

Access

For right or left renal access (Figs. 116–1 and 116–2) a 12-mm incision is made approximately two finger breadths medial and cranial to the anterior superior iliac spine. Other potential sites for initial access include a midclavicular line subcostal approach (as described by M. Stoller) or, in the thin patient, a transumbilical placement. The subcutaneous tissue is spread with a Kelly clamp and the anterior rectus fascia is secured with two Allis clamps. A Veress needle pneumoperitoneum of 25 mm Hg is obtained. Alternatively, the pneumoperitoneum may be obtained using an open or endoscopic cannula technique. A 12-mm trocar is placed at this same site (Fig. 116–1, port site I) and the abdominal pressure is reduced to 15 mm Hg. A 10-mm 30-degree laparoscope is inserted and the underlying viscera and bowel are closely inspected for any injury that may have occurred during Veress needle or initial trocar placement. Subsequently, two additional 12-mm trocars are placed under direct endoscopic vision: 2 cm below the costal margin in the midclavicular line and immediately lateral to the margin of the rectus abdominus muscle approximately three to five finger breadths above the umbilicus. Last, after mobilization of the colon from the abdominal sidewall, a fourth trocar (5 mm) is commonly placed subcostal in the posterior axillary line. For right-sided nephrectomies, a fifth trocar may be placed in the midline approximately 2 to 4 cm below the xiphoid (optional) to help with liver

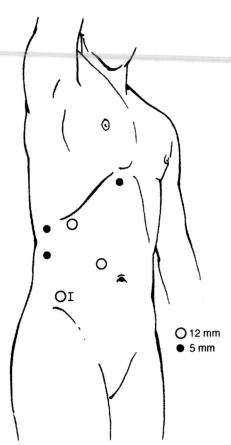

FIG. 116–1. Diagram demonstrating port sites used for right transperitoneal nephrectomy. White circles, 12-mm port sites; I, insufflation port; black circles, 5-mm port sites. The optional upper midline 5-mm port may be used for liver retraction, while the lower lateral optional port is only used if there is difficulty with specimen entrapment in a LapSac.

○ 12 mm
● 5 mm

retraction (Fig. 116–1). Similarly, if at the end of the procedure there is difficulty entrapping the specimen, another port (5 mm) can be placed just above the iliac crest.

With regard to trocars, at present only nonbladed trocars are used at our institutions. The design of these trocars eliminates the need to use any suture to fix them in place and, except for midline ports, precludes fascial closure at the end of the procedure.

Laparoscopic Radical Nephrectomy

Right Side

The peritoneal cavity is closely inspected. The liver is visualized for mass lesions. The outline of the kidney within Gerota's fascia is commonly visible behind the ascending colon.

Step 1. Peritoneal incisions and pararenal dissection. The key to *en bloc* resection of the kidney within Gerota's fascia lies in defining the borders of the dissection. On the right side the dissection follows an anatomic template

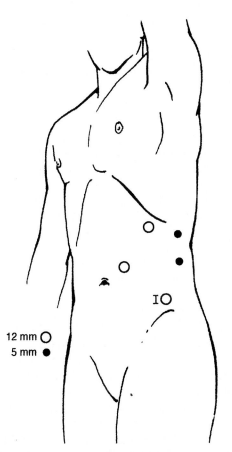

FIG. 116–2. Diagram demonstrating port sites used for left transperitoneal nephrectomy. I, 12-mm insufflation port; white circles, 12-mm port sites; black circles, 5-mm port sites. The lower 5-mm port site is optional; it is only placed if there is difficulty with specimen entrapment in a LapSac.

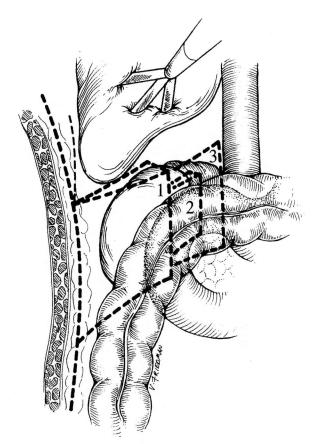

FIG. 116–3. Diagram of the right-sided nephrectomy demonstrating the wedge-shaped configuration. The numbers refer to the three distinct levels of dissection along the medial aspect of the kidney: colon, duodenum, and inferior vena cava. Note that on the right side the line of Toldt paralleling the kidney is left intact; this is done to preclude the kidney from falling medial and obscuring the renal hilum.

with a "wedge-shaped" configuration (Fig. 116–3). The narrow edge of the wedge lies laterally, along the line of Toldt. The dissection is initiated using a 5-mm curved harmonic forceps and atraumatic grasping forceps for countertraction. The harmonic forceps is preferred for the majority of the dissection as it provides excellent hemostasis with minimal associated peripheral thermal injury to surrounding tissues, especially the ascending colon. The line of Toldt is incised beginning at the pelvic brim; this incision is carried upward to the lower pole of the kidney, at which point the incision is continued medially staying approximately 2 to 3 cm away from the ascending colon; this defines the lower border of the wedge as well as the first of three planes of dissection that define the medial broad portion of the "wedge." The colon is thus completely mobilized away from the kidney as the hepatic flexure of the colon is also mobilized medially. As such, the lateral border of the kidney and its lateral retroperitoneal attachments are not disturbed; this results in the kidney remaining firmly attached to the abdominal sidewall, thereby facilitating the hilar dissection later in the procedure. The incision in the line of Toldt is contin-

ued cephalad from the upper pole of the kidney up to the level of the diaphragm. At this time, the triangular ligament of the liver is also divided up to the diaphragm, thereby mobilizing the lateral aspect of the right lobe of the liver and completing the medial-based narrow portion of the wedge.

The broad side of the wedge comprises three distinct levels of dissection along the medial aspect of the kidney (Fig. 116–3): (a) the mobilized ascending colon, (b) Kocher maneuver on the duodenum to move it medially, and (c) dissection of the anterior and right lateral surfaces of the inferior vena cava (IVC). The duodenum may appear flattened against the medial aspect of the kidney; it is important to move slowly during this part of the dissection to clearly identify the duodenum. Also, the surgeon should be cognizant that the duodenum *must* always be dissected away from the kidney *before* the anterior surface of the vena cava can be identified. It is important to identify the cava at this level to orient the surgeon to the path of the cava, which at times can be medial and closely applied to the kidney. To facilitate development of the third and deepest plane of dissection (i.e., the IVC dissection), it is helpful to first define the superior side of the wedge by incising the posterior coronary hepatic ligament from the line of Toldt, laterally, to the level of the IVC, medially; this incision is usually done approximately 1 to 2 cm away from the liver itself. At this cephalad level, the surgeon will come directly onto the lateral and anterior surface of the IVC well above the duodenum and the adrenal gland. At this point, the *en bloc* area of dissection of the specimen has been completely defined, ensuring removal of the kidney within Gerota's fascia, along with the pararenal and perirenal fat, the adrenal gland, and an anterior patch of peritoneum.

Step 2. Securing the gonadal vein. The dissection on the IVC is continued caudally until the entry of the gonadal vein is identified. This vein is circumferentially dissected free from surrounding tissue, secured with four 9-mm vascular clips, and divided between the second and third clips. Alternatively, the 10-mm LigaSure device can be used to divide the gonadal vein. During this portion of the dissection, if one encounters "caval" bleeding it is more than likely due to inadvertent injury to the gonadal vein where it enters the IVC. If this occurs, it is often helpful to raise temporarily the pneumoperitoneum pressure to 25 mm Hg for no more than 10 to 15 minutes; this maneuver appears to effectively decrease venous bleeding significantly and facilitates identification of the venous injury. Also, in the event of a caval injury it is important to notify the anesthesiologist of the problem and request that the patient receive a bolus of intravenous (IV) fluid as, studies by O'Sullivan and colleagues have shown that it is important to keep the patient well hydrated to preclude an air embolus (25).Third, it is helpful to have access to a laparoscopic Satinsky clamp to help control any caval injury.

Step 3. Securing the ureter. The gonadal vein can be traced distally from the vena cava. The right ureter usually lies just posterior and lateral to the right gonadal vein. It is carefully dissected from the retroperitoneal tissues. The ureter can be divided at this point or at the end of the case; four clips are applied and the ureter is divided between clips two and three. During the hilar dissection, it is helpful to grasp the ureter and pull it lateral and anterior, thereby placing the hilum on "stretch." At this point, all of the caudal retroperitoneal attachments to Gerota's fascia can be dissected, thereby freeing the specimen inferiorly.

Step 4. Securing the adrenal vein. Continued cephalad dissection of the IVC exposes the renal hilum and adrenal vein. The adrenal vein is dissected from the surrounding tissue and secured with three 9-mm clips. The adrenal vein is cut such that two clips remain on the caval side. Alternatively, if the supraadrenal area just medial to the IVC has been cleanly dissected down to the diaphragm and the lateral border of the supraadrenal IVC has been identified in this area then once the inferior border of the adrenal has been cleared of tissue an Endo-GIA vascular

load can be used to secure all of the tissue medial to the adrenal and lateral to the IVC, thereby "taking" the adrenal vein in the 3-cm line of vascular staples. Alternatively, the 10-mm LigaSure device can be used to take the adrenal vein.

If one wishes to spare the adrenal gland, then the upper medial border of the kidney needs to be identified. As such, Gerota's fascia in this area is incised. Once the renal capsule of the medial and anterior part of the upper pole is seen, an Endo-GIA stapler can be used to further define the margin of dissection from medial (i.e., IVC side) to lateral below the adrenal gland, thereby preserving the adrenal gland and adrenal vein while rapidly securing and dividing the perirenal fat.

Step 5. The renal hilum. Attention is then turned to the dissection of the right renal vein from the surrounding tissue. At this time it is helpful to place a 5-mm Jarit PEER retractor through the lateral 5-mm subcostal port. The Jarit retractor is placed on the midportion of the kidney at the level of the hilum; the PEER retractor is opened broadly and used to pull the kidney laterally. It is attached to the Endoholder to maintain its position and keep traction on the hilum. This maneuver facilitates the subsequent hilar dissection.

If the IVC has been cleanly dissected, the takeoff of the renal vein is usually evident. The right renal artery is subsequently identified behind the renal vein and dissected circumferentially (Fig. 116–4). The use of the right-angle hook dissector is helpful as tissue can be engaged and lifted away from the underlying vessels prior to its being cut. In this regard, an active electrode monitoring system (Encision, Inc, Boulder, CO) is used to limit the chance of any inadvertent spread of current to the bowel or other structures; with this device, any break in the insulation of the shaft of the hook electrode results in its being disabled. Mobilization of the renal artery must be adequate for comfortable placement of five 9-mm vascular clips; either a linear or right-angle clip applier can be used. The artery is then divided between the second and third clips to leave three clips proximally. If the artery appears to be too broad, 11-mm clips can be used or it can be secured with the Endo-GIA stapler (vascular load). The renal vein is then dissected circumferentially and secured with an Endo-GIA vascular stapler (3-cm load) (Fig. 116–5).

One modification described by Chan and colleagues is to just free the anterior, inferior, and superior borders of the renal artery and then secure it with an Endo-GIA vascular load; however, when doing this it is important for the surgeon to develop the plane of dissection deeply along the upper and lower borders of the renal artery until the muscles of the retroperitoneum can be clearly seen to ensure that the entire width of the artery is secured in the stapler (6). This maneuver saves time by avoiding the dissection of the posterior surface of the renal artery.

On occasion, an adequate length of the renal artery cannot be exposed in the presence of the overlying renal

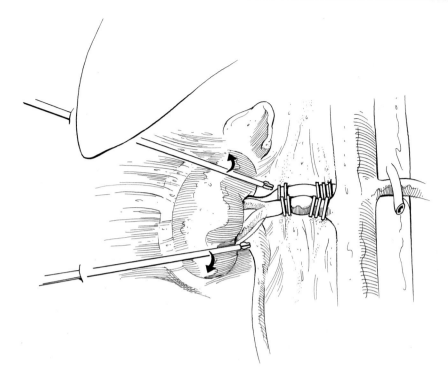

FIG. 116–4. Renal hilar control. The renal artery and vein are individually mobilized and secured with clips on the artery and the Endo-GIA stapler on the vein. Lateral traction on the midportion of the kidney with the Jarit retractor facilitates the hilar dissection.

vein. In this situation one or two clips can be applied across the artery to occlude the artery. Now that the main renal artery is occluded, the renal vein is divided with the Endo-GIA stapler. Then, the artery is further dissected and divided after five clips are applied as previously described, again leaving three clips on the aortic stump of the renal artery.

Rarely, the artery cannot be accessed from the anterior approach. It is then necessary to dissect the kidney laterally, flip the entire specimen medially, and approach the artery posteriorly. In this case, the artery is often dissected further medially, where it crosses beneath the pos-

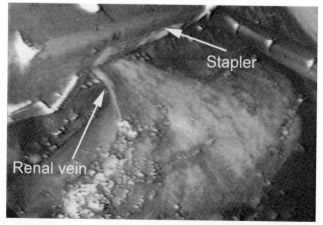

FIG. 116–5. The right renal vein is stapled and cut with an Endo-GIA stapler containing a vascular load.

terior surface of the IVC. Great care must be used in dissecting the anterior surface of the renal artery in this location to not inadvertently injure the IVC.

A third method of approaching the renal artery is to first divide the ureter. The ureter is then held upward, allowing the surgeon to approach the renal artery along its inferior surface first. While this approach is more awkward than the other two, it can be helpful in the case of extensive perihilar adhesions.

Step 6. Freeing the specimen and securing the ureter. The specimen, within Gerota'a fascia, is then freed from the retroperitoneum using electrosurgery, the harmonic dissector, and blunt dissection. At this time, the lateral attachments of the kidney to the abdominal sidewall, which were kept intact at the beginning of the procedure, are incised. At the inferior border of the dissection, if not already done, the ureter is secured with four clips; a locking grasping forceps, passed via the 5-mm subcostal posterior axillary line port, is placed on the ureter above the clips followed by division of the ureter between the second and third clips. Using the locking grasping forceps on the ureter, the entire specimen is moved cephalad until it rests on the anterior surface of the liver. Once in this position, the shaft of the grasping forceps is fixed in place by attaching it to the Endoholder.

Step 7. Entrapment for morcellation. The laparoscope is now moved from the paramedian port to the upper midclavicular line port. An entrapment sack is introduced via the paramedian port and opened just beneath the lower edge of the liver. If specimen morcellation is planned, a LapSac is used. Morcellation should not be performed with any of the other commercially available plastic entrapment sacks as these can be easily perforated with the morcellating forceps; indeed, in a decade the authors have had only two acute bowel injuries during laparoscopic renal surgery: Both occurred when attempting morcellating with the kidney in a plastic sack.

The 8 × 10-in. LapSac is appropriately sized for the majority of renal specimens (i.e., those 1,200 g or smaller). On the back table, a glidewire (i.e., nitinol) is woven through the holes in the edge of the LapSac such that the two free ends exit the edge of the sack at the same point that the blue nylon drawstring exits the edge of the sack. The glidewire greatly facilitates initiation and maintenance of a wide-open entrance to the sack (29). The LapSac is then loaded on the two-tined introducer with the handle aligned with the drawstring and ends of the nitinol guidewire; the tines should stay on the outer surface of the sack. Usually, the sack is rolled counterclockwise from the bottom upward; the handle of the introducer, the two ends of the glidewire, and the nylon drawstring should all be parallel to one another and on the same side of the sack. As the 8 × 10-in. LapSac will not pass through a 12-mm trocar, the trocar is removed and the entrapment sack is passed through the 12-mm abdominal incision, deeply into the abdomen and pelvis, and then unfurled by twirling the introducer clockwise. Following the removal of the LapSac introducer, the 12-mm trocar is replaced. Using two atraumatic grasping forceps, the LapSac is completely unfolded and flattened within the abdomen. Now two traumatic, locking 5-mm grasping forceps are introduced and the upper and lower tabs on the mouth of the LapSac are grasped. The LapSac is opened broadly such that its inferior edge is pulled just beneath the edge of the liver with the traumatic grasper passed via the midline 12-mm port, while the apex of the sack is pulled anterior via the lower midclavicular line port. The laparoscope can be passed into the LapSac, and with circular motions the entrapment sack is further opened. The specimen is then rolled off of the liver into the mouth of the sack; the forceps on the ureter is directed at the forceps holding the upper tab of the sack. As the specimen enters the sack, the forceps on the inferior edge of the sack's mouth is moved slightly cephalad and anterior to trap and push the specimen deeper into the sack.

If entrapment using a two-instrument approach is difficult, then a fifth right trocar (5 mm) is placed just above or at Petit's triangle. Now, the LapSac is opened using three points of fixation; a traumatic locking grasping forceps is then placed on each of the three tabs. When the sack is opened in this manner, the middle grasper pulls the lip of the sack upward against the underside of the abdominal wall, forming the apex of a tent-like opening in the sack; the medial and lateral 5-mm graspers are used to pull the bottom of the sack in either direction, respectively, while displacing the sack posterior, thereby creating the base or floor of the tent, which runs parallel with

the edge of the liver. The base of the sack is then positioned further posterior and cephalad until it lies just under the lower edge of the liver. The surgeon now moves the ureteral grasper toward the grasper on the apex of the sack. In doing this, the specimen rolls off of the liver and into the sack; as this occurs, the assistant holding the medial and lateral graspers on the sack moves the base of the sack anterior, thereby pushing the specimen deeper into the sack (Fig. 116–6). Specimen entrapment in this manner requires three people: the surgeon, who controls the ureteral grasper and thus guides the specimen into the sack; the camera operator to hold the laparoscope and the middle grasper on the sack (apex of the triangle); and an assistant to hold the medial and lateral graspers (base of the triangle) on the sack (Fig. 116–7). While tedious, specimens up to 1,200 g have been successfully entrapped in this manner.

If intact removal is planned, then a 15-mm Endocatch II (US Surgical, Inc, Norwalk, CT) or Endopouch (Ethicon, Inc, Cincinnati, OH) (Fig. 116–8) is introduced and opened just beneath the liver. The self-opening design of this entrapment sack facilitates the entrapment process; however, it should not be used if mechanical morcellation is planned. It is all too easy to perforate the posterior "unseen" section of the plastic sack with even a ring forceps and proceed to "blindly" damage the viscera around the sack. The 15-mm entrapment sack cannot be passed through a 12-mm trocar. As such, the trocar is removed and the barrel of the 15-mm entrapment sack deployment mechanism is gently passed through the trocar incision site under direct endoscopic vision.

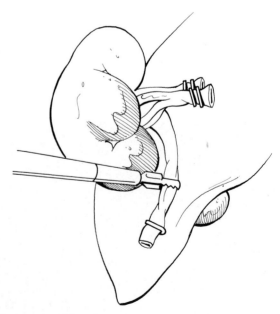

FIG. 116–6. The excised kidney is secured by a locking traumatic forceps on the proximal ureter. The ureter is used as a handle to place the kidney over the liver or spleen in preparation of placement into the LapSac.

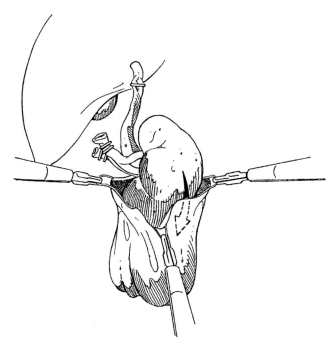

FIG. 116–7. The mouth of the LapSac is triangulated open by three graspers. The kidney is then inserted into the sack.

Step 8. Morcellation versus intact removal. If morcellation of the specimen is planned, then the neck of the LapSac is delivered through the upper midclavicular line port. The surgical field around the port site is further isolated by the sequential placement over the neck of the sack of a sterile adhesive "10,10" drape, a fenestrated absorbent towel, and a nephrostomy drape; the neck of the sack is passed through a hole in each of these drapes. These precautions are taken to help prevent possible wound contamination with any "spilled" tumor cells.

The 12-mm port site through which the neck of the sack has been delivered can be enlarged to 20 mm. Mechanical morcellation with a ring forceps and a Kelly clamp can then be performed. With the 2-cm opening, the tissue can be fragmented under the direct vision of the

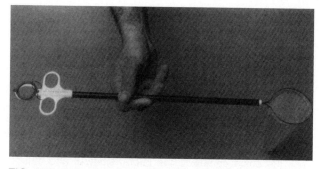

FIG. 116–8. Endocatch device. The polyurethane pouch is attached to the flexible, self-opening metal ring. The Endocatch is available in two sizes; the Endocatch II is larger and more applicable to kidney entrapment.

surgeon. However, again, it is essential for the camera operator to be ever vigilant of any loss of pneumoperitoneum implying puncture of the LapSac. If the LapSac is perforated, then the port site incision is immediately enlarged so the remainder of the specimen within the LapSac can be delivered immediately and intact. At Washington University, this has occurred in only two cases during the past 10 years; in both cases the perforation was identified immediately and the leakage from the sack was scant.

After completion of morcellation the surgeon and all other members of the surgical team who participated during morcellation should regown and reglove. Using this technique over the past decade, the authors have not experienced a wound seed or peritoneal contamination in any of their renal cell cancer patients.

For intact removal, it is recommended to make a lower midline abdominal or a Pfannenstiel incision. The specimen is then extracted intact within the entrapment sack. One should resist the temptation to connect the medial and lateral upper or lower port sites for extraction purposes. The former will result in a more cephalad and possibly more painful incision, while the latter is a "weaker" incision and may result in a delayed postoperative hernia.

Step 9. Exiting the abdomen. At the completion of the procedure, the pneumoperitoneum pressure is reduced to 5 mm Hg. A careful inspection for bleeding is performed; the dissection site is irrigated. The surgeon should be especially attuned to any "rivulets" of red rising through the clear irrigant; this is a definite sign of ongoing bleeding and should result in a careful search to identify and cauterize the bleeding site. A 5-mm laparoscope is placed through the most lateral port. A laparoscopic needle is introduced and 30 cc of 0.25% Marcaine is instilled along the surgical site and the diaphragm for pain control. Now, the other ports are removed under endoscopic control with the 5-mm 30-degree laparoscope.

If 10-mm or larger bladed trocars were used, then the fascia is closed with a 0 Vicryl suture. This is greatly facilitated by using a Carter–Thomason needle grasper and the conical plastic insert. The latter ensures that the closure sutures pass through the fascia 180 degrees from one another, while the former allows for rapid passage and retrieval of the suture. After placement of each fascial suture, the conical plastic insert is pulled off of the suture and the port is replaced. This facilitates closure of the other 10-mm port sites by allowing a grasping forceps to be used to grasp the suture and feed it into the needle grasper at the time of its second passage through the conical plastic insert. For 5-mm ports in adults, no fascial closure is necessary; likewise, if nonbladed trocars were used the fascia of all nonmidline ports do not, in our experience, require closure. Any midline port 10 mm or larger results in a fascial closure. Once all of the fascial sutures have been placed, then each of the ports is removed under endoscopic control via the 5-mm laparoscope. The fascial sutures are tied. The final port is pulled back to the level of the peritoneum. The 5-mm laparoscope is removed and the CO_2 is evacuated from the abdomen. The final 5-mm port is then removed. Skin sites are closed with a subcuticular absorbable 4-0 suture, steristrips, and a bandage.

Left Side

Step 1. Peritoneal incisions and pararenal dissection. The template for anatomic dissection of the left kidney assumes the configuration of an inverted cone (i.e., a water scooper) (Fig. 116–9). The lateral side of the cone is formed by the line of Toldt that is incised from the pelvic brim, cephalad to the level of the diaphragm. On the left side, the colon appears to cover more of the surface area of the anterior portion of the kidney than on the right side; hence, this incision in the line of Toldt is made uninterrupted throughout the length of the retroperitoneum at the outset of the procedure. There are often adhesions from the descending colon at the splenic flexure to the anterior abdominal wall; these attachments need to be sharply released to carry the incision in the line of Toldt cephalad alongside the spleen and up to the diaphragm. This cephalad incision serves to release any splenophrenic attachments, thereby mobilizing the spleen medially away from the abdominal sidewall.

The medial aspect of the cone is then formed by retracting the peritoneal reflection of the descending colon medially and developing the plane between Gerota's fascia and the colonic mesentery. This natural plane between the mesentery of the descending colon and Gerota's fascia is most easily identified and entered along the lower pole of the kidney or just inferior to the kidney. The colon is mobilized medially and cephalad up to the spleen. The anterior upper curve of the cone is formed by the splenocolic ligament, which is incised to fully mobilize the splenic flexure and thereby move the descending colon medially. The posterior upper curve of the cone is formed by the splenorenal ligament, which is incised to further release the spleen and thus preclude any inadvertent tearing of the splenic capsule. The dissection then follows the plane between the spleen and the superior portion of Gerota's fascia. At this point, the *en bloc* area of dissection has been defined and incorporates all of Gerota's fascia, the para- and perirenal fat, and the adrenal gland.

Of note, incision of the splenorenal ligament may be difficult at this early stage of the procedure. Accordingly, it may need to be performed later in the procedure after the renal vessels have been secured.

Step 2. The gonadal vein. The left gonadal vein is the most important structure to identify during a left nephrectomy as it reliably leads the surgeon to the renal vein. The gonadal vein can most easily be exposed inferiorly; it is then traced up to its entry into the renal vein. If need be, the surgeon can carry the dissection down to the level of the inguinal ring to reliably identify the gonadal vein and trace it cephalad; this maneuver is in particular helpful in the morbidly obese patient with a large amount of

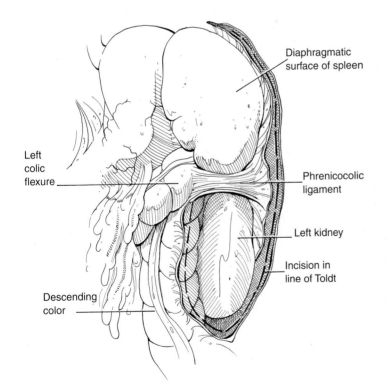

FIG. 116–9. Diagram demonstrating the inverted cone template for *en bloc* dissection during left radical nephrectomy. Unlike on the right side, the reflection of the colon comes to the lateral sidewall and thus an incision in the line of Toldt parallel to the kidney needs to be made; this incision is not carried deeply in an effort to hold the kidney lateral, which helps somewhat with the hilar dissection.

retroperitoneal fat. Anteriorly along the gonadal vein there are rarely any tributaries, thereby providing the surgeon with a safe plane of dissection all the way up to the insertion of the gonadal vein into the main renal vein.

Step 3. Securing the ureter. The left ureter usually lies just posterior and lateral to the gonadal vein. It is carefully dissected from the retroperitoneal tissues and treated in the same manner as the right ureter was for a right nephrectomy.

Step 4. Securing the renal hilum. After tracing the gonadal vein to its junction with the main renal vein, it is secured with four 9-mm vascular clips and divided. Care should be taken to identify the ascending lumbar vein, which may enter the renal vein posteriorly in the area of the gonadal vein or may even join the gonadal vein near its insertion into the renal vein. This vein is likewise secured with four clips and incised. The superior border of the renal vein is then freed by dissection of the adrenal vein; this vein usually lies parallel with or just medial to the insertion of the gonadal vein; the adrenal vein is secured with four 9-mm vascular staples and divided. *It is important to place the clips on these three renal vein tributaries such that they lie at least 1 cm from the main body of the renal vein*; this will facilitate the subsequent safe placement of the Endo-GIA vascular stapler across the renal vein without risking interference of the stapler's function from any of the previously applied clips. If the surgeon inadvertently fires the stapler across a clip, the stapler may "freeze up" and it cannot be properly released (4). In this situation, it may be necessary to convert to an open procedure or proceed to further dissect the renal vein medially to place a second Endo-GIA stapler across the vein; the decision of which way to proceed is dependent upon the surgeon's experience. Alternatively, using the 10-mm LigaSure device, the gonadal, ascending lumbar, and adrenal veins can be occluded and divided; this avoids use of any clips. In the case where the surgeon plans to take the renal artery and renal vein with an Endo-GIA, the LigaSure device replaces the use of a clip applier; the two devices are cost equivalent.

If the surgeon tries to identify the left renal hilum by dissecting the area where it "should be," it is not uncommon for the dissection to drift medially. This can become problematic and, indeed, one may even risk injury to the duodenum, which often lies at the bottom of this "medial hole." Again, the surest way to the renal vein is to trace the left gonadal vein cephalad.

Inferior retraction of the superior border of the renal vein will usually expose the renal artery posterior. The renal artery is dissected free; five 9-mm vascular clips are applied. The artery is then transected between the second and third vascular clips, leaving three clips proximally. Alternatively, the renal artery can be secured using the Endo-GIA vascular stapler following the technique of Chan and Kavoussi (*vide supra*). The renal vein is then secured with the Endo-GIA vascular stapler. Specimen

dissection, entrapment, and morcellation or intact removal are all identical to the description for the right side. The only exception is that the left kidney specimen is displaced onto the anterior surface of the spleen just prior to entrapment.

Transperitoneal Simple Nephrectomy

For right or left simple nephrectomy the approach is similar, however with a triangular, as opposed to a wedge or inverted cone, template. The triangle is based on the line of Toldt on either side. The upper and lower edges of the triangle transect the upper and lower poles of the kidney, respectively; the apex of the triangle is at the vena cava on the right side (origin of the right renal vein) and the aorta on the left side (position where the left renal vein crosses the aorta) (Fig. 116–10).

The dissection is maintained on the renal capsule, thereby separating the adrenal gland from the upper pole. Dissection of the renal hilum on either side is as previously described. The specimen is routinely entrapped and removed intact by extending one of the port sites or morcellated with a ring forceps.

Retroperitoneal Nephrectomy

Access

A 2.0-cm skin incision is created just below and posterior to the tip of the twelfth rib (i.e., in the midaxillary line) and spread further open with a Kelly forceps. The underlying flank musculature is bluntly divided and the underlying thoracolumbar fascia is sharply incised to enter the pararenal fat of the retroperitoneum. It is helpful to use "S"-type or Army–Navy retractors during this portion of the procedure so one can both see and feel the retroperitoneal fat. If the surgeon's index finger is in the retroperitoneal space, he/she should then be able to rotate the finger 180 degrees and assuredly palpate the psoas muscle. Using the index finger, the fat can be further bluntly dissected, following which a balloon dilator is introduced and inflated to 800 cc with room air (Figs. 116–11 and 116–12). During inflation, a 0- or 30-degree, 10-mm laparoscope can be introduced to view the dissection of the tissues by the balloon as it is inflated. If desired, the balloon can then be deflated, repositioned higher or lower in the retroperitoneum, and reinflated to futher increase the available space. The balloon is then deflated and removed. A 10-mm blunt-tip cannula (US Surgical) is inserted and the 30-cc balloon on the distal portion of the cannula is inflated; the soft outer ring of material is then snugged down onto the skin, thereby sealing the body wall between the inner balloon and outer compression ring of the cannula; this tight seal will largely preclude gas leakage into the subcutaneous tissues. The pneumoretroperitoneum is established and the

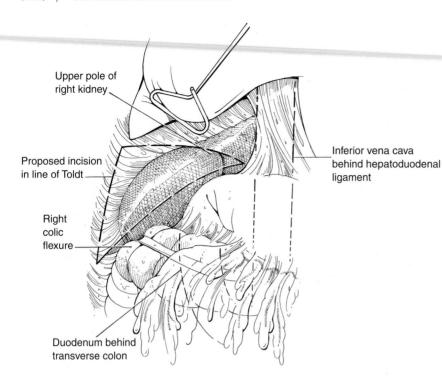

Upper pole of
right kidney

Proposed incision
in line of Toldt

Right
colic
flexure

Duodenum behind
transverse colon

Inferior vena cava
behind hepatoduodenal
ligament

FIG. 116–10. Diagram demonstrating the triangle template used for simple nephrectomy. The lateral border is the line of Toldt. The upper border is the upper pole of the kidney and the lower border is the medial border of the kidney.

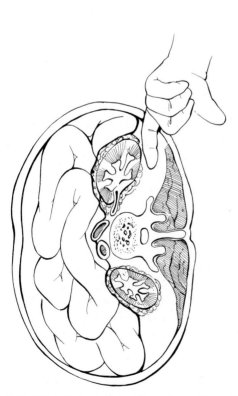

FIG. 116–11. Digital dissection of the retroperitoneal space. This dissection is aimed at creating a space inside Gerota's fascia for subsequent placement of a balloon dilator.

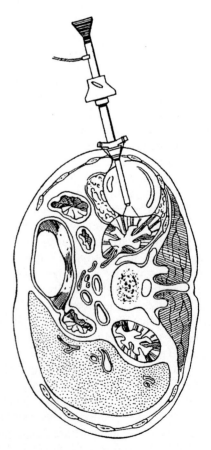

FIG. 116–12. The dissecting balloon is optimally positioned within Gerota's fascia in a posterior direction. Thus, the balloon is placed between the psoas muscle and the kidney or Gerota's fascia as shown.

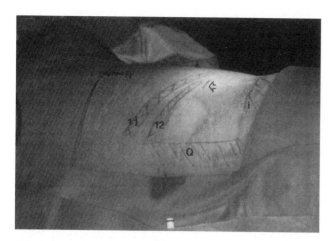

FIG. 116–13. Site of primary trocar placement at the tip of the twelfth rib (black arrow). Patient is placed in the flank position (right side up); the photograph is taken from the patient's back. H, head end of the patient; 11 and 12, 11th and 12th ribs, respectively; Q, quadratus lumborum muscle; I, iliac crest.

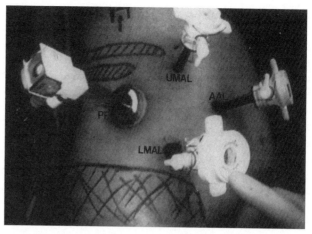

FIG. 116–15. Diamond configuration of port placement during right retroperitoneoscopic nephrectomy. The primary port (PP) is located at the tip of the twelfth rib and is inserted by the open (Hasson) technique. The 12-mm lower midaxillary line (LMAL) port is placed 2 to 3 cm cephalad to the iliac crest. The 5-mm anterior axillary line (AAL) port is placed at the level of the PP. The 5-mm upper midaxillary line (UMAL) port is placed near the tip of the eleventh rib; care must be taken to guard against transpleural placement of this trocar. H, head end of the patient.

10-mm, 30-degree laparoscope is inserted to scan the operative field.

On initial examination, it is usually easy to first identify the psoas muscle. Gerota's fascia and the ureter are typically visible, although this may be difficult in the obese patient or in those patients with any degree of scarring or fibrosis in the retroperitoneal space. A small amount of venous blood overlying the tissues is normal, but there should be no active bleeding.

Accessory ports are placed under endoscopic control (Fig. 116–13). Insertion of additional working ports is performed under endoscopic guidance. Alternatively, Gill described the use of handheld "S" retractors to facilitate digital guidance for placement of additional working ports into the retroperitoneum that may be otherwise difficult to place under direct endoscopic vision (12) (Fig. 116–14).

A 10- or 12-mm port is placed at the lower midaxillary line 2 cm cephalad to the iliac crest, a 5-mm port is placed at the level of the twelfth rib in the posterior axillary line, and a 5-mm port is placed at the level of the eleventh rib on the anterior axillary line. The placement of the ports should form a "T" (Fig. 116–15). Alternatively, ports can be placed only in a subcostal array (three-port approach) or a fifth port can be added anterior to the lower midaxillary line port, thereby creating a "W" array (7). Instrumentation for the laparoscopic retroperitoneoscopic procedure is similar to that for the transperitoneal approach.

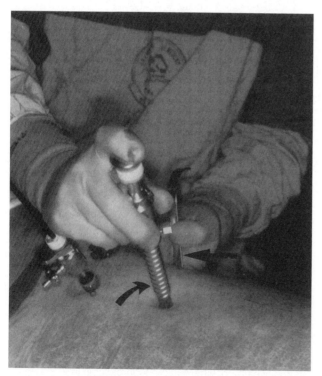

FIG. 116–14. The bimanual technique of secondary trocar (curved arrow) placement during retroperitoneoscopy. The surgeon's finger retracts the peritoneum away from the undersurface of the abdominal wall; the S retractor (straight arrow) prevents trocar injury to the surgeon's finger.

Operative Technique

Visualization of the working field is significantly different than the transperitoneal approach. This field provides few obvious landmarks to orient the surgeon. However, assuming proper dilation of the working space, the kidney will have been displaced anterior. The surgeon should take time to clear the psoas muscle of overlying tissue. As this is done, the surgeon will progress cephalad along the psoas muscle and medially and cephalad the visual pulsation of the renal hilum with the artery presented first should be seen. Gerota's fascia must be incised to gain full access to the hilum; this incision should be created 1 to 2 cm anterior to the psoas muscle.

Dissection is initiated around the renal hilum with sequential control of the renal artery and vein with clip ligation and Endo-GIA stapling, respectively (Fig. 116–16). One caveat is that on the left side the surgeon may encounter the posterior ascending lumbar vein prior to seeing the renal artery; this vein should be dissected, secured with four clips, and then incised. Dependent upon the type of nephrectomy, Gerota's fascia is either left intact (radical/total) or further incised and dissection is continued on the renal capsule (simple). Circumferential mobilization of the kidney is performed. If a radical nephrectomy is planned, then dissection is continued in a cephalad direction that, on the right side, will lead to the adrenal vein, which is secured with three or four clips and divided. On the left side, the adrenal vein is secured with both simple and radical nephrectomies. The ureter is transected between a pair of clips on either side and the

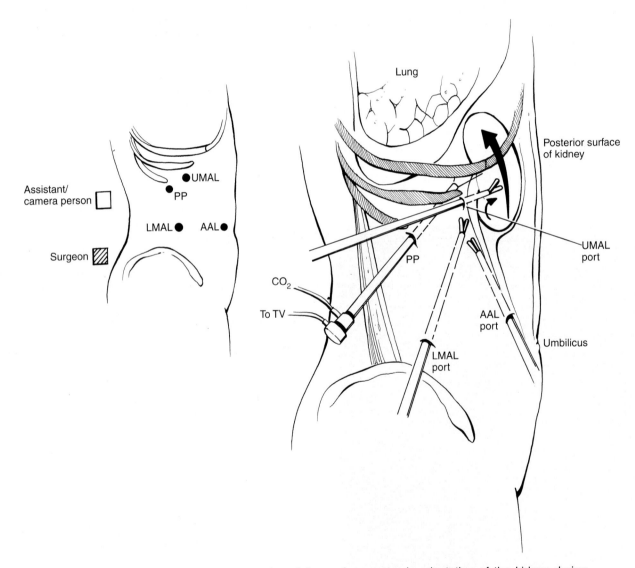

FIG. 116–16. Diagrammatic representation of the end-on anatomic orientation of the kidney during retroperitoneoscopy. Note that the kidney is located above the twelfth rib, whereas the laparoscopic trocars are placed below the twelfth rib. The dark arrow denotes the caudad-to-cephalad direction of retroperitoneoscopic dissection while exposing the kidney. The assistant, working though the upper midaxillary line (UMAL) port, retracts the kidney anteriorly (small arrow). The surgeon works through the lower midaxillary line (LMAL) and anterior axillary line (AAL) ports. The video laparoscope is located in the primary port (PP).

remaining retroperitoneal attachments are divided. Next, if the goal is intact removal then the initial port site is extended, horizontally to 8 to 10 cm, and the entire specimen is retrieved intact after entrapment in a rapidly deployable plastic sack (e.g., Endocatch, US Surgical); alternatively, if morcellation is desired the specimen can be secured in an impermeable sack (i.e., LapSac, Cook Urological, Inc, Spencer, IN). To do the latter, however, often requires opening of the peritoneal cavity to provide sufficient space to maneuver the sack and the specimen.

Entering the peritoneal cavity at some point during the dissection does not require conversion to a transperitoneal technique. The peritoneal cavity is most commonly entered during dissection of the anterior portion of Gerota's fascia. As with the transperitoneal approach to renal surgery, it is important to systematically exit the retroperitoneal space. Following completion of the surgical procedure, the CO_2 pressure in the retroperitoneum is reduced to 5 mm Hg and the operative and port sites are examined to ensure adequate hemostasis. Due to the retroperitoneal approach, the port sites do not require a fascial suture closure. The ports are removed under direct visualization. The port sites are irrigated with saline and the skin closed with a subcuticular 4-0 nonabsorbable suture.

Postoperative Care

Patients receive 15 mg of ketorolac (Toradol) IV every 6 hours as requested, for 36 hours, as well as an oral narcotic as necessary. Diet is resumed immediately with clear fluids and advanced as tolerated. The patient is ambulated on postoperative day 1. Discharge is routinely planned for the evening of postoperative day 1 or the morning of postoperative day 2 provided the patient is passing flatus. Parenteral antibiotics are stopped on postoperative day 1. The patient is discharged on oral analgesics. Of note, it is not uncommon for these patients to develop some constipation postoperatively; as such, use of a Dulcolax suppository as needed and sending the patient home on a stool softener (e.g., Colace, one tablet twice a day) is recommended.

TRANSPERITONEAL RADICAL NEPHROURETERECTOMY

Indications for Surgery

Nephroureterectomy is indicated in cases of TCC of the upper ureter and renal pelvis provided the patient has a normal functioning contralateral kidney. Recently, attention has been given to trying to preserve the affected kidney, even in the face of a normal contralateral kidney, if the disease is papillary and low grade. While highly efficacious for disease control, the open nephroureterectomy results in significant pain and an extended convalescence. Laparoscopic radical nephroureterectomy was introduced by Clayman et al. in 1991 (8).

Patient Preparation and Positioning

The patient preparation is identical to that for laparoscopic radical nephrectomy. However, the patient is informed that an incision will definitely be made to retrieve the specimen intact for staging purposes as high-stage disease would result in a recommendation for postoperative chemotherapy. Patient positioning is similar to that of the transperitoneal laparoscopic nephrectomy. Preoperatively, cystoscopy should be performed to evaluate the lower urinary tract for TCC.

Surgical Technique

Insufflation and Port Placement

Insufflation is performed as described previously for radical, usually in the anterior axillary line three to four finger breadths above the iliac crest. Templates for trocar positioning for both right and left renal access are presented in Figures 116–17 and 116–18. A 10-mm, 30-

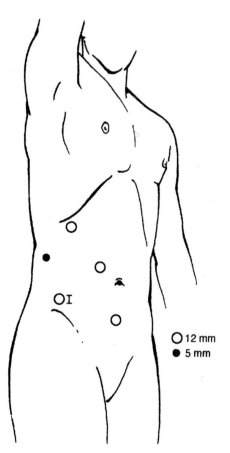

○ 12 mm
● 5 mm

FIG. 116–17. Diagram demonstrating port sites used for right transperitoneal nephroureterectomy. White circles, 12-mm port sites; I, insufflation port; black circles, 5-mm port sites. The optional lateral 5-mm port may be used for liver retraction, while the lower lateral optional port is used for facilitating ureteral dissection.

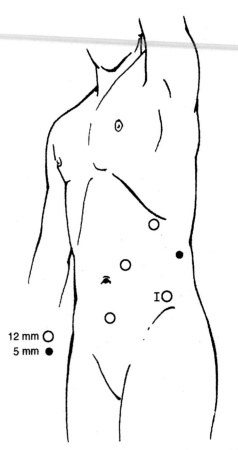

12 mm ○
5 mm ●

FIG. 116–18. Diagram demonstrating port sites used for left transperitoneal nephroureterectomy. I, 12-mm insufflation port; white circles, 12-mm port sites; black circles, 5-mm port sites. The lower 12-mm port site is placed for pelvic dissection.

degree laparoscope is inserted and the underlying bowel is closely inspected for any injury that may have occurred during Veress needle or trocar placement. Subsequently, two additional 12-mm trocars are placed under direct endoscopic vision: 2 cm below the costal margin in the midclavicular line and either at the umbilicus or immediately lateral to the margin of the rectus abdominus muscle approximately three to five finger breadths above the umbilicus. The medial trocar site is used during the majority of cases for the laparoscope as it is midway between the two "working" trocar sites and thus provides the surgeon with an intuitive perspective of the operative field. Last, after mobilization of the colon from the abdominal sidewall a fourth trocar (5 mm) is placed subcostally in the posterior axillary line to aid in retraction. At the end of the procedure, during mobilization of the ureter, another 12-mm port may be placed either in the midline midway between the symphysis pubis and the umbilicus or alternatively in the midclavicular line off the rectus muscle three to four finger breadths below the umbilicus.

Laparoscopic Nephroureterectomy

After access has been obtained the laparoscopic dissection of the kidney proceeds as has been described during the laparoscopic total nephrectomy. The dissection is completed leaving Gerota's fascia intact over the kidney; however, in most cases the adrenal gland is spared. The only exception to this would be for an upper-pole large tumor or if the ipsilateral adrenal gland is not normal on the preoperative CT scan. The nephrectomy is identical to the above descriptions except the ureter is left intact.

After mobilizing all renal attachments and dissecting the proximal and middle ureter, the patient can be placed in the Trendelenburg position, allowing gravity to facilitate the deep pelvic dissection. The ureter is grasped and gently pulled; the harmonic forceps is used to dissect the lower ureter from surrounding tissues. The dissection proceeds caudally over the iliac vessels; the superior vesical vessels that cross the ureter are also secured and divided. The vas or round ligament is identified and divided, as is the ipsilateral medial umbilical ligament. This opens access to the area of the ureterovesical junction.

There are several techniques for distal ureteral management, which are reviewed in subsequent sections. Currently, our preferred technique involves fine dissection of the distal ureter to the level of the intramural ureter or ureteral tunnel. The harmonic shears is especially helpful for this maneuver as it can be used to make a vertical incision through the intramural tunnel at the 12-, 3-, 6-, and 9-o'clock positions, thereby allowing the surgeon to dissect the ureter down to the ureteral tunnel but not through the ureteral tunnel (method of Y. Ono, Nagoya, Japan). An Endo-GIA stapler (tissue load) is then applied to the distal ureter/bladder cuff to free the specimen. This technique can be facilitated by application of the newer Endo-GIA staplers, which have a rotating and articulating head that allows one to more easily come horizontally across the bladder cuff (Fig. 116–19).

The specimen is most easily controlled by grasping the ureter using the subcostal 12-mm trocar site. The patient is maintained in the Trendelenburg position and the kidney placed over the edge of the liver or spleen. The inferior trocar is then removed and a 15-mm Endocatch II (US Surgical) is introduced and opened just beneath the liver or spleen; the self-opening design of this entrapment sack facilitates the entrapment process. The Endocatch II entrapment sack deployment mechanism has a 15-mm diameter and cannot be passed through a 12-mm trocar. As such, the trocar is removed and the barrel of the 15-mm entrapment sack deployment mechanism is gently passed through the trocar incision site under direct endoscopic vision.

For intact specimen removal, the surgeon should fight the urge to "connect the dots" by extending or connecting existing trocar incisions. It is recommended to make a

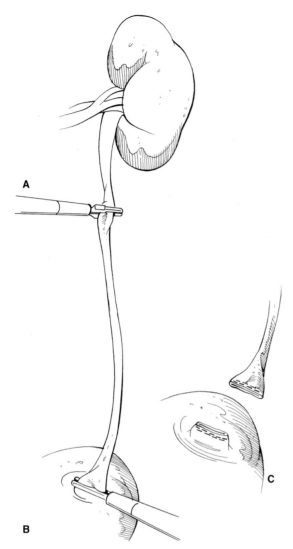

FIG. 116–19. A: Cephalad traction, exerted on the distal ureter, places the ureterovesical junction on stretch. **B:** The Endo-GIA stapler with roticulating head then can be placed across the bladder and fired. **C:** The result is an excision of a 2-cm cuff of bladder *en bloc* with the ureter without any urine leakage. The patient is then placed in a dorsal lithotomy position and the bladder staples are cystoscopically unroofed to prove complete ureteral excision.

lower midline abdominal, Gibson, or Pfannenstiel incision. (*Note:* If a Pfannenstiel incision is planned, the surgeon should mark out the skin incision at the start of the case when the patient is supine as it is difficult to create a symmetrical incision with the patient in the lateral decubitus position.) The specimen is then extracted intact within the entrapment sack. Although all attempts are made to minimize the extraction incision, only gentle traction should be placed on the specimen to avoid rupturing the entrapment sack. Once the specimen is extracted, the entire operative field is inspected for hemostasis. As the pneumoperitoneum is an effective form of venous tamponade, the insufflation pressure is reduced to

5 mm Hg and the entire operative field inspected once again prior to closure of the abdominal incisions. If dilating trocars are used, fascial closure of these sites is not required. All skin incisions are closed with subcuticular sutures.

Cystoscopic Management of the Distal Ureter/Bladder Cuff

After wound closure, the patient is repositioned into a dorsal lithotomy position and flexible cystoscopy is performed. If staples are visualized in the bladder and no ureteral orifice is seen, the procedure can be terminated. More commonly, the ureteral orifice is visualized and a ureteral catheter is gently placed into the remaining short intramural ureteral segment. An Orandi knife or alternatively a 1,000-μ holmium laser fiber is then used to "unroof" the intramural ureter over the ureteral catheter. Unroofing proceeds until the staples are identified. After staple identification, a resectoscope with a rollerball electrode is introduced and the ureteral tunnel and surrounding urothelium are fulgurated for a radius of 1 cm around the site of unroofing. A Foley catheter is left to drain the bladder for 48 hours.

Alternative Approach: Retroperitoneal Laparoscopic Nephroureterectomy

Recently Gill and Ono independently described using a retroperitoneal approach in which the renal dissection is as described for a total retroperitoneoscopic nephrectomy. In the Gill method, the ureter can be plucked cephalad and the specimen delivered via the same method used for total retroperitoneoscopic nephrectomy with intact removal. In the Ono method, the kidney is mobilized downward and an incision is made over the bladder both to excise the cuff of bladder and to deliver the renal specimen (19).

Alternative Management Strategies for the Distal Ureter

Pluck Technique

Transurethral ureteral resection ("pluck" ureterectomy) is performed cystoscopically prior to the laparoscopic component of the procedure with the patient in a dorsal lithotomy position. The ureteral orifice, tunnel, and ureterovesical junction are transurethrally resected out to the perivesical fat. The ureter is thereby released from the bladder. Hemostasis is obtained and a urethral catheter is placed. Early in the laparoscopic portion of the procedure, the ureter is clipped to prevent further leakage of urine into the retroperitoneum. After laparoscopic dissection of the kidney, the surgeon can pluck the ureter cephalad, thereby precluding any pelvic dissection of the ureter. The major drawback of this approach is concern about leakage of malignant cell-laden urine into the retroperitoneum until the ureter is laparoscopically occluded. Instances of seeding after an open pluck procedure have been reported by several urologists (1,15,18).

Needlescopic (Cleveland Clinic) Technique

Application of a needlescopic technique for management of the distal ureter was described by Gill and colleagues in 1999 (14). The patient first undergoes cystoscopy to rule out a concomitant bladder tumor and ensure adequate bladder capacity. Diminished bladder capacity (less than 200 mL) increases the technical difficulty due to limited working space. Cystoscopy is performed with the patient in the 30-degree Trendelenburg position. Two needlescopic trocars (2 mm) are inserted suprapubically into the bladder under cystoscopic vision. A 2-mm Endoloop is inserted through the needlescopic trocar. A 6 Fr ureteral catheter is passed through the loop and into the affected ureter with the assistance of a guide wire. A 24 Fr continuous-flow resectoscope is then passed into the bladder alongside the ureteral catheter. A Collins knife is used to electrosurgically score circumferentially the urothelium around the intramural ureter such that a 2- to 3-cm cuff is outlined.

Using a 2-mm grasper the ureteral orifice and hemitrigone are retracted anteriorly and a full-thickness incision is made with the Collins knife. In this manner approximately 3 to 4 cm of ureter may be dissected free from surrounding tissues. The previously placed Endoloop is then positioned over the ureter and closed tightly, occluding the lumen as the ureteral catheter is withdrawn. The tail of the Endoloop is then cut with 2-mm laparoscopic scissors. The bladder edges about the excised ureter are then coagulated. All instruments are removed from the bladder and a Foley catheter is left indwelling. The laparoscopic retroperitoneal nephrectomy component of the procedure is then performed and the ureter is pulled up and delivered intact with the kidney via a 7- to 10-cm incision.

A concern with this approach is that the ureteral dissection is done at the outset rather than the end of the procedure, thereby exposing the patient to leakage of potentially tumor cell-laden urine. In addition, there can be further leakage along the intravesical port sites.

Myriad other methods for dealing with the distal ureteral cuff during a laparoscopic nephroureterectomy have been described. Nadler describes using the flexible cystoscope and an electrosurgical probe to transurethrally free the ureter from the bladder at the end of the procedure. In this case, the pluck procedure is being done after the ureter has been secured such that leakage of tumor cell-laden urine should be largely precluded. Alternatively, Breda adopted the method of ureteral intussuscep-tion to the laparoscopic approach, thereby avoiding a formal dissection of the distal ureter (10).

Other authors, after completing the nephrectomy portion of the procedure and clip occluding the ureter, make a small Pfannenstiel-type incision and then via a cystotomy perform a formal excision of the ureter and cuff of bladder; the same incision is used to extract the specimen.

Postoperative Care

Postoperative care is identical to the care rendered following a laparoscopic nephrectomy. The only difference is that if a pluck or a formal transvesical resection of a cuff of bladder was completed then the Foley catheter is left in place for 5 to 7 days; a cystogram may be performed prior to removing the catheter. If intussusception was used, then the catheter can be removed routinely on postoperative day 3. In contrast, if the cuff was taken with a stapler and no further treatment of the ureteral orifice or tunnel was required then the Foley catheter can be removed on postoperative day 2; if further transurethral treatment of the ureteral tunnel was needed, then the catheter can be left in place for 5 days.

In these patients, a regimen of routine surveillance cystoscopy (every 3 to 4 months for 2 years, every 6 months for 2 years, and then annually if there has not been a recurrence) is indicated due to the 40% chance of developing a bladder tumor. The role of follow-up IV urograms is more controversial as the 1% to 2% of patients who develop contralateral upper-tract TCC usually present with signs of their disease and it is rare for the IVP to serendipitously reveal an otherwise "silent" occult upper-tract lesion (16). Urine cytology can be obtained at each surveillance visit. The lack of reliability of urine markers for upper-tract TCC mandates against their use (21,30,31).

OUTCOMES

Complications

In series of laparoscopic transperitoneal standard nephrectomy the complication rates have included transfusion, ileus, bowel obstruction, wound infection, medical complications, and other organ injuries. Barrett et al. had two patients requiring transfusion and two bowel obstructions in their series. One patient had a wound infection and another had unstable angina (2). In the Ono group, of 60 patients 2 required blood transfusion. There were intraoperative injuries to the left renal artery, spleen, duodenum, adrenal gland, and a periureteral artery. The duodenal and left renal artery injuries required conversion. Postoperatively two patients suffered an ileus and another suffered a pulmonary embolus (24). The group from Washington University also critically examined their series of 61 laparoscopic nephrectomies and found 2 major complications (ligation of the superior mesenteric artery and bleeding requiring conversion). There were 21 minor complications including congestive heart failure, atelectasis, several nerve palsies due to positioning, ileus, incisional hernia, torn LapSac in two cases, and pleural effusion (11).

Abbou and his group summarized an experience of 50 retroperitoneal laparoscopic nephrectomies. Two patients had minor complications of atelectasis and local inflammation. Two major complications were encountered: one colon injury requiring temporary diversion and one conversion due to bleeding (7). Gill reported on his series of 53 retroperitoneal nephrectomies and had 2 major complications including splenectomy and renal arterial injury requiring conversion. Eight minor complications occurred, including infection, hematoma, ileus, atelectasis, skin rash, and cutaneous hyperesthesia (12).

With regard to nephroureterectomy, Shalhav and colleagues' review of 25 patients revealed 2 major complications and 10 minor complications. This compared favorably with an open cohort that had five major and five minor complications (28). Gill and colleagues reported on 42 patients who underwent a retroperitoneal approach. Complications in this series involved five patients, two of which were considered major: bleeding requiring conversion and excessive retroperitoneal bladder irrigant after cystoscopic disarticulation of the ureter.

Results

The advantages characteristic of minimally invasive procedures have been demonstrated for laparoscopic radical nephrectomy. In this regard there are four areas of importance: efficacy, efficiency, equanimity, and economy. The efficacy of laparoscopic radical nephrectomy has now been documented by a long-term multiinstitutional study showing equivalent cancer-free and recurrence-free survival at greater than 4 years in a cohort of 60 patients (26). Earlier studies by Kavoussi (3-year follow-up) and Ono (2-year follow-up) also showed equivalent results between open and laparoscopic patients (5,20). Next, with time the laparoscopic approach has become more efficient. Indeed, at some institutions (e.g., Cleveland Clinic) the laparoscopic approach is quicker than the open while at other institutions it is on average 1 hour longer. In one area in particular, the laparoscopic approach has proven far superior to the open approach, i.e., the recovery and morbidity for the patient. McDougall and colleagues demonstrated that laparoscopic radical nephrectomy was associated with a significantly decreased postoperative analgesic requirement and a more rapid return of oral intake. In addition, the laparoscopic population had an improved convalescence: a shorter hospital stay and a shorter interval for the return of normal activity and for full recovery. Since their initial report, additional articles have corroborated these findings (Table 116–1). Last, with regard to cost, Cadeddu and colleagues have recently shown that if the laparoscopic procedure is completed in under 4.7 hours, operating room costs are kept to less than $5,500, and the patient leaves the hospital in less than 5 days the overall savings are over $1,000 for the laparoscopic approach (22). In sum, given these results that have been corroborated at multiple centers, laparoscopic radical nephrectomy has truly superseded its open counterpart as the current standard of care.

For nephroureterectomy, due to the paucity of cases the results are less extensive than with nephrectomy. Table 116–2 reviews results of three comparative trials contrasting open nephroureterectomy and laparoscopic or hand-assisted nephroureterectomy. Overall, 66 laparoscopic or

TABLE 116–1. *Laparoscopic radical nephrectomy: worldwide experience, 2002*

Author/reference	Cases	OR time (h)	EBL (cc)	Specimen weight (g)	Stage	Hospital stay (d)	Recovery (wk)	Follow-up (mo.)	Complications (major/minor)	Seeding
Peschel and Janetschek [17]	31	2.4	NS	NS	T1/T2	2.9	NS	18	0%/0%	None
Ono and Kinukawa [24]	91	4.9	300	289	T1/T2	NS	3.0	22	11%	None
Barrett and Rentie [2]	72	2.9	NS	402	T1/T2	4.4	NS	21	1 death 3%/8%	One
Clayman and McDougall [11]	61	5.5	172	452	T1/T2/T3b (r.v.)	3.4	3.6	25	3%/34%	None
Gill [13]	100	2.8	212	403	T1/T2/T3	1.6	4.2	16	3%/11%	None
Kavoussi and Chan [5]	67	4.3	289	NS	T1/T2/T3	3.8	NS	36	15% overall	None
Total	422	3.8	243	387	T1/T2/ T3a/T3b	3.2	3.6	23	Mortalitys 0.3%	0.3%

NS, not significant.

TABLE 116–2. *Comparative nephroureterectomy trials (laparoscopic and hand-assisted laparoscopic versus open trials)*

Author/reference	Operative approach	n	OR time (h)	EBL (mL)	Analgesic (mg MSO$_4$)	Hospital stay (d)	Complete convalescence (wk)
Shalhav et al. [28]	Laparoscopic	25	7.7	199	37	3.6	2.8
	Open	17	3.9	441	144	9.6	10
Seifman et al. [27]	Hand-assisted	16	5.3	557	48	3.9	2.5
	Open	11	3.3	345	81	5.2	7.5
Keeley and Tolley [20]	Laparoscopic	22	2.4	NA	NA	5.5	NA
	Open	26	2.3	NA	NA	10.8	NA
Total	Laparoscopic	66	5.1	339	41.3	4.4	2.7
Total	Open	54	3.0	403	119	9.3	9.0

[a]Alteration in distal ureteral management secondary to recurrences.
NA, Data not available.

hand-assisted laparoscopic procedures were compared to 54 open nephroureterectomies. With regard to efficacy, Shalhav's report, which has follow-up out to 24 months, shows that the overall cancer survival rate appears to be similar and that the bladder recurrence rate also appears similar. However, in that study there was longer follow-up in the open than in the laparoscopic group. This particular area needs further attention over the coming years given the small numbers of patients treated. The efficiency of the procedure favors the open approach by upward of 2 hours. However, the equanimity again favors the laparoscopic approach: Hospital stay and postoperative analgesic requirements were significantly decreased in the cohort undergoing laparoscopic nephroureterectomy. Most strik-

TABLE 116–3. *Laparoscopic instrumentation for standard transperitoneal radical nephrectomy*

Disposable equipment
  5-mm Endoshears (U.S. Surgical)
  12-mm multifire Endo-GIA—vascular and tissue staple with reloads available (U.S. Surgical)
  10-mm Ligasure Atlas device
  Trocars—12-mm (3) (axially dilating clear ports, Ethicon)
  5 × 8 and 8 × 10-inch LapSacs (Cook Urological)
  Veress needles (150-mm) (U.S. Surgical)
  CO$_2$ insufflation tubing
  10 sponges (Raytex)
  5-mm harmonic scalpel (curved jaws) (Ethicon)
Nondisposable equipment
  Trocars—5 mm (2) (Endotip, Storz)
  Endoholder [(Codman (division of Johnson & Johnson)]
  Suction irrigator, extra long, 5-mm (Nezhat system, Storz)
  Laparoscope: 10-mm 0° and a 10-mm 30° lens and a 5-mm 0° lens (Storz)
  3 atraumatic, nonlocking 5-mm smooth-tip (duckbill) grasping forceps (Storz)
  4 traumatic (toothed), locking, 5-mm grasping forceps (Storz)
  LapSac introducer (Cook)
  Electroshield device to attach to electrocautery for active electrode monitoring (Encision)
  5-mm hook electrode (Encision)
  5-mm and 10-mm PEER retractors (J. Jamner Inc.)
  5-mm needleholders (J. Jamner and Storz)
  10-mm soft curved-angled forceps (Maryland dissector) (Storz)
  10-mm right-angle dissector (Storz or J. Jamner)
  Carter Thomason needle suture grasper and closure cones (Inlet Medical)
Available but not opened equipment
  10-mm clip appliers with 9-mm and 12-mm clips (Ethicon)
  Disposable roticulating endoshears (U.S. Surgical)
  Endostitch and all types of suture used (0, 2–0, 4–0, Polysorb, Polydac, and Prolene) (U.S. Surgical)
  Disposable Hasson trocar 12-mm blunt tip (U.S. Surgical)
  3–0 cardiovascular silk (RB-1 needle) and 0-Vicryl suture for fascial closure
  Lapra-ty clips and 10-mm Laparo-Ty clip applier (Ethicon)
  Gauze rolls (5) (Carefree Surgical Specialties)
  10-mm Satinsky clamp with flexible port (Aesculap)

From University of California, Irvine, with permission.

ing, however, full convalescence was expedited by more than 6 weeks with laparoscopic nephroureterectomy. Last, with regard to economy, Meraney and Gill has shown that in their first 14 laparoscopic nephroureterectomy cases there was a 28% greater cost to laparoscopy. However, as operative times have dropped, their last 14 cases were 6% less expensive than for open nephroureterectomy (23). However, in none of the transperitoneal articles has it been shown to be cost effective. As such, unlike laparoscopic radical/total nephrectomy, the laparoscopic nephroureterectomy is still in need of further evaluation to determine its position vis-à-vis open nephroureterectomy. The most important of these aspects remain: efficacy and cost.

Laparoscopic instrumentation for standard transperitoneal radical nephrectomy is listed in Table 116–3.

REFERENCES

1. Arango O, Bielsa O, Carles J, et al. Massive tumor implantation in the endoscopic resected area in modified nephroureterectomy. *J Urol* 1997;157:1893–1896.
2. Barrett PH, Fentie DD, Tarager LA. Laparoscopic radical nephrectomy with morcellation for renal cell carcinoma: the Saskatoon experience. *Urology* 1998;52:23.
3. Bercowsky E, Shalhav AL, Portis A, et al. Is the laparoscopic approach justified in patients with xanthogranulomatous pyelonephritis? *Urology* 1999;54:437–442; discussion 442–433.
4. Chan D, Bishoff JT, Ratner L, et al. Endovascular gastrointestinal stapler device malfunction during laparoscopic nephrectomy: early recognition and management. *J Urol* 2000;164:319–321.
5. Chan DY, Cadeddu JA, Jarrett TW, et al. Laparoscopic radical nephrectomy: cancer control for renal cell carcinoma. *J Urol* 2001;166:2095–2099; discussion 2099–2100.
6. Chan DY, Su LM, Kavoussi LR. Rapid ligation of renal hilum during transperitoneal laparoscopic nephrectomy. *Urology* 2001;57:360–362.
7. Cicco A, Salomon L, Hoznek A, et al. Results of retroperitoneal laparoscopic radical nephrectomy. *J Endourol* 2001;15:355–359.
8. Clayman RV, Kavoussi LR, Figenshau RS, et al. Laparoscopic nephroureterectomy: initial clinical case report. *J Laparoendoscop Surg* 1991;1:343–349.
9. Clayman RV, Kavoussi LR, Soper NJ, et al. Laparoscopic nephrectomy: initial case report. *J Urol* 1991;146:278–282.
10. Dell'Adami G, Breda G. Transurethral or endoscopic ureterectomy. *Eur Urol* 1976;2:156–157.
11. Dunn MD, Portis AJ, Shalhav AL, et al. Laparoscopic versus open radical nephrectomy: a 9-year experience. *J Urol* 2000;164:1153–1159.
12. Gill IS. Laparoscopic radical nephrectomy for cancer. *Urol Clin North Am* 2000;27:707–719.
13. Gill IS, Meraney AM, Schweizer DK, et al. Laparoscopic radical nephrectomy in 100 patients: a single center experience from the United States. *Cancer* 2001;92:1843–1855.
14. Gill IS, Soble J, Miller SD, et al. A novel technique for management of the en bloc bladder cuff and distal ureter during laparoscopic nephroureterectomy. *J Urol* 1999;161:430–434.
15. Hetherington J, Ewing R, Philip N. Modiefied nephroureterectomy: A risk of tumor implantation. *Br J Urol* 1986;58:368–372.
16. Holmang S, Hedelin H, Anderstrom C, et al. Long-term followup of a bladder carcinoma cohort: Routine followup urography is not necessary. *J Urol* 1998;160:45–48.
17. Janetschek G, Jeschke K, Peschel R, et al. Laparoscopic surgery for stage T1 renal cell carcinoma: radical nephrectomy and wedge resection. *Eur Urol* 2000;38:131–138.
18. Jones D, Moisey C: A cautionary tale of the modified "pluck" nephroureterectomy. *Br J Urol* 1993;71:486–487.
19. Kamihira O, Aichi K, Ono Y, et al. Retroperitoneoscopic nephroureterectomy for transitional cell carcinoma of the renal pelvis and ureter: Nayoga experience. *J Urol* 2002;164[Suppl]:20.
20. Keeley FX, Tolley DA. Laparoscopic nephroureterectomy: making management of upper-tract transitional-cell carcinoma entirely minimally invasive. *J Endourol* 1998;12:139–141.
21. Lodde M, Mian C, Wiener H, et al. Detection of upper urinary tract transitional cell carcinoma with ImmunoCyt: a prelimanry report. *Urology* 2001;58:362–366.
22. Lotan Y, Gettman MT, Roehrborn CG, et al. Cost comparison for laparoscopic nephrectomy and open nephrectomy: analysis of individual parameters. *Urology* 2002;59:821–825.
23. Meraney AM, Gill IS. Financial analysis of open versus laparoscopic radical nephrectomy and nephroureterectomy. *J Urol* 2002;167:1757–1762.
24. Ono Y, Kinukawa T, Hattori R, et al. Laparoscopic radical nephrectomy for renal cell carcinoma: a five-year experience. *Urology* 1999;53:280–286.
25. O'Sullivan DC, Micali S, Averch TD, et al. Factors involved in gas embolism after laparoscopic injury to inferior vena cava. *J Endourol* 1998;12:149–154.
26. Portis AJ, Yan Y, Landman J, et al. Long-term followup after laparoscopic radical nephrectomy. *J Urol* 2002;167:1257–1262.
27. Seifman BD, Montie JE, Wolf JS Jr. Prospective comparison between hand-assisted laparoscopic and open surgical nephroureterectomy for urothelial cell carcinoma. *Urology* 2001;57:133–137.
28. Shalhav AL, Dunn MD, Portis AJ, et al. Laparoscopic nephroureterectomy for upper tract transitional cell cancer: the Washington University experience. *J Urol* 2000;163:1100–1104.
29. Sundaram CP, Ono Y, Landman J, et al. Hydrophilic guide wire technique to facilitate organ entrapment using a laparoscopic sack during laparoscopy. *J Urol* 2002;167:1376–1377.
30. Walsh I, Keane P, Ishak L, et al. The BTA stat test: a tumor marker for the detection of upper tract transitional cell carcinoma. *Urology* 2001;58:532–535.
31. Wu W, Liu L, Huang C, et al. The clinical implications of telomerast activity in upper tract urothelial cancer and washings. *Br J Urol* 2000;86:213–219.

CHAPTER 117

Hand-Assisted Laparoscopic Nephrectomy and Nephroureterectomy

James A. Brown and Leonard G. Gomella

Hand-assisted laparoscopic nephrectomy (HALN) was first performed in the pig by Bannenberg et al. in 1996 (1). Nakada and colleagues performed the first HALN in a human the following year, and this modification to the standard laparoscopic technique has been increasingly used worldwide since (8). Narrow profile, non–adhesive-based second-generation HAL devices, Chapter 116, have markedly improved their ease of use and decreased the operative time needed to perform hand-assisted laparoscopic surgery.

This chapter describes the indications, special considerations, technique, and results of HALN and nephroureterectomy (HALNU). We will discuss our surgical technique and also describe other commonly used techniques for HALN and HALNU.

DIAGNOSIS

The diagnosis of conditions that require nephrectomy and nephroureterectomy are described in Chapter 29.

INDICATIONS FOR SURGERY

Simple nephrectomy may be indicated for benign conditions (i.e., nonfunction) and radical nephrectomy for malignancy. Nephroureterectomy is by tradition performed for transitional cell carcinoma of the upper urinary tract. Nephroureterectomy is sometimes needed in cases of upper-tract nonfunction with associated ureteral reflux. HALN is a viable alternative to standard laparoscopic nephrectomy for any case where laparoscopic nephrectomy is indicated (Chapter 116). It is in particular a useful alternative for the urologist with limited laparoscopic experience. HALN is also a useful technique for the patient requiring donor nephrectomy, nephroureterectomy, and radical nephrectomy with removal of an intact kidney. Large kidneys greater than 10 cm and kidneys with perinephric scarring and status following prior surgery may be more easily removed using HALN rather than standard laparoscopy.

ALTERNATIVE THERAPY

Nephrectomy and nephroureterectomy can also be performed by standard transperitoneal and retroperitoneal laparoscopic techniques or a variety of open surgical approaches. Partial nephrectomy and ablative therapy (i.e., radiofrequency and cryotherapy) are also alternative approaches to the management of renal masses (see Chapters 2 and 4).

SURGICAL TECHNIQUE

The obvious difference between HALN and standard transperitoneal laparoscopic and retroperitoneoscopic nephrectomy is the incorporation of a hand-assisted laparoscopic access device. Use of the surgeon's hand as an instrument in the surgical field makes HALN a hybrid technique with most of the advantages of standard laparoscopy while retaining many advantages of open surgery.

After general anesthesia and intravenous access has been obtained and an orogastric tube and Foley catheter have been secured in place, the patient is positioned in the modified flank position with the affected side up. We place a rolled towel under the ipsilateral shoulder and hip with the ipsilateral arm secured with 3-in. cloth tape across the chest on top of folded towels or a pillow. The hips and lower extremities are also secured in place with cloth tape. This allows the patient to be rotated both toward and away from the surgeon as necessary (Fig. 117–1). While we prefer the ipsilateral side elevated approximately 30 degrees on a flat or minimally flexed

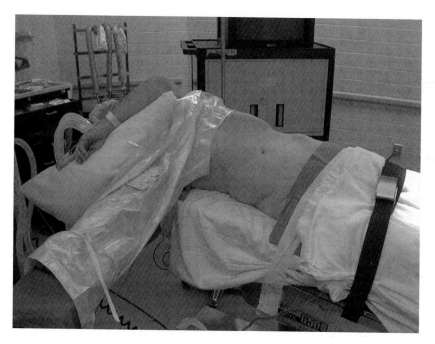

FIG. 117–1. The patient is placed in a modified (30 degree) flank position with a rolled towel under the ipsilateral shoulder and hip.

table, others prefer a more steeply inclined patient (60 degrees) positioned on top of a flexed table. The surgeon stands on the side contralateral to the affected kidney, while the first assistant/camera operator typically stands on the ipsilateral side (Fig. 117–2).

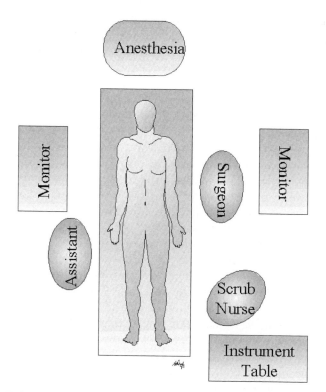

FIG. 117–2. Operating room configuration used during hand-assisted laparoscopic nephrectomy or nephroureterectomy.

Our standard approach is to place a 7-cm supraumbilical incision extending into or skirting the umbilicus for both right- and left-sided procedures. Peritoneal adhesions if present around the insertion site are lysed and the HAL access device placed. We find it helpful to place an interrupted 0 Vicryl suture through the anterior rectus fascia and peritoneum bilaterally at the midpoint of the incision to elevate the body wall when inserting the intraperitoneal portion of the hand-assist port device.

With a trocar through the hand-assist device such as the Lap Disc (Ethicon Endo-Surgery), the peritoneum is insufflated to a pressure of 15 mm Hg. A 12-mm camera port is placed just lateral to the rectus muscle at the level of the HAL device. A second 12-mm port is placed approximately two finger breadths anterior to the tip of the twelfth rib (Fig. 117–3). An additional 5-mm port may be placed as indicated but is rarely necessary in our experience. A mirror of this configuration is used when operating on the contralateral kidney. The hand-port and trocars should ideally be in a diamond configuration and not in a straight line. Others have described creating a nonmidline hand incision in conjunction with upper-abdominal camera and working ports so they may insert their nondominant hand when performing either right or left nephrectomy (Fig. 117–4) (13).

We, by tradition, insert the right hand for the right nephrectomy and the left hand for the left nephrectomy. It is useful if the surgeon trains himself to be ambidextrous as this facilitates the ease of training both right- and left-handed residents and in the performance of simultaneous bilateral nephrectomies. The operating view for a right radical nephrectomy is shown in Figure 117–5.

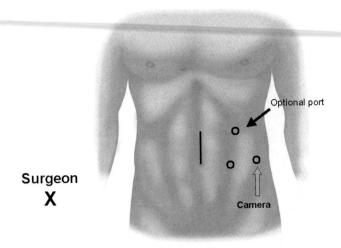

FIG. 117–3. Hand-assisted laparoscopic nephrectomy port placement. The upper 5-mm port is optional.

A damp laparotomy sponge is carried into the peritoneum while inserting the hand and is useful for hemostasis. As in standard laparoscopic nephrectomy, the initial step is to lyse any intraperitoneal adhesions. This is followed by reflection of the ipsilateral ascending or descending colon to gain access to the retroperitoneal space. The incision is made along (or just medial to) the line of Toldt and extended from the iliac vessels to above the splenic or hepatic flexure lateral to the spleen or liver.

Left-Sided Dissection

Similar to standard laparoscopy, the left colon is mobilized by dividing the lienorenal and phrenicocolic liga-

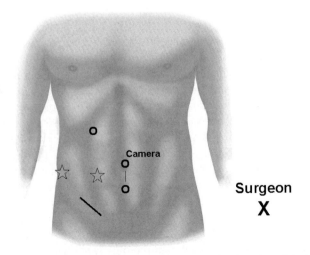

FIG. 117–4. Alternative port placement for hand-assisted laparoscopic nephrectomy.

ments. This allows the splenic flexure to fall medially with gravity and the anterior aspect of Gerota's fascia is exposed by bluntly and sharply separating it from the left colonic mesentery. The left gonadal vein and ureter are identified in the medial aspect tail of Gerota's fascia. The fascia between the gonadal vein and the aorta is divided and this dissection is carried cephalad to the level of the renal hilum; the renal vein and subsequently the renal artery are identified and dissected free of enveloping fascia.

Right-Sided Dissection

During a right HALN, the parietal peritoneal incision along the line of Toldt is extended medially between the liver and the transverse colon, revealing the hepatorenal space of Morrison. The ascending colon and hepatic flexure are mobilized medially, exposing the second stage of the duodenum. The duodenum is then Kocherized, exposing the anterior surface of the inferior vena cava. The incision made in the parietal peritoneum beneath the liver is extended from its medial aspect caudad along the lateral inferior vena cava to below the lower pole of the kidney and then in a curvilinear arc to the right-side wall connecting with the incision along the line of Toldt. The ureter is identified in the tail of Gerota's fascia, and it is clipped and divided. The tail of Gerota's fascia is divided using the harmonic scalpel or the endoscopic scissors, leaving the right gonadal vein or dividing it if necessary. The lower pole is mobilized and the fascia below and overlying the renal vasculature is divided with the hook electrode, harmonic scalpel, or endoscopic scissors.

HALN

The biggest difference between standard laparoscopy and hand-assisted laparoscopy is the use of the surgeon's hand as a mobilizing instrument. Once the renal vein is identified and cleaned of enveloping fascia along its anterior, superior, and inferior surfaces, digital palpation will identify the location of the renal artery. Typically, the artery is most easily mobilized by placing the hand in a "C-shaped" configuration (Fig. 117–6). The index and middle fingers are positioned below the renal vein and used to tilt the lower pole of the kidney laterally and anteriorly if necessary. The fourth finger is placed cephalad to the renal vein to rotate the renal artery beneath the renal vein. The surgeon's thumb is used to depress the vena cava or aorta medially. Of note, during a left HALN the index and middle fingers are typically placed below the renal vein medial to the gonadal vein when depressing the lower pole laterally and anteriorly.

The electrified hook–suction instrument is most useful in dissecting and dividing the fascia enveloping the renal artery and vein. Meticulous care must be taken to identify lumbar veins and to either avoid injury or clip and divide

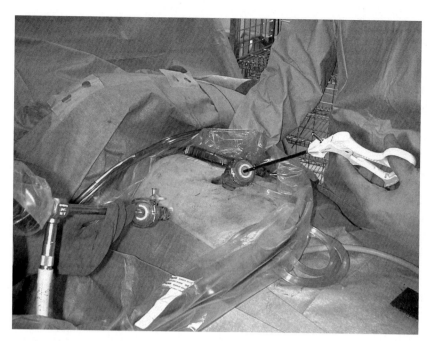

FIG. 117–5. Port and instrument positioning during a right hand-assisted radical nephrectomy.

the vein prior to avulsion. The left adrenal vein must also be avoided or clipped and divided. Once the renal artery and vein have been completely mobilized a minimum of five clips are placed on the artery with at least three on the stay side. Alternatively, the Endo-GIA vascular stapler or locking clips (e.g., hemoclip) may also be used. The vein is usually divided with the Endo-GIA vascular stapler. If the renal hilar dissection is difficult, it may be advantageous to place a single clip on the renal artery with division of the renal vein prior to placing the remaining clips and dividing the renal artery. Great care must be taken to avoid placing the Endo-GIA stapler across clips

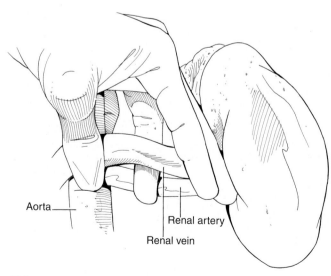

FIG. 117–6. Finger and hand positioning during renal artery and vein dissection.

Aorta

Renal artery

Renal vein

as this can lead to device malfunction and the need for open conversion. As a rule, it is helpful to position clips on the gonadal and adrenal veins at least 1 cm away from the left renal vein to avoid this problem.

After the hilar vasculature has been divided, the remaining lateral and upper pole attachments are divided with the harmonic scalpel or endoscopic scissors. The adrenal gland is removed when necessary, either with the specimen or separately using clips to maintain hemostasis. The adrenal gland or adrenal bed and the renal hilum are inspected for hemostasis. Smaller kidneys can be removed directly through the hand-port site. Larger kidneys require that a laparoscopic entrapment sack (or bowel bag for very large kidneys) be introduced through the hand-port. We prefer to roll the sack prior to insertion, subsequently unrolling it on top of the liver or spleen. Flattening the sack against the psoas musculature facilitates entrapment of the kidney. The sack is opened using a locking grasper to lift the anterior lip of the sack. The upper pole of the kidney is lifted into the sack. Then, the posterior lateral aspect of the sack is grasped with the grasping instrument while the surgeon uses his fingers to hold the medial aspect of the sack and the kidney is pushed into the sack with the thumb. Once entrapped, the specimen is removed through the hand-port, enlarging it if necessary. Following this, the renal bed is thoroughly irrigated and reinspected with the insufflation pressure decreased to approximately 5 mm Hg. Surgicel is placed across the renal hilum or the adrenal bed as necessary to control minimal venous oozing.

We prefer to use the Carter–Thomason instrument to close the 12-mm camera and working ports with 0 Vicryl suture. The patient is rolled supine, replacing the bowel in its normal anatomic position after inspecting it for injury. The laparotomy sponge is removed and the hand incision is closed with running heavy absorbable suture (i.e., no. 1 Vicryl or Maxon). We irrigate the subcutaneous tissue and inject a mixture of 0.25% Marcaine and 1% Lidocaine prior to approximating the subcuticular layer with 4-0 Monocryl. Sterile bandages are applied to the trocar sites. The hand-port incision is covered with a small gauze dressing and Tegaderm.

HALNU

The patient is positioned for nephroureterectomy identically to the position for HALN. The patient is placed in the 30-degree modified flank position with a rolled towel under the ipsilateral shoulder and hip. If a double-J ureteral stent is not indwelling, we perform flexible cystoscopy and place an open-ended 6 Fr catheter into the renal pelvis. The ureteral stent is secured to an indwelling 16 Fr Foley catheter. A 7-cm hand-port incision is made straddling and incorporating the umbilicus in a lower position than for standard hand-assisted nephrectomy (Fig. 117–7). Once the peritoneum has been entered, adhesions are lysed and the hand-port placed. The nephrectomy portion of the case is performed using the techniques described above for HALN. However, the adrenal gland is typically dissected free from the superior pole and spared and the ureter is left intact and doubly clipped at its distal aspect.

Once the nephrectomy portion has been completed, we perform the distal ureteral dissection and bladder cuff excision by simply inserting the opposite hand (left hand for right HALNU and right hand for left HALNU). Hand assistance facilitates the ureteral dissection, in particular for inflamed or adherent ureters. The harmonic scalpel is

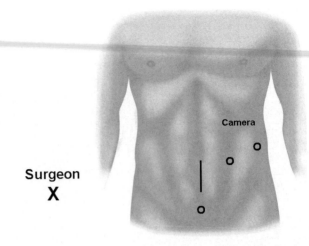

FIG. 117–7. Hand-assisted laparoscopic nephroureterectomy port placement.

in particular useful in dissecting the ureter away from the iliac vessels and down to the level of the level of the bladder. The back of the surgeon's hand is used to mobilize the bladder medially. When necessary, a 5-mm port may be placed in the infraumbilical midline to insert a suction or grasping device for retraction.

While we initially performed cystoscopic excision of the distal ureter, we currently complete the ureteral dissection and bladder cuff excision completely laparoscopically (5). The harmonic scalpel is used to carry the periureteral dissection through the bladder wall into the bladder, where the ureteral vesicle junction and a cuff of bladder mucosa are circumferentially resected. This is done under direct vision to avoid injury to the contralateral orifice (Fig. 117–8A). The cystotomy is closed with

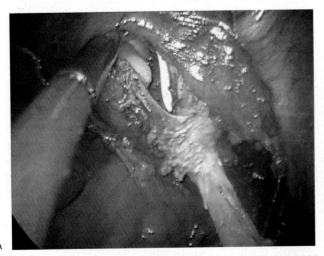

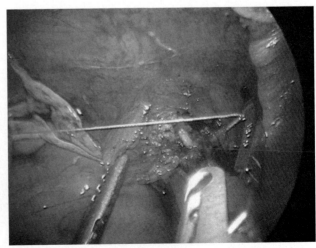

FIG. 117–8. A: Intraoperative view of a right-sided hand-assisted laparoscopic nephroureterectomy. The ureter and cuff of bladder have been partially transected. The indwelling ureteral stent and Foley catheter can be seen. **B:** Use of the Endostitch device for closure of cystotomy during hand-assisted laparoscopic nephroureterectomy.

a running 0 Vicryl suture using the Endostitch device (Fig. 117–8B). We find it helpful to pretie a small loop in the end of the suture and pass the suture through the loop after placing the initial stitch.

Others prefer to cystoscopically manage the intramural ureter (4,12). The techniques described include incising circumferentially around the ureteral orifice to facilitate intramural tunnel excision or unroofing the entire intramural ureter with subsequent ablation of the mucosa with electrocautery. The latter may be performed either prior to or after laparoscopically dividing the distal ureter, typically using the Endo-GIA stapler. This latter technique allows for complete extravesical management of the distal ureter, minimizing the chance of peritoneal tumor contamination. Finally, if total laparoscopic excision of the distal ureter and bladder cuff is performed and the Endostitch is used to close the cystotomy care must be taken to avoid suturing the Foley catheter.

The orogastric or nasogastric tube is removed in the operating room. Ambulation and oral intake is resumed the evening of or the morning after surgery. The pneumatic compression stockings are discontinued on postoperative day 1 and the Foley catheter is removed 1 week after a negative cystogram.

OUTCOMES

Complications

Complications of HAL kidney surgery are similar to those of laparoscopic nephrectomy, including injury to adjacent structures, hemorrhage, and the possibility of open conversion.

Results

HALN compares favorably to and offers many advantages when compared to either open or standard laparoscopic or retroperitoneoscopic nephrectomy. HALN has a shorter learning curve than standard laparoscopic nephrectomy, with most upper-level residents completing their first attempted procedure. Studies comparing HALN to standard laparoscopic nephrectomy have demonstrated statistically similar recovery, morbidity, and cost. A trend toward lower complication rates has also been noted in some HALN series. Most of these series have also demonstrated shorter operative times for patients undergoing HALN (9).

HALN also compares favorably to open radical nephrectomy, with similar negative margin rates and postoperative complication rates but decreased analgesic requirements, hospital stay, and time to complete recovery (7). Compared with standard laparoscopy, hand-assisted laparoscopy appears to be in particular well suited for performing simple nephrectomies on chronically infected kidneys or kidneys that have been operated on previously. HALN also appears to be effective for removing very large tumors (greater than 10 cm) (13). Minimal increases in operative time and estimated blood loss and similar narcotic requirements, complication rates, and convalescence have been seen when removing such large tumors compared with smaller lesions.

HALNU has been compared with open nephroureterectomy and has been noted to be of similar efficacy with similar negative margin rates, but HALNU-treated patients have decreased analgesic requirements, hospital stay, and convalescence (4,12). While some studies have found that HALNU takes longer to perform than open nephroureterectomy (10,12), other studies have demonstrated that HALNU operative times are 1 to several hours shorter (4, 12). This technique is also valuable in that bilateral HALNU can also be performed simultaneously (3).

REFERENCES

1. Bannenberg JJG, Meijer DW, Bannenberg JH, et al. Hand-assisted laparoscopic nephrectomy in the pig: initial report. *Minim Invas Ther Allied Tech* 1996;5:483.
2. Chen J, Chueh SC, Hsu WT, et al. Modified approach of hand-assisted laparoscopic nephroureterectomy for transitional cell carcinoma of the upper urinary tract. *Urology* 2001;86:930.
3. Chueh SC, Chen J, Hsu WT, et al. Hand-assisted laparoscopic bilateral nephroureterectomy in one session without repositioning patients is facilitated by alternating inflation cuffs. *J Urol* 2002;167:44.
4. Landman J, Lev RY, Bhayani S, et al. Comparison of hand-assisted and standard laparoscopic radical nephroureterectomy for the management of localized transitional cell carcinoma. *J Urol* 2002;167:2387.
5. McGinnis DE, Trabalsi EJ, Gomella LG, Strup SE. Hand-assisted laparoscopic nephrouretectomy: description of technique. *Tech Urol* 2001;7:7–11.
6. Lee D, Trabulsi E, McGinnis D, Strup S, Gomella LG, Bagley D. Totally endoscopic management of upper tract transitional-cell carcinoma. *J Endourol* 2002;16:37–41.
7. Mancini GJ, McQuay LA, Klein FA, et al. Hand-assisted laparoscopic radical nephrectomy: comparison to transabdominal radical nephrectomy. *Am Surg* 2002;68:151.
8. Nakada SY, Moon TD, Gist M, et al. Use of a pneumo sleeve as an adjunct in laparoscopic nephrectomy. *Urology* 1997;49:612.
9. Nelson CP, Wolf JS Jr. Comparison of hand-assisted versus standard laparoscopic radical nephrectomy for suspected renal cell carcinoma. *J Urol* 2002;167:1989.
10. Seifman BD, Montie JE, Wolf JS Jr. Respective comparison between hand-assisted laparoscopic and open surgical nephroureterectomy for urothelial cell carcinoma. *Urology* 2001;57:133.
11. Shalhav AL, Dunn MD, Portis AJ, et al. Laparoscopic nephroureterectomy for upper tract transition cell cancer: The Washington University experience. *J Urol* 2000;163:1100.
12. Stifelman MD, Hyman MJ, Shichman S, et al. Hand-assisted laparoscopic nephroureterectomy versus open nephroureterectomy for the treatment of transitional cell carcinoma of the upper urinary tract. *J Endourol* 2001;15:391.
13. Stifelman MD, Sosa RE, Shichman SJ. Hand-assisted laparoscopy in urology. *Rev Urol* 2001;3:63.

CHAPTER 118

Laparoscopic Renal Procedures: Renal Cystectomy, Partial Nephrectomy, Biopsy, and Nephropexy

Stephen E. Strup and Stuart Diamond

Laparoscopic renal surgery is an increasingly popular technique used to treat a wide variety of benign and malignant diseases of the kidney. The benefits of laparoscopic renal surgery, including less postoperative discomfort, shorter hospitalization, and quicker recovery have encouraged surgeons to apply laparoscopic techniques to ablative and reconstructive renal procedures. The management of renal cystic disease and small renal masses has also benefited from the expansion of laparoscopy into renal surgery. Renal biopsy and nephropexy can also be accomplished laparoscopically.

RENAL CYSTECTOMY

Simple cysts are the most common lesions of the kidney. It is estimated that evidence of renal cysts exists in 50% of the adult population (5). The incidence of cysts increases with age; simple renal cysts occur with an incidence of at least 20% by age 40 years and 33% at age 60 years (5).

Diagnosis

The diagnosis of renal cysts was traditionally made during intravenous urography with tomography. Today, ultrasound (US) and computed tomography (CT) are the principal diagnostic tools, and most cysts are found incidentally. Occasionally, a patient with a very large simple cyst may present with vague abdominal or flank discomfort and fullness on physical exam, though most patients are asymptomatic. The sonographic criteria for simple cysts are absence of internal echoes, increased through transmission of sound, and a sharply defined wall.

On CT, cysts are sharply marginated, nonenhancing, and demarcated from surrounding renal parenchyma, with attenuation values in the range of water (-10 to -20 Hounsfield units). On magnetic resonance imaging (MRI) cysts appear as round, homogeneous, and low intensity (dark) on T1-weighted images and increased intensity (lighter) on T2-weighted images.

Indications for Surgery

Occasionally, patients who present with flank pain are discovered to have no other etiology on radiographic evaluation for their complaint other than a large simple cyst, and may be candidates for therapy. Depending on the symptoms, size, site, locations, number, presence of infection, suspicion of malignancy, and other associated pathologic conditions, the following renal cystic disorders can be managed by laparoscopic intervention:

1. Renal cystic masses (i.e., cystic renal cell carcinoma): laparoscopic nephrectomy.
2. Indeterminate cystic masses (Bosniak Type II–IV): evaluation and management.
3. Bosniak Type I and II renal cysts: large (<\>>10 cm) and symptomatic
4. Renal hydatid cysts.
5. Peripelvic or parapelvic cysts.
6. ADPKD-cyst decortication.

Alternative Therapy

Aspiration and injection of sclerosing agents is considered to be the initial course of management for symptomatic renal cysts. Reported success rates range from 75-

97% with complication rates between 1.3–20% (7,8). Another alternative is open surgical marsupialization, which can be performed when more conservative approaches fail or cannot be preformed.

Surgical Technique

Retroperitoneal Approach

Standard positioning and preparation are carried out and the retroperitoneal space is developed with a balloon dissector as previously described. Laparoscopic ultrasound may be used where cysts are difficult to locate. An additional instrument for dissection and countertraction can be placed via a 5-mm trocar midway between the iliac crest and the 12th rib in the posterior axillary line (Figure 118–1).

Once the cyst is exposed, the fluid is aspirated and sent for cytology. The cyst wall is incised with dissecting scissors, harmonic scalpel, or a hook blade and sent for pathologic analysis (Figure 118–2). The base of the cyst is examined for evidence of neoplastic change using cup biopsy forceps to perform frozen section analysis. The edges of the cyst are cauterized and hemostasis is verified after the pneumoretroperitoneum has been lowered to 8 mm Hg. The argon beam coagulator (ConMed Corporation, Utica, NY) can be used to quickly paint over any raw bleeding surfaces. If the argon beam coagulator is used, the retroperitoneum must be vented frequently to prevent buildup of pressure. If bleeding persists fibrin glue with or without Gelfoam can be applied for hemostasis (6).

Transperitoneal Approach

Our approach for treating renal cysts, either simple or multiple, has been laparoscopic marsupialization. This technique has also been reported to treat symptomatic polycystic kidneys (9). Under general anesthesia the patient placed in a 45-degree lateral flank position. An

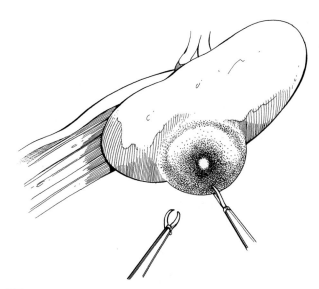

FIG. 118–2. Renal cyst ready to be excised with dissecting scissors.

infraumbilical Hasson trocar is inserted in the peritoneal cavity and the peritoneum insufflated. A 10-mm port is placed under laparoscopic guidance approximately 5 cm lateral and inferior to the umbilicus. A third 5-mm trocar is placed below the costal margin in the anterior axillary line. A fourth port is advocated by some but is rarely necessary in our experience. The white line of Toldt is incised and the colon is reflected medially. Gerota's fascia is then incised. The cysts are then generally readily visualized. Using an Orandi-type needle the cyst can be punctured and cyst fluid sent for cytologic diagnosis. The cyst can then be unroofed with laparoscopic shears and its walls carefully inspected with biopsy sometimes necessary to rule out malignancy. Generally the cyst wall is at least partially resected. Then, using endoscopic clip appliers, we have clipped a portion of the peritoneum to the cyst wall to ensure communication with the peritoneal cavity and decrease the likelihood of recurrence. Occasionally the base of the cyst wall is fulgurated using an argon beam coagulator.

If the cyst is extremely large, another technique is to fashion a window using dissecting scissors. This decompresses the cyst without necessitating the removal of the entire cyst wall. Retroperitoneal fat can be packed into the defect to help maintain window patency. If there is ever any concern that the collecting system has been entered, indigo carmine can be administered. Bleeding is usually minimal. No drains are necessary.

Outcomes

Complications

Bleeding is always a possible complication of marsupialization of a renal cyst. However, this has not been noted in the several series using a laparoscopic approach

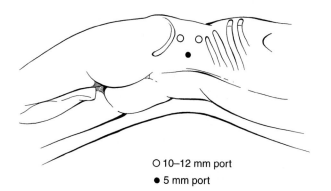

○ 10–12 mm port

● 5 mm port

FIG. 118–1. Patient shown in the flank position from the back. Port sites shown for retroperitoneal laparoscopic procedures such as cyst decortication, renal biopsy and nephropexy. 0 10 to 12-m port by 5-mm port (optional in renal biopsy procedure).

(1,4,8,9,12,13). Reaccumulation of cyst fluid is uncommon but can occur when the window fashioned during marsupialization becomes occluded. Nieh et al demonstrated that the use of fat was helpful in maintaining the patency of the marsupialization window (9). Other complications include prolonged ileus (1%), hemorrhage (3%), urinary fistula (2%), and nerve paresthesia (1%) (1,4,8,9,12,13).

Results

Almost 300 laparoscopic cyst decortications have been reported, for which the indication in nearly three quarters of procedures was a symptomatic simple renal cyst (1,4,8,9,12,13). In most of the cases, a transperitoneal approach was used. Mean operative time was 122 minutes (range 52–240 minutes) for simple peripheral cysts but over 5 hours for peripelvic cysts. Cyst size ranged from 5 cm to 23 cm in diameter. Mean estimated blood loss for simple renal cyst decortication was generally low (93mL), and reported transfusion rates averaged 3.2% (range 0-0011%). The average hospital stay was 2 days and convalescence time was just over 1 week. In most series, pain was relieved in over 75% of patients and was correlated with successful ablation of the cyst.

Laparoscopic renal cyst decortication for symptomatic ADKD has been reported (1,4,8,9,12,13). In all but one case, a transperitoneal approach was used. The mean operating time (165 minutes) was 42 minutes longer than for treatment of simple cysts. The overall complication rate was comparable with that reported for simple cyst ablation. Not unexpectedly, recurrence rates were high for the ADPKD group (15.9%), but comparable with the average of series of simple cyst ablation (16.7%). Though initial relief of pain was achieved in 75 to 100% of patients after laparoscopic cyst ablation, long term follow up showed that pain relief declined over time.

PARTIAL NEPHRECTOMY

Indications for Surgery

Nephron sparing surgery (NSS) is an accepted method of treatment for selected renal masses. The patient must be able to tolerate a laparoscopic procedure. The properly selected renal lesion should be less than 4 cm in size and peripheral in nature. Polar lesions are preferable, especially early in the laparoscopic surgeon's experience with this technique. Renal masses abutting the hilar vessels and central collecting system can be safely resected by the experienced surgeon. Patients with prior renal surgery or history of any inflammatory conditions of the operative kidney should be avoided.

Alternative Therapy

Radical nephrectomy remains the gold standard for renal cell carcinoma and can be performed by a variety of open (retroperitoneal, transabdominal), and laparoscopic (standard, hand assisted, retroperitoneal) techniques. Partial nephrectomy can likewise be approached by these different methods. Ablative procedure (using radiofrequency or cryotherapy) are gaining popularity for smaller lesions (i.e., <4 cm) can be performed by open, laparoscopic and percutaneous approaches.

Surgical Technique

Depending on the planned approach, the patient is placed in a modified 45° flank position (transperitoneal approach) or a flank position (retroperitoneal approach) with all pressure points well padded. The retroperitoneal approach is ideal for posteriorly located tumors which are planned to be treated with a pure laparoscopic technique. Camera and working ports are placed in a similar position as described in retroperitoneal laparoscopic nephrectomy. While typically a three port technique is utilized initially, often an additional 5 mm port is added to aid with suction or retraction.

The transperitoneal approach is ideal for renal masses in nearly any location, but especially those located anteriorly. Traditionally a four port approach is used, with the addition of 5-mm ports as needed for retraction and suction/irrigation.

Hand-assisted laparoscopic surgery is another technique shown to be useful in performing the transperitoneal approach to LPN (11,14). The options for placement of the hand-assist device and ports is shown in Figure 118–3.

After the colon has been mobilized, the kidney is mobilized within Gerota's fascia. If the retroperitoneal approach is used, Gerota's fascia is encountered directly and the kidney is exposed by incising Gerota's fascia widely. During the exposure of the kidney, an attempt is made to leave a portion of fat overlying the renal mass. The remainder of the kidney is then exposed and the ureter identified. The renal hilum is exposed but not extensively dissected. In general, if clamping of the hilum is anticipated, this can be accomplished without risking vascular injury by individually dissecting out the renal artery and vein. If desired, a laparoscopic ultrasound probe can then be inserted (usually via a 12-mm port) and the kidney can be scanned for additional pathology. The depth of the lesion can also be visualized and any underlying vessels or collecting system identified. The fat overlying the mass is then excised and sent for pathological assessment. Additional 5-mm ports are then placed if needed to facilitate resection, aspiration/irrigation, or retraction in preparation for excision of the mass.

Once the mass is completely exposed, a 5-mm margin of normal parenchyma is marked by scoring the renal

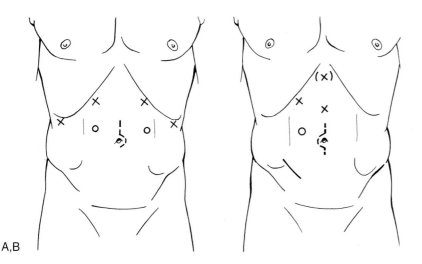

A,B

FIG. 118–3. A: Example of placement of hand device (line) and port placement useful for a right or left hand assisted partial nephrectomy with the hand port in the supraumbilical position. **B:** For right sided tumors, the hand assist device may also be placed in the lower midline across the umbilicus or right lower quadrant to allow the right hand dominant surgeon to use an upper midline port for dissection.

capsule with electrocautery applied through a hook electrode or laparoscopic scissors. The mass is then circumferentially excised using careful blunt dissection directed centrally along the renal pyramids. Small parenchymal vessels are controlled as encountered (Figure 118–4). A variety of tools have been described for this dissection including scissors (10), bipolar cautery (14), and the harmonic scalpel (11). Care is taken to avoid angling the dissection too superficially and entering the capsule of the mass. Once excised, the mass is placed in a specimen bag

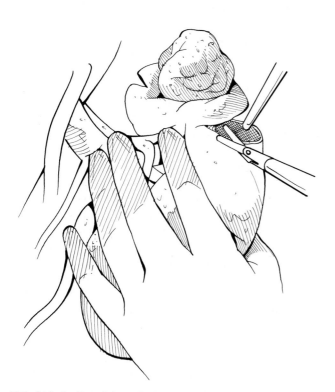

FIG. 118–4. Resection of a left upper pole mass using hand compression and scissors with cautery to resect the mass with a 5-mm margin.

and removed, or placed aside while hemostasis is achieved.

Hemostasis within the surgical defect of the kidney is essential. For larger or more centrally located lesions, clamping of the renal hilum should be considered prior to resection of the mass. If one is utilizing a hand-assisted technique, bulldog clamps or small vascular clamps can be introduced through the hand device and applied prior to resection. With a pure laparoscopic approach, an external vascular pedicle clamp or laparoscopic bulldog clamps can also be utilized (3). We believe that hand assisted laparoscopic partial nephrectomy is the most useful approach since hand compression is a valuable hemostatic tool (Figure 118.4). Parenchymal compression achieves relative hemostasis during the resection of the mass and for application of additional hemostatic techniques. The Argon beam coagulator is a useful adjunct and may be applied through a 5-mm port, with periodic venting of a port necessary to prevent pressure buildup.

A number of maneuvers have been described to control bleeding during laparoscopy and should be familiar to those contemplating partial nephrectomy (6). A useful adjunct for hemostasis is the application of a gelatin sponge and fibrin glue patch (6,10,14). The patch is prepared prior to resection of the lesion, and applied to the resection bed. Additional hemostatic measures can also be used including the placement of pledgeted sutures on either side of the resection bed and tying them over the hemostatic patch with or without a segment of perirenal fat. (Figure 118–5). To check for adequate hemostasis, it is recommended that the insufflation pressure be dropped to inspect for bleeding. A Valsalva maneuver can be done by hyperinflating the lungs to check for bleeding as well. Renal perfusion should be optimized with the use of intravenous mannitol or furosemide and final hemostatic inspection should be done with good renal turgor established.

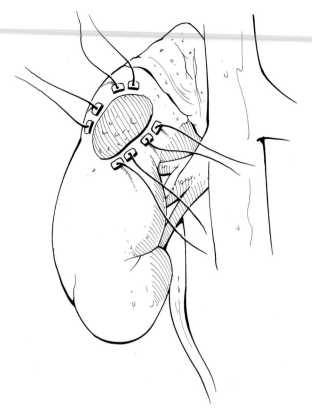

FIG. 118–5. Resection bed of right lateral upper pole lesion with gelatin sponge impregnated with fibrin glue and pledgeted suture in place and ready to be tied down.

The integrity of the collection system can be tested by retrograde distention of the collecting system through a preplaced ureteral catheter using dilute methylene blue or by intravenous administration of indigo carmine. Any defect in the collecting system should be closed using intracorporal suturing techniques. The kidney is then placed back within Gerota's fascia and a retroperitoneal drain is placed and brought out through the most lateral and inferior laparoscopic port.

OUTCOMES

Results

The results of the largest LPN series are shown in Table 1 and includes our institutional series from Thomas Jefferson University.

LAPAROSCOPIC RENAL BIOPSY

Diagnosis

The etiology of intrinsic renal insufficiency is most often sought by nephrologists. Preoperatively, a KUB and renal ultrasound or noncontrast CT can be helpful in locating and characterizing the kidney to be biopsied.

Indications for Surgery

Nephrotic syndrome due to a glomerular pathology, is one of the most common indications for renal biopsy. Patients with a solitary kidney, severe hypertension, bleeding disorders, morbid obesity, and patients who are uncooperative are candidates for alternatives to percutaneous needle biopsy including laparoscopic renal biopsy.

Alternative Treatments

Percutaneous needle biopsy using ultrasound guidance, is the most common method of obtaining renal tissue for diagnostic purposes. Open renal biopsy through a subcostal or dorsal lumbotomy incision can be performed.

Surgical Technique

This procedure is ideally performed through a retroperitoneal approach. Patient preparation and positioning are identical for standard retroperitoneal laparoscopic surgery (Figure 118.1). A 1.5-cm incision is made in the posterior axillary line just lateral to the sacrospinalis muscle 2 cm above the iliac crest. The surgeon stands towards the patients back and finger dissection is carried down to the lumbodorsal fascia where sharp incision is performed to enter the retroperitoneal space. A 10-mm port is placed and a 0 laparoscope is introduced to verify correct anatomic position. Balloon dilation is carried out to dissect the retroperitoneum and create a functional working space.

A pneumoretroperitoneum is maintained at 15 mm to 20 mm Hg and the retroperitoneal space is then inspected visually. A second 10-mm port is placed under direct vision in the posterior axillary line just below the twelfth rib. Further dissection can be carried out using the laparoscope or a 5-mm grasper through the other 10-mm port to identify the lower pole of the kidney, which is usually positioned medially. Cup biopsy forceps or spoon forceps are used to obtain several samples of kidney tissue to be sent to the pathologist for routine and special studies (Figure 118–6). A large core tru-cut type biopsy needle can also be passed percutaneously to obtain the sample.

Hemostasis can be achieved with electrocautery or argon beam coagulator. The retroperitoneal pressure should be reduced to 8 mm Hg and the biopsy site and dissected space examined to make sure of adequate hemostasis. The port site fascial defects can be closed under direct vision with a 2-0 vicryl suture, or left open since the procedure is exclusively retroperitoneal.

A 24-hour observation period is recommended while the patient resumes a regular diet and ambulates since delayed bleeding has been reported. Oral pain medications are utilized depending on the level of the patient's renal function.

TABLE 118-1. *Comparative series of laparoscopic partial nephrectomy*

	Wolf et al. (21)	Stifleman et al. (18)	Gill et al. (6)	Rassweiler et al. (17)	Strup et al. (Thomas Jefferson University unpublished data)
Approach	HALPN transperitoneal	HALPN transperitoneal	Pure lap transperitoneal	Pure lap transperitoneal retroperitoneal	HALPN transperitoneal retroperitoneal
Perioperative parameters					
Number of patients	10	11	50	53	32
Mean tumor size (cm)	2.4	1.9	3.0	2.3	2.6
Central tumors (%)	3 (30%)	NA	9 (18%)	NA	8 (25%)
EBL (cc)	460	319	270	725	400
OR time (mins)	199	273	180	191	217
Hospital stay (days)	2.0	3.3	2.2	5.4	3.8
Final positive margins	0	0	0	0	0
Complications					
Open conversions	0	1	0	4	0
Persistent urine leak	0	0	1	5	1
Intra-op hemorrhage	1	0	1	1	1
Delayed hemorrhage	0	0	1	1	1
Transfusions (%)	1 (10%)	0	2 (4%)	NA	6 (18%)
Reinterventions	0	0	2 (4%)	6 (11%)	1 (3%)
Follow up					
Recurrent disease	0	0	0	0	0
Asynchronous multifocal disease*	NA	NA	NA	NA	1
Mean follow up (mo)	8	8	7.2	24	8.8
Range (mo.)					(4–15)

*One patient who underwent a HALPN for a LLP tumor was found to have a new LUP mass eventually requiring nephrectomy.

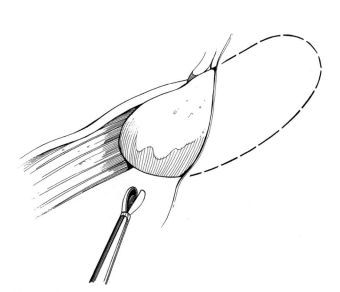

FIG. 118–6. Retroperitoneal view of lower pole of kidney prepared for renal biopsy.

Outcomes

Complications

The frequency of complications difficult to estimate for laparoscopic renal biopsy since there are no large series reported. Gaur, in a series of 17 patients undergoing biopsy, had two cases with bleeding problems (2). If electrocautery is not adequate to control bleeding, then an argon beam coagulator should be available. Fibrin glue and gelfoam hemostatis can also be utilized as for partial nephrectomy for troublesome bleeding (6).

Results

In one series, 100% of patients had an adequate amount of renal tissue obtained for diagnosis (2). Because of the direct visualization using this technique, a biopsy of an adequate amount may be ensured and adequate hemostasis verified.

NEPHROPEXY

The definition of nephroptosis is renal descent of more than two vertebral bodies or greater than 5 cm when the patient moves to the erect position is. The condition is more common in thin women and is demonstrated preferentially on the right side. Nephroptosis is most often an incidental finding and is rarely symptomatic.

Diagnosis

An intravenous pyelogram with the patient in the supine and standing position is the initial test obtained after a careful history suggests symptoms caused by a hypermobile kidney. The flank pain, lower abdominal pain and nausea associated with nephroptosis is thought to be secondary to renal ischemia or acute obstruction. The kidney might become hydronephrotic when it descends into the pelvic position and palpation of the kidney in the lying and standing positions can confirm radiographic test results. A nuclear renal scan is useful in detecting an obstructive pattern after renal descent, as well as diminished blood flow to the kidney when the patient is erect. In addition, the pain associated with obstruction should be relieved in these patients by the placement of a ureteral stent.

Alternative Therapy

The surgical treatment of nephroptosis is varied and controversial. Open nephropexy and its variations are the most commonly utilized procedures.

Surgical Technique

The retroperitoneal approach provides a direct route to the kidney and is the preferred approach. A 10-m trocar is placed in the posterior axillary line just below the twelfth rib. Dissection is carried laterally until the psoas muscle is identified and the kidney visualized medially. The entire posterior and lateral surface of the kidney should be cleared of perirenal fat to allow for accurate placement of tacking sutures. A 5-m port can also be placed midway just lateral to the sacrospinalis muscle (Figure 118).

The operative table is then moved to a head-down position. This causes the hypermobile kidney to be positioned as superiorly as possible. Sutures are then placed in the renal capsule, taking care not to place the sutures too deep, as laceration of the renal parenchyma may cause troublesome bleeding. The sutures placed in the retroperitoneum can be successfully placed in the fascia overlying the quadratus and psoas muscle. Nonabsorbable 3-0 sutures are placed superiorly, laterally and inferiorly for

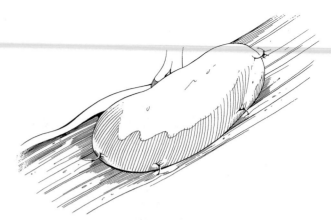

FIG. 118–7. Kidney pexed to the fascia overlying the posterior retroperitoneum. Sutures have been placed to fix the kidney superiorly, laterally, and inferiorly.

•F1•

at least a three-point fixation (Figure 118.4). A regular diet can be written for the patient on the evening of surgery and the patient released after a 24-hour observation period.

REFERENCES

1. Brown JA, Torres, VE, King BF, et al. Laparoscopic marsupialization of symptomatic polycystic kidney disease. *J Urol* 1996; 156:22–27.
2. Gaur DD, Agarwal DK, Khochikar MV, Purhoit KC. Laparoscopic renal biopsy via retroperitoneal approach. *J Urol* 1994;151(4): 925–926.
3. Gill IS, Desai MM, Kaouk JH, et al. Laparoscopic partial nephrectomy for renal tumor: duplication open surgical techniques. *J Urol* 2002;167: 469
4. Guazzoni G, Montorsi F, Berganaschi F, et al. Laparoscopic unroofing of simple renal cysts. *Urology* 1994;43(2):154.
5. Kissane JM. The morphology of renal cystic disease. In: Gardner KD Jr. (ed). *Cystic Diseases of the Kidney.* New York: John Wiley,1976;31.
6. McGinnis, DA, Strup SE, Gomella LG. Management of Hemorrhage During Laparoscopy. *J Endourol* 2000;14(10):915–920.
7. Morgan C Jr, Rader D. Laparoscopic unroofing of a renal cyst. *J Urol* 1992;148:1835–1836.
8. Munch LC, Gill IS, McRoberts JW. Laparoscopic retroperitoneal renal cystectomy. *J Urol* 1994;151:135–138.
9. Nieh PT, Bihrle W. Laparoscopic marsupialization of massive renal cyst. *J Urol* 1993;150:171–173.
10. Rassweiler JJ, Abbou G, Janetschek G, Jeschke K. Laparoscopic partial nephrectomy: The European experience. *Urol Clin North Am* 2000;27 (4):721.
11. Stifelman MD, Sosa RE, Nakada SY, et al. Hand-assisted laparoscopic partial nephrectomy. *J Endourol* 2001;15:161.
12. Stoller ML, Irby PB, Osman M, Carroll PR. Laparoscopic marsupialization of a simple renal cyst. *J Urol* 1992;150:1486–1488.
13. Teichman JMH, Hulbert JC. Laparoscopic marsupialization of the painful polycystic kidney. *J Urol* 1995;153:1105–1107.
14. Wolf JS JR, Seifman BD, Montie JE. Nephron sparing surgery for suspected malignancy: open surgery compared to laparoscopy with selective use of hand assistance. *J Urol* 2000;163:1659.

CHAPTER 119

Laparoscopic Cryoablation and Radiofrequency Ablation of Small Renal Tumors

Michael Wilkin and Stephen Y. Nakada

Recently, minimally invasive needle ablative techniques including cryoablation and radiofrequency ablation (RFA) in the treatment of small, polar renal tumors have received much attention. This heightened interest in nephron-sparing operative techniques can be attributed to the results of long-term studies on patients with renal cell carcinoma (RCC) treated with open partial nephrectomy. Although radical nephrectomy is the current gold standard for RCC therapy, it has been demonstrated that 91% to 98% cancer-specific survival rates can be achieved in patients with tumors smaller than 4 cm treated with partial nephrectomy (1,4).

In addition, widespread usage of ultrasound and computed tomography (CT) has resulted in the detection of small, asymptomatic renal lesions at an increasing frequency (11). Technology has advanced to the point where less invasive techniques such as cryoablation and RFA can be performed safely and more reproducibly. The use of destructive energy to achieve focused tumor ablation is compelling to both urologists and patients.

DIAGNOSIS

The diagnosis of renal masses relies on standard imaging modalities. These include ultrasound, CT, and magnetic resonance imaging (MRI).

INDICATIONS FOR SURGERY

The indications for ablation of small renal masses continues to evolve. Most consider that renal lesions treated in this fashion be less than 4 cm. Patients with a genetic predisposition to recurrent RCC form an optimal subpopulation to study needle ablative, nephron-sparing modalities. Patients with significant comorbidities, soli-

tary kidney, and decreased life expectancies may best benefit from RFA.

ALTERNATIVE THERAPY

The management of small renal masses can include radical and partial nephrectomy performed by a variety of open and laparoscopic (standard transperitoneal, retroperitoneal, or hand-assisted) approaches. Percutaneous cryofrequency ablation and RFA are less commonly utilized approaches.

SURGICAL TECHNIQUE

Laparoscopic Cryoablation

Cryoablation destroys tissue by freezing it. Several animal and human studies have demonstrated the short-term efficacy of cryoablation (Table 119–1). Cryosurgery works at the cellular level via ice formation and solute damage. However, the major mechanism of action involves vascular thrombosis with resultant ischemic necrosis (8). Complete ablation of tissue occurs at temperatures of -19.4°C or lower (3). This target temperature is achieved at a distance of 3.1 mm inside the leading edge of the ice ball (2). Gill et al. routinely seek to extend the ice ball 1 cm beyond the tumor edge to ensure cell kill (6). The ice ball must be controlled using intraoperative ultrasound and thermosensors. The application of cryoablation is logical in treating small polar tumors of the kidney from an anatomic standpoint. The kidney's retroperitoneal position and perinephric fat typically protect adjacent structures such as liver and bowel from the ice ball, thereby decreasing the potential morbidity of the procedure.

TABLE 119–1. *Select renal cryoablation clinical series* •T1•

Author/reference	No. (recurrences)	Contribution
Uchida 1995, Kyoto	2	Percutaneous cryoablation
Delworth 1996, Houston	2	Open cryoablation
Rodriguez 1998, Baltimore	6	Open/laparoscopic cryoablation
Rukstalis 2001, Philadelphia	29 (1)	Open cryoablation
Gill 2001, Cleveland	64 (1)	Laparoscopic cryoablation
Shingleton 2001, Mississippi	45 (5)	Percutaneous cryoablation
Kim 2002, Chicago	12 (1)	Laparoscopic cryoablation
Moon et al. 2002, Wisconsin	15 (0)	Laparoscopic cryoablation

We prefer the modified transperitoneal lateral approach for anteriorly and most superiorly based renal lesions (7). Retroperitoneal access is utilized for all other tumors. The transperitoneal approach allows for excellent viewing of the kidney, an adequate working space within the pneumoperitoneum, and minimal risk of bleeding.

The patient is placed on the operative room table and general endotracheal anesthesia is induced. The patient is placed in the 90-degree lateral position, appropriately padded, and stabilized with padded safety straps. Insufflation is performed via a 12-mm incision in the midclavicular line at or somewhat above the level of the umbilicus dependent upon the patient's body habitus using a Veress technique as described in Chapter 113A. After the pneumoperitoneum is achieved, the Veress needle is removed and a 12-mm port is placed through the same incision using an endoscopic trocar (Optiview, Ethicon Endo-Surgery, Cincinnati, OH) where insufflation is continued. The laparoscope is placed through this port and all additional trocars are placed under direct vision. Additional ports are placed in a diamond configuration as shown in Figure 119–1. The larger cryoprobes require a 5-mm port 6 to 8 cm caudal to the ribs in the anterior axillary line, while the 2-mm cryoprobes can be placed percutaneously, obviating the need for this trocar. Once all ports are placed, the pneumoperitoneum is decreased to 15 mm Hg.

The dissection begins by incising the peritoneum along the white line of Toldt and reflecting the colon medially using blunt and sharp dissection with the harmonic scalpel and atraumatic grasping forceps. Sufficient dissection is performed to allow access to the kidney to target the tumor. Once the kidney is in view, Gerota's fascia is entered using sharp dissection in a longitudinal direction. Blunt dissection is then used to remove some of the perirenal fat overlying the kidney to help expose the tumor. The fat overlying the lesion is left in place.

To localize the lesion, a flexible, steerable laparoscopic ultrasound probe is introduced through a 12-mm port and the kidney is imaged posteriorly to precisely identify the tumor. The tumor size, depth from kidney surface to tumor, and distance from tumor to collecting system are all measured. A needle biopsy of the tumor under ultrasound guidance is taken for pathologic confirmation.

Intrarenal temperatures of -19.4°C or lower are required to achieve uniform cell death. To monitor the temperature of the tumor and the surrounding parenchyma during cryoablation, two 18-gauge thermocouples can be placed percutaneously using the Seldinger technique. Ultrasound guidance is used to position one

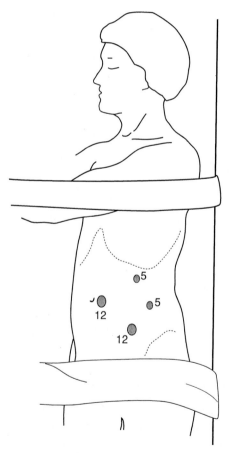

FIG. 119–1. For laparoscopic cryoablation, in the transperitoneal approach we utilize a typical diamond configuration, with ports for the laparoscope, laparoscopic ultrasound probe, and instrument. The fourth port may be substituted if percutaneous cryoprobes are utilized.

thermocouple centrally within the tumor and the second thermocouple peripheral to the tumor. To date, we have been satisfied with adequate results by targeting the ice ball approximately 1 cm beyond the lesion.

Once the tumor is localized and biopsied, a 4.8-mm cryoprobe is introduced through the 5-mm port. Alternatively, a 2-mm cryoprobe may be placed percutaneously through a red rubber catheter guide to protect the skin. After piercing the tumor, the cryoprobe is positioned centrally within the tumor under ultrasound guidance. This ensures complete coverage of the tumor by the ice ball. Cryoablation is performed using the double-freeze technique incorporating two complete freeze–thaw cycles. During the thaw phase, an increase in intraabdominal pressure may be encountered. This should be monitored and controlled by venting the laparoscopic ports. The freeze–thaw cycles are thermally and ultrasonically monitored for appropriate ice ball size, depth, and temperature. To ensure tissue necrosis during the freeze cycles, a target temperature of at least -20°C should be confirmed by the thermocouples (3). A second 2-mm cryoprobe can be utilized to treat small asymmetrical areas seen outside of the ice ball by ultrasound (Fig. 119–2).

After the double-freeze technique is complete and the ice ball has completely thawed, the cryoprobe is removed and hemostasis achieved. Surgicel mesh (Ethicon, Somerville, NJ) or an EndoAvitene plug (Davol, Cranston, RI) may be placed in the cryoprobe site to promote coagulation. Electrocautery may be used to control small areas of bleeding. The pneumoperitoneum should be reduced to 5 mm Hg and the area of operation observed to ensure hemostasis. The colon may be reflected over the kidney and the pneumoperitoneum is then evacuated. The trocars are removed under direct vision to detect any bleeding. The 12-mm port sites are closed by hand or with alternative port site closure devices with 3-0 Vicryl figure-of-eight sutures. Subcuticular 4-0 Vicryl is utilized to approximate the skin edges.

Retroperitoneal Approach

As before mentioned, this approach is best utilized for renal lesions that are posterior and laterally based. For this approach, the patient is placed in the flank position. An incision is made and retroperitoneal access is obtained. Three ports are utilized: one off the tip of the twelfth rib, one 3 cm superior to the iliac crest along the midaxillary line, and one along the posterior axillary line below the twelfth rib (Fig. 119–3).

Once retroperitoneal access is obtained, the procedure progresses stepwise as described above for the transperi-

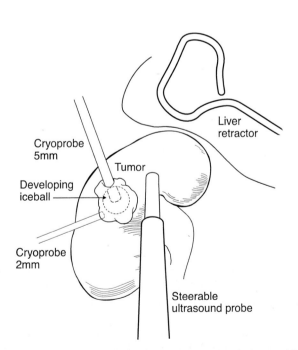

FIG. 119–2. During laparoscopic transperitoneal cryoablation, a 5-mm diamond flex triangle retractor (Genzyme Surgical Products) is utilized while the ultrasound probe and laparoscope monitor the procedure.

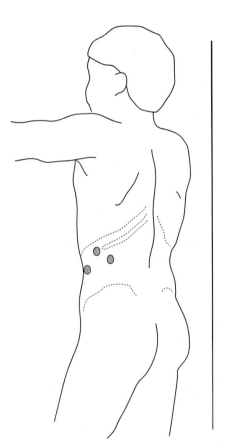

FIG. 119–3. Trocar alignment for retroperitoneal laparoscopic cryoablation. The surgeons stand behind the patient, with the monitors opposite them.

toneal approach once the kidney is in view. Advantages of the retroperitoneal approach include minimal bowel exposure and possibly more rapid convalescence. In addition, risk of adhesion formation may be reduced with this approach. However, bleeding from disrupted vessels following balloon dilation and the smaller working space are disadvantages of this approach.

RFA

RFA utilizes heat to kill tumor cells. Radiofrequency energy has been utilized in surgical settings to achieve hemostasis for many decades. Radiofrequency energy is transmitted to cancerous lesions by direct contact with needle electrodes. Generators deliver alternating current through the needle and into the tumor. Grounding pads are applied to the patient, which completes the electrical circuit. Electrical impedance or tissue resistance to current flow causes local heating. After 10 minutes of RFA, tissue impedance increases sharply to above 100 Ω, shutting down the generator. Investigators have concluded that this drastic rise in impedance indicates tissue desiccation and may correlate to bubble formation (5,10). Tissue destruction results via thermal injury with target temperatures of 80 to 100°C.

Conventional RFA is performed with dry or uninsulated electrodes. A LeVeen RFA electrode (RTC, Sunnyvale, CA) has been designed that consists of about 8 to 10 wires that take the shape of an umbrella when deployed in the tissue. This geometric arrangement secures the electrode within in the tumor and allows for consistent round RFA lesions especially conducive to treating renal lesions. Its design allows current to be automatically transferred from areas of high impedance to ones of low impedance without the use of a coupler solution. Investigators have developed newer types of RFA delivery systems called wet RFA and bipolar RFA. Wet RFA involves adding a continuous infusion coupler of an electrolyte solution to cool the electrode. As a result, larger and more confined lesions are created more quickly and reproducibly. Bipolar RFA has theoretical advantages over conventional RFA due to lack of current dispersion, higher current density, and better control of lesion conformation.

RFA is typically administered percutaneously under ultrasound, MRI, or CT guidance. However, as with cryoablation, anteriorly based lesions are best addressed laparoscopically to minimize intraabdominal organ injuries. To date, the use of RFA in treating renal tumors is limited to animal studies and sporadic clinical reports.

Some investigators have utilized preprocedure embolization of the lesion when performing RFA. RFA procedures for anterior lesions are usually performed laparoscopically as for cryotherapy; posterior lesions are often treated in the interventional radiology suite, usually in conjunction with a radiologist. The image-guided treatment is carried out using MRI or CT guidance with conscious sedation (midazolam and fentanyl), with some patients requiring general anesthesia. A standard dispersive grounding pad is applied to the patient's thigh or buttock.

An electrosurgical generator such as the RITA Model 500 is utilized to deliver 50-W, 460-kHz radiofrequency energy percutaneously via RITA Model 70 15-gauge coaxial probes. Smaller exophytic lesions can be treated with a single electrode whereas larger lesions must be treated with multiple electrodes with overlapping ablation volumes. Target probe temperature is 100°C. Tumors are heated to a maximum wattage of 50 to reach tissue temperatures approaching 70°C for a 10- to 12-minute cycle. Multiple RFA cycles and probe repositioning are performed as necessary to ensure tumor ablation at the target temperature. Some RFA generators feature automatic current pulsing, which decreases the current as impedance rises to maximize the size of the RFA lesion. Energy is applied as the probe is withdrawn from the tumor to coagulate the probe tract to obtain hemostasis and decrease the incidence of tumor tract implantation. Many of these patients can be discharged the same day or on postoperative day 1.

OUTCOMES

Complications

Because long-term data regarding cancer control is lacking at the time of this writing, patients must be informed that laparoscopic cryoablation in the treatment for RCC remains experimental. Explanation of the risks associated with cryoablation must include bleeding, infection, visceral/vascular injury, fistula, hypercarbia, and death. No large-scale studies analyzing laparoscopic cryoablation complications have been performed, but the laparoscopic nephrectomy procedure is associated with a 6% intraoperative complication rate. Bleeding represents the majority of complications. A conversion rate to open surgery of 10% due to bleeding, bowel injury, or difficult dissection has been reported.

Results

Cryoablation

Gill and associates reported a total of 67 patients have been treated with laparoscopic cryoablation and followed prospectively. They reported results of 32 patients (34 tumors) with a mean tumor size of 2.3 cm (7) (Table 119–2). Cryoablation was performed via the transperitoneal approach in 10 and retroperitoneally in 22. Mean surgical time was 2.9 hours, cryoablation time 15.1 minutes, and blood loss averaged 66.8 mL. Hospital stay was less than 23 hours in 69% of patients. During a mean follow-up of 16.2 months, no patient has had radiological

TABLE 119–2. *Features of laparoscopic cryoablation*

Surgical time	2.9 h
Cryoablation time	15.1 min
Blood loss	66.8 mL
Hospital stay	<23 h (24 of 32 patients)
Follow-up term	8.5 mo
Recurrences	None

From Gill IS, Novick AC, Meraney AM, et al. Laparoscopic renal cryoablation in 32 patients. *Urology* 2000;56:748–753, with permission.

evidence of renal fossa, port site, or systemic recurrence. Moreover, no evidence of cancer was found in 23 patients who underwent a 3- to 6-month postprocedure CT-guided biopsy of the cryoablated tumor site. In 20 patients who underwent a 1-year follow-up MRI scan, the cryoablated lesion was no longer detectable in 5. In the remaining 15 patients, the cryolesions had decreased in size by 66%. Recently, 3-year follow-up results have been reported on a cohort of 25 patients. One patient with biopsy-proven RCC recurrence underwent laparoscopic nephrectomy and is currently free of disease (12). Our own experience in 15 cases mirrors the above-noted larger series (Table 119–1).

RFA

Pavlovich and associates at the National Cancer Institute maintain the largest RFA clinical series of 24 ablations in 21 patients with von Hippel–Lindau clear cell RCC or hereditary papillary renal cancer (9). Pavlovich and associates assessed RFA preliminary efficacy with a CT scan 2 months postprocedure. The two radiographic parameters—change in lesion enhancement and change in lesion size—were quantified. The mean tumor size decreased from 2.4 cm to 2.0 cm and 79% of the lesions demonstrated nonenhancement. Five tumors maintained focal areas of persistent enhancement. In addition, mean serum creatinine was unchanged during this interval. No major complications were encountered.

REFERENCES

1. Butler BP, Novick AC, Miller DP, et al. Management of small unilateral renal cell carcinoma. *Urology* 1995;45:34–41.
2. Campbell SC, Krishnamurthi V, Chow G, et al. Renal cryosurgery: experimental evaluation of treatment parameters. *Urology* 1998;52:29–33.
3. Chosy SG, Nakada SY, Lee FT Jr, Warner TF. Monitoring renal cryosurgery: Predictors of tissue necrosis in swine. *J Urol* 1998;159:1370–1374.
4. Fergany AF, Hafez KS, Novick AC. Long term results of nephron sparing surgery for localized renal cell carcinoma: 10-year followup. *J Urol* 2000;163:442–445.
5. Gill IS, Hsu THS, Fox RL, et al. Laparoscopic and percutaneous radiofrequency ablation of the kidney: Acute and chronic porcine study. *Urology* 2000;56:197–200.
6. Gill IS, Novick AC, Meraney AM, et al. Laparoscopic renal cryoablation in 32 patients. *Urology* 2000;56:748–753.
7. Johnson DB, Nakada SY. Laparoscopic cryoablation for renal cell cancer. *J Endourol* 2000;14:873–879.
8. Mazur P. The role of intracellular freezing in the death of cells cooled at supraoptimal rates. *Cryobiology* 1977;14:251–272.
9. Pavlovich CP, Walther MM, Choyke PL, et al. Percutaneous radiofrequency ablation of small renal tumors: Initial results. *J Urol* 2002;167:10–15.
10. Rendon RA, Gertner MR, Sherar MD, et al. Development of a radiofrequency based thermal therapy technique in an in vivo porcine model for the treatment of small renal masses. *J Urol* 2001;166:292–298.
11. Smith SJ, Bosniak MA, Megibow AJ, et al. Renal cell carcinoma: earlier discovery and increased detection. *Radiology* 1989;170:699–703.
12. Steinberg AP, Gill IS, Strzempkowski B, et al. 3-year followup of laparoscopic renal cryoablation in 25 patients. *J Urol* 2002;167:166 (abst).

CHAPTER 120

Laparoscopic Donor Nephrectomy

Deborah Glassman and Stephen C. Jacobs

There are over 50,000 patients in the U.S. on the waiting list for renal allograft transplantation. Only 13,000 of them will be fortunate enough to receive an organ. Living donors provide a bridge over the supply gap; however, only 5,300 live donor nephrectomies were performed in 2000. Laparoscopic donor nephrectomy (LDN) has become the procedure of choice in large renal transplantation centers since it was first performed in 1995 (6). It is a consumer-driven procedure that may ultimately help increase the donor pool and reduce the number of patients awaiting transplantation (4,7). In comparison to open donor nephrectomy, the renal allograft function is equivalent.

This chapter will discuss donor selection and preoperative management, as well as the operative technique of left LDN. It will also briefly cover the postoperative course, right LDN, complications, and results of LDN.

DIAGNOSIS

All selected donors undergo a standard preoperative evaluation. A computed tomography (CT) angiogram is performed to visualize the kidneys and their vascular anatomy. It also verifies that there is no abdominal or renal pathology. The images provide a roadmap to prevent arterial injury at the time of nephrectomy (1). Preferably, the left kidney is used for donation as it provides a longer renal vein for the transplant surgeon, minimizing potential vascular complications in the recipient.

INDICATIONS FOR SURGERY

The criteria for LDN are the same as for open nephrectomy. The donor must be in general good health and free from hypertension, diabetes, renal disease, renovascular disease, heart disease, or cancer. Benign renal masses are not a contraindication for transplantation. Neither is unrelatedness. The age range for donors has increased and

donors as old as 74 years have given a kidney. Relative contraindications for LDN include previous abdominal or retroperitoneal surgery, renal stones, and complicated vascular anatomy.

ALTERNATIVE THERAPY

Open-flank nephrectomy and hand-assisted donor nephrectomy are alternative approaches.

SURGICAL TECHNIQUE

Anesthesia is administered, prophylactic antibiotics are given, and a Foley catheter is placed in the bladder. While the patient is still supine the extraction site is drawn on the skin with an indelible marking pen. In male patients a 6-cm lower midline skin incision is used. In female patients a Pfannenstiel skin incision is created just above the pubic bone. If a patient is markedly obese, an alternate extraction site, such as a port site extension, may be used to avoid poor fascial closure due to technical difficulty with exposure.

The patient is then placed in the lateral decubitus position as if for an open nephrectomy. In contrast to the open positioning, the patient's abdomen is moved close to the ventral edge of the operating table rather than the usual dorsal table edge. This will allow freedom of movement of the instruments. It is also recommended that the patient's uppermost arm rest on pillows rather than a rigid arm support. This will allow the camera-person to gently lean into the patient's arms without causing traction in the axilla. The patient is secured to the table with tape and a leg strap and then sterilely prepped and draped from the xiphoid to the pubic bone.

During the procedure the patient should be well hydrated. Pneumoperitoneum causes a decrease in renal blood flow and it is imperative to maximize diuresis of the donor organ throughout the case. The patient should receive at least 4 to 5 L of intravenous (IV) fluid during the case. The patient should also receive two 25-g doses of Mannitol. The first is given while the colon is being reflected medially and the second during the hilar dissection. The surgeon should periodically check with the anesthesiologist to ensure that the patient has good urine output and blood pressure.

Port Placement

LDN is essentially performed via three ports: a camera port and two working ports (Fig. 120–1). A fourth port is placed through the extraction incision near the end of the case. The initial recommendation is to use 12-mm ports; however, as one becomes more comfortable with the procedure the ports can be downsized to 5 mm. All port sites are marked with ink and infiltrated with 0.5% bupivicaine to provide local anesthesia. Pneumoperitoneum is established with carbon dioxide insufflation via a Veress needle. The initial port is placed 2 cm above the umbilicus, adjacent to the lateral rectus border, using techniques described in chapter on basic laparoscopy. The next two trocars are placed under direct laparoscopic vision using a 30-degree lens. The position of the second port site should be as cephalad as possible 1 cm medial to the costal margin. This will be the camera port for the duration of the procedure. The third trocar is placed midway between the umbilicus and the anterior superior iliac crest. The distance from the first port to the second and third ports should be at least 7 cm each so that the ports form an arc around the kidney.

Operative Procedure

At our center, LDN is performed transperitoneally. The colon is mobilized along the white line of Toldt and the recommended instrument for all sharp dissection is the ultrasonic scalpel in the right port. The left-hand instrument is a blunt-tipped forceps such as a Maryland dissector. However, one must be prepared to use the scalpel in either hand depending on the angle needed to most easily carry out the dissection. The colon must be mobilized from below the iliac vessels to the splenic flexure. The colonic mobilization can be done in a bloodless field as the peritoneal reflection is avascular. Care must be taken, in particular in the thin donor, not to violate the colonic mesentery as this may be a source for internal hernia postoperatively or colonic necrosis. Any mesenteric tears need to be repaired prior to the end of the case. As the colon is rolled medially the kidney can be seen within Gerota's fascia and the hilar vessels will appear.

The line of peritoneal dissection is actually then carried lateral to the spleen so that the spleen, pancreas, and colon all fall medially as a unit. The "splenorenal ligaments" are transected as the dissection is carried cephalad and medially toward the stomach (Fig. 120–2). Once the spleen and pancreas have been mobilized medially the adrenal gland can be seen within Gerota's fascia.

Once the colon has been fully mobilized, Gerota's fascia is entered over the renal vein medially. If the lateral attachments to the kidney have been taken down then it is sometimes necessary to place a lateral port. If another port is necessary to provide further exposure to the renal vessels, a 5-mm trocar can be placed between the costal margin and the anterior superior iliac crest in the midclavicular line. A grasper can then be used to take hold of Gerota's fascia and retract the kidney laterally. The surface of the vein is cleaned off and dissected medially until it crosses the aorta. The adrenal and gonadal branches are identified at their insertion with the renal vein. The branches are dissected free. They are then ligated in continuity with a multifire clip applier through the right port. Four clips are placed on each of the veins. The veins are then divided between clips two and three (Fig. 120–3).

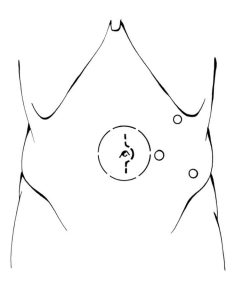

FIG. 120–1. Port placement for left laparoscopic donor nephrectomy. **A:** Camera port (5 to 12 mm): 1 cm medial to the costal margin. **B:** Left-hand working port (5 mm): 2 cm superior to the umbilicus and lateral to the rectus border. **C:** Right-hand working port (5 to 12 mm): Midway between umbilicus and iliac crest. **D:** Extraction site, male (6 to 8 cm): Infraumbilical midline incision. In a female a Pfannenstiel incision is made. **E:** First assistant port (5 mm): Opposite B port in posterior axillary line.

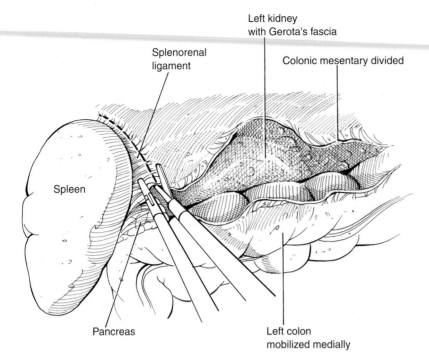

FIG. 120–2. Detachment of "splenorenal ligaments." **A:** Spleen. **B:** Kidney, within Gerota's fascia. **C:** Left colon, mobilized medially. **D:** Pancreas. Dividing the colonic mesentery to rotate the colon medially will develop a plane between the spleen and Gerota's fascia. The line of dissection is carried between the two organs to allow the spleen and pancreas to fall medially. The incision of this plane continues cephalad and medial until the stomach is visualized.

This leaves only a lumbar branch still feeding the renal vein. This will be divided during the arterial dissection. The edges of the gonadal or adrenal vein can be gently retracted toward the renal vein to aid in development of a plane between the vein and artery.

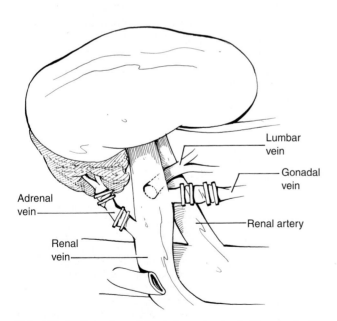

FIG. 120–3. Branches of the left renal vein. **A:** Renal vein. **B:** Adrenal vein. **C:** Gonadal vein. **D:** Lumbar vein. **E:** Renal artery. The gonadal and adrenal branches are identified at their insertion and then dissected circumferentially. Four clips are placed on each branch to ligate them in continuity. Each vein is then divided with Endoshears. The lumbar vein is identified, ligated, and divided later in the procedure.

Cephalad to the renal vein the adrenal gland can be identified. The adrenal must now be dissected away from the superior pole of the kidney. The line of dissection must stay close to the edge of the adrenal gland as the renal artery or an accessory renal artery may lie just lateral to the gland. There is a large amount of fatty lymphatic and ganglionic tissue that lies between the renal hilum and the adrenal gland. Great care must be taken when dividing this tissue as it is friable and can hide small polar branches. As the adrenal gland is retracted medially the upper pole can then be freed. The superior edge of the renal artery may be seen as the adrenal falls medially. The line of dissection can then be carried cephalad from this edge to the superior aspect of the kidney without hitting any major structures.

After identification of the gonadal vein the ureter can be dissected toward the pelvis. A window in the retroperitoneal fat is made medial to the ureter just lateral to the gonadal vein. The psoas muscle and its fascia are identified through the window. In a very thin person the gonadal vein should accompany the ureter to provide a large swath of periureteral tissue around the ureter. In this case the gonadal vein is used as a landmark and the medial window is made between the aorta and the gonadal vein. The ureter may not actually be seen in the periureteral tissue and fat but will be lateral to the gonadal vein. The ureter is retracted laterally and the window is enlarged in the cephalad–caudad direction until the ureter crosses the common iliac vessels. Again, care must be taken to avoid the colonic mesentery. When the ureter is seen crossing the common iliac vessels a window is made lateral to the ureter so the psoas is again seen. The ureter is now encased in a bundle of tissue, which will be divided with it and given to the transplant surgeon.

Once the ureteral packet has been completely defined it can be traced back from the pelvis toward the renal hilum. Gentle retraction of the lower pole and ureter will define the inferior border of the vascular pedicle. There is ganglionic and lymphatic tissue between the gonadal vein and the aorta that must be divided to provide access to the renal artery at its origin. At this point the lumbar vein can usually be identified. It is dissected free from its surrounding tissue clipped in continuity and divided between four clips. This will now allow circumferential freeing of the renal vein. The renal artery will lie posterior to the vein and its inferior aspect can be seen as the renal vein is mobilized. A blunt instrument, usually a suction–irrigator device, can be carefully passed just posterior to the renal vein. A window is developed between the vein and artery to allow placement of the stapler (Fig. 120–4).

It is not necessary to completely free the renal artery of its surrounding tissue. Minimal handling of the artery prevents trauma and vasospasm of the artery. However, it is recommended for the first few procedures that all of the anatomy be clearly identified. Papaverine or another topical vasodilator can be delivered to the renal artery subadventitia with a cholangiogram catheter. This will minimize vasospasm.

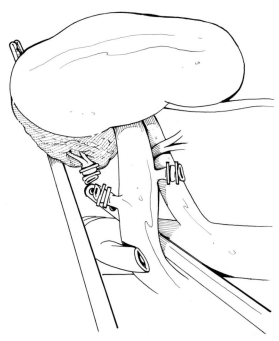

FIG. 120–4. Development of the plane between the renal artery and vein. Dissection of the origin of the artery and division of the lumbar vein allow an instrument to be passed between the two vessels. The suction–irrigator or a blunt grasper can be gently passed in front of the artery. Rotating the instrument will help the dissection. Development of this plane is crucial to allow enough room for placement of the endovascular stapler.

Once the renal artery, vein, and ureter have been freed, the lateral attachments of the kidney can be divided. It is important that the kidney remain fixed in its bed until the vasculature is dissected free so that the kidney does not fall medially. Premature freeing of the kidney from the renal fossa will make exposure difficult and prevent maximal attainable length of the vessels. The ultrasonic scalpel is used to divide the areolar tissue lateral and posterior to the kidney. The left-handed grasper is used to roll the kidney medially as these attachments are freed. Once the renal artery is seen from the posteriolateral aspect the dissection is complete. The kidney is then rolled back into its normal anatomic position. Care must be taken to prevent renal torsion. An instrument is placed each under the superior and inferior poles and the kidney is gently lifted. This ensures that the only remaining attachments are the renal vessels and the ureter. Once the renal dissection is complete it is useful to check with the recipient surgeons that they are going to be ready to accept the organ. The saline ice slush should be fully prepared. A back table for dissection and organ preservation perfusion fluid should be ready in the recipient room.

The previously designated extraction incision site is infiltrated with local anesthetic. In a man the incision is carried down from the skin through the linea alba. The fascial incision must be carried out such that the peritoneal cavity is not entered. Gentle stretching of the musculature and fascial fibers will help ensure smooth organ extraction. In a female the skin incision is made. The superficial tissues are divided in the midline to the level of the fascia. The fascial incision is then made cranial–caudad in the midline, as in a male patient.

Under direct vision, through the extraction site, a 15-mm or 18-mm port with a 15-mm reducer cap is placed. The camera-person through either the left or right ports to retract the small bowel out of the way may use blunt graspers. The port should be angled cephalad and superiorly to minimize small-bowel injury. Once the port has been placed there are two ways to complete the procedure.

Prior to division of the renal vessels the ureter must be divided. If a 12-mm port is being used, an Endo-GIA stapler is place through it to divide the ureter and vessels. The ureter is divided as caudal as possible. The patient should then receive 5000 U of heparin. The heparin should then be allowed to circulate for 2 to 3 minutes as preparation is made to divide the renal artery and vein. There should be enough stapler reloads available to divide the renal artery and vein and any accessory vessels and provide extra as necessary for a stapler misfire or incomplete division.

The extraction bag is placed in the wound through the 15-mm port and the kidney placed in it prior to dividing the vessels. The bag is deployed under the kidney such that the ring provides retraction of the kidney laterally and anteriorly to place the vessels on traction. Prebagging the kidney will also minimize the chance of being unable to place the organ in the extraction bag when it is completely freed of its attachments. An assistant should hold the bag in place so that the surgeon is free to operate with two hands.

After the heparin has been allowed to circulate the endovascular stapler with 2.5-mm staple reload is introduced through the 12-mm port and opened so that the jaws lie on either side of the renal artery. The stapler is levered down close to the origin of the renal artery, but not so close to the renal os as to catch the aortic wall in the staple line. The artery is ligated and divided with the stapler. The patient is then given 50 mg of protamine to reverse the effects of the heparin. The stapler is reloaded and reintroduced to ligate the vein. The bag is again gently retracted to provide length and the stapler is placed low across the vein. The clips from the lumbar, gonadal, and adrenal branches must be avoided to prevent stapler misfire. After the vein has been divided, the kidney is manipulated into the bag by gently shaking the bag and using graspers as necessary.

The bag is closed and the ring pulled back into the handle under direct vision. The ring can cut the kidney or injure small bowel as it is withdrawn. The 15-mm port, Endocatch handle, and ring are all carefully withdrawn through the extraction incision and scissors are used to cut the string of the bag to remove the hardware from the kidney to prevent injury to the organ. The wound is manually stretched to accommodate the kidney. The bag is gently pulled by its string to deliver the kidney from the wound. Excessive compression of the renal parenchyma by a tight extraction incision can cause delayed graft function. The kidney is immediately immersed in the ice saline solution and brought to the back dissection table or recipient room.

If only 5-mm ports are being used then the 15-mm port is used for both stapling and placement of the extraction bag. After the 15-mm port has been introduced a reducer cap is put on it and the stapler introduced through the port. The ureter is divided as described. Grasping forceps are used to hold the kidney in place under its upper and lower poles. Heparin is given and allowed to circulate. The artery and vein are divided as described above. After the vessels have been divided and the stapler removed the reducer cap is removed and the extraction bag is placed so that the bag opens under the kidney. The graspers are slowly withdrawn from under the balancing kidney so that it falls into the bag. The ureter and perinephric tissue are placed in the bag with the graspers and by gently shaking the bag. The bag is withdrawn in the usual manner.

After the kidney has been removed from the bag and placed in saline slush it needs to be perfused with preservation solution, Wisconsin or EuroCollins. The staple lines are cut off the vessels and the solution is perfused in through the renal artery until the venous effluent is clear. The renal vein branches are ligated at their insertion and the Endoclips are removed. The perinephric fat is removed and discarded but the periureteric tissue is left in place so that the ureteral blood supply remains intact. The

ureteral staple line is removed as well. The kidney is then ready for transplantation. While the surgeon is transporting the kidney to the recipient room the assistant can begin the closure process. If there is an immediate concern about bleeding the fascial extraction incision can be approximated with Kocher or Allis clamps and the abdomen can be reinsufflated to examine it. Otherwise, the fascial incision is closed with a running 0-0 absorbable suture. Pneumoperitoneum is then reestablished and the retroperitoneal space is examined. The renal artery and vein stumps are inspected for bleeding, as are the spleen and adrenal gland. The mesentery is examined for tears and repaired if necessary. Irrigation is not necessary but any residual fluid should be removed with the suction–irrigator.

Trocar sites that are greater than 10 mm need to be closed. This can be accomplished under laparoscopic guidance with a fascial closure device and 0-0 absorbable ties or from the superior surface of the fascia if it can be seen through the skin. Instruments are removed from the remaining 5-mm ports and the CO_2 is released. The ports are then withdrawn. It is not necessary to close the fascia of these small sites. The skin incisions are all closed with 4-0 absorbable subcuticular sutures and dressed with steristrips, Band-Aids, or occlusive dressings.

Right Donor Nephrectomy

As stated earlier, the left kidney is most commonly the one chosen for renal donation. Nonetheless, there will be times when it is more opportune to use the right one. Compromised right renal function, benign right renal disease, or simpler vasculature when compared to the left side are all indications for right donor nephrectomy. Right-sided nephrectomy differs from the left by port placement and sequence of dissection.

Four ports are placed at the beginning of the case (Fig. 120–5). The first port is placed lateral to the umbilicus at the rectus border. The second is placed 7 cm inferior to the first, between the iliac crest and the rectus border. The third and fourth ports are positioned 7 and 14 cm, respectively, superior to the first port along the rectus border. The most cephalad port is used for access to place a retractor for the liver. The camera is placed through the second or third port depending on the angle of view needed during the case.

The colon is taken down along the white line of Toldt, as on the left side. The plane between the liver and the superior pole is defined and the peritoneal attachments to the liver are divided so that a fan retractor or blunt grasper can be used to rotate the liver medially. The duodenum is also retracted medially. It is important to hug the duodenum when dividing it away from Gerota's fascia. There may be polar branches that can be easily injured during this part of the dissection. This will expose the inferior vena cava (IVC) and the renal vein should come into view. On occasion, it is

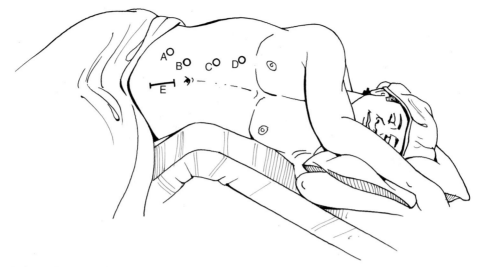

FIG. 120–5. Port placement for a right laparoscopic donor nephrectomy. **A:** Left-hand working port/camera port (5 to 12 mm): 7 cm inferior to the periumbilical port midway between the umbilicus and iliac crest. **B:** Left-hand working port (5 mm): Lateral to the umbilicus at the rectus border. In a patient with a short torso, it may be necessary to place the port slightly inferior to the umbilicus at the rectus border. **C:** Right-hand working port/camera port (5 to 12 mm): 7 cm cephalad to port B, along the rectus border. **D:** Liver retraction port (5 to 12 mm): 14 cm cephalad to port B, medial to the costal margin. **E:** Extraction site, male (6 to 8 cm): Infraumbilical midline incision. In a female a Pfannenstiel incision is made.

necessary to free the lower pole and identify the ureter prior to seeing the renal vein. The ureter can be traced toward the hilum to then find the vein. The renal vein should be freed to its insertion into the IVC. This will allow for maximum length when time for division. The dissection continues cephalad from the superior edge of the renal vein between the kidney and adrenal gland.

Unlike the procedure for left nephrectomy, the posterior and lateral attachments of the right kidney are taken down to facilitate identification of the renal artery. The lower pole is freed and the ureter is retracted medially. The kidney is then rotated medially as the areolar tissue within Gerota's fascia is divided. This will expose the posterior aspect of the right renal artery. A plane is created between the artery and vein, as on the left. This is often more easily accomplished from the posterior aspect of the kidney. The last attachments to be divided are at the superior pole. Once only its vasculature and the ureter hold the kidney, the extraction incision is made. The procedure then continues as for the left-sided LDN.

OUTCOMES

Results

A survey of LDN performed at high-volume renal transplant centers was done by the Program for Advanced Laparoscopic Surgery and Transplantation Services (2). They found that by late 1999 26 of 31 (84%) of the high-volume centers had performed LDN. Concerns of poorer allograft function when compared to open or hand-

assisted techniques have been unfounded (5–7). The length of warm ischemia time is longer for LDN when compared to open donor nephrectomy but this does not seem to affect long-term outcome of allograft function (5). It was initially thought that the rate of ureteral complications might be higher in LDN compared to open nephrectomy (3). This has not been borne out in high-volume centers, suggesting that the ureteral complications were related to the inadequate periureteral tissue and vascular supply accompanying the ureter rather than the operative procedure itself. To date, there are no long-term studies specific to laparoscopic donor outcomes.

REFERENCES

1. Del Pizzo JJ, Sklar GN, You-Cheong JW, et al. Helical computerized tomography arteriography for evaluation of live renal donors undergoing laparoscopic nephrectomy. *J Urol* 1999;162:31–34.
2. Finelli FC, Gongora E, Sasaki TM, et al. A survey: the prevalence of laparoscopic donor nephrectomy at large U.S. transplant centers. *Transplantation* 2001;71:1862–1864.
3. Philosophe B, Kuo PC, Schweitzer EJ, et al. Laparoscopic versus open donor nephrectomy: comparing ureteral complications in the recipients and improving the laparoscopic technique. *Transplantation* 1999;68:497–502.
4. Ratner LE, Hiller J, Sroka M, et al. Laparoscopic live donor nephrectomy removes disincentives to live donation. *Transplant Proc* 1997;29:3402–3403.
5. Ruiz-Deya G, Cheng S, Palmer E, et al. Open donor, laparoscopic donor and hand assisted laparoscopic donor nephrectomy: a comparison of outcomes. *J Urol* 2001;166:1270–1273; discussion 1273–1274.
6. Schulam PG, Kavoussi LR, Cheriff AD, et al. Laparoscopic live donor nephrectomy: the initial 3 cases. *J Urol* 1996;155:1857–1859.
7. Schweitzer EJ, Wilson J, Jacobs S, et al. Increased rates of donation with laparoscopic donor nephrectomy. *Ann Surg* 2000;232:392–400.

CHAPTER 121

Hand-Assisted Laparoscopic Donor Nephrectomy

J. Stuart Wolf, Jr.

Transplantation of the kidney from a living donor is associated with a shorter waiting time, better allograft function, and better survival than transplantation from a cadaveric donor. In an attempt to minimize the pain and suffering of the living kidney donor, and possibly to increase the donor pool, laparoscopic techniques have been introduced. Originally described using standard laparoscopic techniques with subsequent intact removal of the kidney through an abdominal incision, the hand-assisted laparoscopic approach to laparoscopic donor nephrectomy has recently been popularized because it is technically simpler, has a shorter learning curve, and may provide better intraoperative control of vascular injury.

DIAGNOSIS

Potential donors undergo evaluation based on the transplant team's institutional protocols.

INDICATIONS FOR SURGERY

Prospective donor evaluation starts with a complete medical history and physical examination. Any systemic or genitourinary diseases that might pose a risk to future renal function are most strongly considered. A full discussion of the entire donor evaluation process is beyond the scope of this chapter, but mention will be made of anatomic considerations in the selection of a prospective donor for laparoscopic versus open surgical donor nephrectomy. Laparoscopic donor nephrectomy, whether with the standard or the hand-assisted approach, is technically simpler on the left side. The endoscopic stapler that is typically used to control the renal vein does sacrifice some vein length, and for a short right renal vein this might be problematic. With experience and technical modifications, however, right-sided kidneys can safely be removed laparoscopically. In general, multiple renal arteries are no more a liability with laparoscopy than they are with open surgery. A small lower-pole artery should always be avoided, regardless of the approach, because of potential risk to the ureteral blood supply. A substantial lower-pole artery located well caudal from the hilum is more difficult to manage with laparoscopy than with open surgery because it tends to get in the way of the hilar dissection.

ALTERNATIVE THERAPY

Other options for living renal donation include standard open surgery, video-assisted minilaparotomy techniques where special retractors and visualization through a laparoscope allow the open surgical procedure to be done through a small open incision, and standard transperitoneal or retroperitoneal laparoscopic approaches.

SURGICAL TECHNIQUE

On the preoperative day, the patient drinks only clear liquids and a magnesium citrate bowel preparation. Antibiotics are administered. Pre- and intraoperative intravenous (IV) fluid administration should be aggressive. Run in one to two leaders of normal saline in the preoperative area and during induction. Maintain a high IV fluid rate such that six to eight liters of fluid are administered during the operation.

After induction of general anesthesia and endotracheal intubation, insert a urethral catheter and orogastric tube. For a left nephrectomy, turn the patient to a partial right flank position (45 degrees). Flexion of the table is not necessary. Subsequent rotation of the table can provide near-supine or near-flank position. Prepare and drape the abdomen and flank sterilely.

Make the incision for the hand-assistance device in the midline around the umbilicus. For a larger patient, move the incision a bit cephalad and for a smaller patient move it caudal. For patients concerned about cosmesis, consider a Pfannenstiel incision, although the reach up to the kidney with the intraabdominal hand is a stretch.

Laparoscopic ports can be placed with the intraabdominal hand suspending the abdominal wall. Noncutting trocars are preferred with this technique. Insert the 12-mm primary video laparoscope port 2 to 3 cm lateral to the hand-assistance device, inline with the umbilicus. Insert the main working laparoscopic port, also 12 mm, in a line connecting the primary video laparoscope port and the ipsilateral shoulder, 2 to 3 cm subcostal. This is usually in the anterior to midaxillary line. Finally, insert a 5-mm assisting port 2 to 3 cm above the iliac crest, in the midaxillary line (Fig. 121–1). This spatial relationship of the hand-assistance site and the port sites allows easy visualization of the operative site on either side of the working instrument, using a 30-degree video laparoscope. The surgeon inserts the left hand into the hand-assistance device, bringing in a laparotomy pad that can be used to soak up fluid and blood. The surgeon stands cephalad to the assistant, with both to the right of the patient.

Using monopolar scissors, incise the peritoneum at the line of Toldt, extending from the spleen to the iliac vessels. Once the incision has been taken down to the surface of Gerota's fascia, grasping the colon with the intraabdominal hand and exerting traction medially and anteriorly will put the flimsy connections of the peritoneum and mesentery to Gerota's fascia on stretch, exposing

them for further medial reflection. Lateral retraction of the kidney within Gerota's fascia using an instrument through the 5-mm assisting port facilitates this step. After the initiation of this dissection, a right-angle electrocautery probe is more useful than the scissors and is the instrument used for most of the remainder of the procedure. If the plane of dissection has been defined well, the intraabdominal hand can be used to perform bluntly the final reflection of the visceral contents (including the pancreas) medially. Below the lower pole of Gerota's fascia, the surface of the psoas muscle is exposed. At the upper pole, the degree of splenic mobilization depends on the relationship of the spleen to the kidney. If the spleen covers just the tip of the upper pole, then all that is needed is incision of the lienorenal attachments. If the spleen covers the kidney more extensively, then incision of all lateral attachments of the spleen may be required to allow complete medial rotation of the spleen off of the kidney. The goal of this initial dissection is to reflect the spleen and colon off of the kidney such that minimal if any manual retraction is needed to maintain complete exposure.

Next, open Gerota's fascia and the underlying perinephric tissue widely from the upper to lower poles, on the anterior surface. Traction on the perinephric tissue caudal to the kidney puts the attachments at the lower pole on stretch, allowing them to be incised easily. Once the tip of the lower pole has been dissected out, use the forefinger of the intraabdominal hand to elevate the lower pole, putting the lateral and posterior perinephric attachments on stretch. Use an instrument through the 5-mm assisting port to retract tissue laterally. With the intraabdominal hand grasping the kidney, the remainder of the

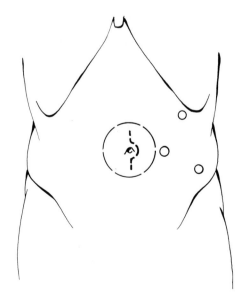

FIG. 121–1. Sites of hand-assistance device and ports. **1:** Hand-assistance device, placed through periumbilical midline incision (dotted line). **2:** The 12-mm primary laparoscope port. **3:** The 12-mm working port. **4:** The 5-mm assisting port.

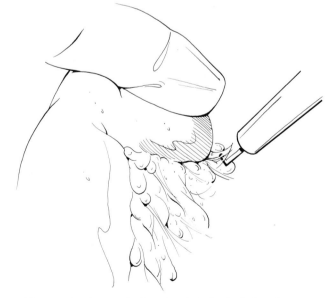

FIG. 121–2. Removal of perinephric fat includes the upper pole of the kidney, which is facilitated by caudal traction and rotation of the kidney medially.

lateral and posterior perinephric attachments can be incised quickly. Pull the kidney caudal with the intraabdominal hand to address the perinephric attachments at the upper pole of the kidney (Fig. 121–2). Freeing the upper pole is often a challenging part of the procedure, involving working back and forth between the anterior and posterior surfaces of the kidney at the limits of the hand and instruments.

At this point, the kidney is completely mobilized except for its medial attachments. Medial perinephric tissue is maintained until near the conclusion of the procedure to prevent the kidney from twisting about the hilum during vascular dissection. Now, incise the reflection of Gerota's fascia over the renal vein. If the renal vein is not easily identified, first identify the gonadal vein and follow it cephalad. Clear all tissue off of the renal vein, and its adrenal and the gonadal branches, using the right-angle electrocautery probe. Use bipolar electrocautery to coagulate the gonadal vein for a distance of about 2 cm below the renal vein and divide it. Coagulate the adrenal vein with bipolar electrocautery in a similar fashion, but also place two clips on the adrenal gland side of the vein and incise just below the clips. The purpose of using bipolar electrocautery on the renal vein branches, rather than clips, is to obviate entanglement of the endoscopic stapler with clips on the renal vein when it is ligated at the conclusion of the procedure (Fig. 121–3).

Attention is now directed to the gonadal vein just below the lower pole of the kidney. Sharply incise tissue at the medial aspect of the vein until just deep to the posterior leaf of Gerota's fascia. Insert one finger of the intraabdominal hand medial and then underneath the gonadal vein, moving it laterally on top of the psoas muscle until the entirety of the tissue below the kidney has been encircled with the finger. By gathering the gonadal vein and ureter into a single packet of tissue, devascularization of the ureter is prevented. Reflect excess perinephric tissue off of this gonadal–ureteral packet later-

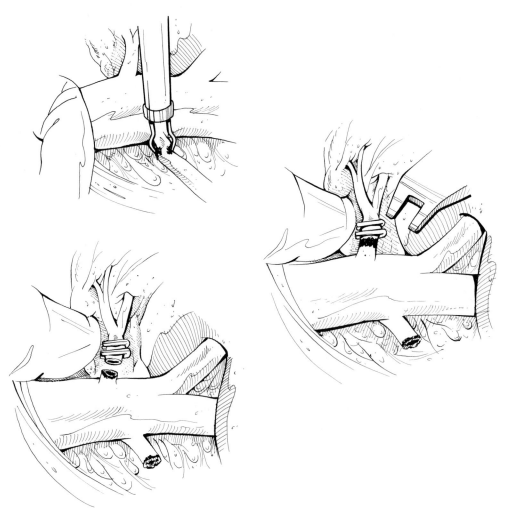

FIG. 121–3. Bipolar cautery of the gonadal vein (*top*) is followed by bipolar cautery, then clipping of the adrenal side of the adrenal vein (*middle*), with the end result being a renal vein freed of its branches without any clips on the vein.

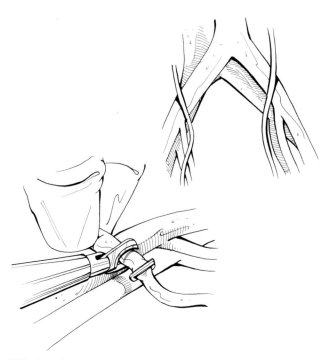

FIG. 121–4. The ureter is incised above clips, at the level of the iliac vessels.

ally up to the lower pole of the kidney. Using sharp and blunt dissection, mobilize the gonadal–ureteral packet distally to the level where the ureter crosses over the external iliac artery. Only at this distal end of the dissection is the gonadal vein separated off of the packet of tissue and then coagulated and divided. Apply one or two clips to the ureter at or below its crossing over the external iliac artery and incise above the clips to leave the proximal end of the ureter open (Fig. 121–4). A healthy squirt of urine should be immediately apparent. If not, continue IV fluid administration even more vigorously, and administer 20 mg of furosemide.

Flip the ureter onto the anterior surface of the kidney and use an instrument through the 5-mm assisting port to

elevate the lower pole of the kidney anteriorly and laterally. Using the intraabdominal hand to both dissect and retract, and with careful use of the right-angle electrocautery probe, gradually incise the tissue between the lower pole of the kidney and the aorta until the renal hilum is encountered (Fig. 121–5). A lumbar vein is usually present inferior to the renal artery. Manage this in a similar fashion to the adrenal vein, with bipolar electrocoagulation and incision above two clips placed on the stay (posterior) side. Use the right-angle electrocautery probe to lift and incise tissue off of the renal artery and between the renal artery and renal vein. Although we have avoided its use because of the cost, an ultrasonic shears does have the advantage at this step of obviating electrical current spread to the artery, which may induce vasospasm. Now, incise the remainder of the perinephric attachments on the posteromedial surface of the kidney such that the kidney is held in place only by the renal vasculature, perihilar tissues, and the attachments between the kidney and adrenal gland. Place caudal traction on the kidney with the intraabdominal hand (or retract the kidney caudally with an assisting instrument and gently retract periadrenal tissue cephalad) and carefully reflect the adrenal gland off of the kidney from an anterior approach. As the caudal aspect of the adrenal gland is addressed, take care not to injure an anterior branch of the renal artery that is commonly at this location (Fig. 121–6).

Now, elevate the kidney with the intraabdominal hand, with fingers under the upper pole and the thumb underneath the lower pole and lifting the kidney directly anteriorly, to put the hilum on stretch. The final perihilar attachments can be incised with the right-angle electrocautery probe such that the kidney is held in place now only by the renal artery and vein. As this final portion of the dissection is being performed, administer 12.5 g of mannitol. Move the laparoscope to the upper 12-mm port and place the working instruments through the medial 12-mm port. This provides an angle for the instruments that

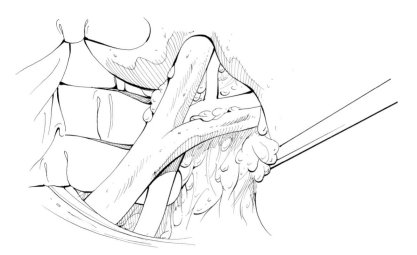

FIG. 121–5. With the kidney retracted anteriorly and laterally by an instrument through the assisting port, both the intraabdominal hand and the primary working instrument are free to address the well-exposed hilum.

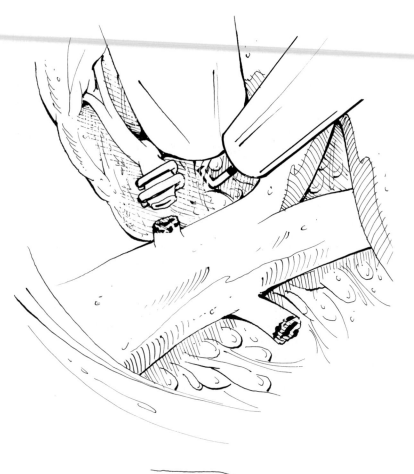

FIG. 121–6. Careful dissection at the caudal aspect of the adrenal gland to avoid injury to any anterior branch of the renal artery.

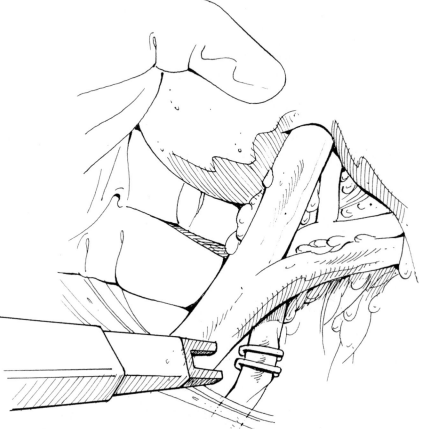

FIG. 121–7. With the kidney elevated using the intraabdominal hand, in rapid succession apply three clips to the base of the renal artery.

is more perpendicular to the renal artery and vein, thus maximizing vessel length. Test fit the clip applier around the base of the renal artery and test for easy passage of the endoscopic stapler around the renal vein at or just medial to the adrenal vein branch. The large size clip applier (11-mm clips) will often be sufficient for control of the renal artery when medium to large clips (9 mm) are too short. On occasion, even the 11-mm clips are not large enough for safe control of the renal artery, and in such cases an endoscopic stapler can be used to control the artery as well.

Squirt papaverine solution onto the renal artery using an endoscopic needle. Place the kidney back into its anatomic position and desufflate the abdomen. Waiting at least 5 minutes without pneumoperitoneum and manipulation of the kidney should allow resolution of any spasm in the renal arterial vasculature. Upon returning the intraabdominal hand and reinsufflating, the kidney should feel extremely firm. If it is not, then wait even longer. An engorged kidney with full vascular inflow will be unlikely to suffer from acute tubular necrosis in the recipient.

With the kidney elevated using the intraabdominal hand, in rapid succession apply three clips to the base of the renal artery (Fig. 121–7), incise above the clips, and control the renal vein with the linear cutting endoscopic stapler. With hand assistance, warm ischemia times between 1 and 2 minutes are typical. As the kidney is removed to the back table for cold perfusion, apply a laparotomy pad intraabdominally at the operative site until pneumoperitoneum is reachieved. Inspect the operative site carefully at normal and low pneumoperitoneum pressure, controlling any bleeding sites with electrocautery or application of clips. Inspect carefully the clips on the artery without manipulating them. Close the 12-mm ports sites in the fascial layer with a single suture, close the fascia of the hand-assistance incision site, and then close the skin.

For a right-sided kidney, options for placement of the hand-assistance device include the same midline location or an ipsilateral lower-quadrant incision. The former requires that the right hand be placed into the abdomen. This is our preferred technique, but some right-handed surgeons opt to use only their left hand intraabdominally, which is facilitated by the ipsilateral lower-quadrant incision. In this case port sites would be moved more medially than the locations described above. The right-sided renal vein is much shorter, and an endoscopic stapling device that lays down only three rows of staples without cutting, as opposed to the usual linear cutting endoscopic stapler (which provides six rows of staples with incision between the third and fourth rows), will provide slightly more length on the renal vein in the transplanted kidney, albeit with slightly longer warm ischemia time because the vein has to be cut sharply with scissors for kidney removal. Another option for a right-sided kidney is to use a laparoscopic Satinsky clamp to control the side of the vena cava just medial to the renal vein. The renal vein is resected sharply right on the surface of the vena cava, and then the vena cavotomy is closed with laparoscopic suturing.

Postoperatively, parenteral narcotics are used the afternoon and evening after the procedure. Use IV ketorolac around the clock (not p.r.n.) for the first 24 hours, including a dose at skin closure in the operating room. Start a clear liquid diet postoperatively, with instructions to the patient that if nausea develops to stop taking liquids for a few hours before trying again. On the morning of postoperative day 1, advance to regular diet as tolerated and switch from parenteral to oral pain medication. Most patients take solid food on postoperative day 1. Get the patient up to a chair on the day of the operation and start ambulation in the hallway the next day. Most patients are ready for discharge on postoperative day 1 or 2.

OUTCOMES

Complications

The spectrum of complications following hand-assisted donor nephrectomy is similar to that of all laparoscopic nephrectomies. Complications listed in the hand-assisted laparoscopic donor nephrectomy series to date (Table 121–1) include transient urinary retention, fever, cellulitis, ileus, transfusion of blood products, neuralgia, minor wound herniation, conversion to open surgery, postoperative exploration for bleeding and small-bowel obstruction, and hospital readmission. The overall rate of minor complications among the series listed in Table 121–1 is 13%, with a 2.1% major complication rate. Of the procedures, 2.3% were converted to open surgery. Allograft complications that are pertinent to the method of harvesting include delayed allograft function, ureteral leakage or obstruction, and allograft loss. The table indicates that the aggregate incidences of these allograft complications are 3.3%, 2.1%, and 2.3%, respectively.

Results

Of the harvested kidneys in the series listed in Table 121–1, 15% had multiple renal arteries. Not surprisingly, only 5% of kidneys were harvested from the right side. The mean operating time was 231 minutes and the mean warm ischemia time was 2 minutes. Hand-assisted laparoscopic donor nephrectomy appears to maintain the benefits of minimally invasive surgery in terms of minimizing the duration and intensity of donor convalescence. Only 35 mg of morphine sulfate equivalents were required parenterally during the mean hospital stay of 2.9 days. The mean time to return to normal nonstrenuous activity was 10.3 days.

TABLE 121–1. Results of hand-assisted laparoscopic donor nephrectomy

Author/reference	No. of patients	No. of kidneys >1 renal artery	No. of right kidneys	Mean operating time (min)	Mean warm ischemis time (min)	Mean parenteral narcotics (mg MSO₄ equivalents)	Mean hospital stay (d)	Mean recovery (d)	No. of minor complications	No. of major complications	No. of conversions to open surgery	No. Loss of allograft	No. Uteral Complication	No. Delayed Allograft Function
Wolf et al. [5]	10	2	0	215	2.9	36	1.8	9.9	3	0	0	0	0	1
Kercher et al. [2]	30	0	0	275	1.2	—	3.4	—	7	0	1	0	0	0
Buell et al. [1]	30	—	3	246	2.2	—	2.9	—	—	—	2	1	—	2
Wolf et al. [6]	23	7	0	206	3.1	59	1.7	8	4	0	0	3	2	1
Stifelman et al. [4]	60	10	2	240	2	35.5	3.5	11.2	3	3	0	0	1	1
Ruiz-Deya et al. [3]	23	—	4	165	1.6	7.5	2	—	2	0	1	0	0	—
Totals	176	15%	5%	231.3	2.0%	34.7%	2.9	10.3	13%	2.1%	2.3%	2.3%	2.1%	3.3%

REFERENCES

1. Buell JF, Alverdy J, Newell K, et al. Hand-assisted laparoscopic live-donor nephrectomy. *J Am Coll Surg* 2001;192:132–136.
2. Kercher K, Dahl D, Harland R, et al. Hand-assisted laparoscopic donor nephrectomy minimizes warm ischemia. *Urology* 2001;58:152–156.
3. Ruiz-Deya G, Cheng S, Palmer E, et al. Open donor, laparoscopic donor and hand assisted laparoscopic donor nephrectomy: a comparison of outcomes. *J Urol* 2001;166:1270–1274.
4. Stifelman MD, Hull D, Sosa RE, et al. Hand assisted laparoscopic donor nephrectomy: a comparison with the open approach. *J Urol* 2001; 166:444–448.
5. Wolf JS Jr, Marcovich R, Merion RM, et al. Prospective, case-matched comparison of hand-assisted laparoscopic and open surgical live donor nephrectomy. *J Urol* 2000;163:1650–1653.
6. Wolf JS Jr, Merion RM, Leichtman AB, et al. Randomized controlled trial of hand-assisted laparoscopic versus open surgical live donor nephrectomy. *Transplantation* 2001;72:284–290.

CHAPTER 122

Laparoscopic Management of Calculus Disease

Stephen R. Keoghane and Francis X. Keeley, Jr.

Although the indications for laparoscopic ureterolithotomy are limited, it nevertheless can be a useful tool in the minimally invasive, urologic surgeon's armamentarium. Ureteral stones can be managed using a variety of methods, including watchful waiting, extracorporeal shock wave lithotripsy (ESWL), rigid and flexible ureteroscopy, antegrade ureteroscopy via a percutaneous approach, and open ureterolithotomy. Each of these methods may have a significant role to play in the routine management of ureteral stones, depending on the availability of local equipment and expertise.

DIAGNOSIS

Routine imaging studies such as excretory urography, retrograde pyelograms, ultrasound, and computed tomography urography are used in the diagnosis of renal and ureteral calculus disease.

INDICATIONS FOR SURGERY

Open ureterolithotomy has become a rare procedure in departments with access to modern equipment, yet a recent 10-year review of over 1,000 patients treated at a university hospital quoted an 8% incidence for open surgery in the 1990s (1). The authors' indications for open surgery included high-risk patients who could not tolerate multiple general anesthetics, difficult ureteric anatomy, difficult patient anatomy such as fixed hips, very large stones, and failure of minimally invasive techniques. These are essentially the patients with whom laparoscopic ureterolithotomy should be discussed. Laparoscopic ureterolithotomy is a procedure associated with relatively high conversion and complication rates and is most commonly indicated only as a salvage procedure or for very large ureteral stones. Disadvantages of the technique include the potential for adjacent organ injury, urinary leakage, or fistula. In addition, patients

should be counseled that this procedure has a recognized risk of conversion, while this risk is essentially zero for other common treatments for ureteral stones, such as ESWL and ureteroscopy.

ALTERNATIVE THERAPY

Open lithotomy and a variety of other minimally invasive approaches (ESWL, laser lithotripsy, percutaneous nephroscopy, and others) are alternatives to laparoscopic techniques.

SURGICAL TECHNIQUE

The retroperitoneal laparoscopic approach was first described in 1979 by Wickham (18), but it took until the early 1990s for the description and popularization of the transperitoneal approach. Over the past two decades the world literature on the subject has remained scarce, reinforcing the limited application of this technique.

Laparoscopic ureterolithotomy can be carried out via a transperitoneal or retroperitoneal approach, each of which has unique advantages and disadvantages. Transperitoneal laparoscopy is the authors' technique of choice, by virtue of familiar anatomy and increased space, and will be the method described. An advantage of the transperitoneal approach is that it is less likely to be affected by retroperitoneal infection or inflammation that may result from impacted stones and/or previous interventions.

Preoperative consent should include the risk of conversion to open surgery as well as the complications noted later. The procedure is performed under general anesthesia using routine urologic antibiotic prophylaxis. Compression stockings and pneumatic boots are essential. The patient is placed in the lithotomy position initially and a retrograde ureteropyelogram and stent placement is carried out. If the stent will not pass beyond an impacted stone, a guide wire should be advanced to the stone through an open-ended ureteral catheter. These are then secured to a urethral catheter and draped in the sterile field so that a stent can later be placed under direct vision.

The patient is then placed in the lateral decubitus position as used for the flank approach to the kidney in open surgery. The legs are lowered 20 degrees from the horizontal and the table rotated slightly back to allow the colon to drop away from the ureter. Gel pads are placed under the patient to cushion pressure areas as skin trauma during prolonged laparoscopic cases is a rare but concerning complication.

Access to the Peritoneal Cavity

Figure 122–1 demonstrates the site of port placement. Turning down the theater lights following camera insertion may allow identification of abdominal wall vessels outlined by the endoscopic light. This luxury may not be available in the obese patient.

Identifying the Ureter and Stone

The colon is reflected medially and the ureter identified from vermiculation and the bulge caused by the

stone. The ureter may be difficult to identify because of tortuosity and inflammation from obstruction and previous interventions. It is helpful to utilize landmarks such as the lower border of the kidney and the iliac vessels, especially in obese patients, and compare the intraoperative images to an intravenous ultrasonography (IVU) or retrograde. Finally, intraoperative fluoroscopy, while rarely necessary, can be useful.

Ureterolithotomy

Once the ureter is identified, blunt dissection is performed, preserving periureteric vasculature. Lack of ureteric fixation prior to ureterotomy can sometimes cause difficulty, which can be addressed by either fixing the ureter with a suture through the complete thickness of the abdominal wall, using a Babcock clamp, or, when performing the ureterotomy, cutting from inside out with a curved blade (6). The ureter may otherwise be opened with scissors, diathermy, a neodynium:YAG laser fiber (4), or a laparoscopic scalpel, taking the incision proximal to the stone and ensuring that it is large enough to extract the calculus.

The surgeon should remember that the ureter proximal to the stone may be dilated, which is sometimes a source of anatomic confusion as well as a risk for proximal migration of the stone. Calculi can be removed from the ureter using leverage or a grasper (Fig. 122–2) or by angling and compressing the ureter. Fragmentation is the main concern during this phase of the operation, and the grasper should probably be reserved for hard stones. Thereafter, the calculi should be removed from the peritoneal cavity via a 12-mm port for relatively small stones or placed in a retrieval bag.

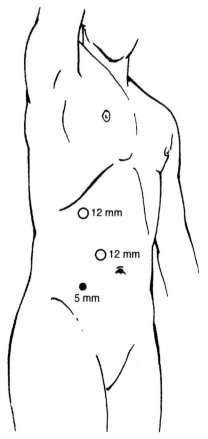

FIG. 122–1. Site of port placement.

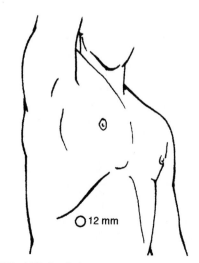

FIG. 122–2. Calculi can be removed from the ureter using leverage or a grasper or by angling and compressing the ureter.

Closing the Ureterotomy

When a guide wire and ureteric catheter has been placed to, but not past, the stone as mentioned above, the guide wire can be used to place a double-pigtail ureteral stent under direct vision. Its placement should be confirmed with fluoroscopy if the proximal coil cannot be visually confirmed to be in the renal pelvis. Interrupted sutures of 4-0 Vicryl or Monocryl should be placed to approximate the ureteral wall. Suturing the edematous inflamed ureter is technically challenging. Closure may be deferred in cases with severe edema or a small (less than 1 cm) ureterotomy, but prolonged urinary leakage can occur if the ureter is left open. If the ureterotomy is not closed properly and the ureter not stented, a ureteral fistula may develop. A nonsuction drain should be placed via the inferior port site and left alongside the ureterotomy.

POSTOPERATIVE CARE

Postoperatively, the urethral catheter is removed after 48 hours if the patient is clinically well. The drain is removed 24 hours later if no additional drainage has occurred. If an increase in drainage occurs, the catheter should be replaced for an additional 24 hours and the process repeated.

OUTCOMES

Complications

The risk of conversion appears to be higher for the retroperitoneal approach. Li et al. reported a conversion rate of up to 60% with their initial retroperitoneal experience, although this fell markedly after the first 40 cases (11). Goel and Hemal reported an 18% conversion rate in 55 patients with mid- or upper-ureteric stones treated with retroperitoneal laparoscopic ureterolithotomy (7). Reasons for conversion included stone migration, severe periureteric fibrosis, vascular injury, and loss of the pneumoperitoneum due to a peritoneal tear. Other authors have reported a lower conversion rate of 0 to 9.5% using the transperitoneal route (10,16).

Complications in Goel and Hemal's series (7) were not uncommon and included damage to the external iliac artery, wound infection, and fever. Perhaps more concerning, the authors reported a 70% ureteric stricture rate in the laparoscopic group as demonstrated on excretory urogram. Although "no complications" were reported in Turk et al.'s series of 21 patients (16), two patients had a prolonged ureteric leak as demonstrated on IVU. Prolonged urinary leakage is the most common "procedure-specific" complication, reported in just under 20% of one large series (6), and this complication has been reported despite ureteric suturing and the use of a ureteric stent (2). Further, major complications including bleeding, fever, ureteric avulsion, hypercarbia, and ureteric strictures are not unknown (6). Hospital stay (Table 122–1) is not that dissimilar from an open ureterolithotomy and is related predominantly to the duration of urinary leakage.

Results

Given the limited indications for the procedure, it is unlikely that laparoscopic ureterolithotomy will be subjected to the rigors of a randomized controlled trial. Prospective, observational studies may help define its role within the context of overall stone management, especially for large upper-ureteral stones. Small ureteral stones are best managed by either watchful waiting, ESWL *in situ*, or ureteroscopy.

The role of laparoscopic ureterolithotomy is essentially as an alternative to open surgery for salvage procedures or for massive stones that may require multiple endoscopic procedures. A recent review of the literature points to success rates between 90% and 100%, but not without a risk of complications and conversions to open surgery (6) (Table 122–1). In some hospitals without access to or

TABLE 122–1. *Results of laparoscopic ureterolithotomy*

Author/Reference	Nhalyong and Taweemonkongasp [13]	Turk et al.[16]	Keeley et al. [10]	Bauer et al. [2]	Chang TD, and Dretler [3]	Goel and Hemal [7]
Procedures	10	21	14	24	9	101
Access						
Transperitoneal	10	20	14	0	8	1
Retroperitoneal	0	1	0	24	1	101
Stone Size (mm)	10		27		13.2	16
Operating Time (min)	181	90	105	61	158	79
Mean Hospital Stay (range)	9.2 (5–23)	(2–7)	5.6 (4–8)	3.6	5.2 (2–13)	3.5
Success (%)	100	90	100	100	100	92
Complications (%)						
Early			14		11	7
Late			7			4

From Gaur et al. Laparoscopic ureterolithotomy: Technical considerations and long term follow-up. *BJU Int* 2002;89:339–343, with permission.

expertise in flexible ureteroscopy and the holmium:YAG laser, it may be used as an alternative to ureteroscopy for large (greater than 1 cm) proximal ureteral stones.

REFERENCES

1. Ather MH, Paryani A, Memon A, Sulaiman N. A ten year experience of managing ureteric calculi: changing trends towards endourological intervention—is there a role for open surgery? *BJU Int* 2001;88: 173–177.
2. Bauer JJ, Schulam PG, Kaufman HS, Moore RG, Irby PB, Kavoussi LR. Laparoscopy for the acute abdomen in the postoperative urologic patient. *Urology* 1998;51:917–919.
3. Chang TD, Dretler SP. Laparoscopic pyelolithotomy in an ectopic kidney. *J Urol* 1996;156:1753.
4. Fahlenkamp D, Schonberger B, Liebetruth L, Lindkee A, Loening S. Laparoscopic laser ureterolithotomy. *J Urol* 1994;152:1549–1551.
5. Gaur DD, Agrawal DK, Purohit KC, Darshane AS. Retroperitoneal laparoscopic pyelolithotomy. *J Urol* 1994;151:927–929.
6. Gaur DD, Triverdi S, Prabhudesai MR, Madhusudhana HR, Gopichand M. Laparoscopic ureterolithotomy: Technical considerations and long term follow-up. *BJU Int* 2002;89:339–343.
7. Goel A, Hemal AK. Upper and mid-ureteric stones: A prospective unrandomised comparison of retroperitoneoscopic and open ureterolithotomy. *BJU Int* 2001;88:679–682.
8. Harmon WJ, Kleer E, Segura JW. Laparoscopic pyelolithotomy for calculus removal in a pelvic kidney. *J Urol* 1996;155:2019–2020.
9. Hoenig DM, Shalhav AL, Elbahnasy AM, McDougall EM, Clayman RV. Laparoscopic pyelolithotomy in a pelvic kidney: a case report and review of the literature. *J Soc Laparoendoscop Surg* 1997;1:163–165.
10. Keeley FX, Gialas I, Pillai M, Chrisofos M, Tolley DA. Laparoscopic ureterolithotomy: the Edinburgh experience. *BJU Int* 1999;84:765–769.
11. Li S, Hou S, Li KM. Retroperitoneoscopic ureterolithotomy (RPU): an effective treatment for large proximal ureteral stone. *Eur Urol* 2000;37[Suppl]:20(abst 500).
12. Micali S, Moore RG, Averch TD, Adams JB, Kavoussi LR. The role of laparoscopy in the treatment of renal and ureteral calculi. *J Urol* 1997; 157:463–466.
13. Nualyong C, Taweemonkongasp T. Laparoscopic ureterolithotomy for upper ureteric calculi. *J Med Assoc Thai* 1999;82:1028–1033.
14. Ramakumar S, Lancini V, Chan DY, Parsons JK, Kavoussi LR, Jarrett TW. Laparoscopic pyeloplasty with concomitant pyelolithotomy. *J Urol* 2002;167:1378–1380.
15. Sinha R, Sharma N. Retroperitoneal laparoscopic management of urolithiasis. *J Laparoendoscop Adv Surg Tech* 1997;7:95–98.
16. Turk I, Deger S, Roigas J, Fahlenkamp D, Schonberger B, Loening SA. Laparoscopic ureterolithotomy. *Tech Urol* 1998;4:29–34.
17. Turk I, Deger S, Winkelmann B, Schonberger B, Loening SA. Laparoscopic bilateral pyelolithotomy in a horseshoe kidney. *BJU Int* 2001; 88:442.
18. Wickham JEA. The surgical treatment of renal lithiasis. In: *Urinary calculus disease*. New York: Churchill Livingstone, 1979:145–198.

CHAPTER 123

Laparoscopic Pyeloplasty

Fernando J. Kim and Thomas W. Jarrett

After the first successful reconstructive procedure was performed by Kuster in 1891, a variety of procedures (open and minimally invasive surgeries) have been described for management of the obstructed ureteropelvic junction (UPJ). Laparoscopic pyeloplasty was first described in 1993 by Schuessler et al. (8) as a less invasive means of reconstructing the ureteropelvic junction under direct visualization, preserving the principles of open pyeloplasty without the associated morbidity of a large flank incision.

DIAGNOSIS

The diagnosis of a UPJ obstruction in general can be made by intravenous urogram or diuretic renal scan. Preoperative computed tomography may be helpful in identifying patients with a crossing vessel who are being considered for an endopyelotomy procedure. Retrograde pyelography has an important role in confirmation of the diagnosis and for exact delineation of the obstruction. This can usually be performed in conjunction with the procedure.

INDICATIONS FOR SURGERY

Laparoscopic pyeloplasty is effective for all most types of UPJ obstruction but should be strongly considered in instances where a less invasive procedure is less likely to be successful. Such situations include renal ptosis, crossing vessels, strictures greater than 2 cm in length, failed previous endoscopic procedures, concomitant renal stones, and poor renal function.

ALTERNATIVE THERAPY

Open pyeloplasty has been considered "the gold standard" intervention for correcting UPJ obstruction with a success rate exceeding 90% (6,7), but it is associated with significant postoperative morbidity related with open flank surgery. Several minimally invasive procedures for repairing UPJ obstruction have been developed to minimize the postoperative morbidity but these techniques (percutaneous antegrade and endoscopic retrograde approaches) yield a lower success rate of 66% to 90% when compared to open pyeloplasty (4,5).

SURGICAL TECHNIQUE

The patient is admitted the same day of surgery. After antibiotic administration and induction of general anesthesia, an orogastric tube and sequential compression devices are placed on the lower extremities. Using a flexible cystscope (frog-legged position for women and supine for men) a retrograde pyelogram is performed to confirm the diagnosis and demonstrate the exact site and nature of the obstruction. A 7 Fr × 28-cm (double-pigtail) stent is placed and correct position confirmed with fluoroscopy. A longer than usual stent is used to minimize the possibility of stent displacement out of the bladder during surgical manipulation of the UPJ.

A Foley catheter is then inserted before the patient is placed in a 45° lateral decubitus position. A roll is placed under the ipsilateral shoulder down to the ipsilateral pelvis to keep the operating site elevated and stable. The ipsilateral arm is placed across the chest, protecting the pressure points with foam, and the contralateral arm rests in anatomic position. The lower knee is bent slightly, and the ipsilateral leg is kept almost straight with pillows or foam placed between them to prevent pressure ulcers and neurological injury. Wide cloth tape is placed across the upper shoulder, arm, and hip and secured to the operative table. The table is tested tilting maximally to the left and right. The entire abdomen and flank from the xiphoid to the pubis is shaved carefully and then scrubbed.

Trocar Placement

This procedure is performed by the transperitoneal approach. Pneumoperitoneum is established by inserting a Veress needle into the umbilicus. After an insufflation pressure of 20 mm Hg is established three midline trocars are placed (Fig. 123–1). The umbilical trocar is 10 mm to allow for the camera and 30° lens. The remaining trocars are placed 2 finger breadths above the symphysis pubis and 8 cm above the umbilicus. Trocars are either 5 or 12 mm depending on surgical side (right or left) and dominant hand of the surgeon. The larger trocar would be placed in the dominant hand of the surgeon to allow for passage of the needle driver and/or Endostitch device during the repair of the UPJ.

The surgeon operates from the opposite side of the affected renal unit and uses the supra- and infraumbilical sites as the working ports. The assistant or the robot arm (AESOP) stands on the same side of the operating room table as the surgeon and manipulates the camera by the umbilical port.

The table is rotated with the ipsilateral side up and the lateral peritoneal reflection overlying the kidney is incised along the white line of Toldt from the upper pole

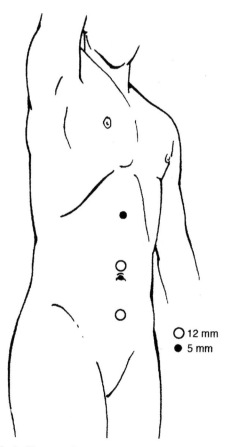

○ 12 mm
● 5 mm

FIG. 123–1. Trocar placement for transperitoneal laparoscopic pyeloplasty.

to approximately 3 cm below the lower pole. The renocolic ligaments are then divided sharply and the colon is retracted medially with a sweeping motion, further exposing the retroperitoneum. On the right side, a Kocher maneuver may be necessary to mobilize the duodenum off the medial aspect of the kidney.

The ureter is identified just medial to the lower pole of the kidney and usually lies lateral and posterior to the gonadal vessels. Gentle palpation of the indwelling stent confirms the structure to be the ureter. A plane between the psoas muscle and the ureter is created using gentle sweeping motions and the ureter is dissected cephalad until the ureteropelvic junction is identified. It is important to dissect the ureter with its adjacent tissue attached to maximize the blood supply. The ureter should only be skeletonized in the area of the UPJ for delineation of the anatomy. Extra attention should be made for lower pole-crossing vessels, which can be damaged with overzealous dissection. In the presence of crossing vessels, the renal pelvis and ureter are carefully dissected free so that the ureter can be easily transposed anteriorly as needed. The ureter and renal pelvis are then mobilized as needed to allow for a subsequent tension-free repair.

At this point the surgeon must commit to the type of repair to be used depending on the nature of the UPJ obstruction. Any renal calculi can be removed using a combination of direct extraction using forceps through the pyelotomy or with the aid of a flexible cystoscope passed through the upper trocar.

Anderson–Hynes Dismembered Pyeloplasty

Dismembered pyeloplasty is our preference in most clinical circumstances (Fig. 123–2). It is especially preferable with crossing vessels and a large redundant renal pelvis. Scissors are used to transect the UPJ, taking care not damage the ureteral stent. The renal pelvis is first incised circumferentially above the area of stenosis, and the stent is then delivered through this incision. Again, care must be taken to avoid transecting the internal stent. The posterior wall is transected, thus completely freeing the ureter from the renal pelvis. The proximal ureter is spatulated on the lateral aspect using laparoscopic scissors with attention not to spiral the incision. When a crossing vessel is present the ureter must be transposed anteriorly to these vascular structures prior to reanastomosis to the renal pelvis. A reduction pyeloplasty is performed at this point when necessary.

Next, 4-0 absorbable stay sutures are placed at the apex of the spatulated ureter and then through the most dependent portion of the reduced renal pelvis and tied using intracorporeal techniques. This suture is then used in a running fashion to approximate the anterior portions of the renal pelvis and ureter. Sutures can be placed using

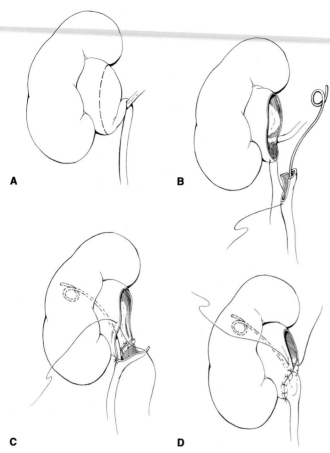

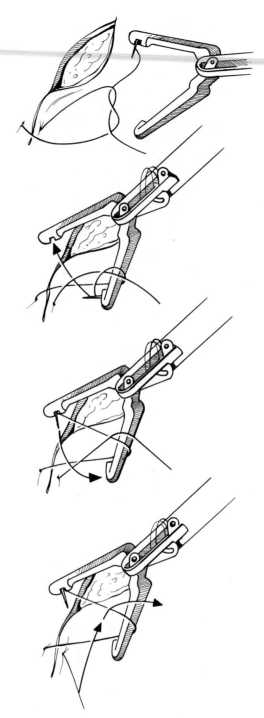

FIG. 123–2. Hynes–Anderson dismembered pyeloplasty technique.

the free-hand technique or the Endostitch device (Fig. 123–3) (1).

The same technique is performed to close the posterior aspect of the anastomosis. The cephalad portion of the pyelotomy is sutured and tied with continuous 4-0 absorbable sutures using the Endostitch or free-hand technique. Before the last knot is tied down the stent is placed back into the renal pelvis and up into an upper calyx. The remainder of the renal pelvis can be similarly closed using a running absorbable suture

Foley V–V Pyeloplasty

The Foley Y-V pyeloplasty (Fig. 123–4) may be considered in the absence of crossing vessels when there is a small renal pelvis or a high ureteral insertion into the renal pelvis. Using laparoscopic scissors, a wide-based V-shaped flap is constructed from the anterior pelvis. The proximal ureter is spatulated anteriorly. Using 4-0 absorbable sutures, the apex of the V flap is sutured to the apex of the spatulated ureteral incision and tied intracorporeally with the Endostitch or free-hand techniques. The lower wall is completed first using the Endostitch to place the sutures and the anastomosis is completed with

FIG. 123–3. Endostitch device.

sutures that are placed from the apex out toward the upper pelvis.

Fenger Nondismembered Pyeloplasty (Heinecke–Mickolicz)

The Fenger pyeloplasty (Fig. 123–5) may be considered for a short stenotic segment in the absence of crossing vessels or a high insertion. The principle of this pro-

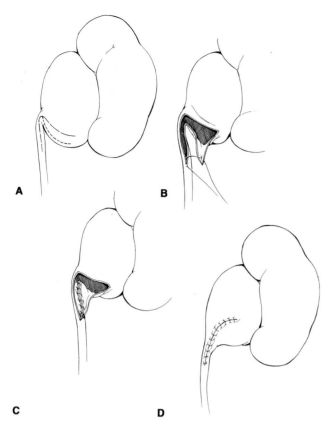

FIG. 123–4. Foley V–V pyeloplasty technique.

versely in a Heineke–Mickolicz fashion over the stent using one continuous 4-0 absorbable suture.

After the chosen anastomosis is completed fibrin glue may be used to help seal the anastomotic site. Then, the pneumoperitoneum pressure is dropped to 5 mm Hg and the operative sites are examined for bleeding. After hemostasis is adequately obtained a small closed-bulb suction drain (Jackson–Pratt) is positioned carefully in the retroperitoneum to lie adjacent to the newly completed anastomosis but never in direct contact. The drain is brought out through a small stab incision in the posterior axillary line and then secured with a 2-0 silk stitch.

All trocars are then removed under direct vision. The abdominal fasciae of all 5/12-mm port sites are closed with interrupted 2-0 absorbable sutures using the Carter–Thomas closure device. The drain is connected to the bulb suction. The CO_2 pneumoperitoneum is removed to decrease postoperative shoulder irritation. The skin incisions are closed with subcuticular 4-0 polyglactin sutures and adhesive skin tape.

POSTOPERATIVE CARE

The orogastric tube is removed just before extubation. On the floor, vigilant records of the outputs must be kept to dictate drain management. The Foley catheter is removed on postoperative day 1 or 2 if the drain fluid output is consistently less than 30 to 50 cc per 8 hours. A drain fluid creatinine is obtained if output is greater than this. Following removal of the Foley, the retroperitoneal drain outputs must be monitored for increased output. If the outputs increase, the Foley should be replaced until which time they drop to acceptable levels. The retroperitoneal drain may be removed when the drainage is negligible after the Foley removal, which is usually postoperative day 2. In some cases, patients are sent home with the drains in place if they have met all other criteria for discharge.

A clear liquid diet is started on postoperative day 1 and advanced following the passage of flatus. The intravenous antibiotics are continued for 24 hours, and then switched to an oral agent. The ureteral stent is removed in the office in 4 to 6 weeks. The anastomosis is then radiologically re-evaluated with an intravenous urogram (IVU) or renal nuclear scan 6 weeks after stent removal unless the patient has recurrent symptoms. A follow-up diuretic renal scan is obtained at 6 months postoperatively and compared with the previous study. Thereafter, an IVU or a renal scan is obtained at yearly intervals.

cedure is a longitudinal incision and transverse closure. This technique has the potential advantage of a shorter operative time because fewer intracorporeal sutures are needed. A longitudinal incision is made with laparoscopic scissors from the renal pelvis distally to 1 to 2 cm below the UPJ segment. The initial pyelotomy incision, just above the UPJ, can be made with a laparoscopic knife or scissors. The longitudinal incision is then closed trans-

OUTCOMES

Complications

All complications of abdominal laparoscopy are possible and consideration for injury to adjacent organs should

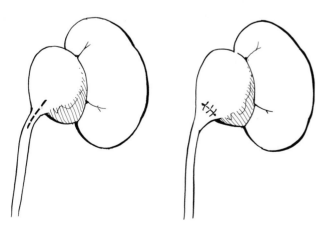

FIG. 123–5. Fenger nondismembered pyeloplasty (Heinecke–Mickolicz) technique.

be considered when the clinical situation is deteriorating. The most common complications are usually due to persistence of urinary leak or urinoma. The possibility of urinoma requiring revision of drains can be minimized with vigilant placement at the time of surgery. Most controlled urinary leaks can be managed as an outpatient with continued-suction drainage with or without a Foley catheter. Most will close with time. Failure to drain the urine or urinoma requires either percutaneous or surgical drainage.

Results

Laparoscopic pyeloplasty retains the benefits of open pyeloplasty while minimizing the morbidity of incisional trauma. This approach should be considered especially in those instances where endopyelotomy is either contraindicated or has compromised results. Such situations include renal ptosis with renal kinking, poor renal function, strictures longer than 2 cm, concomitant nonobstructing renal stones, and crossing lower-pole vessels. The major disadvantage of the laparoscopic approach is the learning curve. The technique requires not only laparoscopic expertise but also experience with intracorporeal suturing and tying.

Results have been promising. In a series of 100 consecutive laparoscopic pyeloplasty cases from the Johns Hopkins Hospital, 96% were successful with a mean radiographic follow-up of 2.2 years (3). Fifty-six of 100 patients were found, intraoperatively, to have lower-pole crossing vessels and thus underwent dismembered pyeloplasty. In patients with calculi, concomitant laparoscopic pyeloscopy with extraction of the stones was performed. Recently, a French multicenter study examined 55 retroperitoneal laparoscopic pyeloplasty cases and found that 95% of cases were successfully completed laparoscopically. All patients were pain free and radiographically unobstructed by 3 months (9). The overall complication rate was 12.7%. Complications in seven patients included hematoma in three, urinoma in one, severe pyelonephritis in one, and anastomotic stricture in two requiring open pyeloplasty at 3 weeks and delayed balloon incision at 13 months, respectively.

The largest comparative series between laparoscopic and open pyeloplasties was reported on a retrospective series of 42 patients who underwent laparoscopic pyeloplasty and 35 who underwent open repair in regard to outcome and complications (2). Follow-up ranged up to 22 months in the laparoscopic group and 58 months in the open series. The complication rate for the laparoscopic group was 12% (five patients) while the open group had 11% (four patients). No significant difference in pain-free rates between both groups was observed (laparoscopic, 62% versus open, 60%). Objective success was based on radiographic findings. Radiological failure was observed in one patient in the laparoscopic group (within 24 hours after the stent was removed) and in two patients in the open group.

Laparoscopic pyeloplasty is a feasible but technically demanding procedure. This surgical technique maintains the advantages of open reconstruction of the ureteropelvic junction while decreasing the morbidity due to a large flank incision. Improvements in laparoscopic technique and instrumentation have led to acceptable procedure times. Moreover, longer follow-up has shown durable success rates comparable to open surgery.

REFERENCES

1. Adams JB, Schulam PG, Moore RG, et al. New laparoscopic suturing device: Initial clinical experience. *Urology* 1995;46:242–245.
2. Bauer JJ, Bishoff JT, Moore RG, et al. Laparoscopic versus open pyeloplasty: Assessment of objective and subjective outcome. *J Urol* 1999; 163:692–695.
3. Jarrett TW, Chan DY, Charambura TC, Fugita O, Kavoussi LR. Laparoscopic pyeloplasty: The first 100 cases. *J Urol* 2002;167:1253–1256.
4. Motola JA, Badlani GH, Smith AD. Results of 221 consecutive endopyelotomies: an eight-year follow-up. *J Urol* 1993;149:453.
5. Nakada SY, Johnson M. Ureteropelvic junction obstruction: retrograde endopyelotomy. *Urol Clin North Am* 2000;27:677.
6. Notely RG, Beaugie JM. The long-term follow-up of Anderson–Hynes pyeloplasty for hydronephrosis. *Br J Urol* 1973;45:464.
7. Persky L, Krause JR, Boltuch RL. Initial complications and late results in dismembered pyeloplasty. *J Urol* 1977;118:162.
8. Schuessler WW, Grune MT, Tecuanhuey LV, et al. Laparoscopic dismembered pyeloplasty. *J Urol* 1993;150:1795.
9. Soulié M, Salomon L, Patard JJ, Mouly P, Manunta A, Antiphon P, Lobel B, Abbou CC, Plante P. extraperitoneal laparoscopic pyeloplasty: A multicenter study of 55 procedures. *J Urol,* 2001;166:48–50.

CHAPTER 124

Laparoscopic Adrenalectomy

Jihad H. Kaouk and Inderbir S. Gill

First performed by Gagner and colleagues (5) in 1992, laparoscopic adrenalectomy has evolved to become the standard of care for most surgical adrenal diseases. It is widely accepted that laparoscopic adrenalectomy is safe, reproducible, and effective (6). Advantages over open surgery include shorter hospital stay, less postoperative pain, quicker convalescence, better cosmesis, and lower complication rate. With increasing worldwide experience, several approaches for laparoscopic adrenalectomy have been described, including transperitoneal, retroperitoneal, and recently transthoracic laparoscopic approaches (7). To further minimize morbidity, laparoscopic adrenalectomy using needlescopic instruments (2 mm) has been performed (9).

INDICATIONS

Laparoscopic adrenalectomy is indicated for surgical management of both functional and nonfunctional benign adrenal lesions (Table 124–1). With experience, laparo-

TABLE 124-1. *Indications and contraindications for laparoscopic adrenalectomy*

Indications
  Aldosteromas
  Pheochromocytoma
  Adrenal cyst/Myelolipoma
  Cushing's disease or Cushing's adenoma
  Nonfunctioning adenoma >4 cm, increasing in size, or
    with abnormal MRI characteristics
  Solitary adrenal metastasis/small cancer
Contraindications
  General
    Unacceptable cardiopulmonary risk
    Uncorrectable coagulopathy
    Suspected bowel obstruction
  Specific
    Adrenal tumor with local invasion
    Adrenal tumor with venous thrombus
    Adrenal tumor >10–12 cm (relative contraindication)

scopic adrenalectomy may be indicated for selected patients with a small adrenal carcinoma; however, large adrenal malignancy with evidence of local infiltration or venous invasion remains the main adrenal-specific contraindication to laparoscopic adrenalectomy today.

DIAGNOSIS

Imaging using computed tomography (CT) or magnetic resonance imaging (MRI) is the usual method for the diagnosis of adrenal mass. Preoperative serum and urine metabolic panel identifies functional adrenal tumors, which are treated accordingly.

ALTERNATIVE THERAPY

Open adrenalectomy, either by the transabdominal or retroperitoneal approach, is the standard. Various techniques have been described for laparoscopic adrenalectomy, including transperitoneal (11), retroperitoneal (17), needlescopic (9), and, recently, transthoracic transdiaphragmatic technique (7) in selected patients.

SURGICAL TECHNIQUES

Patients with pheochromocytoma are given calcium channel blocker and/or alpha-adrenergic blockers preoperatively and admitted the day before surgery for intravenous hydration. A parenteral broad-spectrum antibiotic is given on call to the operating room. Bowel preparation is limited to clear fluids and two bottles of magnesium citrate administered the evening before surgery. A Foley catheter is inserted and antiembolism stockings are placed on both legs.

The choice of laparoscopic technique (transperitoneal versus retroperitoneal) depends primarily on the experience and preference of the individual laparoscopic surgeon. The transperitoneal approach is commonly

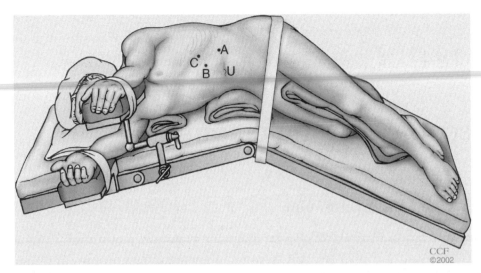

FIG. 124–1. The patient is positioned in the 45-degree modified flank position. The operative table is flexed and the kidney rest is elevated. The arms are placed on a double arm board in a neutral position. The patient is taped to the operating table after adequate padding of all pressure points. Port placement is shown. **A:** A 12-mm secondary port is placed along the midclavicular line at the umbilicus level. **B:** A 12-mm primary port is placed at the lateral edge of the ipsilateral rectus muscle along the level of the twelfth rib. **C:** A 5-mm secondary port is placed at the angle of the costal margin with the lateral edge of the ipsilateral rectus muscle. On occasion, a 2-mm port is placed along the lateral subcostal margin for additional traction. During right adrenalectomy, an additional 5-mm port is inserted at the subxiphoid location for cephalad retraction of the liver.

employed during laparoscopic adrenalectomy especially for larger tumors measuring over 10 cm. Keeping in mind the unique high retroperitoneal location of the adrenal glands, we believe there are two specific indications wherein the laparoscopic retroperitoneal approach may be superior: previous multiple transperitoneal procedures and morbid obesity.

Transperitoneal Laparoscopic Adrenalectomy

The patient is placed in the 45-degree modified flank position for the transperitoneal approach (Fig. 124–1). The kidney rest is elevated and the operation table is flexed. This maximizes the space between the twelfth rib and the iliac crest. Care must be taken to eliminate all pressure points so foam padding is liberally used at all bony pressure points and the extremities are placed in neutral position. The surgeon and assistant stand facing the abdomen of the patient during the transperitoneal approach.

Initially, peritoneal insufflation is performed by inserting a Veress needle into the abdomen at the umbilicus level along the midclavicular line. CO_2 insufflation is started and pneumoperitoneum is achieved to a pressure of 15 mm Hg. The Veress needle is replaced by a 12-mm laparoscopic port, into which a 10-mm laparoscopic telescope with a 30-degree angle lens is inserted. A total of three to four ports are used. Under direct vision, a 12-mm port is placed at the lateral edge of the ipsilateral rectus muscle along the level of the twelfth rib and a 5-mm port

at the angle of the costal margin with the lateral edge of the ipsilateral rectus muscle. The laparoscope is then shifted to the middle port (Fig. 124–1). During right adrenalectomy, an additional 5-mm port is inserted at the subxiphoid location for cephalad retraction of the liver.

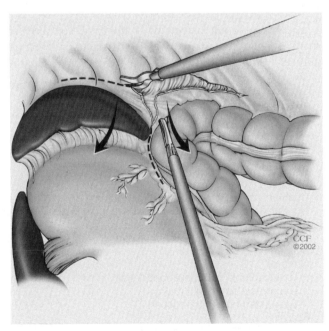

FIG. 124–2. Left transperitoneal adrenalectomy. The descending colon is mobilized medially and the spleen is mobilized superomedially (arrows) to expose Gerota's fascia covering the left kidney and adrenal gland.

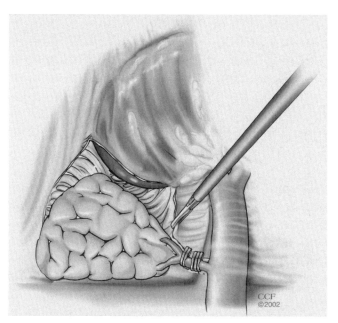

FIG. 124–3. Left transperitoneal adrenalectomy. The left renal vein is identified and traced to the main left adrenal vein, which is clipped and cut. Gerota's fascia covering the upper pole of the left kidney is incised and the left adrenal gland is exposed.

Transperitoneal Left Adrenalectomy

By incising along the line of Toldt, the descending colon is mobilized medially and the spleen is mobilized superomedially to expose Gerota's fascia covering the left kidney (Fig. 124–2). The left renal vein is identified and traced to the main left adrenal vein, which is clipped and cut. On occasion, the gonadal vein may be traced cephalad to allow rapid identification of the left renal vein and thereby the left adrenal vein. Gerota's fascia covering the upper pole of the left kidney is incised and the left adrenal gland, covered by the periadrenal fat, is exposed (Fig. 124–3). The plane between the adrenal gland and the aorta is then meticulously dissected with care to control multiple small arteries to the adrenal gland (Fig. 124–4). The adrenal gland is then mobilized from the undersurface of the diaphragm and the inferior phrenic vessels are controlled (Fig. 124–5). Finally, the adrenal gland is mobilized off the kidney upper pole, taking care not to injure any aberrant upper-pole renal segmental artery. Care is taken to mobilize the adrenal gland along with its surrounding fat, thereby avoiding direct manipulation of the adrenal gland itself, to prevent rupture of the adrenal capsule, adrenal fragmentation, and troublesome hemorrhage.

Transperitoneal Right Adrenalectomy

The initial peritoneotomy is created high, immediately along the undersurface of the liver, in a horizontal manner, extending from the sidewall of the abdomen laterally up to the inferior vena cava medially. This high peritoneotomy exposes the right adrenal gland immediately. The right colon and the hepatic flexure do not require mobilization (Fig. 124–6). The adrenal gland surrounded by the periadrenal fat is retracted laterally, and the space between it and the inferior vena cava is developed gently with hook electrocautery. This dissection is carried cephalad until the right main adrenal vein is identified (Fig. 124–7). Following dissection and clipping of the adrenal vein, dissection of the adrenal gland is similar to left adrenalectomy (Fig. 124–8). The specimen is placed in a bag and extracted intact through an extended laparo-

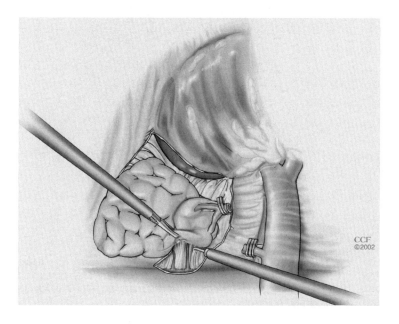

FIG. 124–4. Left transperitoneal adrenalectomy. The adrenal gland is then meticulously dissected off the aorta with care to control multiple small arteries to the adrenal gland.

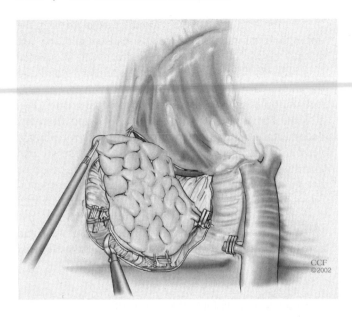

FIG. 124–5. Left transperitoneal adrenalectomy. The adrenal gland is mobilized from the undersurface of the diaphragm and the inferior phrenic vessels are controlled.

scopic port incision. Laparoscopic exit is performed in a routine fashion.

Retroperitoneal Laparoscopic Adrenalectomy

The patient is positioned in the standard 90-degree full flank position during the retroperitoneal approach. The kidney rest is elevated and the operation table is flexed minimally. Care is taken to pad all positional pressure points as described for the transperitoneal approach. The

surgeon and assistant stand facing the patient's back during retroperitoneoscopy (Fig. 124–9).

A three-port technique is routinely employed. The initial retroperitoneal access is achieved using the open (Hasson) technique (8). A 1.2-cm transverse skin incision is created just below the tip of the twelfth rib, and flank muscles are bluntly split. The thoracolumbar fascia is

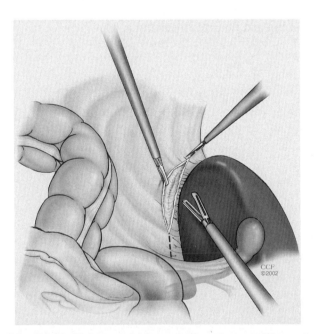

FIG. 124–6. Right transperitoneal adrenalectomy. The peritoneal reflection over the vena cava and along the liver edge is incised. The liver is retracted cephalad and the adrenal gland is exposed. The right colon is not routinely mobilized.

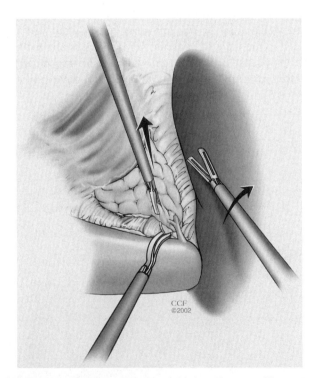

FIG. 124–7. Right transperitoneal adrenalectomy. The anterior border of the vena cava is identified and dissected cephalad toward the right main adrenal vein, which is identified and secured.

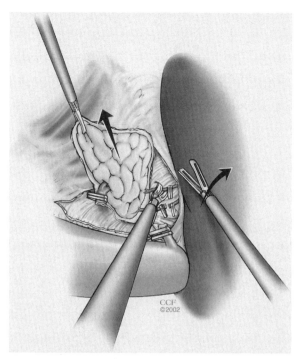

FIG. 124–8. Right transperitoneal adrenalectomy. Following dissection and clipping of the adrenal vein, the adrenal gland is mobilized from the undersurface of the diaphragm and the inferior phrenic vessels are controlled.

air. The balloon is deflated, repositioned higher toward the kidney upper pole, and reinflated. Such secondary dilation creates an adequate working space along the undersurface of the diaphragm. The balloon is deflated then replaced with a 10-mm blunt-tip cannula with a 30-cc balloon mounted tip (US Surgical, Norwalk, CT) and cinched against the undersurface of the abdominal wall in an airtight fashion. After CO_2 pneumoretroperitoneum (15 mm Hg) is established, a 30-degree lens laparoscope is introduced and the anatomic landmarks are examined: the psoas muscle, the anteriorly displaced kidney with its surrounding Gerota's fascia, and the diaphragm muscle fibers. Under direct vision, two secondary laparoscopic ports are placed. An anterior port is inserted near the anterior axillary line, 3 cm cephalad to the iliac crest (10-mm port), and a posterior port is inserted at the junction of the lateral border of the erector spinae muscle with the undersurface of the twelfth rib (5- or 10-mm port).

Retroperitoneoscopic Left Adrenalectomy

The left main adrenal vein is longer, located along the inferomedial border of the adrenal gland, and drains into the left renal vein. The posterior aspect of Gerota's fascia is incised at the level of the renal upper pole/adrenal gland. The avascular plane between the renal upper pole and the inferior and lateral edges of the adrenal is dissected, and the upper renal pole is completely mobilized within the Gerota's fascia (Fig. 124–10). Dissection is continued along the medial aspect of the upper pole of the kidney toward the renal hilum and the main left adrenal vein is identified and secured along the inferomedial

exposed and incised to enter the retroperitoneum. Using blunt finger dissection, a retroperitoneal space is developed immediately anterior to the psoas muscle and posterior to Gerota's fascia. A balloon dilator is inserted in the created retroperitoneal space, then inflated with 800 cc of

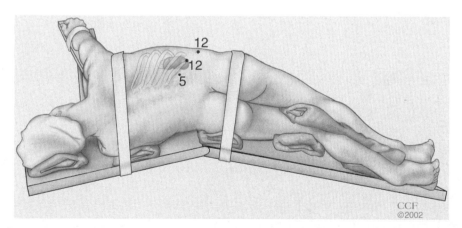

FIG. 124–9. The patient is positioned in the standard 90-degree full flank position during the retroperitoneal approach. The kidney rest is elevated and the operation table is flexed. The arms are placed on a double arm board in a neutral position. The patient is taped to the operating table after adequate padding of all pressure points. Port placement is shown. **A:** A 1.2-cm transverse skin incision is created just below the tip of the twelfth rib and the initial retroperitoneal access is achieved using the open (Hasson) technique. The retroperitoneal working space is developed using a balloon dissector. A 10-mm balloon mounted port is placed and cinched against the abdominal wall in an airtight fashion. **B:** An anterior port is placed along the anterior axillary line, 3 cm cephalad to the iliac crest. **C:** A posterior port is inserted at the junction of the lateral border of the erector spinae muscle with the undersurface of the twelfth rib.

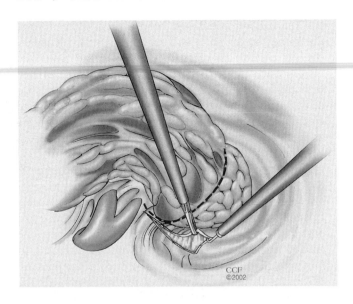

FIG. 124–10. Left retroperitoneal adrenalectomy. The posterior aspect of Gerota's fascia is incised at the level of the renal upper pole/adrenal gland (dotted line) and from the undersurface of the diaphragm.

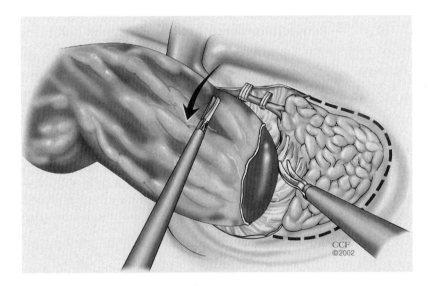

FIG. 124–11. Left retroperitoneal adrenalectomy. The avascular plane between the renal upper pole and the inferior and lateral edges of the adrenal is dissected, and the upper renal pole is completely mobilized within Gerota's fascia. Dissection is continued along the medial aspect of the upper pole of the kidney toward the renal hilum and the main left adrenal vein is identified and secured along the inferomedial edge of the left adrenal gland.

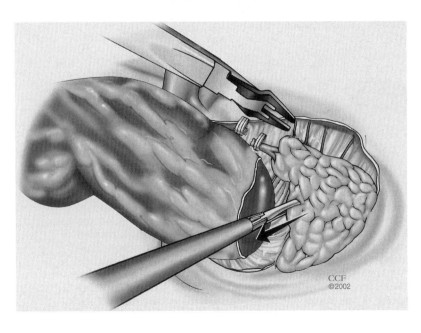

FIG. 124–12. Left retroperitoneal adrenalectomy. Anterolateral retraction of the adrenal gland is applied and dissection is continued in the area between the aorta and the adrenal gland and adrenal branches arising from the aorta are dissected and controlled. Sequentially, the adrenal gland is mobilized along its superior border from under the diaphragm where adrenal branches of the inferior phrenic vessels are controlled.

edge of the left adrenal gland (Fig. 124–11). Alternatively, the main left adrenal vein may be identified along the superior border of the left main renal artery. Anterolateral retraction of the adrenal gland is applied and dissection is continued in the area between the aorta and the adrenal gland and adrenal branches arising from the aorta are dissected and controlled. Sequentially, the adrenal gland is mobilized along its superior border from under the diaphragm where adrenal branches of the inferior phrenic vessels are controlled (Fig. 124–12). The specimen is extracted intact using an Endocatch bag (US Surgical) from the primary port site, which may require enlargement accordingly.

Retroperitoneoscopic Right Adrenalectomy

The main right adrenal vein is short and stubby, located along the superomedial border of the adrenal gland, and drains directly into the vena cava. Initially, the right renal artery is identified, and dissection performed along its superior edge to identify the anterolateral border of the inferior vena cava. This usually requires careful control of multiple small blood vessels, running obliquely from the renal hilum and inferior vena cava toward the inferior edge of the adrenal gland. Dissection is carried cephalad along the vena cava until the main right adrenal vein is identified and controlled (Fig. 124–13). The adrenal gland is then mobilized from the undersurface of the diaphragm where the phrenic vessels are controlled (Fig. 124–14). Finally, the plane between the kidney and the adrenal gland is dissected where multiple small arterial

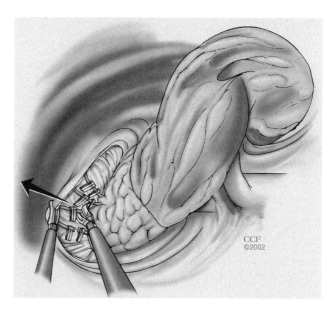

FIG. 124–14. Right retroperitoneal adrenalectomy. The adrenal gland is mobilized from the undersurface of the diaphragm and phrenic vessels are controlled.

and venous branches from the renal hilum entering the adrenal gland along its inferomedial border are encountered and controlled (Fig 124–15).

Needlescopic Approach

Needlescopic (2-mm) laparoscopic adrenalectomy is performed using the transperitoneal approach (9), partially incorporating 2-mm instrumentation. To minimize skin scars yet preserve the excellent visualization provided by a 10-mm laparoscope, the primary port is cosmetically placed within the umbilicus and a 10-mm laparoscopic with a 45-degree lens is used. Two secondary ports (2 and 5 mm) are placed along the lateral surface of the ipsilateral rectus muscle. An additional 2-mm port is on occasion positioned laterally for better retraction. The surgical steps follow the same technique described above for the transperitoneal approach.

Transthoracic Approach

Transthoracic transdiaphragmatic laparoscopic adrenalectomy has been successfully described for the highly select patient who has undergone previous extensive ipsilateral transperitoneal and retroperitoneal open surgery (7). In this infrequent clinical scenario, the extensive transperitoneal and retroperitoneal postsurgical adhesions preclude an efficient subsequent transperitoneal laparoscopic approach to the adrenal gland. The virgin thoracic cavity provides a transdiaphragmatic minimally invasive approach to the adrenal gland. In brief, double lumen endotracheal intubation, which allows deflation of

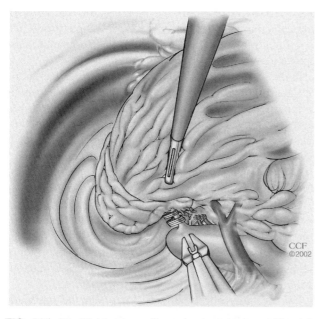

FIG. 124–13. Right retroperitoneal adrenalectomy. The lateral border of the inferior vena cava is identified and dissection is carried cephalad until the main right adrenal vein is identified and controlled.

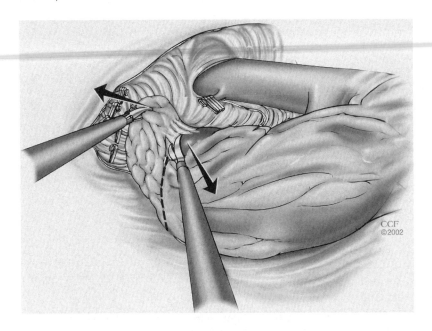

FIG. 124–15. Right retroperitoneal adrenalectomy. The plane between the kidney and the adrenal gland is dissected where multiple small arterial and venous branches from the renal hilum entering the adrenal gland along its inferomedial border are encountered and controlled.

the ipsilateral lung, is achieved and the patient is placed in the prone position. A four-port transthoracic approach is used without pneumoinsufflation. Under laparoscopic ultrasound guidance, the adrenal gland is localized and the diaphragm is incised precisely at the site. Adrenalectomy is achieved and the diaphragm is sutured laparoscopically.

OUTCOMES

Complications

In a Medline review by Brunt (1), complications were tabulated from 50 studies of laparoscopic adrenalectomy involving 1,522 patients and 48 studies of open adrenalectomy involving 2,273 patients, published from 1980 through 2000. The total reported complication rate was 10.9% for laparoscopic adrenalectomy versus 25.2% for open adrenalectomy. The most common complication during laparoscopic adrenalectomy was intraoperative bleeding (4.7% versus 3.7 % for the open group); however, open surgery had more incidence of organ injury (0.7% versus 2.4%). The incidence of other complications reported during laparoscopic adrenalectomy was lower than during open adrenalectomy: wound problems (2.5% versus 6.9%), gastroenterologic (0.7% versus 1.2%), pulmonary (0.9% versus 5.5%), cardiac (0.3% versus 1.6%), and deep vein thrombosis (0.5% versus 0.6%). Overall mortality was 0.3% versus 0.9% for the laparoscopic and open adrenalectomy groups, respectively.

Results

Multiple studies have demonstrated the feasibility, effectiveness, and safety of laparoscopic adrenalectomy. For this chapter, we performed a Medline search of the English literature (1995–2002), identifying various articles comparing laparoscopic and open adrenalectomy (Table 124–2). Overall, 349 cases of laparoscopic adrenalectomy were compared to 340 cases of open adrenalectomy. Operative time was 3.1 hours versus 2.4 hours, estimated blood loss was 142 cc versus 364 cc, hospital stay was 4.1 days versus 8.6 days, and convalescence was 18 days versus 33 days for the laparoscopic versus open adrenalectomy, respectively. The laparoscopic group had significantly fewer complications (9.7%) compared to the open adrenalectomy group (42%).

In the literature, it is still unclear as to which technique of laparoscopic adrenalectomy, transperitoneal versus retroperitoneal, is superior. In a prospective randomized study, we found no significant difference in terms of surgical time (2.6 hours versus 2.3 hours), blood loss, analgesic requirements, and hospital stay (25 hours vs 27.5 hours) when comparing transperitoneal versus retroperitoneal laparoscopic adrenalectomy, respectively.

For pheochromocytomas, laparoscopic adrenalectomy is a feasible and safe option. Induction of pneumoperitoneum does not increase the risk of a hypertensive crisis (16). In addition, early control of the adrenal vein prior to adrenal mobilization minimizes the chances of uncontrolled catecholamine release.

For morbidly obese patients, we prefer the retroperitoneal laparoscopic approach to adrenalectomy. Compared to open surgery performed on the same subset of

TABLE 124-2. *Comparative studies: open versus laparoscopic adrenalectomy*

Author	No. of patients Laparoscopic	No. of patients Open	Diagnosis Laparoscopic	Diagnosis Open	Surgical approach Laparoscopic	Surgical approach Open	Operative time (h) Laparoscopic	Operative time (h) Open	Blood loss (mL) Laparoscopic	Blood loss (mL) Open	Hospital stay (d) Laparoscopic	Hospital stay (d) Open	Specimen size (cm) Laparoscopic	Specimen size (cm) Open	Convalescence (d) Laparoscopic	Convalescence (d) Open	Complication % Laparoscopic	Complication % Open
Guzzoni (1)	20	20	Pheo, 7 Conn's, 10 Cushing, 3	Pheo, 10 Conn's, 7 Cushing, 3	Trans.	Various	2.8	2.4	100	450	3.4	9	3.0	3.1	9.7	16	5	25
Brunt (2)	24	42	Pheo, 11 Conn's, 6	Pheo, 19 Conn's, 8	Trans.	Anterior, 25 Posterior, 17	3.1	2.4	104	400	3.2	7.7	2.7	3.4	10.6	NA	16	67
Thompson (18)	50	50	Other, 7 Pheo, 10 Conn's, 24 Cushing, 10 Adenoma, 6	Other, 15 Pheo, 7 Conn's, 25 Cushing, 10 Adenoma, 8	Trans.	Dorsal	2.8	2.1	NA	NA	3.1	5.7	2.9	2.9	27	49	6	18
Vargas (19)	20	20	Pheo, 6 Conn's, 11 Cushing, 2 Carcinoma, 1	Pheo, 6 Conn's 11 Cushing, 2 Carcinoma, 1	Trans.	Subcostal, 7 Flank, 13	3.2	3.0	245	283	3.1	7.2	4.6	3.8	21	49	10	25
Winfield (20)	21	17	Conn's, 16 Adenoma, 3 Metastasis, 2	Pheo, 7 Conn's, 6 Other, 4	Trans.	Various	3.7	2.3	183	266	2.7	6.2	1.8	2.5	22	46	14	65
Dudley (3)	36	23	Pheo, 13 Conn's, 5 Cushing, 11	Pheo, 1 Conn's, 2 Cushing, 19	Trans.	Posterior	2.6	1.4	194	426	3.5	8.5	4.0	3.2	NA	NA	5.6	52
Imai (14)	40	40	Other, 7 Pheo, 8 Conn's, 16 Cushing, 6 Adenoma, 10	Other, 1 Pheo, 7 Conn's, 17 Cushing, 7 Adenoma, 9	Trans.	Flank	3	2.1	40	162	12	18	2.8	2.7	NA	NA	5	50
Gill (12) Hazzan (13)	110 28	100 28	NA Pheo, 10 Conn's, 12 Cushing, 4 Adenoma, 2	NA Pheo, 11 Conn's, 11 Cushing, 5 Adenoma, 1	NA Trans.	NA Flank	3.3 3.1	3.65 2.3	125 NA	563 NA	1.9 4	7.6 7.5	NA 3.6	NA 2.9	NA 15	NA 39	10 16	33 39

NA, not available.

patients; laparoscopy was associated with shorter operating times, reduced blood loss, fewer complications, and more rapid recovery (4).

Large adrenal masses have been excised laparoscopically. We reviewed the data of 14 patients who underwent laparoscopic adrenalectomy for large adrenal masses and compared them to 14 comparable patients undergoing similar open adrenalectomy (13). The mean tumor size for the laparoscopic and open groups was comparable (8 cm versus 7.8 cm). Operative time and blood loss was comparable for both groups; however, laparoscopy provided shorter hospital stays (2.4 days versus 7.7 days), less analgesic requirement, early feeding (1.3 days versus 3.8 days), and less complications (21% versus 50%).

In experienced hands, adrenal cancer can be approached laparoscopically in select patients. We reviewed 25 adrenalectomies for cancer (transperitoneal, 12; retroperitoneal, 13). Mean size of adrenal tumors was 4.8 cm (1.8 to 9 cm). Mean operative time was 3 hours, blood loss 233 cc, and hospital stay 2.3 days. Two cases were electively converted to open surgery due to local invasion into the inferior vena cava wall. At 20-month follow-up, three patients developed local recurrence.

REFERENCES

1. Brunt LM. The positive impact of laparoscopic adrenalectomy on complications of adrenal surgery. *Surg. Endoscop* 2002;16:252–257.
2. Brunt LM, Doherty GM, Norton JA, et al. Laparoscopic adrenalectomy compared to open adrenalectomy for benign adrenal neoplasms. *J Am Coll Surg* 1996;183:1–10.
3. Dudley NE, Harrison BJ. Comparison of open posterior versus transperitoneal laparoscopic adrenalectomy. *Br J Surg* 1999;86:656–660.
4. Fazeli-Matin S, Gill IS, Hsu THS, Tak Sung G, Novick AC. Laparoscopic renal and adrenal surgery in obese patients: comparison to open surgery. *J Urol* 1999;162:665–669.
5. Gagner M, Lacroix A, Bolte E. Laparoscopic adrenalectomy in Cushing's syndrome and pheochromocytoma. *N Engl J M* 1992;327:1033.
6. Gill IS. The case for laparoscopic adrenalectomy. *J Urol* 2002;166:429–436.
7. Gill IS, Meraney AM, Thomas JC, et al. Thoracoscopic transdiaphragmatic adrenalectomy: the initial experience. *J Urol* 2001;165:1875–1881.
8. Gill IS, Munch LC, Grune MT. Access for retroperitoneal laparoscopy. *J Urol* 1996;156:1120.
9. Gill IS, Soble JJ, Tak Sung G, et al. Needlescopic adrenalectomy—the initial series: comparison with conventional laparoscopic adrenalectomy. *Urology* 1998;52:180–186.
10. Guazzoni G, Montorsi F, Bocciardi L, et al. Transperitoneal laparoscopic versus open adrenalectomy for benign hyperfunctioning adrenal tumors: A comparative study. *J Urol* 1995;153:1597–1600.
11. Hamilton BD. Transperitoneal laparoscopic adrenalectomy. *Urol Clin North Am* 2001;28:61–70.
12. Hazzan D, Shiloni E, Golijanin D, et al. Laparoscopic vs open adrenalectomy for benign adrenal neoplasm. *Surg Endoscop* 2001;15:1356–1358.
13. Hobart MG, Gill IS, Schweizer D, et al. Laparoscopic adrenalectomy for large-volume (τ5cm) adrenal masses. *J Endourol* 2000;14:149–154.
14. Imai T, Kikumori T, Ohiwa M, et al. A case-controlled study of laparoscopic compared with open lateral adrenalectomy. *Am J Surg* 1999;178:50–54.
15. Mann C, Millat B, Boccara G, Atger J, Colson P. Tolerance of laparoscopy for resection of phaeochromocytoma. *Br J Anesth* 1996;77:795–801.
16. Sung GT, Gill IS, Hobart M, Soble J, Schweizer D, Bravo EL. Laparoscopic adrenalectomy: prospective, randomized comparison of transperitoneal vs retroperitoneal approaches. *J Urol* 1999;161[Suppl]:abst 69.
17. Suzuki K. Laparoscopic adrenalectomy: retroperitoneal approach. *Urol Clin North Am* 2001;28:85–95.
18. Thompson GB, Grant CS, van Heerden JA, et al. Laparoscopic versus open posterior adrenalectomy: a case-control study of 100 patients. *Surgery* 1997;122:1132–1136.
19. Vargas HI, Kavoussi LR, Bartlett DL, et al. Laparoscopic adrenalectomy: a new standard of care. *Urology* 1997;49:673–678.
20. Winfield HN, Hamilton BD, Bravo EL, Novick AC. Laparoscopic adrenalectomy: the preferred choice? A comparison to open adrenalectomy. *J Urol* 1998;160:325–329.

CHAPTER 125

Laparoscopic Radical Prostatectomy

Michael D. Fabrizio, Serdar Deger, and Ingolf A. Türk

Among the various treatment alternatives, radical prostatectomy offers definitive pathologic staging and prognostic information while removing the affected organ. This procedure has been shown to provide excellent long-term cancer control in those patients with pathologically confirmed and organ-confined prostate cancer (2,4). The radical prostatectomy has been by tradition performed using a retropubic or perineal approach. Following the progression of other open urologic procedures, the laparoscopic approach is now being performed at many centers worldwide.

Since the first radical prostatectomy, around the turn of the century, there has been a refinement in technique, culminating with the nerve-sparing approach described by Walsh in 1983 (6). The laparoscopic radical prostatectomy (LRP) was first reported by Schuessler et al. in 1997 and has been further refined by Guillonneau, Vallancien, Abbou, and Tuerk (1,3,5). While early in evolution, the LRP has proven to be an effective surgical option in the treatment of adenocarcinoma of the prostate.

DIAGNOSIS

Adenocarcinoma of the prostate is typically diagnosed through routine medical screening, which includes a digital rectal examination and serum prostate-specific antigen (PSA). An abnormal digital rectal examination, elevated PSA level, or PSA velocity should prompt a transrectal ultrasound-guided biopsy of the prostate.

Once the diagnosis of cancer is made, the patient should undergo appropriate preoperative counseling and a thorough discussion of treatment options. Preoperative staging studies including computerized tomography of the abdomen and pelvis are typically not performed in a patient with clinical staged T1c prostate cancer and a PSA less than 10 ng per mL. A radioisotope bone scan is usually performed if the PSA level is greater than 10 ng per mL. Of course, either of these studies is obtained if the surgeon determines that they are clinically appropriate.

INDICATIONS FOR SURGERY

A laparoscopic radical prostatectomy is indicated in patients who would have a life expectancy of at least 10 years. The same indications apply to the laparoscopic, open, and perineal approaches. Patients should have organ-confined prostate cancer at the time of presentation.

The choice of a nerve-sparing or a non–nerve-sparing approach should be mutually agreed upon by the surgeon and patient. In general, contraindications to nerve sparing include palpable disease at the apex, Gleason grade 5 disease, markedly elevated PSA (i.e., greater than 20 ng per mL), and a preoperative impotence. Although unable to palpate induration at the time of the LRP, any intraoperative difficulties with mobilization of the neurovascular bundle including fixation should be a relative contraindication to a nerve-sparing approach.

Previous abdominal surgery is no longer a contraindication to the laparoscopic radical prostatectomy. The type of previous abdominal procedure, however, may change the approach. The authors have performed laparoscopic radical prostatectomies on patients with previous colon resections and a history of elective abdominal procedures, but caution should be used when there is a history of peritonitis. In addition, pelvic lipomatosis is an absolute contraindication to the LRP. Finally, due to the extreme Trendelenburg position typically employed during the procedure any known intracranial pathology such as arteriovenous malformations, cerebral aneurysms, or a history of cerebral vascular accidents should serve as a contraindication to the LRP. Laparoscopic pelvic lymph node dissection is reserved for those patients with Gleason grade 4 or 5 disease, high-volume disease, or a PSA greater than 10.

ALTERNATIVE THERAPY

Treatment options for localized prostate cancer include observation, cryotherapy, brachytherapy, external beam radiation therapy, and radical prostatectomy. Radical prostatectomy can be performed through a retropubic or perineal approach..

SURGICAL TECHNIQUE

In addition to the normal preoperative laboratory and radiographic studies, the patient receives a mechanical bowel prep the day before surgery. On the morning of surgery, the patient is typed and screened, undergoes a 500-cc neomycin enema, and receives a cephalosporin antibiotic. We use sequential pneumatic compression devices throughout the procedure.

LRP is preformed with the patient in the supine position with the arms tucked and the table slightly flexed. A rectal bougie is placed and the abdomen/genitalia are prepped and draped in the usual sterile fashion. A 20 Fr Foley catheter is inserted into the urinary bladder after the sterile field has been established. At this point, a Veress needle is used to insufflate the abdominal cavity to 20-cm pressure. After a pneumoperitoneum has been established, five trocars are placed. The first 12-mm trocar is placed at the level of the umbilicus (Fig. 125–1). This can be placed using an optical port, employing an open technique, or by gently applying pressure to the 12-mm trocar and introducing it into the abdomen. We use a zero-degree lens throughout the procedure and inspect the abdominal cavity after placement of our first trocar. Our next two 12-mm trocars are placed just lateral to the rectus on the right and left sides, respectively. These 12-mm trocars are placed 2 to 4 cm inferior to the umbilicus. Finally, two 5-mm trocars are placed off the anterior iliac spine on the right and left sides, respectively. Thus, a total of five ports are utilized throughout the procedure (Fig. 125–1). The patient is now placed into the extreme Trendelenburg position. At this point, a laparoscopic pelvic lymph node dissection can be performed if warranted.

If available, the Aesop (Computer Motion, Inc., Goleta, CA) is placed on the patient's right side of the table and used to control the zero-degree laparoscope and camera through the umbilical port. The assistant stands on the patient's right side and the surgeon stands on the patient's left side throughout the procedure. A fan retractor is used through the right 12-mm port to provide retraction of the bowel. Once the cul-de-sac is clearly identified and any sigmoidal attachments are incised, the vas deferens is identified on both the right and left hand sides at the level of the internal ring. The peritoneum is scored in a line along the vas deferens down to the *cul-de-sac* (Fig. 125–2). This incision is carried down to the second peritoneal fold in the *cul-de-sac*. The vas deferens is skeletonized on the right and left sides. The surgeon holds bipolar cautery in his left hand (through the left 5-mm port) and the scissors enter through the left 12-mm port. The vas deferens is dissected down to the level of the seminal vesicles on both right and left sides. Hemostasis is maintained with the bipolar cautery. Once the seminal vesicles are identified, the assistant retracts the vas deferens anteriorly using a grasper through the 5-mm right port (Fig. 125–3) and using the irrigator–aspirator through the 12-mm right port. The surgeon now proceeds to dissect the seminal vesicles using a combination of

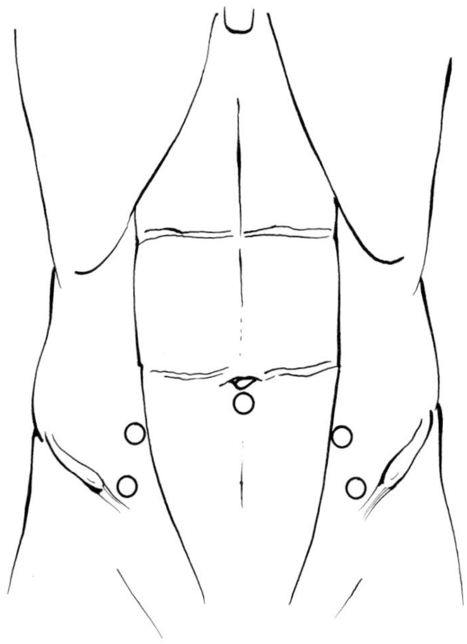

FIG. 125–1. Port placement for laparoscopic prostatectomy. Five ports are utilized.

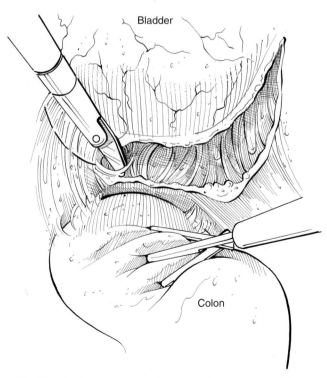

FIG. 125–2. Scoring the peritoneum along the vas deferens into the *cul-de-sac*.

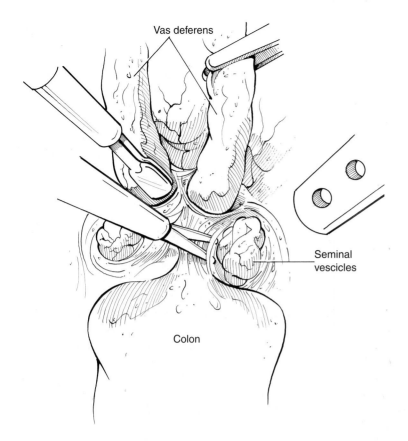

FIG. 125–3. The vas deferens is lifted anteriorly by the assistant and the seminal vesicles are dissected free.

sharp and blunt dissection with the bipolar cautery and scissors. The seminal vesicles are completely mobilized to their tips (Fig. 125–3). In the next step, the surgeon and assistant retract the seminal vesicles and Denonvillier's fascia is incised, which creates a plane between the posterior surface of the prostate and the rectum. The perirectal adipose tissue should be clearly identified. If necessary, a rectal bougie can be manipulated by an assistant to confirm the exact location of the rectum.

Attention is now focused at the level of the bladder. The bladder is filled with 200 cc of saline, and using the bipolar cautery and laparoscopic scissors through the left ports the lateral aspect of the bladder is dissected off the anterior abdominal wall by connecting the points between the incised median and umbilical ligaments and the lateral peritoneal reflection (Fig. 125–4). The bladder is emptied and now has been mobilized. The endopelvic fascia can be seen on both the left and right sides without

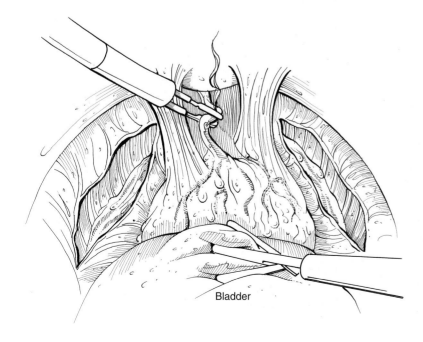

FIG. 125–4. The bladder is freed off the anterior abdominal wall by incising the umbilical ligaments and lateral attachments.

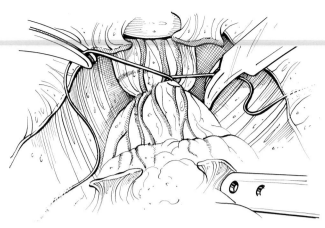

FIG. 125–5. The endopelvic fascia is incised and the dorsal vein complex identified.

difficulty. The surgeon incises the endopelvic fascia bilaterally and the fatty tissue overlying the prostate is carefully dissected away using the bipolar cautery. The superficial dorsal vein is cauterized using the bipolar forceps (Fig. 125–5). Thus, the anterior surface of the prostate is exposed and the puboprostatic ligaments on the right and left sides are sharply divided with the laparoscopic scissors. The deep dorsal venous complex runs parallel to the urethra at the level of the prostatic apex and is now ligated with a 0 Vicryl suture ligature on a CT-1 needle. The needle is slightly straightened and passed through the right 12-mm port using a laparoscopic needle driver. A laparoscopic grasper is used from the left 12-mm port site. The assistant uses a 5-mm irrigator–aspirator through the right 5-mm port for retraction. Using the 0 Vicryl, the dorsal vein complex is ligated with a figure-of-eight suture passed anterior to the urethra and posterior to this deep venous dorsal complex (Fig. 125–6). The suture is tied intracorporeally and the

dorsal vein complex is secured but not divided at this point.

The next step involves division of the prostatic base from the bladder neck. This is one of the more difficult portions of the LRP. However, with experience the plane is easily visualized. The authors prefer to use a curved harmonic scalpel for this portion of the procedure. The assistant retracts the bladder using a fan retractor from the right 12-mm port and using a 5-mm irrigator–aspirator outlines the Foley catheter balloon down toward the level of the prostatic base. The surgeon uses a bipolar cautery from the left 5-mm port and a curved harmonic scalpel from the left 12-mm port to begin division of the prostatic base from the bladder neck (Fig. 125–7). The detrusor fibers are often seen at this point and the prostatic base is developed anteriorly. The bladder is entered and the Foley catheter is identified. The balloon is deflated and the assistant retracts the Foley catheter cephalad using a grasper from the right 5-mm port site. The posterior bladder mucosa is scored with the harmonic scalpel, and this is carried through the posterior surface of the prostate (Fig. 125–8). The seminal vesicles and accompanying vas deferens, which have been dissected posteriorly, are now brought anteriorly and grasped by the assistant using the laparoscopic 5-mm grasper.

The next sequence of maneuvers is determined by the decision to perform a nerve-sparing approach. If a nerve-sparing approach is attempted, a right-angled dissector can be utilized through the right 12-mm port site to free the neurovascular bundle on the lateral surface of the prostate. Apically, the neurovascular bundle can be sharply dissected from the apex of the prostate prior to division of the dorsal venous complex and at the base the neurovascular bundle can be dissected free with a combination of right-angle dissection and laparoscopic scissors. With the assistant lifting the seminal vesicle anteriorly,

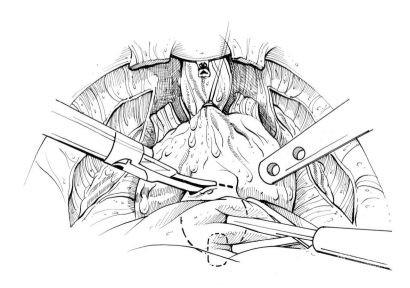

FIG. 125–6. Ligation of the deep dorsal vein complex using 0 Vicryl on CT-1 needle.

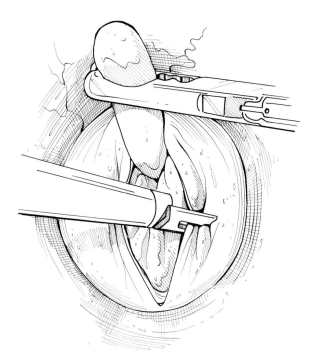

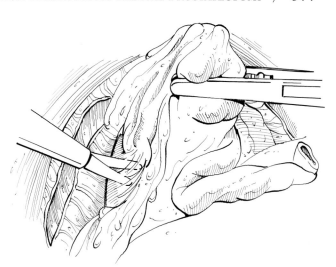

FIG. 125–8. Division of the posterior bladder neck and identification of the previously dissected seminal vesicles and vas deferens.

FIG. 125–7. Division of the anterior bladder neck and prostatic base using the harmonic scalpel.

the vascular pedicle can be divided using the harmonic scalpel. Sharp dissection can be used to free the remaining reflection of endopelvic fascia off the lateral surface of the prostate (Fig. 125–9). The rectum is gently pushed posteriorly while working toward the apex of the prostate. A rectal bougie can be utilized to identify the rectum if necessary. Small perforating blood vessels may be encountered and are best left alone.

If a non–nerve-sparing approach is performed, the assistant grasps the seminal vesicle, lifting anteriorly, and the surgeon divides the entire vascular pedicle and neurovascular bundle with the harmonic scalpel, working

toward the apex of the prostate (Fig. 125–10). At this point, the prostate is attached posteriorly by the rectourethralis muscle and the urethra. The dorsal vein complex is sharply incised and the apical notch of the prostate developed. The anterior urethra is now sharply divided, exposing the catheter, which is gently retracted, and the posterior urethra is subsequently divided (Fig. 125–11). The assistant provides gentle cephalad retraction by grasping the base of the prostate to allow maximum exposure of the urethra. The rectourethralis muscle is sharply incised with either the harmonic scalpel or scissors and the prostate can be rolled to both the left and right sides to facilitate this maneuver. Again, a rectal bougie can facilitate visualization of the rectum. The prostate with the accompanying seminal vesicles and vas deferens is now placed into the left lower quadrant, and

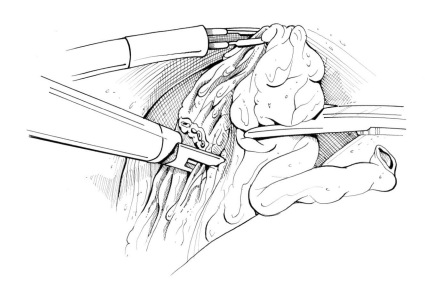

FIG. 125–9. Sharply dissecting the neurovascular bundle of the lateral aspect of the prostate.

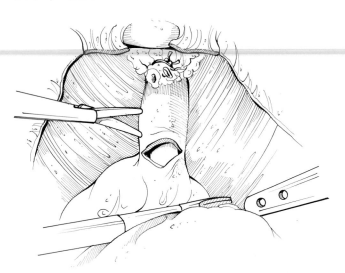

FIG. 125–10. Division of the entire vascular pedicle and neurovascular bundle.

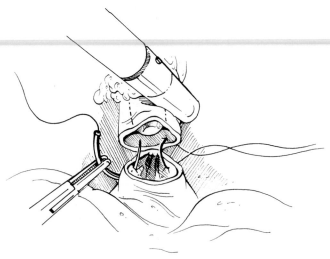

FIG. 125–12. Urethral anastomosis beginning with the posterior sutures.

the pelvis is copiously irrigated. Any bleeding is addressed with the bipolar cautery.

The rectal bougie is used to manipulate the rectum to inspect the anterior surface of the rectum, and if necessary a 20 Fr Foley catheter can be gently placed in the rectum and the pelvis filled with saline. Air is injected into the Foley catheter. If there is no evidence of leak, it can be assumed that there is no immediate rectal injury.

Next, the bladder neck is identified and the ureteral orifices are observed for efflux of urine. A urethral sound is placed. Urethral or bladder neck margins maybe sent for frozen section if necessary. Once the ureteral orifices are identified, the urethral–vesical anastomosis is begun (Fig. 125–12). Using a 2-0 Vicryl on a UR-6 needle through the right 12-mm port, the anastomosis is begun by placing a stitch through the posterior bladder neck from outside the bladder. The needle is grasped and using

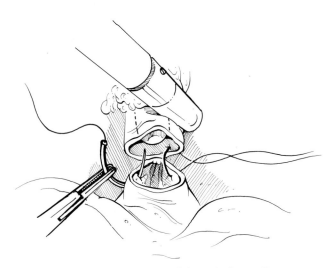

FIG. 125–11. Division of the anterior urethra.

the right 12-mm port, the posterior stitch on the right side of the urethra is placed. Next, a second suture is introduced through the left 12-mm port and, in similar fashion, the posterior bladder neck is sutured outside in followed by the posterior urethra inside out. Thus, the knots are tied on the outside of the bladder (Fig. 125—12). The table is reflexed and the bladder is reapproximated to the urethra. The assistant may facilitate this maneuver by grasping the posterior bladder from the right side and holding it in place while the sutures are tied intracorporeally. At this point, the remaining portion of the anastomosis is completed. Using the 2-0 Vicryl suture, the sutures are placed circumferentially from either the right or left 12-mm port as determined by the patient's anatomy. On occasion, it is necessary to place a backhanded suture from the left 12-mm port.

If necessary, bladder neck reconstruction can be performed anteriorly using a 2-0 Vicryl on a UR-6 needle; the bladder neck can be reconstructed by placing a suture through the anterior portion of the bladder neck in interrupted fashion. The sutures are tied intracorporeally. The remaining anterior sutures can be placed. Typically, the left anterior bladder neck and the urethral sutures are placed through the right 12-mm port and visa versa. This allows for more effective needle positioning. A new 20 Fr Foley catheter is placed under direct visualization prior to completing the anastomosis and the final anterior sutures are tied intracorporeally. The bladder is tested by instilling 60 cc of saline, and if a leak is detected another suture can be placed. In general, seven to eight sutures are used for the urethral–vesical anastomosis. Next, the right 5-mm port site incision is extended to accompany a 10-mm Endocatch device (Auto Suture, Norwalk, CT). Once the Endocatch is deployed, the accompanying needles and prostate with accompanying seminal vesicles and vas deferens are delivered into the bag. The bag is closed and brought through the right 5-mm port site. The external oblique fascia and muscle are incised with electrocautery and the bag removed. This small incision is closed using a two-layer technique of 0 Vicryl for the muscle followed by the oblique fascia. The abdomen is reinsufflated, and then a Jackson–Pratt drain is placed through the left 5-mm port. It is secured in place with a 3-0 Nylon suture. The remaining port sites are closed in standard fashion using 0 Vicryl. The authors prefer to use a Carter-Thomason (Inlet Medical, Eden Prairie, MN) instrument. All wounds are copiously irrigated and a 4-0 Monocryl is used for the skin. The Foley catheter is left to gravity drainage and the Jackson–Pratt drain left to bulb suction.

OUTCOMES

Results

Patients are started on a clear liquid diet on postoperative day 2 and advanced accordingly. The Jackson–Pratt drain is typically left in place for 2 days. Excessive drainage is rare. The catheter is typically removed on postoperative day 5 to 7. Our average blood loss is 175 cc. At present, patients appear to have comparable continence rates to an open cohort using the validated UCLA quality of life questionnaire, which is administered to all of our patients pre- and postoperatively. Our margin status is comparable to most open series, with a 13% posi-

tive margin rate with those patients with pT2 disease. Of those patients with pT3 disease, 45% have positive margins. As with the European experience, our early procedures were non-nerve sparing. It is still early, but potency rates are not equivalent to the open procedure. However, we have performed only a limited number of nerve-sparing procedures in the last 6 months. Thus, long-term data is lacking. Finally, intraoperative and postoperative complication rates are comparable to most open series.

Although early in evolution, recent data has demonstrated that the laparoscopic radical prostatectomy is technically feasible and can be comparable to traditional avenues of surgical extirpation. Long-term data will continue to be important to determine whether the laparoscopic radical prostatectomy remains an effective alternative to the open or perineal approaches.

REFERENCES

1. Abbou CC, Salomon L, Hoznek P, et al. Laparoscopic radical prostatectomy: Preliminary results. *Urology* 2000;55:631.
2. Catalona WJ, Smith DS. Cancer recurrence and survival rates following anatomic radical retropubic prostatectomy for prostate cancer. *J Urol* 1998;160(6, Pt 2):2428–2434.
3. Guillonneau B, Vallancien G. Laparoscopic radical prostatectomy: The Montsouris technique. *J Urol* 2000;163:1643.
4. Han M, Partin AW, Pound CR, et al. Long term biochemical disease-free and cancer-specific survival following anatomic radical retropubic prostatectomy. *Urol Clin North Am* 2001;28:3.
5. Turk I, Deger S, Winkelmann B, et al. Laparoscopic radical prostatectomy. Technical aspects and experience with 125 cases. *Eur Urol* 2001;40:46.
6. Walsh PC, Donker PJ. Impotence following radical prostatectomy: Insight into etiology and prevention. *J Urol* 1982;128:492–497.

CHAPTER 126

Robot-Assisted Anatomic Laparoscopic Prostatectomy: Vattikuti Institute Prostatectomy

Ashutosh Tewari and Mani Menon

Surgery in the future will not be about blood and guts, but rather...bits and bytes.

Ashutosh Tewari

Advances in laparoscopic techniques have resulted in minimally invasive surgery replacing several previously open operations such as cholecystectomy. However, counterintuitive movements, flat resolution in 2D mode, limited range of motion, lack of tactile feedback because of long instruments, and difficulty in intracorporeal suturing all contribute to a reluctance in the widespread application of laparoscopic surgery to complex reconstructive procedures. However, recent developments in the field of surgical robotics have ushered in a new era of minimally invasive surgery that now challenges the bastions of conventional open surgery. Currently available telemanipulation devices allow the performance of complex surgical tasks with dexterity and minimal fatigue due to their ergonomic design, expanded degree of movements, tremor filtering, and 3D stereoscopic visualization. They provide an unsurpassable view of the operative field and unrestricted ability to execute any surgical task. Robotic surgery has been applied to complex surgical procedures such as pyeloplasty, radical cystectomy, donor nephrectomy, and radical prostatectomy (1–3).

We have developed a minimally invasive robot-assisted radical prostatectomy by standardizing a unique sequence of surgical steps, appropriate visual angles using different lenses, optimal retraction strategies, precise suturing steps, anatomic sparing of the neurovascular structures, and incorporating time-tested open surgical principles (4,9). Due to its origin from Vattikuti Institute of Urology, we term this procedure Vattikuti Institute prostatectomy (VIP) (5–11).

DIAGNOSIS

Standard procedures to diagnose and stage prostate cancer are described in Chapter 125 (Radical prostatectomy)

ALTERNATIVE THERAPY

Treatment options for localized prostate cancer include observation, cryotherapy, brachytherapy, external beam radiation therapy, and radical prostatectomy. Radical prostatectomy can be performed through a retropubic or perineal approach. The standard laparoscopic radical prostatectomy is presented in Chapter 125.

INDICATIONS FOR SURGERY

Men with clinically localized prostate cancer who choose surgical treatment are candidates for this procedure. Patients are excluded if their life expectancy is less than 10 years or their Charlson comorbidity score is 3 or above. Patients undergo a thorough preoperative evaluation including serum prostate-specific antigen (PSA), international prostate symptom score (IPSS), sexual function inventory, quality of life score, and incontinence questionnaire. We also record information about other comorbidities, such as stroke, cerebral aneurysm, diabetes mellitus, hypertension, cardiopulmonary disorder (COPD), and history of myocardial infarctions. A history of stroke or cerebral aneurysm is a relative contraindication for this procedure as the patient would be placed in a pronounced Trendelenburg position for 1 to 3 hours. Previous abdominal surgery is not a contraindication.

SURGICAL TECHNIQUE

Patients are admitted on the day of surgery and receive deep vein thrombosis (DVT) prophylaxis (Heparin 5000 IU subcutaneously on call to the operating room) and antibiotic in the preoperative holding. Venodyne boots are placed and the abdomen is shaved from the nipple to the groin.

Da Vinci Robotic Technology

The da Vinci system (Figs. 126–1, 126–2) uses a sophisticated master–slave robot that incorporates 3D visualization, scaling of movement, and wristed instrumentation. The system has three multijoint robotic arms with one controlling a binocular endoscope and the other two controlling articulated instruments. Two lenses—0 degrees or 30 degrees—are used. Two finger-controlled handles (the "masters") housed in a mobile console control the two robotic arms and together with a foot pedal control camera movement. Instrument movement can be scaled from 1:1, which allows exact finger movements to be transmitted to the instrument tip, to 1:3 and 1:5, which scale down the movements to allow precise and delicate dissection (5,6,9).

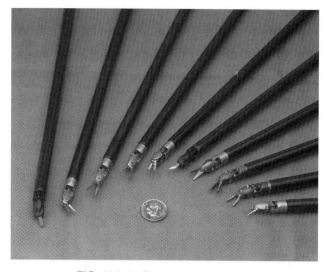

FIG. 126–2. The da Vinci system.

Surgical Team

The VIP team includes one console-side and two patient-side surgeons. The operating surgeon sits at the console, and is not scrubbed. The patient-side team is scrubbed, and places the ports, presents the operative field to the operating surgeon and uses suction to keep the filed clean. This team should be facile with laparoscopy.

Patient Positioning

We place the patient in the Trendelenburg position, padding all pressure points. The legs are placed in a lithotomy position in patients over 6 feet tall. Otherwise, we partially abduct the legs over a few pillows. The arms are tucked in and the patient is secured to the table using cloth tapes.

Port Placement

A pneumoperitoneum is created with a Veress needle introduced through a upper left periumbilical puncture. We then place a 12-mm port on the left upper side of the umbilicus and introduce the binocular scope (Fig. 126–3). The remaining ports are placed under direct vision, using the stereoscopic 30-degree lens looking up to inspect the peritoneal cavity. Two 8-mm da Vinci ports are placed approximately 10 to 12 cm from the midline slightly below the camera port and are used for the instrument arms. Two additional conventional ports are placed on the right side for retraction, suction, and the insertion of sutures. The lateral one is a 10-mm and the medial one is a 5-mm port. A sixth port (5 mm) is placed below and lateral to the left robotic port. The robot is now docked in

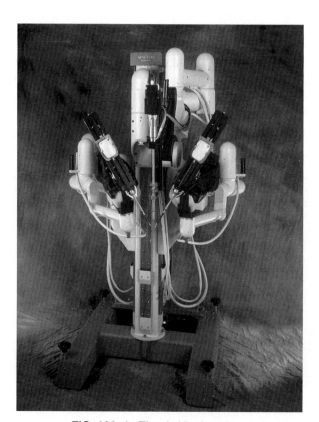

FIG. 126–1. The da Vinci system.

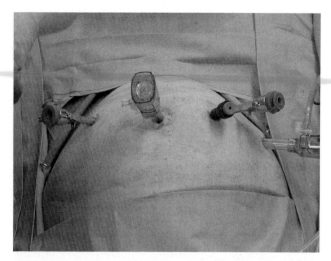

FIG. 126–3. A 12-mm port is placed on the left upper side of the umbilicus and the binocular scope introduced.

position. With experience, this step—Veress needle to docking of the robot—can be accomplished in approximately 15 minutes.

Development of the Extraperitoneal Space

Although the ports are placed intraperitoneally, the rest of the operation is performed extraperitoneally (Fig. 126–4). The peritoneal cavity is inspected using a 30-degree upward-looking lens. The extraperitoneal space is entered through a transverse peritoneal incision extending from the left to the right medial umbilical ligament. The incision is extended in an inverted U to the level of the vasa on either side. The medial and median umbilical ligaments are transected and the extraperitoneal space is

developed. This approach allows the bladder, prostate, and bowel to drop posteriorly, avoiding the cumbersome retraction that is necessary sometimes when the initial dissection is in the *cul-de-sac*.

Lymph Node Dissection

We use a 0-degree lens for visualization and a 1:3 scaling for lymphadenectomy (Fig. 126–5). Lymphadenectomy is performed if the preoperative serum PSA is more than 10 ng per mL, the biopsy Gleason score is greater than 6, or if more than 50% of the biopsy cores are positive for cancer (7). The medial and lateral surface landmarks for the lymph node dissection include the medial umbilical ligament medially and the testicular vessels traversing the internal inguinal ring laterally. Exposure of the external iliac arteries is sometimes facilitated by mobilization of the sigmoid colon or cecum. The initial incision is be made through the posterior peritoneal membrane beginning just lateral to the medial (obliterated) umbilical ligament, high over the pubic bone, and extended just medial to the external iliac artery back toward the bifurcation of the common iliac artery, where the ureter may be identified. The vas deferens crossing in a medial direction from the internal ring toward the region of the bladder and prostate is isolated, coagulated, and then transected. Traction to the vas is avoided because it may result in postoperative testicular pain. Using the medial edge of the external iliac artery as a guide, the external iliac vein is located and cleared of all fibrolymphatic tissue off its anterior and medial surfaces. This essentially creates the lateral border of the obturator lymph node packet. The dissection proceeds beneath the external iliac vein out to the pelvic sidewall and then inferiorly to the femoral canal, where the lymphatic channels are ligated at a convenient point. The dissection then pro-

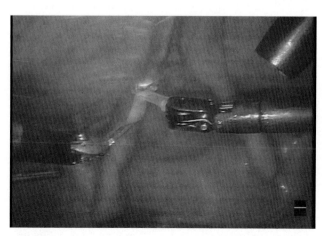

FIG. 126–4. The rest of the operation is performed extraperitoneally.

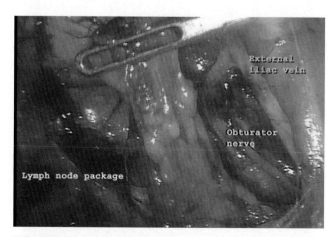

FIG. 126–5. A 0-degree lens is used for visualization and a 1:3 scaling for lymphadenectomy.

ceeds superiorly along the pelvic sidewall to the bifurcation of the common iliac artery, where the lymph nodes in the angle between the external iliac and hypogastric arteries are removed. Next, the obturator lymph nodes are removed with care to avoid injury to the obturator nerve. The obturator artery and vein are skeletonized but are usually left undisturbed and are not ligated unless excessive bleeding occurs. At the completion of the dissection, the vasculature in the hypogastric and obturator fossa should be neatly skeletonized.

Incision of the Endopelvic Fascia and Exposure of the Prostatic Apex

The 0-degree lens with a 1:3 scaling is used for this part of the dissection (Fig. 126–6). The endopelvic fascia often has a weak area through which we can expose the levator fibers. This fascia is incised using the da Vinci hook or spatula. Dissection is carried out inferiorly until the urethra with the surrounding puboperinealis muscle is exposed (8), and superiorly until the prostatovesical junction is identified, by the detection of a subtle tongue of retroperitoneal fat. The puboprostatic ligaments are not transected but left intact to anchor the urethral stump after prostatectomy.

Dorsal Vein Stitch

The nonscaled setting is used for this step (Fig. 126–7). A 6-inch suture on a CT-1, 0 braided, polyglactin, 36-mm taper needle (Ethicon) is used to control the dorsal venous plexus. The suture is placed about 2 cm distal to the prostatic apex. The needle is passed horizontally from the right to the left, anterior to the urethra and behind the dorsal vein complex. It is then passed backward anterior to the complex and behind the puboprostatic ligaments.

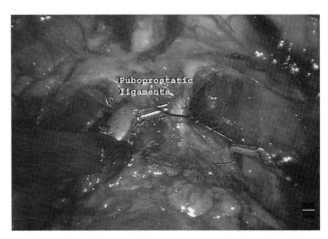

FIG. 126–7. Dorsal vein stitch.

The suture is knotted, securing the dorsal vein complex. An additional suture is placed midway between the apex and base of the prostate for traction and rotation of the prostate during posterior dissection.

Retroapical Dissection and Release of the Neurovascular Bundles

The plane between the prostatourethral junction and the rectourethralis/rhabdosphincter is developed using blunt dissection with the da Vinci hook or scalpel. Because the field is bloodless at this stage of operation and the prostate is in its normal anatomic position, it is easy and safe to develop this plane. This maneuver not only releases the neurovascular bundles at the apex but helps enormously in precisely identifying the posterior apical margin of the prostate at the time of final detachment of the specimen. It divides the tethering of the posterior urethra to the rectum, enabling us to transect the urethra cleanly at a later stage. Because the neurovascular bundles are close to the prostatic apex, electrocautery must not be used at this stage of the operation.

Bladder Neck Transection

This is one of the more difficult steps of conventional laparoscopic prostatectomy because of the lack of anatomic landmarks (Fig. 126–8). We find that the 30-degree lens looking down and the 3D visualization aid in the delineation of the prostatovesical junction. The junction is usually at the point at which loose fat can no longer be swept off the prostate. Another visual clue is provided by looking at the lateral, convex borders of the prostate, where a tongue of retroperitoneal fat identifies the prostatourethral junction. The left-side assistant pulls the prostatic traction suture to the foot of the patient. The surgeon provides firm countertraction with the da Vinci

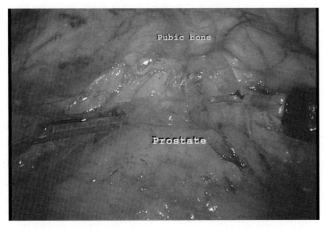

FIG. 126–6. The 0-degree lens with a 1:3 scaling is used for this part of the dissection.

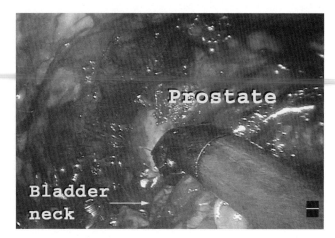

FIG. 126–8. Bladder neck transection.

forceps. The bladder neck is incised using an electrocautery hook and 1:3 scaling for adequate coagulation of the bleeders. We start the dissection laterally on either side, where it is easy to identify the prostatovesical junction. No attempt is made to preserve the anterior bladder neck. Rather, it is incised eccentrically so that the posterior lip is slightly longer than the anterior. This helps in better visualization of the posterior suture line during the anastomosis.

Identification of the Foley catheter ensures that the anterior bladder neck has been incised appropriately. The Foley balloon is deflated now and the left-side assistant grasps the tip of the catheter with firm anterior traction. Using the shaft of the catheter as a landmark, the mucosa at the posterior bladder neck is incised precisely. The posterior detrusor muscle is cleanly incised in the midline. Using the da Vinci long-tip forceps for countertraction, the surgeon grasps the cut end of the posterior bladder neck in the midline and gradually dissects it away from the prostate, maintaining a clean detrusor margin for the subsequent urethrovesical anastomosis. It is important that the field should be bloodless and the visualization superb to perform this step accurately. The assistant uses short bursts of gentle suction to avoid loss of the pneumoperitoneum. Vigorous and injudicious suctioning can tear the bladder neck and urethra, increasing the difficulty of the anastomosis. The catheter is removed and the left-side assistant retracts the posterior prostatic base anteriorly. This exposes the anterior layer of Denonvillier's fascia. The fascia is incised, exposing the vasa and the seminal vesicles. The vasa and the seminal vesicles are grasped and pulled upward individually. The vasa are transected and the seminal vesicles skeletonized, avoiding damage to the neurovascular bundles. When preservation of potency is paramount, the tips of the seminal vesicles may be left *in situ*. In such instances, we get frozen sections of the margins of the seminal vesicles.

Control of the Lateral Pedicles and Preservation of the Neurovascular Bundles

The lateral pedicles are controlled using hem-o-lock clips (Weck, Research Triangle Park, NC) (Figs. 126–9 and 126–10). The clips are applied close to the prostate and the pedicle is divided between them. We avoid use of electrocautery from this point on. The neurovascular bundles are enclosed within the layers of the periprostatic fascia (3,10,11). This fascia is composed of two thin layers, which split posteriorly to enclose the neurovascular bundles. The layers of the periprostatic fascia fuse with the anterior layers of Denonvillier's fascia lateral to the prostate, forming a triangular tunnel. The inner layer of periprostatic fascia (also called prostatic fascia) forms the medial vertical wall of this triangle, the outer layer of periprostatic fascia (also called levator fascia) forms the lateral wall, and the anterior layer of Denonvillier's fascia forms the posterior wall. This triangular space is wide near the base and gets narrower near the apex. The medial wall of the triangle (prostatic fascia) is intimately attached to the prostatic capsule and is pierced by multiple neurovascular branches, or micropedicles, that enter the prostate. The micropedicles (tiny arteries, veins, and nerves) have no consistent pattern and tether the neurovascular bundles to the posterolateral surface of the prostate.

We use an articulated robotic scissors to incise the prostatic fascia anterior and parallel to the neurovascular bundles. Once the correct plane is entered, most of the dissection occurs in a relatively avascular plane. Two to three micropedicles are usually present that enter the prostate. These pedicles will bleed when cut, but the bleeding usually stops when the prostate is completely freed. Anatomic studies have shown that the neurovascular bundle is 3 to 7 mm away from the fascia, or about 5 to 9 mm from the plane of dissection that we use (3).

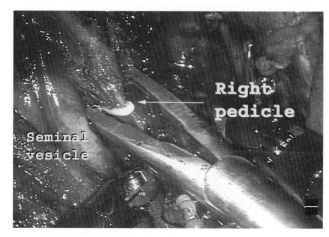

FIG. 126–9. The lateral pedicles are controlled using hem-o-lock clips.

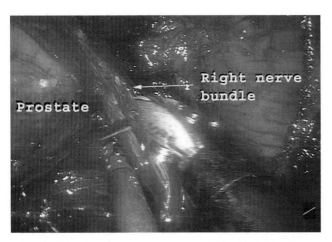

FIG. 126–10. The lateral pedicles are controlled using hem-o-lock clips.

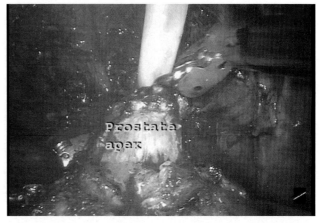

FIG. 126–12. Incision of dorsal venous complex and urethra.

Posterior Dissection

At the bladder neck, Denonvillier's fascia is thick and composed of multiple layers. The plane between the prostate and rectum is developed with the articulated scissors, using a combination of blunt and sharp dissection (Fig. 126–11). The plane of dissection leaves the posterior-most layer(s) of Denonviller's fascia on the rectum. We feel that this lessens the likelihood of rectal injury. Venous tributaries between the prostate and rectum are coagulated only when necessary as minor bleeding will stop once the urethra is transected. Dissection is carried down to the apex of the prostate.

Incision of Dorsal Venous Complex and Urethra

We use a 0-degree lens with 1:3 scaling here (Fig. 126–12). The dorsal venous complex is incised tangen-

tial to the prostate to avoid capsular incision. A plane between urethra and dorsal venous complex is gently developed to expose the anterior urethral wall. A van Buren urethral sound identifies the anterior surface of the urethra at the urethroprostatic junction. The anterior wall of the urethra is transected with the scissors a few millimeters distal to the apex of the prostate. The urethral sound is removed and a Foley catheter is placed. The left-side assistant applies firm anterior traction to the catheter, exposing the posterior wall of the urethra at the prostatic apex. The posterior wall of the urethra and the rectourethralis muscle are cut under direct vision. Because the posterior apex has been dissected at an earlier stage of the operation, the rectum falls away and the rectourethralis can be transected with impunity. The freed specimen is then placed in a specimen retrieval bag.

Parietal Biopsies

Using the articulated scissors, biopsies are obtained from the periurethral tissues anterior and posterior to the prostatic apex, from the prostatovesical junction, and from tissues anterior to the neurovascular bundles, where indicated (Fig. 126–13). The biopsies are sent for frozen section. In the rare instance that the biopsies show cancer, additional tissue is removed from the appropriate location.

Urethrovesical Anastomosis

We use one dyed and one undyed 3-0 Monocryl sutures on a 17-mm taper needle (RB-1, Ethicon) for the anastomosis (Figs. 126–14 and 126–15). The needle is small enough to make the rotation in even the narrowest pelvis, and the suture is strong enough to bring the tran-

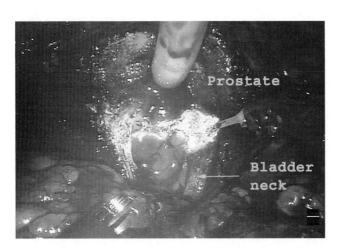

FIG. 126–11. Posterior dissection.

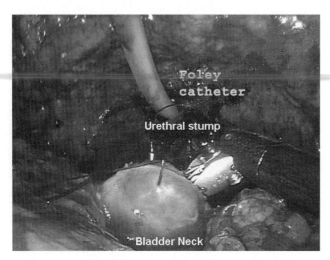

FIG. 126–13. Parietal biopsies.

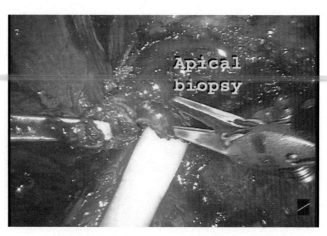

FIG. 126–15. Urethrovesical anastomosis.

sected urethra and the bladder neck together. The two suture tails are tied together with multiple throws of knots, leaving a 6-inch length of suture on either side with an attached needle. A tissue pledget—usually a piece of the vas or umbilical ligament—is placed over the knot. The left-side assistant pulls the Foley catheter anteriorly, exposing the posterior urethral wall. The needle of the dyed suture is passed at the 4-o'clock position outside in on the bladder. We then pass the needle inside out at 4-o'clock on the urethra. We continue suturing clockwise along the posterior cut ends, ending at the 8-o'clock position inside the bladder. The suture is then passed inside out through the bladder at the 9-o'clock position, turning the corner. One or two more throws are placed from the urethra to the bladder, ending with the suture exiting at around 10-o'clock, inside out on the bladder. The suture is pulled snug, completing the posterior layer of the anastomosis. The tissue pledget provides enough tension to approximate the edges and pre-

vents the knot from pulling through the bladder. It is important to understand that no intracorporeal knotting has been done for the anastomosis. The left-side surgeon places the catheter in the bladder and holds the end of the dyed suture with traction. Now, we pass the needle of the undyed end (which is on the outside surface of the bladder at 4-o'clock) outside in on the urethra. Suturing proceeds counterclockwise, ending where it meets the first suture. The left hand is used for the urethral pass and the right hand for the vesical pass. The assistant replaces the Foley catheter with a new one and advances it into the bladder. The balloon is tested and the two ends of the suture are tied. With the balloon of the catheter away from the bladder neck, the bladder is filled with 250 cc of saline to test the integrity of the anastomosis.

Retrieval of Specimen and Completion of Surgery

When the anastomosis is not watertight, a suction drain is placed through one of the 5-mm ports. The entrapped

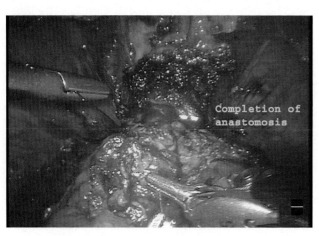

FIG. 126–14. Urethrovesical anastomosis.

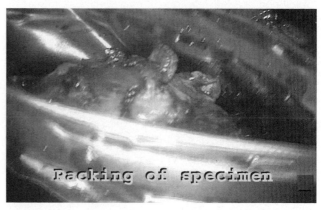

FIG. 126–16. Retrieval of specimen and completion of surgery.

specimen is removed after enlarging the umbilical port incision as required (Fig. 126–16). The incision is closed in layers.

POSTOPERATIVE CARE AND DISCHARGE

The patients are sent to recovery on intravenous fluids, antibiotics, and pain medications. They either go home on the same day or next morning. The catheter is removed anyway between 4 to 7 days depending on the quality of anastomosis.

OUTCOMES

See Tables 126–1 through 126–3.

Results

For our last 250 patients, the mean operating time was around 2.5 hours (165 minutes with lymphadenectomy and135 minutes without it) and the average blood loss was 150 mL. The median specimen Gleason score was 7, and the mean tumor volume was 7.0 mL. Four patients had a positive surgical margin (three unifocal, one multifocal). Ninety-five percent of patients were discharged within 23 hours and mean catheterization time was 4.2 days. The complication rate was 4%. These results compare well with "best-in-class" results for open or laparoscopic radical prostatectomy (2,4).

VIP is a safe, effective, and reproducible technique for removing the prostate. The procedure incorporates principles of both laparoscopic and open radical prostatectomy. We find the operation to be technically challenging, but less so than conventional laparoscopic prostatectomy. VIP is a feasible alternative to nonrobotic laparoscopic prostatectomy.

TABLE 126–1. *Baseline variables in contemporary patients undergoing prostatectomy*

Variable	RRP N = 135	VIP N = 440	P value
Age in years	63.1 (42.8–72)	59.9 (40–72)	NS
Serum PSA (ng/ml)	7.3 (1.9–35)	6.4 (0.6–41)	NS
Prostate Volume (cc)	48.4 (24.2–70)	58.8 (18–140)	NS
Clinical Stage:			
T1a	0%	(0.5%)	NS
T1c	58.8%	49%	
T2a	9.8%	10.0%	
T2b	35.3%	39%	
T3a	3.9%	1.5%	
Gleason Mean	6.6	6.5	NS
2–4	0%	0%	
5	3%	0%	
6	49%	66.5%	
7	35%	27.6%	
8	10%	3.9%	
9–10	3%	1.9%	
BMI	27.6 (17–41)	27.7 (19–38)	NS
Previous abdominal and hernia surgery	19%	20%	NS
Charlson Score	2.5	2.3	NS

TABLE 126–2. *Operative and postoperative variables in 300 contemporary patients undergoing prostatectomy*

Variable	RRP N = 100	VIP N = 200	P value
Operative time (H)	163 (86–395)	160 (71–315)	NS
EBL (cc) (Range)	910 (200–5000)	153 (25–750)	<0.001
Intraoperative Blood Transfusion	*Autologous*	*Autologous*	
	56	0%	<0.001
	Banked	*Banked*	
	11	0%	
Total	67%	0%	
Post op pain score Mean (Range)	7 (4–10)	3 (1–7)	P<0.05
Discharge Hemoglobin	10.1 g/l (6.9–14.6)	13 g/dl (7.3–15.1)	P<0.05
Mean Hospital Stay (Days)	3.5 (3–6)	1.2 (<1–5)	P<0.05
Discharged within 24 hours	0%	93%	P<0.001
Duration of catheterization (Mean in days) (Range)	15.8 (7–28)	7 (1–18)	P<.05
Mean Follow-up (days)	556	236	p<0.05
Undetectable PSA (%)	85%	92%	NS
Percentage Cancer in specimen	18.3 (5–90)	19 (1–80)	NS
Gleason score			
Mean	6.6	6.9	NS
2–4	0%	0%	
5	1%	.5%	
6	41%	43%	
7	38%	40%	
8	18%	8%	
9–10	2%	2.5%	
Path stage			
T2a	18%	14.7%	NS
T2b	75%	72%	
T3a	4%	6.8%	
T3b	3%	6.3%	
Positive Node incidence	2%	1%	NS
Margin positivity in Organ confined cancers (PT2a–T3a)	15%	1%	P<0.05
Extensive (>1 mm)	8%	5%	
Focal (<1 mm)			

TABLE 126–3. *Complications in 300 patients undergoing prostatectomy*

Variables	RRP (N = 100)	VIP (200)	P value
Aborted	1 (1%)	2 (1%)	
Conversion	NA	0	NS
Rectal injuries	1 (1%)	0	NS
Post operative ileus	3 (3%)	3 (1.5%)	NS
Wound dehiscence/Hernia	1 (1%)	2 (1.5%)	NS
Post operative (Fever/Pneumonia)	4 (4%)	0	P<0.05
Lymphocele	2 (2%)	0	NS
Obturator Neuropathy	2 (2%)	0	NS
DVT	1 (1%)	1 (0.5%)	NS
Post operative MI	1 (1%)	0	
Post operative bleeding/Reexploration	4 (4%)	1 (0.5%)	NS
Total	20%	5%	<0.05

REFERENCES

1. Cleary K, Nguyen C. State of the art in surgical robotics: clinical applications and technology challenges. *Comput Aided Surg* 2001;6: 312–328.
2. Guillonneau B, Rozet F, Cathelineau X, et al. Perioperative complications of laparoscopic radical prostatectomy: the Montsouris 3-year experience. *J Urol* 2002;167:51–56.
3. Lepor H, Gregerman M, Crosby R, Mostofi FK, Walsh PC. Precise localization of the autonomic nerves from the pelvic plexus to the corpora cavernosa: a detailed anatomical study of the adult male pelvis. *J Urol* 1985;133:207–212.
4. Lepor H, Nieder AM, Ferrandino MN. Intraoperative and postoperative complications of radical retropubic prostatectomy in a consecutive series of 1,000 cases. *J Urol* 2001;166:1729–1733.
5. Menon M, Shrivastava A, Tewari A, et al. Laparoscopic and robot assisted radical prostatectomy: Establishment of a structured program and preliminary analysis of outcomes. *J Urol* 2002;168: 945–949.
6. Tewari A, Shrivastava A, Menon M. Prospective Comparison of Robotic and Radical Prostatectomy in 300 patients. *BJU Int* 2003;92: 205–210.
7. Menon M, Tewari A, El-Galley R, et al. Genetic adaptive neural network model to predict PSA progression following radical prostatectomy: A multiinstitutional study. *J Urol* 1999;161:359.
8. Myers RP. Practical surgical anatomy for radical prostatectomy. *Urol Clin North Am* 2001;28:473–490.
9. Tewari A, Peabody J, Sarle R, et al. Technique of da Vinci robot-assisted anatomic radical prostatectomy. *Urology* 2002;60:569–572.
10. Menon M, Tewari A, Peabody J. Vathkuti Institute prostatectomy:technique. *J Urol* 2003;169:2289–2292.
11. Tewari A, Menon M. Editorial debate—point counterpoint:radical prostatectomy—retropubic, perineal or robotic. *Contemp. Urol* 2004; 16(2):38–58.

CHAPTER 127

Laparoscopic Management of Lymphoceles

Larry C. Munch

Persistent leakage of lymph following procedures that interrupt the normal lymphatic drainage channels in the retroperitoneum or pelvis can develop into collections within an epithelialized cavity. These lymphoceles can become large and symptomatic. Procedures from which lymphoceles might develop include renal transplantation (1% to 12%) and pelvic lymph node dissection for prostate cancer (0.5% to 10%). Factors contributing to the formation of lymphoceles following transplantation include unligated hilar lymphatic channels from the donor kidney and acute allograft rejection, while general factors include the addition of anticoagulants in the early postoperative period. Other complications that can occur as a result of lymphocele formation include allograft ureteral obstruction, vascular compression leading to thrombosis of the transplanted kidney, and the development of severe lower-extremity edema from pelvic venous obstruction.

With the development of laparoscopic techniques, transperitoneal marsupialization of lymphoceles became a feasible, minimally invasive alternative to the open approach. McCullough et al. (5) published the first report of laparoscopic drainage of a lymphocele in 1991. Other series followed and it appeared that the laparoscopic approach was a viable alternative. Gill et al. (1) in 1995 published a two-center report comparing laparoscopic versus open marsupialization of lymphoceles in contemporary groups of patients with pelvic lymphoceles. They found a statistically significant decrease in analgesic requirements, hospital stay, and time to resumption of normal activities in patients undergoing the laparoscopic approach, while operative times, complications, and success rates were comparable. They concluded that the laparoscopic approach should be the preferred initial definitive therapy in patients with symptomatic pelvic lymphoceles.

DIAGNOSIS

A lymphocele must be differentiated from urinoma, hematoma, or abscess preoperatively. A urinoma is detected by evidence of extravasation on radionuclide scan. A hematoma has a dense, nonhomogeneous echogenic pattern and an abscess is usually identified by clinical signs of infection or sepsis. Lymphoceles are characterized ultrasonographically as fluid-filled, on occasion loculated cystic cavities.

INDICATIONS FOR SURGERY

Asymptomatic lymphoceles usually require no definitive therapy. Deep venous thrombosis (and pulmonary embolus) from compression of iliac vein, lower-extremity/genital edema, compromised function of renal allograft, and obstructive/irritative voiding dysfunction are all indications that a symptomatic lymphocele should be repaired.

ALTERNATIVE THERAPY

When lymphoceles become symptomatic, initial treatment options can include percutaneous aspiration with or without sclerosis using agents such as tetracycline or povidone iodine. Due to high recurrence rates with these techniques, it is usually necessary to perform a more definitive procedure. Prior to the development of current laparoscopic techniques, the recommended approach was marsupialization of the lymphocele wall via a transperitoneal open approach, often with the interposition of omentum to maintain patency of the "window." In this way, lymph is absorbed via secondary channels and symptoms are relieved.

SURGICAL TECHNIQUE

Preoperative noncontrast computed tomography (CT) scanning provides optimal information regarding the size, location, and anatomic relationships of surrounding structures of the lymphoceles. These images should be present in the operating suite at the time of surgery to facilitate the planning of the port placement sites. Ultrasonography performed at the time of the procedure will confirm the boundaries of the lymphocele.

Patients should undergo general endotracheal anesthesia with placement of an orogastric tube to decompress the stomach. A urethral catheter should be placed and be available in the operating field. Patients are positioned supine with the entire abdomen prepped and draped. The surgeon stands on the side opposite the lymphocele with the assistant on the same side. Intraoperative ultrasonography should be performed prior to abdominal insufflation to avoid entering the lymphocele with the initial puncture and plan the optimal port placement.

The camera port should be placed at least 10 cm cephalad to the most superior aspect of the lymphocele near the midline. The abdomen is insufflated with CO_2 via a Veress needle or with a blunt-tip direct-vision trocar. In renal transplant patients having a peritoneal dialysis catheter present, insufflation can be rapidly accomplished via this catheter. The two working ports (5 mm) should be placed at least 10 cm apart from each other along an axis parallel to the upper edge of the lymphocele (Fig. 127–1).

In most cases, the lymphocele is identified by its appearance as a bulging, thin-walled blue-gray mass within the pelvis, often distorting other nearby structures. In cases where the overlying peritoneum precludes easy recognition of the wall, transabdominal ultrasonography with simultaneous intraabdominal depression of the peritoneum may identify the location of the lymphocele. If the lymphocele size is somewhat smaller or cannot be identified with the laparoscopic camera, ultrasound-guided percutaneous puncture of the lymphocele can be carried out with a long spinal needle. Dilute methylene blue can be introduced to overdistend the lymphocele. Subsequent transabdominal ultrasound-guided puncture of the suspected lymphocele will drain methylene blue solution and identify the boundaries of the lymphocele. If the lymphocele cannot be differentiated from the bladder, the bladder can be externally drained and refilled via the catheter to identify its boundaries under ultrasonographic guidance and localize the lymphocele.

Once identified, 3 to 4 cm of lymphocele wall is excised with electrocautery scissors or ultrasonic dissectors. Care is taken to examine the interior of the lymphocele for possible presence of the allograft ureter, significant blood vessels, or bladder to prevent injury to them. The allograft ureter can be located cephalad or caudad, anterior or posterior. The bladder is usually located medially, iliac vessels and native ureter posteriorly, and the

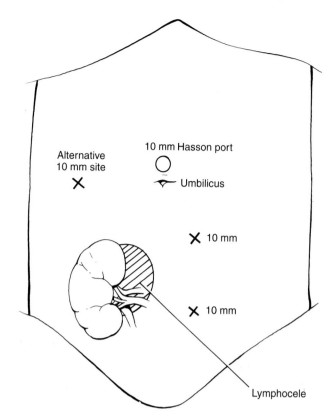

FIG. 127–1. Trocar positioning to approach a right-side lymphocele.

renal allograft laterally. Internal septations should be bluntly disrupted. Meticulous attention to hemostasis of the wall is imperative.

These maneuvers create the peritoneal "window" that will allow continuous drainage of lymphatic fluid into the central lymphatic channels within the peritoneal cavity. Although traditional dogma states that a pedicled segment of omentum should be secured to the base of the lymphocele, Gill et al. (1) found no significant difference in the recurrence of lymphoceles based on the presence of the omental tongue in their series. If indicated, the omentum can be fixated to the base of the lymphocele with standard laparoscopic stapling devices or intracorporeal sutures.

After completing the marsupialization and drainage of the lymphocele, the abdominal cavity is desufflated and hemostasis is verified. All ports should be removed under direct vision and the fascia of all ports greater than 5 mm should be closed. Subcuticular closure of the skin with placement of sterile strips completes the procedures.

Most patients can be discharged on the same or following day. Oral cephalosporin antibiotic coverage for 1 or 2 days is sufficient. In cases where significant distal peripheral edema is present, care should be taken in the immediate postoperative period to identify and treat the potentially massive movement of fluid from the extremities into the vascular spaces, which could result in acute pulmonary edema and respiratory failure.

Although the majority of symptomatic lymphoceles following renal transplantation or pelvic lymph node dissection are superficial and can be managed in the previously described manner, instances can occur in which the lymphocele is located caudal, posterior, or inferomedial to the allograft or in close association with the bladder, ureter, or iliac vessels not immediately adjoining the peritoneal cavity. An adequate peritoneal window cannot be created with standard techniques and placement of an omental tongue may not be possible. Lucas and colleagues (3) described a technique in the open treatment of lymphoceles meeting these criteria whereby an internalized peritoneal dialysis catheter was employed to bridge the gap between the lymphocele cavity and the intraperitoneal cavity. The "cuff" of this catheter was secured to the common wall to prevent migration of the catheter. Lymph fluid can freely drain into the peritoneal cavity even if the "window" otherwise becomes obliterated. No evidence of recurrence or infectious complications occurred in their series during a mean follow-up of more than 5 years.

Matin and colleagues (4) reported on the application of a similar laparoscopic technique on two patients who developed remote posttransplant lymphoceles by "cabling" two internal peritoneal dialysis catheters through the limited peritoneal window to maintain lymphoperitoneal drainage. Both procedures were successful with 20-month follow-up.

Complications are minimal if care is taken throughout the procedure but can include injury to the bladder, bowel, vascular structures, or allograft ureter. Many of these complications, if recognized, can be treated laparoscopically without long-term morbidity. The more serious complications including bowel perforation, injury to vascular structures, or allograft ureter may require conversion to an open approach for repair.

OUTCOMES

Results

Success rates are excellent in both the laparoscopic and open surgical groups. With the significantly reduced hospital stay and overall decreased costs, the transperitoneal laparoscopic lymphocelectomy should be considered the standard approach in postrenal transplant or radical prostatectomy cases of lymphocele formation.

REFERENCES

1. Gill IS, Hodge EE, Munch LC, Goldfarb DA, Novick AC, Lucas BA. Transperitoneal marsupialization of lymphoceles: a comparison of laparoscopic and open techniques. *J Urol* 1995;153:706–711.
2. Hsu THS, Gill IS, Grune MT, Andersen R, Eckhoff D, Goldfarb DA, Gruessner R, Hodge EE, Munch LC, Nghiem DD, Nye A, Reckard CR, Shaver T, Stratter RJ, Taylor RJ. Laparoscopic lymphocele: a multi-institutional analysis. *J Urol* 2000;163:1096–1099.
3. Lucas BA, Gill IS, Munch LC. Intraperitoneal drainage of recurrent lymphoceles using an internalized Tenckhoff catheter. *J Urol* 104: 970–972.
4. Matin SF, Gill IS. Laparoscopic marsupialization of the difficult lymphocele using internalized peritoneal dialysis. *J Urol* 2000 1498–1500.
5. McCullough CS, Soper NJ, Clayman RV, So SSK, Jendrisak MD, Hanto DW. Laparoscopic drainage of a post-transplant lymphocele. *Transplantation* 1991;51:725–727.

CHAPTER 128

Laparoscopic Bladder Procedures: Radical Cystectomy, Partial Cystectomy, and Urachal Cyst Excision

Ingolf A. Türk and Stefan A. Loening

Radical cystectomy with urinary diversion remains the gold standard treatment for muscle-invasive bladder carcinoma. Constant advances in anesthesiology and surgical technique and a more sophisticated postoperative care decreased the risk of such major surgery. However, radical cystectomy remains an aggressive procedure with significant morbidity and mortality. The complication rate in the early postoperative period after radical cystectomy and urinary diversion is still 25% to 35% (7). This remaining morbidity of open cystectomy has stimulated interest in treatment alternatives with less morbidity without compromising the oncological outcome.

Advances in laparoscopic surgery have resulted in a notable decrease in patient morbidity with speedier recovery and a shorter hospital stay. Laparoscopic application in the field of cystectomy started in 1992 when Parra et al. (10) reported a laparoscopic simple cystectomy for symptomatic pyocystitis. The first cystectomy for cancer was performed in 1993 and subsequently others have reported their technique involving laparoscopic-assisted techniques. Our group started with laparoscopic radical cystectomy and urinary diversion in March 2000 to treat patients with muscle-invasive bladder cancer.

DIAGNOSIS

The diagnosis of bladder pathology relies upon cystoscopy, transurethral biopsy, and selected imaging studies.

INDICATIONS

Radial cystectomy is in general indicated for the definitive management of muscle-invasive bladder carcinoma or in patients with high-risk bladder cancer who have failed standard intravesical therapies. Partial cystectomy can be considered for small lesions located away from the base of the bladder in patients who are not considered optimum candidates for radical surgery or for conditions such as extensive extravesical endometriosis.

ALTERNATE THERAPY

Open radical cystectomy remains the standard of care for muscle-invasive bladder cancer. Protocols combining radiation and chemotherapy are available for bladder preservation strategies.

SURGICAL TECHNIQUE

Preoperative preparation includes a bowel preparation of clear liquids only starting preoperative day 2, 3 L of mechanical bowel preparation fluid on preoperative day 1, and a cephalosporin and metronidazole on call to the operating room. The patient is placed supine with a steep Trendelenburg position, and a six-port transperitoneal laparoscopic access is established (Fig. 128–1). As in the open procedure, the right-handed surgeon stands to the patient's left. Camera monitors are positioned at the patient's feet. In our experience, the surgeon's dissection is best accomplished via laparoscopic scissors attached to monopolar cautery in one hand and graspers attached to bipolar cautery in the other. The first assistant utilizes suction in one hand and graspers for retraction in the other. We commonly utilize the Aesop robotic arm and voice recognition to give control of the camera to the surgeon.

Bilateral pelvic lymph node dissections are performed, removing tissue from the obturator fossa and external

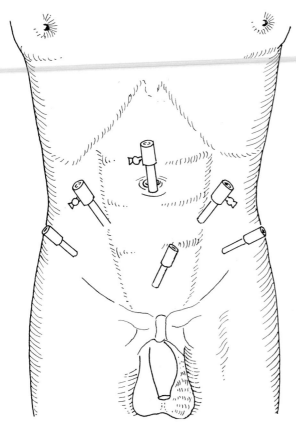

FIG. 128–1. Number and placement of the trocars for laparoscopic cystectomy.

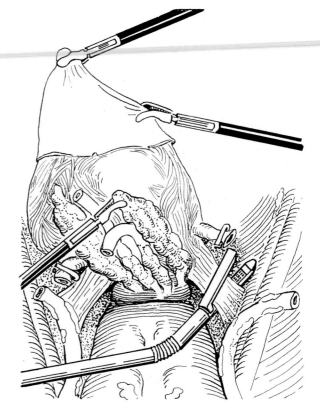

FIG. 128–2. Transection of the bladder pedicles with Endo-GIA.

iliac vein and artery from the obturator fossa up to the bifurcation of the aorta. The ureters are mobilized from the iliac vessel crossover to their entry into the bladder. Next, the peritoneum over the pouch of Douglas is incised and the vasa deferentia (in male) identified. Each vas is dissected toward the seminal vesicles, which are completely mobilized. The vasa and seminal vesicles are lifted anterior–superiorly so that the Denonvillier's fascia can be incised and the plane between the prostate and the rectum developed. In females, the pouch of Douglas is incised and the posterior wall of the vagina is mobilized from the rectum. Also, both ovaries are mobilized after transsection of the ovarian vessels.

The dissection now turns anteriorly, where the peritoneum over the umbilical ligaments is incised and the ligaments transected. The space of Retzius is developed as in the open procedure, with the urinary bladder dissected off the anterior abdominal wall and the endopelvic fascia exposed. The endopelvic fascia is incised bilaterally and the puboprostatic or pubourethral (women) ligaments divided. The dorsal vein complex is sutured with a 0-Vicryl pursestring suture but not divided at this point.

The posterior and anterior pedicles of the bladder and the pedicles of the prostate or uterus are divided by serial applications of the Endo-GIA stapler (Fig. 128–2). The

dorsal vein complex is now divided just proximal to the suture. The urethra is divided close to the pelvic floor, the catheter is removed, and the bladder neck is sutured closed to avoid leakage of urine in the peritoneal cavity with the risk of tumor spelling. In men, the remaining attachments are divided to completely free the specimen (bladder, prostate, and seminal vesicles), and it is secured in an endobag for later removal during the urinary diversion. In women, the bladder and the anterior wall of the vagina are removed to complete the dissection and the specimen immediately entrapped in an endobag for immediate removal through the vaginal opening. The vagina is then closed by a running 0-Vicryl suture.

Laparoscopic Mainz II Pouch (Rectum–Sigma Pouch)

The ileal loop urinary diversion has been the standard type of urinary diversion since 1950. The procedure has been developed into a laparoscopic procedure and provides a suitable form of diversion. (12). To date, most authors perform a laparotomy after lap cystectomy to remove the specimen and construct the urinary diversion (ileal conduit).

The most noticeable benefit of the sigma–rectum pouch diversion is the easy construction and the nearly

100% day- and nighttime continence of properly selected patients. The rectum–sigma pouch is a modification of the ureterosigmoidostomy and was first described by Fisch et al. as an alternative continent urinary diversion (4). To our knowledge, we performed in April 2000 the first continent urinary diversion completely laparoscopically using the Mainz-pouch II technique (13). Another issue of the laparoscopic procedure is how to remove the cystectomy specimen. Until now laparoscopists have made a minilaparotomy incision for specimen removal. The opening of the sigmoid and rectum or the vagina also allows us to remove the specimen without enlarging any of the abdominal port sites.

Prior to surgery, patients undergo outpatient sigmoidoscopy to exclude diverticulosis.

Further selection criteria included a competent anal sphincter, assessed by the ability to hold a 200- to 300-mL water enema for 2 hours, and adequate renal function (serum creatinine less than 1.5).

An antimesenteric enterotomy is made with an electric hook at the rectosigmoid junction and extended 10 cm proximally and 10 cm distally (Fig 128–3). In men, this allows for transanal removal of the specimen (Figure 128–4). The posterior walls of the rectum and sigmoid are then anastomosed side to side with a running 3-0 Maxon suture to form the posterior wall of the pouch (Fig. 128–5). Nonrefluxing ureteral anastomoses are formed by preparing a 3-cm submucosal bed in the posterior

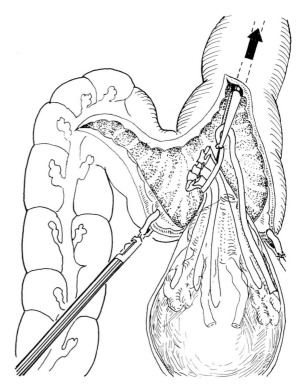

FIG. 128–4. Removal of the specimen in the endobag via the opened rectum.

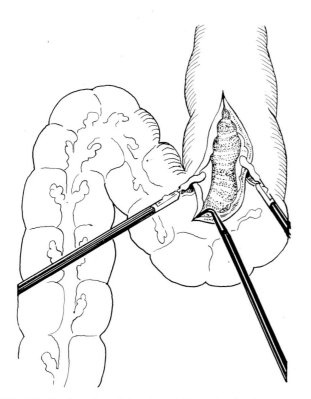

FIG. 128–3. Opening of the sigmoid intestine (antimesenterically) with electric hook.

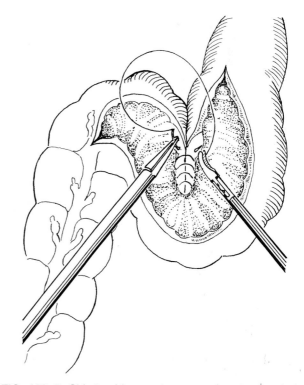

FIG. 128–5. Side-to-side anastomoses of rectum and sigmoid to form the posterior wall of the pouch.

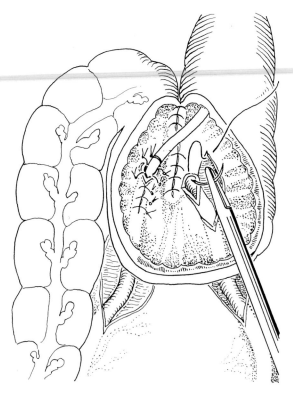

FIG. 128–6. Suturing of the mucosa of the sigmoid over the already implanted ureter to create the submucosal tunnel (nonrefluxing anastomoses).

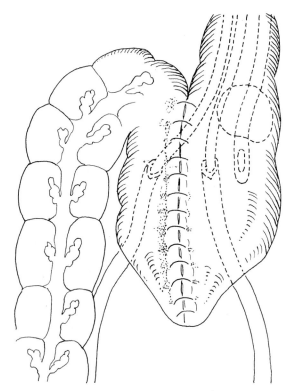

FIG. 128–7. The anterior wall of the pouch is closed with running sutures (3-0 Maxon) and both ureters were stented with 8 Fr ureteral catheters and the pouch was drained with a 26 Fr Nelaton catheter.

plate of the pouch, and then drawing the mobilized ureters through the pouch plate and securing with three to four sutures in this previous formed bed. After insertion of 8 Fr monopigtail ureteral catheters (via the opened rectum), the submucosal tunnels are completed by suturing the mucosa over the ureters (Fig. 128–6). The ureteral stents are brought out of the anus and the pouch is drained with a transanal 26 Fr Nelaton catheter. The anterior wall of the pouch is closed with a running 3-0 Maxon suture (Fig. 128–7). The pelvis is drained with a single Jackson–Pratt (JP) through one of the lateral 5-mm trocar incisions. Hemostasis is checked, all trocars are removed under vision, and the trocar sites closed with running sutures.

OUTCOMES

Complications

From April 2000 to June 2002, 12 patients (6 male, 6 female) diagnosed with clinical T2N0M0 transitional cell carcinoma (TCC) of the bladder were selectively offered laparoscopic radical cystectomy with continent urinary diversion—the Mainz II sigma-rectum pouch. All 12 procedures were completed laparoscopically without intraoperative complications. Conversion to open surgery was not required in any case. The median operating time was 6.3 hours (range, 5.5 to 7.9 hours). The median estimate blood loss was 220 cc (range, 150 to 300 mL, 0 transfusions), and approximately 1,500 mL of combined crystalloid/colloid intravenous fluids were required per the discretion of the anesthesiologist. The only complication was a pouch leak at 3 weeks follow-up, repaired by open suturing.

Results

In general, liquids were tolerated on postoperative day (POD) 2, the JP drain was removed on POD 4, the ureteral stents were removed on POD 8, and the pouch drain was removed on POD 9. On POD 10, intravenous pyelographys were performed, demonstrating normal upper tracts and no leakage from the pouch. Patients were discharged on PODs 10 to 12 (median, 11), significantly earlier than patients after comparable open surgery. All patients are fully continent (day/night) of urine and stool. Histopathologic examination of the specimens revealed transitional cell carcinoma: pT1 G3 + CIS (n = 1), pT2b G2-3 (n = 4), pT3a G3 (n = 4), and pT3b G3 (n = 3). The resection margins were free of tumor in all specimens. Positive lymph nodes were revealed in one patient, who was treated with adjuvant chemotherapy. Follow-up ranges 2 to 25 months and has shown no local or systemic recurrence so far. In follow-up, all upper tracts are normal with no evidence of hydronephrosis. The renal function is normal and a mild hyperchloraemic acidosis compensated with oral sodium bicarbonate has been required in 9 of 12 cases.

BLADDER RECONSTRUCTION AND PARTIAL CYSTECTOMY

Reconstructive bladder surgery includes the two extremes of either enlargement of the bladder or reduction of bladder size. Bladder enlargement procedures include autoaugmentation, enteric augmentation, or augmentation with biodegradable materials. Bladder reduction procedures are usually done for limited bladder tumors, symptomatic bladder diverticula, or for bladder endometriosis.

Laparoscopic bladder augmentation has been performed in patients with small-capacity or contracted bladders. Ehrlich reported the first laparoscopic autoaugmentation in an 8-year-old child with neurogenic bladder (3). The procedure took 70 minutes and after 1 year follow-up the symptoms were improved, with rare incontinence. With advances in laparoscopic suturing techniques most of the work in laparoscopic bladder reconstruction has centered on the problem of augmentation using either bowel or biologically inert substances.

Docimo et al. presented a case of laparoscopic bladder augmentation using stomach. In a 17-year-old girl with a sacral agenesis a wedge of stomach was obtained (staple technique) and sutured to the opened bladder using an Endostitch (2). Gill et al. performed in three patients a laparoscopic enterocystoplasty using ileum, sigmoid, and right colon. The bowel was exteriorized to facilitate the bowel reanastomosis and ileal patch construction. The circumferential enterovesical anastomosis was performed intracorporeally. The operative time was 5.3 to 8 hours, without any intraoperative or postoperative complications (5). The first complete laparoscopic enterocystoplasty was done by Meng et al. (8). The ileal loop mobilization, bowel reanastomosis, and enterovesical anastomosis were performed completely intracorporeally using staple and freehand suturing techniques. The operative time was 9 hours, and 4 weeks postoperatively the bladder capacity was with 250 cc improved.

A promising area for the future might be the segmental or complete replacement of the bladder with biodegradable graft material. There are several animal studies where the authors could demonstrate that a laparoscopic technique for partial bladder wall replacement using a free graft is feasible. The biodegradable grafts are tolerated by host bladder and are associated with predominantly mucosal regeneration at 12 weeks postoperatively (11).

There have been several case reports with regard to laparoscopic bladder reduction procedures, most commonly diverticulectomy. The transsection of the diverticulum was performed either using an Endo-GIA device or intracorporeal suturing techniques.

The role of partial cystectomy in the management of bladder carcinoma is still controversial. So far there is no report in the literature about using the laparoscopic approach for partial cystectomy in the case of bladder cancer. Kozlowski et al. successfully treated a patient with bladder pheochromocytoma by laparoscopic partial cystectomy (6).

Bladder endometriosis is a rare disease and partial cystectomy is mostly the treatment of choice for these patients. There have been several reports about successful use of the laparoscopic approach for this purpose (9). Chapron et al. reported eight women on whom they performed a laparoscopic partial cystectomy in cases of muscle-invasive endometriosis of the bladder. The bladder resection was carried out transperitoneally under cystoscopic control and the closure of the bladder was achieved with one layer of a running suture and intracorporeal knotting. The mean follow-up was 31.6 months and all patients were symptom free, with no recurrence in any patient (1).

URACHAL CYST MANAGEMENT

The urachus is the allantoic duct that obliterates at month 2 to 4 of gestation. It becomes the so-called median umbilical ligament and runs as a fibrous cord from the dome of the bladder to the umbilicus. In some patients the urachal or allantoic tract may persist and appears in several anomalies, like a patent urachus with free communication between the bladder and the umbilicus or a urachal cyst. In most cases these anomalies are asymptomatic and discovered incidentally.

The most common urachal anomaly is a urachal cyst and becomes symptomatic when it becomes infected. The typical symptoms are periumbilical inflammation, tenderness, and erythema. When a symptomatic urachal cyst or remnant is suspected the standard workup includes the cystoscopy with inspection of the bladder dome and computed tomography, which usually reveals the cystic structure. There have been several reports of successful management of urachal cysts or remnants by means of laparoscopy, and the authors' department has experience with two patients.

After the induction of general anesthesia and placement of a Foley catheter and nasogastric tube, the patient is positioned supine. Through a small incision in the left epigastrium a Veress needle is inserted to establish a pneumoperitoneum. A 7-mm optical trocar is inserted via the same incision. After clearly visualizing the urachus, cyst, and bladder another two 5-mm working trocar is placed. The urachus were detached just caudal to the umbilicus, maximizing the resection margin. Sometimes, an intubation of the patent urachus with a ureteral catheter will be helpful for better identification. The urachal cord and cyst are mobilized toward the bladder using sharp dissection with a bipolar grasper and monopolar scissors. The bladder is then distended and the peritoneum is incised along the plane between the urachus or cyst and bladder dome. In cases of significant attachments of the urachal cyst to the bladder a resection of bladder cuff is recommended. The bladder defect is closed with one layer of running suture with Vicryl 2-0 and intracorporeal tying. The specimen is placed in an Endobag and removed through one of the small extended trocar sites.

A 3-year-old boy and a 19-year-old girl presented to our department, both with a symptomatic urachal cyst. Both patients had recurrent periumbilical inflammation, an "oozing umbilicus," and pain. After the above-mentioned workup we performed the laparoscopic urachal cyst resection in both cases with resection of a bladder cuff. Both specimens were removed intact. Operating time was 45 and 56 minutes, respectively. The Foley catheter remained in place for 8 days. No intraoperative complications were observed and in both cases the postoperative course was uneventful. The final pathologic evaluation confirmed the diagnosis of benign urachal remnant. Both patients are asymptomatic and void without difficulty.

REFERENCES

1. Chapron C, Dubuisson JB. Laparoscopic management of bladder endometriosis. *Acta Obstet Gynecol Scand* 1999;78:887–890.
2. Docimo SG, Moore RG, Adams J, et al. Laparoscopic bladder augmentation using stomach. *Urology* 1995;46:565–569.
3. Ehrlich RM, Gershman A. Laparoscopic seromyotomy (auto-augmentation) for non-neurogenic bladder in a child: initial case report. *Urology* 1993;42:175–178.
4. Fisch M, Wammack R, Steinbach F, et al. Sigma–rectum pouch (Mainz pouch II). *Urol Clin North Am* 1993;20:561–569.
5. Gill IS, Rackley RR, Merany AM, et al. Laparoscopic enterocystoplasty. *Urology* 2000;55:178.
6. Kozlowski PM, Mihm F, Winfield HN. Laparoscopic management of bladder pheochromocytoma. *Urology* 2001;57:365.
7. Malavaud B, Vaessen C, Mouzin M, et al. Complications for radical cystectomy. *Eur Urol* 2001;39:79–84.
8. Meng MV, Anwar HP, Elliot SP, et al. Pure laparoscopic enterocystoplasty. *J Urol* 2002;167:1386.
9. Nezhat C, Nezhat F, Nezhat CH, et al. Urinary tract endometriosis treated by laparoscopy. *Fertil Steril* 1996;66:920–924 .
10. Parra RO, Andrus CH, Jones JP, et al. Laparoscopic cystectomy: initial report on a new treatment for retained bladder. *J Urol* 1992;148:1140–1144.
11. Portis AJ, Elbahnasy AM, Shalhav AL, et al. Laparoscopic augmentation cystoplasty with different biodegradable grafts in an animal model. *J Urol* 2000;164:1405–1411.
12. Puppo P, Perachino M, Ricciotti G, et al. Laparoscopically assisted transvaginal radical cystectomy. *Eur Urol* 1995;27:425–428.
13. Turk I, Deger S, Winkelmann B, et al. Laparoscopic radical cystectomy with continent urinary diversion (rectal sigmoid pouch) performed completely intracorporeally: the initial 5 cases. *J Urol* 2001;165:1863–1866.

CHAPTER 129

Laparoscopic Colposuspension

Jerilyn M. Latini and Karl J. Kreder

Stress urinary incontinence (SUI) is typically defined as the involuntary leakage of urine with coughing, laughing, sneezing, exercising, or any sudden increase in intraabdominal pressure. This leakage is objectively demonstrable.

DIAGNOSIS

SUI can be subdivided based on the physical exam and urodynamic findings. In anatomic SUI (types I and II) there is laxity of the urethropelvic and pubourethral ligaments, leading to hypermobility of the urethra and rotational descent of the bladder neck to varying degrees. The degree of urethral hypermobility should be determined during the video component of a video-urodynamic study. Appropriate and effective treatment for uncomplicated urethral hypermobility associated with types I and II SUI is best initiated once intrinsic deficiency and a detrusor cause for the urinary incontinence have been ruled out.

In intrinsic sphincter deficiency (ISD, or type III SUI), the continence mechanism of the urethra itself is deficient, leading to incompetence. The urethra and bladder neck are in the correct anatomic position and there is no hypermobility present. The urethral sphincter's ability to resist increases as intraabdominal pressure is decreased, leading to urinary incontinence. Urethral sphincteric deficiency is quantified during urodynamic testing by measuring the mean urethral closing pressure (MUCP) and/or the abdominal leak point pressure (aLPP). The aLPP is the lowest intraabdominal pressure at which leakage occurs in the absence of any detrusor activity. An aLPP of less than 100 cm water and/or MUCP of less than 20 cm water are suggestive of ISD. Intrinsic sphincter deficiency and urethral hypermobility are two distinct clinical entities but are not mutually exclusive and frequently coexist in women with SUI.

INDICATIONS FOR SURGERY

Indications for treatment of SUI include significant loss of urine leading to social and/or hygienic problems. The overall aim of surgical correction is to lift, support, and anchor the urethrovesical junction, thereby preventing excessive urethral mobility. Securing the endopelvic fascia and anterior vaginal wall to a strong supportive structure corrects and maintains the retropubic position of the proximal urethra and bladder neck. The precise mechanism by which continence is achieved is debated. The currently accepted theory of continence is that the urethra is compressed against a supportive hammock of tissue during stress maneuvers that increase urethral closing pressure. Fixation of the endopelvic fascia to the posterior pubic symphysis via postoperative fibrosis may also be involved. Laparoscopic incontinence procedures were first introduced to reduce the operative morbidity associated with conventional open surgery: shorten the patient's hospital stay, time of recuperation, length of catheterization, and return to presurgical level of functioning, and still provide the long-term, high rate of treatment success.

ALTERNATIVE THERAPY

Surgical procedures for female SUI can be categorized into transabdominal, transvaginal, combined, or traditional versus minimally invasive. Major categories of antiincontinence procedures include: open abdominal retropubic urethropexy or colposuspension (e.g., Burch colposuspension, Marshall–Marchetti–Krantz [MMK]), laparoscopic retropubic colposuspension, anterior colporrhaphy, bladder buttress operation or vaginal wall repair (Kelly plication), suburethral sling procedures (pubovaginal sling, bone-anchored transvaginal sling, tension-free vaginal tape), bladder neck needle suspensions without endoscopic control (Pereyra), bladder neck needle suspensions under endoscopic control (Raz–Stamey), periurethral injections (collagen, carbon), and artificial urinary sphincters.

SURGICAL TECHNIQUE

Laparoscopic colposuspension may be performed via extraperitoneal or transperitoneal approach. Both methods will be described in this section in an abbreviated manner.

Extraperitoneal or Retroperitoneal Approach

This is the technique described by McDougall and coworkers (14). Intravenous (IV) antibiotics are administered prior to beginning the procedure. With the patient under general endotracheal anesthesia and in a low lithotomy position in slight Trendelenburg, a nasogastric tube and Foley catheter are placed. The retropubic space of Retzius is entered and dilated through a 2-cm midline transverse incision halfway between the umbilicus and the pubic symphysis. The anterior rectus fascia is identified, secured, and incised to allow entry of the operator's finger and digital creation of a space behind the pubic symphysis in the midline. A dilating balloon catheter fashioned from the finger of a surgical glove and a red rubber catheter is inserted into the retropubic space and inflated with saline to create the retroperitoneal laparoscopic working space. The dilating balloon catheter is replaced with a Hasson-type laparoscopic port. Pneumoretroperitoneum is attained via insufflation of the retropubic space with CO_2 at 15 mm Hg pressure. The 30-degree laparoscope is inserted and two other 10-mm working ports are inserted at the left lateral border of the rectus muscle (Fig. 129–1). This allows the right-handed surgeon to operate the laparoscopic instrument using one's dominant hand and place the nondominant index finger in the vagina during the procedure, just as one would do during an open colposuspension. The endopelvic fascia at the junction of the proximal urethra with the bladder neck and the Cooper's ligament are identified. With the operator's finger elevating the vaginal fornix up toward Cooper's ligament, the endopelvic fascia is secured to the ipsilateral ligament. The same maneuver is repeated on the contralateral side (Fig. 129–2). Depending on the laparoscopic surgeon's technical preference, this can be accomplished by intracorporeal suturing with or without laparoscopic suture clips or by using mesh and endosurgical staples or bone anchors. Elevation of the bladder neck and proximal urethra behind the pubic symphysis corrects the urethral hypermobility.

After securing the endopelvic fasciae to the ipsilateral Cooper's ligaments, IV indigo carmine is administered. The Foley catheter is removed and cystourethroscopy is performed to confirm that there has not been entry of the bladder or urethra by suture or other fixation material and to check for bilateral ureteral patency. Withdrawing the

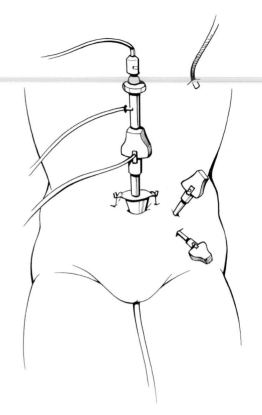

FIG. 129–1. Port placement for laparoscopic bladder neck suspension by a right-handed surgeon.

cystourethroscope into the urethra allows the surgeon to laparoscopically visualize that the bladder neck and proximal urethra have been elevated and well supported (Fig. 129–3). Following removal of the cystourethroscope, the Foley catheter is replaced to gravity drainage.

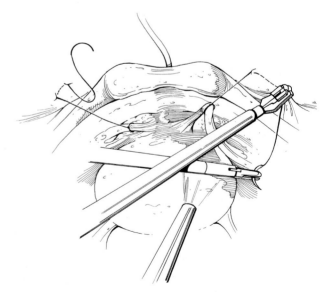

FIG. 129–2. A suture incorporates paravaginal tissue and the ipsilateral Cooper's ligament on both sides. With the assistant elevating the bladder neck, the suture is fixed at Cooper's ligament.

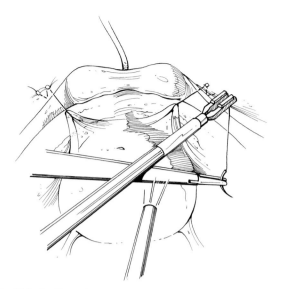

FIG. 129–3. Completed repair with well-supported bladder neck.

The two lateral ports are removed under direct laparoscopic vision, as per usual, followed by removal of the Hasson cannula and laparoscope. The fascia of the two lateral port sites need not be closed as there is no risk of hernia formation given that the procedure is retroperitoneal. Tying the previously placed holding sutures reapproximates the fascia of the midline transverse incision.

Transperitoneal Approach

IV antibiotics are administered prior to beginning the procedure. With the patient under general endotracheal anesthesia and in a low lithotomy position in slight Trendelenburg, a nasogastric tube and Foley catheter are placed. The peritoneal cavity is entered through a small infraumbilical incision using either the Veress needle or Hasson-type trocar. Pneumoperitoneum is established. Two other 10-mm working ports are placed similarly to the retroperitoneal approach, along with a third port in the midline halfway between the pubis and umbilicus. To enter the retropubic space of Retzius intraabdominally, the umbilical ligaments are identified laterally, marking the lateral aspects of the bladder. The anterior parietal peritoneum over the bladder is incised transversely directly under the pubic symphysis. This is dissected from the anterior abdominal wall to enter the retropubic space of Retzius. The remainder of the procedure is similar to that described for the extraperitoneal approach.

Modifications in Laparoscopic Techniques

It must be kept in mind that most all of the reported series of laparoscopic bladder neck suspensions provide evidence that deviations from the original description of a given surgical technique (here, the open Burch colpo-

suspension) need to be assessed in their own right. Three recent series evaluated the results of the laparoscopic colposuspension as Burch described (7,16,17). Most others addressed modifications of the originally described procedure and therefore are difficult to compare to the open Burch procedure.

Endoscopic suture placement adds a degree of complexity and increases the operative time during laparoscopic colposuspension. Endoscopic suturing in the space of Retzius can be difficult due to the limitations of monocular vision, instrument mobility, and angle of freedom in lower accessory cannula positions (7). Modifications such as fixing strips of polypropylene (Prolene) hernia mesh to the paraurethral tissues and Cooper's ligament using a surgical tacking device, that is, bone anchors (5) or surgical titanium staples (6,20,24), have been described. The use of fibrin glue/sealant has also been described (8). The use of polydioxanone suture clips simplifies intracorporeal knot tying and facilitates securing the suture and tissues under the appropriate amount of tension (14,18). These techniques have been designed to shorten the length of the procedure and lower the level of complexity while maintaining the necessary surgical maneuvers. Other series also addressed these issues and an exhaustive discussion will not be presented here.

One Versus Two Sutures

Laparoscopic colposuspension can be performed using one suture on each side (usually nonabsorbable suture with a double bite) or two single-bite sutures on each side. Ideally, using one suture would lower operating time while not compromising efficacy. In a single randomized comparison of the number of paravaginal polytetrafluoroethylene sutures placed during laparoscopic colposuspension, significantly higher objective and subjective measures of cure were found in those women undergoing the two-suture technique at 1 year of follow-up: 83% objective cure rate (pad test) for two sutures versus 58% for one suture and 89% subjective cure rate for two sutures versus 65% for one suture (17). This trial was stopped prematurely when an interim analysis revealed significant differences in the cure rate for the two study arms.

Sutures Versus Mesh and Staples

One trial attempted to address this in a prospective, randomized fashion in 69 women who underwent laparoscopic colposuspension using either polytetrafluoroethylene sutures or polypropylene mesh fixed by an Endostapler (20). At 6 weeks and 12 months, there appeared to be no difference in objective cure rates. However, due to issues with the methodology, the true effectiveness of these two techniques remains unclear. Another small prospective, randomized study of 20 patients addressed this issue but was of poor quality, with short follow-up of 2 to 12 months (24). Upon preliminary analysis, no valid conclusions could be drawn. A third prospective, randomized controlled series (25) involved 53 women who underwent laparoscopic colposuspension using sutures (27 women) or nonabsorbable mesh fixed with tacks or staples (26 women). At short-term follow-up of 12 months, the subjective failure rate was not significantly different between the two groups (7.4% with sutures and 15.4% with mesh/tacks/staples). The objective failure rate was significantly lower in the suture group (11.1%) compared with the mesh/tacks/staples group (26.9%). Whether any of these results will be durable over time remains to be determined. Given the apparent time-dependent decline in cure rate following antiincontinence procedures, the authors appropriately state that studies with 5 or more years of follow-up and larger numbers of patients are needed to accurately evaluate any relevant issues.

Extraperitoneal Versus Transperitoneal Laparoscopic Colposuspension

The extraperitoneal approach is associated with disadvantages such as impaired instrument mobility with lower accessory cannula positions and obstruction of the space of Retzius if a pneumoperitoneum is inadvertently created by peritoneal entry. On the other hand, advantages of this approach include unhindered entry into the retropubic space in the setting of intraabdominal adhesions, avoidance of peritoneal entry with the associated postoperative pain and ileus, a decreased risk of injury to the bladder and intraabdominal organs, and essentially no risk of herniation at the cannula sites. This issue also remains to be determined. A small study (24) with short-term follow-up attempted to address this issue, but upon critical analysis no valid conclusions could be drawn.

POSTOPERATIVE MANAGEMENT

Postoperative antibiotics are administered for 7 days. The Foley catheter is removed on the morning after surgery. Postvoid residual (PVR) urines are obtained after each void for 48 to 72 hours. The patient is taught to perform clean intermittent catheterization (CIC) until the PVR is consistently less than 100 cc. The majority of patients' postoperative pain is well managed with oral pain medication. Patients are typically discharged home the day after surgery.

OUTCOMES

Complications

Reviews of reported comparative series has shown that there was no difference in perioperative complications

between the open and laparoscopic procedures, including injury to the bladder. (2,3,22) The estimated blood loss was higher in the open procedure in all studies. Laparoscopic colposuspension took longer than the open procedure in four of the five studies, whereas in one (22) laparoscopic times were shorter. Although a quantitative analysis could not be performed, pain and analgesic requirement seemed to be less in the laparoscopic group. The length of hospital stay and time to return to activities, where reported, were longer for the open colposuspension group. A longer duration of catheterization was also reported in most series.

Results

Several authors reported encouraging early success rates results in treating stress incontinence. These studies are remarkable in that most were retrospective reviews including small numbers of patients with short-term (less than 12 to 18 months) follow-up and utilized subjective outcome methods.

Lose reviewed the laparoscopic colposuspension literature between January 1991 and January 1997 (11). The one prospectively randomized trial found that laparoscopic colposuspension was not as effective in the treatment of genuine stress incontinence as the open procedure at 12 months of follow-up. The four nonrandomized comparative studies did not show a difference in cure rate between the two colposuspension techniques (5,14,18,19).

An excellent analysis by Moehrer et al. was designed to determine the effects of laparoscopic colposuspension surgery on urinary incontinence (15). The Cochrane Incontinence Group Specialized Register of Controlled Trials of the Incontinence Review Group was searched through April 2001 for randomized or quasirandomized controlled trials studying effects of treatment in women with symptomatic or urodynamic evidence for stress or mixed urinary incontinence. Follow-up did not exceed 18 months in any study other than Burton (2), who reports a 5-year follow-up. Eight eligible trials were identified, and although the inclusion and exclusion criteria varied in some respects all participants were judged to have SUI based on urodynamic investigation. Laparoscopic colposuspension was performed via the transperitoneal approach in six studies and extraperitoneally in two. There is a recognized learning curve associated with laparoscopic surgical procedures, and it should be noted that the number of laparoscopic colposuspensions performed by each surgeon varied between the eight studies from less than 20 to more than 30. Various operative techniques for laparoscopic colposuspension were compared by three groups and the numbers and types of sutures used were not consistent between the studies.

After 6 to 18 months follow-up, women's subjective cure rates ranged from 85% to 96% in the open and 85%

to 100% in the laparoscopic group (P = NS). Quantified symptoms using voiding diaries and pad tests showed significant improvement following both open and laparoscopic colposuspension, but less so for the laparoscopic group. At 18 months follow-up, there was no difference seen in the number of incontinence episodes. In one study with longer follow-up, there was marked deterioration in the laparoscopic group and the mean number of incontinent episodes approached the preoperative level over 3 to 5 years.

Longer-term comparative trials have also found that the effectiveness of laparoscopic bladder neck suspension procedures declines more rapidly with time than an open repair (12,13). At 45 months mean follow-up, 30% of those in the laparoscopy group were continent, similar to the results with the transvaginal Raz group at a mean follow-up of 59 months, with 35% of women remaining continent.

el-Toukhy and Davies (6) prospectively investigated laparoscopic colposuspension (49 patients) using Prolene mesh and titanium tacks to open Burch colposuspension (38 patients) in a nonrandomized fashion. The mean follow-up was 32 months (range, 25 to 40 months). At 3 months postoperatively, the objective cure rate was 70% for the laparoscopic and 87% for the open group of patients (P < 0.05). Efficacy in both groups fell over time and by the end of follow-up this decline was more marked in the laparoscopic group. Objective cure rates were 62% for the laparoscopic versus 79% for the open Burch group (P < 0.05). Subjectively, 77% of women in the laparoscopic group versus 89% of those in the open group reported cure or symptomatic improvement and satisfaction with the procedure and would recommend it to a friend.

REFERENCES

1. Burton G. A randomized comparison of laparoscopic and open colposuspension. *Neurourol Urodynam* 1994;13:497–498.
2. Burton G. A three-year prospective randomized urodynamic study comparing open and laparoscopic colposuspension. *Neurourol Urodynam* 1997;16:353–354.
3. Carey M, Rosamilia A, Dwyer P, et al. Laparoscopic versus open colposuspension: a prospective multicentre randomized single-blind comparison. *Neurourol Urodynam* 2000;19:389–391.
4. Cutner AS. A randomized trial of open versus laparoscopic colposuspension for genuine stress incontinence. *Natl Res Reg* 2002;3 (www.update-software.com).
5. Das S, Palmer JK. Laparoscopic colposuspension. *J Urol* 1995;154:1119–1121.
6. el-Toukhy TA, Davies AE. The efficacy of laparoscopic mesh colposuspension: results of a prospective controlled study. *BJU Int* 2001;88:361–366.
7. Fatthy H, El Hao M, Samaha I, et al. Modified Burch colposuspension: laparoscopy versus laparotomy. *J Am Assoc Gynecol Laparoscop* 2001;8:99–106.
8. Kiilholma P, Haarala M, Polvi H, et al. Sutureless endoscopic colposuspension with fibrin sealant. *Tech Urol* 1995;1:81–83.
9. Kitchener HC. A randomised trial of open versus laparoscopic colposuspension for genuine stress incontinence. *Natl Res Reg* 2002;3 (www.update-software.com).
10. Korram MM. Laparoscopic colposuspension operation. *J Gynecol Surg* 1995;10:205–206.
11. Lose G. Laparoscopic Burch colposuspension. *Acta Obstet Gynecol Scand* 1998;77:29–33.
12. McDougall EM. Laparoscopic management of female urinary incontinence. *Urol Clin North Am* 2001;28:145–149.
13. McDougall EM, Heidorn CA, Portis AJ, et al. Laparoscopic bladder neck suspension fails the test of time. *J Urol* 1999;162:2078–2081.
14. McDougall EM, Kluke CG, Carnell T. Comparison of transvaginal versus laparoscopic bladder neck suspension for stress urinary incontinence. *Urology* 1995;45:641–649.
15. Moehrer B, Ellis G, Carey M, et al. Laparoscopic colposuspension for urinary incontinence in women. *Cochrane Database System Rev* 2002;2.
16. Persson J, Bossmar T, Wolner-Hanssen P. Laparoscopic colposuspension: a short term urodynamic follow-up and a three-year questionnaire study. *Acta Obstet Gynecol Scand* 2000;79:414–420.
17. Persson J, Wolner-Hanssen P. Laparoscopic colposuspension for stress urinary incontinence: a randomized comparison of one or two sutures on each side of the urethra. *Obstet Gynecol* 2000;95:151–155.
18. Polascik TJ, Moore RG, Rosenberg MT, et al. Comparison of laparoscopic and open retropubic urethropexy for treatment of stress urinary incontinence. *Urology* 1995;45:647–652.
19. Ross JW. Laparoscopic Burch repair compared to laparotomy Burch for cure of urinary stress incontinence. *Int Urogynecol J* 1995;6:323–328.
20. Ross JW. Two techniques of laparoscopic Burch repair for stress incontinence: a prospective randomized study. *J Am Assoc Gynecol Laparoscop* 1996;3:351–357.
21. Smith AR, Stanton SL. Laparoscopic colposuspension. *Br J Obstet Gynaecol* 1998;105:383–384.
22. Su TH, Wang KG, Hsu CY, et al. Prospective comparison of laparoscopic and traditional colposuspensions in the treatment of genuine stress incontinence. *Acta Obstet Gynecol Scand* 1997;76:576–582.
23. Summitt RL, Lucente VL, Karram MM, et al. Randomized comparison of laparoscopic and transabdominal Burch urethropexy for the treatment of genuine stress incontinence. *Obstet Gynecol*, 2000;95[4, Suppl 1]:S2.
24. Wallwiener D, Grischke EM, Rimbach S, et al. Endoscopic retropubic colposuspension: "Retziusscopy" versus laparoscopy—a reasonable enlargement of the operative spectrum in the management of recurrent stress incontinence? *Endoscop Surg Allied Tech* 1995;3:115–118.
25. Zullo F, Palomba S, Piccione F, et al. Laparoscopic Burch colposuspension: a randomized controlled trial comparing two transperitoneal surgical techniques. *Obstet Gynecol* 2001;98:783–788.

CHAPTER 130

Laparoscopic Retroperitoneal Lymph Node Dissection

Howard N. Winfield and Vincent G. Bird

Advances in surgical technique and the availability of newer chemotherapeutic agents have allowed for highly successful treatment of testicular cancer. As the majority of patients can now be cured with use of one or a combination of these modalities, the focus of care has shifted toward attaining cure with least morbidity. Due to its minimally invasive approach, laparoscopic retroperitoneal lymph node dissection (L-RPLND) may be part of a new treatment paradigm for patients with clinical stage I nonseminomatous germ cell tumors. L-RPLND offers a highly accurate and reliable method of evaluating the extent and presence of lymph node metastases. Refinements in laparoscopic surgical technique and instrumentation have allowed for the performance of this minimally invasive procedure with low morbidity.

DIAGNOSIS

Testicular cancer is diagnosed by history and physical examination. Assessment of the serum tumor markers, alpha-fetoprotein (αFP), beta-human chorionic gonadotropin (βHCG), and lactate dehydrogenase, along with radiologic imaging, typically consisting of computerized tomography of the retroperitoneum and plain-film radiography of the chest, aid in the clinical staging of the tumor

INDICATIONS FOR SURGERY

The use of RPLND primarily involves patients found to have nonseminomatous germ cell tumors, as 20% to 30% of these patients with clinical stage I disease will have retroperitoneal lymph node metastases. Of more concern are patients with stage T2 to T4 primary tumors, evidence of lymphovascular invasion, and embryonal cell carcinoma, who are in general believed to be at an even higher risk of retroperitoneal and systemic relapse (1,4,9). Although the literature is replete with controversy concerning the use of chemotherapy versus RPLND, surgery is often advocated as a staging, and possibly curative, procedure for such patients. Under these circumstances RPLND is performed in a unilateral template fashion to preserve antegrade ejaculation. L-RPLND has been used as an alternative to open RPLND in this select patient group. However, upon pathologic confirmation of metastatic disease following L-RPLND patients are then upstaged and in general given chemotherapy. Thus, the therapeutic effectiveness of L-RPLND in such cases is untested. As such, L-RPLND should currently be considered a diagnostic procedure. However, used as such, this minimally invasive procedure may greatly aid in identifying patients with pathologic stage I nonseminomatous testis tumors that can be spared chemotherapy and obviate the need for surveillance protocol alone. The general indications for L-RPLND are shown in Table 130–1.

ALTERNATIVE THERAPY

Alternative treatment approaches for patients with stage I nonseminomatous germ cell tumors include open RPLND, chemotherapy, and surveillance.

TABLE 130–1. *Indications for laparoscopic retroperitoneal lymph node dissection*

Clinical Stage I Nonseminomatous Testicular Cancer
Negative Testis Tumor Markers
No Absolute Contraindications to Laparoscopic Surgery
Residual Isolated Abdominal or Pelvic Mass After Chemotherapy in the Presence of Negative Testis Tumor Markers

SURGICAL TECHNIQUE

On the day prior to surgery the patient undergoes a mechanical bowel preparation, which includes a clear liquid diet and one gallon of Go-Lytely. This preparation cleanses and decompresses the bowel, which may improve laparoscopic exposure. Type and crossmatching is done for 2 U of blood. Janetschek et al. also recommend that a low-fat diet be started 1 week prior to and continued for 2 weeks after surgery to minimize chylous ascites. The patient should have nothing by mouth after midnight on the night prior to surgery.

RPLND for patients with stage I nonseminomatous germ cell tumors involves either right- or left-sided template surgery, depending on the testis involved with disease. Nerve-sparing templates are now used, which yield virtually a 100% chance of maintaining antegrade ejaculation (see Fig. 130–1) (2). Surgery for each template will be described.

Transperitoneal Approach

Right-Sided Template

The patient is positioned on the operating table with the right side elevated 45 degrees upward. This allows for both supine and lateral decubitus positioning as needed. The table is slightly flexed at the level of the umbilicus. Trendelenburg or reverse Trendelenburg positioning can

then be used as needed. In general, trocar ports are 5 to 12 mm and placed in a midline vertical arrangement (Fig. 130–2).

The initial step in L-RPLND is to gain wide exposure of the retroperitoneum. Dissection is begun along the white line of Toldt from the level of the cecum to the hepatic flexure. Cephalad, this incision is carried above the level of the transverse colon and lateral to the duodenum (Kocher maneuver) along the vena cava up to the level of the hepatoduodenal ligament.

The duodenum and the head of the pancreas are further mobilized medially until the anterior surfaces of the vena cava, aorta, and left renal vein crossing the aorta are completely exposed. The peritoneal incision is also carried laterally around the liver toward the triangular ligaments, allowing for medial and superior retraction of the liver. This mobilization is necessary to ensure adequate exposure of the inferior vena cava and renal vessels.

Inferiorly, the incision is extended along the spermatic vessels to the level of the internal inguinal ring. Dissection is also extended around the cecum and upward along the root of the mesentery, allowing for medial mobilization of these structures.

At this point, the dissection has exposed the entire right-sided template. This template includes all preaortic tissue between the left renal vein and the inferior mesenteric artery, the interaortocaval nodes, and all tissue on the ventral and lateral surfaces of the vena cava extending

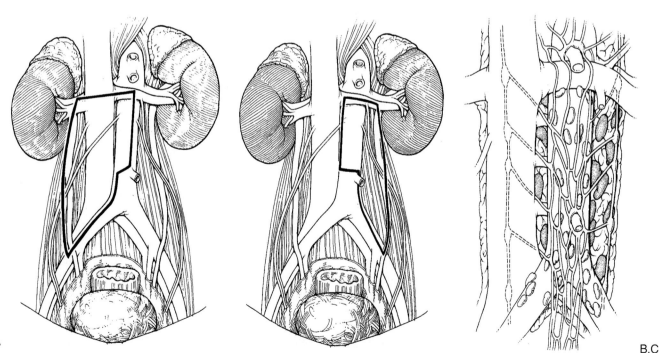

A   B,C

FIG. 130–1. A: Template for right modified nerve-sparing retroperitoneal lymph node dissection (RPLND). **B:** Template for left modified nerve-sparing RPLND. **C:** Anterior view of retroperitoneal sympathetic fibers. (From Foster RS, Donohue JP. *Nerve sparing RPLND. AUA update series*, vol. 15. Dallas, TX: AUA, 1993:lesson 15, with permission.)

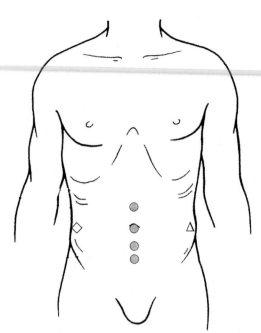

Legend

⬤ = 10/11 mm port.

◇ = 5 mm port for right L-RPLND in anterior axillary line.

△ = 5 mm port for left L-RPLND in anterior axillary line.

FIG. 130–2. Trocar placement for transperitoneal laparoscopic retroperitoneal lymph node dissection. (From Clayman RV, ed. *Laparoscopic urology.* St. Louis, MO: Quality Medical Publishing, 1993:272–308, with permission.)

laterally to the ureter. The template is bounded superiorly by the right renal vessels and inferiorly by where the ureter crosses the iliac vessels. The template extends posteriorly to the level of the lumbar vessels. There is recent evidence to suggest that dissection posterior to the lumbar vessels within the template is not necessary in clinical stage I patients as no tumor was found in any patients undergoing laparoscopic lymphadenectomy that included this region (5). However, this finding requires corroboration by further studies.

After the entire template has been exposed, dissection is begun inferiorly where the spermatic vessels enter the internal inguinal ring. Typically, one should identify a nonabsorbable stitch, left at the time of radical orchiectomy, that signifies the distal margin of this dissection. The testicular vein is then dissected up to its insertion with the vena cava. Careful dissection is required where the spermatic vein joins the inferior vena cava to prevent inadvertent disruption and bleeding. The testicular artery is clipped and transected where it crosses the inferior vena cava.

After this has been done the lymphatic tissue overlying the great vessels is dissected free. The lymphatic tissue on the anterior surface of the inferior vena cava is divided, and the anterior and lateral surfaces of the inferior vena cava are dissected free of lymphatic tissue from the level of the renal vessels going inferiorly to where the ureter crosses the iliac vessels. It is important that the left renal vein has already been clearly identified and exposed to prevent injury to this structure during this part of the dissection. The lymphatic tissue overlying the common iliac artery, starting at the level where the ureter crosses it, is dissected free, going in a cephalad direction

until the origin of the inferior mesenteric artery is reached. Cephalad to this artery the lymphatic tissue is divided toward the lateral border of the aorta so that all tissue anterior to this vessel is freed and included with the specimen. If not already done so, during this part of the dissection the testicular artery is clipped at its insertion into the aorta. This dissection is continued cephalad until the right renal artery, traversing the interaortocaval space, is identified, which marks the superior border of the template. The interaortocaval lymphatic tissue is now excised, with its posterior border being the level of the lumbar vessels. Great care must be taken with retraction of the great vessels as vascular injury may result in hemorrhage that is difficult to control by laparoscopic means. Lumbar vessels may need to be sacrificed to ensure retrieval of all lymphatic tissue. All sympathetic nerve fibers should be spared, if possible.

With the medial and superior borders of the template freed, attention is paid to the lateral border along the ureter. After the ureter has been identified, all lymphatic tissue medial to it is freed, beginning where the ureter crosses over the common iliac artery, and proceeding cephalad to the level of the renal vessels, where the most cephalad portion of the dissection has already been completed.

The posteriorly located lumbar vessels may also be encountered during this portion of the dissection. They should only be clipped and divided when needed to facilitate removal of lymphatic tissue. At this point the lymphatic packages are completely free. They are placed in a specimen bag and removed. Obvious tumor or suspicious fibrolymphatic tissue should be sent for pathologic frozen section interpretation. The colon and duodenum are then repositioned to their normal anatomic positions.

Left-Sided Template

The patient is placed on the operating table with the left side elevated 45 degrees upward. All other aspects of positioning and port placement (except now for left-sided dissection) are similar to that as described for right-sided dissection. Dissection is begun by incising the white line of Toldt on the left side, from the splenic flexure to the pelvic brim. The incision is extended distally along the spermatic vein all the way to the internal inguinal ring, where a nonabsorbable stitch, left at time of radical inguinal orchiectomy, should be identified. Superiorly, the dissection is carried medially around the splenic flexure just below the edge of the spleen. At this point the colon is mobilized medially until the entire anterior surface of the aorta is exposed. At this point the entire length of the spermatic vein, from the renal vein to the internal inguinal ring, is dissected free and removed. The left renal vein is identified and freed along its anterior and inferior surface at this point of the dissection. The ureter, which defines the lateral border of the dissection, is then identified. All lymphatic tissue is dissected free from the ureter from the level of the renal hilum to where the ureter crosses the common iliac artery. Then, starting where the ureter crosses (the inferior border of the template) the common iliac artery, all lymphatic tissue is dissected free from the lateral surface of this blood vessel. From here the dissection is continued cephalad along the lateral surface of the aorta to the level of the inferior mesenteric artery. This artery is preserved during this dissection. Cephalad to the inferior mesenteric artery all lymphatic tissue on the anterior and lateral surfaces of the aorta is removed. Dissection is continued in this manner up to the level of the renal vein. All lymphatic tissue associated with the renal vein is now dissected free. If there is a lumbar vein inserting into the posterior surface of the renal vein it must be divided to dissect free all lymphatic tissue. As a final step, the lymphatic package is dissected free posteriorly. The lymphatic tissue is separated from the lumbar vessels. The lymphatic package is then removed.

L-RPLND for Stage II or III Disease After Chemotherapy

L-RPLND has in general only been performed in a unilateral fashion, and there is only limited experience of L-RPLND being performed for stage II or III tumors after chemotherapy. In such cases L-RPLND may be performed when there has been a good response to chemotherapy where only smaller tumors/masses (5 cm or less) remain, and tumor markers have returned to normal. In such cases, dissection is carried out in a similar fashion as described for the unilateral templates involved but focusing primarily on resection of the residual tumor mass. Those with experience in such cases have noted that, due to chemotherapy, although tissue planes are more difficult to identify, mobilization of the bowel and identification of the tumor is possible. Due to the desmoplastic reaction typically seen after treatment with chemotherapy, careful dissection is required as tumor/residual tissue may be adherent to blood vessels. Janetschek et al. noted that teratomas are usually well delineated, but other types of tumor-free residual tissue may be adherent to surrounding venous structures (7). All vascular branches from the tumor must also be carefully dissected out, clipped, and transected.

Retroperitoneal Approach

Since the introduction of the balloon dissecting technique by Gaur, the laparoscopic retroperitoneal approach has been used for a variety of urologic procedures (3). Rassweiler et al. reported use of this technique for L-RPLND in eight cases (8). This technique differs from transperitoneal L-RPLND in how access and exposure are obtained. The essential features of this technique include placing the patient in the flank position without Trendelenburg. On the side of dissection a small incision is made in the lumbar triangle between the twelfth rib and iliac crest. Blunt dissection is then used to identify the retroperitoneal space (see Fig. 130–3). The retroperitoneal space is then expanded by use of one of a variety of commercial or homemade balloon dilating devices. Placement of secondary trocars is shown in Figure 130–4. A wide longitudinal incision of Gerota's fascia is recommended for optimal exposure of the retroperitoneum. L-

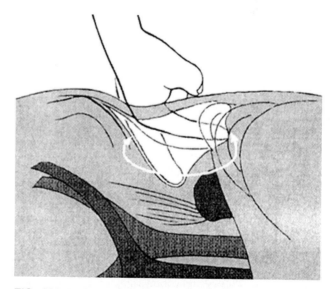

FIG. 130–3. Blunt dissection of retroperitoneal space with index finger pushing peritoneum medially; the working space is created between the lumbar aponeurosis and renal (Gerota's) fascia. (From Janetsckek G. Laparoscopic retroperitoneal lymph node dissection. *Urol Clin North Am* 2001;28:107–114, with permission.)

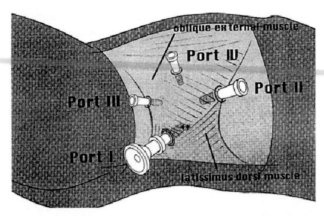

FIG. 130–4. Port placement for laparoscopic retroperitoneal lymph node dissection (L-RPLND). Surgeon stands at the backside. *Port I*, 12 mm for laparoscope; *port II*, 10 mm for right hand of surgeon; *port III*, 5 mm for left hand; *port IV*, 5 mm for assistant.

RPLND is then performed using the same template and landmarks as described for transperitoneal L-RPLND.

Use of this approach for L-RPLND, to date, is limited. Authors with considerable experience with retroperitoneoscopy reporting on use of this technique classified retroperitoneal L-RPLND as difficult. Others have also explored extraperitoneal L-RPLND by a more anterior approach.

POSTOPERATIVE CARE

In an otherwise uncomplicated case the orogastric tube may be removed at the end of the operation. Ambulation is initiated on the following morning, after which time the indwelling urethral catheter and pneumatic compression stockings may be discontinued. Diet is advanced on postoperative day 1. After the first 24 hours oral analgesics ordinarily suffice for pain control.

OUTCOMES

Complications

The predominant approach to L-RPLND has been by a transperitoneal route. The data presented here relates to L-RPLND performed by this technique. Potential complications associated with L-RPLND most often relate to intraoperative hemorrhaging. Other complications specifically related to this procedure include lymphocele formation and chylous ascites. The cumulative major (0.7%) and minor (7.8%) complication rates of this minimally invasive procedure are reasonable (Table 130–2) (5). Patients undergoing L-RPLND are likely to experience fewer pulmonary complications than those undergoing open surgery by midline or thoracoabdominal incision. Janetschek et al. noted the presence of chylous ascites in

21% of patients who underwent L-RPLND for persistent stage IIb tumor/mass (7). The authors believe that this complication is not related to surgical technique, as all lymphatic tissue was clipped, but rather due to the brief time to oral intake after L-RPLND compared to open RPLND. All such cases resolved with conservative measures (low-fat/medium-chain triglyceride diet). In the hands of experienced laparoscopists, complications specifically related to laparoscopy, such as bowel injury due to trocar insertion or intraoperative manipulation, are less likely.

In one of the largest contemporary series, 76 patients, the authors report that only 2 patients required conversion to an open procedure, one of which involved a patient with a horseshoe kidney (5). There were three intraoperative vascular complications: lacerations of the vena cava, renal vein, and a lumbar vein. The authors noted that these three complications were all laparoscopically controlled with compression, clips, and fibrin glue. Minor postoperative complications included lymphocele in three patients and genitofemoral nerve irritation in one patient. Normal antegrade ejaculation was reported in 73 of 74 patients.

Results

A summation of the worldwide experience with L-RPLND is shown in Table 130–2. The rarity of testicular cancer and the relative paucity of centers with sufficient laparoscopic expertise for this procedure in part explain the limited size of these series. A 5% open conversion rate is reasonable for this complex procedure. Only one local recurrence is noted in this summation (9). In this situation the tumor had recurred in the contralateral field. Longer follow-up of a larger number of patients is still needed to assess the diagnostic efficacy of this procedure.

A major point of discussion relating to L-RPLND is whether this procedure is simply a diagnostic procedure or may also be considered a therapeutic procedure. As the vast majority of patients found to have retroperitoneal tumors at the time of L-RPLND received adjunctive chemotherapy, it is not possible to determine the potential therapeutic efficacy of this procedure. L-RPLND has been used in a therapeutic fashion for a limited number of patients who underwent chemotherapy and had a persistent retroperitoneal mass. Janetschek et al. described a group of 49 patients (stage IIb, 35 patients; stage IIc, 14 patients) who underwent chemotherapy, had persistent retroperitoneal mass, and subsequently underwent L-RPLND (5). These patients all had normalization of tumor markers and a reduction of tumor size after chemotherapy. Of these patients, 18 had mature teratomas, 1 had active tumor, and 30 had necrosis and fibrosis only. The one patient with active tumor received two additional cycles of chemotherapy and has remained disease free. L-RPLND is believed

TABLE 130-2. *Worldwide experience with laparoscopic retroperitoneal lymph node dissection for clinical stage I disease*

Study	Number of patients	Mean operating time (min)	Conversion rate (%)	Complication rate (%)		Antegrade ejaculation (%)	Recurrences (%)		Follow-up (range, mean months)
				Minor	Major		Local	Distant	
Rukstalis and Chodak (3)	1	510	0	0	0	—	—	—	—
Stone et al. (2)	1	360	0	0	0	—	—	—	—
Gerber et al.	20	480	10.0	20.0	0	100.0	0	10.0	2–25, 10
Klotz (15)	4	285	25.0	0	0	—	—	—	—
Rassweiler et al. (5)	17	291	5.9	5.9	5.9	94.1	0	11.8	4–43, 27
Giusti et al. (16)	6	325	0	16.7	0	100.0	0	0	12–42, 27
Nelson et al. (17)	29	258	6.9	6.9	0	96.6	0	6.9	1–65, 16
Janetschek et al. (18)	76	294	2.6	5.3	0	98.7	1.3	0	10–87, 45
Total	154	314	5.2	7.8	0.7	98.0	0.7	4.1	1–87, 31

to be therapeutic in the 18 patients with mature teratoma. At a mean follow-up of 35 months, there have been no relapses in this group.

REFERENCES

1. Bosl GJ, Bajorin DF, Sheinfeld J, et al. Cancer of the testis. In: DeVita VF Jr, Hellman S, Rosenberg SA, eds. *Cancer*. Philadelphia: Lippincott Williams & Wilkins, 2001:1491–1518.
2. Donohue JP, Foster R, Rowland R, et al. Nerve-sparing retroperitoneal lymphadenectomy with preservation of ejaculation. *J Urol* 1990;144: 287–291.
3. Gaur D. Laparoscopic operative retroperitoneoscopy: Use of a new device. *J Urol* 1992;148:1137–1139.
4. Heidenreich A, Sesterhenn IA, Mostofi FK, et al. Prognostic risk factors that identify patients with clinical stage I nonseminomatous germ cell tumors at low risk and high risk for metastases. *Cancer* 1998;83: 1002–1011.
5. Janetschek G. Laparoscopic retroperitoneal lymph node dissection: *Urol Clin North Am* 2001;28:107–114.
6. Janetschek G, Hobisch A, Peschel R, et al. Laparoscopic retroperitoneal lymph node dissection for clinical stage I nonseminomatous testicular carcinoma: Long-term outcome. *J Urol* 2000;163:1793–1796.
7. Janetschek G, Peschel R, Bartsch G. Laparoscopic retroperitoneal lymph node dissection. *Atlas Urol Clin North Am* 2000;8:71–90.
8. Rassweiler JJ, Seemann O, Frede T, et al. Retroperitoneoscopy: Experience with 200 cases. *J Urol* 1998;160:1265–1269.
9. Sogani PC, Perrotti M, Herr HW, et al. Clinical stage I testis cancer: Long term outcome of patients on surveillance. *J Urol* 1998;159: 855–858.

CHAPTER 131

Pediatric Laparoscopic Nephrectomy

Ricardo González and María Fernanda Lorenzo Gómez

Nephrectomy and heminephrectomy for benign conditions have specific indications in children. It is in general agreed that open nephrectomy is the procedure of choice for pediatric renal neoplasms. Benign diseases are in particular well suited for laparoscopic intervention in children.

DIAGNOSIS

The diagnosis of congenital and acquired upper-tract lesions is primarily based on imaging studies with the appropriate clinical correlation.

INDICATIONS FOR SURGERY

Laparoscopic intervention of symptomatic multicystic renal dysplasia, renal atrophy, or hypoplasia leading to hypertension, pain, or infections is gaining momentum among pediatric urologists. This is also true for upper-pole nephrectomy performed to treat duplication anomalies with a nonfunctioning upper moiety. The advantages of the laparoscopic approach, which include improved cosmesis, shorter hospitalization, and less postoperative pain, may be more apparent in older children than in infants. When complete ureterectomy is necessary, the laparoscopic route may also avoid the second incision (5).

Relative contraindications to a laparoscopic approach to the pediatric kidney include neoplastic processes, severe inflammatory reactions that may make the dissection difficult, and a large kidney. The inconveniences of previous intraperitoneal surgery can be avoided using the retroperitoneal approach.

ALTERNATIVE THERAPY

Open surgical intervention is the standard alternative approach to laparoscopic intervention. Some authors prefer the transperitoneal and others the retroperitoneal accesses. The transperitoneal approach has the advantage of a larger working space but the retroperitoneal approach offers theoretical protection against postoperative adhesions and injury to intraabdominal organs (3).

SURGICAL TECHNIQUE

Transperitoneal Nephrectomy

The child is prepared with an enema the day before surgery. The patient is typed and screened for possible blood transfusion. General anesthesia with endotracheal intubation is necessary. The stomach is decompressed via an orogastric tube and the bladder is catheterized.

The child is positioned at a 45-degree angle with the operated side elevated. A bag or kidney rest is used to increase the space between the ribs and iliac crest. Pressure points are adequately padded. Access to the abdomen to establish pneumoperitoneum is gained by the Bailez modification of the Hasson technique, in which a semicircumferential incision is used to lift the umbilical skin to the point where it joins the peritoneum. This technique allows direct vision and blunt access to the peritoneal cavity without risk of intestinal lesion (Fig. 131–1) (4).

A 5- or 10-mm trocar is introduced and the abdomen is insufflated with CO_2. The pressure is maintained at 10 to 12 mm Hg. Two additional 5-mm ports are placed at the midclavicular line below the costal margin and above the iliac crest for the operating instruments. For right nephrectomy an additional epigastric port may occasionally be needed for liver retraction. (refer to figure in other chapter) The white line of Toldt lateral to the colon is incised and the colon is reflected medially. On the right side care is exercised not to injure the duodenum. The ureter is isolated in its middle segment and grasped for traction. Cephalad mobilization of the ureter leads to the renal hilum. Gerota's fascia is entered and the kidney is

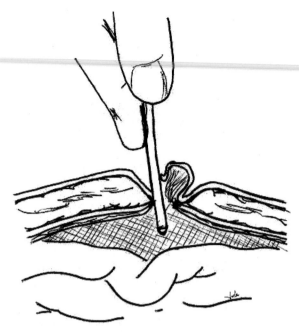

FIG. 131–1. The Bailez technique for laparoscopic access in children. A semicircumferential incision is used and the umbilical skin lifted to the point where it joins the peritoneum. This technique allows direct vision and blunt access to the peritoneal cavity and minimizes intestinal injury.

mobilized and elevated in a cephalad and lateral direction. Division of the ureter between clips facilitates this maneuver. The artery and vein are isolated. In the majority of pediatric cases the vessels are small enough to be clipped with two proximal clips and one distal clip. The vessels are then divided between the clips. The use of the bipolar coagulator (5) facilitates the sealing of vessels up to 5 mm in diameter.

Large cysts of a multicystic kidney or a large hydronephrotic kidney are drained via a needle aspirator to facilitate the dissection and removal of the specimen.

In most cases the decompressed kidney can be removed using an endoscopic bag through a 10-mm port. Larger specimens may require enlargement of the periumbilical incision. Larger kidneys that may require morcellation are best removed through an open extraperitoneal approach.

The instruments are removed one at a time, inspecting the sites for possible bleeding. The umbilical port site and 10-mm port sites are closed with PDS or Vicryl sutures. Five-millimeter port sites other than at the umbilicus may not need fascial closure.

Transperitoneal Upper-Pole Nephrectomy

The common indication for this procedure is a duplication anomaly with a nonfunctioning upper moiety (7). The distal upper-pole ureter may be ectopic or enter a ureterocele. In ureteral ectopia, complete removal of the distal ureter is seldom necessary. The management of ureteroceles is beyond the scope of this chapter. If a cystoscopy was performed immediately prior to the procedure, a ureteral stent may be left indwelling in the lower-pole ureter to assist in its identification. We find that the rigidity provided by the catheter aids in the detection. However, in most cases there is a marked discrepancy in the diameter of the ureters, with the upper pole being dilated (6,7).

The patient is positioned as for a total nephrectomy. The same ports are used. A fourth lower-abdominal port for the assistant is often useful. After exposing the ureters, the dilated one corresponding to the upper-pole moiety is transected between clips. The upper moiety ureter is dissected in a cephalad direction until it passes posterior to the main renal hilum. The ureter to be excised is dissected close to the adventitia to avoid injury to the lower moiety ureter. At this point Gerota's fascia is opened and the upper pole of the kidney dissected. The demarcation between the upper and lower segments is usually clearly seen. The upper-pole ureter is identified in the suprahilar region and gently pulled in a cephalad

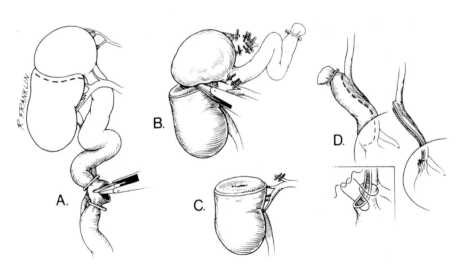

FIG. 131–2. Laparoendoscopic right upper-pole partial nephroueterectomy. **A:** The ureter is clipped and divided in the region of the midureter. **B, C:** The ureter has been dissected from beneath the main renal pedicle and the upper-pole vasculature has been clipped. The hydronephrotic cap is dissected off with the parenchyma minimally divided. **D:** The ureter is dissected to the common sheath and there is a strip of the ureter left attached as the remaining wall of the ureter is dissected and ligated at the bladder wall.

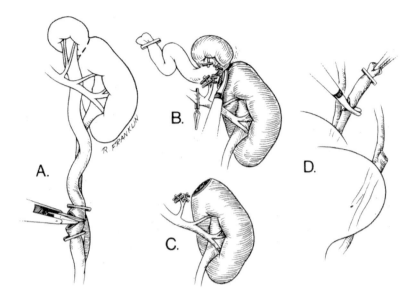

FIG. 131–3. Laparoendoscopic left upper-pole partial nephroureterectomy. **A:** The ureter is clipped and divided in the region of the midureter and dissected in a rostral direction. **B, C:** The upper-pole segmental vessels are clipped and the cap of the kidney allowed to demarcate. The plane of amputation is marked, an endoscopic bulldog is applied to the major pedicle, and the upper-pole cap is amputated. **D:** The ureter is dissected in a caudal direction to the point of the common vascularity and there amputated with the stump left open.

direction until it is completely delivered above the main renal vessels. Traction on the ureter will allow identification of the vessels (usually small) supplying the upper pole. They are dissected, clipped, and divided.

If the upper pole is hydronephrotic, it can be opened. This maneuver provides a clear view of the demarcation between the segments. The thin parenchyma of the upper pole is divided with diathermy scissors, as one would decorticate a renal cyst. Bleeding at the edge is controlled with coagulation. The urothelium at the floor of the upper moiety can be left attached to the lower renal segment. The attachment of this urothelial surface to the ureter is divided and the specimen is removed through the 10-mm port.

Laparoscopic heminephrectomy can be combined with an open procedure in the lower ureter, such as reimplantation or ureterocele removal. In these cases the specimen can be removed through the lower-abdominal incision used to perform such an operation. An illustrative example of partial nephrectomy in the pediatric patient is demonstrated in Figures 131–2 and 131–3.

Retroperitoneal Approach

Some surgeons favor the retroperitoneal approach for both total and partial nephrectomy. The patient can be placed in the lateral (3,9) or prone position (1). The more commonly used lateral position will be described. The patient is placed in a full lateral position, slightly tilted forward with flexion to maximize the space between the ribs and the iliac crest. The table is also tilted forward to allow the peritoneum to fall away from the kidney. Two methods to create the retroperitoneal space have been described. Those favoring the use of a balloon start creating a space at the posterior axillary line above the iliac crest, bluntly dissecting with a finger the space. A balloon constructed with a glove finger attached to a

catheter and filled with cold saline is then introduced in this space. (6). Two additional ports are placed under vision. The most important landmark in retroperitoneoscopy is the psoas muscle. Following it in a cephalad direction the posterior aspect of the kidney is encountered. Others prefer to gain retroperitoneal access at the tip of the twelfth rib and then create the space first with finger dissection and then with the tip of the lens and by insufflation. Either method appears to be satisfactory (3).

Once the kidney is identified in the retroperitoneum, Shanberg et al. recommend division of the ureter and complete mobilization of the kidney prior to clipping and dividing the vessels (9). In contrast, El-Ghoneimi et al. prefer to leave the anterior surface of the kidney attached to the posterior peritoneum until after the vessels are divided (3).

OUTCOMES

Results

Pediatric laparoscopic nephrectomy and heminephrectomy are reasonable alternatives to open procedures in children. The cosmetic advantages for older children in whom larger incisions are required for open surgery are clear. For upper-pole heminephrectomy, in older children the laparoscopic approach deserves serious consideration. The role of laparoscopic surgery in infant renal surgery is less evident because in this age group both nephrectomy and heminephrectomy can be accomplished through small incisions with minimal hospitalization (2,8).

REFERENCES

1. Borzi P. A comparison of the lateral and posterior retroperitoneoscopic approach for complete and partial nephrectomy in children. *BJU Int* 2001;87:517–520.

2. Elder J, Hladky D, Selzman A. Outpatient nephrectomy for nonfunctioning kidneys. *J Urol* 1995;154(2, Pt 2):712–714.

3. El-Ghoneimi A, Sauty L, Maintenant J, Macher M, Lotttmann H, Aigrain Y. Laparoscopic retroperitoneal nephrectomy in high risk children. *J Urol* 2000;164:1076–1079.

4. Franc-Guimond J, Kryger J, González R. Experience with the Bailez technique for laparoscopic access in children. *BJU Int* 2002.

5. Hamilton B, Gatti J, Cartwright P, Snow B. Comparison of laparoscopic versus open nephrectomy in the pediatric population. *J Urol* 2000;163: 937–939.

6. Horowitz M, Shah S, Ferzli G, Glassberg K. Laparoscopic partial upper pole nephrectomy in infants and children. *BJU Int* 2001;87:514–516.

7. Janetcschek G, Seibold J, Radmayr C, Bartsch G. Laparoscopic heminephrectomy in pediatric patients. *J Urol* 1997;158:1928–1930.

8. Jednak R, Kryger J, Barthold J, Gonzalez R. A simplified technique of upper pole heminephrectomy for duplex kidney. *J Urol* 2000;164: 1326–1328.

9. Shanberg A, Sanderson K, Rajpoot D, Duel B. Laparoscopic retroperitoneal renal and adrenal surgery in children. *BJU Int* 2001; 87:521–524.

CHAPTER 132

Laparoscopic Management of the Nonpalpable Testicle

Linda A. Baker and Gerald H. Jordan

The term *cryptorchidism* refers to the absence of a testicle in the scrotum. During embryonic life, the testis differentiates adjacent to the mesonephric kidneys and normally descends via the inguinal canal to its scrotal position. However, in 0.8% to 1.8% of 1-year-old boys this process is faulty, resulting in cryptorchidism. In the majority of cryptorchid boys, a testicle is palpable in the groin, but in approximately 20% a testicle is nonpalpable. In these cases, the gonad might be absent, intraabdominal (along the normal path of descent or ectopic), or within the inguinal canal (canicular). By tradition, open exploration through the groin or abdomen was performed. However, in 1976 Cortesi described diagnostic laparoscopy to localize the nonpalpable testicle and techniques for therapeutic laparoscopy rapidly followed.

DIAGNOSIS

A history of palpable gonads, hypospadias, genital surgery, or inguinal herniorrhaphy should be obtained at the time of initial physical exam. The use of warm lubricant facilitates the often difficult exam. Contralateral compensatory hypertrophy may indicate the lack of functioning testicular tissue on the nonpalpable side, but is not absolutely accurate and necessitates surgical exploration. Preoperative testing to identify the presence or absence of a nonpalpable testis (hormonal stimulation or radiological evaluations) is usually not productive and therefore not recommended. Hormonal therapy [i.e., β-human chorionic gonadotropin (hCG)] has promoted testicular descent in some nonpalpable cases but is best applied to the patient with bilateral nonpalpable testes. Ultrasound, venography, herniography, angiography, computed tomography (CT) and magnetic resonance imaging (MRI) have been employed to locate the nonpalpable testis, but unfortunately all lack sufficient sensitivity to be solely relied upon. While MRI or gadolinium-enhanced magnetic resonance angiography has better sensitivity, it requires an anesthetic, is costly, and is still not nearly as accurate as laparoscopy. Only laparoscopy uniformly and unequivocally determines the presence or absence of gonadal tissue and localizes it.

The differential diagnosis of bilateral nonpalpable cryptorchidism includes anorchidism, undescended testicles (bilateral or unilateral with contralateral absence), and ambiguous genitalia due to female pseudohermaphroditism or another intersex condition. Life-threatening congenital adrenal hyperplasia (CAH) must be ruled out. A karyotype, endocrine testing, radiographic studies, and, if indicated, laparoscopy usually provide the necessary information to make an intersex diagnosis. A normal appearing masculinized phallus does not eliminate this possibility. Routine neonatal screening for CAH has aided detection of this entity.

INDICATIONS FOR SURGERY

To maximize the opportunity for spontaneous testicular descent during the first 6 months of life, while preventing the histological changes that occur in those testicles that remain undescended beyond the first year of life, we recommend surgery between ages 6 to 12 months. Data supporting this "early orchiopexy" recommendation is being reported with improved testicular growth and Leydig cell function. The goals of laparoscopic orchiopexy are identical to the goals of open orchiopexy, namely, to improve fertility (and possibly diminish malignant transformation potential), relocate the testicle to the scrotum for easier examination, correct the associated inguinal hernia, prevent testicular torsion, and alleviate possible psychological trauma resulting from an empty hemiscrotum.

ALTERNATIVE THERAPY

Traditional open surgical techniques include inguinal exploration with the extension of the inguinal incision proximally to explore the abdomen or primary open abdominal approach. Open inguinal exploration is not 100% reliable at ruling out an intraabdominal testis. Pooling data from five series (1,2,6–9), laparoscopy has identified 40 testicles in 78 "negative" open explorations for a nonpalpable testicle.

SURGICAL TECHNIQUE

Unilateral Nonpalpable Testis

Preoperatively, the family is counseled of the possible surgical scenarios. If a testicle is palpable under anesthesia (18%), then an inguinal orchiopexy is performed. If it remains nonpalpable under anesthesia, then diagnostic laparoscopy is performed. If an atrophic testicular remnant is identified, a laparoscopic orchiectomy might be performed (surgeon's bias). If a subjectively good testicle is found, a laparoscopic orchiopexy is performed. Figure 132–1 illustrates the approach to management of the nonpalpable undescended testicle.

Diagnostic Laparoscopy

After adequate anesthesia is attained, the patient is secured to the bed in the supine, frog-legged position with arms tucked. Preparation and draping must be suitable for an open abdominal procedure, be it planned or necessary. A urethral Foley catheter and an oral gastric tube are passed. Given that most patients are between 6 to 24 months of age, safety concerns have led most surgeons to abandon blind-access techniques (Veress needle) and to use open-access techniques. Holding sutures are placed in the fascia to help elevate it for the peritonotomy. The authors use the InnerDyne Step introducer system, a radially dilating access sheath, to achieve 5- or 10-mm access. Alternatively, exclusively needlescopic 2-mm access (and working ports) can be used, but they provide less light and a smaller visual field. After insufflation to 14 cm of water, a 5-mm 0-degree camera is used to inspect the abdomen for injury. The patient is then placed in the Trendelenburg position and each internal ring is inspected bilaterally. On the unaffected side, the testicular vessels and vas are easily identified, leaving the closed internal ring (Fig. 132–2). Caudal traction on the descended testis can help visualization of its cord struc-

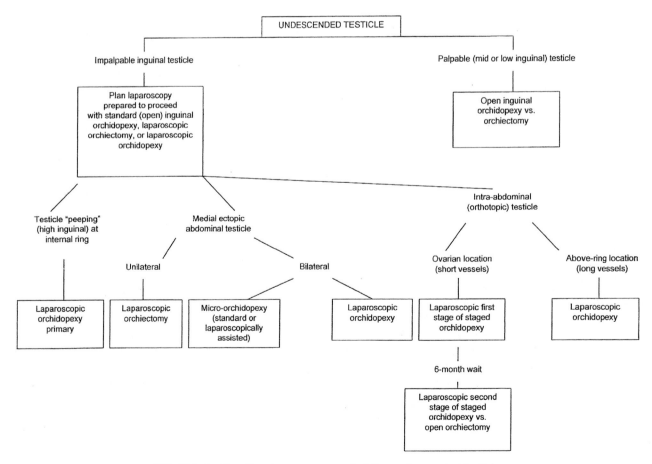

FIG. 132–1. Algorithm for management of the undescended testicle.

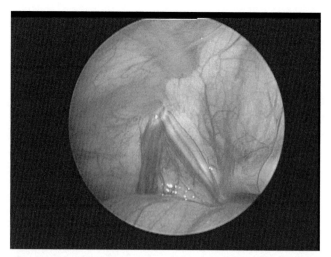

FIG. 132–2. The laparoscopic appearance of a normal left groin. The spermatic vessel leash can be seen joined by the vas deferens passing through a closed internal ring. Traction is on the testicle, emphasizing the location of the ring.

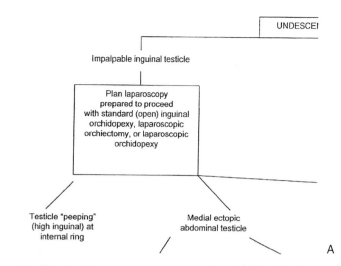

tures. On the affected side, the internal ring is noted and the testicle, vas, and testicular vessels are sought.

If the ring is closed with a normal vas and normal testicular vessels exiting (Fig. 132–2), the groin is explored for the testis or nubbin by a laparoscopic or open approach. The removal of any remaining testicular nubbin is controversial because 10% of nubbins may contain viable germ cells and theoretically could undergo malignant change. If normal appearing vas and testicular vessels exit an open internal ring (Fig. 132–3), the inguinal canal can be "milked" retrograde in an attempt to push a canalicular (peeping) testicle or nubbin into the abdomen (Figs. 132–4A and 132–4B). In any case, if the gonad is not found the groin must be explored either by open or laparoscopic techniques. If blind-ending vessels are

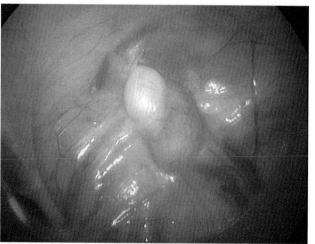

FIG. 132–4. A: Laparoscopic appearance of the right groin; the spermatic vessel leash joined by the vas can be seen passing adjacent the open internal ring (patent processus vaginalis). **B:** With gentle pressure on the groin, the testicle can be seen delivered into the abdomen.

clearly identified, ending in a "horsetail" appearance and often within proximity to a blind ending vas, the testis is not viable and the procedure is terminated, although some surgeons again would remove any testicular nubbin found (Fig. 132–5).

An intraabdominal testis could be found (Fig. 132–6) where an orchidopexy will be performed. If a blind-ending vas can be seen without testicular vessels in the vicinity, the laparoscopic exploration is not complete and must continue rostrally toward the aortic origin of the testicular vessels until either the gonad is found (gonadal disjunction) or blind-ending vessels are found. Another finding might be a medially ectopic testis where the ectopic abdominal testicle comes to rest medial to its respective medial umbilical artery. The vas deferens is short; most of these testicles have not been noted to have looping vas or disassociation of the paratesticular tubular structures; and, by definition, the spermatic vessel leash

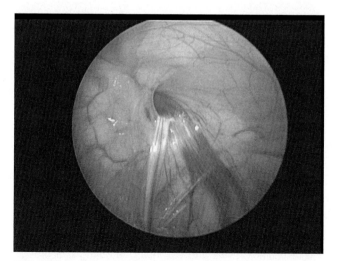

FIG. 132–3. The laparoscopic appearance of the right groin in which there is a patent processus vaginalis (hernia).

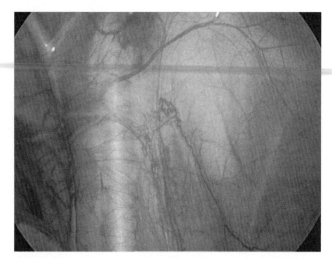

FIG. 132–5. The laparoscopic appearance of the right groin, with the classic blind-ending vas and blind-ending testicular vessels in proximity to each other.

is short. These testicles are difficult to place in the scrotum and in some cases may require orchiectomy.

Primary Laparoscopic Orchiopexy

To perform a primary laparoscopic orchiopexy, the patient is placed in the Trendelenburg position with the ipsilateral side of the bed tilted upward. Two 2–5 mm working ports are passed just inferior to the umbilicus and lateral to the inferior epigastric vessels (Fig. 132–7). A peritonotomy is made just lateral to the testicular vessels. It is carried over the top of the internal ring and continued lateral and superior to the vas, with care to not injure the inferior epigastric vessels or the bladder and leaving the peritoneal area medial and between the testicular vessels and the vas undisturbed. Once the peritonotomy is completed, the testicular vessels, testicle, and vas

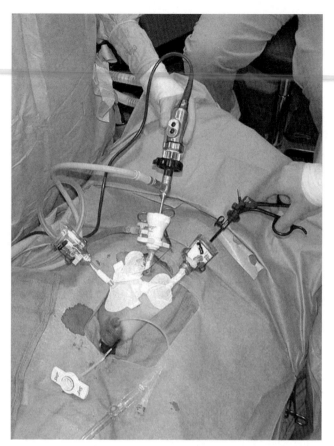

FIG. 132–7. Typical cannula placement for left laparoscopic orchiopexy.

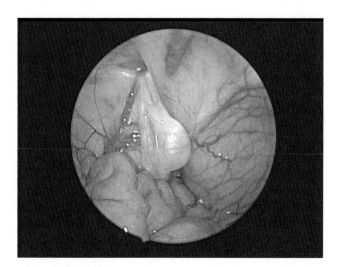

FIG. 132–6. The laparoscopic appearance of the low left abdominal testicle.

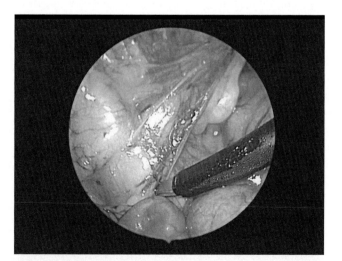

FIG. 132–8. The peritonotomies have been completed and the gubernaculum was transected. The testis is retracted medially and ventrally, with the sheet of peritoneum medial to the testicular vessels and vas intact. Tethering attachments on the dorsal side of the peritoneum can be divided as the testis is pulled toward the contralateral internal ring.

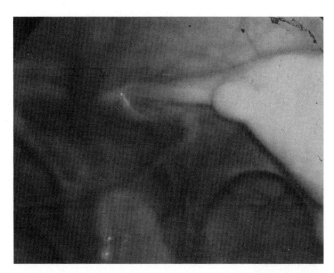

FIG. 132–9. Laparoscopic appearance of the right groin; the testicle is retracted into the abdomen and a looping vas is seen extending adjacent to the inferior (gubernacular) attachment.

are elevated on this peritoneal pedicle, thereby dissecting the plane between these structures and the external iliac vessels (Fig. 132–8). Care is taken to not harm the external iliac vessels, inferior epigastric vessels, or a long looping vas (Fig. 132–9). The testicle is then retracted rostrally, inverting the processus vaginalis and the gubernaculum. The gubernaculum is thinned and cut across with Bovie cautery (Fig. 132–10), taking care to watch for a long looping vas. Cautery is necessary because the gubernacular attachments are highly vascular. The testicle is then retracted toward the contralateral internal ring to assess length. In most cases, if the testicle can reach the contralateral internal ring, length is sufficient to place the testicle well in the respective hemiscrotum. While

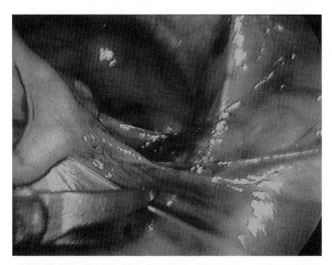

FIG. 132–10. Laparoscopic appearance of right testicle being retracted into the abdomen; gubernacular attachments are being divided with electrocautery.

vigorous mobilization of the vas should be avoided for fear of testicular atrophy, the vas must be sufficiently mobilized to prevent ureteral kinking from the paravasal attachments. Any remaining attachments preventing testicular mobility are carefully dissected, and, once adequate length is assured, the testicle can be transferred to the scrotum.

In some instances, length is inadequate. One option is to incise the peritoneum parallel to the testicular vessels as far proximal as is safe. Then, the peritoneal incision is extended perpendicular over the testicular vessels without their injury. Often this perpendicular incision significantly "relaxes" the vessels, allowing scrotal positioning. If length still remains an issue and the peritoneum medial to the vas and vessels is intact, the spermatic vessels can be divided (Fowler–Stephens approach; see below).

Several techniques are described to deliver the testis into the scrotum, including retrograde placement of a clamp or port. By placing a port, the pneumoperitoneun can be maintained in the event the testis is "fumbled." The authors use the InnerDyne Step 10 mm for the transfer. The Maryland grasper in the ipsilateral abdominal port is passed medial to the inferior epigastric vessels just over the top of the superior pubic ramus. A scrotal skin incision is made in the ipsilateral hemiscrotum and a subdartos pouch is generated. The laparoscopic Maryland is then guided out through the scrotal incision. The 10-mm Step introducer is then passed on the Maryland (Fig. 132–11A). The 10-mm trocar is introduced through the Step introducer (Fig. 132–11B). The Maryland graspers are then transferred down to the scrotal port, the gubernaculum of the testis is grasped, and the testis is delivered via the port into the scrotum (Fig. 132–12A). The testis is secured intrascrotally in the subdartos pouch by the fixation technique preferred by the surgeon (Fig. 132–12B). The intraabdominal pressure is lowered to 4 mm Hg and the surgical field assessed for bleeding (Fig. 132–12C).

In children, the fascia of any 5- or 10-mm port site is closed, as hernias have been reported. All CO_2 is evacuated and skin wounds are closed and dressed. These children do profit from adjuvant caudal anesthesia and local injection of cannula sites using bupivacaine (Marcaine). The children are discharged with instructions to advance diet as tolerated and to prevent straddle toy use. Recovery is usually less than 24 hours.

One-Stage Fowler–Stephens Laparoscopic Orchiopexy

If the maneuvers outlined above result in inadequate length of the testicular vessels preventing scrotal positioning, a one-stage Fowler–Stephens procedure can be performed. Via a contralateral 5-mm port, the testicular artery and vein are clipped and transected, preserving the vasal blood supply to the testicle, thus allowing the testicle to be placed in the scrotum with one laparoscopic pro-

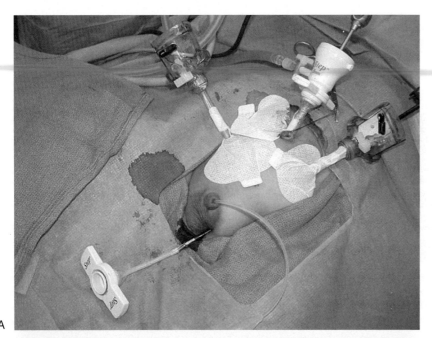

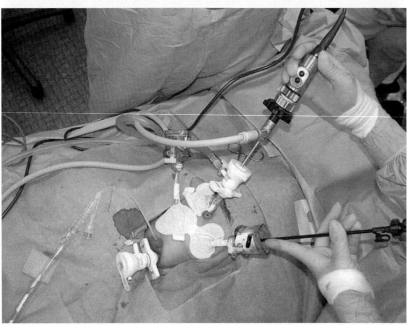

FIG. 132–11. A: Via the ipsilateral abdominal port, a laparoscopic Maryland dissector is passed medial to the ipsilateral inferior epigastric vessels, over the anterior pubic ramus, and out thru the scrotal skin incision. The 10-mm Step introducer is loaded on the Maryland and pushed intraperitoneally as the Maryland is drawn back into the abdomen. Note the Maryland in the ipsilateral port exiting the scrotum. **B:** The trocar is advanced into the introducer with visualization via the intraabdominal camera.

cedure. However, this technique has a higher risk of testicular atrophy.

Two-Stage Fowler–Stephens Laparoscopic Orchiopexy

If, at the time of diagnostic laparoscopy, a high testis is found that stands little chance of reaching the scrotum without transection of the testicular vessels, a two-stage Fowler–Stephens laparoscopic orchiopexy is a good approach. In this case, a contralateral 5-mm port is placed and the only peritonotomy performed is parallel and immediately medial to the testicular vessels, a safe distance proximal to the iliac vessels. Via this peritonotomy, the vessels are encircled and a 5-mm vascular clip applier is used to ligate the vessels. The vessels are transected and the procedure is terminated. Six months later, a second laparoscopy is performed following the steps outlined in the primary laparoscopic orchiopexy. The vessels are mobilized to the clips and the mobilized testis is transferred into the scrotum. During the 6-month interval, collateral blood supply via the paravasal arteries ostensibly is enhanced.

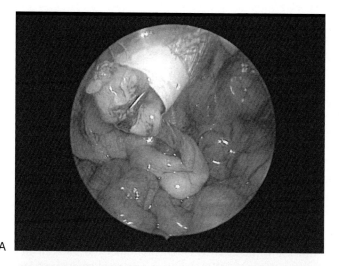

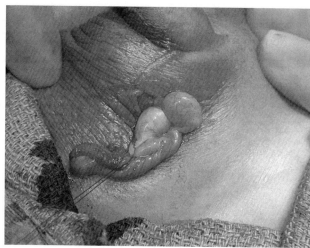

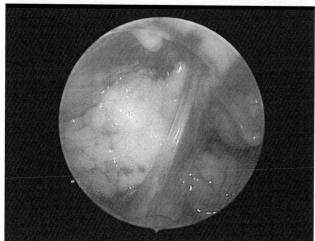

FIG. 132–12. A: Intraabdominal testicle being pulled into the 10-mm laparoscopic cannula using testicular grasping forceps. The testicle is then delivered to the right hemiscrotum. **B:** The outside appearance with the testicle delivered to the level of the scrotum. **C:** Intraabdominal view after the left testicle has been transferred to the scrotum.

Some authors have suggested that testicles that have been managed with staged division of the spermatic vessel leash be evaluated with color Doppler in an effort to evaluate the viability of the testicle prior to undertaking the second stage. Realistically, however, even if by Doppler the testicle does not appear to be viable the remaining gonadal tissue should be removed as atrophy by ultrasound criteria cannot be felt to be pathognomonic of complete atrophy of the gonadal tubular structures. Ostensibly, these structures could continue to carry the risk of malignant transformation.

Bilateral Nonpalpable Testes

Bilateral *palpable* undescended testes are managed in the same fashion as unilateral palpable undescended testes. However, some pediatric urologists agree that for the child with bilateral nonpalpable testicles laparoscopic management is imperative, irrelevant of the laboratory results after hCG stimulation or serum MIS sampling. In

patients with high bilateral intraabdominal testes, most pediatric urologists perform staged reconstructions. Surgery is completed on one side, confirming unilateral testis survival prior to embarking on the contralateral side, because in many of these complex cases a Fowler–Stephens approach must be used.

Laparoscopic Orchiopexy for Intersex States

Therapeutic laparoscopic techniques including laparoscopic gonadal biopsy, gonadectomy (for dysgenetic gonads or when contrary to sex assignment), orchiopexy, and in some cases removal of ductal structures have a prominent place in the management of intersex children (male pseudohermaphrodites, true hermaphrodites, or XX males with genital ambiguity and nonpalpable gonads). Minimalization of physical scarring from surgery is paramount in this patient population, who often suffer from poor body and sexual self-esteem.

TABLE 132-1. *Comparison of open versus laparoscopic orchiopexy success rates from two large published series*

	1° orchiopexy		One-stage F-S		Two-stage F-S	
	n	%	n	%	n	%
Open orchiopexy [Docimo (5)]	80	81.3	321*	66.7*	56*	76.8*
Laparoscopic orchiopexy [Baker (1)]	178	97.2	27	74.1	58	87.9

Success was defined as scrotal position and lack of atrophy.
n = number of testes.
* = likely includes a significant number of palpable testes

OUTCOMES

Outcomes analyses always compare to a "gold standard." In the case of orchiopexy, open surgical techniques are the gold standard, with the early postoperative outcome variables being testis position (scrotal) and lack of testicular atrophy. A 1995 metaanalysis of open surgical results (5) found an overall 76.1% success rate with open orchiopexy for the intraabdominal testicle. By procedure,

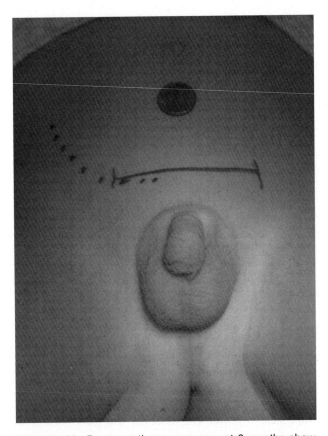

FIG. 132–13. Postoperative appearance at 6 months showing a patient following laparoscopic right orchidopexy for a right intraabdominal testicle. Note the complete normal appearance of the right hemiscrotum. A penny is placed on the child's abdomen for reference. Note that the laparoscopic cannula sites are virtually invisible. Drawn on the child's abdomen are what could have been the abdominal incisions for an open abdominal orchidopexy.

open one-stage Fowler–Stephens orchiopexy yielded a 67% success rate while the two-stage Fowler–Stephens yielded 77%. Transabdominal orchiopexy was successful in 81% while microvascular orchiopexy worked in 84%. In comparison, a 2001 multiinstitutional analysis of laparoscopic orchiopexy was performed, collating the results from 10 US centers (1). Of 310 laparoscopic orchiopexies performed over 9 years, 263 testes in 227 patients were seen in follow-up. Primary laparoscopic orchiopexy was successful in 97.2% of 178 testes. One-stage Fowler–Stephens laparoscopic orchiopexy was successful in 74.1% of 27 testes while two-stage Fowler–Stephens laparoscopic orchiopexy was successful in 87.9% of 58 testes. Comparing these two studies, the laparoscopic approach yielded higher success rates than the same approach performed open (Table 132–1). In addition, both analyses revealed that one-stage Fowler–Stephens approaches had a significantly higher atrophy rate than the two-stage repair. Early experience with needlescopic orchiopexy suggests excellent safety, speed, cosmetic results, and testicular outcomes.

The higher the testicle, the more profound the anatomic aberrances. The long-term function of these testes with respect to malignant degenerative potential and fertility will be outcomes analyzed by the next generation of pediatric urologists. The development of sperm aspiration techniques associated with various applications of assisted fertilization seems to favor orchiopexy.

Laparoscopy for the nonpalpable testis, combining diagnosis and therapy, has become the standard approach at many US and European centers. A consistent definitive diagnosis by laparoscopy is imperative and outweighs the price of its invasiveness. The experienced laparoscopic surgeon can accomplish identical or even improved surgical results (1) with similar operative time and diminished surgical morbidity (Fig. 132–13). Laparoscopic orchiopexy is associated with the highest testicular success rate (scrotal position without testicular atrophy) (1). This fact alone should lead "nonlaparoscopists" to critically reevaluate management strategies.

REFERENCES

1. Baker LA, et al. A multi-institutional analysis of laparoscopic orchidopexy. *BJU Int* 2001;87:484–489.

2. Boddy SA, Corkery JJ, Gornall P. The place of laparoscopy in the management of the impalpable testis. *Br J Surg* 1985;72:918–919.
3. Carr MC. *The non-palpable testis. AUA update series*, vol. 20(29). Baltimore: AUA Office of Education, 2001:226–231.
4. Diamond DA, Caldamone AA. The value of laparoscopy for 106 impalpable testes relative to clinical presentation. *J Urol* 1992;148(2, Pt 2):632–634.
5. Docimo SG. The results of surgical therapy for cryptorchidism: a literature review and analysis. *J Urol* 1995;154:1148–1152.
6. Koyle MA, et al. The role of laparoscopy in the patient with previous negative inguinal exploration for impalpable testis. *J Urol* 1994;151:236 (abst 35).
7. Koyle MA Rajfer J, Ehrlich RM. The undescended testis. *Pediatr Ann* 1988;17:39, 42–46.
8. Lakhoo K, Thomas DF, Najmaldin AS. Is inguinal exploration for the impalpable testis an outdated operation? [see comments]. *Br J Urol* 1996;77:452–454.
9. Perovic S, Janic N. Laparoscopy in the diagnosis of non-palpable testes. *Br J Urol* 1994;73:310–313.

SECTION XII

Frontiers in Urology

Section Editor: Louis Kavoussi

CHAPTER 133

Robotics in Urologic Surgery

Matthew T. Gettman and Jeffrey A. Cadeddu

The English word "robot" is derived from the Czech word "robota," which is defined as obligatory servitude. In the industrial revolution, the benefits of automation were realized in a variety of manufacturing roles. The invention of the transistor in 1948, which allowed robots to be developed in conjunction with computers, was a major factor that provided the foundation of modern robotic technology. The performance characteristics of robotic devices have enabled a variety of industrial applications in that they can perform repetitive tasks quickly with excellent precision and do not fatigue. Based on the success of robotic devices for industrial applications, robots have also been developed for medical applications as couriers, laboratory analysis, rehabilitation, and in the operating room.

All robotic devices involve an integrated system of mechanical and computer-based components. Most robots used for manufacturing or surgical applications incorporate the use of a mechanical arm. The complexity of the mechanical arm, in part, determines the function of the robot and the range of motion (ROM) boundary (working envelope). A mechanical arm, in similar fashion as the human arm, consists of multiple appendages (links) that are connected in series with joints. In similar fashion as a human hand holding conventional surgical instruments, the last appendage of a robotic arm also holds an end effector (surgical instrument). The type of end effector ultimately determines the function of the mechanical arm (Fig. 133–1). Depending on the type of robotic system, a variety of reusable or nonreusable end effectors have been developed for mechanical arms in surgery. In addition, the end effectors of some mechanical arms are interchangeable, thereby increasing the versatility of the robotic device. The links of the mechanical arm can be actively or passively driven at each joint.

The number of joints determines the translational or rotational degrees of freedom (DOF) for the mechanical arm. For instance, a human elbow has one rotational

degree of freedom, whereas the wrist has three rotational degrees of freedom. The overall motion capabilities of the mechanical arm (i.e., total robotic DOF) are defined as the sum of the total number of DOF for each joint. As such, the human palm has seven DOF (sum of the wrist, elbow, and shoulder). For a mechanical arm to have complete freedom of motion, at least six DOF are required. For coordination of complex robotic movements and for safety purposes, sensors can be placed at all joints, thereby permitting computerized control of the mechanical arm. In addition, the ability to override the computerized control of a mechanical arm is another important safety feature.

Robots are broadly classified as offline or online systems. Offline robots are preprogrammed for autonomous repetitive function. On the other hand, online robots require the use of human judgment and perception. With

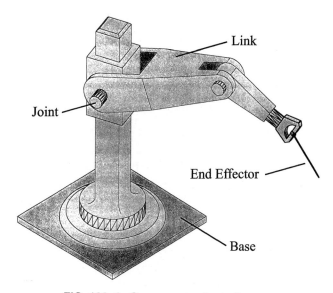

FIG. 133–1. Components of robotic arm.

online robots, the operator controls each movement of the robot and, conversely, the robot enhances or simplifies the task of the operator. Some online robots are designed with a haptic interface that provides the operator with important tactile and force-feedback information. Given the risks and complexity of surgery, most robots designed for applications in the operating room are considered online robots. For laparoscopic applications, the increasingly popular master–slave robotic systems are an example of an online robot. With these systems, motions of the surgeon at a remote control station are replicated by robotic arms positioned at or within the patient.

ENDOUROLOGIC APPLICATIONS

Transurethral Resection of the Prostate

Davies et al. first developed a robotic system capable of accurate and rapid resection of the prostate called PROBOT (5). The original PROBOT provided seven DOF for computerized resection that was performed with a small cutting blade rotating at 40,000 repetitions/minute (5). To improve the safety of resection and limit the boundaries of resection to those of a cone, a modified PROBOT was subsequently introduced with only four DOF (10) (Fig. 133–2). After the PROBOT safety frame

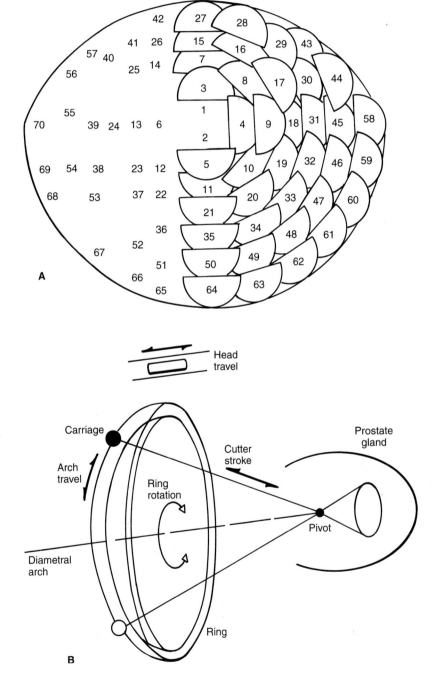

FIG. 133–2. A: Resection pattern for robotic-assisted transurethral resection of the prostate (TURP). **B:** Safety frame modification of TURP robot to restrict resection to boundaries of a cone.

was further modified, five patients were successfully treated with an unaided offline robotic system that incorporated preoperative prostatic mapping with transrectal ultrasound. Although all PROBOT cases were successful, transrectal US did not provide sufficient accuracy to map the prostate before transurethral resection of the prostate (TURP) (10).

Ho et al. recently evaluated in human cadavers the feasibility of robotic-assisted transurethral laser resection of the prostate (CALRP) (11). By numerically calculating the motion sequence plan of the laser fiber and profiling the prostate tissue removal rate, the authors concluded CALRP may improve the repeatability and reliability of laser TURP (11).

Flexible Endoscopy

Bowersox and Cornum used an experimental master–slave robotic system to successfully navigate a 15.5 Fr flexible cystoscope through a 25-cm segment of porcine small intestine plicated to a diameter of 5 to 6 mm (2). The system included two manipulators (tip deflector and torque/advancement), a remote control unit, and a 3D vision system.

Percutaneous Renal Access

Prior iterations of robots for percutaneous renal access have included a robotic system consisting of a passive mechanical arm with five DOF with a C-arm for imaging. Registration between the manipulator and C-arm was coordinated with a personal computer that also displayed the needle trajectory on the fluoroscopic images. A second attempt was a prototype system for percutaneous

renal access using a modified Laparoscopic Assistant Robotic System (LARS) robot with three DOF and biplanar fluoroscopic imaging.

The Johns Hopkins group later introduced a modified robot for percutaneous renal access called PAKY (Percutaneous Access of the Kidney) that also incorporates an active system for positioning and driving the access needle (Fig. 133–3) (3). The novel needle injection stage has a low radiographic profile that, to minimize needle deflection, holds the needle on the barrel rather than proximally, thereby stabilizing needle insertion (14). After manually targeting the calyx, the manipulator is locked allowing the surgeon to rotate the C-arm freely to a lateral view. The insertion depth and pathway are then continuously monitored during access, thereby increasing the safety and accuracy of the procedure. When access was performed with PAKY in laboratory experiments and in nine clinical cases, Cadeddu et al. reported in both groups a 100% "one-stick" success rate and a mean access time of 8.2 minutes (3).

Prostate Biopsy

Rovetta et al. described an image-guided robotic system for transperineal prostatic biopsy with an accuracy of 3D needle positioning within 1 to 2 mm (13). Although they reported the system was faster than the conventional biopsy technique, the system is still considered experimental because of high costs and prolonged set-up time (13).

LAPAROSCOPIC APPLICATIONS

Commercially Available Robots

Endoscope Manipulator

The Automated Endoscope System for Optimal Positioning (AESOP) (Computer Motion, Goleta, CA) is designed specifically for holding and manipulating the laparoscope and incorporates an active mechanical arm with six DOF that is directly attached to the operating room table. The AESOP robot is manipulated using a foot or hand control or a voice activation system. AESOP can maintain a steady image throughout the entire surgical procedure and can also eliminate the necessity of an assistant surgeon. The primary advantage of the AESOP robot is the excellent 2D image quality that is possible during laparoscopy. With the AESOP robot, the surgeon is less dependent on human second assistants to provide the optimal view during the laparoscopic procedure.

Master–Slave Robotic Systems

With all master–slave systems, the surgeon uses remote controls to move robotic arms operating on the patient; this requires judgment and perception of the sur-

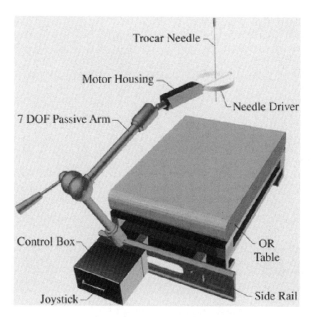

FIG. 133–3. PAKY robot utilized for percutaneous access.

geon, although the operative motions of the surgeon can be enhanced. As such, the goals of telerobotic surgery are a decreased learning curve and increased surgical precision. In particular, master–slave systems enhance surgical performance by filtering physiological tremors and by providing motion scaling. For instance, with motion scaling of 5:1 a movement of 5-mm by the surgeon would result in a 1-mm movement of the end effector.

The Zeus robotic system (Computer Motion) consists of a remote control unit, two robotic manipulator arms, and a camera arm (AESOP robot). Both robotic manipulators are mounted on the operating room table and each can move freely through conventional trocars using a proprietary "free-pivot technology." The standard Zeus robotic manipulators provide four DOF; however, the recently introduced Microwrist instruments provide five DOF (scissors and graspers only). All instruments are reusable and incorporate a durable pull-rod design with a diameter of 3.5 to 5 mm. From a sitting position, the surgeon controls the robotic system by viewing a standard 2D video monitor. At the control panel, the surgeon maneuvers both robotic manipulators with joystick-like controls and controls the AESOP robot (i.e., laparoscope) with a voice activation system. Although the original imaging capabilities with the Zeus robotic system were

2D, a 3D imaging system is now available. A variety of Zeus-specific instruments are available because the designs are easily adapted from conventional laparoscopic instruments. In addition, an effective haptic interface is not available with the Zeus system. Another disadvantage is the high initial capital investment for the robotic system, although the end effectors for the Zeus robotic system are reusable.

The da Vinci robotic system (Intuitive Surgical, Mountain View, CA) also consists of a remote control unit, two robotic manipulators, and a robotic camera arm (Fig. 133–4). All robotic arms are mounted on a portable base that is independent of the operating room table. Each robotic manipulator is attached to the patient via reusable laparoscopic ports, whereas the camera arm is positioned via a standard laparoscopic port. End effectors for the da Vinci system have limited reusability. The end effectors, however, incorporate a proprietary Endowrist technology that provides six DOF plus grip. This mimics the motions of the human wrist with similar up-and-down and side-to-side flexibility. Because of constraints with the Endowrist technology, fewer end effectors are currently available for the da Vinci robotic system. Similar to the Zeus robotic system, control of the entire system is performed with the surgeon sitting at an ergonomic remote control unit. The

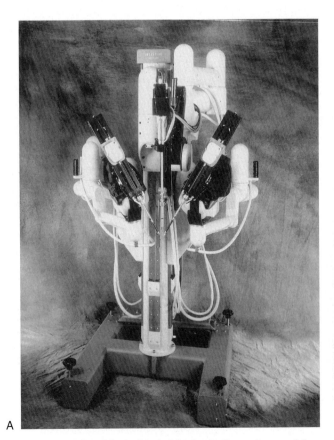

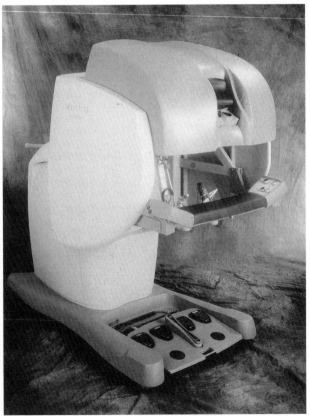

A

B

FIG. 133–4. A: da Vinci robotic system mobile surgical arm unit consisting of camera arm and two robotic manipulators. **B:** Remote control unit.

surgeon holds master grips and controls the movement of the robotic arms by looking into a standard 3D imaging system. Other performance enhancements, similar to the Zeus robotic system, include the capabilities of motion scaling and tremor filtering. Disadvantages of the da Vinci robotic system are lack of an effective haptic interface, occasional problems with installation and positioning of the robot relative to the patient, limitations on instruments designed specifically for urologic applications, impaired direct communication between the surgeon and operating room team, and high initial and individual procedural costs. In contrast to the Zeus robotic system, the end effectors for the da Vinci robotic systems are associated with a predetermined number of "uses." Upon attaching an end effector to the robotic arm, the computer automatically removes a use from the end effector. As such, the individual procedural costs include a proportional cost of the end effectors plus the cost of any required conventional laparoscopic equipment.

TECHNICAL ISSUES

With the recent introduction of advanced telerobotic systems, technical concerns with port placement, installation of the robot, coordination of the operating surgeon and assistants, dissection, and the learning curve have appeared.

1. *Port placement.* Effective port placement is one of the most important aspects of robotic surgery. In general, the laparoscopic ports should be arranged so that the robot is best positioned for the more challenging tasks (i.e., intracorporeal suturing) of the case. With the da Vinci robotic system, for example, the working trocars should ideally be placed at least 7 cm from the camera port to avoid the possibility of intraoperative robotic arm collisions and facilitate intracorporeal suturing. Similar precautions should be taken in trocar and mechanical arm positioning with the Zeus robotic system to assure optimal robotic function. Further, the free pivot technology and the ability to independently position each of the robotic arms can facilitate positioning with the Zeus robotic system. Suboptimal trocar or robotic positioning can make robotic-assisted laparoscopy much more cumbersome than conventional laparoscopy, regardless of the robotic system. When the optimal port position for suturing is less effective for other aspects of the planned procedure (i.e., initial dissection), preparation may be performed with conventional laparoscopic instruments before installing the robot for suturing.

2. *Installation of the robotic device.* Accurate installation of the robotic device can impact the performance of the laparoscopic procedure. As a time-savings measure, the robotic arms of the da Vinci robotic sys-

tem can be sterilely prepared away from the operative field before the patient enters the operating room. Because the robotic arms are independent of the operating room table, the patient should be properly positioned before installing the robotic device. With the Zeus robotic system, these time-savings measures are not possible as the robotic manipulators are directly mounted to the operating room table. Regardless of the robotic system, the mechanical arms of the robot should be installed in such a manner that maximizes the range of motion for all end effectors.

3. *Coordination of the operating surgeon and assistant surgeon.* With telerobotic surgery, the surgeon is positioned remotely from the operating room table. Regardless of the laparoscopic application being performed, the scrubbed assistants are therefore critical to the success of the procedure. After assisting with trocar placement and robot positioning, the scrubbed assistants are responsible for exchange of end effectors on the robotic arms. In addition, the assistants also use conventional laparoscopic instruments for introduction/removal of suture, countertraction, suction, and assistance with hemostasis. The role of the assistant is especially important when nonrobotic laparoscopic instruments are required. Further, the preferential use of conventional laparoscopic instruments may be faster and also more advantageous from a standpoint of cost-effectiveness. Most importantly, the scrubbed assistant is also available in the event that emergent laparotomy is required.

Because of the physical distance separating the surgeon and assistants, intraoperative communication can be impaired. In this regard, the open design of the Zeus remote control unit may be advantageous to the periscope-type design of the da Vinci robotic system.

4. *Dissection.* The commercially available robotic systems were initially developed preferentially for intracorporeal suturing in cardiac surgery. When using the robotic systems for intraabdominal laparoscopy, dissection can sometimes be slower and more cumbersome than standard laparoscopy. Decreased efficiency is influenced by a number of factors, including design of the robotic arms for precise rather than gross movements, difficulty in attaining adequate countertraction to facilitate dissection, limitations with the current availability of surgical instruments for robotic systems, or poor coordination between the surgeon and operative team. In addition, because an effective force-feedback system is not a characteristic of the current robotic technologies, laparoscopic maneuvers with either robotic system requires increased attention to visual rather than tactile cues.

5. *Learning curve of telerobotic systems.* Similar to conventional laparoscopy, a learning curve is also

present with telerobotic surgical procedures; however, the learning curve is thought to be less steep using the robotic technology. Because tactile feedback is extremely limited with both the Zeus da Vinci robotic systems, a learning curve exists with performing surgery preferentially with visual cues. As such, the lack of tactile feedback can contribute to inadvertent tissue damage or inadvertent suture breakage. A learning curve can also exist when using magnified 3D imaging systems, especially for surgeons accustomed to performing conventional laparoscopy using a standard video monitor.

RENAL AND ADRENAL APPLICATIONS

Using the Zeus robotic system, Gill et al. first reported feasibility of laparoscopic telerobotic nephrectomy and adrenalectomy in the animal model (7). In the study, the performance of standard laparoscopic nephrectomy and adrenalectomy was compared to the corresponding telerobotic procedures. The robotic-assisted techniques required longer operative times, but the adequacy of surgical dissection and blood loss were equivalent (7). The initial report of a telerobotic laparoscopic nephrectomy in humans was reported by Guillonneau et al. using the Zeus robotic system (9). The procedure was safely performed with an operative time of 200 minutes and an estimated blood loss of less than 100 cc (9).

Telerobotic laparoscopic pyeloplasty has also been performed clinically and in the animal model (8). In humans, robotic-assisted laparoscopic pyeloplasty has subsequently been described with the da Vinci robotic system and the Zeus robotic system. When patients undergoing da Vinci-assisted laparoscopic Fengerplasty or Anderson–Hynes pyeloplasty were compared to patients undergoing the corresponding procedures without the robot, the da Vinci-assisted procedures were associated with shorter operative times and decreased suturing times (6). Further, the magnitude of improvement was greatest for patients treated with the more difficult Anderson–Hynes repair.

LAPAROSCOPIC PROSTATE APPLICATIONS

Laparoscopic radical prostatectomy (RP) has been performed using the da Vinci robotic system. In an initial experience of five patients, the mean operative time was 222 minutes for the da Vinci-assisted procedures. The researchers concluded the da Vinci robotic system simplified the vesicourethral anastomosis; however, the higher operating room cost was considered a disadvantage (12).

LAPAROSCOPIC BLADDER APPLICATIONS

Building on the clinical experience with da Vinci-assisted laparoscopic RP, Beecken et al. reported the first case of da Vinci-assisted laparoscopic cystectomy and ileal neobladder (1). The procedure was performed with an overall operative time of 510 minutes and estimated blood loss was less than 200 cc. The da Vinci robot was used to facilitate intracorporeal suturing for the urethral anastomosis, construction of the neobladder, and the ureteroileal anastomoses (1). Bowel continuity was reestablished after a minilaparotomy was performed for specimen removal.

Finally, Cho et al. compared the performance of extravesical ureteral reimplantations with or without the Zeus robotic system in an animal model (4). Procedures performed with the Zeus robotic system required significantly more operative time, but all anastomoses were immediately watertight and suturing characteristics were comparable between treatment groups.

FUTURE DIRECTIONS

Despite the recent development in advanced robotic devices, a paucity of information exists regarding the advantages, applicability, and cost-effectiveness of these surgical systems. Similar to other types of advanced technology (i.e., shockwave lithotripsy, laser) that have been introduced to the practice of urology, the clinical benefits must be demonstrated. Future technical modifications will likely improve robotic surgical systems, including an effective haptic interface and improved instrumentation. New types of robotic devices will likely expand beyond the current boundaries, driven by the continued development of nanotechnology and microrobots where robots could be placed into the body and directed to the area of pathology.

Virtual reality will also impact robotic surgery. Because telerobotic surgery is already performed via a video monitor, it is likely that virtual reality simulators will be introduced that allow unlimited life-like instruction and practice for telerobotic surgical systems. In addition, an increased emphasis on the preoperative planning of robotic surgery also appears feasible. In the future, a capability may exist whereby the radiographic images of the patient could be imported to a virtual reality laparoscopic robotics simulator. In this manner, the surgeon or trainees could review and practice the intended surgical procedure in virtual reality, using the patient's 3D images, before the patient even entered the operating room.

Telecommunication may have the biggest impact on robotic surgery. With the current technology, telementoring is an accepted discipline in laparoscopic and endourologic surgery. However, the hurdles of physician licensure for telerobotics and liability must also be resolved before telerobotics can flourish.

Finally, the cost of advanced robotic technology will also need to be addressed in the future. For example, the da Vinci robotic system costs approximately $800,000 and is estimated to cost up to $1,000 for equipment charges for each individual case. With the current rising health care costs, few institutions can afford the routine use of telerobotic surgery in urology. To this end, the benefit of all new advanced technologies should be carefully evaluated.

REFERENCES

1. Beecken WD, Wolfram M, Bentas W, et al. Laparoscopic radical cystectomy and intra-abdominal formation of an orthotopic ileal neobladder: report of the initial case. *Eur Urol* 2003;44:337–339.
2. Bowersox JC, Cornum RL. Remote operative urology using a surgical telemanipulator system: preliminary observations. *Urology* 1998;52: 17–22.
3. Cadeddu JA, Stoianovici D, Chen R, et al. Stereotactic mechanical percutaneous renal access. *J Endourol* 1998;12:121–125.
4. Cho WY, Sung GT, Meraney AM, et al. Remote robotic laparoscopic extravesical ureteral reimplantation with ureteral advancement technique. *J Urol* 2001;165[Suppl]:V640.
5. Davies BL, Hibbard RD, Coptcoat MJ, et al. A surgeon robot prostatectomy—laboratory evaluation. *J Med Eng Tech* 1989;13:273–277.
6. Gettman MT, Peschel R, Neururer R, et al. Laparoscopic pyeloplasty: comparison of procedures performed with the da Vinci robotic system versus standard techniques. *Eur Urol* 2002;1[Suppl]:58.
7. Gill IS, Sung GT, Hsu TH, et al. Robotic remote laparoscopic nephrectomy and adrenalectomy: initial experience. *J Urol* 2000;164: 2082–2085.
8. Graham RW, Graham SD, Bokinsky GB, et al. Urological upper tract surgery with the da Vinci robotic system, pyeloplasty. *J Urol* 2001; 165[Suppl]:V74.
9. Guillonneau B, Jayet C, Tewari A, et al. Robot assisted laparoscopic nephrectomy. *J Urol* 2001;166:200–201.
10. Harris SJ, Arambula-Cosio F, Mei Q, et al. The Probot—an active robot for prostate resection. *Proc Inst Mech Eng* 1997;211:317–325.
11. Ho G, Ng WS, Teo MY, et al. Computer-assisted transurethral laser resection of the prostate (CALRP): theoretical and experimental motion plan. *IEEE Trans Biomed Eng* 2001;48:1125–1133.
12. Pasticier G, Rietbergen JBW, Guillonneau B, et al. Robotically assisted laparoscopic radical prostatectomy: feasibility study in men. *Eur Urol* 2001;40:70–74.
13. Rovetta A. Tests on reliability of a prostate biopsy telerobotic system. *Stud Health Tech Info* 1999;62:302–307.
14. Stoianovici D, Cadeddu JA, Demaree RD, et al. An efficient needle injection technique and radiological guidance method for percutaneous procedures. *Proceedings of the First Joint Conference Computer Vision, Virtual Reality and Robotics in Medicine and Medical Robotics and Computer-Assisted Surgery*, Grenoble, France, 1997:295.

CHAPTER 134

Telesurgery

Michael W. Phelan, Kent Perry, and Peter G. Schulam

Urology has historically been at the forefront when employing technology to advance surgical practice; however, it has been slow to embrace laparoscopy. Arguments against laparoscopy in urology included longer operative times and lack of evidence supporting effectiveness and utility. Moreover, unlike general surgery, urology did not have less challenging, commonly performed cases such as laparoscopic cholecystectomy to advance surgical skills and confidence prior to tackling more advanced cases.

There have been several technological advances that have allowed laparoscopy to become more widely accepted. Improved laparoscopic instrumentation as well as hand-assisted laparoscopic procedures allow surgeons without formal laparoscopic training to perform complex cases by introducing tactile and 3D perception to laparoscopy. The many procedures now commonly performed gives testimony to the current popularity of the technique (Table 134–1).

TABLE 134–1. *Urologic laparoscopic surgery procedures*

Adrenalectomy
Bladder Augmentation
Cystectomy
  Partial
  Radical
Lymphadenectomy
  Pelvic
  Retroperitoneal
Nephrectomy
  Simple
  Radical
  Partial
  Donor
Orchidopexy and Orchiectomy
Prostatectomy
Pyeloplasty
Renal Biopsy
Renal Ablation Techniques
Ureteroneocystostomy
Ureterotomy (Stone Impaction)
Urethropexy
Varicocelectomy

Exponential advances in powerful computers, multimedia programs, telecommunication, and robotic technology parallel advances in minimally invasive surgery. Combining all of these technologies to further advance surgery is the natural extension of laparoscopy. This new discipline, known as telesurgery, integrates laparoscopy, multimedia, telecommunication, and robotic technology to provide surgical care from a distance (1). A widespread definition of telesurgery encompasses teleconsultation, telementoring, and teleproctoring as well as remote surgery. However, the more narrow definition of telesurgery refers solely to the act of remote surgery. The introduction of robotic technology to the existing telesurgery repertoire was the next logical progression of telesurgery. Like its laparoscopic predecessor, the long-term viability of telesurgery will depend upon its ability to improved surgical outcomes.

TELESURGERY

Radiology and pathology were among the first disciplines to employ technology and telemedicine. Due to the relative simplicity of image-only working environments, they were able to provide consultation from remote sites via the Internet. However, the initial long transmission times of these images limited its usefulness due to a lack of bandwidth. With the development of broadband Internet via cable modems and digital subscription lines (DSL), clinical images can now be transmitted in reasonable amounts of time.

In its simplest form, urologists have used telesurgery extensively over the past two decades. The videomonitor in the cystoscopy suite has greatly improved resident education in performing endoscopic procedures. Remote mentoring, the origins of telesurgery, was an easy transition from existing teaching methods.

In the surgical community, broadband development allowed telemedicine to move beyond teleconsultation and proceed to telementoring. Telementoring involves supervising surgery in real time from remote sites, requiring real-time exchange of video and audio images between local and remote surgeons.

However, unlike business videoconferencing, telesurgery is a more complex entity. In telesurgery, there is a real patient whose outcome depends on the skill of the local surgeon. With the existing technology, telesurgery is not a substitute for a competent local surgeon who must have reasonable surgical skills to correct a surgical mishap or complete the surgery if communication breaks down. Telesurgery as it exists today is a tool that can enhance the performance of local surgeons but requires the local surgeon to have the skills necessary to complete the desired procedure. In addition, unlike local telementoring, there is lag time between transmitting/receiving an image. This lag time presents a problem in advising a remote surgeon because an undesirable maneuver may be performed before it can be stopped.

The initial experience with telementoring occurred in 1994 at the Johns Hopkins Hospital in Baltimore. First, the authors performed telementoring from a remote site within the same hospital as the operating surgeons (5,9). These initial successful experiences with telementoring provided proof of concept. The next step in the progression of telemedicine involved mentoring from a physical distance (3.5 miles) with indirect link established with a Trunk-1 (T1) line (4,10). In this series (3) seven successful laparoscopic procedures were performed, including orchiopexy, internal spermatic vein ligation, two pelvic lymphadenectomies, a renal biopsy, and two radical nephrectomies.

The next step in the evolution of laparoscopic telementoring involved proctoring surgery from overseas. The group from Johns Hopkins in Baltimore applied these proven concepts and similar operative links to interact with various groups in Europe and Southeast Asia (6–8). The images were transmitted via three integrated services digital network (ISDN) lines that resulted in a 1-second lag time. However, even with this limitation, the mentoring of less experienced surgeons at great distances occurred without complication.

The next advancement in telesurgery involved the progression from telementoring to the actual surgical procedure being performed by a remote surgeon. Laparoscopic techniques, equipment, and the development of robotic technology have allowed this progression to take place. Remote telesurgery involves utilization of a robotic slave at the remote site acting as a surrogate surgeon. The robotic slave will perform the surgery as instructed by the remote surgeon, the master. The first successful telesurgical procedure occurred in Rome via a link to the Johns Hopkins Hospital (2). In this procedure, successful percutaneous renal access was obtained in Rome by a surgeon in Baltimore.

There remain many technical barriers that have slowed widespread use of telesurgery, specifically image quality and lag time, which are directly related to bandwidth. Bandwidth is defined as the amount of information that can be transmitted over communication lines in a given period of time. In telesurgery the image quality is very important to successfully mentor or perform remote robotic surgery, and with limited bandwidth image quality suffers. With conventional telephone lines it is necessary to compress images for transmission. The compression–decompression process (CODEC) degrades image quality and, in the process, slows transmission rates. Increased errors and frustration occur in task assignments when the lag time increases. The lag time that results from this processing and limited bandwidth presents problems for both telementoring and remote surgery with respect to patient safety and surgical outcomes. With the propagation of improved bandwidth such as DSL, cable modems, and fiber optic networking, faster transmission can be expected. Unfortunately, the improved networks must exist from the site of surgery to the remote surgical station. Frequently, there are technological gaps in the lines that ultimately slow the transmission.

Another fundamental flaw in telesurgery is the potential to drop the signal during the procedure. Loss of signal would be disastrous unless there is an experienced surgeon at the surgical site to take over and perform the surgery. The most reliable system would be a direct high-speed line between remote and local surgical sites. This is difficult and expensive to accomplish. Potentially, satellite communication could eliminate gaps in existing telecommunication lines. However, even with satellite technology the potential to drop a signal would not be eliminated.

Currently, a combination of four ISDN lines at 128 Kb per second each (512 Kb per second send and receive total) are used for a secure point-to-point connection. This results in a reasonable lag time of approximately 400 milliseconds. This time is, of course, somewhat dependent on the distance that the signal must travel at the speed of light. Other more common Internet connection types are also available (Table 134–2). However, these connection types are not point to point and must be routed through multiple points and are not secure. In addition, all of the other Internet connection types—

TABLE 134–2. *Internet connection speeds*

Technology	Max speed (Mb/sec) Send	Max speed (Mb/sec) Receive
56-k Modem	0.056	0.056
ISDN	0.128	0.0128
DSL	1.5*	0.512*
Cable	Highly Variable	Highly Variable
T1	1.544	1.544
Ethernet	10	10
T3	44.736	44.736
OC-3	155.52	155.52
OC-12	622.08	622.08

TABLE 134–3. *Telesurgery definitions*

Bandwidth: Amount of Data Transmitted Over a Line or Channel per Unit Time. Units are Expressed as Bits per Second (bps), Kilobits per Second (Kbps), or Megabits per Second (Mbps). Higher Bandwidth Results in Higher Information-Carrying Capacity.

Broadband: High-Speed, High-Capacity Transmission Channels. Signals Transmitted Over Coaxial or Fiberoptic Lines Rather Than Conventional Telephone Lines.

Cable Modems: Broadband Internet Access Via Coaxial Cable Provided by Cable Television Providers. Bandwidth Equals 2 Mbps.

DSL (Digital Subscriber Lines): Modulation Schemes of Existing Conventional Copper Telephone Wires to Provide High-Speed Internet Connections. Bandwidths Reaching 32 Mbps Possible.

ISDN (Integrated Services Digital Network): International Standard for Transmitting Data Over Digital Telephone Lines. Supports Transfer Rates in Increments of 64 Kbps.

Time Lag: Time Delay Experienced from the Translation of a Local Instruction, Propagation of Instruction Over a Line to a Remote Site, Decoding Instruction, and, Finally, Execution of Instruction.

including DSL, cable modem, T1, and T3—exhibit a degradation of data transmission speed as one moves further from the source to the router. Thus, at this time many places would not be able to reliably utilize one of these faster connection types. Further, these technologies are subject to Internet congestion, which can delay signal transmission significantly. A protocol for these other types of connections to be used as a point-to-point technology is currently being developed; this has the potential to offer very large and secure bandwidth but is not yet available for general use.

Table 134–3 defines common telesurgery terms.

ROBOTIC SURGERY

The initial push to develop robotic surgery was driven by the potential use in the battlefield. In addition to battlefield hazards, surgeons face biohazards such as exposure to human immunodeficiency virus and hepatitis, as well as other contagious diseases. Operating from a remote site with a robotic device would allow some protection to the surgeon and the operating staff in high-risk patients by minimizing direct contact time with an infectious source.

In addition to operating at safe distance from harm's way it was also recognized that robotic surgery could provide benefits over both open surgery and laparoscopic surgery in other ways. In industrial assembly, robots provide precise, reproducible tasks without developing fatigue. These characteristics are certainly desirable in surgery. However, surgery involves very complex maneuvering through variable anatomy. This makes preprogrammed robotic surgery nearly impossible.

In developing robotic minimally invasive surgery, one must improve on the existing laparoscopic technology. Existing laparoscopic instruments are not always comfortable for the surgeon to use. In addition, laparoscopic procedures tend to involve longer operative times. The combination of longer operative times and lack of ergonomic instruments can lead to surgeon fatigue, which in turn can result in less precision, more tremors, and, in general, a less desirable surgical outcome. Robotic surgery may improve on these limitations by providing an ergonomic environment and precise, reproducible movements with the ability to filter tremors without fatigue. In traditional laparoscopic surgery there are limitations that make the learning curve very steep. In addition, the surgical instrumentation for laparoscopy is not as facile as the human hand due to loss of several degrees of freedom. Some of these gaps can be closed with the use of robotic surgery. Robotic surgery provides better dexterity and flexibility than the existing laparoscopic instrumentation. The improved dexterity can be explained with the concept of *degrees of freedom* (DOF). Degrees of freedom is defined as the number of possible movements provided by a joint (Fig. 134–1). If the joints are arranged in a series the DOF is equal to the sum of all the DOFs provided by each joint. For example the elbow (1 DOF), the wrist (3 DOFs), and the shoulder (3 DOFs) allow the human palm to experience 7 DOFs, although only 6 DOFs are really afforded (3). Whereas traditional laparoscopic instruments provide only 4 DOFs, robotic instruments can provide 6 DOFs. The additional DOFs provided by robotic surgery allow the remote surgeon more flexibility in performing tasks and allow more complex maneuvers than standard laparoscopic surgery. These more complex maneuvers may close the gap that exists between standard laparoscopic instruments and the human hand.

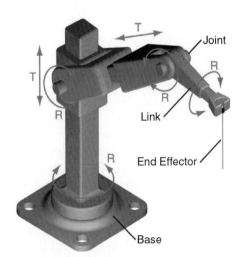

FIG. 134–1. Robotic arm demonstrating concept of degrees of freedom. (From Computer Motion Goleta, CA, with permission.)

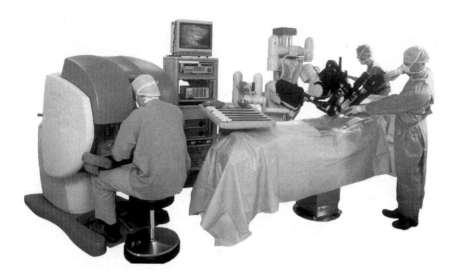

FIG. 134–2. The da Vinci robotic system setup.

The translation of these DOFs takes place through a master–slave system. The master is the surgeon at the remote site. The slaves are the robotic arms that are within the surgical field. The master is seated at a console with his hands attached to a device controlling the remote robotic arms. Software translates the surgeon's hand movements into commands relayed to the robotic arms.

There are certainly benefits that result form the use of robotic surgery. However, this system is not perfect and there are certainly drawbacks. As with any new technological advancement there is a learning curve that must be overcome. Robotic surgery also lacks good tactile sensation. With the current technology robotic surgery is completely performed through visual clues only. Finally, the current surgical robotic equipment is expensive and the start-up cost and service costs may be prohibitive for some hospitals. Longer setup and operative times add substantial costs to the surgical procedure as well as the high cost of the disposal.

The first robotic device to win US Food and Drug Administration (FDA) approval for surgical procedures was AESOP, or *a*utomated commercial *e*ndoscopic *s*ystem for *o*ptimal *p*ositioning (Computers in Motion, Goleta, CA). AESOP functioned initially as a laparoscopic camera holder and later as a retracting assistant. AESOP is very useful while working in confined areas with little movements of the camera. However, AESOP does not move as fast as a human assistant and this may be a disadvantage if frequent camera repositioning is necessary. Another disadvantage of AESOP is the lack of camera rotation.

The HERMES control system is a voice recognition technology. The surgeon prerecords commands onto a voice card and these voice commands are recognized by the HERMES system. In the operating room the surgeon wears a microphone and vocalizes commands to the HERMES system. With the HERMES system the surgeon can control ASEOP, operating lights, the endo-

scope's light source, the insufflator, and the camera printer.

The two most common robotic systems in use for minimally invasive surgery are the ZEUS (Computers in Motion) and da Vinci (Intuitive Surgical, Sunnyvale, CA). These two systems share many similarities in that both employ a remote workstation and hand input devices and use high-quality image projectors. The robotic endoscopic instruments provide additional DOFs, which makes port placement less crucial. With less experienced laparoscopic surgeons this may save on additional unplanned port placements. However, there are several differences in the design of the equipment—such as hand control design, instrument design, and display design—that make the two systems functionally distinct.

The da Vinci consists of a surgeon console or workstation, a 3D monitor, and a patient side cart with robotic instruments. In the da Vinci system the surgeon sits at a remote console (Fig. 134–2 and looks at a 3D image of the surgical field that is transmitted from a dual-lens 12-mm endoscope. Each lens is equipped with its own three-chip digital video camera, which provide the 3D image. With this configuration the camera port must be positioned between the two working ports to generate the stereoscopic image. The master control is designed to accommodate the surgeon's fingers (Fig. 134–3). The da Vinci endoscopic instruments are a modification of the standard instruments. In addition to open and close motions the system allows wrist articulation. The surgeon's hand motions are translated by computer software and carried out by the robotic instruments within the patient. The hand movements can be scaled, which minimizes fatigue and hand tremor. For example, a 5:1 scale will translate 5 mm of movement by the surgeon's hand in 1 mm of robotic arm movement. The da Vinci robotic instruments provide 6 DOFs.

The ZEUS system consists of a surgeon console, computer controller, and three interactive robotic arms (Fig.

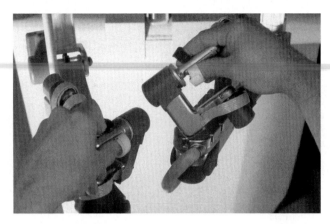

FIG. 134–3. The da Vinci system master control.

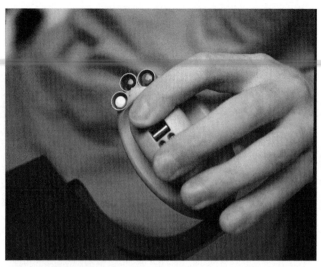

FIG. 134–5. ZEUS robotic system handles. (From Computers in Motion, Goleta, CA, with permission.)

134–4). One of the robotic arms, the AESOP arm, holds a standard laparoscope. The other two robotic arms are modifications of the AESOP and act as the working arms. All three of the robotic arms attach to the rails of a standard surgical table. This allows the surgeon to freely rotate and tilt the table without repositioning the robotic devices. With the use of a standard laparoscope one can be flexible in port placement. In contrast to the immersed display of the da Vinci system, the ZEUS system's display is more like a computer workstation. The surgeon sits in front of a vertical display; a high-definition image magnifies the operative field 10× for the surgeon. The master control is designed to accommodate the surgeon's fingers (Fig. 134–5). With the ZEUS system the surgeon

does not experience stereoscopic vision. Instead, he views the surgical field in the standard 2D laparoscopic view. However, the ZEUS system can provide 3D views if special glasses are worn.

The late 1990s marked the transition from the dream of robotic surgery to the reality of robotic surgery. Robotic surgery has now been used to perform pelvic lymph node dissection, radical nephrectomy, radical prostatectomy, pyeloplasty, and renal transplant.

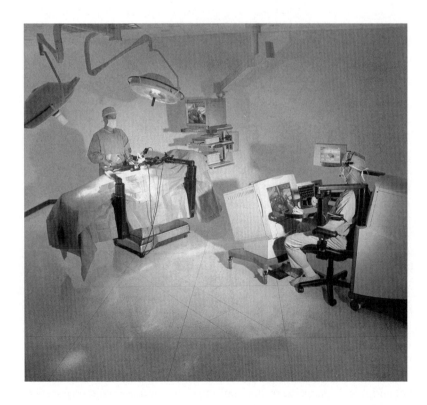

FIG. 134–4. The ZEUS robotic system.

ETHICAL AND LEGAL ISSUES

Patient confidentiality with telesurgery remains a concern. Transmission of medical information and images of actual procedures across the Internet and telecommunication lines exposes patients to potential violations of privacy. Secure lines and encryption devices will aid in minimizing patient exposure, but no system will be foolproof and some patient confidentially might be compromised.

The legal issues surrounding telemedicine are potentially very complex, in particular given the litigious environment in which we must operate in the United States. For example, what is the legal and professional relationship of the remote surgeon to the patient? Who is responsible if a bad clinical outcome results from telesurgery, the remote or local surgeon? Are local surgeons negligent if they are not utilizing remote experts?

Moreover, if surgery or mentoring occurs over state lines or abroad what medical licensures are required? These are questions that have yet to be answered, but if telesurgery becomes more common and more complex procedures are performed guidelines will need to be established. At a minimum, patients must be informed of all the potential problems associated with telesurgery.

REFERENCES

1. Abbou C, et al. Laparoscopic radical prostatectomy with a remote robot. *J Urol* 2001;165:1964.
2. Caddedu J, et al. Stereotatic mechanical percutaneous renal access. *J Endourol* 1998;12:121–125.
3. Caddedu J, Stoianovicci D, Kavoussi L. Robotics in urologic surgery. *Urology* 1997;49:501–507.
4. Cheriff A, et al. Telesurgery consultation. *J Urol* 1996;156:1391–1393.
5. Docimo SG, et al. Early experience with telerobotic surgery in children. *J Telemed Telecare* 1996;2:48–50.
6. Janetschek G, Bartsch G, Kavoussi L. Transcontinental interactive laparoscopic telesurgery between the United States and Europe. *J Urol* 1998;160:1413.
7. Lee B, et al. A novel method of surgical instruction: International telementoring. *World J Urol* 1998;16:367–370.
8. Lee B, et al. International telesurgical: Our initial experience. *Stud Health Tech Info* 1998;50:41–47.
9. Moore RG, et al. Telementoring of laparoscopic procedures: initial clinical experience. *Surg Endoscop* 1996;10:107.
10. Schulam PG, et al. Telesurgical mentoring: Initial clinical experience. *Surg Endoscop*, 1997;11:1001–1005.

CHAPTER 135

Novel Tissue Ablation Technology

Jay T. Bishoff and Steven M. Baughman

Frequent abdominal imaging using ultrasound, computed tomography (CT) scan, and magnetic resonance imaging (MRI) has led to the increased detection of small, incidental renal tumors (10). The resulting stage migration toward lower stage at the time of initial diagnosis has fostered an increased interest in minimally invasive treatments in the kidney. The long-term results established by radical nephrectomy have set the standard of care to which all newer therapies are compared. Nephron-sparing techniques for small tumors have joined radical nephrectomy as safe and effective means of treating small tumors of the kidney (9). Following this recent trend, laparoscopic and ablative procedures have been pursued as treatment options for small renal tumors, especially in patients of advanced age or with significant comorbidities. This chapter discusses novel ablative therapies for management of small renal tumors.

CRYOABLATION THERAPY

Clinical experience with cryotherapy for urologic applications was first gained in prostate cancer therapy, where its use has been complicated by the prostate' proximity to the urethra and rectum. The kidney is better suited for this and other ablative techniques because of its location near the retroperitoneum and surrounding retroperitoneal fat and Gerota's fascia. Further, the tumors that arise within the kidney are often unifocal.

In cryoablation, target tissue destruction is literally achieved through rapid freezing after placing cryoprobes directly into the tumor and cooling with liquid nitrogen or argon to a central, core temperature of less than -180°C. Rapid freezing causes crystal formation in the microvasculature, extracellular spaces, and within the cells, eventually resulting in uncoupling of oxidative phosphorylation and rupturing of plasma cell membranes with subsequent solute shifts. Progressive failure of the microvasculature

The views expressed in this article are those of the author and do not reflect the official policy of the US Department of Defense or other departments of the US Government.

results in endothelial cell damage, edema, and platelet aggregation with thrombosis and vascular occlusion. In an animal model, Chosy et al. demonstrated that a renal tissue temperature of less than -20°C was necessary to create tissue necrosis (3). Temperatures as low as -40°C may be needed for destruction of tumor cells. Despite the low temperatures at the center of the probe, there is rapid warming of surrounding tissue, toward the periphery of the "ice ball." Baust et al. found temperatures to be approximately -40°C 5 to 6 mm inside the edge of the ice ball (1). Based upon these studies, most surgeons extend the ice ball to a minimum of 1 cm beyond the edge of the target lesion.

Percutaneous, open, and laparoscopic approaches have been utilized to deliver cryoablation. Adequate cryodestruction requires intraoperative monitoring of the resultant ice ball that can be performed utilizing ultrasound and thermocouples. On ultrasound the cryoablated region appears hypoechoic and demonstrates loss of normal flow characteristics on color-flow Doppler that closely approximates the size and location of the ice ball. Intraoperative laparoscopic ultrasound is used to monitor the progression of the ice ball, achieve adequate margin, avoid injury to the collecting system, and evaluate the kidney for other possible lesions not apparent on preoperative imaging. Larger lesions (greater than 1 cm) require multiple passes or multiple probes to achieve adequate ablation.

Ideal lesions for cryoablation are small T1 lesions less than 3 cm in size, in particular in patients with solitary kidneys. In our series of eight patients with small (mean, 2.0 cm) renal tumors, the tumors in seven patients were successfully ablated (3). One patient at 9 months follow-up was found to have an enhancing lesion in the area of cryoablation and radical nephrectomy showed a small focus of viable tumor. Similar results were reported by Levin, who performed laparoscopic cryoablation in 39 patients with 1 patient who developed a recurrence at 9 months (10). MRI-guided ablation has also shown a high rate of success (14). The results of reported series are shown in Table 135–1. These series are all small and there

TABLE 135–1. *Summary of cryoablation series*

Senior author/reference	No. of patients	No. of lesions	Mean tumor diameter (cm)	Mean OR time (min)	Ablation time	Mean EBL (cc)	Mean probe temp.	Hospital stay (d)	Follow-up	Recurrence
Uchida. *Br J Urol* 1995;75:132	2 (Both with Advanced Disease)	2	NR	NR	Single 22 min	NR	−20°C	NR	CT	Both Died of Metastatic Disease
Dalworth. *J Urol* 1996;155:252	2	3	4.3	240	NR	450	−180°C	5	MRI or CT at 1–3 mo	10% enlargement of AML at 3 mo
Gill. *Urol* 1998;52:543	10	11	1.9	135	Double Freeze 13 min	75	−186°C	<<1	CT or MRI	Biopsy Negative
Zegel. *J Ultrasound Med* 1998;17:571	6	14	NR	NR	7–15 min	NR	−180°C	NR	CT or MRI	None 3–22 mo postoperative
Bishoff. *J Endourol* 1999;13:233	8	8	2.0	210	Single 15 min or Double 5 min	140	−180°C	3.5	CT at 5 mo	None
Rodriguez. *Urol* 2000;55:25	7	7	2.2	234	15 Minutes Double or Single	111	−180°C	4.4	14 mo	None
Gill. *Urol* 2000;56:748	32	34	2.3	170	15 min	67	−185°C	<<23 h	MRI/CT Guided Biopsy	None at 16 mo
Remer. *Am J Radiol* 2000;174:635	21	23	<<4 cm	NR	NR	NR	−180°C	NR	MRI	None at 6 mo
Rukatalis. *Urol* 2001;57:34	29	29	2.2	NR	Double Cycle	150	−140°C 180°C	3	CT/MRI	1/29
Shingleton. *J Urol* 2001;165:773	20	22	3	97	Triple Cycle	NR	NR	<<23 h	MRI	1 Patient at 9 mo
Kim. *J. Urol* 2002;167:1	12	12	2.2	NR	Double Cycle	60	NR	3.25	CT	2/12 Biopsy Proven at Mean 305 d

NR, not reported; EBL, estimated blood loss.

is, in general, short-term follow-up such that any definitive conclusions will require larger prospective studies.

Potential complications of cryosurgery include urinary fistula formation, posttreatment hemorrhage, and injury to adjacent structures to include the collecting system, bowel, and liver. Even brief contact of the cooling cryoprobe to surrounding structures can lead to necrosis and fibrosis. In our animal studies, we noted severe adhesions between cryoablated kidney and overlying bowel in non-retroperitonealized kidneys, although without any evidence of bowel injury or fistulas (3).

THERMAL ABLATION

Radiofrequency Interstitial Tissue Ablation

Radiofrequency ablation (RFA) has been utilized in a number of different clinical applications, ranging from cardiac dysrhythmias to primary and metastatic liver lesions, as well as tumors of the nervous system and bone. Urologists have used this technology to treat benign prostatic hypertrophy (BPH) through a transurethral approach and prostate cancer through a transperineal approach. The radiofrequency (RF) energy can be intro-

duced percutaneously, laparoscopically, or through an open approach using ultrasound, fluoroscopic, CT, or MRI guidance (Fig. 135–1). The RF energy returns to the RF generator via a series of skin grounding pads that complete the electrical circuit. The probe carries an alternating current of high-frequency radiowaves that causes the local ions to vibrate, and the resistance in the tissue creates heat to the point of desiccation (thermal coagulation). Microscopic examination immediately after RFA reveals intense stromal and epithelial edema with marked hypereosinophilia and pyknosis. This is replaced in the matter of days to weeks by coagulative necrosis with concentric zones of inflammatory infiltrate, hemorrhage, and fibrosis (17).

Precise control of the lesion size can be achieved by temperature-based or impedance-based monitoring. Temperature-based systems depend upon thermocouples imbedded within the tips of the electrodes. Sufficient amounts of RF energy (10 to 90 W) are applied to raise the tissue temperature to the minimum 60°C required to induce coagulative necrosis. However, temperatures recorded at the periphery of the ablation area have been found to be 20 to 30°C cooler than temperatures recorded at the thermocouples. For this reason, some authors favor

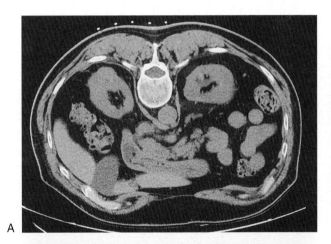

A

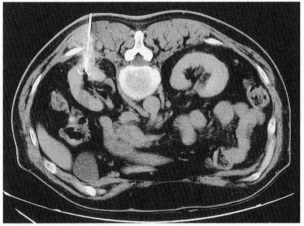

B

C

FIG. 135–1. A. Preradiofrequency amblation. **B.** Needle electrode placed into renal mass and deployed. **C.** Post ablation CT shows no enhancement in area of radiofrequency treatment.

TABLE 135–2. *Summary of radiofreqnency ablation series*

Senior author/ reference	No. of patients	Lesions ablated	Tumor size (cm)	Mean OR time	RFA time	Mean EBL (cc)	Probe temp.	Hospital stay	Mean follow-up	Recurrence
J Endourol 1998;11:251	3	3	3,2.5,5	NR	12 min	NR	NR	NR	1 Week CT	NR
Radiology 2000;217:665	8	9	3.3	NR	12 min	NR	NR	NR	10.3 mo	5 Lesions Have XXXX Enhancement
Walther. *J Urol* 2000; 163:1424–1428	4	14	NR	NR	Single 5 min or Double 5 min	NR	Tissue temperature 60°C	NR	NR	No Metastasis in Tumors << 3
Pavlovitch. *J Urol* 2002;167:10	21	24	2.4	NR	Double 10–12 min	NR	70°C	<<24 h	2 mo	None
Revidon. *J Urol* 2001;166:292	10	11	2.4	NR	17 min	NR	NR	<<24 h	Nephrectomy Performed After RFA	64% Had Residual Tumor After Removal of Kidney
Su. *J Urol* 2002; 167:1424(abst)	17	22	2.0	NR	NR	NR	NR	NR	3.2 mo	1/22 Had Enhancement at 3 mo

NR, not reported; EBL, estimated blood loss.

an impedance-based system, which applies RF energy until the tissue becomes sufficiently desiccated as to become an insulator. In this manner, the flow of RF energy back to the return pad is blocked, causing a gradual decrease in tissue impedance that suggests that the thermal lesion is continuing to evolve; a rise in impedance (to approximately 200 Ω) suggests that the tissue is desiccated and that further thermal lesion growth is unlikely.

While ultrasound, fluoroscopy, CT, and MRI have all been used for patient positioning and for percutaneous placement of the RFA probe, none of these modalities has proven reliable for the intraoperative monitoring of the RFA lesion. On ultrasound imaging, there is no immediate change in the echotexture in the area of RFA, and color and power Doppler are of no added benefit secondary to variable and inconsistent findings. Moreover, RFA can sometimes disturb ultrasound imaging. In a series of animal experiments, we found CT to be excellent for positioning of the patient and probe and for immediate posttreatment imaging, but it was not helpful for intraoperative monitoring (4). Lewin et al. used MRI to monitor real-time tissue destruction during RFA. This group demonstrated a zone of decreased signal surrounded by a rim of hyperintensity on T_2-weighted and STIR (turbo *s*hort inversion-*t*ime *i*nversion *r*ecovery) images. However, confirmatory images obtained after conclusion of the ablation session revealed a propensity for these T_2-weighted images to underestimate the size of the RF lesion (12). Thus, insofar as intraoperative monitoring for RF is concerned, there is no imaging modality that can ensure a sufficient extent of tissue ablation in real time while avoiding injury to normal, adjacent parenchyma.

The clinical efficacy of RFA on renal tumors has been reported in several series (Table 135–2). Walther et al. explored 14 tumors less than 5 cm in four patients with multiple renal lesions and performed RFA just prior to surgical excision. Complete immediate treatment effect was noted in 10 of 11 patients; in the final case, only 35% of the tumor was ablated, without any discussion by the authors to explain this exception (17). Excluding any technical inconsistencies, as with the early results of cryoablation, early treatment failure needs to be put into the context of long-term, prospective clinical trials. While the current short-term data are encouraging, only long-term follow-up will determine the ultimate place of RF in treating renal tumors.

MICROWAVE TISSUE COAGULATION

Tissue absorption of microwaves (30 to 3,000 MHz) results in increased temperatures through production of kinetic energy and heat. Probes placed directly into the target tissue increase temperatures according to the frequency used, time of application, and the inherent properties of the tissue being ablated. Urologic applications include the treatment of benign prostatic hyperplasia and renal tumors. In the kidney microwave tissue coagulation (MTC) has been used clinically to assist with hemostasis during partial nephrectomy. In four patients, Maito et al. inserted a MTC needle probe into the kidney during partial nephrectomy without vascular occlusion. Using microwaves generated at 2,450 MHz, 15 to 20 areas around the mass were treated with MTC and the tumor excised. Tumor extirpation without significant bleeding was accomplished in all four cases. In one case a positive surgical margin prompted radical nephrectomy (13). No patient in this small series had delayed bleeding or urinoma formation. Future advances in determining the ideal settings, cycles, and ablation times may allow use of microwave coagulation technology to perform extensive resection of renal tissue with minimal blood loss and avoid warm ischemic injury to the kidney.

INTERSTITIAL LASER THERMOABLATION

Laser ablation of target tissue using one or several laser fibers has been described in the treatment of head and neck, liver, brain, and kidney tumors as well as treatment of benign hyperplasia of the prostate and uterine fibroids. Using MRI-guided interstitial laser thermoablation (ILT) De Jode et al. treated kidney tumors in three patients. Laser energy from a neodymium:YAG source was percutaneously delivered to the tumors under real-time MRI guidance in an open-access scanner. Follow-up gadolinium-enhanced MRI confirmed necrosis in the target tissue. One patient showed areas of enhancement consistent with viable tumor and underwent an additional ablation of the enhancing areas (5). Additional investigation is needed to determine the ultimate use of lasers in tissue ablation.

HIGH-INTENSITY FOCUSED ULTRASOUND

For over a half a century the biologic effects of high-intensity focused ultrasound (HIFU) have been known. In modern clinical medicine, it has been used in the treatment of glaucoma and as an alternative therapy for BPH and prostate cancer (6). By focusing ultrasound waves in a very narrow focal zone, high-intensity ultrasound fields may be created. Temperatures as high as 65°C can be generated by a pulse wave of only 5 seconds. Tissue at the focal point is ablated while superficial layers are in general spared. Unlike RFA, the tissue destruction is almost instantaneous—an ablative intensity of 1,500 W/cm^2 for 1 second will produce a lesion roughly 0.5 cm^2 per exposure.

HIFU causes tissue destruction by five mechanisms: thermal effects, cavitation, mechanical forces, chemical reactions, and accelerations. Cavitation refers to the development of a shock wave that occurs when a rapidly formed bubble suddenly collapses (the basic principle behind ESWL). Thermal effects and cavitation are the predominant forms of tissue ablation in HIFU. The same physical considerations that are required for diagnostic ultrasound imaging also apply here: A fluid or soft-tissue path is necessary for the propagation of the soundwave with the absence of bony or gaseous obstructions. Like ultrasound, the technique is completely noninvasive, obviating the need to access the kidney percutaneously or surgically.

There are three main features of HIFU that make lesion creation unpredictable: (a) Cavitation itself is a phenomenon whose effects are difficult to predict; (b) the high acoustic pressures induced by HIFU create nonlinearity of the propagated soundwave; (c) the preexistence of one thermal lesion may perturb the intended placement of subsequent lesions, the so-called "lesion–lesion interaction."

There are limited reports of clinical use of HIFU for the treatment of renal tumors. Susani et al. treated healthy tissue and renal tumors in two patients prior to radical nephrectomy. They found necrosis of tumor in the ablated areas at the time of harvest (15). Vallancien et al. treated kidney tumors in eight patients, resulting in coagulation necrosis at the site of ablation. No subcapsular or perirenal hematomas were seen and there was no evidence of renal pelvis or ureter injury. However, several patients suffered second- and third-degree skin burns (16). Kohrmann et al. reported using HIFU in 24 patients immediately prior to nephrectomy. In 19 of 24 cases hemorrhage and necrosis was discovered macroscopically (7). More recently the same investigators reported the use of HIFU to treat three different tumors in a single patient. Each lesion was treated on three different occasions approximately 30 days apart. Three months after the last treatment session an MRI showed significant regression in two tumors, while one tumor in the upper pole of the kidney appeared unaffected. The authors attributed the failure to absorption of the ultrasound energy by interposed ribs (8).

Although HIFU by its nature is prepared for real-time monitoring of evolving tissue changes during treatment, the ablative lesion cannot be reproducibly imaged during the procedure. Accurate delivery of HIFU is limited by movement during respiration and blocked by ribs and other bony structures. There are no temperature sensors in the tissue to ensure that all portions of the target lesion reach temperatures sufficient for tissue necrosis. As a minimally invasive technique, HIFU holds great promise, but full realization is currently limited by adequate visualization of the target tissue and destructive lesion, thermal injury to the skin, and its unpredictable effect on tissues.

INTERSTITIAL PHOTON RADIATION ENERGY

Using radiation as the energy source, this technology also uses the basic mode of thermotherapy to ablate tissue. The photon radiosurgery system (PRS) delivers precise, focused, and controllable local radiation therapy without exposing intervening layers of tissue. In contrast to RFA, PRS may not be as sensitive to the dissipating effect of vascular flow and as such may be effective in ablating tissue near the renal hilum.

Chan et al. reported a PRS feasibility trial in a canine model. Through a midline laparotomy, 12 mongrel dogs received photon radiation to the left lower pole kidney and right hilum with 15 Gy at a radius of 1.3 cm for 10 minutes, resulting in a 2.5-cm lesion. Histopathologic examination revealed coagulation necrosis, gradually replaced by organizing necrosis and fibrosis (2). To date there no clinical or human trials where renal tumors are ablated with PRS. One would expect this technology, like RF and HIFU, to be similarly limited in its ability for real-time monitoring of the ablative lesion.

CONCLUSION

Feasibility studies in animal and human models and a few clinical trials document that novel ablative technologies can be safely applied to the treatment of small renal lesions. What remains of great concern is the long-term success of these technologies as alternatives to definitive and established surgical cancer treatments. Open nephron-sparing surgery enjoys the endorsement of numerous clinical trials with sufficient long-term follow-up to document its equivalent safety and efficacy compared to radical nephrectomy in the treatment of small renal tumors. Prospective clinical trials that would yield a similar endorsement for ablative technologies are ongoing, but have not yet achieved the same status as radical nephrectomy or nephron-sparing techniques.

Given the uncertain nature of these incidental lesions (benign or malignant), precise pathologic diagnosis is critical for determining appropriate clinical and radiographic follow-up. Most ablative techniques do not permit the collection of tissue specimen after treatment in all patients. Although most of the clinical trials perform renal biopsy prior to ablation, Dechet et al. has shown that renal biopsy can be fraught with inaccuracies, with 26% of the biopsies reported as nondiagnostic and 16% biopsies of malignant tumors reported as benign (18). To determine the long-term efficacy of new technologies precise pathologic diagnosis is critical.

The precise anatomic characteristics that are amenable to ablative techniques (lesion size, location within the kidney, proximity to the renal hilum and collecting system) have not been clearly defined. Similarly, limited data exist on the propriety of using ablative techniques for the treatment of complex cystic lesions that may harbor cystic renal cell carcinoma. These minimally invasive ablative techniques with novel energy sources await the support of clinical trials that demonstrate rates of local

tumor recurrence and long-term survival comparable to nephron-sparing surgery and radical nephrectomy, whose success has already been established.

REFERENCES

1. Baust J, Gage AA, Ma H, Zhang CM. Minimally invasive cryosurgery: technological advances. *Cryobiology* 1997;34,373–384.
2. Chan DY, Koniaris L, Magee C, et al. Feasibility of ablating normal renal parenchyma by interstitial photon radiation energy: Study in a canine model. *J Endourol* 2000;14:111–116.
3. Chosy SG, Nicety SO, Lee FT. Thermosensor-monitored renal cryosurgery in swine: predictors of tissue necrosis. *J Urol* 1996:157:250.
4. Crowley JD, Shelton J, Iverson AJ, Burton MP, Dalrymple NC, Bishoff JT. Laparoscopic and computed tomography-guided percutaneous radio-frequency ablation of renal tissue: acute and chronic effects in an animal model. *Urology* 2001;57:976–980.
5. De Jode MG, Vale JA, Gedroyc WM. MR-guided laser thermoablation of inoperable renal tumors in an open-configuration interventional MR scanner: preliminary clinical experience in three cases. *J Magn Reson Imag* 1999;10:545–549.
6. Hill CR, ter Haar GR. Review article: High intensity focused ultrasound—potential for cancer treatment. *Br J Radiol* 1995;68:1296–1303.
7. Korhmann KU, Michel MS, Back W. Non-invasive thermoablation in the kidney: first results of the clinical feasibility study. *J Endourol* 2000[Suppl 14]:A34(abst).
8. Kohrmann KU, Michel MS, Gaa J, et al. High intensity focused ultrasound as noninvasive therapy for multilocal renal cell carcinoma: case study and review of the literature. *J Urol* 2002;167:2397–2403.
9. Lau W, Blute ML, Spotts B, et al. Matched comparison of radical nephrectomy versus nephron sparing surgery for renal cell carcinoma with a normal contralateral kidney: Long term follow up. *Mayo Clin Proc* 2000;75:1236–1242.
10. Lee CT, Katz J, Shi W, et al. Surgical management of renal tumors 4 cm or less in a contemporary cohort. *J Urol* 2000;163:730–736.
11. Levin HS, Meraney AM, Novick AC, et al. Needle biopsy histology of renal tumors 3–6 months after laparoscopic renal cryoablation. *J Urol* 2000;163:S682, 153(abst).
12. Lewin JS, Connell CF, Duerk JL, et al. Interactive MRI-guided radiofrequency interstitial thermal ablation of abdominal tumors: Clinical trial for evaluation of safety and feasibility. *J Magn Reson Imag* 1998;8:40–46.
13. Maito S, Nakashima M, Kimoto Y, et al. Application of microwave tissue coagulation in partial nephrectomy for renal cell carcinoma. *J Urol* 1998;159:960–962.
14. Shingleton WB, Sewell P. Renal tumor cyroablation utilizing interventional magnetic resonance imaging. *J Urol* 2000;163:S689, 155(abst).
15. Susani M, Madersbacher S, Kratzik C, et al. Morphology of tissue destruction induced by focused ultrasound. *Eur Urol* 1993;23:34–37.
16. Vallancien G, Harouni M, Veillon B, et al. Preliminary results of a phase I dose escalation clinical trial using focused ultrasound in the treatment of localized tumours. *Eur J Ultrasound* 1999;9:11–15.
17. Walther MM, Shawker TH, Libutti SK, et al. A phase 2 study of radiofrequency interstitial tissue ablation of localized renal tumors. *J Urol* 2000;163:1424–1428.
18. Dechet CB, Zincke H, Sebo TJ, et al. Prospective analysis of computerized tomography and needle biopsy with permanent sectioning to determine the nature of solid renal masses in adults. *J Urol* 2003;169(1):71–74.

CHAPTER 136

Tissue Sealing and Hemostasis

Eugene L. Park and Sanjay Ramakumar

Techniques for wound management have been around as long as there have been wounds. The ancient Egyptians recognized the hemostatic properties of raw meat for traumatic wounds. Medicine men of Native American tribes understood wound packing, suturing, healing by secondary intention, and cautery on bleeding vessels (1).

In the modern era, surgical methods of hemostasis start with physical compression or ligation. This includes simple methods such as direct pressure, suture ligation, and packing, to more complex compression devices, hemostatic clips, and stapling devices. These methods provide both a physical barrier to blood loss as well as permitting the body's own coagulation cascade to take effect.

Urology has its own particular hemostatic problems, and the retroperitoneum does not contain bleeding well once violated. The partial nephrectomy is a procedure that lends itself to innovation. Open procedures allow hypothermia and clamping of the renal hilum, or manual compression by an assistant. The traditional method for achieving hemostasis is placement of transcapsular U-shaped sutures across the parenchyma. As minimally invasive techniques are applied to more and more urologic procedures the hemostatic systems and instruments need to meet the particular requirements of the specialty. With laparoscopy, the technical challenges can be intimidating, and advanced laparoscopic skills are necessary for suturing. Laparoscopic compression devices have ranged from kidney tourniquets to cable ties and compression tapes, and though these techniques may be feasible they are not yet been widely used.

While advances in instrument engineering will likely improve traditional systems, future techniques will build on this and several other modalities: energy sources, coagulation enhancement, and tissue adhesives.

ENERGY SOURCES

Electrocautery is a near universal energy source in surgery for dissection and hemostasis. The generator can be adjusted for coagulation, cutting or blended mode at differing power settings. Cutting current is high-frequency electrical current that disintegrates cells at the wound edge. Mild thermal injury occurs locally and small blood vessels are thrombosed. Coagulation current results when the oscillation is dampened, and hemostasis occurs without cutting. The cells are rapidly desiccated, and the neighboring vessels coagulate. Current can be applied in monopolar or bipolar mode via a variety of tools including scissors, blunt or hook electrodes, or forceps.

Safety starts with controlling the entry and exit points of the current. Proper large area grounding is of primary importance. The active electrode can harm adjacent organs by unintentional direct contact, or contact with another conductive instrument. Proper insulation and energy settings can circumvent capacitative coupling injuries, where the current jumps insulation or gaps. The Ligasure Vessel Sealing System (Valleylab, Boulder, CO) is an electrosurgical unit which forms a seal dubbed an autologous clip, effective for vessels up to 7-mm in diameter. The energy fuses the vessel walls together, forming a permanent bond. It has been applied to cystectomy, prostatectomy, and laparoscopic assisted nephrectomy successfully.

A newer electrosurgical unit is PlasmaKinetic Tissue Management System (Gyrus Medical, Inc., Maple Grove, MN) which offers improvements in hemostatic control over traditional electrosurgical instruments. The system can be utilized as an open surgical tool, resectoscope, or endoscopic probe via a 5F working channel. Delivering bipolar energy used as easily as monopolar instruments, it provides more reliable hemostasis by forming an ionized plasma corona around the active zone of the device. This localized energy causes tissue vaporization which is immediately washed away by irrigation. The degree of local energy control allows procedures such as transurethral resection of the prostate to be performed with normal saline irrigation. With minimal concern for

TUR syndrome, larger glands can be treated transurethrally. When used for hemostasis, vessel sealing capabilities are touted to be up to 7 mm.

Argon beam coagulation is a form of electrocautery providing thermal coagulation of tissue surfaces without direct contact. The system uses a stream of argon gas, an inert noncombustible element, to blow away blood from the surface while monopolar current is applied. This forms a plasma beam that is especially suited for hemostasis of surface bleeding with a typical coagulation depth of 1 mm to 2 mm, and a maximal depth of 3 mm to 4 mm under good control. It has been applied to urologic surgery in open, endoscopic and laparoscopic cases. Particular precautions should be taken in laparoscopy because of the gas flow rates as high as 4 L/min. Careful monitoring of insufflation pressure by the surgeon is necessary with manual venting as needed. Pressure release safety valves can be applied to laparoscopic ports as well.

Ultrasonic cutting and coagulating devices were reported for surgical use since the 1970's2. The Ultracision Harmonic Scalpel by (Johnson & Johnson, Somerville, NJ) is widely available for cutting and sealing tissues. High frequency vibration (55.5 kHz) causes friction, heating and denaturing proteins with thermal destruction of tissue. The power settings vary the amplitude of the excursion from 50 microns to 100 microns, with the lower setting yielding more thermal coagulation, and the higher more tissue cutting. It is approved for vessel sealing up to 3 mm to 4 mm, however good technique may be effective for larger vessels. The control and therefore the safety margin is much better that with traditional monopolar electrocautery, although thermal injury is still possible. Multiple centers have reported successful experience with the device, including for such procedures as laparoscopic partial nephrectomy. The Cavitron Ultrasonic Surgical Aspirator (Valleylab) is more specific for fine dissection. It provides tissue fragmentation, irrigation, and aspiration in procedures requiring precise tissue removal. It has been applied to urosurgical animal models, however its clinical use in urology has been limited.

Various laser sources ranging from argon, CO2, Nd:YAG, Ho:YAG, Er:YAG, KTP, and tunable dye have been utilized in surgery. Laser light is monochromatic, that is being emitted in a single wavelength, and coherent with the light waves in phase and parallel with each other.

Argon lasers emit blue-green light (488 nm to 514 nm) that is absorbed by hemoglobin and transformed to heat. The result is a superficial thermal coagulation. CO2 lasers emit at 10,600 nm, and this is strongly absorbed by water. Due to the high water content of most tissues, the generated steam and carbonization of water has a very shallow depth of penetration. Neodymium-Yttrium Aluminum Garnet Lasers emit in the infrared range (1060nm), and penetrates better than CO2 and argon lasers. The holmium-YAG laser has a wavelength of 2.1 nm and is highly absorbed by water. It causes a minimal amount of thermal coagulation and necrosis, and can cut and ablate tissues easily. The erbium-YAG laser (2.94 nm) is extremely shallow in its penetration, allowing for highly precise control. The potassium-titanyl-phosphate (KTP) laser (0.532 nm) is absorbed by red and black pigments, and is absorbed by hemoglobin and melanin. It is a superficial photocoagulator up to a depth of 2 mm. The tunable dye laser (577 nm) has been used successfully in treatment of port-wine stains.

The use of lasers in urologic surgery specifically for tissue sealing has been for laser welding(4). Laser light is absorbed by tissue pigments, water, or protein solders to produce thermal destruction and alteration. It is thought that extracellular matrix proteins such as collagen and fibrinogen are initially affected, succeeded by alteration in electrostatic and covalent bonding between structural proteins. Various studies examined success with vasovasostomy, hypospadias repair, bladder and ureteral repair with favorable results(4).

TISSUE ADHESIVES

Tissue adhesives are being developed and used for adjuncts or in place of traditional hemostatic methods. Informally called glues, these substances represent an area of intense scientific examination.

Cyanoacrylates, first described in 1940s, are the basis for many super glues however they are not useful surgically. Short chain forms such as methyl alpha-cyanoacrylate and polymethacrylate caused acute and chronic inflammation, rapid tissue necrosis, and extensive adhesion formation. This intense necrotizing reaction makes it unsafe for internal use. Longer chain molecules such as hexyl-, octyl and decyl-cyanoacrylates appear less toxic and are currently used for skin closure.

Many simple collagen matrices exist for the use of coagulation enhancement. They range from collagen sponges, pads, foams or fibrillar powders, to oxidized regenerated cellulose. Coagulation factors such as thrombin, fibrinogen, specific clotting factors, and calcium have been added to synergize the effect. A representative group of commercial products is listed in Table 136.1.

What will probably enhance current surgical technique the most in the future is the use of tissue glues and sealants. Fibrin glues and polyethylene glycol (PEG)-based hydrogels are two of the most promising.

The basic components of fibrin glues are fibrinogen and thrombin. Thrombin is a specific protease that transforms fibrinogen to fibrin, forming a crosslinked matrix. This is in a sense the natural clotting mechanism purified. Current applications of this technology derive the clotting factors from plasma from bovine, donor human, pooled human and even the patient's own plasma sources.

Fibrin sealant Tisseel VH (Baxter Healthcare Corporation, Fremont, CA) is one commercially available preparation. The indication for use is as an adjunct to hemosta-

TABLE 136.1

Trade names	Type	Source	Mechanism of action	Biodegradation	Application	Indication
Gelfoam[1]	Porcine skin gelatin sponge or powder	Porcine	Clotting cascade	4–6 weeks	Apply sponge with pressure or saturate powder with saline and apply with pressure. Remove excess	Adjunct to hemostasis
INSTAT[2] MCH Microfibrillar Collagen Hemostat	Collagen pad or powder	Bovine	Clotting cascade and platelet activation	8–10 weeks	Apply with pressure and remove excess	Adjunct to hemostasis in surgical procedures
Helistat[3] Helitene[3]	Collagen hemostatic sponge or powder	Bovine	Clotting cascade and platelet aggregation		Straight from package and remove excess.	Sponge or fibrillar form. Adjunct to hemostasis in surgical procedures
Ultrafoam[4] Avitene UltraWrap™	Collagen Hemostatic sponge	Bovine	Clotting cascade and platelet aggregation	<90 days	Cut to area, apply with moderate pressure	Adjunct to hemostasis in surgical procedures
Avitene[4] Avitene UltraWrap™	Collagen hemostatic sheet or flour	Bovine	Clotting cascade and platelet aggregation		Single syringe applicator, remove excess, and compress area	Adjunct to hemostasis in surgical procedures
Surgifoam[5]	Collagen gelatin sponge	Porcine	clotting cascade	4–6 weeks	Cut to size and apply with compression. Remove excess	Hemostasis when conventional methods impractical
Surgicel[6] Fibrillar absorbable hemostat	Oxidized regenerated cellulose (ORC)	Plant	Clotting cascade and platelet activation	7–14 days	Straight from package and remove excess	
CoStasis[6] Surgical Hemostat	Collagen, thrombin, fibrinogen	Bovine, bovine, patient plasma	Coagulum formation, clotting cascade and platelet activation	Few weeks	Draw patient blood and centrifuge. Dual syringe applicator with plasma and thrombin mixture	Vascular anastomosis reinforcement, cancellous bone and capillary bed bleeding
FloSeal[7] Matrix Hemostatic Sealant	Collagen, thrombin	Bovine, bovine	Gel formation at site, clotting cascade	6–8 weeks	Reconstitute 1 syringe and apply, direct compression recommended for heavy bleeding	Adjunct to hemostasis in surgical procedures
Plasmaseal[8]	Human plasma concentrate, thrombin	Patient plasma	Coagulum formation, clotting cascade		Draw patient plasma and centrifuge. Dual chamber applicator with plasma and thrombin	
FibRx[9]	Fibrinogen, Factor XIII, and modified thrombin	Human plasma	Coagulum formation, clotting cascade		Single syringe applicator	
Tisseel[7] VH fibrin sealant	Fibrinogen, aprotinin, thrombin, and calcium chloride	Human plasma, bovine protein	Coagulum formation, clotting cascade		Reconstitute 2 syringes. Dual syringe applicator. Gas sprayer applicator also available	Adjunct to hemostasis in surgical procedures
CoSeal[6]	Polyethylene glycol (PEG) polymer	Synthetic hydrogel	Gel polymerized at site	Within 30 days	Reconstitute 2 syringes. Dual syringe applicator	Vascular anastomosis reinforcement
FocalSeal-L[10] AdvaSeal-S	Peg-based hydrogel	Synthetic hydrogel	Gel polymerized at site	<30 days	Reconstitute 1 syringe, two syringe application	Pulmonary suture line reinforcement, Dural sealant
BioGlue[9]	Bovine serum albumin and glutaraldehyde	Bovine	Adherence		Dual chamber applicator	Vascular anastomosis reinforcement

1. Pharmacia & Upjohn Company, Kalamazoo, MI.
2. Johnson & Johnson Wound Management, Somerville, NJ.
3. Integra LifeSciences Corporation, Plainsboro, NJ.
4. Davol, Inc., Cranston, RI.
5. Ethicon, Inc., Somerville, NJ.
6. Cohesion Technologies, Inc., Palo Alto, CA.
7. Baxter Healthcare Corporation, Fremont, CA.
8. Plasmaseal San Francisco.
9. CryoLife, Inc., Kennesaw, GA.
10. Genzyme Corporation, Cambridge, MA.

sis in surgeries involving cardiopulmonary bypass, and treatment of splenic injuries. Investigational use for a multitude of applications, including partial nephrectomy and ureteral repair, is ongoing. The sealant comes in four separate vials. The freeze-dried sealer protein and fibrinolysis inhibitor solution are reconstituted as the sealer protein solution. The human thrombin is reconstituted with the calcium chloride solution to form the Thrombin Solution. The two solutions are applied with a dual syringe applicator, and the parts are fixed in place for 3 to 5 minutes to ensure adherence to the surrounding tissues. The solidified fibrin glue reaches full strength in about 2 hours.

PEG-based hydrogels are synthetic, nontoxic, water soluble materials not recognized by the immune system. The various formulations are currently indicated to reinforce vascular and pulmonary suture lines, as well as dura mater closure. Their specific swelling and degradation properties are tailored to each application. Current investigation is underway for its application for sealing the cut surface of the kidney to control hemostasis and urinary leakage(6).

AdvaSeal-S (Genzyme Biosurgery, Lexington, MA) is one biodegradable preparation currently being investigated for urologic use. The sealant comes in two vials and a preloaded syringe (Figure 136.1). The vials contain a photoinitiator and some macromer in a powder form in one, and water, fructose and ferrous gluconate in the other. These are reconstituted in a syringe to form the primer solution. The sealant syringe is preloaded with the viscous PEG macromers. The primer is applied first via syringe to promote good adherence. The sealant is applied in an uninterrupted layer over the primed area. A green-light wand waved 1 to 2cm from the sealant delivers light for 40 seconds to photopolymerize the gel in

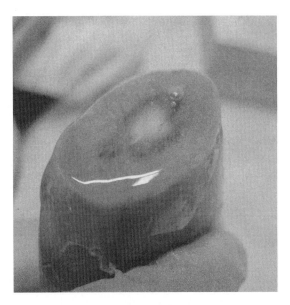

FIG. 136–2.

place. The result is a strong, clear, adherent, flexible matrix that is bioabsorbable (Figure 136.2).

PEG-based hydrogels are being investigated for its hemostatic and tissue sealing potential. Coseal (Cohesion Technologies, Palo Alto, CA) is a PEG-based hydrogel system which has been approved for intraabdominal use as a hemostatic agent.

SUMMARY

Compression, electrocautery, and energy sources have been the mainstay of hemostatic surgical techniques because of availability and effectiveness. Newer generators and delivery systems may increase the ease of use and enhance safety; however there are inherent boundaries to this technology. Improvements in biological glues and sealants are likely candidates to overcome some of the current limitations, especially in the realm of minimally invasive surgery.

The ideal sealant would be safe and effective. Desirable characteristics include biodegradability with minimal inflammatory tissue reaction, safe clearance of breakdown products and low adhesion potential. It is unlikely that any sealant product alone will be effective in controlling massive hemorrhage, but may be effective in combination with existing techniques. The ideal use would be for diffuse hemorrhage, or bleeding from small vessels and organ parenchyma. These sealants will preferably prevent, contain, or minimize urinary leakage as well. It may prove useful in aiding closure of urinary fistulas, or to reinforce a repair of a urinary anastomosis

It should be stressed that newer technology contributes the most benefit by adding to rather than outdating current techniques. It is unlikely that any sealant or glue will

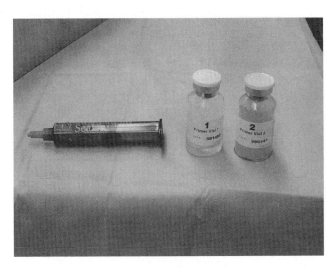

FIG. 136–1.

replace meticulous and proper surgical technique. Future technological developments will undoubtedly contribute to the available tools and methods, and hopefully will improve outcomes.

REFERENCES

1. Stone E. *Medicine Among the American Indians.* New York: Hoeber, 1932;78–79.
2. Hodgson WJ. The ultrasonic scalpel. *Bull NY Acad Med* 1979;55(10): 908–915.
3. Quinlan DM, Naslund MJ, Brendler CB. Application of argon beam coagulation in urological surgery. J Urol 1992;147(2):410–412.
4. Scherr DS, Poppas DP. *Laser Tissue Welding in Urological Surgery.* AUA Update Series, Volume 17, Lesson 22, 1998.
5. Spotnitz, WD, Dalton MS, Baker JW, Nolan SP. Reduction of perioperative hemorrhage by anterior mediastinal spary application of fibrin glue during cardiac operations. *Ann Thorac Surg* 1987;44:529–531.
6. Ramakumar S. Colegrove PM. Nelson JR. Slepian MJ. Photopolymerized PEG-lactide hydrogels: an effective means for hemostasis during laparoscopic partial nephrectomy. *J Urol* 167(4) Suppl: 2.

CHAPTER 137

Tissue Engineering

Ramakrishna Venkatesh and Jaime Landman

With traditional reconstructive techniques, the healing of body tissues is optimized by creating a local microenvironment that is rich in oxygen and nutrients and eliminating hostile factors such as necrotic tissue and debris and reducing the local inflammatory response. Replacement of body structures with tissue engineering techniques is dependent on similar factors. Typically, a scaffolding is provided and efforts are focused on optimizing the local microenvironment to give local viable tissues structural cues for organized growth and differentiation. It is through greater understanding of the normal mechanisms of growth, differentiation, and healing that tissue engineering will address the patient's needs.

The term "tissue engineering" was first used by Wolter and Meyer in 1985 in reference to a corneal tissue prosthesis (20). Specifically, tissue engineering describes the fabrication of functional living tissue in the laboratory using living cells to replace a lost or damaged tissue or organ. Technologies of tissue engineering integrate cell culture, scaffolds, and specific signals (i.e., autocrine and paracrine factors) to create new functional tissues. Successful replacement of native tissues with tissue engineering techniques thus relies on an understanding of the native function of the tissue being replaced, the healing and integration process, and the biology of the local environment.

By tradition, lost or damaged organs or tissues have been replaced by alloplastic prosthetic materials, reconfiguration of innocent and functional local healthy structures (i.e., bowel segments), tissue flaps, or allograft transplantation. The limitations of each of these techniques has placed great interest and hope in the field of tissue engineering.

THE TISSUE ENGINEERING TRIAD

The three basic components of biologic tissues are the cells, the extracellular matrix, and the signaling systems, whose secreted products, through activation of genes, are responsible for cellular proliferation and differentiation. The principles of tissue engineering reproduce natural processes and structures and adopt the laws of developmental biology and morphogenesis. The three key components of tissue engineering are inductive morphogenetic signals, responding stem cells, and the extracellular matrix scaffolding. To date, tissue engineering technologies have typically used an organism's regenerative capacity by providing assistance in the form of a bioabsorbable scaffold with or without cells grown in tissue culture. Recently, there has been considerable interest in the application of stem cells due to their ability to differentiate into different cell types and their great proliferative potential.

TISSUE ENGINEERING STRATEGIES IN THE GENITOURINARY SYSTEM

The development of urogenital biologic substitutes to restore and maintain normal function involves two types of tissue engineering techniques: *in vivo* and *in vitro* technologies. *In vivo* technology is guided tissue regeneration and involves deployment of a biodegradable scaffold without cells into the host, relying on the body's natural ability to regenerate new tissue growth. *In vitro* technology uses biodegradable membranes that are seeded *in vitro* with primary cultured cells derived from a biopsy specimen of the host's native tissue. This composite graft is deployed in the host, relying on the native regenerative capacity for incorporation and continued growth.

Many initial limitations of *in vitro* tissue culture of genitourinary-associated cells have been overcome, and studies over the last decade have indicated that it is possible to harvest autologous urothelial cells and bladder smooth-muscle cells from patients, expand them in culture, and return them to the human or large animals in sufficient quantities for reconstructive purposes (4,16) (Fig. 137–1).

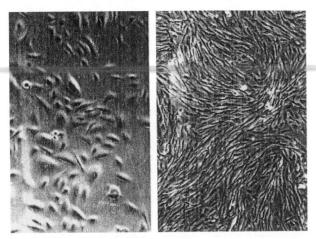

FIG. 137–1. *In vitro* culture of (left) bladder urothelial cells and (right) smooth-muscle cells.

To practically apply cells grown in culture, growth scaffolds are required. The design and selection of the scaffold biomaterials are critical in the development of engineered genitourinary tissues. Scaffolds are structures fabricated from either natural materials like collagen or synthetic polymers (Fig. 137–2). Scaffolds for use in tissue engineering have been designed from three classes of biomaterials: naturally derived materials (e.g., collagen and alginate), synthetic polymers [e.g., polyglycolic acid (PGA), polylactic acid (PLA), and polylactic-co-glycolic acid (PLGA)], and acellular tissue matrices (e.g., bladder submucosa and small intestinal submucosa). The scaffold functions as an artificial extracellular matrix and provides a predefined configuration to the tissue and also promotes the development of new tissues. The tissue-specific function of an engineered material can be maintained by providing an appropriate combination of specific signals (e.g., growth factors) during the process of tissue development. The scaffold biomaterial must be capable of controlling the structure and function of the engineered tissue in a predesigned manner by interacting with transplanted cells and/or host cells. This also provides mechanical support until the engineered tissue has sufficient mechanical integrity to support itself.

Acellular tissue matrices are collagen-rich matrices prepared by removing cellular components from tissues. These matrices have proven to support cell ingrowth and regeneration of genitourinary tissues, including urethra and bladder, with no evidence of immunogenic rejection. The mechanical properties of the collagen matrices are quite similar to that of native bladder submucosa.

ENGINEERING GENITOURINARY TISSUES

Bladder

Clinically, bladder augmentation or replacement is commonly performed using nonurologic tissues such as gastrointestinal segments. However, complications such as infection, metabolic disturbances, urolithiasis, mucus production and plugging, perforation, and malignant transformation have been described. Use of synthetic materials such as porous and nonporous alloplasts for bladder reconstruction is also associated with significant limitations such as stone formation, fibrous capsule induction, and mechanical failures.

Acellular matrix, prepared from allogenic bladder tissue after removing all the cellular components, was used for bladder augmentation following partial cystectomy in rats by Probst and coworkers (15). They reported mucosal regeneration in 10 days and muscle regrowth in 4 weeks following augmentation, with contractile activity to electric and carbochol stimulation. However, there was 26% to 63% incidence of bladder stone formation. Yoo and coworkers showed in their study on supratrigonal bladder augmentation in dogs using allogeneic bladder submucosa that there was a significant increase (100%) in bladder volume in scaffolds seeded with cells compared to scaffolds without prelined cells (30%) (22). Also, the

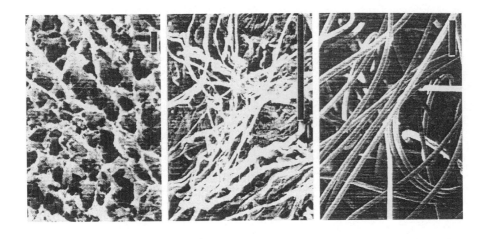

FIG. 137–2. Biomaterials on scanning electron micrography (size of bars=100μm): (left) collagen sponge, (center) acellular matrix from pig bladder submucosa, and (right) polyglycolic acid matrix.

augmented bladders showed normal cellular organization consisting of urothelium and smooth muscle with normal tissue compliance.

Small intestinal submucosa (SIS) is a collagen-based biodegradable thin translucent membrane prepared from pig small intestine by mechanically removing the mucosa and the seromuscular layers. Depending on the mechanism of preparation of SIS, it may also contain growth factors, cytokines, and structural proteins, all of which may facilitate cell migration and cell–cell interaction for growth and differentiation. Kropp and colleagues have shown bladder augmentation using SIS following partial cystectomy in rats produced complete epithelialization in 2 weeks and partial smooth-muscle regeneration of implants occurred by 12 weeks postoperatively (10). At 48 weeks, all three layers of normal bladder were present. They also reported that the regenerated bladder exhibited functional cholinergic and purinergic innervation similar to the normal rat bladder (19). However, *in vitro* studies showed reduction in the maximal contractility of SIS bladder tissue by 50% compared to those of normal bladder tissue. A subsequent study by the same authors in a dog model showed that at 15 months following augmentation similar results were noted in the augmented bladder with normal compliance (10).

Acellular biomaterials for bladder augmentation or substitution produce normal regeneration of urothelial layer but incomplete muscle layer development. However, bladders augmented with the matrix seeded with cells showed a 99% increase in capacity compared with bladders augmented with the cell-free matrix showing 33% increase in capacity. Atala and coworkers showed that composite tissue-engineered structures could be created *de novo* by implanting polymers with human bladder smooth-muscle cells on one surface and urothelial cells on the other surface (2). It has been hypothesized that building a 3D structure *in vitro* prior to implantation would facilitate the eventual terminal differentiation of the cells after implantation *in vivo* and decrease graft contracture due to inflammatory response to the matrix. In a study using a dog model, a trigone-sparing cystectomy and reconstruction with and without a polymer scaffold and also with a polymer with seeded cells was performed (13). At 11 months postoperative evaluation, 95% of the precystectomy volume was preserved in tissue-engineered bladders with preimplanted cells. However, only 22% and 46% of preoperative bladder capacity was maintained in the cystectomy-only controls and polymer-only grafts, respectively. Clinical trials applying the above technology for bladder augmentation are in progress.

Urethra and Ureters

Urethral reconstruction is performed for hypospadias, epispadias, and urethral injuries with stricture formation.

Nongenital skin, local genital skin, or buccal mucosa are commonly used for reconstruction or replacing the urethral tissue. These grafts are associated with complications. Similarly, donor site pain and morbidity are also problematic. PGA tubular scaffolds seeded with cultured urothelial cells implanted into athymic mice resulted in polymer degradation and evidence of tubular urothelial development (3).

Kropp and coworkers compared SIS onlay patch graft urethroplasty to full-thickness preputial skin grafts in a rabbit model (11). Histological evaluation after 12 weeks demonstrated that SIS promoted urethral regeneration with three to four layers of stratified columnar epithelium with evidence of circular smooth-muscle regeneration underneath the urothelium. There was no evidence of diverticulum formation in the SIS group, but all grafts in the preputial skin group had evidence of diverticulum formation. Although long-term studies need to be conducted to determine the clinical applicability of SIS for urethral reconstructive surgery, SIS could prove to be very valuable in cases in which penile skin is not available.

Cultured sheets of autologous urethral epithelium obtained from a biopsy have been used for hypospadias repair in humans. The transplanted cells formed the new urethra with a well-organized epithelium (17). Acellular collagen matrix derived from porcine bladder has proved to be a suitable graft for urethral defects experimentally and clinically. The neourethras created from the matrix demonstrated a normal urothelial luminal lining and organized muscle bundles, without any signs of strictures or complications. Over 60 pediatric and adult patients with urethral disease have been reported to be treated successfully with the human bladder collagen-based matrix (8).

Ureteral reconstruction has been performed by seeding human urothelial cells and smooth-muscle cells onto PGA tubular scaffolds (2). The urothelial cells proliferated to form a multilayered luminal lining and the smooth-muscle cells organized into multilayered structures surrounding the urothelial cells. Shalhav and colleagues performed segmental ureteral replacement with a free biodegradable scaffold without autologous cells in a porcine model (18). A 1.5- to 2.8-cm upper ureteric segment was excised and laparoscopically replaced by a stented (6 Fr double-J stent) tube graft made of acellular matrix prepared from porcine ureters and from minipig SIS. At 12 weeks, all animals had complete ureteric obstruction at the level of graft, although urothelial regeneration was observed in the ureteral segments.

Bioengineered materials have also been used to repair vesicoureteric reflux. Endoscopic injection therapy using injectable chondrocyte–alginate gel for the treatment of vesicoureteral reflux has been clinically investigated. Twenty-nine patients with vesicoureteral reflux were injected with autologous chondrocytes harvested from the patient's ears. At 3 months postprocedure, 79% showed no reflux after one or two injections (5).

Renal Function Replacement

Renal transplantation is currently the preferred method of treatment for end-stage renal disease (ESRD). Major problems associated with renal allograft transplantation are the shortage of suitable organs and the morbidity associated with immunosuppressive therapy. Other problems include chronic allograft failure, operative complications, increased infections, and cardiovascular and bone diseases. The kidney, with its complex structure and function, is a very challenging structure to reconstruct by tissue engineering technology. Bioengineering attempts to either replace isolated kidney function parameters through the use of extracorporeal units or replacement of total renal function by tissue-engineered bioartificial structures are being pursued.

An extracorporeal hemofilter or bioartificial glomerulus has been created with the use of polysulfone fibers with high hydraulic permeability (Fig. 137–3) (7). This property allows for a convective hemofiltration that is predominantly dependent on hydraulic pressure gradient across the membrane. This process is unlike a diffusive movement that is mainly dependent on solute concentration gradient that occurs across conventional hemodialysis membrane. The convective process imitates the normal glomerular process of toxin removal with distinct advantages of increased clearance of higher molecular weight solutes and removal of all solutes up to a molecular weight cutoff at the same rate. The hollow fiber of small caliber is prone for thrombotic occlusion. Lining of the filtration surfaces with autologous endothelial cells expressing anticoagulant factors through gene transfer can minimize clot formation in these hollow fibers. Nondegradable, stable substrate, ProNectin F, is coated inside the hollow fiber surface for seeded endothelial cell attachment. Endothelial cell seeding of the unit resulted in a decrease in the leak rate for albumin; the leak rate was 83% without cells and 3% with endothelial cell coverage. In this prototype, thrombosis resulted in the loss of filtration. However, thrombotic complications may be prevented by transfer of genes that continuously express anticoagulant proteins. Although this experimental unit has a low filtration rate (2.2 mL per min), it has significantly improved selectivity to albumin.

The bioartificial renal tubule model for reabsorbing much volume of ultrafiltrate was designed by applying porcine renal proximal tubular cells lining hollow fibers. Blood was allowed to flow on the outside of the fibers. In this model, active transport properties of sodium, bicarbonate, glucose, and organic anions were demonstrated.

A combination of extracorporeal hemofilter and bioartificial renal tubules in an extracorporeal unit was assessed in acutely uremic dogs (7). It was shown that the levels of potassium and blood urea nitrogen were controlled during treatment with the device. The fractional resorption of sodium and water reached 40% to 50% of the ultrafiltrate volume. This demonstrated the technological feasibility of an extracorporeal assist device reinforced by proximal tubular cells. Immunocompetent cells would be impermeable through the hollow fiber, thereby preventing the rejection of the transplanted cells within the device. Conceivably, this device could be used either extracorporeally or implanted within a patient.

In another attempt at renal reconstruction, Atala and coworkers isolated kidney cells from a rabbit model, performed an *in vitro* cell expansion using traditional tissue culture techniques, seeded these cells on 3D polymer scaffolds, and implanted them subcutaneously into athymic mice (1). The cells proliferated and organized into glomeruli and highly organized tubular structures (Fig. 137–4). The resulting structure produced fluid containing high levels of uric acid and creatinine. These initial results demonstrate that cells derived from the nephron seeded onto a biodegradable polymer and reimplanted into a host animal gave rise to renal tubular structures.

Porcine cells are currently considered the best source for reconstruction of organs for both human xenotransplantation and immunoisolation cell therapy due to anatomic and physiological similarities to human tissue. Animal studies have demonstrated the technical feasibility of this form of cell therapy in the acute uremic state due to ischemic or nephrotoxic renal failure, where replacement of proximal tubule cell function with a cell therapy device would be a logical therapy (7).

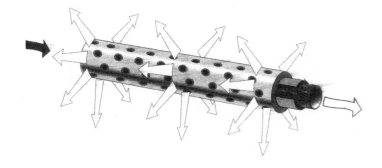

FIG. 137–3. Diagram of a tissue-engineered hemofilter consisting of microporous synthetic hollow fiber, extracellular matrix (preadhered), and a confluent layer of autologous endothelial cells lining the luminal surface of the fiber.

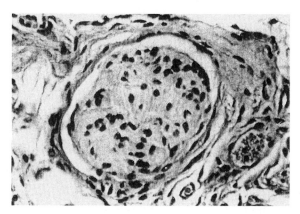

FIG. 137–4. Glomerulus formation in the tissue-engineered renal units (hematoxylin & eosin stain; magnification ×400).

Genital Tissue

Kershen and colleagues described the creation of autologous corporeal tissue for phallus reconstruction (9). Initial experiments in athymic mice have shown that cultured human corporal smooth-muscle cells, obtained by corporal biopsy from individuals during penile surgery, applied to biodegradable polymers can create corpus cavernosum tissue *de novo*. The endothelial cells isolated from corpus cavernosum express functional vascular endothelial growth factor and have the capability to form a 3D capillary network.

Park et al. have shown that human corporal smooth-muscle cells and endothelial cells seeded on biodegradable polymer scaffolds are able to form vascularized cavernosal muscle when implanted *in vivo* (14). Human cavernosal smooth-muscle and endothelial cells seeded on acellular collagen matrices derived from rabbit corpora are able to form vascularized corporal structures *in vivo*. For clinical application, further studies including the cell delivery vehicles and functional and biomechanical studies of the neocorpora must be performed. In a subsequent study, Yoo and coworkers used chondrocytes harvested from rabbit ears to construct a penile prosthesis. The animals did well and could copulate and impregnate their female partners. Further functional studies needs to be done before this can be applied in the clinical setting (23).

Machluf and coworkers have shown in an animal model that isolated Leydig cells encapsulated in alginate/poly-L-lysine microspheres can secrete testosterone. The protective covering prevents the relatively large host immune cells from attacking the cells (12).

STEM CELL AND FETAL TISSUE ENGINEERING

When extensive tissue reconstruction is required, a tissue biopsy from a failed end-stage organ may not yield adequate normal cells for expansion using conventional tissue culture technologies. In this situation use of pluripotent stem cells may be used to create a sufficient quantity of different cell types. Stem cells are able to multiply to a higher degree *in vitro* than fully differentiated cells of specialized tissues. These progenitor cells can be induced to differentiate and function after several generations *in vitro*. They also have the ability to differentiate into many of the specialized cells required to reconstruct a complex tissue.

Once a prenatal diagnosis of a pathologic condition is made, such as bladder exstrophy, a small tissue biopsy could be obtained under ultrasound guidance and expanded *in vitro*. This could then be used at the time of birth for reconstruction. Fauza and coworkers showed in a lamb exstrophy model that the tissue-engineered bladders were more compliant 2 months postoperatively compared to the native exstrophy bladders that were closed without additional tissue-engineered bladder tissue (6).

FUTURE DIRECTIONS

Replacement of lost tissue through tissue engineering has resulted from advances in associated fields of cell biology and material sciences. Currently, clinical trials involving partial bladder replacement using tissue engineering methods are in progress. Tissue engineering techniques for replacement of other urologic tissues may soon have clinical applicability.

Improvements in the understanding of the immune system may allow for implantation of allograft or even xenograft cells to generate functional tissue. Similarly, application of gene therapy technology by transfection of cultured cells with viral and nonviral transducing agents may greatly expand our ability to replace native tissues and organs by manipulation of healing, proliferation, and differentiation processes. Gene therapy also has the potential to allow bioengineered tissues the ability to be resistant to malignancy, ischemia, and perhaps aging.

Current advances in technology are only beginning to reach clinical fruition. However, the limitations of current allograft harvesting will continue to drive interests in producing replacement tissues using bioengineering techniques.

REFERENCES

1. Atala A, Schlussel RN, Retik AB. Renal cell growth in vivo after attachment to biodegradable polymer scaffolds. *J Urol* 1995;153:4.
2. Atala A, Freeman MR, Vacanti JP, et al. Implantation in vivo and retrieval of artificial structures consisting of rabbit and human urothelium and human bladder muscle. *J Urol* 1993;150:608–612.
3. Atala A, Vacanti JP, Peters CA, et al. Formation of urothelial structures in vivo from dissociated cells attached to biodegradable polymer scaffolds in vitro. *J Urol* 1992;148:658–662.
4. Cilento BG, Freeman MR, Schneck FX, et al. Phenotypic and cytogenetic characterization of human bladder urothelia expanded in vitro. *J Urol* 1994;152:665–670.
5. Diamond DA, Caldamone AA. Endoscopic correction of vesicoureteral reflux in children using autologous chondrocytes: Preliminary results. *J Urol* 1999;162:1185–1188.

6. Fauza DO, Fishman S, Mehegan K, et al. Videofetoscopically assisted fetal tissue engineering: Bladder augmentation. *J Pediatr Surg* 1998; 33:7–12.

7. Humes HD, Buffington DA, MacKay SM, Funke AJ, Weitzel WF. Replacement of renal function in uremic animals with a tissue-engineered kidney. *Nat Biotech* 1999;17:451–455.

8. Kassaby EA, Yoo J, Retik A, Atala A. A novel inert collagen matrix for urethral stricture repair. *J Urol* 2000;308S:70.

9. Kershen RT, Yoo JJ, Moreland RB, et al. Novel system for the formation of human corpus cavernosum smooth muscle tissue in vivo. *J Urol* 1998;159[Suppl]:156.

10. Kropp BP. Small-intestinal submucosa for bladder augmentation: a review of preclinical studies. *World J Urol* 1998;16:262–267.

11. Kropp BP, Ludlow JK, Spicer D, et al. Rabbit urethral regeneration using small intestinal submucosa onlay grafts. *Urology* 1998;52: 138–142.

12. Machluf M, Boorjian S, Caffaratti J, et al. Microencapsulation of Leydig cells: A new system for the therapeutic delivery of testosterone. *Pediatrics* 1998;102S:32.

13. Oberpenning F, Meng J, Yoo J, Atala A. De novo reconstitution of a functional urinary bladder by tissue engineering. *Nat Biotech* 1999;17: 149–155.

14. Park HJ, Kershen R, Yoo J, et al. Reconstitution of human corporal smooth muscle and endothelial cells in vivo. *J Urol* 1999;162: 1106–1109.

15. Probst M, Dahiya R, Carrier S, Tanagho EA. Reproduction of functional smooth muscle tissue and partial bladder replacement. *Br J Urol* 1997;79:505–515.

16. Puthenveettil JA, Burger MS, Reznikoff CA. Replicative senescence in human uroepithelial cells. *Adv Exp Med Biol* 1999;462:83–91.

17. Romagnoli G., Luca MD, Faranda F, et al. Treatment of posterior hypospadias by the autologous graft of cultured urethral epithelium. *N Engl J Med* 1990;323:527–530.

18. Shalhav AL, Elbahnasy AM, Bercowsky, Clayman RV, et al. Laparoscopic replacement of urinary tract segments using biodegradable materials in a large animal model. *J Endourol* 1999;13:241–244.

19. Vaught JD, Kropp BP, Sawyer BD, Rippy MK, Badylak SF, Shannon HE, Thor KB. Detrusor regeneration in the rat using porcine small intestinal submucosal grafts: functional innervation and receptor expression. *J Urol* 1996;155:374–378.

20. Wolter JR, Meyer RF. Sessile macrophages forming clear endothelium-like membrane of successful keratoprosthesis. *Trans Am Ophthalmol Soc* 1985;82:187–202.

21. Yoo JJ, Ashkar S, Atala A. Creation of functional kidney structures with excretion of urine-like fluid in vivo. *Pediatrics* 1996;98S:605.

22. Yoo JJ, Meng J, Oberpenning F, Atala A. Bladder augmentation using allogenic bladder submucosa seeded with cells. *Urology* 1998;51: 221–225.

23. Yoo JJ, Park HJ, Lee I, et al. Autologous engineered cartilage rods for penile reconstruction. *J Urol* 1999;162:1119–1121.

CHAPTER 138

Image-Guided Therapy

David Y. Chan and Stephen B. Solomon

Technological advancements have allowed for the development of minimally invasive image-guided therapies for the treatment of urologic diseases. By tradition, imaging served to diagnose and plan surgical interventions. Today, real-time imaging has revolutionized medicine. Image-guided minimally invasive procedures performed on an outpatient basis are now competing with open surgical procedures. The most successful examples of the image-guided therapy include extracorporeal shock wave lithotripsy and brachytherapy for clinically localized prostate cancer. The ability to focus powerful shock waves on a renal calculus has forever changed the management and treatment of urologic stone disease. Similarly, with improved techniques in prostate implantation of radionuclides early cancer control rates for brachytherapy have been reported to be similar to radical retropubic prostatectomy series. These procedures have resulted in more rapid patient recovery, fewer complications, reduced costs, and improved comesis. As technology continues to advance, so will image-guided therapies. Surgeons must continue to understand the availability, advantages, and limitations of these novel techniques (1).

Image-guided therapy is a new frontier. As such, what is novel and en vogue today may be obsolete and history tomorrow. Rather than listing all image-guided therapies currently performed, it is more appropriate and important to understand the basic principles of image-guided therapy: accurate real-time image guidance and effective ablative therapy. Percutaneous renal tumor ablation for the treatment of small renal tumors will serve as an example.

Increased abdominal imaging has resulted in the increase detection of small incidental renal tumors. This has posed a dilemma for many urologists as these small lesions (less than 3 cm) are found in asymptomatic patients. Some of these patients are older, with significant comorbidities, and are not candidates for surgery, while others may not desire surgery.

DIAGNOSIS

Renal masses are often found either during evaluation of hematuria or flank pain or identified serendipitously during routine abdominal imaging. Typically, computed tomography (CT) scan will demonstrate a solid parenchyma mass with heterogeneous density and enhancement after administration of intravenous contrast. A chest x-ray is usually performed to rule out metastatic disease. Bone scan is obtained if patients complain of bony pains, if there is an elevation of serum alkaline phosphatase, or if there is hypercalcemia.

INDICATIONS FOR PROCEDURE

As the efficacy of image-guided therapy for small renal tumors remains to be defined, the indications for percutaneous management of renal tumors continue to evolve. Currently, they include patients with multiple comorbidities that contraindicate traditional open or laparoscopic surgery, solitary kidney, renal insufficiency, congenital malignant syndromes such as Von Hippel–Lindau, and patient preference.

Patients must understand that to date percutaneous ablation of renal tumors is still under investigation and not proven. After percutaneous ablation, these patients must undergo frequent radiographic follow-up and possible postprocedure biopsy. They must also understand they may ultimately need partial or total nephrectomy if there is evidence of recurrence after percutaneous ablation.

ALTERNATIVE THERAPY

The gold standard for the treatment of renal tumors is radical nephrectomy. For patients with small renal tumors (less than 4 cm), partial nephrectomy is the preferred approach to maximize preservation of renal function. Expectant management has also been recommended in older patients who are more likely to succumb to their comorbidities than to a small incidental renal tumor. It cannot be overemphasized that the percutaneous approach is still under investigation and patients must be counseled at length of the various options available. Percutaneous ablation of small renal tumors is an alternative treatment when the patient is not a candidate for surgery.

SURGICAL TECHNIQUE

An interdisciplinary approach with the radiologist and surgeon is essential. A thorough history and physical examination is performed. Pertinent preoperative imaging is reviewed to guide approach and treatment window. Preoperative laboratory tests, that is, serum creatinine, complete blood count, prothrombin time, and partial thromboplastin time, are obtained. Informed consent is obtained with detailed discussion of the risks and various alternatives.

Patients with contrast enhancing renal masses less than 4 cm are candidates for the procedure. Standard supine CT scans are obtained preoperatively. Exophytic and endophytic lesions are eligible for treatment, although exophytic ones are preferred due to the limited collateral damage of normal renal parenchyma. Anterior lesions, large tumors, or tumors with renal sinus component may be less amenable for percutaneous ablation.

Most patients tolerate the procedure with intravenous or conscious sedation with fentanyl and midazolam. All patients should be under cardiac and pulmonary monitoring with telemetry and pulse oximetry. Patients with narcotic tolerance and airway issues may require general anesthesia.

Successful image-guided therapy requires the union of accurate real-time imaging with effective ablative therapy. With high-speed array parallel processing and new image reconstruction algorithms, real-time CT fluoroscopy or continuous imaging CT is now possible. Rapid processing CT scanners are available that allow intraoperative guidance. This dynamic image monitoring during urologic procedures is the epitome of current image-guided therapy. Although real-time magnetic resonance imaging (MRI) is available, material incompatibilities and access issues have currently limited its clinical utility. Although economic, ultrasonography has the most operator variability of cross-sectional imaging techniques. CT fluoroscopy is our preferred choice of image guidance in percutaneous renal tumor ablation.

Multiple investigations using cryoablation (9), radiofrequency (3,6,11,12) and high-intensity focused ultrasound (4) as renal ablative modalities have been described. To focus this discussion, percutaneous radiofrequency ablation (RFA) is described. Radiofrequency interstitial tissue ablation devices (RITA Medical Systems, Mountain View, CA), Cool-tip electrodes (Radionics, Burlington, MA), and LeVeen Needle Electrodes (Boston Scientific, Natick, MA) are approved by the US Food and Drug Administration as radiofrequency ablation devices.

An alternating electrical current delivered at high frequency (460,000 Hz) by a needle electrode is applied to the target tissue. Ions within the tissue follow the alternating current and the process results in ionic agitation and frictional heating. This leads to protein denaturation and desiccation. Secondary endpoints of tissue necrosis are currently used. Target tissue necrosis is achieved as the tissue gradually desiccates and eventually loses its ability to conduct current. As temperature and impedance increase the lesion becomes more resistant to electrical current flow. Tissue necrosis is suggested once the tissue impedance reaches a clinically relevant level or when temperature of the tines reaches the targeted temperature. This results in volume ablation, resulting in coagulative necrosis. Radiofrequency ablation has been applied with good success in advanced, unresectable hepatocellular carcinoma (8) and hepatic metastases. Several investigators have been examining the safety and feasibility of applying interstitial RF energy to patients with renal cell carcinoma (3,5–7,11,12).

The patient is usually placed in the prone position and CT imaging is performed. Grounding pads are placed. Care is taken to avoid prosthetic implants during pad placement. Patient with cardiac pacemakers may require pacer adjustment to prevent spontaneous activation during RF ablation. The appropriate entry site that avoids critical structures such as bowel and lung is identified on the CT images, and the CT table is moved to that position. The CT scanner laser light reflecting off the patient's skin is used to identify the location of the desired CT slice. Fiducials, or 1-mm metallic bead stickers, are placed on the patient's skin along the CT scanner laser light slice selected. Another CT image is obtained at the laser light position. The fiducials seen on the image can then guide the appropriate needle entry site and angle of trajectory. The skin is cleaned with Betadine solution, and the patient is draped. Local lidocaine is administered at the entry site and along the expected trajectory path. A scalpel blade is used to nick the skin allowing for the needle to pass more smoothly.

Under CT fluoroscopy, an 18-gauge core biopsy needle is inserted into the renal mass and a biopsy specimen is obtained. CT fluoroscopy scans allow visualization of the needle as it passes through the body and allows real-time adjustments to reach the final target.

After the biopsy is completed, the RF probe is inserted. Again, CT fluoroscopy may be used to provide real-time guidance of probe placement. Some CT scanner manufacturers with multislice detectors allow for imaging the slice above and below the slice selected. This gives more 3D information to allow optimal placement for 3D volume ablation.

If the LeVeen Needle Electrode is used, the probe is inserted to the center of the tumor, as the tine configuration is umbrella shaped when fully deployed (Fig. 138–1a). If the RITA StarBurst probe is used, the probe is advanced just within the peripheral tumor margin, as the

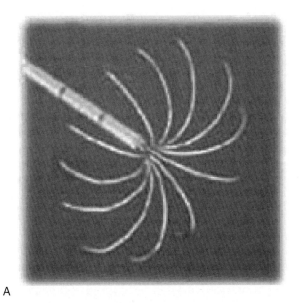

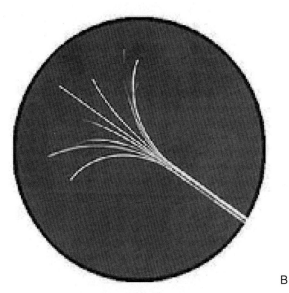

FIG. 138–1. Radiofrequency array probes **A:** LeVeen Needle Electrode (Bos Scientific, Natick, MA) **B:** Starburst XL (RITA Medical, Mountain View, CA).

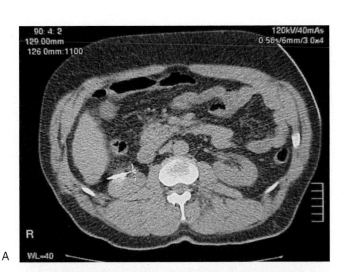

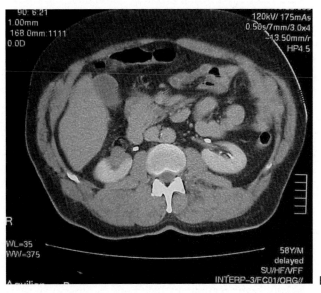

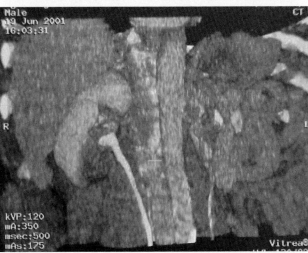

FIG. 138–2. A: Percutaneous radiofrequency ablation of a small right renal tumor. **B:** Follow-up contrast computed tomography (CT) immediately demonstrates absence of contrast enhancement, suggesting successful ablation. **C:** 3D CT reconstruction immediately revealing ablated tumor.

tines of probe protrude forward (Fig. 138–1b). Regardless of probe, the tissue ablation diameter should ideally exceed the CT measured tumor diameter by 5 to 10 mm. This ensures that the margins of the tumor are treated adequately.

The LeVeen Needle Electrode is impedance controlled. In this system, tissue necrosis is completed when the tissue impedance reaches a clinically relevant level. The clinical endpoint or completion of treatment occurs when there is "roll-off," or reduction in power concurrent with an increase in impedance. A second phase ablation is usually performed with this system (Figs. 138–2a to –2c).

The RITA electrosurgical device delivers up to 150 W and treatment is temperature based as measured by the five thermocouples. The tumor is treated until the average temperature of the thermocouples reaches the target temperature of 105C. The lesions are usually treated for one or two, 5- to 8-minute cycles, depending on tumor size. If there is inadequate treatment, the probe may be repositioned and the tumor retreated. After treatment is completed the, the probe is slowly withdraw in the "track ablate" mode to prevent bleeding and reduce the risk of tumor seeding.

As percutaneous RFA is still under investigation, these patients require close follow-up. Serial imaging is obtained every 3 months for the first 2 years, then every 6 months for the second 2 years, then annually thereafter. If there is renal mass enhancement or growth of tumor is evident, the patient should be counseled regarding possible retreatment or surgical extirpation of the lesion.

OUTCOMES

Complications

One patient developed moderate pain during the procedure and the procedure was terminated. That patient underwent repeat procedure under general anesthesia. Twenty-seven of 29 patients completed the procedure under intravenous sedation.

Major complications included one perioperative mortality on postprocedure day 2. Autopsy demonstrated aspiration pneumonia. The coagulative necrosis was found at the treated tumor site. One patient was readmitted with an ileus and minimal thermal ablation of the adjacent liver. He was treated conservatively. Minor complications included eight small perinephric hematoma related to treatment. All were managed conservatively without need for transfusion.

Results

We performed 37 renal RFA procedures in 29 patients with 35 renal tumors (6). These patients were considered high risk for surgery and/or anesthesia. Three patients had VHL disease with previous multiple partial nephrectomies. The average lesion size was 2.2 cm (range, 1 to 4

cm). In most cases, the procedure was performed as an outpatient procedure. Five patients were admitted overnight for observation. With a mean follow-up of 9 months, 94% of treated tumors demonstrated no evidence of enhancement on follow-up imaging. Two patients required retreatment secondary to persistent enhancement on follow-up imaging. Other groups have found similar success and recurrence rates in percutaneous RFA (6,11).

Percutaneous radiofrequency ablation for small renal tumor is a novel image-guide therapy. It is dependent on accurate real-time imaging and effective ablative therapy. Although our initial experience is promising, with any novel technique it is important to balance enthusiasm with evidence. Successful image-guided therapy relies on evolution of technology with careful evaluation of current techniques. Further investigations and refinements into high-intensity focused ultrasound (4), intraoperative treatment monitoring with MRI thermometry (2), and more accurate tissue targeting with robotic guidance (10) will overcome some of the current doubts and deficiencies in current ablative therapy and image guidance and reduce operator radiation exposure.

REFERENCES

1. Chan DY, Solomon S, Kim FJ, Jarrett TW. Image-guided therapy in urology. *J Endourol* 2001;15:105–110.
2. Chen JC, Moriarty JA, Derbyshire JA, Peters RD, Trachtenberg J, Bell SD, Doyle J, Arrelano R, Wright GA, Henkelman RM, Hinks RS, Lok SY, Toi A, Kucharczyk W. Prostate cancer: MR imaging and thermometry during microwave thermal ablation—initial experience. *Radiology* 2000;214:290–297.
3. Gervais DA, McGovern FJ, Arellano RS, McDougal WS, Mueller PR. Renal cell carcinoma: clinical experience and technical success with radio-frequency ablation of 42 tumors. *Radiology* 2003;226:417–424.
4. Kohrmann KU, Michel MS, Gaa J, Marlinghaus E, Alken P. High intensity focused ultrasound as noninvasive therapy for multilocal renal cell carcinoma: case study and review of the literature. *J Urol* 2002;167: 2397–2403.
5. Michaels MJ, Rhee HK, Mourtzinos AP, Summerhayes IC, Silverman ML, Libertino JA. Incomplete renal tumor destruction using radio frequency interstitial ablation. *J Urol* 2002;168:2406–2409.
6. Ogan K, Jacomides L, Dolmatch BL, Rivera FJ, Dellaria MF, Josephs SC, Cadeddu JA. Percutaneous radiofrequency ablation of renal tumors: technique, limitations, and morbidity. *Urology* 2002;60: 954–958.
7. Rendon RA, Kachura JR, Sweet JM, Gertner MR, Sherar MD, Robinette M, Tsihlias J, Trachtenberg J, Sampson H, Jewett MA. The uncertainty of radio frequency treatment of renal cell carcinoma: findings at immediate and delayed nephrectomy. *J Urol* 2002;167:1587–1592.
8. Seidenfeld J, Korn A, Aronson N. Radiofrequency ablation of unresectable primary liver cancer. *J Am Coll Surg* 2002;194:813–828.
9. Shingleton WB, Sewell PE Jr. Percutaneous renal tumor cryoablation with magnetic resonance imaging guidance. *J Urol* 200;165:773–776.
10. Solomon SB, Patriciu A, Bohlman ME, Kavoussi LR, Stoianovici D. Robotically driven interventions: a method of using CT fluoroscopy without radiation exposure to the physician. *Radiology* 2002;225: 277–282.
11. Su LM, Jarrett TW, Chan DY, Kavoussi LR, Solomon, SB. Percutaneous computed tomography-guided radiofrequency ablation of renal masses in high surgical risk patients: preliminary results. *Urology* 2003 61:26–33.
12. Walther MC, Shawker TH, Libutti SK, Lubensky I, Choyke PL, Venzon D, Linehan WM. A phase 2 study of radio frequency interstitial tissue ablation of localized renal tumors. *J Urol* 2000;163:1424–1427.

CHAPTER 139

Management of Ureteral Obstruction: Novel Stents and Prosthetics

Paulos Yohannes and Benjamin R. Lee

The management of extrinsic ureteral compression due to a malignancy may present a dilemma to the practicing urologist. By tradition, urinary diversion was accomplished by open surgical techniques—an approach that carries significant morbidity to the terminally ill patient; in addition, as most cases were diagnosed late the overall survival rate was dismal and such surgical endeavors became very controversial and ethically unacceptable. With the advent of minimally invasive surgery, new techniques and devices have facilitated urinary diversion with less morbidity.

The use of ureteral stents for the management of ureteral obstruction in the cancer patient was first reported by Gibbons et al. in 1976 (8). However, single indwelling ureteral stents in patients with extrinsic malignant obstruction have been associated with high failure rate (5). Nephrostomy tubes, often placed after failed management with single ureteral stents, are cumbersome and have an adverse effect on the quality of life; in addition, nephrostomy tubes are associated with recurrent urinary tract infections (UTIs) as well as sepsis and intermittent hematuria.

In the last two decades, various modifications of the single-J ureteral stents have been made to minimize the incidence of stent blockage from tumor overgrowth. Schlick and associates developed the "tumor stent" and Tligui et al. introduced a "cloverleaf" double-J stent (26,31). Metallic stents have found a place in the treatment of malignant obstruction of the ureter as well, and further experience is being accumulated. Extraanatomic urinary diversion or subcutaneous ureteral prostheses have also been investigated as an alternative to percutaneous nephrostomy (29). The use of two parallel ureteral double-pigtail stents has also shown promising results in patients when a single stent has failed (7,16,24).

In this chapter, we will discuss the advancements made in the management of malignant ureteral obstruction. Current treatment options include multiple ureteral stents in a single ureter, subcutaneous urinary diversion, extraanatomic nephrovesical bypass, and self-expandable endoluminal metallic stents.

MULTIPLE URETERAL STENTS IN A SINGLE URETER

Docimo and Wolf demonstrated that the success rate of single, double-pigtail stent in the management of extrinsic ureteral compression due to malignancies is short lived (5). The biomaterial makeup of ureteral stents is easily obstructed and not rigid enough to keep the stent lumen open despite tumor overgrowth. As a result, Lui and Hebrinko introduced the use of multiple double-pigtail stents in a single ureter for the management of ureteral obstruction when single pigtail stent has failed (16). Two stents in a single ureter would not only double the intraluminal stent diameter but also create a groove between the stents that facilitates urinary drainage; this groove is not as easily prone to obstruction by tumor overgrowth—on the contrary, the space between a single stent and ureteral wall can easily be compressed with external compression from tumor.

Different stent-size combinations have been used in this technique. The original clinical experience with Lui and Hebrenko (16) used two 4.7 Fr pigtail stents. Recently, the use of two 8 Fr stents and a combination of 8/6 Fr stents have also been reported (7,24). The size of the ureteral stent employed depends on the elasticity of the ureter and degree of external tumor compression. The use of two stents in a single ureter for the management of ureteral obstruction due to a malignancy has been shown to be clinically safe and effective. Experience with this approach, however, is limited to few institutions (7,16,24).

Recently, Rotariu and colleagues (24) reported their experience with this approach. Seven patients with malignant obstruction of the ureter, after having failed treatment with a single stent, underwent placement of two double-pigtail stents in a single ureter. The etiology of extrinsic compression included cervical cancer, transitional cell cancer of the bladder, and non-Hodgkin's lymphoma. In one patient, obstruction was bilateral. The stents were changed every month. With a mean follow-up of 16 months, all surviving patients tolerated the stents; three patients died within 3 months of treatment. Surprisingly, irritative voiding symptoms from the stents were minimal. Similarly, Fromer and colleagues (7) reported on the use of two 8 Fr double-pigtail catheters in five patients with cervical cancer (three), pelvic sarcoma (one), and transitional cell carcinoma (one). At a mean follow-up of 12 months, two patients had complete resolution of hydronephrosis and symptoms at 10 and 18 months; two other patients died at 8 and 12 months with patent and functioning stents. The fifth patient developed pyonephrosis and died from disease progression within 3 weeks of stent placement.

Multiple stents can be placed in a retrograde or antegrade fashion. Because placement of two stents simultaneously may present a technical dilemma, the use of a peel-away sheath (Cook, Spencer, IN) or ureteral access sheath (Applied Medical, Laguna Hills, CA) is helpful. The use of these sheaths allows for a smooth advancement of stents simultaneously. The sheath also serves as a barrier to the already compromised ureteral wall. Often, it is necessary to dilate the strictured segment of ureter using a balloon dilator to facilitate insertion of the sheath.

Both stents can also be placed after balloon dilatation, without the aid of a ureteral sheath. Because of limited experience with the use of multiple stents in a single ureter, the incidence of encrustations and infection with this approach is not known.

SUBCUTANEOUS URINARY DIVERSION

Extraanatomic bypass (also known as subcutaneous urinary diversion, circumventing nephrocystostomy) for relief of ureteral obstruction, especially due to a malignancy, has been reported with encouraging preliminary results in patients with a short life expectancy (Table 139–1). The clinical experience with this approach is limited to only few centers worldwide. The extraanatomic prosthesis obviates the need for an external appliance, thereby improving the quality of life in patients with advanced malignancies. It also allows patients to void naturally. Subcutaneous urinary diversion is indicated when management with single or multiple double-pigtail stents has failed.

Placement can be performed wither under general or local anesthesia. Patients are positioned in the lateral or prone position if a single side or bilateral subcutaneous urinary diversion is desired, respectively. The prosthesis is inserted into the renal pelvis percutaneously and tunneled subcutaneously into the bladder, where a small suprapubic incision is made to introduce the prosthesis inside the bladder. The nephrostomy and suprapubic bladder catheters can also be placed separately and subsequently connected to each other subcutaneously. The composition, size, and length of the stents are variable from one institution to another. A nephrostomy tube may be left in place in the ipsilateral kidney until proper functioning of the extraanatomic bypass has been confirmed.

TABLE 139–1. *Clinical experience with subcutaneous urinary diversion; contemporary series*

Senior author/ reference	No. of patients	Diagnosis	Follow-up	Complications	Type of prosthesis
DiLelio 1991	9	Cervical (2), Ovarian (1), Vulvar (1), Prostatic (1), Sigmoid (3), Ureteral Necrosis (1)	44 d–24 mo	Orchitis (1), Recurrent Cystitis (1), Obstruction (2), Wound Dehiscence (1), Urinary Leak (1)	Polyvinyl Chloride, Polyurethane, Silicone, Size Not Listed
Lingam 1994	5	Colon (3), Uterine Sarcoma (1)	15 mo	3/5 Patent	7 Fr Double-Pigtail Stent Biliary RF (1)
Nakada 1995	2	Pancreas (1), Breast (1) 6 wk	9 wk	None	8.5 Fr, 70-cm Double-Pigtail Stent
Cockburn. *AJR* 1997;169: 1588	1	N/A	5 mo	None	Two 8 Fr, 25-cm Single-Loop Catheters
Nissen Korn. *J Urol* 2000; 163:528	8	Prostate (6), Bladder (2)	5.5 mo	None	Two 14 Fr, 50-cm polyurethane J Stents
Jabbour. *J Endourol* 2001;15:611	27	22 Neoplastic, 5 Benign	6.3 mo	Parietal (8.5%), Skin Erosion (1), Local Tumor Progression (2)	Composite: Inner, Silicone; Outer, PTFE

Complications with subcutaneous urinary diversion include skin erosion, orchitis, secondary parietal complications, and recurrent cystitis (14). Difficulties in placing the prosthesis can occur at an incidence of 19% (14). Bladder fistula can occur and may necessitate placement of a nephrostomy tube. Stent change every 4 to 12 months is recommended. Changing the ureteral stent may be tricky; a long guide wire is needed to prevent loss of subcutaneous nephrovesical access. Although subcutaneous nephrovesical bypass stents have been shown to be safe and effective, it will be difficult to assess its long-term feasibility due to the indication of its use.

EXTRAANATOMIC BYPASS

Extracorporeal urinary bypass was introduced by Tomooka et al. (29). In this technique, nephrostomy and suprapubic catheters are placed in the usual fashion and connected to each other externally; this approach obviates the need for creating a subcutaneous tunnel. It is relatively easy to manage and the external appliances can be concealed. To date, this simplistic approach has only been reported by one institution, but it represents a feasible alternative for patients with limited life expectancy.

METALLIC STENTS

Self-expandable endoluminal metallic stents (SPESs) were first introduced in biliary and vascular surgery (9,11). In 1988, Milroy et al. introduced the use of expandable metallic stents in the management of urethral stricture disease; the use of metallic stents has also been reported in the treatment of lower urinary tract symptoms secondary to benign prostatic hyperplasia and detrusor sphincter dyssynergia (18). In 1990, Gort further expanded its application by using SPESs for the treatment of ureteroileal stricture. Subsequently, SPESs were used in the ureter (Table 139–2). The indications for SPESs include malignant or benign extrinsic ureteral compression, benign intrinsic ureteral strictures, ureteroileal strictures, primary malignant disease of the ureter, and stricture disease that has failed other techniques of intervention (ureterolysis, double-J stent insertion, hormone therapy, etc.) (1,2,17,22,23).

Different types of self-expanding metallic stents have been described in the literature. The Wallstent (Schneider, Zurich), the most common SPES, consists of cobalt chromium molybdenium iron alloy and has great flexibility; it is available in 8 mm (24 Fr) and 10 mm (30 Fr) diameter and 42 and 68 mm length (1,17,22,23).

The use of Memotherm (NovoMed, Inc., Mannheim, Germany) and Sinus stent (Optimed, Germany), a nickel titanium alloy, was first reported by Pauer et al. (23). Their study used all three types of metallic stents (including Wallstent) and demonstrated that all three appear to be equally effective. The Accuflex (Meditech, Boston Scientific Corp., Boston, MA), a self-expandable metallic stent made of woven titanium-based metal alloy, is associated with a significant decrease in length after deployment (2). It is highly flexible and contains two flares in both ends to secure it to the ureter. Finally, the Strecker (Meditech, Boston Scientific) stent, the only balloon-expandable metal stent, consists of knitted tantalum monofilament wire. It is less flexible, highly radioopaque, and can be delivered to the strictured segment easily and accurately (2). Studies have shown that there was no difference in outcome with either the Strecker or Accuflex stent (2). Most SPESs can accommodate 7 Fr ureteroscopes after complete epithelialization. Placement of a combination of different types of SPESs in one patient is not recommended due to the theoretical risk of electrolytic reaction between alloys.

The use of an SPES in the distal ureter can be technically challenging. The stent should be deployed at the proper location to prevent obstruction or reflux/incrustation. In addition, the distal end of the SPES should be positioned within the intramural ureter; too proximal or too distal positioning may case kinking of the ureter or reflux, respectively (17).

Radiographic evaluation of the ureter in the end of the procedure often reveals a disproportion of SPES to ureter—a finding referred to as "the Stocking phenome-

TABLE 139–2. *Clinical series of self-expanding endoluminal metallic stents in malignant extrinsic compression of the ureter*

Senior author/reference	No. of patients ureters	Site of stricture	Previous measures	Patency rate (%)	Follow-up (mo)
Pauer (1992)	12/15	N/A	N/A	83	1–12
Lugmayr. *Radiology* 1996;198:105	40/54	N/A	D-J Chemotherapy	63.8[a] 31[b]	1–44 (10.5)
Barbalais. *J Urol* 1997;158:54	12/14	N/A	D-J (12)	78	8–16
Lopez-Martinez (1997)[c]	8/8	DU-8	N/A	75[d]	1–48
Ahmed. *J Endourol* 1999;13:221[c]	3/3	DU-3	Hormone (3)	0	5

DU, distal ureter; N/A, not available; D-J, double-pigtail ureteral stent.
[a]Success rate after 6 mo.
[b]Success rate after 12 mo.
[c]Prostate cancer.
[d]100% patent at 12 mo; 60% patent at 24 mos.

non" (23). This finding is normal and should not lead to further intervention. At the end, a double-J ureteral stent is placed through the SPES for a period of 4 weeks until edema and hyperplastic reaction resolves. Transabdominal color Doppler sonogram can be used to document urine flow through the stent (2). Finally, perioperative antibiotic coverage is important to prevent stent colonization.

After placement of the SPES, hyperplasia of the regenerating urothelium is notable. The hyperplastic reaction can create obstruction to urinary drainage; therefore, insertion of a ureteral stent is recommended. The degree of hyperplasia is proportional to the amount of force exerted on the wall of the ureter; therefore, the ureter should not be overdistended (30). Moreover, reactive hyperplasia is uncommon in patients who have undergone radiation therapy (17). The time it takes for complete coverage of SPES by urothelium is between 8 weeks and 6 months (18). The advantages of epithelialization include prevention of incrustations, migration, and UTI.

Familiarity with the SPES-related complications is important. In the early postoperative period (less than 8 weeks), the most common cause of obstruction is reactive edema and hyperplasia; obstruction from reactive hyperplasia has been reported as early as 24 hours (2). In some cases, epithelialization may take longer secondary to peristalsis and constant flow of urine. If epithelialization is incomplete, incrustations may form a stone causing obstruction and UTI; the incidence of incrustations is 5% (17). Therefore, coverage with perioperative antibiotics is imperative. On occasion, a mucus plug may cause transient obstruction. Migration of a SPES has been reported only once and is best treated by placement of an additional SPES (2).

Obstruction of an SPES from tumor progression or local recurrence usually presents late (greater than 4 months). Although endoscopic resection of tumor may be attempted, the best therapeutic option is either a second expandable metallic stent, double-J ureteral stent, or a nephrostomy tube (1,2,17). Ingrowth of scar tissue causing obstruction has been reported in one patient; this was successfully treated by a second SPES (22). Stone formation above the stricture 2 years after SPES placement has also been described (22). Endoscopic manipulation of urinary tract pathology above the SPES is safe and should not deter the urologist from implementing rapid care. Gross hematuria after placement of a metallic stent is rare and transient (2,17). Finally, erosion of an SPES has not been reported.

The application of SPESs in patients with locally advanced prostate cancer has been reported by several investigators with varying patency rates (0% to 100%) (1,2,17). Patients with non–organ-confined prostate cancer who present with ureteral obstruction are all candidates for SPESs; however, patency rate in patients with hormone refractory cancer is poor, with most stents obstructing from tumor overgrowth within the first 1 to 3 months (1). In the event that SPES fails in these patients, the only other alternative is placement of nephrostomy tube. Therefore, proper patient selection plays a major role in the success rate of metallic stents in prostate cancer. In most cases, the endoluminal stents are placed using the antegrade approach because visualization of the ureteral orifices is difficult due to local invasion of tumor (1). In addition, the stents have to project into the bladder, increasing the likelihood of worsening hematuria, incrustations, and irritative bladder symptoms such as hematuria.

Currently, the Wallstent is not approved by the US Food and Drug Administration for use in the ureter in the United States. In malignant extrinsic compression of the ureter, clinical experience of metallic stents has been variable.

FUTURE OUTLOOK

The search for the ideal biocompatible material continues. There are several major limiting factors for the long-term use of biomaterials within the urinary tract. Device-related encrustations and UTIs cause significant morbidity and mortality. According to Reid (1998), over 90% of retrieved stents are covered with pathogens. In addition, 50% of patients with long-term indwelling catheters will experience recurrent encrustations and blockage, and stent encrustation is a time-related phenomenon (6).

The ideal stent or other type of prosthetic is yet to be developed. The development of a prosthetic that is in constant contact with urine presents a challenge unlike prosthetics that are not exposed to urine (testicular and penile prostheses, pubovaginal slings, and artificial sphincters). Currently, the synthetic polymer compounds used in the urinary tract have included polyethylene, silicone, polyurethane, and proprietary polymers such as Silitek, C-Flex, and Percuflex. The ideal prosthetic stent should be composed of a nonionic polymer. The inherent properties of nonionic polymers that makes this group of biomaterials ideal for stent–urine interface include less platelet adhesion, superior resistance to encrustation and intraluminal blockage, and lower coefficient of friction, with ease of insertion and less discomfort (10,15).

There are several areas of research oriented to minimize, if not eliminate, the morbidity associated with ureteral stents. These efforts have focused on the different properties of the stent covering that promote bacterial adherence. Hydrogel catheters promote surface translocation of *Proteus*, while silicone stents slows bacterial translocation (2). In addition to frequent stent changes, protective covering of the biomaterials with biocides has also been demonstrated to minimize the incidence of colonization. The use of silver alloy, nitrofurazone, and surfacine has been shown to reduce the incidence of UTIs in patients with indwelling stents (25,28). Finally, bioabsorbable ureteral stents are currently being investigated. Placing a biomaterial that will dissolve within a few days to weeks will eliminate the need for a second procedure. However, the clinical role of this novel device is not only under active investigation but its role in the management of malignant ureteral obstruction is in question.

REFERENCES

1. Ahmed M, Bishop MC, Bates CP, et al. Metal mesh stents for ureteral obstruction caused by hormone-resistant carcinoma of prostate. *J Endourol* 1999;13:221–224.
2. Barbailas GA, Siablis D, Liatsikos EN, et al. Metal stents: a new treatment of malignant ureteral obstruction. *J Urol* 1997;158:54–58.
3. Cockburn JF, Borthwick CA, Hanaghan J, et al. Radiologic insertion of subcutaneous nephrovesical stent for inoperable ureteral obstruction. *AJR* 1997;169:1588–1590.
4. Denstedt JD, Wollin TA, Reid G. Biomaterials used in urology: current issues of biocompatibility, infection, and encrustation. *J Endourol* 1998;12:493–500.
5. Docimo SG, DeWolf WC. High failure rate of indwelling ureteral stents in patients with extrinsic obstruction: experience at two institutions. *J Urol* 1989;142:277–279.
6. El-Faqih SR, Shamsuddin AB, Chakrabarti A, et al. Polyurethane internal ureteral stents in treatment of stone patients: morbidity related to indwelling times. *J Urol* 1991;146:1487–1491.
7. Fromer DL, Shabsigh A, Benson M, et al. Simultaneous multiple double pigtail stents for malignant ureteral obstruction. *Urology* 2002;59:594–596.
8. Gibbons RP, Correa RJ, Cummings KB, et al. Experience with indwelling ureteral stent catheter. *J Urol* 1976;115:22–26.
9. Gillams S, Dick R, Dooley JS, et al. Self-expandable stainless braided endoprosthesis for biliary strictures. *Radiology* 1990;174:137–140.
10. Groman SP, Tunney MM, Keane PF, et al. Characterization and assessment of a novel poly(ethylene oxide)/polyurethane composite hydrogel (Aquavene) as a ureteral stent biomaterial. *J Biomed Mater Res* 1998;39:642–649.
11. Günther RW, Vorwerk D, Bohndorf K, et al. Iliac and femoral artery stenosis and occlusions treatment with intravascular stents. *Radiology* 1989;172:785–730.
12. Hepperlen TW, Mardis HK, Kammandel H. The pigtail ureteral stent in the cancer patient. *J Urol* 1979;121:17–18.
13. Herrero JA, Lezana A, Gallego J, et al. Self-expanding metallic stents in the treatment of ureteral obstruction after renal transplantation. *Nephrol Dialysis Transplant* 1996;11(5):887–889.
14. Jabbour ME, Desgrandchamps F, Angelescu E, et al. Percutaneous implantation of subcutaneous prosthetic ureters: long term experience. *J Endourol* 2001;15:611–614.
15. Kulik E, Ikada Y. In vitro platelet adhesion to nonionic and ionic hydrogels with different water contents. *J Biomed Mater Res* 1996;30:295–304.
16. Liu JS, Hrebinko RL. The use of 2 ipsilateral ureteral stents for relief of ureteral obstruction from extrinsic compression. *J Urol* 1998;159:179–181.
17. Lugmayr HF, Pauer W. Wallstents for the treatment of extrinsic malignant ureteral obstruction: midterm results. *Radiology* 1996;198:105–108.
18. Milroy EJG, Chapple CR, Cooper JE, et al. A new treatment for urethral strictures. *Lancet* 1988;1:1424–1427.
19. Nakada SY, Gerber AJ, Wolf JS, et al. Subcutaneous urinary diversion utilizing a nephrovesical stent: a superior alternative to long-term external drainage. *Urology* 1995;45:538–541.
20. Nissenkorn I, Gdor Y. Nephrovesical subcutaneous stent: an alternative to permanent nephrostomy. *J Urol* 2000;163:528–530.
21. Paterson PJ, Forrester A. Extra-anatomic urinary diversion. *J Endourol* 1997;11:411–412.
22. Pauer W, Eckerstorfer GM. Use of self-expanding permanent endoluminal stents for benign ureteral strictures: mid-term results. *J Urol* 1999;162:319–322.
23. Pauer W, Kerbl K. Self-expanding permanent endoluminal stents in the ureter: technical considerations. *Tech Urol* 1995;1(2):67–71.
24. Rotariu P, Yohannes P, Alexianu, et al. Management of malignant extrinsic ureteral obstruction by two double-J stents in a single ureter. *J Endourol* 2001;15:979–983.
25. Saint S, Elmore JG, Sullivan SD, et al. The efficacy of silver alloy-coated urinary catheters in preventing urinary tract infections: a meta-analysis. *Am J Med* 1998;105:236–241.
26. Schlick R, Seidel EM, Kalem T, et al. New endoureteral double-J stent resists extrinsic ureteral compression. *J Endourol* 1998;12:37–40.
27. Stickler D, Highes G. Ability of *Proteus mirabilis* to swarm over urethral catheters. *Eur J Clin Microbiol Infect Dis* 1999;18:206–208.
28. Subramanyam S, Yurkovetsiky A, Hale D, et al. A chemically intelligent antimicrobial coating for urologic devices. *J Endourol* 2000;14:43–48.
29. Tamooka Y, Yokoyama M, Takeuchi M. Extracorporeal urinary bypass for malignant ureteral obstruction. *Urology* 1994;43:878–879.
30. Thijssen AM, Millward SF, Mai KT. Ureteral response to the placement of metallic stents: an animal model. *J Urol* 1994;151:268–270.
31. Tligui M, Nouri M, You R, et al. Value of cloverleaf double-J ureteral stent in the treatment of extrinsic ureteral compression. *Progr Urol* 2000;10:92–94.

CHAPTER 140

Lasers In Urologic Surgery

Michael J. Manyak and John W. Warner

A laser is a light source that is most often used in medicine to provide controlled thermal energy to tissue. The term LASER is an acronym for light amplification by stimulated emission of radiation. Therefore, lasers are amplified light identified by the medium used to generate light. Lasers are capable of providing adjustable wavelengths, extremely short pulse durations, and intense power delivery to cause unique alteration of tissues and structures. The precision in control of the spatial and temporal properties of lasers in combination with minimally invasive access has made possible several diagnostic and therapeutic applications (11).

Although the application of lasers to urologic problems most commonly is in laser lithotripsy, thermal use of lasers remain an option for management of other disorders such as benign prostatic hyperplasia, papillary bladder cancer, urogenital cutaneous lesions, and urethral strictures. Lasers can also be used for diagnostic purposes where photosensitization of epithelial tumors followed by exposure to ultraviolet or blue wavelengths of light allows fluorescent detection or treatment. Other intriguing potential uses of lasers, such as for tissue welding, remain investigational at this time.

LIGHT AND TISSUE EFFECTS

Laser light characteristics depend on the medium used to generate light, with different wavelengths emitted by a wide variety of solid, liquid, and gas laser media. Lasers possess three striking properties that separate them from other light sources. The typical incandescent light produces light of various wavelengths in all directions. Lasers, by comparison, produce light of specific wavelengths (monochromatic) with wavelength peaks and valleys in phase (coherent) in one direction (collimated). Because of these properties, lasers are capable of producing light of extreme brightness and singularity of wavelength that can be directed.

The tissue effects of laser energy are a function of the laser wavelength, tissue absorption characteristics, power delivered, and time of exposure. Thermal tissue destruction can be accomplished by either coagulation or vaporization. As tissue temperature increases from 50°C to 100°C, tissue effects progress from protein denaturation to DNA destruction and changes in membrane permeability. Capillary coagulation occurs around 60 to 65°C. If the tissue temperature exceeds 100°C, the fluid content of the tissue will vaporize in a plume containing fluid vapor and charred tissue components. A zone of coagulation necrosis surrounds the surgical lesion created.

By adjusting the wavelength, power, and time of exposure, the degree of thermal conduction and local tissue repair mechanisms can be controlled. As the laser energy is increased, removal of tissue occurs. Applying focused energy above this ablation threshold is in general useful for incising tissue while a lower-power, defocused beam results in coagulation and hemostasis. The presence of water will shift the ablation energy to a higher threshold because it cools the tissue. This impedes surface ablation and simultaneously cools the laser fiber to allow a higher-wattage delivery without damage to the fiber. This concept is relevant to urologic use of lasers because these procedures, with the exception of treatment of external genitalia lesions, occur in an aqueous environment. Thus, a higher laser wattage is needed to achieve efficient ablation of the same tissue under water than in air.

Currently, the most frequent urologic uses of lasers are for therapeutic applications but some of the most diverse uses may very well be for diagnosis. Diagnosis using a laser varies in one fundamental respect from therapeutic applications of lasers: Diagnostic uses in general detect changes that result from the *effect of tissue on light* while therapeutic uses rely on the *effect of light on tissue* (15). Diagnostic methods under active clinical investigation include fluorescent detection and optical coherence tomography (4,9). Continued progress in image resolution holds great promise for incorporation of these types of techniques into daily practice.

UNIQUE SAFETY CONSIDERATIONS

Surgical use of lasers does require safety measures unique to their respective characteristics. Proper training is imperative for both physicians and operating room personnel to ensure the safety of both patient and personnel. Precautions unnecessary for other modalities include protective eyewear appropriate to filter the wavelength in use, telescopic lens covers for endoscopic use, and proper draping techniques to prevent fire. Use of photodynamic therapy requires eye and skin protection for the patient to avoid inadvertent intense light exposure during treatment. Intravesical use of lasers causes less concern for some of these precautions but it is important that all personnel involved with the procedures understand the potential for complications related to laser use.

TYPES OF LASERS

Several lasers provide thermal energy for tissue destruction so the selection of laser type to achieve a desired result requires some understanding of individual laser capabilities. Depth of light penetration in tissue depends on several local tissue factors that contribute to the scatter and absorption of the energy (17). In general, a longer wavelength will correspond to greater depth of penetration (Fig. 140–1). Absorption by water or blood will likewise limit the depth of penetration. These penetration characteristics frequently dictate the type of laser to be used for thermal ablation of tissue.

Another component of optimal laser selection is the light delivery system. Light is directed to the desired target in general with an optical fiber composed of quartz

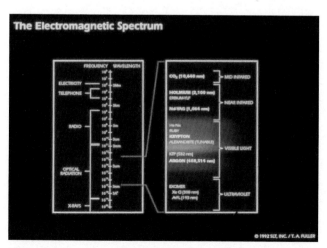

FIG. 140–1. The electromagnetic spectrum. Each laser emits a very specific wavelength depending on the substance that is excited (lased).

and silica that directs the laser beam along the long axis of the fiber by internal reflectance. In this "free-beam" method, the laser beam is offset from the tissue for exposure. In cases where penetration is desired, the deeper penetration characteristics of an Nd:yttrium–aluminum–garnet (YAG) laser can be enhanced by use of a contact or interstitial laser optical fiber. Other modifications of optical fiber tips provide diffuse rather than focused light distribution when that attribute is required.

Carbon Dioxide (CO_2) Laser

The CO_2 laser has an invisible infrared wavelength of 10,600 nm and is usually coupled to a visible helium–neon beam to highlight the target area. The CO_2 beam is directed through an articulating arm by a series of mirrors and is focused on the tissue to be vaporized. The infrared CO_2 beam is absorbed by water, which usually limits its use to surface applications although the CO_2 beam can be directed through a waveguide to allow for use through the laparoscope. Depth of tissue penetration is less than 0.1 mm with a small area of coagulation necrosis. Disadvantages of the CO_2 laser include production of a plume with potential vaporization of infectious viral particles, necessitating use of a high-filtration mask for all cutaneous applications. In addition, the CO_2 laser has poor coagulative properties for vessels over 1.0 mm and development of oxidized char impedes vaporization of underlying tissue.

Argon Laser

The argon laser produces wavelengths in the blue–green spectrum that are absorbed by pigmented molecules such as hemoglobin. The argon beam may be transmitted through a flexible quartz fiber and penetrates 1 to 2 mm in tissue. Advantages include flexible application, minimal plume with vaporization, and excellent hemostatic properties. Disadvantages include the need for a dedicated water supply for cooling the laser and the requirement for tinted filters to protect the eyes of operating room staff and patient.

Nd:YAG Laser

The Nd:YAG laser is a solid-state laser utilizing a crystal seed with neodymium ions to furnish the active medium. The beam is in the near-infrared portion of the light spectrum (1064 nm) and requires a helium–neon aiming beam for illumination of the target tissue. The Nd:YAG laser is absorbed poorly by water, tissue proteins, and blood and therefore produces relatively high tissue penetration of 3 to 5 mm with good coagulation. This degree of tissue penetration clearly can be a disadvantage as well. A sapphire tip limits backscatter and enhances the laser cutting properties but caution is advised due to the extremely high temperatures produced at the tip.

Potassium–Titanyl Phosphate (KTP) Crystal Laser

The KTP crystal laser is generated by passing a rapidly pulsed Nd:YAG beam through a potassium thiophosphate crystal, which doubles the frequency and halves the wavelength to 532 nm. The coagulative properties of this visible green light source are similar to the argon laser with comparable depths of tissue penetration (1 to 2 mm).

Holmium:YAG Laser

Holmium is a rare earth element that, when doped with YAG, can emit laser radiation at a wavelength of 2,100 nm with normal pulse duration of 250 ms. This laser operates in the near-infrared portion of the electromagnetic spectrum and is therefore invisible to the human eye. The holmium laser is especially suited for endoscopic procedures because the 2,100-nm wavelength can be transmitted through standard optical fibers. At this wavelength, the pulse is strongly absorbed by water in superficial tissue and provides excellent incisive and tissue ablation properties. Recently, holmium lasers have largely supplanted the use of pulsed dye lasers for lithotripsy of urinary calculi due to their reliability and ease of maintenance.

Erbium:YAG Laser

Erbium is another rare earth metal used in combination with YAG to produce laser light. This laser emits light at 2,940 nm, which coincides with the water absorption peak in the infrared spectrum. Because of this close approximation with the absorption peak of water, it has been claimed that Er:YAG lasers produce more precise and efficient ablation with less thermal damage than Ho:YAG lasers (2). This laser has been used for tissue ablation as well as lithotripsy with an optical fiber.

Semiconductor Lasers

Semiconductor lasers are smaller, less expensive, and have significantly less energy and cooling requirements than traditional lasers (Fig. 140–2). Diode lasers have recently gained increasing popularity because these qualities provide an affordable, cost-effective light source. Diode lasers can be better understood by comparison to a light-emitting diode (LED). In an LED, an electrical current is directed through an appropriate semiconductor with spontaneous light emitted. A laser light is produced by applying the same principles except a reflective resonator is added to continuously reflect the stimulated light. The very specific light emitted from the laser

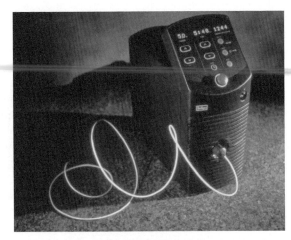

FIG. 140–2. Semiconductor diode laser that is easily portable, inexpensive, and stable.

passes through an aperture designed to allow emission of only a certain wavelength. The wavelength is determined by the semiconductor compound and can be transmitted easily along an optical fiber.

Dye Lasers

Dye lasers employ an organic liquid dye as the active medium that is optically excited by another light source. Liquid dyes have complex sets of electronic and vibrational energies and the wavelength emitted depends on the type of dye used. The primary advantage of dye lasers is that the wavelength can be changed by changing the dye used for excitation. Pulsed dye lasers have been used for lithotripsy of urinary calculi and for photodynamic therapy. The need to change the dye in these lasers at a regular interval makes them more difficult and expensive to maintain compared to other lasers.

DIAGNOSTIC USE OF LASERS

Lasers have long been considered tools for ablative therapy but the endoscopic application of light for diagnosis is increasing. Fluorescent properties of tumors in combination with photosensitizing agents have long been of interest for diagnosis of occult malignancy, with the bladder the primary urologic focus for this application (1). Fluorescence is the emission of light from an excited molecule as it returns to its ground state and occurs at wavelengths longer than those of excitation. The most common compounds used for fluorescent detection are porphyrins, which produce a characteristic reddish hue in tissue after exposure to ultraviolet or blue-green visible light. The most promising agent, 5-aminolevulinic acid (5-ALA), avoids the skin photosensitivity associated with most photosensitizers because it can be administered

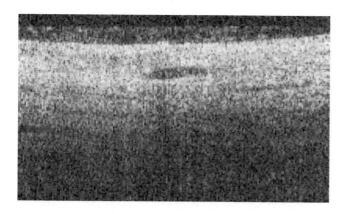
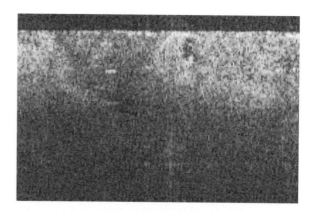

A

B

FIG. 140–3. Optical coherence tomography (OCT) of (**A**) normal bladder epithelium and muscularis compared to (**B**) transitional cell carcinoma. OCT allows real-time visualization of structures below the epithelium. (From Zagaynova EV, Streltsova OS, Gladkova ND, Nizhny Novgorod State Medical Academy and Institute of Applied Physics of the Russian Academy of Sciences, with permission.)

directly into the bladder. Fluorescence with 5-ALA has reportedly improved sensitivity for transitional cell carcinoma (TCC) compared to conventional endoscopy with white light (97% vs. 73%) and has been used to improve tumor-free rates with transurethral resection (10).

Optical coherence tomography (OCT) uses inexpensive solid-state red diodes to create a cross-sectional tomographic image based on optical scattering within tissue (7). OCT is similar to ultrasound pulse–echo imaging but uses optical rather than acoustic reflectivity. Unlike ultrasound, however, OCT does not require a conducting medium and can image through air or water with far greater resolution than ultrasound (4). In combination with endoscopy, OCT permits imaging of the epithelial surface of internal organs with visualization beneath the surface. Preliminary imaging of bladder malignancies suggests that this technology will be useful for staging superficial malignancies and determining extent of tumor boundaries (21) (Fig. 140–3).

UROLOGIC LASER PROCEDURES

Laser Applications for Benign Prostatic Hyperplasia

The treatment for benign obstruction of the urinary flow from an enlarged prostate has undergone a revolution in the past decade. The search for techniques that improve outcomes or increase safety over standard electrocautery resection has led to many applications of thermal energy to vaporize or coagulate prostate tissue. Lasers were the first of these technologies applied to benign prostatic hyperplasia (BPH) and remain a viable option for thermal destruction of obstructive prostate tissue.

Coagulation and Vaporization

The Nd:YAG laser was first utilized in urology because of its availability, ease of endoscopic transmission by optical fiber, and minimal absorption of the 1064-nm wavelength by either water or hemoglobin. This transmission through an aqueous medium is important because the irrigant used in urologic endoscopic procedures does not interfere with energy delivery. On the contrary, the fluid allows higher-wattage tolerance by the optical fiber, cools the surface of the prostate tissue, and shifts the ablation threshold to a higher wattage. This produces greater tissue penetration without surface ablation, producing deeper coagulation and larger tissue defects. Tissue destruction is most often accomplished with Nd:YAG laser energy by aiming the laser beam from a short distance (free-beam method) to cause coagulation. Higher energies than the 60 W used for coagulation have been used to cause an immediate defect by vaporization. Contact optical fibers, which deliver the laser energy only at the tissue–fiber interface (contact method), for tissue vaporization have been used less often.

Visual laser ablation of the prostate (VLAP) is the free-beam method of treatment that uses a fiber with a right-angled tip for beam direction (Fig. 140–4). This was the most commonly employed method dating from the first report in 1991 (3). Larger series reported 3-year follow-up with high patient satisfaction rates, minimal acute perioperative morbidity, very low complication rates from strictures and contractures (1% to 2%), and acceptable durability of results (8). Longer-term follow-up for these coagulative procedures is lacking. These and other reports did establish the safe performance of laser coagulation in high-risk patients with severe coexisting medical problems including systemic anticoagulation.

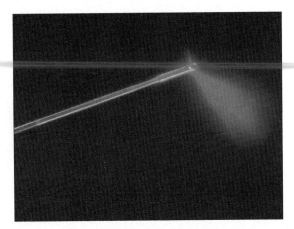

FIG. 140–4. Optical fiber with light deflected 90 degrees for free-beam laser ablation of prostate tissue.

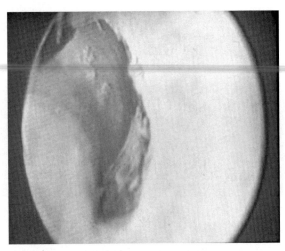

FIG. 140–5. Enucleation of prostate adenoma by Ho:yttrium–aluminum–garnet laser vaporization.

These procedures differ significantly from conventional electroresection, however, in the lack of acute tissue removal, which contributes to delayed symptom relief. The coagulative necrosis causes secondary atrophy and regression of these lesions, rather than sloughing of the necrotic tissue, resulting in shrinkage of prostatic adenoma. Clinical results usually are not manifested for several weeks to months following laser coagulative procedures, similar to results obtained with other thermal prostate treatments that use radiofrequency or microwave technology to deliver energy. Patients in general are catheterized for several days posttreatment due to prostatic edema and potential for acute urinary retention. Despite proper patient selection, about one-third of patients will not have sufficient symptom relief, a similar but slightly less common characteristic of other thermal procedures.

Interstitial Laser Coagulation

Another method of laser ablation evolved with transurethral insertion of interstitial diode laser fibers into the prostate (14). Interstitial laser coagulation (ILC) differs by causing an ellipsoid coagulation necrosis inside the adenoma rather than at its urethral surface. Flexibility of insertion allows easy treatment of intravesical prostate tissue, unlike the free-beam approach. While the durability and long-term retreatment rates are yet to be established beyond 3 years, the procedure carries no serious morbidity and has been done under local anesthesia.

Enucleation

Enucleation of the obstructing adenoma, rather than vaporization or coagulation, can also be performed with laser technology (Fig. 140–5). The holmium laser has been most adaptable to this approach, which has achieved results comparable to transurethral resection (TURP) (5).

In this procedure, holmium laser resection of the prostate (HoLRP), like electroresection, accomplishes immediate relief of obstruction in a similar operative time. However, HoLRP differs from TURP because the enucleated adenoma requires morcellation to extract the tissue. Despite this limitation, very large glands can be transurethrally extracted in experienced hands (13).

Laser Lithotripsy

The most widespread clinical impact of lasers in urology has been in the domain of calculus management. The advent of small rigid and flexible ureteroscopes in conjunction with holmium laser use has rendered open surgical management of ureteral stones practically obsolete. The earliest reports of calculus fragmentation with a ruby laser were impractical due to heat generation but revealed that surrounding the calculus with fluid improved fragmentation by confining the laser energy. Further investigation demonstrated that stone pigmentation affected laser light absorption and that the stress wave energy could be increased significantly with heat reduction by confinement of the laser energy.

Laser lithotripsy with pulsed dye lasers occurs by both photoacoustic and photomechanical mechanisms. The discharge of laser energy on the stone produces a focus of microscopic heating that results in thermal expansion. Further heating leads to ionization of stone material and the formation of plasma, seen as a bright flash of white light (Fig. 140–6). Water is essential for confining the plasma and enhances fragmentation rates approximately 10×. A cavitation bubble is created that first expands and then collapses. Shock waves generated at expansion and collapse of this bubble create stone fragmentation (Fig. 140–7). Lithotripsy with the holmium:YAG laser appears to be predominantly by a photothermal mechanism that

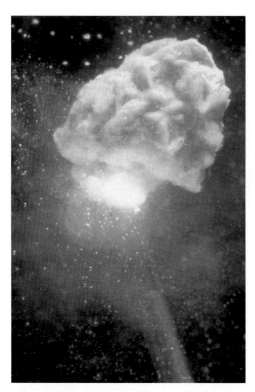

FIG. 140–6. Plasma formation from Ho:yttrium–aluminum–garnet laser at urinary calculus interface. Plasma propagates shock wave energy from cavitation.

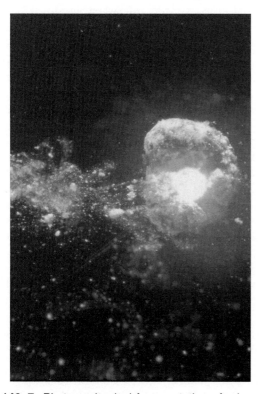

FIG. 140–7. Photomechanical fragmentation of urinary calculus following plasma formation.

causes chemical decomposition rather than cavitation. This unique mechanism of action allows the holmium laser to be used effectively on all types of stones, including cystine calculi that do not absorb pulsed dye laser energy.

Holmium laser energy may be delivered via several size fibers with the smaller fibers ideal for both flexible and rigid ureteroscopes. Multiple large series have confirmed both the effectiveness and safety of holmium lithotripsy (6). Stone-free rates after laser lithotripsy of upper urinary calculi are in the mid-90% range for all ureteral calculi and 85% for renal calculi. The safety profile of holmium laser lithotripsy is well documented with very low perforation and stricture rates. A further advantage to holmium lithotripsy is its efficacy in morbidly obese patients, whose body habitus precludes effective extracorporeal shock wave lithotripsy or percutaneous nephrolithotomy. Holmium lithotripsy has also proven successful in cases of failed electrohydraulic lithotripsy and creates significantly smaller fragments than pneumatic lithotripsy, pulsed dye laser, or electrohydraulic lithotripsy (19). In addition, pediatric urolithiasis and urolithiasis of pregnancy are safely treated with this technology.

Laser Treatment of TCC of the Renal Pelvis and Ureter

The improvement in endoscopic access to the upper urinary tract has allowed intraluminal laser ablation of papillary transitional cell malignancies. Both the Nd:YAG and Ho:YAG lasers can be delivered via small-diameter optical fibers and have been used for tumor ablation. In contrast to lower urinary tract tumors, where direct laser exposure may be easier, upper-tract lesions are in general irradiated at an oblique angle. The most common laser energy used is 25 W with the Nd:YAG laser for ureteral lesions, less than that used in the lower urinary tract. The lower energy decreases the chance of ureteral perforation due to the incident angle of exposure and thinner ureteral musculature. This is less of an issue in the renal pelvis and higher energies may be used more safely in that location. Less scarring and stricture formation has been noted in the upper urinary tract after the use of laser compared to electrofulguration. Local recurrence is reported in 33% of patients with renal pelvic and ureteral tumors. Recurrence and progression of disease correlates closely with higher grade and stage, so laser thermal destruction of tumors is best reserved for lower-grade, superficial lesions. In patients with specific indications for conservative therapy, however, laser ablation of upper-tract transitional cell carcinoma (TCC) with close ureteroscopic surveillance is now considered a reasonable alternative to surgical removal. This form of treatment may be especially well suited for patients with lesions in a solitary kidney.

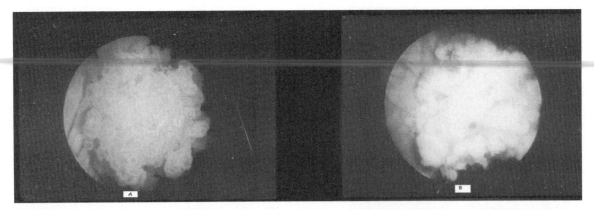

FIG. 140–8. A: Papillary transitional cell carcinoma before coagulation necrosis from Nd:yttrium–aluminum–garnet laser exposure. **B:** Typical tumor discoloration signifying adequate thermal treatment.

Laser Treatment of TCC of the Lower Urinary Tract

Destruction of bladder malignancies by laser thermal treatment does not provide tissue for histological evaluation and any laser therapy should be preceded by appropriate biopsies to determine tumor grade and stage. Laser therapy was initially restricted to patients with recurrent tumors where the pathologic diagnosis was determined; it is now reasonable to treat the first occurrence with a laser if the tumor appears as a well-pedunculated, low-grade, papillary tumor and a biopsy of the tumor base is obtained. Lesions that are poorly accessible for transurethral resection, such as on the anterior bladder wall, may be best addressed with a laser alone or in combination with standard resection. Thermal laser treatment is not in particular effective for carcinoma in situ (Tis) because of its extent and multifocality.

Treatment of superficial bladder cancer by the Nd:YAG laser has proven effective in long-term studies (16). Papillary tumors are in general treated with 30 to 40 W directed from close proximity to the tumor until the color of the treatment area blanches (Fig. 140–8). Adjacent areas are treated similarly until the entire lesion has been covered. Suspicious areas adjacent to the tumor base often are painted with the laser beam. Reports of recurrence rates after laser exposure are similar to rates after standard transurethral resection. However, Nd:YAG laser use may prove advantageous because vascular coagulation decreases bleeding and may obviate the need for posttreatment catheterization. Further, stimulation of the obturator reflex does not occur with thermal lasers. Flexible endoscopic instruments can be used with the small-diameter optical fibers to allow treatment of lesions in locations otherwise inaccessible to rigid instruments. A disadvantage of this technique is the inability to sample tissue from the tumor base for accurate staging. Safety of laser ablation of bladder tumors is evidenced by the extremely low risk of bladder perforation (16).

Photodynamic Therapy

Photodynamic therapy (PDT) is an intriguing modality that has been used to treat high-grade, diffuse, and recurrent transitional cell bladder tumors (12). Rather than destruction by thermal energy, PDT tumorcidal effects result from production of a highly reactive oxygen species produced by absorbance of specific visible light wavelengths by a photosensitizing agent. Lasers are the most efficient light source for PDT, with diode lasers being more cost effective and reliable than the previously more often used tunable dye variety.

Porphyrin sensitizers delivered by intravenous injection have been the most commonly used photosensitizers but intravesical instillation of 5-ALA (which causes porphyrin accumulation in tumors) is gaining significant interest for its therapeutic use in addition to its use for fluorescent tumor detection (10) (Fig. 140–9). TCC of the bladder is responsive to PDT, with better responses in general noted for treatment of carcinoma *in situ*. Reports of patients treated with PDT for bladder carcinoma demonstrate an overall response rate of 51% for papillary TCC and 66% for patients with Tis (20). Whole-bladder PDT is a potential alternative to cystectomy in selected patients refractive to conventional intravesical therapy for superficial disease but it has failed to gain widespread acceptance despite reasonable efficacy because of technical issues and potentially unacceptable side effects. Treatment in general consists of 20 to 30 J per cm^2 of light to the target area after calculation of surface area. Although no system for bladder surface area calculation is felt to be exact, triplanar transabdominal sonography may provide the least crude method for surface area calculation because overdistention and contour distortion are evident and can be avoided. Other technical aspects peculiar to bladder PDT include choice of optical fiber tip for light distribution, optical fiber placement, and stabilization of the optical fiber to prevent movement during treatment.

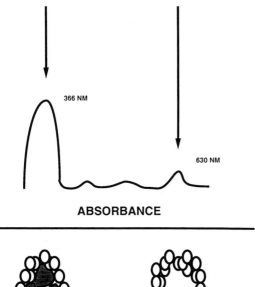

FIG. 140–9. Principles of photosensitization using a typical porphyrin sensitizing agent. Wavelengths in the ultraviolet range provide characteristic fluorescence while longer wavelengths are used for photodynamic therapy.

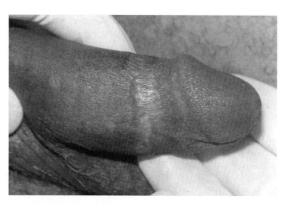

FIG. 140–10. An excellent cosmetic effect following Nd: yttrium–aluminum–garnet laser treatment of superficial penile squamous cell carcinoma.

Laser Treatment of Urethral Strictures and Posterior Urethral Valves

Despite initial enthusiasm for thermal laser ablation of urethral strictures, no definitive long-term advantage over traditional urethrotomy has been demonstrated. Recurrence rates do not appear to be lessened with laser use compared to conventional methods. Recent reports with Ho:YAG and diode lasers note good short-term results but longer-term evaluation is lacking. One advantage of this technique, as with tumor ablation, is the relative lack of bleeding.

Nd:YAG laser ablation of congenital posterior urethral valves has been demonstrated to be effective in the pediatric population. Precise destruction of valve tissue with no complications has been reported as an outpatient procedure without need for postoperative indwelling catheterization.

Laser Treatment of External Genitalia

Lasers are a good tool for precise, controlled ablation of human papilloma virus (HPV) on the external genitalia. Excellent therapeutic and cosmetic results have been obtained with the CO_2 and Nd:YAG laser treatment of large penile lesions. Magnification with loupes or an operating microscope is required for multiple smaller lesions. Safety precautions for operating room personnel are imperative because viral particles remain viable in the laser plume; a dedicated suction apparatus must be used to capture the laser plume. Nd:YAG treatment of condyloma requires irrigation to cool the tissue during treatment. The efficacy of current topical antiviral agents and labor-intensive nature of laser treatment make this procedure much less cost effective than use of topical ointments (18). Laser procedures are very effective, however, for cases of refractive disease or large villous lesions. Treatment of urethral condyloma proximal to the meatus is not amenable to CO_2 therapy because this laser energy cannot be transmitted via a fiber. Both the Nd:YAG and holmium lasers have been used for urethral condyloma with good results and very few complications.

In addition to benign penile lesions, lasers are currently used for treatment of superficial squamous cell carcinoma of the penis. Successful treatment of premalignant or low-grade penile malignancy (Bowen's disease, erythroplasia of Queyrat, bowenoid papulosis) can be achieved using many of the common surgical lasers (Fig. 140–10). Because these lesions are superficial, are often multifocal, and require precise treatment, the CO_2 laser in combination with an operating microscope is often considered the ideal approach. The Nd:YAG and CO_2 lasers are well suited to treat superficial squamous cell penile lesions with good results reported but not recommended for T1 and T2 squamous cell carcinoma of the penis. Reports of effective local treatment of Kaposi's sarcoma with the Nd:YAG laser have been beneficial for urethral meatal obstruction.

REFERENCES

1. Benson RC Jr, Farrow GM, Kinsey JH, et al. Detection and localization of in situ carcinoma of the bladder with hematoporphyrin derivative. *Mayo Clin Proc* 1982:548–555.
2. Chan KF, Lee H, Teichman JMH, et al. Erbium:YAG laser lithotripsy mechanism. *J Urol* 2002;168:436–441.
3. Costello AJ, Johnson DE, Bolton DM. Nd:YAG laser ablation of the prostate as a treatment for benign prostatic hypertrophy. *Lasers Surg Med* 1992;12:121.

4. Feldchtein FI, Gelikonov GV, Gelikonov VM, et al. Endoscopic applications of optical coherent tomography. *Optics Express* 1998;3: 257–269.

5. Gilling PJ, Kennett KM, Fraundorfer MR. Holmium laser resection of the prostate (HoLRP) versus transurethral resection of the prostate (TURP): results of a randomised trial with 2 years follow-up. *J Endourol* 2000;14:757–760.

6. Gould DL. Holmium:YAG laser and its use in the treatment of urolithiasis: our first 160 cases. *J Endourol* 1998;12:23–26.

7. Huang D, Swanson EA, Lin CP, et al. Optical coherence tomography. *Science* 1991;254:1178–1181.

8. Kabalin J, Gunars B, Doll S. Nd:YAG laser coagulation prostatectomy: 3 years of experience with 227 patients. *J Urol* 1996;155:181–185.

9. Kreigmaier M, Baumgartner R, Knuechel R, et al. Detection of early bladder cancer by 5-aminolevulinic acid induced porphyrin fluorescence. *J Urol* 1996;155:105–110.

10. Kreigmaier M, Zaak D, Rothenberger K-H, et al. Transurethral resection for bladder cancer using 5-aminolevulinic acid induced fluorescence endoscopy versus white light endoscopy. *J Urol* 2002;168: 475–478.

11. Manyak MJ. Endoscopic future perspectives: light as a diagnostic tool. In: Sosa RE, ed. *Textbook of endourology*. Philadelphia: WB Saunders, 1996:206–214.

12. Manyak MJ. Photodynamic therapy for urologic malignancies. *AUA Update* 1995;12:94–104.

13. Moody JA, Lingeman JE. Holmium laser enucleation for prostate adenoma greater than 100 gm: comparison to open prostatectomy. *J Urol* 2001;165:459–462.

14. Muschter R, Hofstetter A, Hessel S, et al. Hi-tech of the prostate: interstitial laser coagulation of benign prostatic hypertrophy. In: Anderson RR, ed. Laser surgery: advanced characterization therapeutics and systems. *SPIE Proc* 1992;1643(111):25–34

15. Parrish JA, Wilson BC. Current and future trends in laser medicine. *Photochem Photobiol* 1991;53:731–738.

16. Smith JA Jr. Endoscopic applications of laser energy. *Urol Clin North Am* 1986;13:405–419.

17. Stein BS. Laser–tissue interaction. In: Smith JA Jr, Stein BS, Benson RC Jr, eds. *Lasers in urologic surgery*, 3rd ed. St. Louis: Mosby–Year Book, 1994:10–25

18. Strauss MJ, Khanna V, Koenig JD, et al. The cost of treating genital warts. *Int J Dermatol* 1996;35:345–348.

19. Teichman JM, Vassar GJ, Bishoff JT, et al. Holmium:YAG lithotripsy yields smaller fragments than lithoclast, pulsed dye laser or electrohydraulic lithotripsy. *J Urol* 1998;159:17–23.

20. Walther MM. The role of photodynamic therapy in the treatment of recurrent superficial bladder cancer. *Urol Clin North Am* 2000;27: 163–170.

21. Zagaynova EV, Streltsova OS, Gladkova ND, et al. In vivo optical coherence tomography feasibility for bladder disease. *J Urol* 2002;167: 1492–1496.

Index

Page numbers in *italics* indicate figures. Page numbers followed by "t" indicate tables.